MW00635427

NEW YORK SCHOOL OF REGIONAL ANESTHESIA

# Hadzic's Peripheral Nerve Blocks and Anatomy for Ultrasound-Guided Regional Anesthesia

## NOTICE

Medicine is an ever-changing science. As new research and clinical experience broaden our knowledge, changes in treatment and drug therapy are required. The authors and the publisher of this work have checked with sources believed to be reliable in their efforts to provide information that is complete and generally in accord with the standards accepted at the time of publication. However, in view of the possibility of human error or changes in medical sciences, neither the authors nor the publisher nor any other party who has been involved in the preparation or publication of this work warrants that the information contained herein is in every respect accurate or complete, and they disclaim all responsibility for any errors or omissions or for the results obtained from use of the information contained in this work. Readers are encouraged to confirm the information contained herein with other sources. For example and in particular, readers are advised to check the product information sheet included in the package of each drug they plan to administer to be certain that the information contained in this work is accurate and that changes have not been made in the recommended dose or in the contraindications for administration. This recommendation is of particular importance in connection with new or infrequently used drugs.

NEW YORK SCHOOL OF REGIONAL ANESTHESIA

# Hadzic's Peripheral Nerve Blocks and Anatomy for Ultrasound-Guided Regional Anesthesia

**SECOND EDITION**


Editor

**Admir Hadzic, MD, PhD**

Professor of Anesthesiology
Department of Anesthesiology
St. Luke's–Roosevelt Hospital Center
College of Physicians and Surgeons
Columbia University
New York, New York

Associate Editors

**Ana Carrera, PhD, MD**
**Thomas B. Clark, DC, RVT**
**Jeff Gadsden, MD, FRCPC, FANZCA**
**Manoj Kumar Karmakar, MD, FRCA, FHKCA, FHKAM**
**Xavier Sala-Blanch, MD**
**Catherine F. M. Vandepitte, MD**
**Daquan Xu, MD, MSc, MPH**



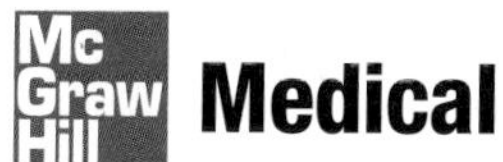


New York Chicago San Francisco Lisbon London Madrid Mexico City
Milan New Delhi San Juan Seoul Singapore Sydney Toronto

The McGraw-Hill Companies

**Hadzic's Peripheral Nerve Blocks and Anatomy for Ultrasound-Guided Regional Anesthesia, Second Edition**



5 6 7 8 9 0 CTP/CTP 18 17 16 15

Set ISBN 978-0-07-154961-5
Set MHID 0-07-154961-7
Book ISBN 978-0-07-154963-9
Book MHID 0-07-154963-3
DVD ISBN 978-0-07-154964-6
DVD MHID 0-07-154964-1

This book was set in Minion Pro by Cenveo Publisher Services.
The editors were Brian Belval and Robert Pancotti.
The production supervisor was Catherine H. Saggese.
Project management was provided by Deepti Narwat Agarwal, Cenveo Publisher Services.
The text designer was Alan Barnett; the cover designer was Brian Barsoom.
China Translation & Printing Services, Ltd. was printer and binder.

**Library of Congress Cataloging-in-Publication Data**

Hadzic's peripheral nerve blocks and anatomy for ultrasound-guided regional anesthesia/editor, Admir Hadzic.—2nd ed.
p. ; cm.
Peripheral nerve blocks and anatomy for ultrasound-guided regional anesthesia
Rev. ed. of: Peripheral nerve blocks : principles and practice.
c2004.
Includes bibliographical references and index.
ISBN-13: 978-0-07-154961-5 (set : hardcover : alk. paper)
ISBN-10: 0-07-154961-7 (set : hardcover : alk. paper)
ISBN-13: 978-0-07-154963-9 (hardcover : alk. paper)
ISBN-10: 0-07-154963-3 (hardcover : alk. paper)
[etc.]
1. Nerve block. I. Hadzic, Admir. II. New York School of Regional Anesthesia. III. Peripheral nerve blocks. IV. Title: Peripheral nerve blocks and anatomy for ultrasound-guided regional anesthesia.
[DNLM: 1. Nerve Block—methods. 2. Peripheral Nerves—anatomy & histology. 3. Peripheral Nerves—ultrasonography. 4. Ultrasonography—methods. WO 300]
RD84.P458 2012
617.9'6—dc23

2011025098

# DEDICATION

I dedicate this book to Dr. Jerry Darius Vloka,
a peerless scholar whose contribution to and teaching of
regional anesthesia have provided an educational platform and
inspiration for generations of practitioners and academicians alike.
You are a beacon of light and a paragon of scholarship and virtue.
I am profoundly privileged to number you among my closest friends.
May many generations of students slake their thirst at the well of your wisdom,
and may our friendship outpace the ravages of time.

With love and respect,
*Admir*

"Tell me what company thou keepst, and I'll tell thee what thou art."

*Cervantes*

# CONTENTS

# CONTRIBUTORS

**Marina Alen, MD**
Fellow, Regional Anesthesia
St. Luke's–Roosevelt Hospital Center
New York, New York

**Honorio T. Benzon, MD**
Professor
Department of Anesthesiology
Feinberg School of Medicine
Northwestern University
Chicago, Illinois

**Rafael Blanco, MD**
MBBS, F.R.C.A., D.E.A.A. & Intensive Care
Consultant Anaesthesiologist
Complexo Hospitalario Universitario A Coruña
Spain

**Ana Carrera, PhD, MD**
Lecturer of Human Anatomy
Faculty of Medicine
University of Girona
Girona, Spain

**Lorenzo Casertano, CSCS**
Physical Therapy
Columbia University, New York, New York

**Junping Chen, MD**
Fellow, Regional Anesthesia
St. Luke's–Roosevelt Hospital Center
New York, New York

**Thomas B. Clark, DC, RVT**
Adjunct Professor of Radiology
Department of Radiology
Logan College of Chiropractic
St. Louis, Missouri

**Adam B. Cohen, MD**
Attending Physician
Department of Orthopedic Surgery
St. Luke's–Roosevelt Hospital Center
New York, New York

**Jose De Andrés, MD, PhD**
Head of Department
Department of Anesthesia
Hospital General Universitario
Valencia. Spain

**Belen De Jose Maria, MD, PhD**
Senior Pediatric Anesthesiologist
Department of Pediatric Anesthesia
Hospital Sant Joan de Deu
Barcelona, Spain

**Jeffrey Dermksian, MD**
Assistant Clinical Professor
Department of Orthopaedic Surgery
Columbia University
New York, New York

**Steven A. Dewaele, MD**
Associate Consultant
Department of Anesthesiology and Intensive Care
AZ St Lucas
Ghent, Belgium

**Tomás Domingo, MD**
Pain Unit, Department of Anaesthesiology
Hospital Universitari de Bellvitge
Associate Professor, Human Anatomy
Universitat de Barcelona, Campus de Bellvitge
Barcelona, Spain

**F. Kayser Enneking, MD**
Professor and Chair
Department of Anesthesiology
University of Florida
Gainesville, Florida

**Carlo D. Franco, MD**
Professor
Department of Anesthesiology and Anatomy
J.H.S. Hospital Cook County
Rush University Medical Center
Chicago, Illinois

**Ashton P. Frulla, BS**
Research Assistant
Department of Anesthesiology
St. Luke's–Roosevelt Hospital
New York, New York

**Jeff Gadsden, MD, FRCPC, FANZCA**
Assistant Professor of Clinical Anesthesiology
Department of Anesthesiology
College of Physicans and Surgeons
Columbia University
New York, New York

**Philippe E. Gautier, MD**
Head of Department
Department of Anaesthesia
Clinique Ste Anne-St Remi
Brussels, Belgium

**Kimberly Gratenstein, MD**
Regional Anesthesia Fellow
Department of Anesthesiology
St. Luke's–Roosevelt Hospital
New York, New York

**Fermin Haro-Sanz, MD**
Associate Professor
Anestesiologia Reanimación Terapia del Dolor
Universidad de Navarra
Navarra, Spain

**Paul Hobeika, MD**
Assistant Professor of Orthopedic Surgery
Department of Orthopedics and Orthopedic Surgery
St. Luke's–Roosevelt Hospital
College of Physicians and Surgeons Columbia University
New York, New York

**Patrick Horan, MPH**
Research Fellow
Department of Anesthesiology
St. Luke's–Roosevelt Hospital Center
New York, New York

**Brian M. Ilfeld, MD, MS (Clinical Investigation)**
Associate Professor in Residence
Department of Anesthesiology
University of California, San Diego
San Diego, California

**Manoj Kumar Karmakar, MD, FRCA, FHKCA, FHKAM**
Associate Professor and Director of Paediatric Anesthesia
Department of Anaesthesia and Intensive Care
The Chinese University of Hong Kong
Prince of Wales Hospital
Shatin, New Territories
Hong Kong

**Kwesi Kwofie, MD**
Fellow, Regional Anesthesia
St. Luke's–Roosevelt Hospital Center
New York, New York

**Wing Hong Kwok, FANZCA**
The Chinese University of Hong Kong
Prince of Wales Hospital
Shatin, New Territories
Hong Kong

**Manuel Llusa, MD, PhD**
Associate Professor
Department of Human Anatomy and Embryology
University of Barcelona
Barcelona, Spain

**Ana M. López, MD, PhD**
Senior Specialist
Department of Anesthesiology
Hospital Clínic
Barcelona, Spain

**Philippe B. Macaire, MD**
Senior Consultant
Department of Anesthesiology and Pain Management
Rashid Hospital
Dubai, United Arab Emirates

**Thomas Maliakal, MD**
Resident
Department of Anesthesiology
St. Luke's–Roosevelt Hospital Center
New York, New York

**Josep Masdeu, MD**
Department of Anesthesia
Hospital Moisés Broggi
Consorci Sanitari Integral
Barcelona, Spain

**Colleen E. McCally, DO**
Regional Anesthesia Fellow
St. Luke's–Roosevelt Hospital Center
New York, New York

**Carlos Morros, MD, PhD**
Associate Professor
Department of Anesthesia
Clínica Diagonal. Barcelona. Spain

**Alberto Prats-Galino, MD, PhD**
Professor
Laboratory of Surgical Neuro-Anatomy
Human Anatomy and Embryology Unit
Faculty of Medicine
University of Barcelona
Barcelona, Spain

**Miguel Angel Reina, MD, PhD**
Associate Professor
Department of Clinical Medical Sciences and Research
Laboratory of Histology and Imaging
Institute of Applied Molecular Medicine
CEU San Pablo University
School of Medicine
Madrid, Spain

**Wojciech Reiss, MD**
Fellow, Regional Anesthesia
St. Luke's–Roosevelt Hospital Center
New York, New York

**Elizabeth M. Renehan, MD, MSc, FRCPC**
Department of Anesthesiology
University of Florida
Gainesville, Florida

**Teresa Ribalta, MD, PhD**
Professor of Pathology
Department of Anatomical Pathology
Hospital Clínic
University of Barcelona Medical School, IDIBAPS
Barcelona, Spain

**Vicente Roqués, MD, PhD**
Consultant Anaesthetist
Anesthesia and Intensive Care
Hospital Universitario Virgen de la Arrixaca
Murcia, Spain

**Xavier Sala-Blanch, MD**
Staff Anesthesiologist
Department of Anesthesia
Hospital Clinic
University of Barcelona
Barcelona, Spain

**Carlos H. Salazar-Zamorano, MD**
Attending Anesthesiologist
Anesthesia Resident Coordinator
Department of Anesthesiology
Hospital de Figueres
Figueres, Spain

**Gerard Sanchez-Etayo, MD**
Department of Anesthesiology
Hospital Clinic
Barcelona, Spain

**Alan C. Santos, MD, MPH**
Professor of Anesthesiology
College of Physicians and Surgeons
Columbia University
New York, New York
Chairman of Anesthesiology
St. Luke's–Roosevelt Hospital Center
New York, New York

**Luc A. Sermeus, MD**
Lector, Department of Anesthesiology
University of Antwerp
Wilrijk, Belgium

**Ali Nima Shariat, MD**
Clinical Instructor
Department of Anesthesiology
St. Luke's–Roosevelt Hospital Center
New York, New York

**Uma Shastri, MD**
Fellow, Regional Anesthesia
St. Luke's–Roosevelt Hospital Center
New York, New York

**Sanjay K. Sinha, MBBS**
Director of Regional Anesthesia
Department of Anesthesiology
St. Francis Hospital and Medical Center
Hartford, Connecticut

**Dr. rer. nat. Martin Sippel**
Senior Vice President
Center of Excellence in Pain Control and CVC
B. Braun Melsungen AG
Melsungen, Germany

**Leroy Sutherland, MD**
Fellow, Regional Anesthesia
St. Luke's–Roosevelt Hospital Center
New York, New York

**Douglas B. Unis, MD**
Assistant Clinical Professor
Department of Orthopaedic Surgery
College of Physicians and Surgeons
Columbia University
New York, New York

**Catherine F. M. Vandepitte, MD**
Consultant Anesthesiologist
Katholieke Universiteit Leuven
Leuven, Belgium

**André van Zundert, MD, PhD, FRCA, EDRA**
Professor of Anesthesiology
Catharina Hospital
Eindhoven, Netherlands
University Maastricht
Maastricht, Netherlands
University of Ghent
Ghent, Belgium

**Chi H. Wong, MS, DO**
Anesthesiology Resident
Department of Anesthesiology
Yale New Haven Hospital
New Haven, Connecticut

**Daquan Xu, MD, MSc, MPH**
Research Associate
Department of Anesthesiology
St. Luke's–Roosevelt Hospital Center
New York, New York

**Tatjana Stopar Pintaric, MD, PhD, DEAA**
Associate Professor of Anesthesiology
University Medical Center Ljubljana
Ljubljana, Slovenia

# PREFACE

*Peripheral Nerve Blocks and Anatomy for Ultrasound-Guided Regional Anesthesia,* second edition, is being published at an exciting time in the development of regional anesthesia. Reflecting on the first edition of the book,* we believe its success was due largely to the tried-and-true nature of the material taught. It would not be an overstatement to say that the first edition of this book influenced professional lives of many colleagues and ultimately benefited patients worldwide. The success helped garner the New York School of Regional Anesthesia (NYSORA) additional esteem that it enjoys today. In line with the philosophy of the first edition, this second edition minimizes presentation of theoretical considerations. Instead, the featured techniques and teachings are gleaned directly from the trenches of the clinical practice of regional anesthesia.

In recent years, the field of regional anesthesia, and in particular peripheral nerve blockade, has entered an unprecedented renaissance. This renaissance is due primarily to the widespread introduction of ultrasound-guided regional anesthesia. The ability to visualize the anatomy of interest, the needle–nerve relationship, and the spread of the local anesthetic has resulted in significant growth of interest in and use of peripheral nerve blocks. Regardless, many aspects of ultrasound-guided regional anesthesia still require clarification and standardization. Examples include dilemmas regarding the ideal placement of the needle for successful and safe blockade, the number of injections required for individual techniques, the volume of local anesthetic for successful blockade, the integration of additional monitoring tools such as nerve stimulation and injection pressure monitoring and many others. For these reasons, we decided to defer publication of the second edition and opted to wait for clarification from clinical trials or collective experience to provide more solid recommendations. As a result, just as with the first edition, the second book features only tried-and-true descriptions of peripheral nerve block techniques with wide clinical applicability rather than a plethora of techniques and modifications that have mere theoretical considerations. Where the collective experience has not reached the necessary level to recommend teaching a certain technique (e.g., neuraxial blocks), we opted to feature anatomic considerations rather than vague or inadequately developed technique recommendations, which may lead to disappointments, or possibly complications, if they are adopted without careful consideration.

*The first edition was titled *Peripheral Nerve Blocks: Principles and Practice.*

The second edition is organized as a collection of practical introductory chapters, followed by detailed and unambiguous descriptions of common regional anesthesia block procedures rather than an exhaustive theoretical compendium of the literature. Although ultrasound guidance eventually may become the most prevalent method of nerve blockade globally, most procedures world-wide are still performed using the methods of peripheral nerve stimulation and/or surface landmarks, particularly in the developing world. Because this book has been one of the main teaching sources internationally, we decided to retain the section on the traditional techniques of nerve blockade in addition to the new section on ultrasound-guided regional anesthesia. Since knowledge of surface anatomy is essential for practice of both traditional and ultrasound regional anesthesia procedures, we decided to also add an Atlas of Surface Anatomy (Section 8).

The book is organized in eight sections that progress from the foundations of peripheral nerve blocks and regional anesthesia to their applications in clinical practice. Ultrasound-guided regional anesthesia is a field in evolution, and many of its aspects still lack standardization and clear guidance. For this reason, we decided to produce this new edition as an international collaborative effort. This collaboration resulted in teaching that is based not only on our experience at NYSORA but also is endorsed by a number of opinion leaders in the field from around the globe. I would like to thank them for the contributions, enthusiasm, and passion that they invested in creating the second edition of *Peripheral Nerve Blocks*. This book also would not be what it is without the large extended family of educators and trainees, who took part in the numerous NYSORA educational programs, including our educational outreach program in developing countries in Asia. I thank you immensely for your input, which inspired us to deliver this updated edition, and for your multiple contributions through e-mails, suggestions, and discussion on the NYSORA.com website.

There are no standards of care related to peripheral nerve blocks, despite their widespread use. With this edition, we have tried to standardize the techniques and the monitoring approach during local anesthetic delivery, for both greater consistency and greater safety of peripheral nerve blocks. Different institutions naturally may have different approaches to techniques that they customize for their own needs. The material we present in this volume however, comes from the trenches of clinical practice, so to speak. Most procedures described are accompanied by carefully developed flowcharts to facilitate decision making in clinical practice that the authors themselves use on an everyday basis.

The successful practice of ultrasound-guided regional anesthesia and pain medicine procedures depends greatly on the ability to obtain accurate ultrasound images and the ability to recognize the relevant structures. For these reasons, we decided to add an atlas of ultrasound anatomy for regional anesthesia and pain medicine (Section 7) procedures to this volume. The anatomy examples consist of a pictorial guide with images of the transducer position needed to obtain the corresponding ultrasound image and the cross-sectional gross anatomy of the area being imaged. Once the practitioner absorbs this material, he or she can extrapolate the knowledge of the practical techniques presented to practice virtually any additional regional anesthesia technique. We have expended painstaking efforts to provide cross-sectional anatomy examples where possible. Perfecting the matching of ultrasound and anatomy sections is not always possible because the sonograms and cross-sectional anatomy views are obtained from volunteers and fresh cadavers, respectively. The reader should keep in mind that the ultrasound images are obtained from videos during dynamic scanning. For this reason, the labeled ultrasound images are accurate to the best of our abilities and within the limitations of the ultrasound equipment even when they do not perfectly match the available paired cross-sectional anatomy.

Due to popular demand, we decided to include a DVD containing videos of the most common ultrasound-guided nerve block procedures. Assuming that videos are the most beneficial method for novices and trainees, we decided to include videos of well-established ultrasound-guided nerve blocks that should cover most indications for peripheral nerve blocks. Once trainees have mastered these techniques, they typically require only knowledge about the specific anatomy of the block(s) to be performed to apply the principles learned in the videos to any other nerve block procedure. This is another example of how the atlas of ultrasound anatomy (Section 7) included in the book will be useful. With the wealth of information presented in a systematic fashion, we believe that the Atlas also will be of value to anyone interested in the ultrasound anatomy of peripheral nerve and musculoskeletal systems, including radiologists, sonographers, neurologists, and others.

With this edition of *Peripheral Nerve Blocks and Anatomy for Ultrasound-Guided Regional Anesthesia,* we have tried to provide a wealth of practical information about the modern practice of peripheral nerve blocks and the use of ultrasound in regional anesthesia and to present multiple pathways to troubleshoot common clinical problems. We hope this book will continue to serve as one of the standard teaching texts in anesthesiology, and we thank the readership of previous edition their support and encouragement.

Sincerely,
Admir Hadzic, MD

# ACKNOWLEDGMENTS

This book would not be possible without the contributions and support from a number of remarkable people and top professionals in their respective fields.

Most notably, special thanks to Professor Alan Santos, MD, the chair of the Department of Anesthesiology at St. Luke's–Roosevelt Hospitals, where a significant part of the clinical teaching and research of the New York School of Regional Anesthesia (NYSORA) has taken place over the years. Alan's commitment to education and academics, and his leadership have created a unique milieu where faculty and staff drawn to academics can excel and pursue their academic goals with a remarkable departmental support.

Hats off to our current and past fellows in regional anesthesia. You have been immeasurably helpful and a continuing source of inspiration for many projects and NYSORA endeavors, and you have been so much fun to work with as well. In particular, thanks and love go to "NYSORA Angels" Drs. Kim Gratenstein and Colleen Mitgang for the all-around help and positive vibe. I also extend gratitude to our residents who have helped create teaching ideas and a multitude of didactic algorithms through our daily interactions in clinical practice.

Many thanks to my numerous U.S. and international collaborators, whose support, relentless challenges, and innovative didactic material have made a palpable contribution to this project. A bow to you, my colleagues at St. Luke's–Roosevelt Hospital, New York, and our site director, Dr. Kurian Thomas, whose daily organizational skills and clinical leadership made many of our endeavors possible—often magically so—in these times of increasing financial and manpower strain.

Many thanks to my family: foremost, my son Alen Hadžić, my parents Junuz and Safeta Hadžić, my sister Admira, and the entire family for allowing me to work on this book project while depriving them of my presence.

Special thanks to the illustrator, Lejla Hadžić. Her artistic vision and talent adorns this book with a plethora of detailed illustrations. Lejla has been spearheading multiple projects in her own primary area of expertise, restoration of war- and weather-ravaged cultural monuments with a Swedish-based organization, Cultural Heritage Without Borders (CHWB), for which she has received much international acclaim. Many thanks also to Emma Spahic for lending her artistic eye and Photoshop skills to the project.

This book owes a great deal to a number of gifted clinicians, academicians, and regional anesthesia teams from around the globe. Many thanks to Dr. Catherine Vandepitte, who has spent countless hours editing and collating the material. Daquan Xu, MD, has contributed his unmatched organizational skills and knowledge of anatomy and ultrasonography. At the peak of our efforts to produce this book, Daquan actually moved in with me in my apartment on the Hudson River in Lincoln Harbor, across from the Midtown section of Manhattan. While enduring 16- to 18-hour days working on the book in the winter of 2011, Daquan would take five-minute breaks on the balcony to gaze over the skyline of New York. We would stop working only when Daquan became so tired that he could not see the Empire State Building any more. This sign became known as "The Daquan Sign to Quit Working". Boundless appreciation to Dr. Sala-Blanch and his team, Miguel Reina, Ana Carrera, Ana Lopez, and many others, for their support, contribution in vision, and, in particular, original anatomic material. Thank you to Dr. Manoj Karmakar and his team for their cutting-edge contributions to various sections of the atlas of ultrasound anatomy. Thank you to Thomas Clark, who used his unmatched skills in musculoskeletal imaging to muster some great ultrasound anatomy in the Atlas section of the book. Many thanks to Dr. Jeff Gadsden for his contribution and best wishes for success as he takes over the leadership of the Division of Regional Anesthesia at St. Luke's–Roosevelt Hospital, a position I have held for the past 15 years. As he continues to build the division and the regional anesthesia fellowship, I have moved on to multiple other teaching and publishing endeavors. In particular, I will focus on keeping our two textbooks on regional anesthesia current in years to come.

Special thanks to a truly inspiring video team, the Ceho Brothers of *Film Productions Division* of *Stone Tone Records, Inc.* Aziz and Mirza Ceho are award-winning documentary filmmakers who have contributed their immense artistic talent to the accompanying DVD, ***5 Nerve Blocks for 95% of Indications.*** Making a good instructional DVD has proved to be an incredibly time-consuming task. However, we believe our efforts have been justified and we have created a uniquely detailed and true-to-life educational tool. This DVD should be particularly helpful to clinicians who need to adopt a few, uniquely effective nerve block techniques that can be used to provide regional anesthesia to a wide variety of patients.

Many thanks to Brian Belval, senior editor at McGraw-Hill Medical. Brian is one of the most inspirational and insightful managing editors I have ever worked with. I will admit without reservation that this book would not be what it is without his vision and personal touch. Likewise, the unmatchable attention to detail of Robert Pancotti, senior project development editor, has much to do with the quality of this project.

Special thanks to Lorenzo Casertano for loaning his ripped fencing body for the Atlas of Surface Anatomy that adorns Section 8 at the end of the book. Likewise, thank you to Alecia Yufa and Alen Hadžić for modeling for the Atlas and the techniques.

Finally, a word of gratitude to my bandmates from *Big Apple Blues Band* (www.bigappleblues.com), who contributed the original music on all tracks on the ***5 Nerve Blocks for 95% of Indications*** DVD. Barry Harrison, Anthony Kane, Hugh Pool, Zach Zunis, Rich Cohen, Tom Papadatos, and Bruce Tylor are some of the very top cats in the NYC music scene. Their talent and passion have been an important source of inspiration for me on the band stage, in the studio, and in life in general.

## *Disclosure*

I have served as an industry advisor over the course of my career and have received consulting honoraria and research grants in the past from GE, Baxter, Glaxo Smith-Kline Industries SkyPharma, Cadence, LifeTech, and others. I hold an equity position at Macosta Medical USA. Macosta Medical USA owns intellectual property related to injection pressure monitoring and several other patents related to the field of anesthesiology. Finally, I have invested a lifetime's worth of energy and love into building NYSORA over the past 15 years. My passion for regional anesthesia and undying commitment to these multiple endeavors undoubtedly has created biases that may have influenced the teaching in this book; I take full responsibility and stand by all of them.

SECTION 1

# Foundations of Peripheral Nerve Blocks

# 1 Essential Regional Anesthesia Anatomy

*Admir Hadzic and Carlo Franco*

A good practical knowledge of anatomy is important for the successful and safe practice of regional anesthesia. In fact, just as surgical disciplines rely on surgical anatomy, regional anesthesiologists need to have a working knowledge of the anatomy of nerves and associated structures that does not include unnecessary details. In this chapter, the basics of regional anesthesia anatomy necessary for successful implementation of various techniques described later in the book are outlined.

## Anatomy of Peripheral Nerves

All peripheral nerves are similar in structure. The *neuron* is the basic functional unit responsible for the conduction of nerve impulses (Figure 1-1). Neurons are the longest cells in the body, many reaching a meter in length. Most neurons are incapable of dividing under normal circumstances, and they have a very limited ability to repair themselves after injury. A typical neuron consists of a cell body (soma) that contains a large nucleus. The cell body is attached to several branching processes, called dendrites, and a single axon. Dendrites receive incoming messages; axons conduct outgoing messages. Axons vary in length, and there is only one per neuron. In peripheral nerves, axons are very long and slender. They are also called nerve fibers.

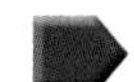

## Connective Tissue

The individual nerve fibers that make up a nerve, like individual wires in an electric cable, are bundled together by connective tissue. The connective tissue of a peripheral nerve is an important part of the nerve. According to its position

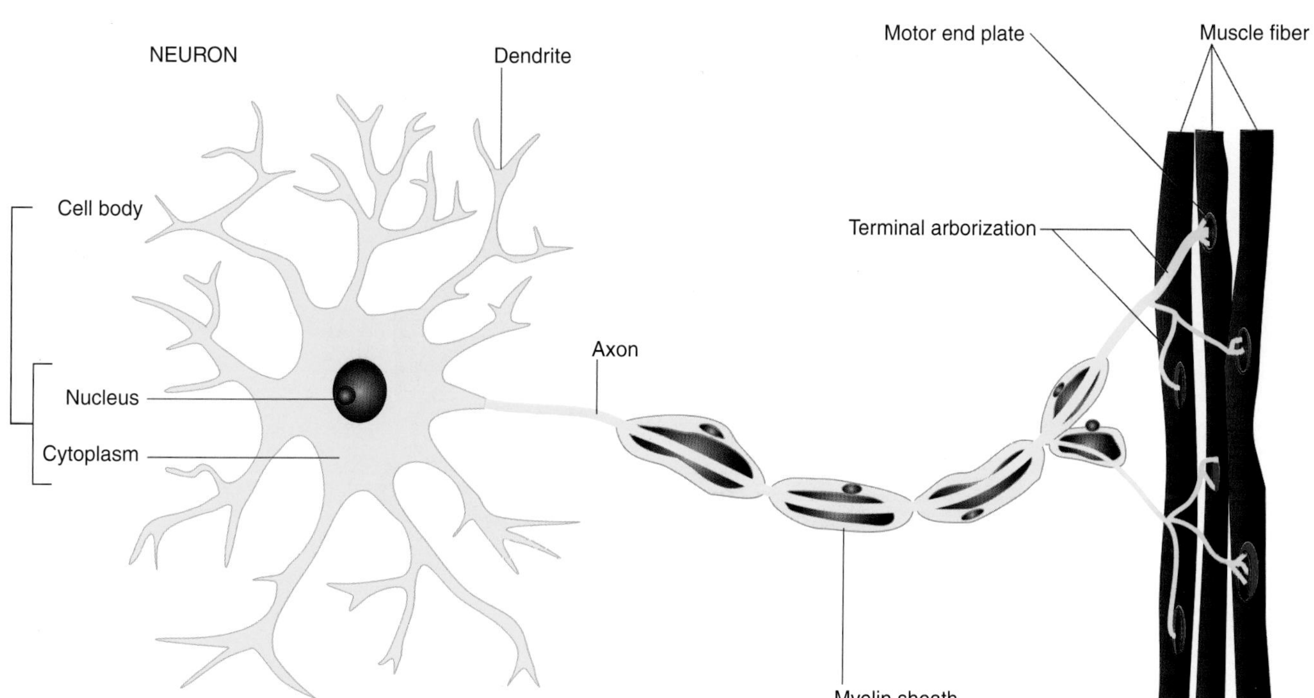


**FIGURE 1-1.** Organization of the peripheral nerve.

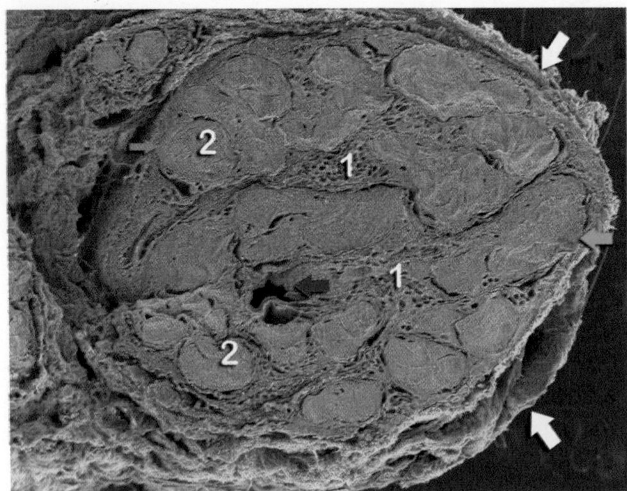


**FIGURE 1-2.** Histology of the peripheral nerve and connective tissues. *White arrows*: External epineurium (epineural sheath), 1 = Internal epineurium, 2 = fascicles, *Blue arrows*: Perineurium, *Red arrow*: Nerve vasculature *Green arrow*: Fascicular bundle.

in the nerve architecture, the connective tissue is called the epineurium, perineurium, or endoneurium (Figure 1-2). The *epineurium* surrounds the entire nerve and holds it loosely to the connective tissue through which it runs. Each group of axons that bundles together within a nerve forms a fascicle, which is surrounded by perineurium. It is at this level that the nerve–blood barrier is located and constitutes the last protective barrier of the nerve tissue. The *endoneurium* is the fine connective tissue within a fascicle that surrounds every individual nerve fiber or axon.

Nerves receive blood from the adjacent blood vessels running along their course. These feeding branches to larger nerves are macroscopic and irregularly arranged, forming anastomoses to become longitudinally running vessel(s) that supply the nerve and give off subsidiary branches.

## Organization of the Spinal Nerves

The nervous system consists of central and peripheral parts. The central nervous system includes the brain and spinal cord. The peripheral nervous system consists of the spinal, cranial, and autonomic nerves, and their associated ganglia. Nerves are bundles of nerve fibers that lie outside the central nervous system and serve to conduct electrical impulses from one region of the body to another. The nerves that make their exit through the skull are known as cranial nerves, and there are 12 pairs of them. The nerves that exit below the skull and between the vertebrae are called spinal nerves, and there are 31 pairs of them. Every spinal nerve has its regional number and can be identified by its association with the adjacent vertebrae (Figure 1-3). In the cervical region, the

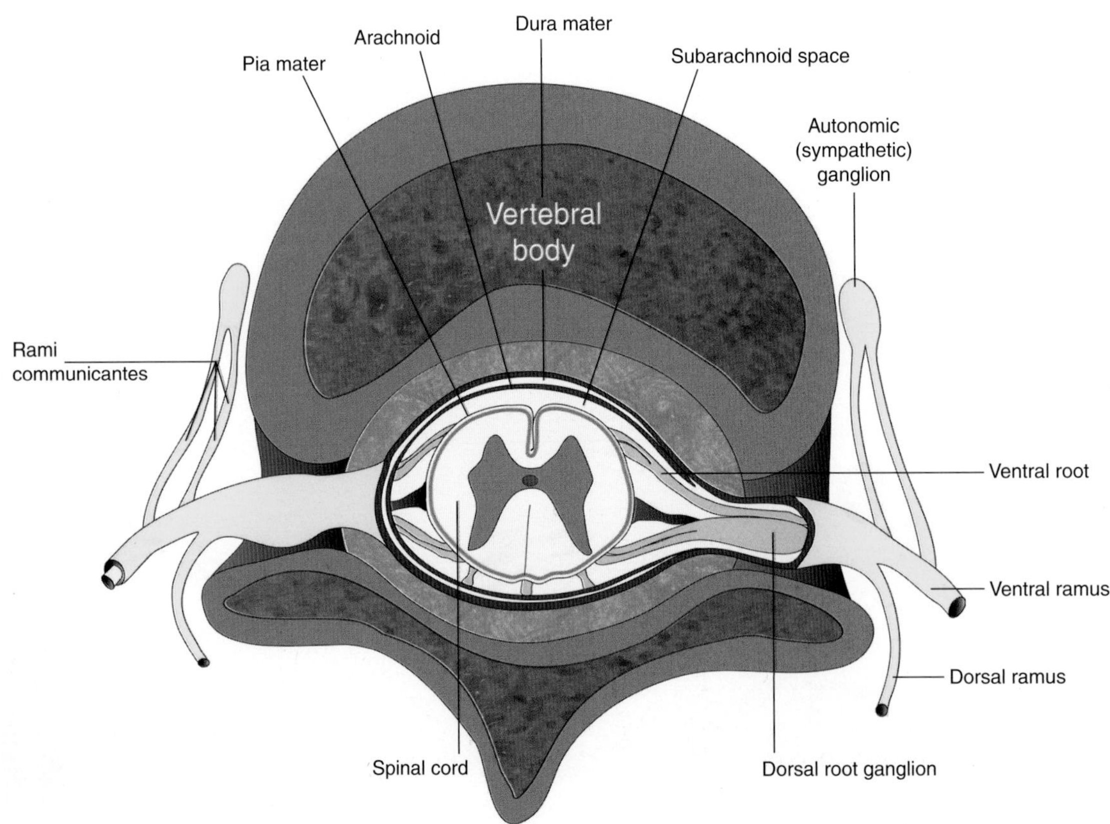


**FIGURE 1-3.** Organization of the spinal nerve.

first pair of spinal nerves, C1, exits between the skull and the first cervical vertebra. For this reason, a cervical spinal nerve takes its name from the vertebra below it. In other words, cervical nerve C2 precedes vertebra C2, and the same system is used for the rest of the cervical series. The transition from this identification method occurs between the last cervical and first thoracic vertebra. The spinal nerve lying between these two vertebrae has been designated C8. Thus there are seven cervical vertebrae but eight cervical nerves. Spinal nerves caudal to the first thoracic vertebra take their names from the vertebra immediately preceding them. For instance, the spinal nerve T1 emerges immediately caudal to vertebra T1, spinal nerve T2 passes under vertebra T2 and so on.

## Origin and Peripheral Distribution of Spinal Nerves

Each spinal nerve is formed by a dorsal and a ventral root that come together at the level of the intervertebral foramen (Figure 1-3). In the thoracic and lumbar levels, the first branch of the spinal nerve carries visceral motor fibers to a nearby autonomic ganglion. Because preganglionic fibers are myelinated, they have a light color and are known as white rami (Figure 1-4). Two groups of unmyelinated postganglionic fibers leave the ganglion. Those fibers innervating glands and smooth muscle in the body wall or limbs form the gray ramus that rejoins the spinal nerve. The gray and white rami are collectively called the rami communicantes. Preganglionic or postganglionic fibers that innervate internal organs do not rejoin the spinal nerves. Instead, they form a series of separate autonomic nerves and serve to regulate the activities of organs in the abdominal and pelvic cavities.

The dorsal ramus of each spinal nerve carries sensory innervation from, and motor innervation to, a specific segment of the skin and muscles of the back. The region innervated resembles a horizontal band that begins at the origin of the spinal nerve. The relatively larger ventral ramus supplies the ventrolateral body surface, structures in the body wall, and the limbs. Each spinal nerve supplies a specific segment of the body surface, known as a dermatome.

### *Dermatomes*

A dermatome is an area of the skin supplied by the dorsal (sensory) root of the spinal nerve (Figures 1-5 and 1-6). In the head and trunk, each segment is horizontally disposed, except C1, which does not have a sensory component.

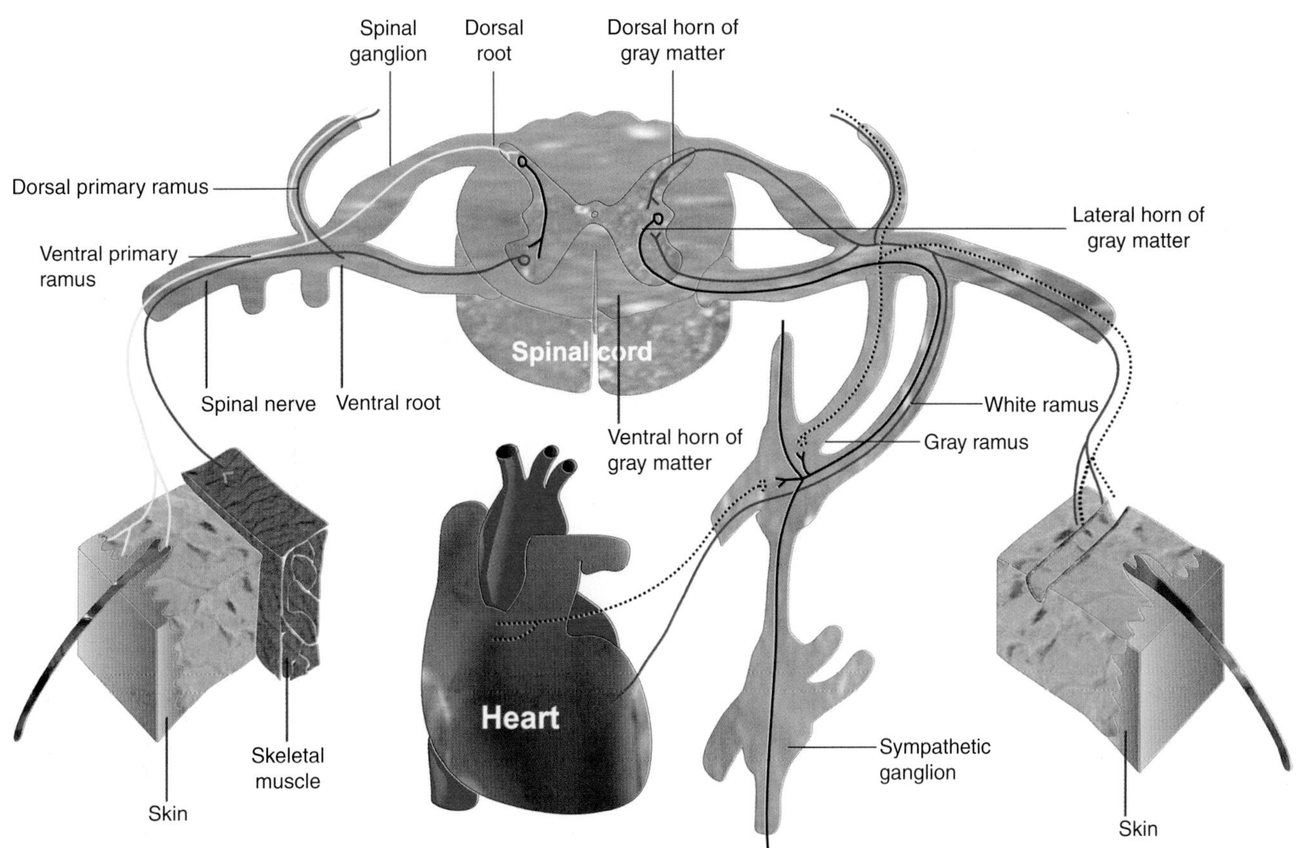


**FIGURE 1-4.** Organization and function of the segmental (spinal nerve).

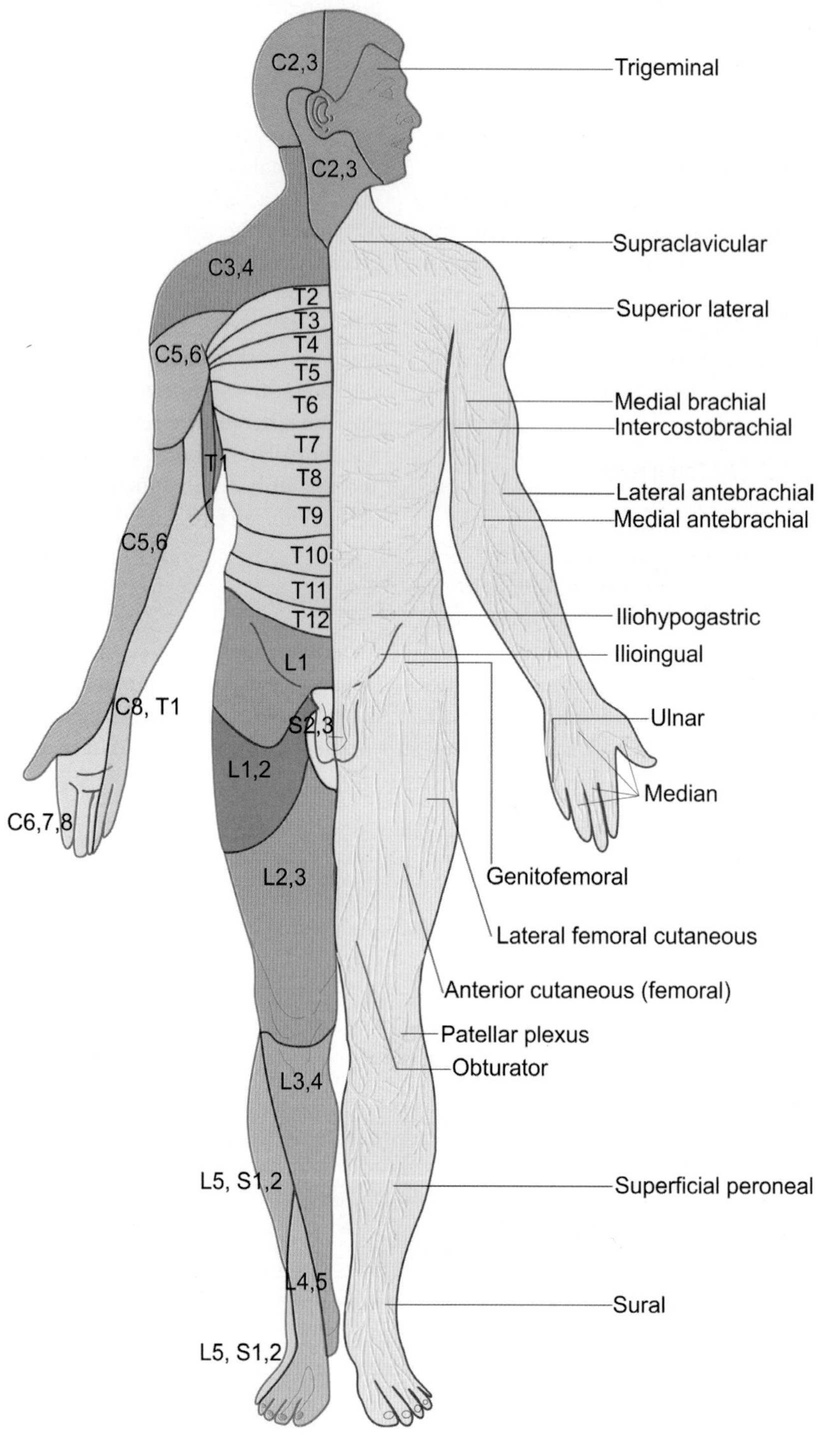


**FIGURE 1-5.** Dermatomes and corresponding peripheral nerves: front.

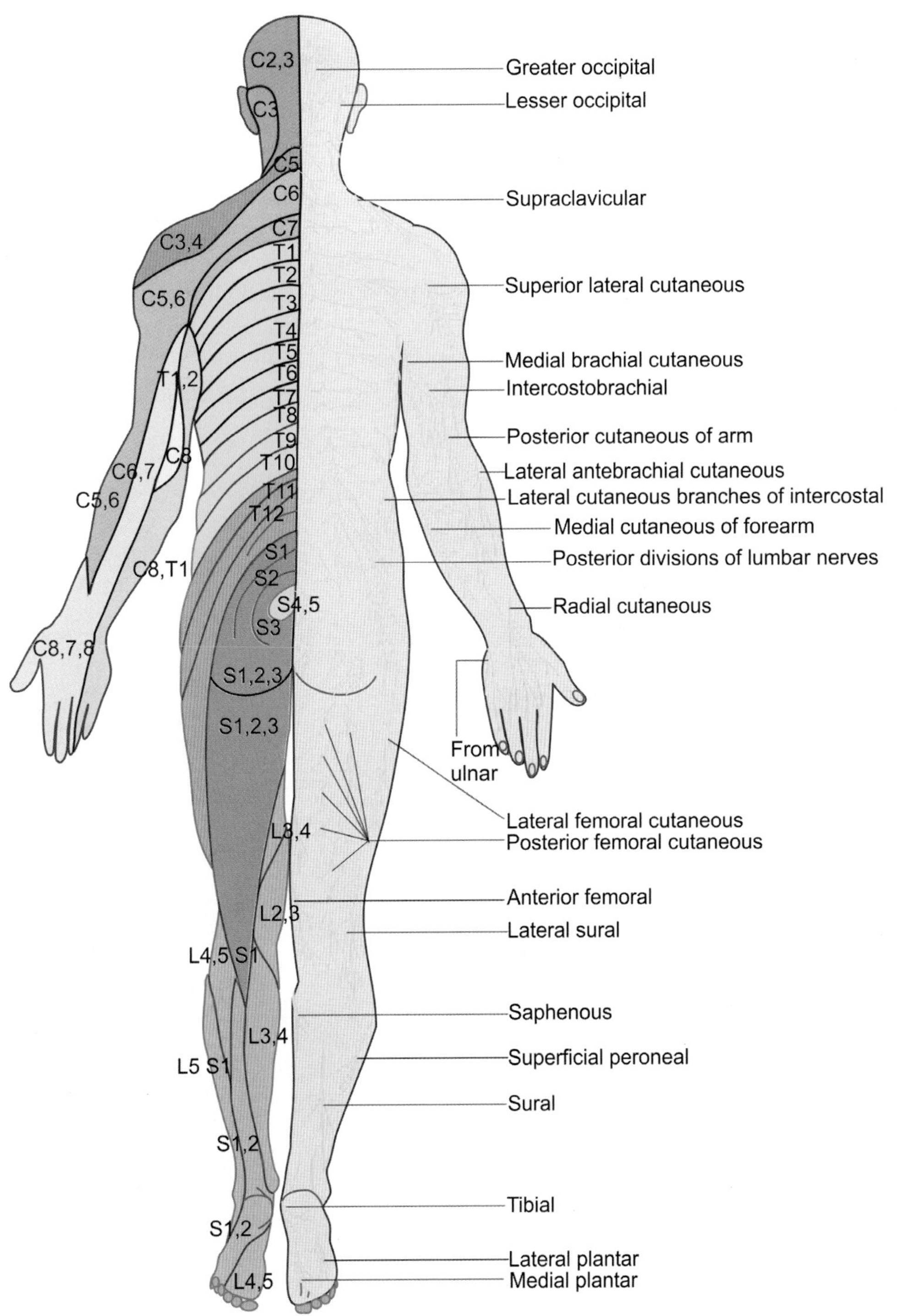


**FIGURE 1-6.** Dermatomes and corresponding peripheral nerves: back.

The dermatomes of the limbs from the fifth cervical to the first thoracic nerve, and from the third lumbar to the second sacral vertebrae, form a more complicated arrangement due to rotation and growth during embryologic life. There is considerable overlapping of adjacent dermatomes; that is, each segmental nerve overlaps the territories of its neighbors. This pattern is variable among individuals, and it is more of a guide than a fixed map.

### *Myotomes*

A myotome is the segmental innervation of skeletal muscle by a ventral root of a specific spinal nerve (Figure 1-7).

## TIPS

- Although the differences between dermatomal, myotomal, and osteotomal innervation are often emphasized in regional anesthesiology textbooks, it is usually impractical to think in those terms when planning a regional block.
- Instead, it is more practical to think in terms of areas of the body that can be blocked by a specific technique.

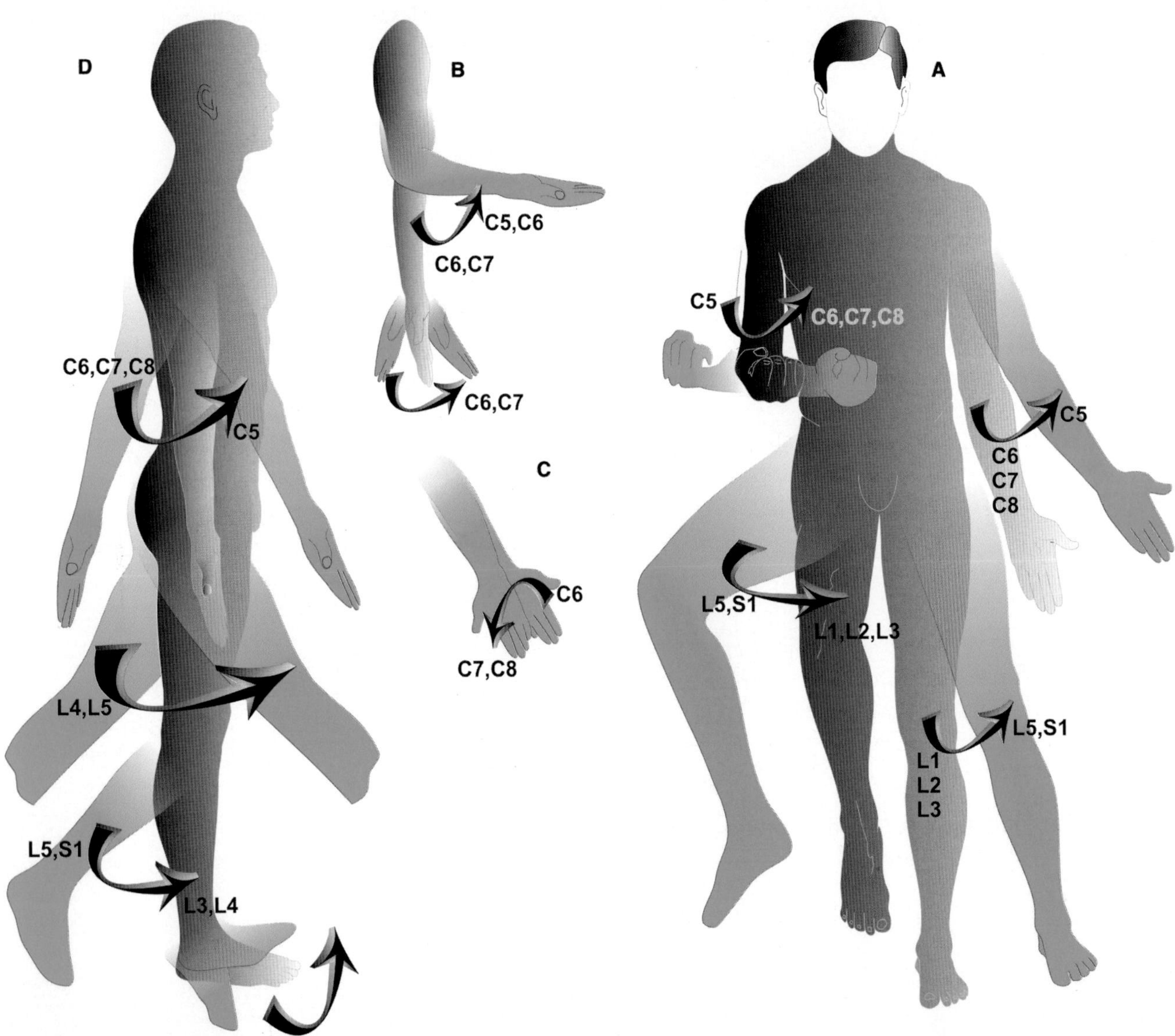


**FIGURE 1-7.** Motor innervation of the major muscle groups. (A) Medial and lateral rotation of shoulder and hip. Abduction and adduction of shoulder and hip. (B) Flexion and extension of elbow and wrist. (C) Pronation and supination of forearm. (D) Flexion and extension of shoulder, hip, and knee. Dorsiflexion and plantar flexion of ankle, lateral views.

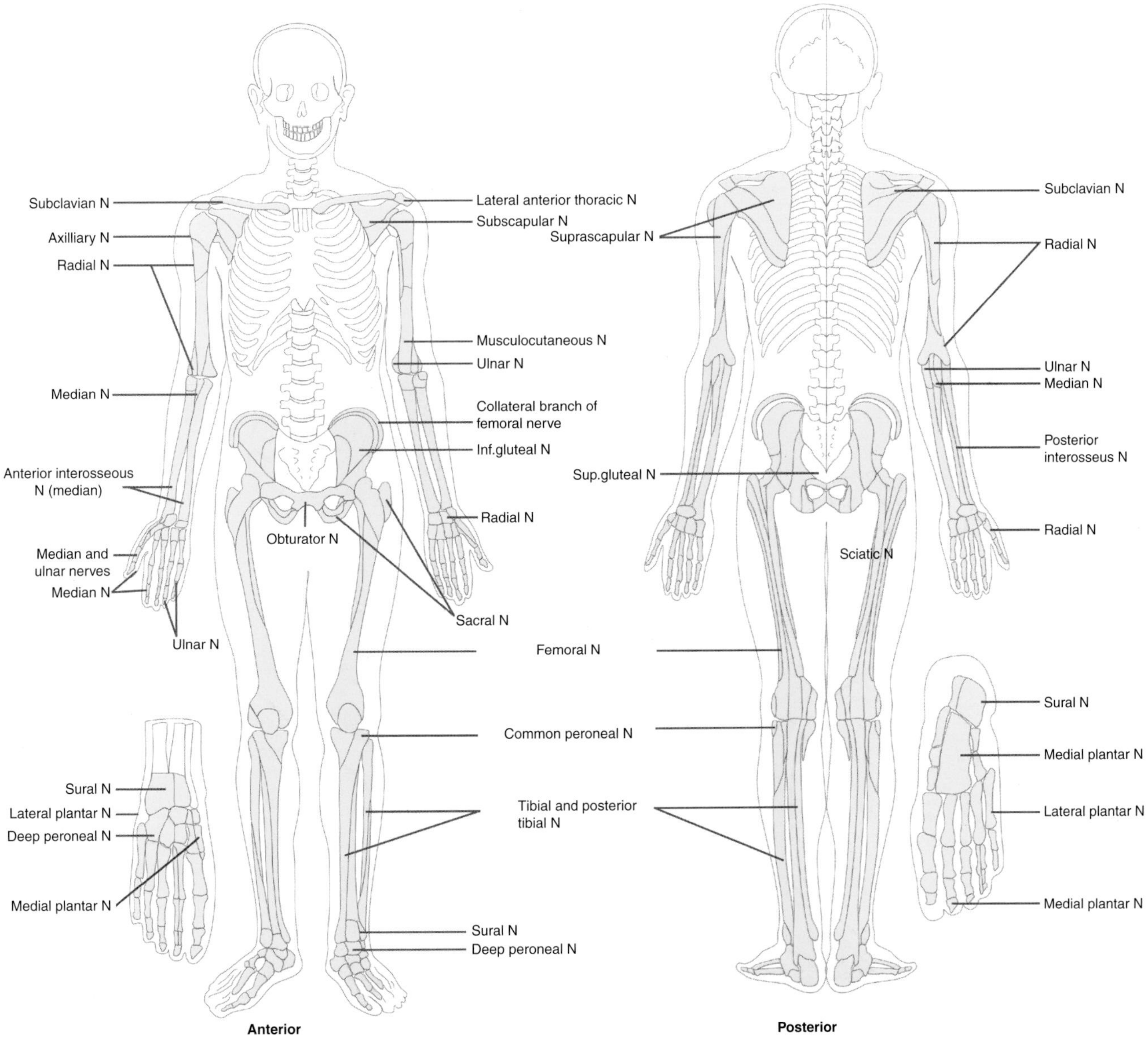

Subclavian N
Axilliary N
Radial N
Median N
Anterior interosseous N (median)
Median and ulnar nerves
Median N
Ulnar N
Obturator N
Lateral anterior thoracic N
Subscapular N
Suprascapular N
Musculocutaneous N
Ulnar N
Collateral branch of femoral nerve
Inf.gluteal N
Sup.gluteal N
Radial N
Sacral N
Femoral N
Common peroneal N
Tibial and posterior tibial N
Sural N
Deep peroneal N
Sural N
Lateral plantar N
Deep peroneal N
Medial plantar N
Subclavian N
Radial N
Ulnar N
Median N
Posterior interosseus N
Radial N
Sciatic N
Sural N
Medial plantar N
Lateral plantar N
Medial plantar N
Anterior
Posterior

**FIGURE 1-8.** Osteotomes.

*Osteotomes*

The innervation of the bones follows its own pattern and does not coincide with the innervation of more superficial structures (Figure 1-8).

## Nerve Plexuses

Although the dermatomal innervation of the trunk is simple, the innervation of the extremities, part of the neck, and pelvis is highly complex. In these areas, the ventral rami of the spinal nerves form an intricate neural network; nerve fibers coming from similar spinal segments easily reach different terminal nerves. The four major nerve plexuses are the cervical plexus, brachial plexus, lumbar plexus, and sacral plexus.

## The Cervical Plexus

The cervical plexus originates from the ventral rami of C1-C5, which form three loops (Figures 1-9 and 1-10). Branches from the cervical plexus provide sensory innervation of part of the scalp, neck, and upper shoulder and motor innervation to some of the muscles of the neck, the thoracic cavity, and the skin (Table 1-1). The phrenic nerve, one of the larger branches of the plexus, innervates the diaphragm.

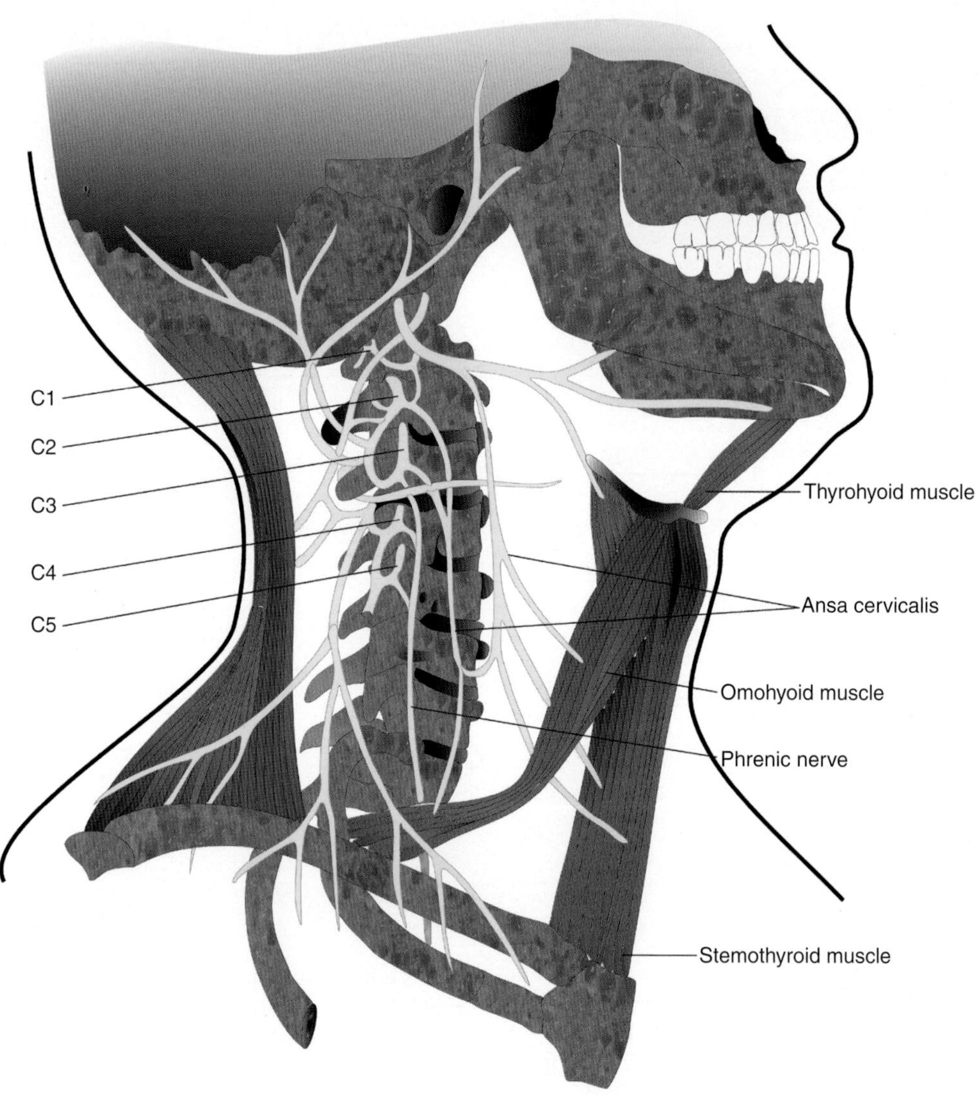


**FIGURE 1-9.** Organization of the cervical plexus.

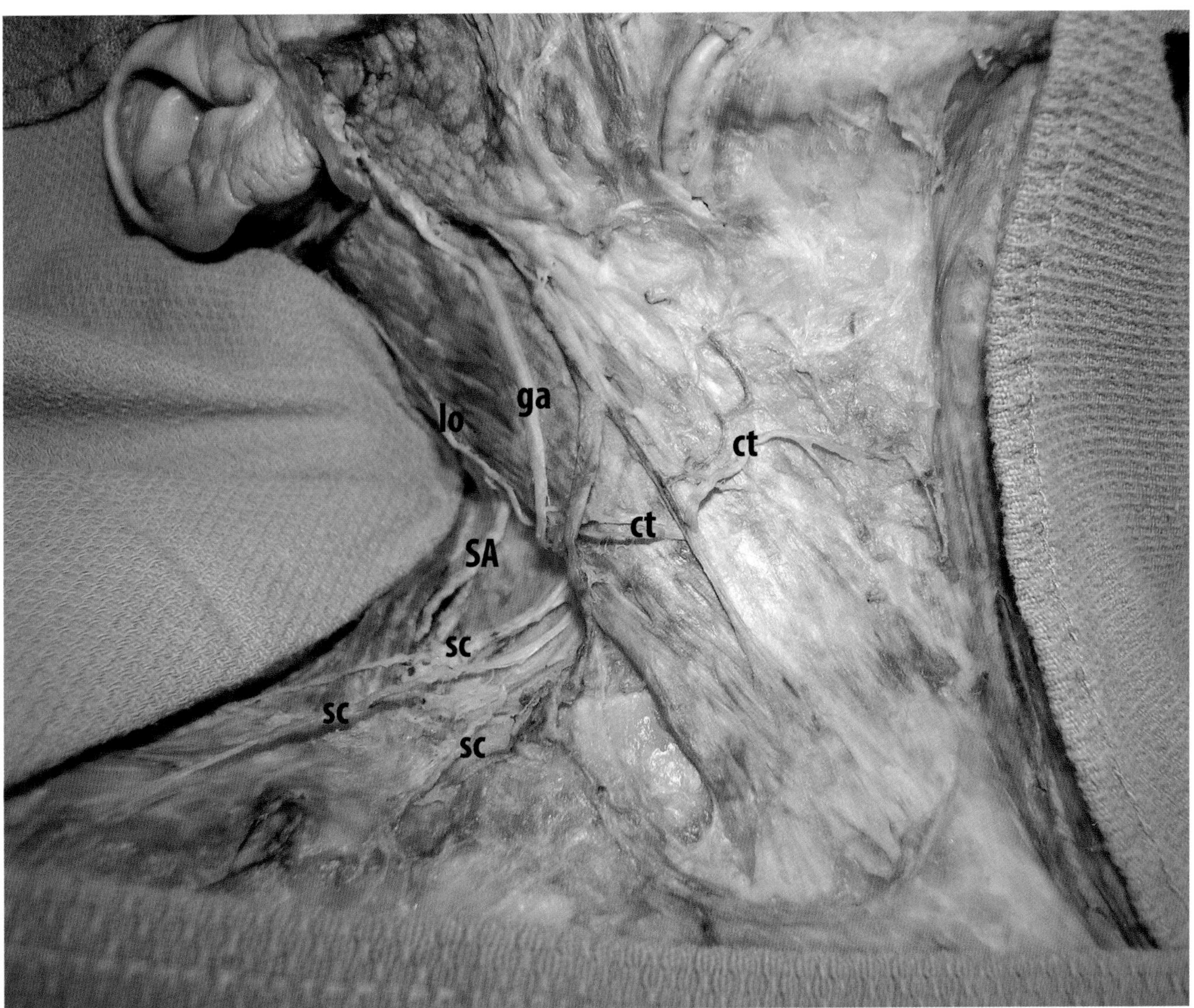


**FIGURE 1-10.** Superficial cervical plexus branches. ct, transverse cervical; ga, greater auricular; lo, lesser occipital; sc, supraclavicular. Also shown is the spinal accessory nerve (SA).

**TABLE 1-1 Organization and Distribution of the Cervical Plexus**

| NERVES | SPINAL SEGMENTS | DISTRIBUTION |
|---|---|---|
| Ansa cervicalis (superior and inferior branches) | C1-C4 | Five of the extrinsic laryngeal muscles (sternothyroid, sternohyoid, omohyoid, geniohyoid, and thyrohyoid) by way of N XII |
| Lesser occipital, transverse cervical, supraclavicular, and greater auricular nerves | C2-C3 | Skin of upper chest, shoulder, neck, and ear |
| Phrenic nerve | C3-C5 | Diaphragm |
| Cervical nerves | C1-C5 | Levator scapulae, scalene muscles, sternocleidomastoid, and trapezius muscles (with N XI) |

## The Brachial Plexus

The brachial plexus is both larger and more complex than the cervical plexus (Figures 1-11, 1-12, 1-13, 1-14A,B, 1-15A,B, and 1-16). It innervates the pectoral girdle and upper limb. The plexus is formed by five roots that originate from the ventral rami of spinal nerves C5-T1. The roots converge to form the superior (C5-C6), middle (C7), and inferior (C8-T1) trunks (Table 1-2). The trunks give off three anterior and three posterior divisions as they approach the clavicle. The divisions rearrange their fibers to form the lateral, medial, and posterior cords. The cords give off the terminal branches. The lateral cord gives off the musculocutaneous nerve, and the lateral root of the median nerve. The medial cord gives off the medial root of the median nerve and the ulnar nerve. The posterior cord gives off the axillary and radial nerves.

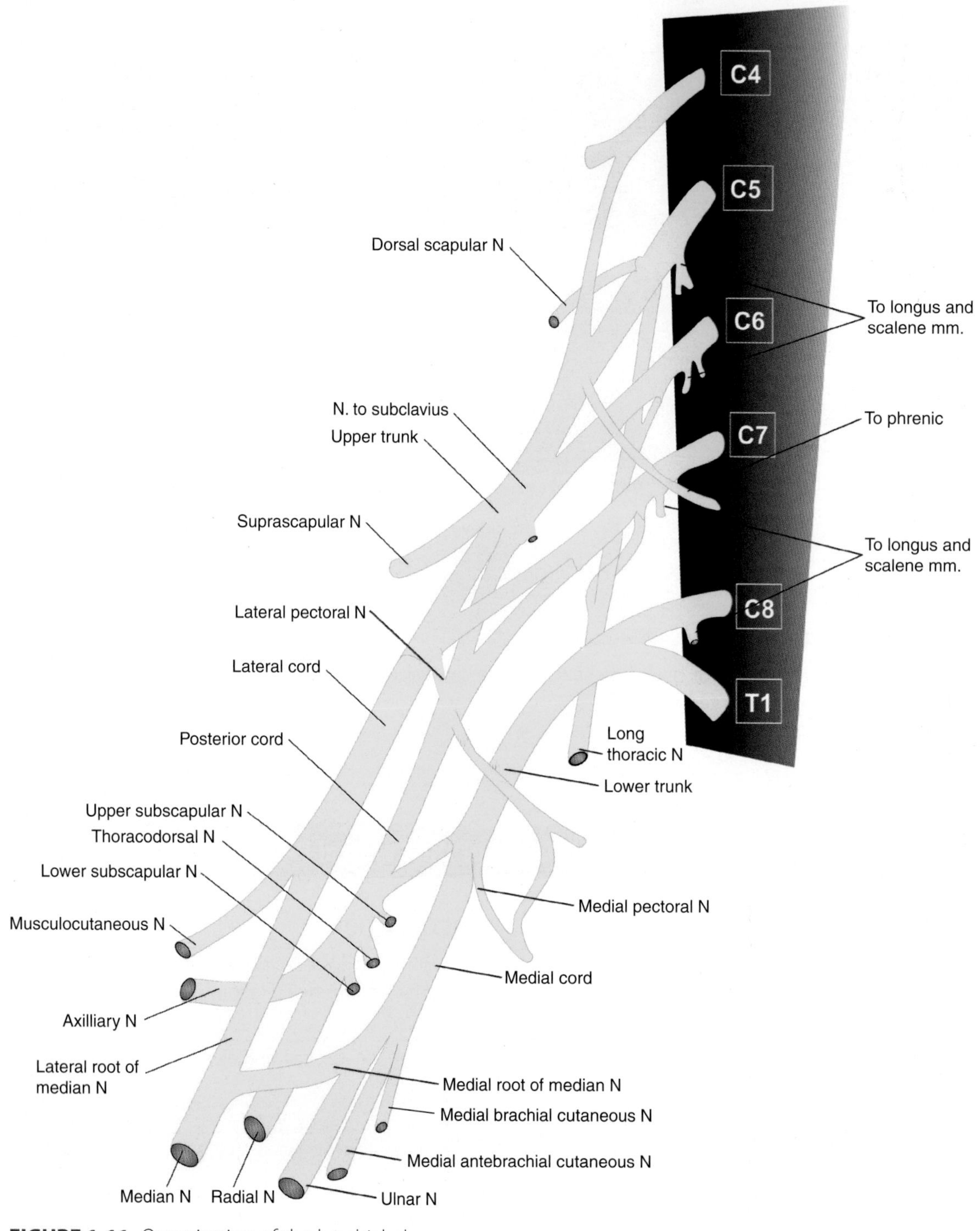


**FIGURE 1-11.** Organization of the brachial plexus.

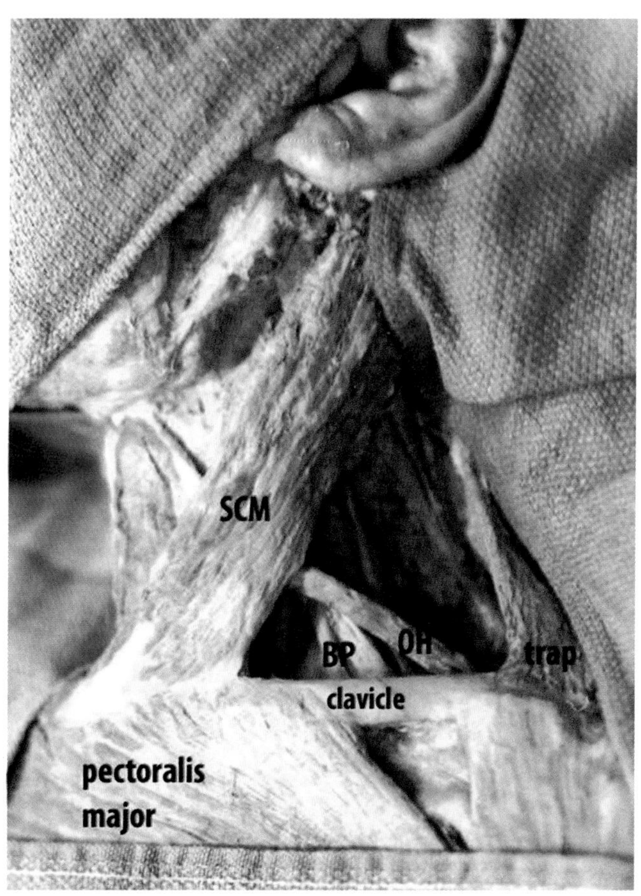


**FIGURE 1-12.** View of the posterior triangle of the neck, located above the clavicle between the sternocleidomastoid (SCM) in front and the trapezius (trap) behind. It is crossed by the omohyoid muscle (OH) and the brachial plexus (BP).

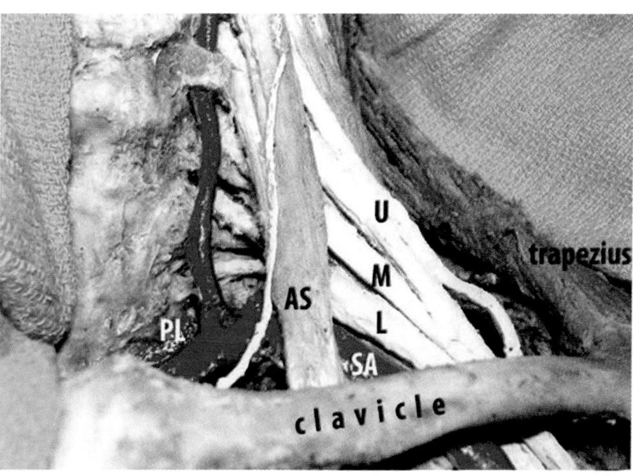


**FIGURE 1-13.** The brachial plexus (in yellow) at the level of the trunks (U, M, and L) occupies the smallest surface area in its entire trajectory. Also shown are the dome of the pleura (PL) in blue, the subclavian artery (SA) and the vertebral artery, both in red. The phrenic nerve, in yellow, is seen traveling anterior to the anterior scalene muscle (AS).

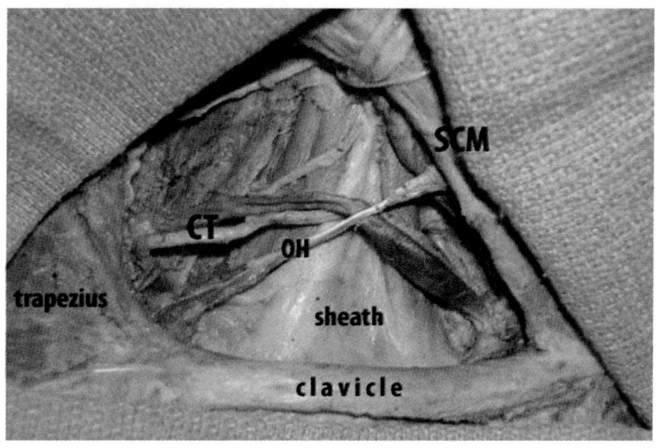


A

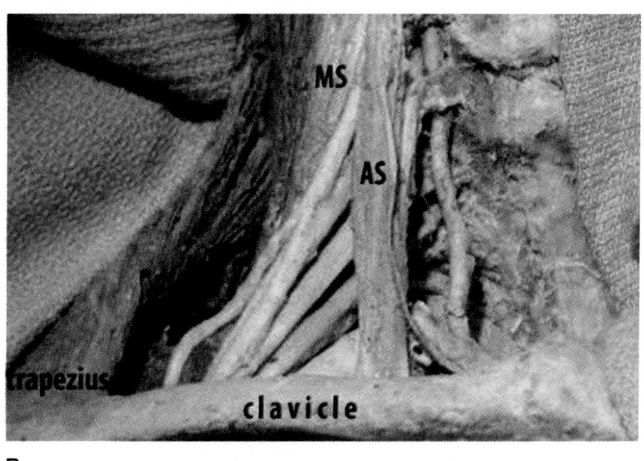


B

**FIGURE 1-14.** (A) A thick fascia layer (sheath) covers the brachial plexus in the posterior triangle. Also seen is part of the sternocleidomastoid muscle (SCM), the cervical transverse vessels (CT), and the omohyoid muscle (OH). (B) Once the sheath is removed, the brachial plexus can be seen between the anterior scalene (AS) and middle scalene (MS) muscles. (Part A reproduced with permission from Franco CD, Rahman A, Voronov G, et al. Gross anatomy of the brachial plexus sheath in human cadavers. Reg Anesth Pain Med. 2008;33(1):64-69. Part B reproduced from Franco CD, Clark L. Applied anatomy of the upper extremity. *Tech Reg Anesth Pain Mgmt.* 2008;12(3):134-139, with permission from Elsevier.)

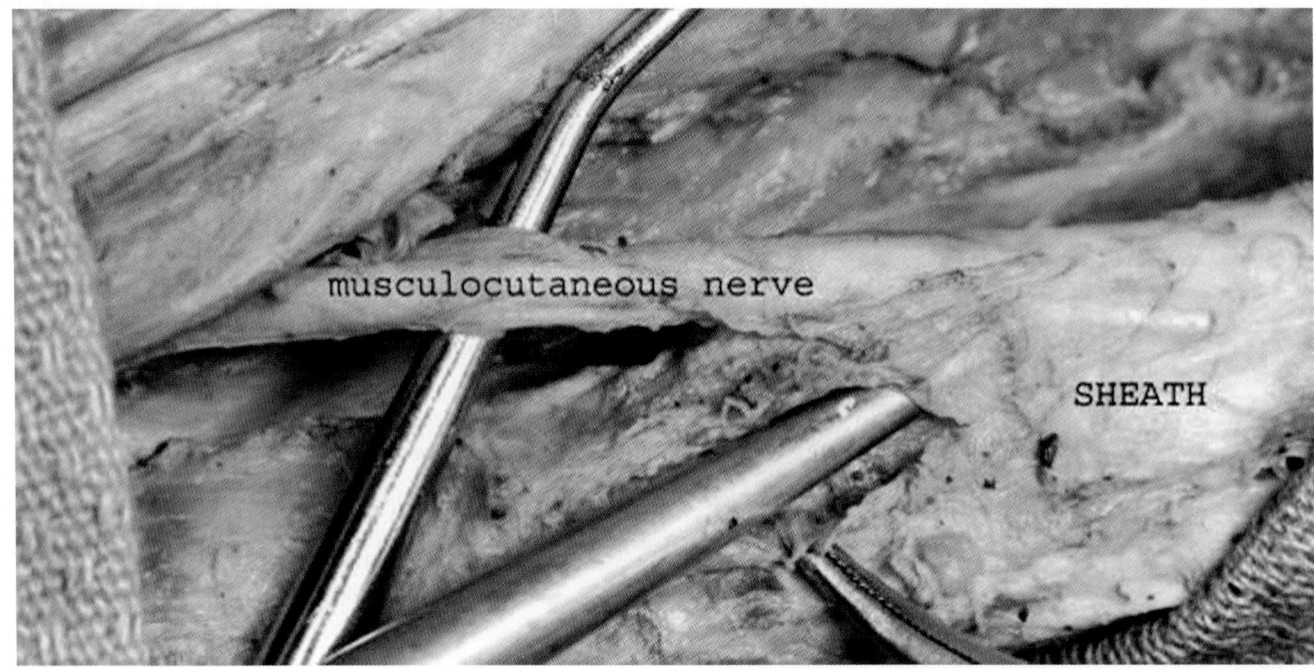


A

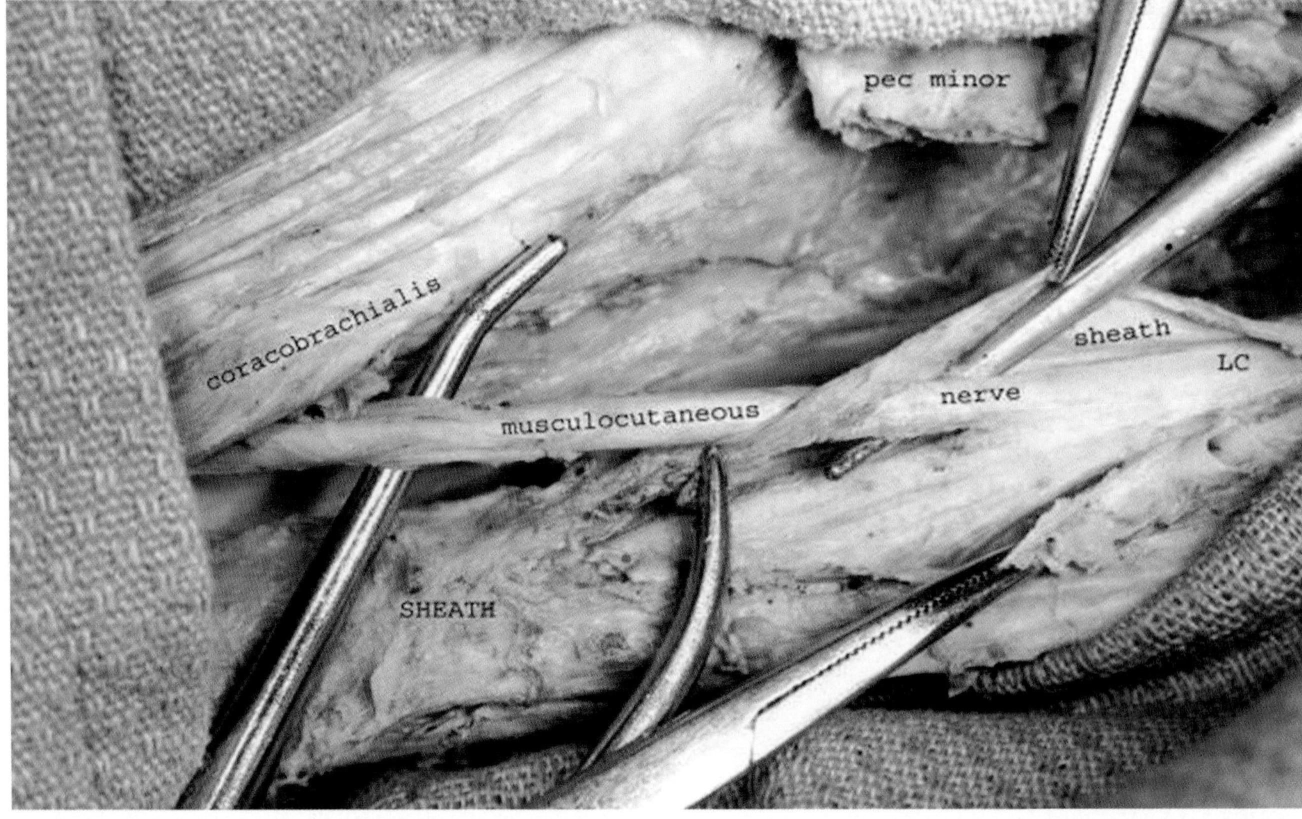


B

**FIGURE 1-15.** (A) In the axilla the brachial plexus is also surrounded by a thick fibrous fascia that here is shown partially open with a metal probe inside. The musculocutaneous nerve can be seen exiting the sheath and entering the coracobrachialis muscle. (B) The sheath has been open. Pectoralis minor (pec minor) has been partially resected. The takeoff of the musculocutaneous nerve from the lateral cord (LC) inside the sheath is clearly visible. (Reproduced with permission from Franco CD, Rahman A, Voronov G, et al. Gross anatomy of the brachial plexus sheath in human cadavers. *Reg Anesth Pain Med.* 2008;33(1):64-69.)

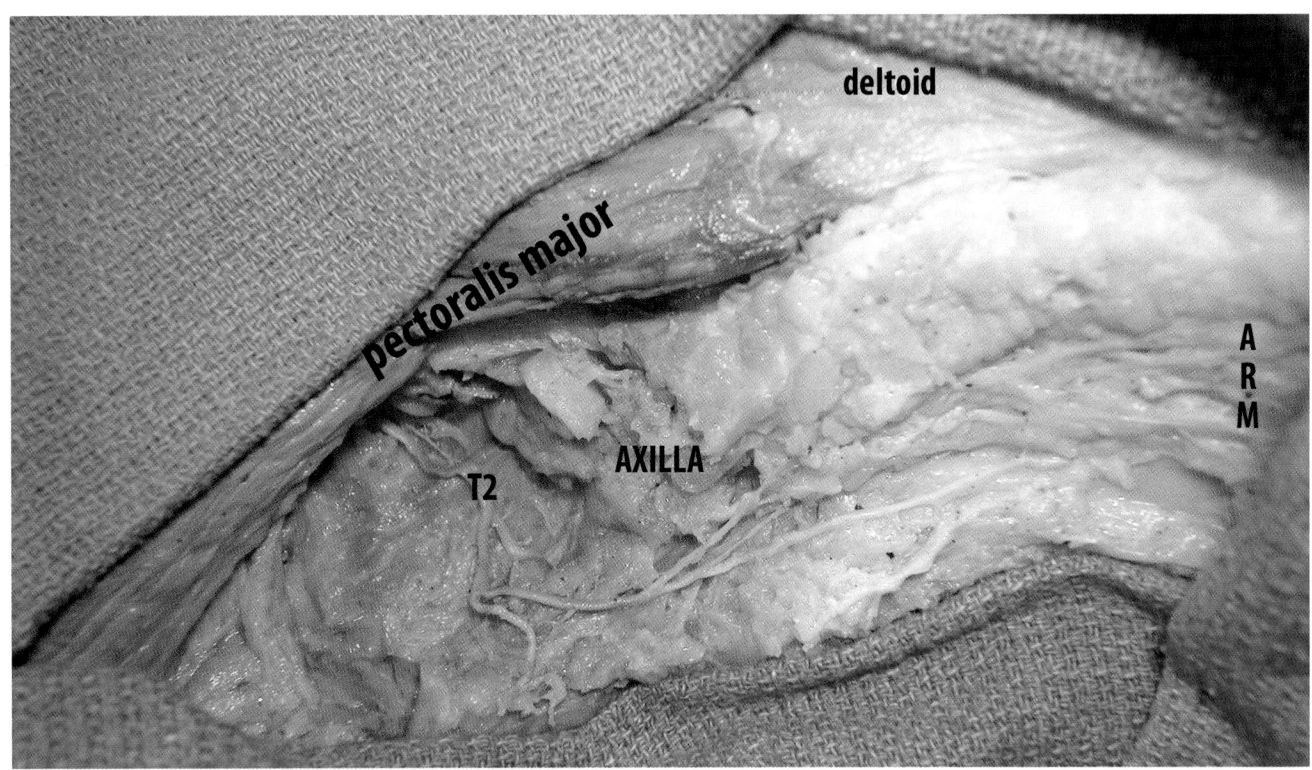


**FIGURE 1-16.** Intercostobrachial nerve (T2) is the lateral branch of the second intercostal nerve that supplies sensory innervation to the axilla and upper medial side of the arm.

**TABLE 1-2 Organization and Distribution of the Brachial Plexus**

| NERVE(S) | SPINAL SEGMENTS | DISTRIBUTION |
|---|---|---|
| Nerves to subclavius | C4-C6 | Subclavius muscle |
| Dorsal scapular nerve | C5 | Rhomboid muscles and levator scapulae muscle |
| Long thoracic nerve | C5-C7 | Serratus anterior muscle |
| Suprascapular nerve | C5, C6 | Supraspinatus and infraspinatus muscles |
| Pectoralis nerve (median and lateral) | C5-T1 | Pectoralis muscles |
| Subscapular nerves | C5, C6 | Subscapularis and teres major muscles |
| Thoracodorsal nerve | C6-C8 | Latissimus dorsi muscle |
| Axillary nerve | C5, C6 | Deltoid and teres minor muscles; part of skin of shoulder |
| Radial nerve | C5-T1 | Extensor muscle of the arm and forearm (triceps brachii, extensor carpi radialis, and extensor carpi ulnaris muscles) and brachioradialis muscle; digital extensors, and abductor pollicis muscle; skin over the posterolateral surface of the arm. |
| Musculocutaneous nerve | C5-C7 | Flexor muscles on the arm (biceps brachii, brachialis, and coracobrachialis muscles); skin over lateral surface of forearm |
| Median nerve | C6-T1 | Flexor muscles on the forearm (flexor carpi radialis and palmaris longus muscles); pronator quadratus and pronator teres muscles; digital flexors (through the palmar interosseous nerve); skin over anterolateral surface of hand |
| Ulnar nerve | C8, T1 | Flexor carpi ulnaris muscle, adductor pollicis muscle and small digital muscles; skin over medial surface of the hand |

## The Lumbar Plexus

The lumbar plexus is formed by the ventral rami of spinal nerves L1-L3 and the superior branch of L4 (Figures 1-17, 1-18A,B, and 1-19). In about 50% of the cases, there is a contribution from T12. The inferior branch of L4, along with the entire ventral rami of L5, forms the lumbosacral trunk that contributes to the sacral plexus.

Because the branches of both the lumbar and sacral plexuses are distributed to the lower limb, they are often collectively referred to as the lumbosacral plexus. The main branches of the lumbar plexus are the iliohypogastric, ilioinguinal, genitofemoral, lateral femoral cutaneous, obturator, and femoral nerves (Figures 1-19, 1-20A,B; Table 1-3).

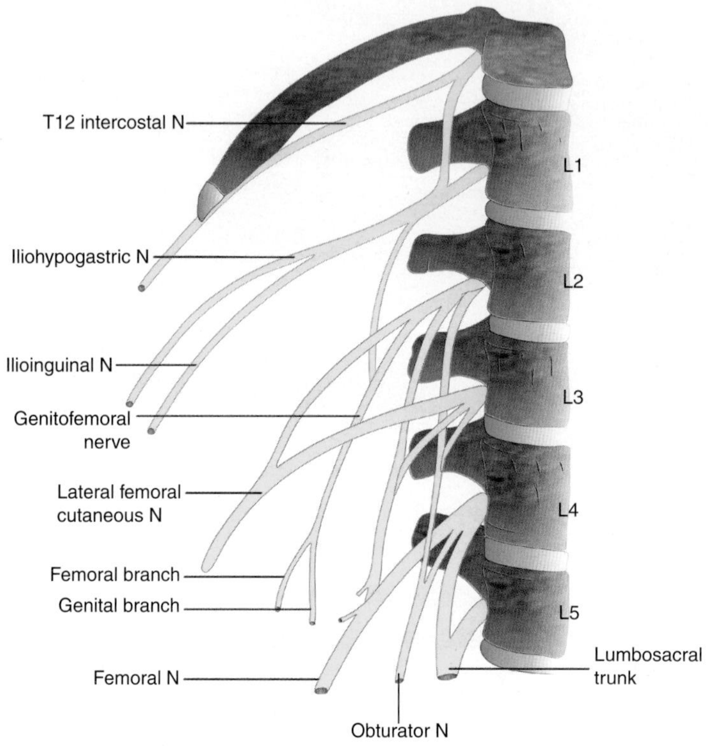


**FIGURE 1-17.** Organization of the lumbar plexus.

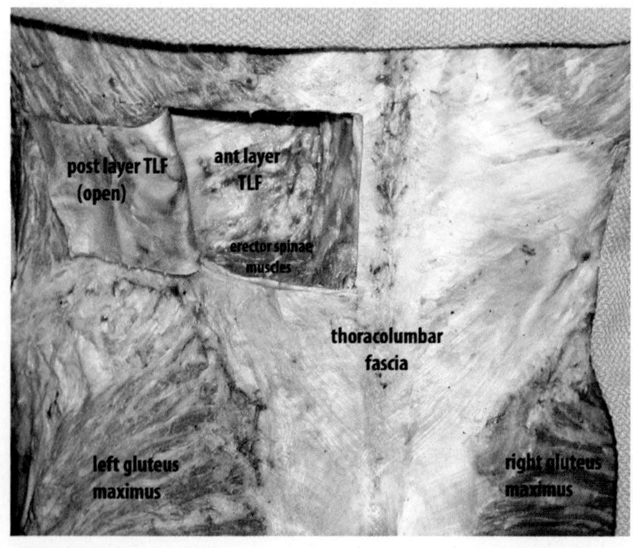


A

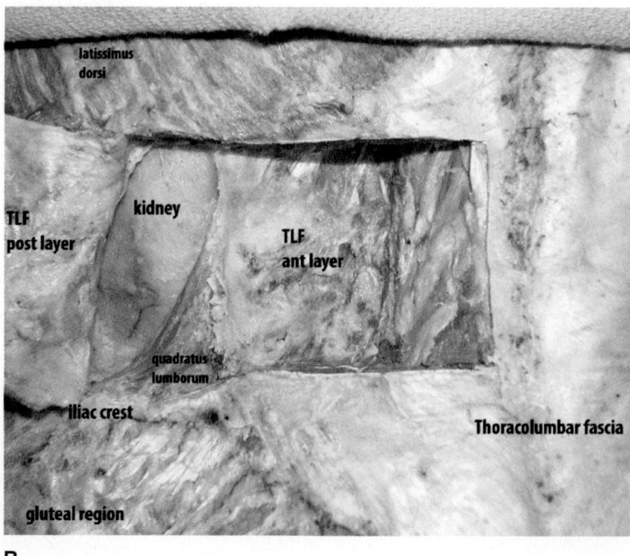


B

**FIGURE 1-18.** (A) Posterior view of the back to show the thoracolumbar fascia (TLF), whose posterior layer has been open as a small window through which part of the erector spinae muscles has been resected to show the anterior layer of the thoracolumbar fascia. (B) One step further in the dissection shows part of the quadratus lumborum muscle.

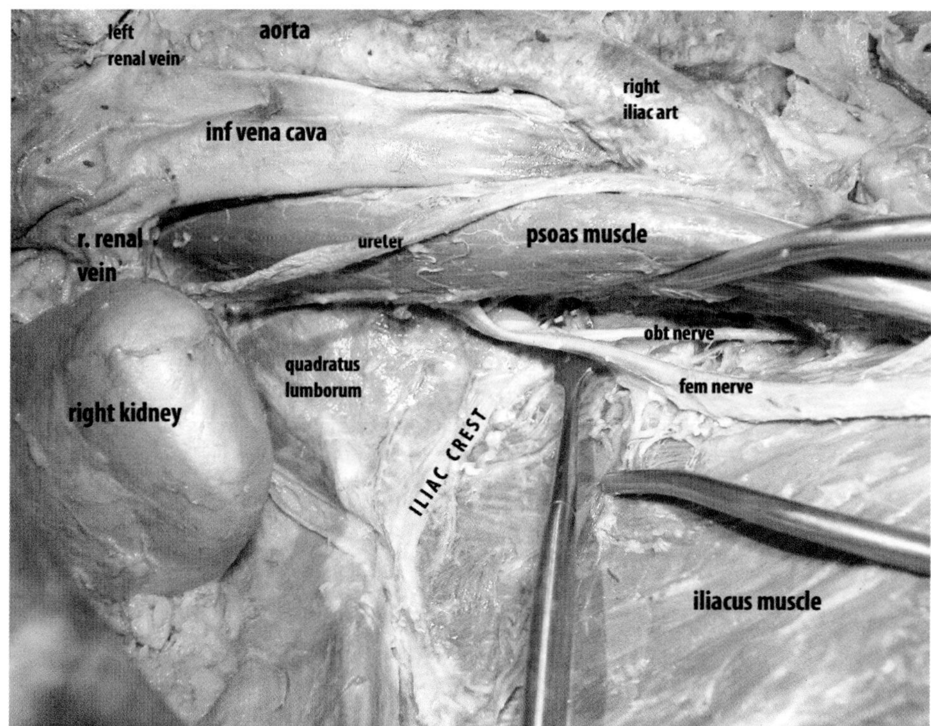


**FIGURE 1-19.** Two branches of the lumbar plexus, the femoral nerve and obturator, are seen between the quadratus lumborum and psoas muscles in the right retroperitoneal space.

**TABLE 1-3 Organization and Distribution of the Lumbar Plexus**

| NERVE(S) | SPINAL SEGMENTS | DISTRIBUTION |
|---|---|---|
| Iliohypogastric nerve | T12-L1 | Abdominal muscles (external and internal oblique muscles, transverse abdominis muscles); skin over inferior abdomen and buttocks |
| Ilioinguinal nerve | L1 | Abdominal muscles (with iliohypogastric nerve); skin over superior, medial thigh, and portions of external genitalia |
| Genitofemoral nerve | L1, L2 | Skin over anteromedial surface of thigh and portions over genitalia |
| Lateral femoral cutaneous nerve | L2, L3 | Skin over anterior, lateral, and posterior surfaces of thigh |
| Femoral nerve | L2-L4 | Anterior muscles of thigh (sartorius muscle and quadriceps group); adductor of thigh (pectineus and iliopsoas muscles); skin over anteromedial surface of thigh, as well as the medial surface of leg, and foot through the saphenous nerve |
| Obturator nerve | L2-L4 | Adductors of thigh (adductors magnus, brevis, and longus); gracilis muscle; skin over medial surface of thigh<br>Note: Writing about a branch of a branch of the lumbar plexus may produce some confusion. |

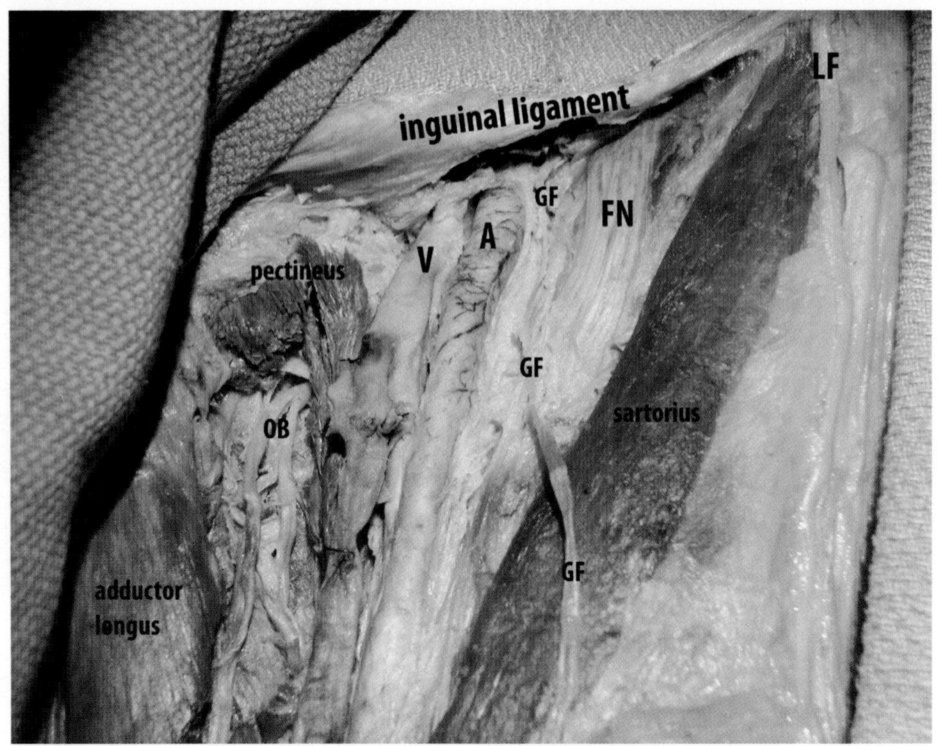


A

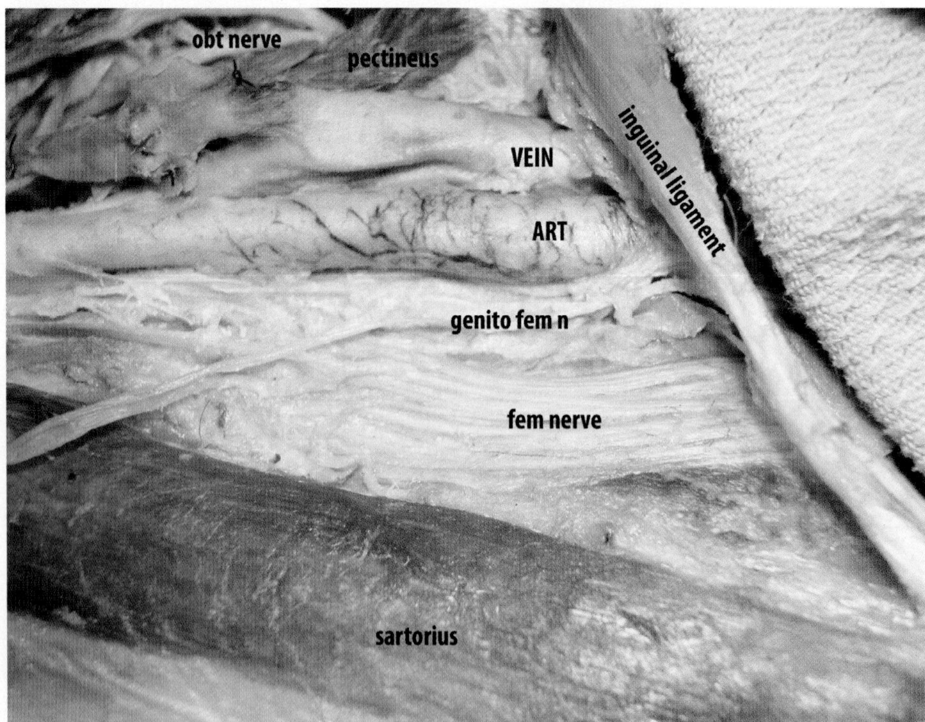


B

**FIGURE 1-20.** (A) Frontal view of the upper anterior thigh showing the inguinal ligament and some branches of the lumbar plexus: FN, femoral nerve; GF, femoral branch of genitofemoral nerve; LF, lateral femoral cutaneous nerve; OB, obturator nerve. The femoral vein (V) and artery (A) are also shown. (B) The same nerves of (A) are shown from the lateral side.

## The Sacral Plexus

The sacral plexus arises from the lumbosacral trunk (L4-L5) plus the ventral rami of S1-S4 (Figures 1-21,1-22A,B, 1-23, and 1-24). The main nerves of the sacral plexus are the sciatic nerve and the pudendal nerve (Table 1-4). The sciatic nerve leaves the pelvis through the greater sciatic foramen to enter the gluteal area where it travels between the greater trochanter and ischial tuberosity. In the proximal thigh it lies behind the lesser trochanter of the femur covered superficially by the long head of the biceps femoris muscle. As it approaches the popliteal fossa, the two components of the sciatic nerve diverge into two recognizable nerves: the common peroneal and the tibial nerve (Figures 1-25 and 1-26).

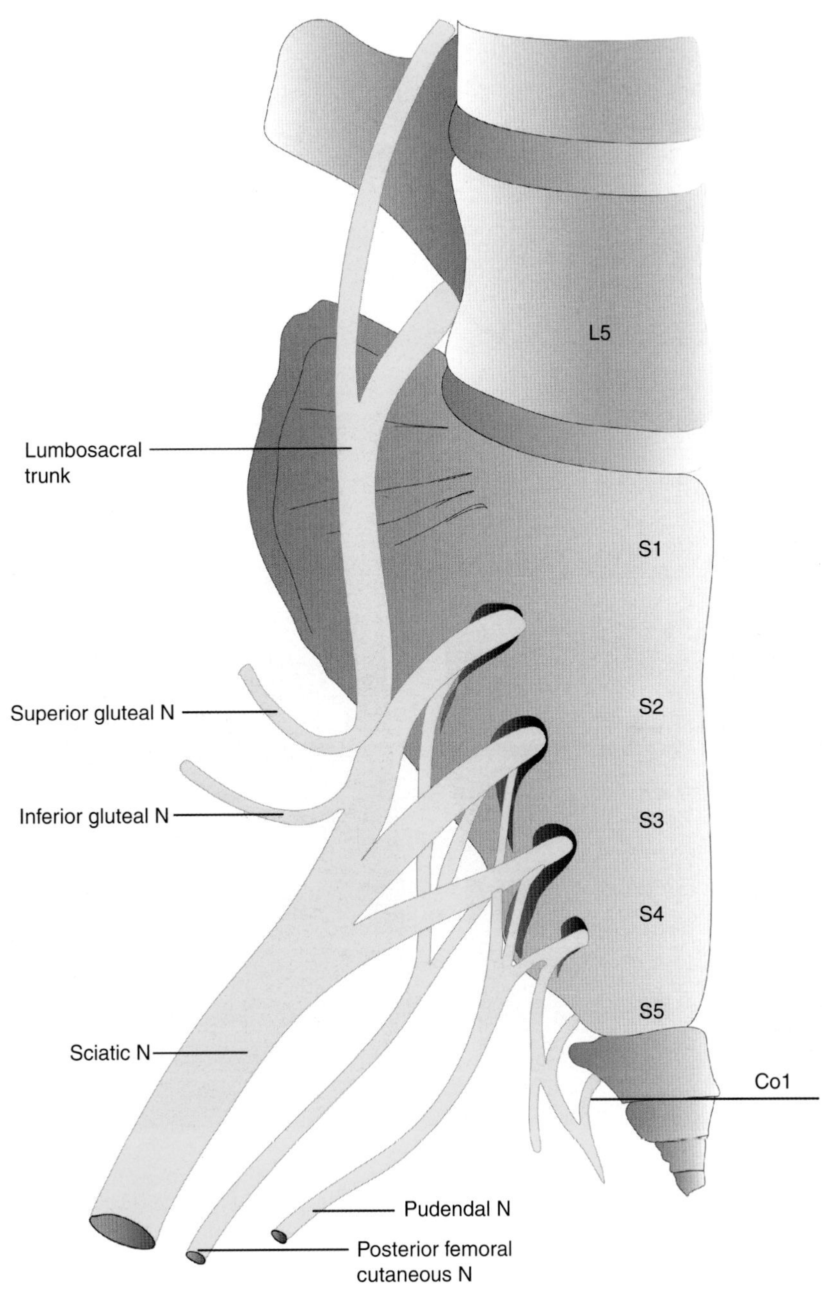


**FIGURE 1-21.** Organization of the sacral plexus.

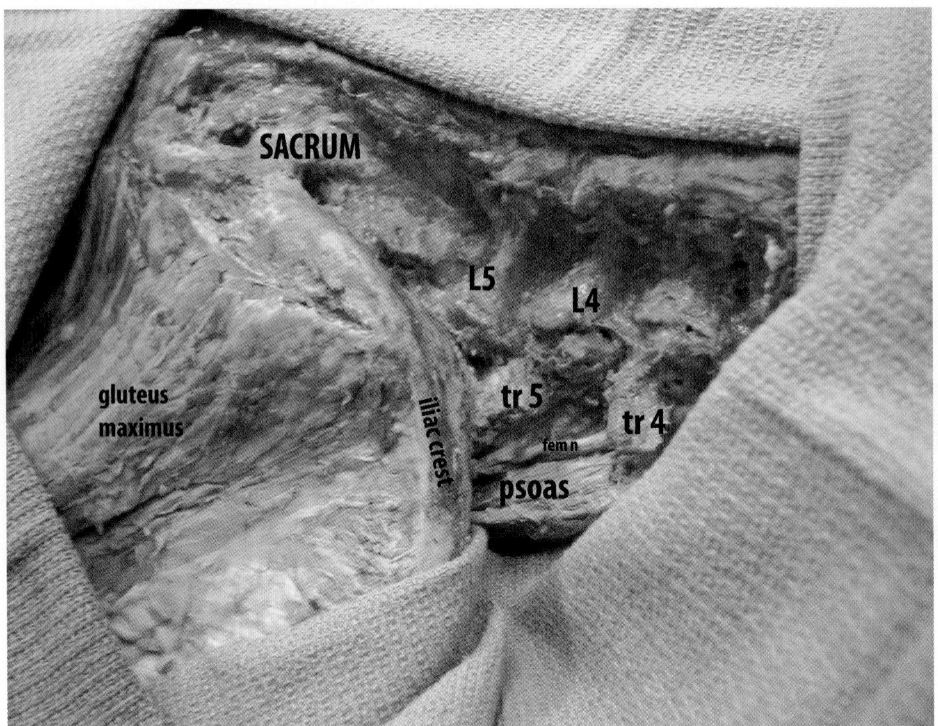


A

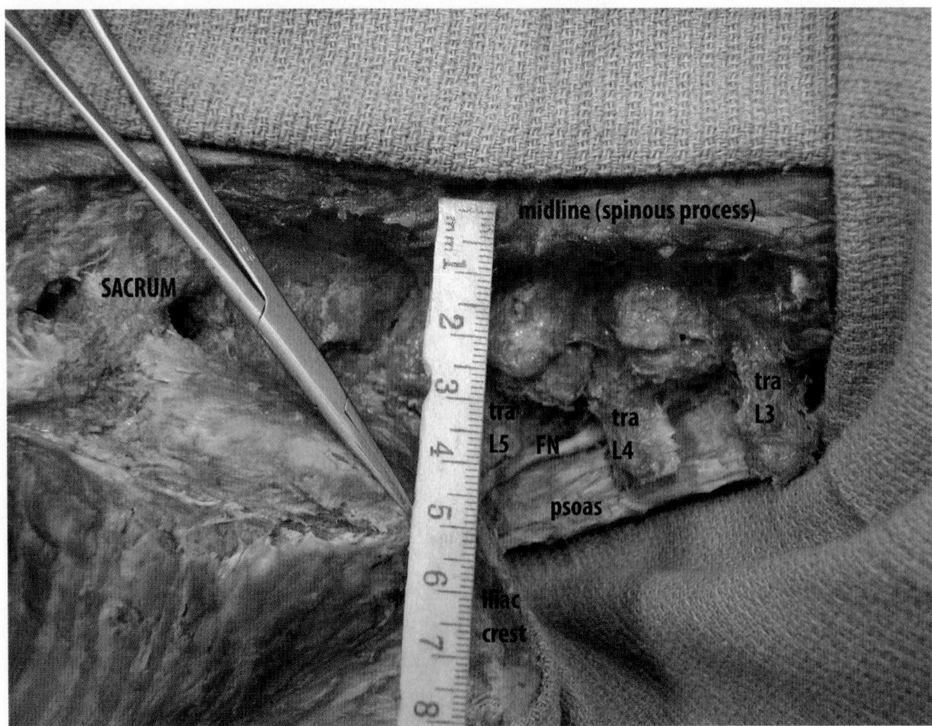


B

**FIGURE 1-22.** (A) The back and paraspinal muscles have been removed to show the transverse processes of the last lumbar vertebra, the psoas muscle, and the femoral nerve. (B) Same as (A) showing that the lateral edge of the psoas muscle at the iliac crest is between 4 and 5 cm from the midline. fem, femoral.

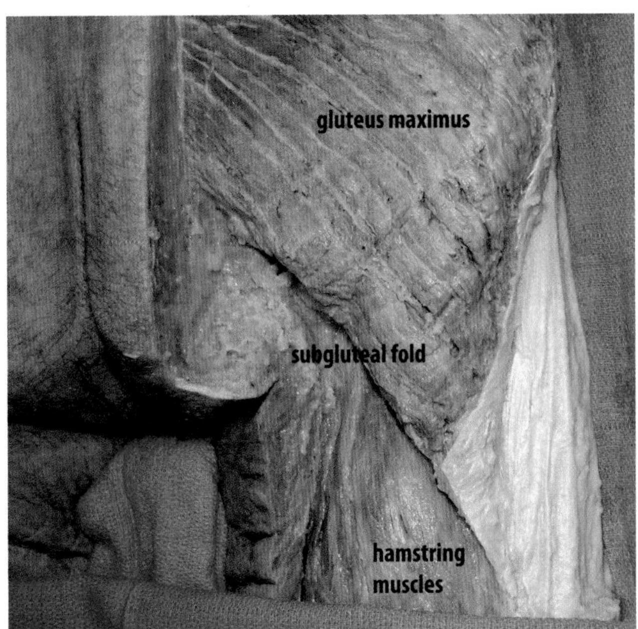


**FIGURE 1-23.** Dissection of the right gluteal area demonstrates that the inferior border of the gluteus maximus does not correspond superficially with the subgluteal fold; instead both cross each other diagonally. (Reproduced from Franco CD. Applied anatomy of the lower extremity. *Tech Reg Anesth Pain Mgmt.* 2008;12(3):140-145, with permission from Elsevier.)

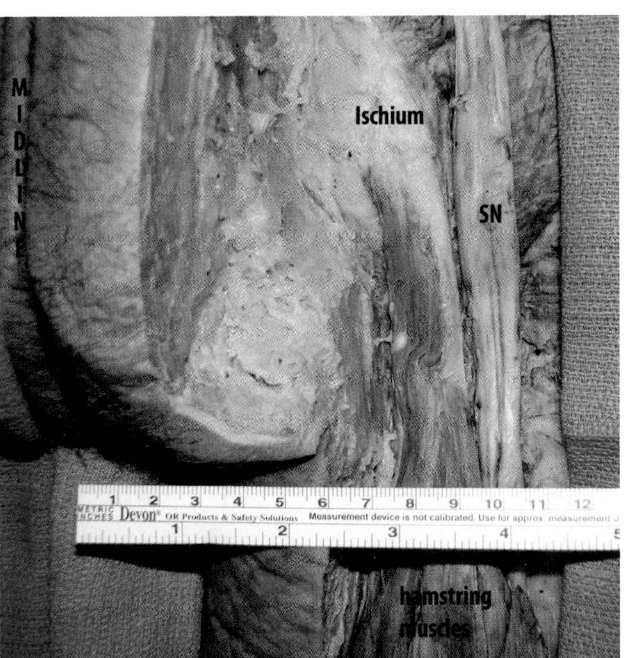


**FIGURE 1-24.** The sciatic nerve (SN) from the gluteal area to the subgluteal fold is located about 10 cm from the midline in adults. This distance is not affected by gender or body habitus. (Reproduced with permission from Franco CD, Choksi N, Rahman A, Voronov G, Almachnouk MH. A subgluteal approach to the sciatic nerve in adults at 10 cm from the midline. *Reg Anesth Pain Med.* 2006;31(3):215-220.)

**TABLE 1-4 Organization and Distribution of the Sacral Plexus**

| NERVE(S) | SPINAL SEGMENTS | DISTRIBUTION |
|---|---|---|
| Gluteal nerves<br>Superior<br>Inferior | L4-S2 | Abductors of thigh (gluteus minimus, gluteus medius, and tensor fasciae latae); extensor of thigh (gluteus maximus) |
| Posterior femoral cutaneous nerve | S1-S3 | Skin of perineum and posterior surface of thigh and leg |
| Sciatic nerve | L4-S3 | Two of the hamstrings. Note: All three hamstrings are innervated by the sciatic nerve (only motor nerve of the posterior thigh), especially the long head of biceps (semitendinosus and semimembranosus); adductor magnus (with obturator nerve) |
| Tibial nerve | | Flexor of knee and plantar flexors of ankle (popliteal, gastrocnemius, soleus, and tibialis posterior muscles and long head triceps of biceps femoris muscle); flexors of toes; skin over posterior surface of leg, plantar surface of foot |
| Common peroneal nerve | | Biceps femoris muscle (short head); peroneus (brevis and longus), and tibialis anterior muscles; extensors of toes, skin over anterior surface of leg and dorsal surface of foot; skin over lateral portion of foot (through the sural nerve) |
| Pudendal nerve | S2-S4 | Muscles of perineum, including urogenital diaphragm and external anal and urethral sphincter muscles; skin of external genitalia and related skeletal muscles (bulbospongiosus, ischiocavernosus muscles) |

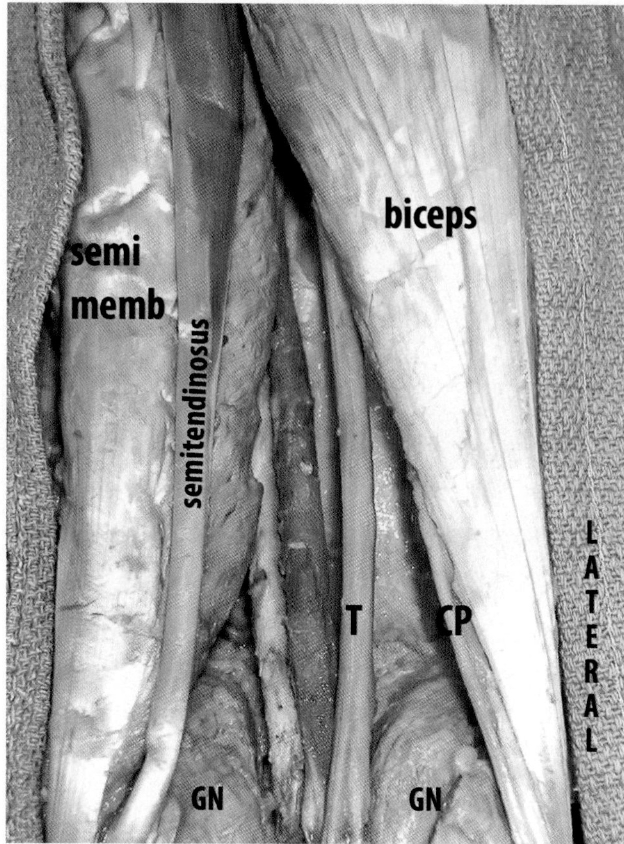


**FIGURE 1-25.** Both components of the sciatic nerve, common peroneal (CP) and tibial (T) nerves diverge from each other at the popliteal fossa. Lateral and medial gastrocnemius muscles (GN) are also shown.

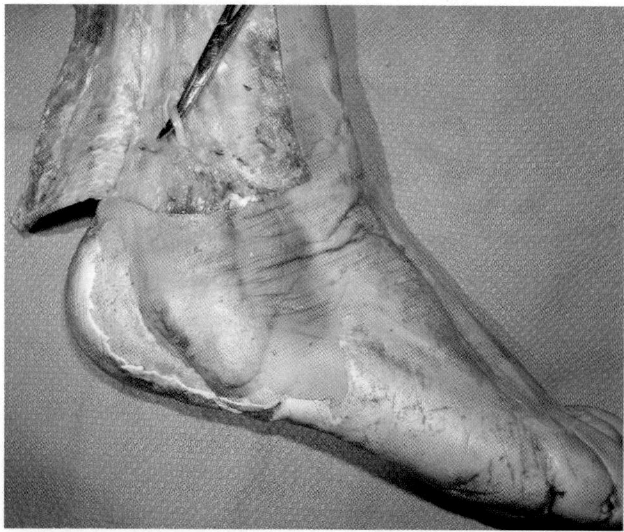

**FIGURE 1-26.** The sural nerve is shown behind the lateral malleolus.

# Thoracic and Abdominal Wall

## Thoracic Wall

The intercostal nerves originate from the ventral rami of the first 11 thoracic spinal nerves. Each intercostal nerve becomes part of the neurovascular bundle of the rib and provides sensory and motor innervations (Figure 1-27). Except for the first, each intercostal nerve gives off a lateral cutaneous branch that pierces the overlying muscle near the midaxillary line. This cutaneous nerve divides into anterior and posterior branches, which supply the adjacent skin. The intercostal nerves of the second to the sixth spaces reach the anterior thoracic wall and pierce the superficial fascia near the lateral border of the sternum and divide into medial and lateral cutaneous branches. Most of the fibers of the anterior ramus of the first thoracic spinal nerve join the brachial plexus for distribution to the upper limb. The small first intercostal nerve is in itself the lateral branch and supplies only the muscles of the intercostal space, not the overlying skin. The lower five intercostal nerves abandon the intercostal space at the costal margin to supply the muscles and skin of the abdominal wall.

## Anterior Abdominal Wall

The skin, muscles and parietal peritoneum, or the anterior abdominal wall, are innervated by the lower six thoracic nerves and the first lumbar nerve. At the costal margin, the seventh to eleventh thoracic nerves leave their intercostal spaces and enter the abdominal wall in a fascial plane between the transversus abdominis and internal oblique muscles. The seventh and eighth intercostal nerves slope upward following the contour of the costal margin, the ninth runs horizontally, and the tenth and eleventh have a somewhat downward trajectory. Anteriorly, the nerves pierce the rectus abdominis muscle and the anterior layer of the rectus sheath to emerge as anterior cutaneous branches that supply the overlying skin.

The subcostal nerve (T12) takes the line of the twelfth rib across the posterior abdominal wall. It continues around the flank and terminates in a similar manner to the lower intercostal nerves. The seventh to twelfth thoracic nerves give off lateral cutaneous nerves that further divide into anterior and posterior branches. The anterior branches supply the skin as far forward as the lateral edge of rectus abdominis. The posterior branches supply the skin overlying the latissimus dorsi. The lateral cutaneous branch of the subcostal nerve is distributed to the skin on the side of the buttock.

The inferior part of the abdominal wall is supplied by the iliohypogastric and ilioinguinal nerves, both branches of L1.The iliohypogastric nerve divides, runs above the iliac crest, and splits into two terminal branches. The lateral cutaneous

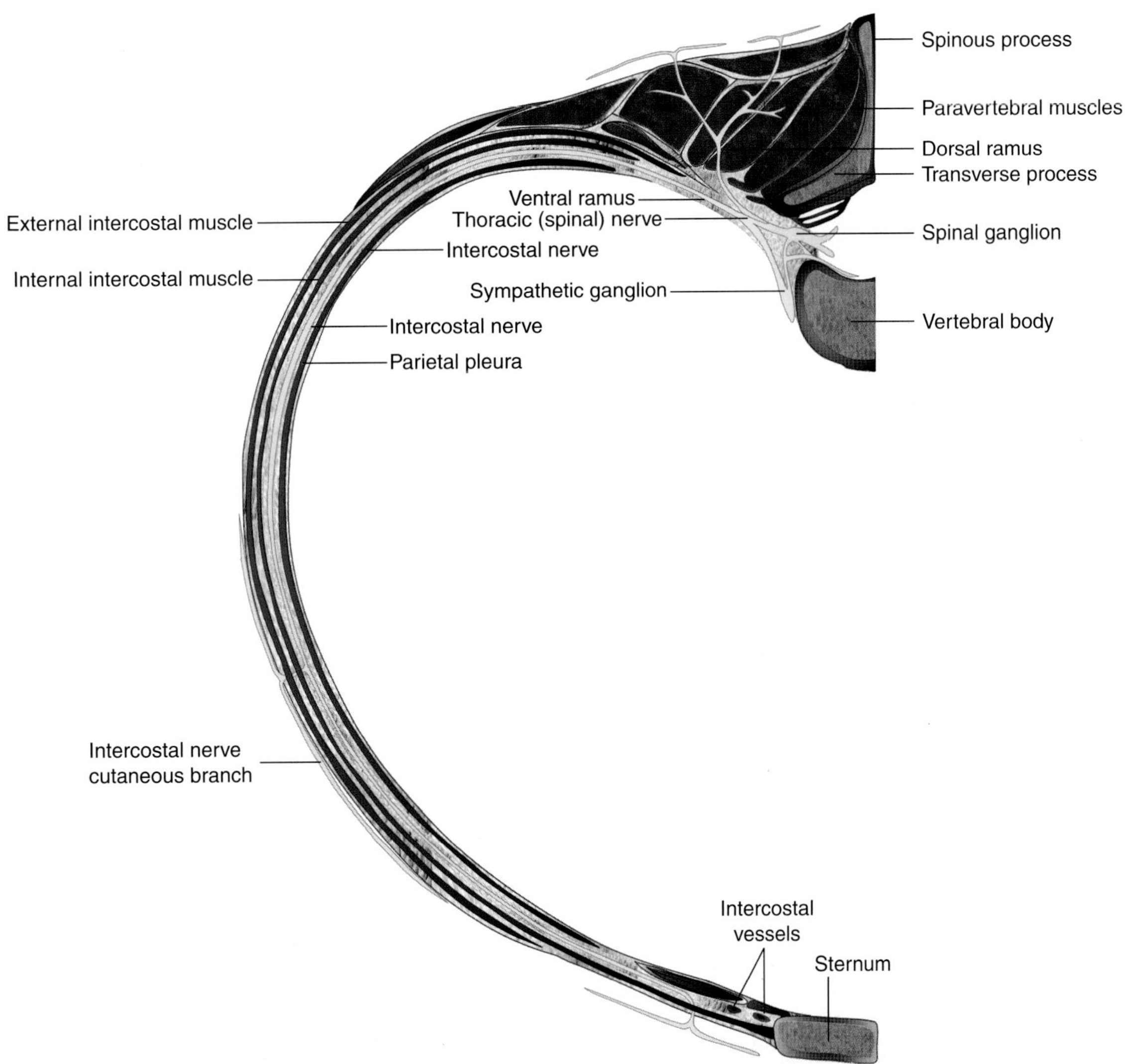


**FIGURE 1-27.** Organization of the segmental spinal nerve, intercostal nerve, and innervations of the chest wall.

branch supplies the side of the buttock; the anterior cutaneous branch supplies the suprapubic region.

The ilioinguinal nerve leaves the intermuscular plane by piercing the internal oblique muscle above the iliac crest. It continues between the two oblique muscles eventually to enter the inguinal canal through the spermatic cord. Emerging from the superficial inguinal ring, it gives cutaneous branches to the skin on the medial side of the root of the thigh, the proximal part of the penis, and the front of the scrotum in males and the mons pubis and the anterior part of the labium majus in females.

## Nerve Supply to the Peritoneum

The parietal peritoneum of the abdominal wall is innervated by the lower thoracic and first lumbar nerves. The lower thoracic nerves also innervate the peritoneum that covers the periphery of the diaphragm. Inflammation of the peritoneum gives rise to pain in the lower thoracic wall and abdominal wall. By contrast, the peritoneum on the central part of the diaphragm receives sensory branches from the phrenic nerves (C3, C4, and C5), and irritation in this area may produce pain referred to region of the shoulder (the fourth cervical dermatome).

# Innervation of the Major Joints

Because much of the practice of peripheral nerve blocks involves orthopedic surgery, it is important to review the innervation of the major joints to have a better understanding of the nerves involved for a more rational approach to regional anesthesia.

## Shoulder Joint

Innervation to the shoulder joints originates mostly from the axillary and suprascapular nerves, both of which can be blocked by an interscalene block (Figure 1-28).

## Elbow Joint

Nerve supply to the elbow joint includes branches of all major nerves of the brachial plexus: musculocutaneous, radial, median, and ulnar nerves.

## Hip Joint

Nerves to the hip joint include the nerve to the rectus femoris from the femoral nerve, branches from the anterior division of the obturator nerve, and the nerve to the quadratus femoris from the sacral plexus (Figure 1-29).

## Knee Joint

The knee joint is innervated anteriorly by branches from the femoral nerve. On its medial side it receives branches from the posterior division of the obturator nerve while both divisions of the sciatic nerve supply its posterior side (Figure 1-30).

## Ankle Joint

The innervation of the ankle joint is complex and involves the terminal branches of the common peroneal (deep and superficial peroneal nerves), tibial (posterior tibial nerve), and femoral nerves (saphenous nerve). A more simplistic view is that the entire innervation of the ankle joint stems from the sciatic nerve, with the exception of the skin on the medial aspect around the medial malleolus (saphenous nerve, a branch of the femoral nerve) (Figure 1-31).

## Wrist Joint

The wrist joint and joints in the hand are innervated by most of the terminal branches of the brachial plexus including the radial, median, and ulnar nerves (Figure 1-32).

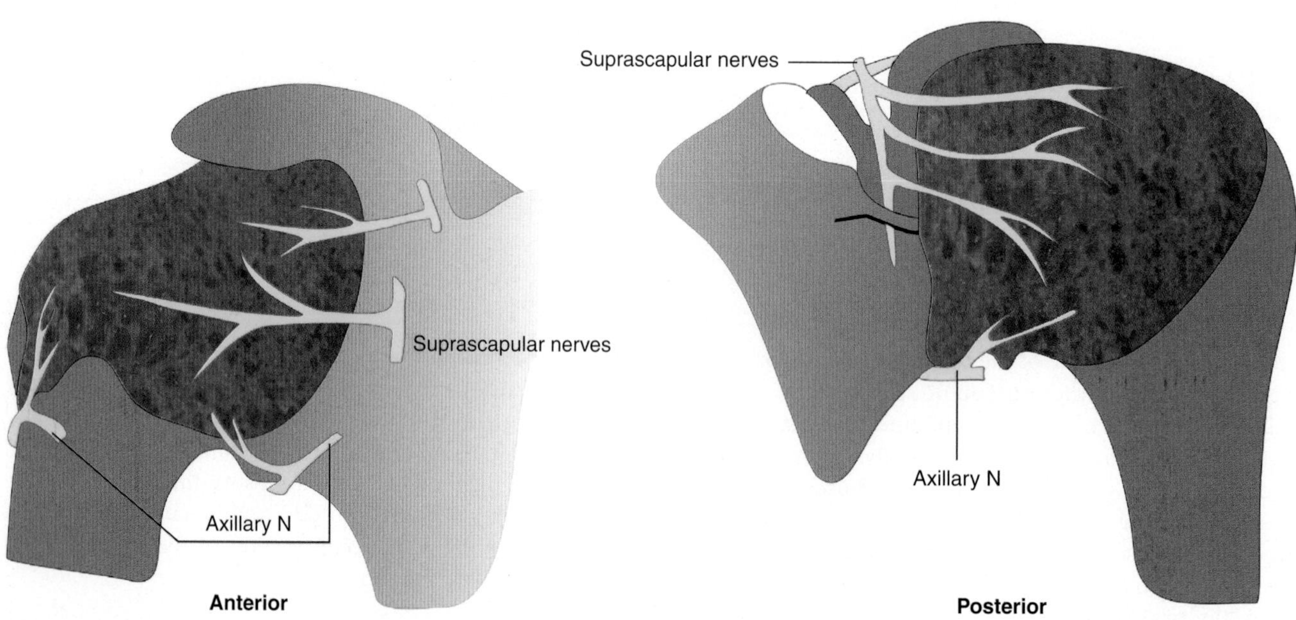


**FIGURE 1-28.** Innervation of the shoulder joint.

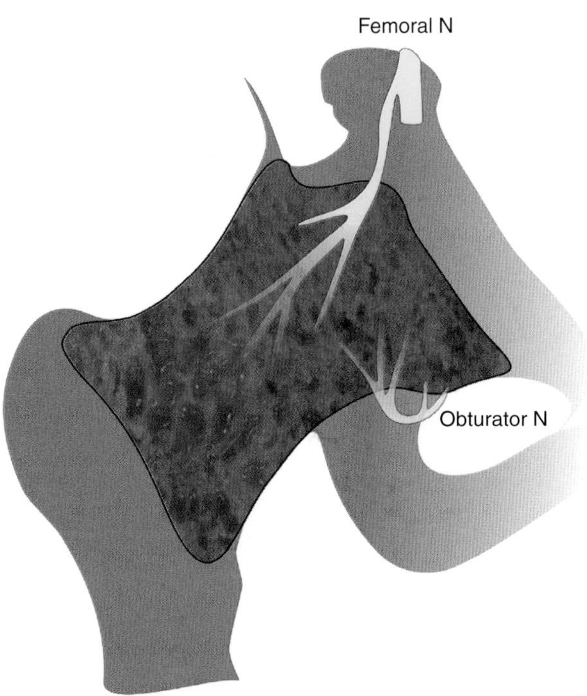


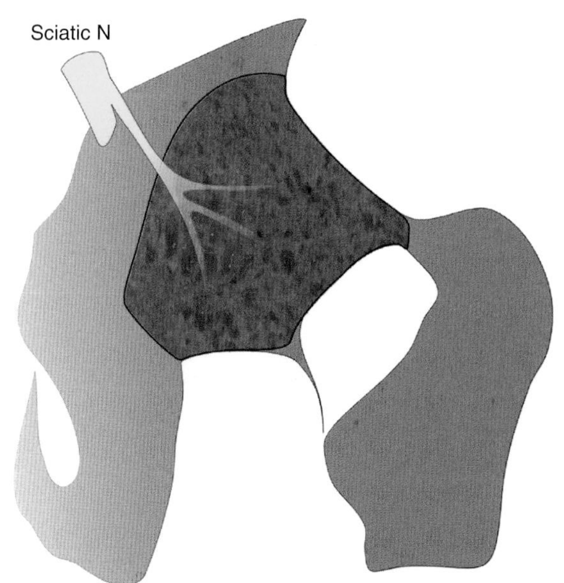


**FIGURE 1-29.** Innervation of the hip joint.

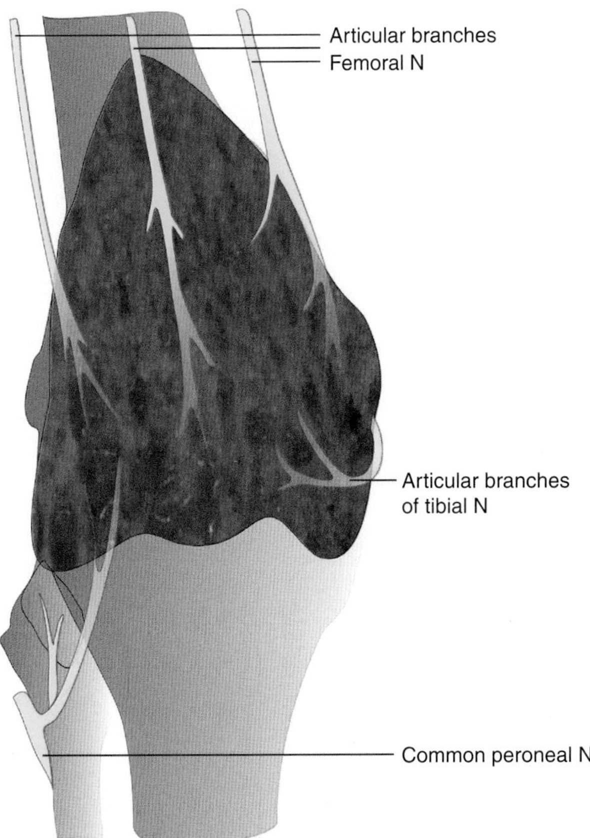


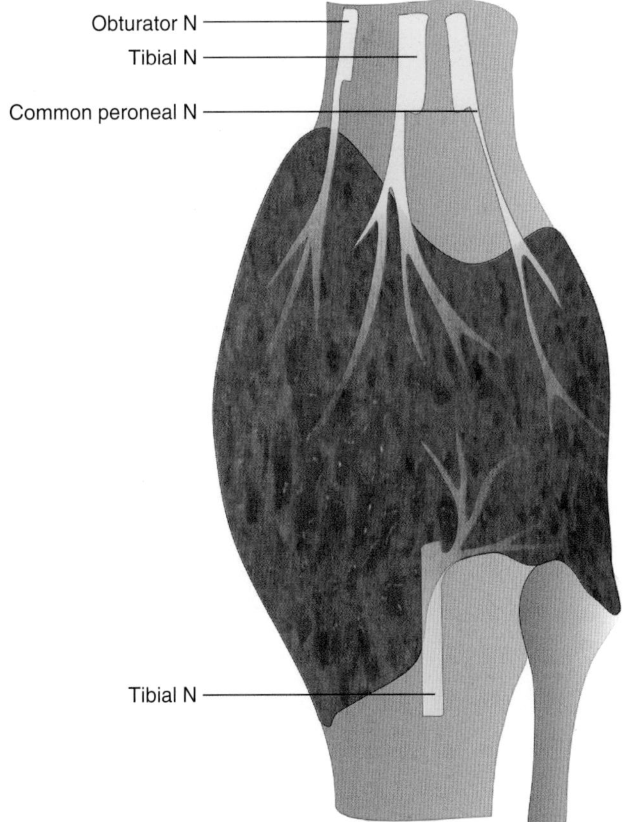


**FIGURE 1-30.** Innervation of the knee joint.

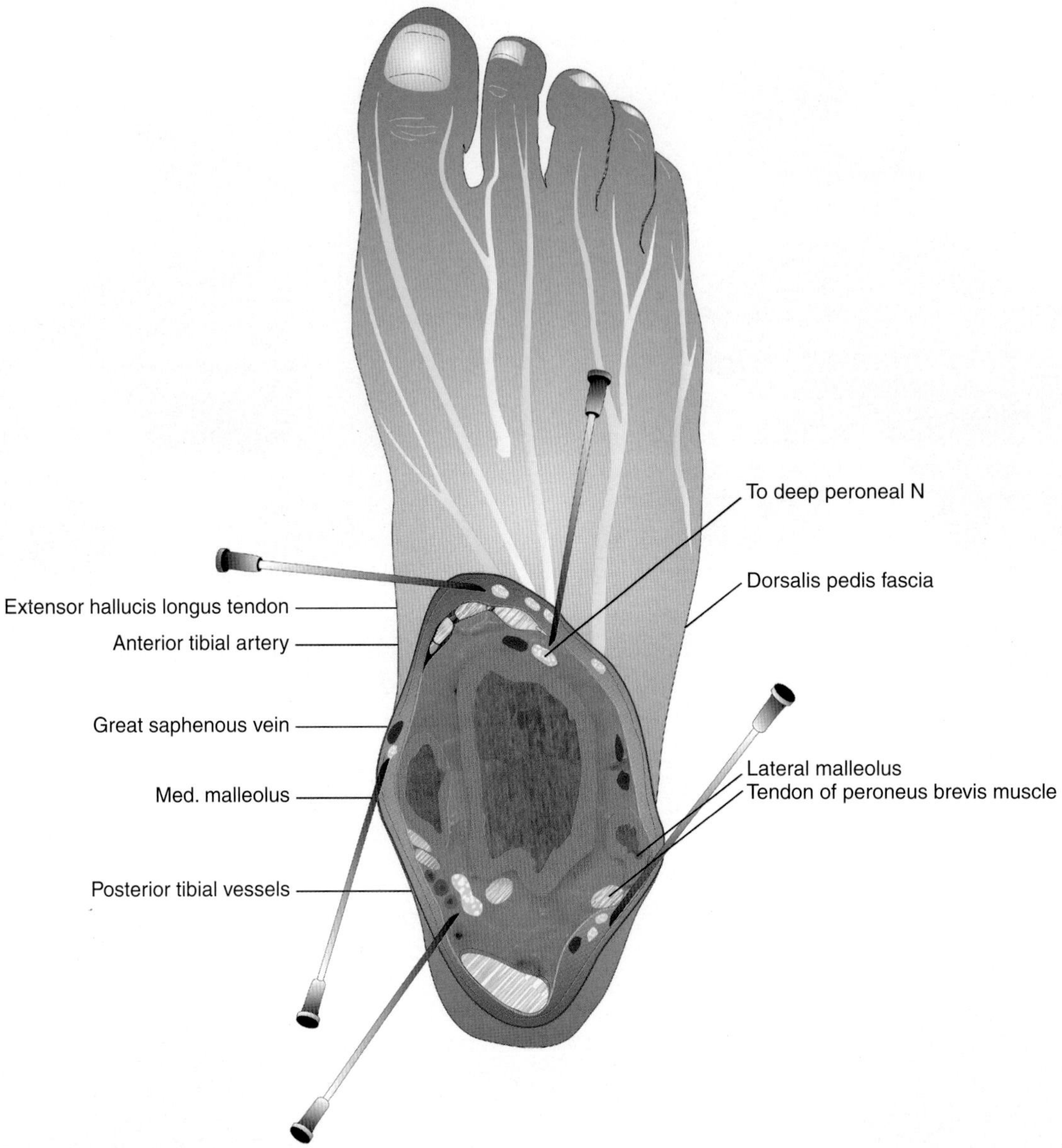

To deep peroneal N
Dorsalis pedis fascia
Extensor hallucis longus tendon
Anterior tibial artery
Great saphenous vein
Med. malleolus
Posterior tibial vessels
Lateral malleolus
Tendon of peroneus brevis muscle

**FIGURE 1-31.** Innervation of the ankle joint and foot.

Extensor pollicis longus
Radius
Extensor pollicis brevis
Superficial radial N
Base of first metacarpal

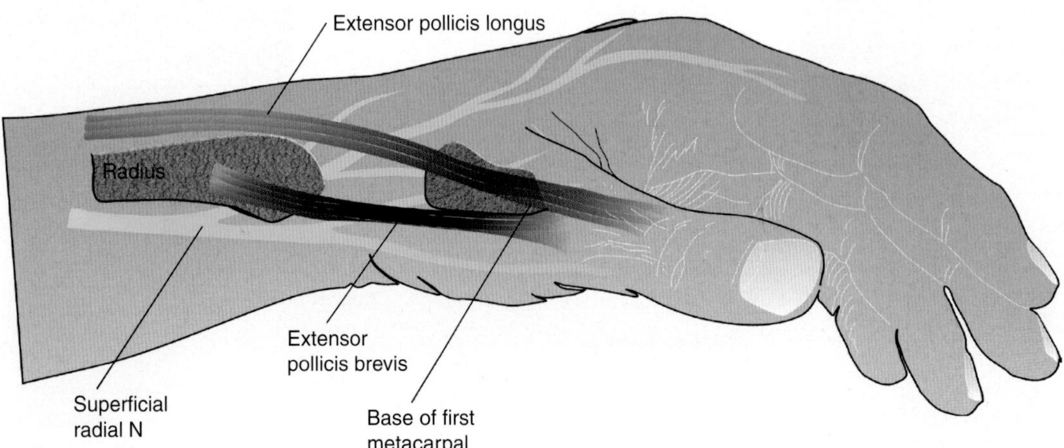

**FIGURE 1-32.** Innervation of the wrist and hand.

## SUGGESTED READINGS


Clemente CD. *Anatomy: A Regional Atlas of the Human Body.* 4th ed. Philadelphia, PA: Lippincott; 1997.

Dean D, Herbener TE. *Cross-Sectional Human Anatomy.* Philadelphia, PA: Lippincott; 2000.

Gosling JA, Harris PF, Whitmore I, Willan PLT. *Human Anatomy: Color Atlas and Text.* 5th ed. London, UK: Mosby; 2008.

Grey H. *Anatomy, Descriptive and Surgical.* Pick TP, Howden R, eds. New York, NY: Portland House; 1977.

Hahn MB, McQuillan PM, Sheplock GJ. *Regional Anesthesia: An Atlas of Anatomy and Techniques.* St. Louis, MO: Mosby; 1996.

Martini FH, Timmons MJ, Tallitsch RB. *Human Anatomy.* 7th ed. Upper Saddle River, NJ: Prentice Hall; 2011.

Netter FH. *Atlas of Human Anatomy.* Summit, NJ: Ciba-Geigy; 1989.

Pernkopf E. *Atlas of Topographical and Applied Human Anatomy.* 2nd ed. Munich, Germany: Saunders; 1980. *Head and Neck*; vol 1.

Pernkopf E. *Atlas of Topographical and Applied Human Anatomy.* 2nd ed. Munich, Germany: Saunders; 1980. *Thorax, Abdomen and Extremities*; vol 2.

Rohen JW, Yokochi C, Lütjen-Drecoll E. *Color Atlas of Anatomy.* 4th ed. Baltimore, MD: Williams and Wilkins; 1998.

Rosse C, Gaddum-Rosse P. *Hillinshead's Textbook of Anatomy.* 5th ed. Philadelphia, PA: Lippincott-Raven; 1997.

Vloka JD, Hadžić A, April EW, Geatz H, Thys DM. Division of the sciatic nerve in the popliteal fossa and its possible implications in the popliteal nerve blockade. *Anesth Analg.* 2001;92:215-217.

Vloka JD, Hadžić A, Kitain E, et al. Anatomic considerations for sciatic nerve block in the popliteal fossa through the lateral approach. *Reg Anesth.* 1996;21:414-418.

Vloka JD, Hadžić A, Lesser JB, et al. A common epineural sheath for the nerves in the popliteal fossa and its possible implications for sciatic nerve block. *Anesth Analg.* 1997;84:387-390.

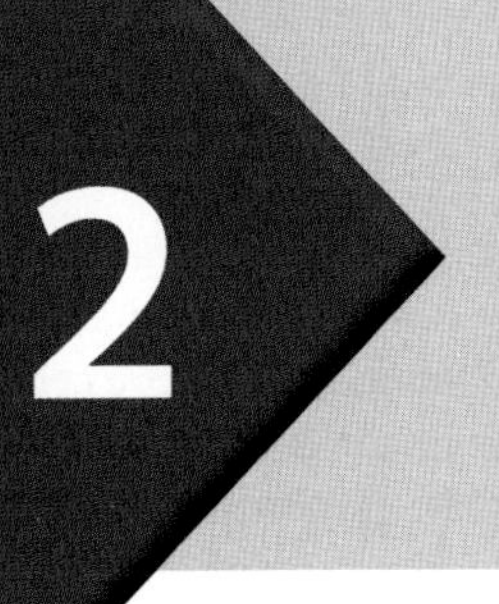

# Local Anesthetics: Clinical Pharmacology and Rational Selection

*Jeff Gadsden*

Local anesthetics (LAs) prevent or relieve pain by interrupting nerve conduction. They bind to specific receptor sites on the sodium ($Na^+$) channels in nerves and block the movement of ions through these pores. Both the chemical and pharmacologic properties of individual LA drugs determine their clinical properties. This chapter discusses the basics of the mechanism of action of LAs, their clinical use, and systemic toxicity prevention and treatment.

## Nerve Conduction

Nerve conduction involves the propagation of an electrical signal generated by the rapid movement of small amounts of several ions ($Na^+$ and potassium $K^+$) across a nerve cell membrane. The ionic gradient for $Na^+$ (high extracellularly and low intracellularly) and $K^+$ (high intracellularly and low extracellularly) is maintained by a $Na^+$-$K^+$ pump mechanism within the nerve. In the resting state, the nerve membrane is more permeable to $K^+$ ions than to $Na^+$ ions, resulting in the continuous leakage of $K^+$ ions out of the interior of the nerve cell. This leakage of cations, in turn, creates a negatively charged interior relative to the exterior, resulting in an electric potential of 60–70 mV across the nerve membrane.

Receptors at the distal ends of sensory nerves serve as sensors and transducers of various mechanical, chemical, or thermal stimuli. Such stimuli are converted into minuscule electric currents. For example, chemical mediators released with a surgical incision react with these receptors and generate small electric currents. As a result, the electric potential across a nerve membrane near the receptor is altered, making it less negative. If the threshold potential is achieved, an action potential results, with a sudden increase in the permeability of the nerve membrane to $Na^+$ ions and a resultant rapid influx of positively charged $Na^+$ ions. This causes a transient reversal of charge, or depolarization. Depolarization generates a current that sequentially depolarizes the adjacent segment of the nerve, thus "activating" the nerve and sending a wave of sequential polarization down the nerve membrane.

Repolarization takes place when sodium permeability decreases and $K^+$ permeability increases, resulting in an efflux of $K^+$ from within the cell and restoration of the electrical balance. Subsequently, both ions are restored to their initial intracellular and extracellular concentrations by the $Na^+$-$K^+$-adenosine triphosphate pump mechanism. Because the rapid influx of $Na^+$ ions occurs in response to a change in the transmembrane potential, $Na^+$ channels in the nerve are characterized as "voltage gated." These channels are protein structures with three subunits that penetrate the full depth of the membrane bilayer and are in communication with both the extracellular surface of the nerve membrane and the axoplasm (interior) of the nerve. LAs prevent the generation and conduction of nerve impulses by binding to the $\alpha$ subunit of the $Na^+$ channel and preventing the influx of $Na^+$ into the cell, halting the transmission of the advancing wave of depolarization down the length of the nerve.

A resting nerve is less sensitive to a LA than a nerve that is repeatedly stimulated. A higher frequency of stimulation and a more positive membrane potential cause a greater degree of transmission block. These frequency- and voltage-dependent effects of LAs occur because repeated depolarization increases the chance that a LA molecule will encounter a $Na^+$ channel that is in the activated, or open, form—as opposed to the resting form—which has a much greater affinity for LA. In general, the rate of dissociation from the receptor site in the pore of the $Na^+$ channel is critical for the frequency dependence of LA action.

## Structure–Activity Relationship of Local Anesthetics

The typical structure of a LA consists of hydrophilic and hydrophobic domains separated by an intermediate ester or amide linkage. The hydrophilic group is usually a tertiary amine, and the hydrophobic domain is an aromatic moiety. The nature of the linking group determines the pharmacologic properties of LA agents. The physicochemical properties of these agents largely influence their potency and duration of action. For instance, greater lipid solubility increases both the potency and duration of their action. This is due to a greater affinity of the drug to lipid membranes and therefore greater proximity to its sites of action. The longer the drug remains in the vicinity of the membrane, rather than being replaced by the blood, the more likely the drug will be to effect its action on the $Na^+$ channel in the membrane. Unfortunately, greater lipid solubility also increases toxicity, decreasing the therapeutic index for more hydrophobic drugs.

**TIP**

- A common misconception is that block duration is related to protein binding. In fact, dissociation times of local anesthetics from $Na^+$ channels are measured in seconds and do not have a bearing on the speed of recovery from the block. More important is the extent to which local anesthetic remains in the vicinity of the nerve. This is determined largely by three factors: lipid solubility; the degree of vascularity of the tissue; and the presence of vasoconstrictors that prevent vascular uptake.

The $pK_a$ (the pH at which 50% of the drug is ionized and 50% is present as base) of the LA is related to pH and the concentrations of the cationic and base forms by the Henderson-Hasselbalch equation: $pH = pK_a + \log([\text{base}]/[\text{cation}])$.

The $pK_a$ generally correlates with the speed of onset of action of most amide LA drugs; the closer the $pK_a$ to the body pH, the faster the onset. The coexistence of the two forms of the drug—the charged cation and the uncharged base—is important because drug penetration of the nerve membrane by the LA requires the base (unionized) form to pass through the nerve lipid membrane; once in the axoplasm of the nerve, the base form can accept a hydrogen ion and equilibrate into the cationic form. The cationic form is predominant and produces a blockade of the $Na^+$ channel. The amount of base form that can be in solution is limited by its aqueous solubility.

An ester or an amide linkage is present between the lipophilic end (benzene ring) and the hydrophilic end (amino group) of the molecule. The type of linkage determines the site of metabolic degradation of the drug. Ester-linked LAs are metabolized in plasma by pseudocholinesterase, whereas amide-linked drugs undergo metabolism in the liver.

## The Onset and Duration of Blockade

### Local Anesthetic Diffusion

A mixed peripheral nerve or nerve trunk consists of individual nerves surrounded by an investing epineurium. When a LA is deposited in proximity to a peripheral nerve, it diffuses from the outer surface toward the core along a concentration gradient. Consequently, nerves located in the outer mantle of the mixed nerve are blocked first. These fibers are usually distributed to more proximal anatomic structures than those situated near the core of the mixed nerve and often are motor fibers. When the volume and concentration of LA solution deposited in the vicinity of the nerve are adequate, the LA eventually diffuses inward to block the more centrally located fibers. In this way, the block evolves from proximal structures to distal structures. Smaller amounts and concentrations of a drug only block the nerves in the mantle and smaller and more sensitive central fibers.

### Onset of Blockade

In general, LAs are deposited as close to the nerve as possible, preferably into the tissue sheaths (e.g., brachial plexus, lumbar plexus) or epineurial sheaths of the nerves (e.g., femoral, sciatic). The actual site of local anesthetic injection and its relationship to the nerve structures is much better understood since the advent of the use of ultrasound guidance during nerve blockade. Intraneural or sub-epineural injections reportedly occur relatively frequently with some peripheral nerve blocks. The available data indicate that such injections result in faster onset of blockade, most likely due to the intimate proximity of LA to the nerve tissue. This is hardly surprising because the LA must diffuse from the site of injection to the nerve, the site of action. However, intraneural injections should not be recommended as a safe practice despite limited reports suggesting that intraneural injections do not inevitably lead to nerve injury. These data must be interpreted with caution because the term *intraneural injection* is often used loosely to denote injections within epineurium or even tissue sheaths that envelop the peripheral nerves or plexi. However, neurologic injury is much more likely to occur should an intraneural injection occur intrafascicularly.

The rate of diffusion across the nerve sheath is determined by the concentration of the drug, its degree of ionization (ionized LA diffuses more slowly), its hydrophobicity, and the physical characteristics of the tissue surrounding the nerve.

**TIP**

- The relationship between concentration and block onset is logarithmic, not linear; in other words, doubling the concentration of LA will only marginally speed up the onset of the block (although it will block the fibers more effectively and prolong the duration).

### Duration of Blockade

The duration of nerve block anesthesia depends on the physical characteristics of the LA and the presence or absence of vasoconstrictors. The most important physical characteristic is lipid solubility. In general, LAs can be divided into three categories: short acting (e.g., 2-chloroprocaine, 45–90 minutes), intermediate duration (e.g., lidocaine, mepivacaine, 90–180 minutes), and long acting (e.g., bupivacaine, levobupivacaine, ropivacaine, 4–18 hours). The degree of block prolongation with the addition of a vasoconstrictor appears to be related to the intrinsic vasodilatory properties of the LA; the more intrinsic vasodilatory action the LA has, the more prolongation is achieved with addition of a vasoconstrictor.

Although this discussion is in line with current clinical teaching, it is really more theoretical than of significant clinical relevance. For instance, dense blocks of the brachial plexus with 2-chloroprocaine are likely to outlast weak poor quality blocks with bupivacaine. In addition, classical teaching does not take into account the nerve to be anesthetized. As an example, a sciatic nerve block with bupivacaine lasts almost twice as long as an interscalene or lumbar plexus block with the same drug dose and concentration. These differences must be kept in mind to time and predict the resolution of blockade properly.

## Differential Sensitivity of Nerve Fibers to Local Anesthetics

Two general rules apply regarding susceptibility of nerve fibers to LAs: First, smaller nerve fibers are more susceptible to the action of LAs than large fibers (Figure 2-1). Smaller fibers are preferentially blocked because a shorter length of axon is required to be blocked to halt the conduction completely. Second, myelinated fibers are more easily blocked than nonmyelinated fibers because local anesthetic pools near the axonal membrane. This is why C-fibers, which have a small diameter (but are unmyelinated), are the most resistant fibers to LA.

The sensitivity of a fiber to LAs is not determined by whether it is sensory or motor. In fact, muscle proprioceptive afferent (A-beta) and motor efferent fibers (A-alpha) are equally sensitive. These two types of fibers have the same diameter, which is larger than that of the A-gamma fibers that supply the muscle spindles. It is the more rapid blockade of these smaller A-gamma fibers, rather than of the sensory fibers, that leads to the preferential loss of muscle reflexes. Similarly, in large nerve trunks, motor fibers are often located in the outer portion of the bundle and are more accessible to LA. Thus motor fibers may be blocked before sensory fibers in large mixed nerves.

The differential rate of blockade exhibited by fibers of varying sizes and firing rates is of considerable practical importance. Fortunately, the sensation of pain is usually the first modality to disappear; it is followed by the loss of sensations of cold, warmth, touch, deep pressure, and, finally, loss of motor function, although variation among patients and different nerves is considerable.

## Local Anesthetics and pH

LA drugs, as previously described, pass through the nerve membrane in a nonionized lipid-soluble base form; when they are within the nerve axoplasm, they must equilibrate into an ionic form to be active within the $Na^+$ channel. The rate-limiting step in this cascade is penetration of the LA through the nerve membrane. LAs are unprotonated amines and as such tend to be relatively insoluble (Figure 2-2). For this reason, they are manufactured as water-soluble salts, usually

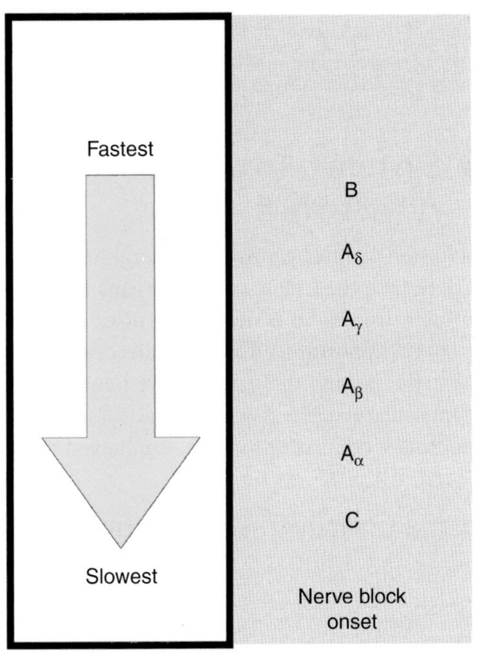


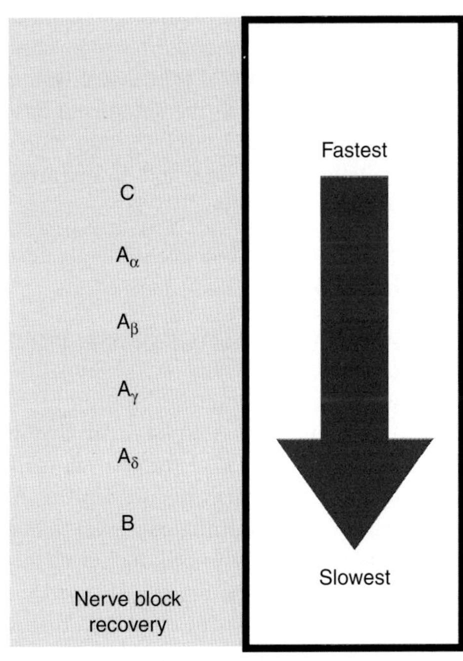


**FIGURE 2-1.** Differential rate of nerve blockade.

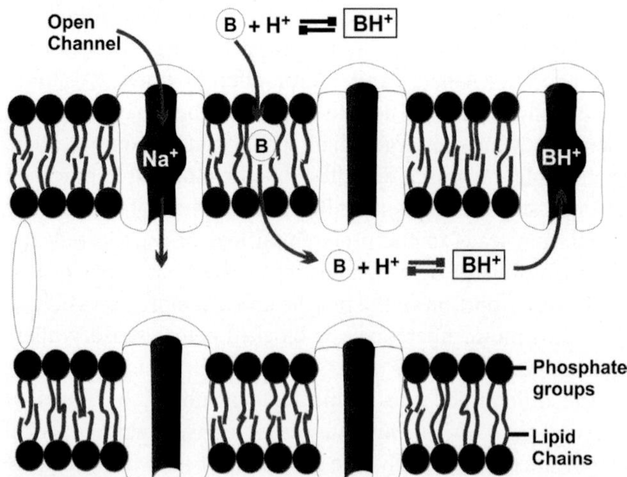


**FIGURE 2-2.** Local anesthetics and pH. Local anesthetics pass through the nerve membrane in a nonionized, lipid-soluble base form. When they are within the nerve axoplasm, they must equilibrate into an ionic form to exert their action on the $Na^+$ channel.

hydrochlorides. Although LAs are weak bases (typical $pK_a$ values range from 7.5–9), their hydrochloride salts are mildly acidic. This property increases the stability of LA esters and any accompanying vasoconstrictor substance. However, this means that the cationic form predominates in solution.

For this reason, sodium bicarbonate ($NaHCO_3$) is often added to LA. This increases the amount of drug in the base form, which slightly shortens the onset time. Obviously, the limiting factor for pH adjustment is the solubility of the base form of the drug. Unfortunately, only small changes in pH can be achieved by the addition of bicarbonate because of the limited solubility of the base. As such, only small decreases in onset time are realized. For instance, with the alkalinization of bupivacaine, an increase in the amount of base in solution is limited by the minimal solubility of free base in solution. For each LA, there is a pH at which the amount of base in solution is maximal (a saturated solution). Further increases in pH result in precipitation of the drug and do not produce an additional shortening of onset time.

## Protein Binding

LAs are in large part bound to plasma and tissue proteins. However, they are pharmacologically active only in the free, unbound state. The most important binding proteins for LAs in plasma are albumin and alpha$_1$-acid glycoprotein (AAG). The binding to AAG is characterized as high-affinity but low-capacity binding; hence LAs bind to AAG preferentially compared with albumin. However, binding to AAG is easily saturated with clinically achieved blood levels of LA. Once AAG saturation occurs, any additional binding is to albumin. Albumin can bind LA drugs in plasma in concentrations many times greater than those clinically achieved.

**TIP**

- Local anesthetic solutions containing epinephrine are made acidic to prevent breakdown of the vasoconstrictor. There appears to be an onset advantage to alkalinizing these solutions due to their low pH (e.g., lidocaine with epinephrine, pH 3.5). Alkalinizing plain lidocaine results in a slightly faster onset but also a shortened duration. However, the clinical relevance of 1–2 minutes of onset difference is of questionable practical relevance.

Note that the fraction of drugs bound to protein in plasma correlates with the duration of LA activity: bupivacaine > etidocaine > ropivacaine > mepivacaine > lidocaine > procaine and 2-chloroprocaine. However, no direct relationship exists between LA plasma protein binding and binding to specific membrane-bound $Na^+$ channels. Rather, there is a direct correlation between protein binding and lipid solubility, as there is for all drugs. The more lipid soluble the drug, the more likely it will remain in the lipid-rich environment of the axonal membrane where the $Na^+$ channel resides.

The degree of protein binding of a particular LA is concentration dependent and influenced by the pH of the plasma. The percentage of drug bound decreases as the pH decreases. This is important because with the development of acidosis, as may occur with LA-induced seizures or cardiac arrest, the amount of free drug increases. The magnitude of this phenomenon varies among LAs, and it is much more pronounced with bupivacaine than with lidocaine. For instance, as the binding decreases from 95% to 70% with acidosis, the amount of free bupivacaine increases from 5% to 30% (a factor of 6), although the total drug concentration remains unchanged. Because of this increase in free drug, acidosis renders bupivacaine markedly more toxic.

## Systemic Toxicity of Local Anesthetics

In addition to interrupting peripheral nerve conduction, LAs interfere with the function of all organs in which the conduction or transmission of nerve impulses occurs. For instance, they have important effects on the central nervous system (CNS), the autonomic ganglia, the neuromuscular junction, and musculature. The risk of such adverse reactions is proportional to the concentration of LA achieved in the circulation.

### Plasma Concentration of Local Anesthetics

The following factors determine the plasma concentration of LAs:

- The dose of the drug administered
- The rate of absorption of the drug

- Site injected, vasoactivity of the drug, use of vasoconstrictors
- Biotransformation and elimination of the drug from the circulation

Noted that although the peak level of a LA is directly related to the dose administered, administration of the same dose at different sites results in marked differences in peak blood levels. This explains why large doses of LA can be used with peripheral nerve blocks without the toxicity that would be seen with an intramuscular or intravenous (IV) injection. It is also for this reason that the adherence to strictly defined maximum doses of LAs is nonsensical. As an example, 150 mg of ropivacaine at the popliteal fossa will result in a markedly different plasma level than the same dose administered intercostally. Careful consideration of patient factors and the requirements of the block should precede selection of LA type and dose for peripheral nerve block.

Short-acting ester local anesthetics are inherently safer with respect to systemic toxicity due to their clearance by pseudocholinesterase. In the case of 2-chloroprocaine, peak blood levels achieved are affected by the rate at which the LA drug undergoes biotransformation and elimination (plasma half-life of about 45 seconds–1 minute). In contrast, peak blood levels of amide-linked LA drugs are primarily the result of absorption.

## Central Nervous System Toxicity

The symptoms of CNS toxicity associated with LAs are a function of their plasma level (Figure 2-3). Toxicity is typically first expressed as stimulation of the CNS, producing restlessness, disorientation, and tremor. As the plasma concentration of the LA increases, tonic-clonic seizures occur; the more potent the LA, the more readily convulsions may be produced. With even higher levels of LA, central stimulation is followed by depression and respiratory failure, culminating in coma.

The apparent stimulation and subsequent depression produced by applying LAs to the CNS presumably are due to depression of neuronal activity. Selective depression of inhibitory neurons is thought to account for the excitatory phase in vivo. However, rapid systemic administration of a LA may produce death with no, or only transient, signs of CNS stimulation. Under these conditions, the concentration of the drug probably rises so rapidly that all neurons are depressed simultaneously. Airway control and support of respiration constitute essential treatment. Benzodiazepines or a small dose of propofol (e.g., 0.5–1.0 mg/kg) administered IV in small doses are the drugs of choice for aborting convulsions. The use of benzodiazepines as premedication is often recommended to elevate the seizure threshold; however, they must be used with caution because respiratory depression with excessive sedation may produce respiratory acidosis with a consequent higher level of free drug in the serum.

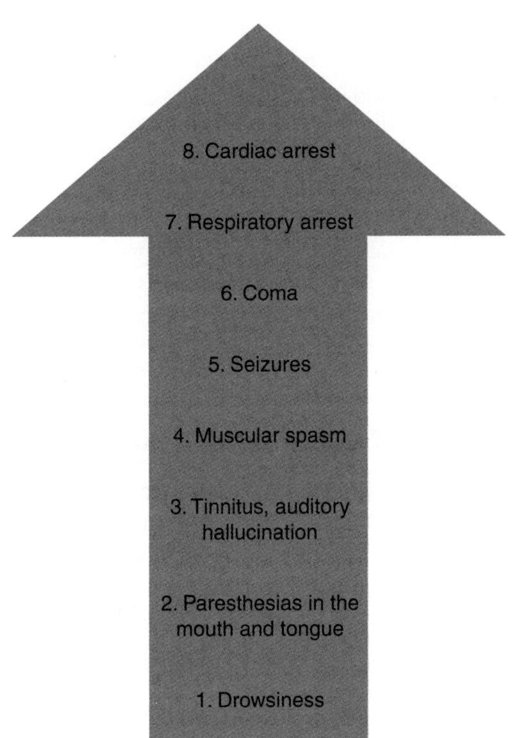


**FIGURE 2-3.** Progression of local anesthetic toxicity.

## Cardiovascular Toxicity

The primary site of action of LAs in the cardiovascular system is the myocardium, where they decrease electrical excitability, conduction rate, and the force of myocardial contraction. Most LAs also cause arteriolar dilatation, contributing to hypotension. Cardiovascular effects typically occur at higher systemic concentrations than those at which effects on the CNS are produced. However, note that it is possible for cardiovascular collapse and death to occur even in an absence of the warning signs and symptoms of CNS toxicity. It is believed that this is probably the result of action on the pacemaker cells or the sudden onset of ventricular fibrillation. In animal studies on LA cardiotoxicity, all caused dose-dependent depression of the contractility of cardiac muscle. This depressant effect on cardiac contractility parallels the anesthetic potency of the LA in blocking nerves. Therefore, bupivacaine, which is four times more potent than lidocaine in blocking nerves, is also four times more potent in depressing cardiac contractility. Deaths caused by a bupivacaine overdose have been associated with progressive prolongation of ventricular conduction and widening of the QRS complex, followed by the sudden onset of arrhythmia such as ventricular fibrillation.

## Pregnancy and Local Anesthetic Toxicity

Plasma concentrations of AAG are also decreased in pregnant women and in newborns. This lowered concentration effectively increases the free fraction of bupivacaine in plasma, and it may have been an important contributing factor to the bupivacaine toxicity in pregnant patients and to the number of cardiac arrests that have been reported with inadvertent overdoses of bupivacaine in pregnant women. However, with intermediate-duration LAs (e.g., lidocaine and mepivacaine), smaller changes in protein binding occur during pregnancy, and the use of these LAs is not associated with an increased risk of cardiac toxicity during pregnancy.

### Pharmacodynamics and Treatment of Local Anesthetic Toxicity

Blood levels of lidocaine associated with the onset of seizures appear to be in the range of 10 to 12 μg/mL. At these concentrations, inhibitory pathways in the brain are selectively disabled, and excitatory neurons can function unopposed. As the blood levels of lidocaine are increased further, respiratory depression becomes significant and at much higher levels (20–25 μg/mL), cardiotoxicity is manifested. In contrast, for bupivacaine, blood levels of approximately 4 μg/mL result in seizures, and blood levels between 4 and 6 μg/mL are associated with cardiac toxicity. This is reflective of a much lower therapeutic index for bupivacaine compared with lidocaine in terms of cardiac toxicity. In the setting of neurotoxicity without cardiac effects, high levels of LA in the brain rapidly dissipate and are redistributed to other tissue compartments. However, with the onset of significant cardiotoxicity, cardiac output diminishes, resulting in impairment in redistribution.

**TIP**

- No current monitoring method can prevent systemic toxicity. Cases have been reported despite (1) negative aspiration for blood, (2) the use of recommended dosages, and (3) the observation of local anesthetic spread in a tissue plane and not intravascularly. This is a reminder that constant vigilance and preparation for treatment is essential during all regional anesthetic procedures.

The long-acting LAs, such as bupivacaine and etidocaine, carry a significantly higher risk of cardiac arrest and difficult resuscitation. Note that such complications do not always occur immediately on injection of a LA and may be delayed up to 30 minutes. Many of these toxic effects occur following inadvertent intravascular injection of large amounts of drugs via an epidural catheter or from tourniquet failure during IV administration of a regional anesthetic. In patients with systemic neurotoxicity, treatment consists of halting the seizure by administering a benzodiazepine (midazolam 0.05–0.1 mg/kg) or a small dose of propofol (0.5–1.0 mg/kg) while preventing the detrimental effects of hypoxia and hypercarbia by ventilating with 100% oxygen. Providing that the hemodynamics are adequate, this can be achieved through bag-mask ventilation or the use of a laryngeal mask airway: Tracheal intubation is not always necessary (or always desirable) because these episodes are fortunately often short lived. However, it is extremely important to oxygenate and ventilate the patient because hypoxia, hypercarbia, and acidosis all potentiate the negative inotropic and chronotropic effects of LA toxicity. If ventilation is inadequate with the measures just described, tracheal intubation with the aid of a muscle relaxant is indicated.

For patients exhibiting signs of cardiotoxicity (widened QRS complex, bradycardia, hypotension, ventricular fibrillation, and/or cardiovascular collapse), standard cardiac resuscitative measures should apply. Of primary importance in cardiac arrest is the maintenance of some degree of circulation and perfusion of vital organs by closed chest massage while electrical and pharmacologic therapies are being instituted. Drugs that have little value or indeed worsen the resuscitative efforts include bretylium, lidocaine, and calcium channel blockers. The use of lipid emulsion in LA toxicity has been reported to result in remarkably successful resuscitation, despite the fact that its mechanism remains obscure. Several theories exist, such as its role as a "lipid sink," that draws the drug out of solution, as well as its possible role in overriding the inhibition of mitochondrial carnitine-acylcarnitine translocase, thereby providing the myocardium with fatty acid for fuel. Although neither theory has been proven, the vast majority of experimental evidence suggests that lipid emulsion therapy is a low-risk, high-yield intervention that can only benefit the otherwise moribund patient (see Table 2-1 for directions for use).

The use of vasopressor agents, such as epinephrine and vasopressin, has long been a standard part of the management of cardiac arrest, and at the moment, guidelines have not changed. However, experimental evidence involving animals has shown worsened outcomes when combined with lipid emulsion, perhaps due to increased myocardial intracellular acidosis. Further work in this area needs to be done before any recommendation can be made, and at present, the inclusion of these agents as standard resuscitative drugs is warranted. Finally, in cases of severe toxicity with large doses of long-acting LAs, timely institution of cardiopulmonary bypass may prove lifesaving. The information on local anesthetic toxicity was briefly presented here for the sake of clarity; an entire chapter is devoted to the toxicity of local anesthetics (Chapter 10).

## Types of Local Anesthetics

As previously mentioned, LA drugs are classified as esters or amides (Figure 2-4). A short overview of various LAs with comments regarding their clinical applicability in peripheral blockade is provided in this section.

### Ester-Linked Local Anesthetics

Ester-linked LAs are hydrolyzed at the ester linkage in plasma by pseudocholinesterase. The rate of hydrolysis of ester-linked LAs depends on the type and location of the substitution in

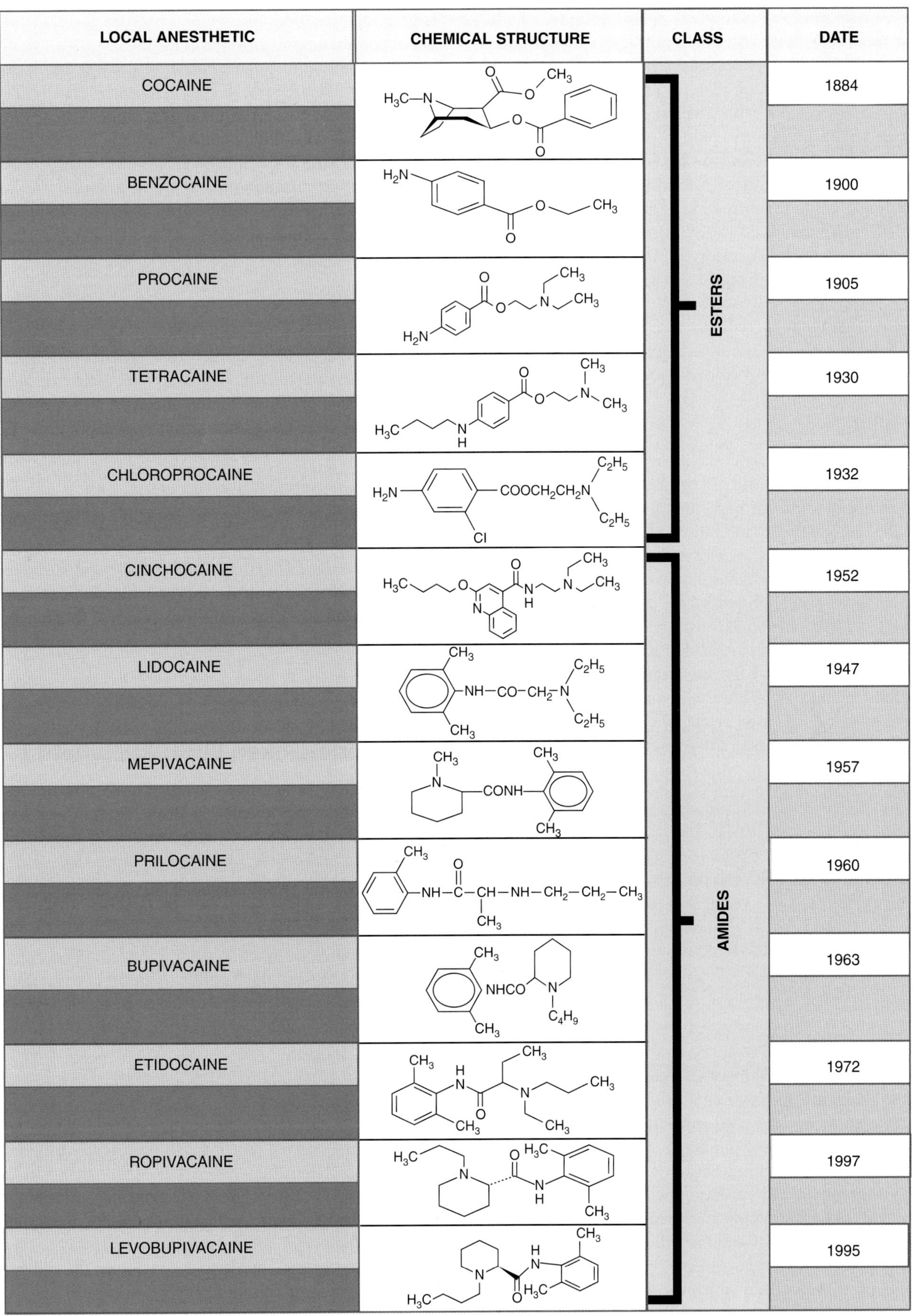

| LOCAL ANESTHETIC | CHEMICAL STRUCTURE | CLASS | DATE |
|---|---|---|---|
| COCAINE | | ESTERS | 1884 |
| BENZOCAINE | | ESTERS | 1900 |
| PROCAINE | | ESTERS | 1905 |
| TETRACAINE | | ESTERS | 1930 |
| CHLOROPROCAINE | | ESTERS | 1932 |
| CINCHOCAINE | | AMIDES | 1952 |
| LIDOCAINE | | AMIDES | 1947 |
| MEPIVACAINE | | AMIDES | 1957 |
| PRILOCAINE | | AMIDES | 1960 |
| BUPIVACAINE | | AMIDES | 1963 |
| ETIDOCAINE | | AMIDES | 1972 |
| ROPIVACAINE | | AMIDES | 1997 |
| LEVOBUPIVACAINE | | AMIDES | 1995 |

**FIGURE 2-4.** Local anesthetics, their classification, chemical structure, and approximate time of introduction.

the aromatic ring. For example, 2-chloroprocaine is hydrolyzed about four times faster than procaine, which in turn is hydrolyzed about four times faster than tetracaine. However, the rate of hydrolysis of all ester-linked LAs is markedly decreased in patients with atypical plasma pseudocholinesterase, and a prolonged epidural block in a patient with abnormal pseudocholinesterase has been reported. Another hallmark of metabolism of ester-linked LAs is that their hydrolysis leads to the formation of para-aminobenzoic acid (PABA). PABA and its derivatives carry a small risk potential for allergic reactions. A history of an allergic reaction to a LA should immediately suggest that a current reaction is due to the presence of PABA derived from an ester-linked LA. However, although exceedingly rare, allergic reactions can also develop from the use of multiple-dose vials of amide-linked LAs that contain PABA as a preservative.

### Cocaine

Cocaine occurs naturally in the leaves of the coca shrub and is an ester of benzoic acid. The clinically desired actions of cocaine are blockade of nerve impulses and local vasoconstriction secondary to inhibition of local norepinephrine reuptake. However, its toxicity and the potential for abuse have precluded wider clinical use of cocaine in modern practice. Its euphoric properties are due primarily to inhibition of catecholamine uptake, particularly dopamine, at CNS synapses. Other LAs do not block the uptake of norepinephrine and do not produce the sensitization to catecholamines, vasoconstriction, or mydriasis characteristics of cocaine. Currently, cocaine is used primarily to provide topical anesthesia of the upper respiratory tract, where its combined vasoconstrictor and LA properties provide anesthesia and shrinking of the mucosa with a single agent.

### Procaine

Procaine, an amino ester, was the first synthetic LA. Procaine is characterized by low potency, slow onset, and short duration of action. Consequently, although once widely used, its use now is largely confined to infiltration anesthesia and perhaps diagnostic nerve blocks.

### 2-Chloroprocaine

An ester LA introduced in 1952, 2-chloroprocaine is a chlorinated derivative of procaine. Chloroprocaine is the most rapidly metabolized LA used currently. Because of its rapid breakdown in plasma (<1 minute), it has a very low potential for systemic toxicity. Enthusiasm for its use in spinal anesthesia was tempered by reports of neurologic deficits during the 1980s. Such toxicity appeared to have been a consequence of low pH and the use of sodium meta-bisulfite as a preservative in earlier formulations. A newer 2-chloroprocaine commercial preparation from which the preservatives have been removed has been released, and the initial studies appear to be promising, with no reports of toxicity. This drug has largely replaced lidocaine in our practice for short-acting spinal anesthetics for procedures lasting less than 1 hour.

A 3% 2-chloroprocaine solution is also our LA of choice for surgical anesthesia of short duration that results in relatively minor tissue trauma and postoperative pain (e.g., carpal tunnel syndrome, knee arthroscopy, muscle biopsy). Its characteristics in peripheral nerve blockade include fast onset and short duration of action (1.5–2 hours). The duration of blockade can be extended (up to 2 hours) by the addition of epinephrine (1:400,000).

### Tetracaine

Tetracaine was introduced in 1932, and it is a long-acting amino ester. It is significantly more potent and has a longer duration of action than procaine or 2-chloroprocaine. Tetracaine is more slowly metabolized than the other commonly used ester LAs, and it is considerably more toxic. Currently, it is used in spinal anesthesia when a drug of long duration is needed, as well as in various topical anesthetic preparations. Because of its slow onset and potential for toxicity, tetracaine is used rarely for peripheral nerve blocks in our practice. Some centers, however, have used tetracaine in combination with other local anesthetics, commonly lidocaine, with success. The combination is often known by the nickname "supercaine." The prevalence of the use of supercaine in modern regional anesthesia is not known.

## Amide-Linked Local Anesthetics

As opposed to ester-linked drugs, amide-linked LAs are metabolized in the liver by a dealkalization reaction in which an ethyl group is cleaved from the tertiary amine. The hepatic blood flow and liver function determine the hepatic clearance of these anesthetics. Consequently, factors that decrease hepatic blood flow or hepatic drug extraction both result in an increased elimination half-life. Renal clearance of unchanged LAs is a minor route of elimination, accounting for only 3% to 5% of the total drug administered.

### Lidocaine

Lidocaine was introduced in 1948 by the Swedish drug manufacturer Astra, and it remains one of the most versatile and widely used LAs. It is the prototype of the amide class of LAs. Lidocaine is absorbed rapidly after parenteral administration and from the gastrointestinal and respiratory tracts. Lidocaine can be used in almost any peripheral nerve block in which a LA of intermediate duration is needed. A concentration of 1.5% or 2% with or without the addition of epinephrine is most commonly used for surgical anesthesia. More diluted concentrations are suitable in pain management, particularly for diagnostic blocks.

## Mepivacaine

Mepivacaine, introduced in 1957, is an intermediate-duration amino amide LA. Its pharmacologic properties are similar to those of lidocaine. Although it was suggested that mepivacaine is more toxic to neonates (and as such is not used in obstetric anesthesia), it appears to have a slightly higher therapeutic index in adults than lidocaine. Its onset of action is similar to that of lidocaine, but it enjoys a slightly longer duration of action than lidocaine. Our first choice in any peripheral nerve block technique is 1.5% mepivacaine when an intermediate-duration blockade is desired (3–6 hours, depending on the type of nerve block and addition of a vasoconstrictor).

## Prilocaine

Prilocaine is an intermediate-duration amino amide LA with a pharmacologic profile similar to that of lidocaine. The primary differences are a lack of vasodilatation and an increased volume of distribution, which reduces its CNS toxicity. However, it is unique among amide LAs for its propensity to cause methemoglobinemia, an effect of metabolism of the aromatic ring to o-toluidine. The development of methemoglobinemia depends on the total dose administered (usually requires 8 mg/kg) and does not have significant consequences in healthy patients. If necessary, it is treated by IV administration of methylene blue (1–2 mg/kg). Prilocaine is used infrequently in peripheral nerve blockade.

## Etidocaine

Etidocaine is a long-acting amino amide introduced in 1972. Its neuronal blocking properties are characterized by an onset of action similar to that of lidocaine and a duration of action comparable with that of bupivacaine. Etidocaine is structurally similar to lidocaine, with alkyl substitution on the aliphatic connecting group between the hydrophilic amine and the amide linkage. This feature increases the lipid solubility of the drug and results in a drug more potent than lidocaine that has a very rapid onset of action and a prolonged duration of anesthesia. A major disadvantage of etidocaine is its profound motor blockade over a wide range of clinical concentrations, which often outlasts sensory blockade. For these reasons, etidocaine is not used for peripheral nerve blockade.

## Bupivacaine

Since its introduction in 1963, bupivacaine has been one of the most commonly used LAs in regional and infiltration anesthesia. Its structure is similar to that of lidocaine, except that the amine-containing group is a butylpiperidine. Bupivacaine is a long-acting agent capable of producing prolonged anesthesia and analgesia that can be prolonged even further by the addition of epinephrine. It is substantially more cardiotoxic than lidocaine. The cardiotoxicity of bupivacaine is cumulative and substantially greater than would be predicted by its LA potency. At least part of the cardiotoxicity of bupivacaine may be mediated centrally because direct injection of small quantities of bupivacaine into the medulla can produce malignant ventricular arrhythmias. Bupivacaine-induced cardiotoxicity can be difficult to treat.

Bupivacaine is widely used both in neuraxial and peripheral nerve blockade. The blocking property is characterized by a slower onset and a long, somewhat unpredictable duration of blockade. Because of its toxicity profile, large doses of bupivacaine should be avoided.

## Ropivacaine

The cardiotoxicity of bupivacaine stimulated interest in developing a less toxic, long-lasting LA. The development of ropivacaine, the *S*-enantiomer of 1-propyl-2′, 6′-pipecolocylidide, is the result of that search. The *S*-enantiomer, like most LAs with a chiral center, was chosen because it has a lower toxicity than the *R*-enantiomer. This is presumably because of slower uptake, resulting in lower blood levels for a given dose. Ropivacaine undergoes extensive hepatic metabolism after IV administration, with only 1% of the drug eliminated unchanged in the urine. Ropivacaine is slightly less potent than bupivacaine in producing anesthesia when used in lower concentrations. However, in concentrations of 0.5% and higher, it produces dense blockade with a slightly shorter duration than that of bupivacaine. In concentrations of 0.75%, the onset of blockade is almost as fast as that of 1.5% mepivacaine or 3% 2-chloroprocaine, with reduced CNS toxicity and cardiotoxic potential and a lower propensity for motor blockade than bupivacaine. For these reasons, ropivacaine has become one of the most commonly used long-acting LAs in peripheral nerve blockade.

**TIP**

- Bupivacaine has fallen out of favor in many centers due both to its potential for serious toxicity, as well as the availability of ropivacaine, a LA characterized by a slightly decreased duration of action than bupivacaine but an improved safety profile. However, the advent of ultrasonography has allowed for a dramatic reduction in the volumes of LA necessary to achieve many nerve blocks. Consequently, some practitioners have begun to use bupivacaine again, albeit in smaller doses, to maximize the duration of blockade.

## Levobupivacaine

Levobupivacaine contains a single enantiomer of bupivacaine hydrochloride, and is less cardiotoxic than bupivacaine. It is extensively metabolized with no unchanged drug detected in the urine or feces. The properties of levobupivacaine in peripheral nerve blockade are less well studied than those of ropivacaine, however, research results suggest that they seem to parallel those of bupivacaine. Therefore, levobupivacaine is a suitable, less toxic alternative to bupivacaine.

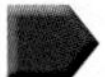

## Additives to Local Anesthetics

### Vasoconstrictors

The addition of a vasoconstrictor to a LA delays its vascular absorption, increasing the duration of drug contact with nerve tissues. The net effect is prolongation of the blockade by as much as 50% and a decrease in the systemic absorption of LA. These effects vary significantly among different types of LAs and individual nerve blocks. For example, because lidocaine is a natural vasodilator, the effect is pronounced for those blocks compared with blocks using ropivacaine, which has its own slight vasoconstricting effect. Epinephrine is the most commonly used vasoconstrictor in peripheral nerve blockade. A decrease in nerve blood supply has been associated with epinephrine when combined with local anesthetics. However, this effect was not seen when concentrations of epinephrine were maintained at 1:400,000 (2.5 μg/mL). As such, this is the recommended concentration when used as an adjuvant.

**TIP**

- Epinephrine also serves as a marker of intravenous injection of local anesthetic. An increase in heart rate of 20 bpm or greater and/or an increase in systolic blood pressure of 15 mmHg or greater after a dose of 15 μg of epinephrine is should raise a suspicion of intravascular injection.

### Opioids

The injection of opioids into the epidural or subarachnoid space to manage acute or chronic pain is based on the knowledge that opioid receptors are present in the substantia gelatinosa of the spinal cord. Thus combinations of a LA and an opiate are often successfully used in neuraxial blockade to both enhance the blockade and prolong analgesia. However, in peripheral nerves, similar receptors are absent or the effects of opiates are negligibly weak. For this reason, opiates do not have a significant clinical role in peripheral nerve blockade.

### Clonidine

Clonidine is a centrally acting selective partial $\alpha_2$-adrenergic agonist. Because of its ability to reduce sympathetic nervous system output from the CNS, clonidine acts as an antihypertensive drug. Preservative-free clonidine, administered into the epidural or subarachnoid space (150–450 μg), produces dose-dependent analgesia and, unlike opioids, does not produce depression of ventilation, pruritus, nausea, or vomiting. Clonidine produces analgesia by activating postsynaptic $\alpha_2$ receptors in the substantia gelatinosa of the spinal cord. Much less research has been done on the effects of clonidine in peripheral nerve blockade. A recent meta-analysis showed that clonidine prolongs the duration of both the sensory and motor block by approximately 1.5 to 2 hours. Of note, there appears to be no benefit to using clonidine in continuous perineural infusions. In addition, side effects, notably sedation, orthostatic hypotension, and fainting, should be considered when using clonidine. The latter two effects, in particular, can interfere with mobilization postoperatively. Although life-threatening hypotension or bradycardia has not been reported when clonidine is used with peripheral nerve blocks, its circulatory effects may complicate resuscitation in a setting of LA toxicity.

## Selecting Local Anesthetics for Peripheral Nerve Blocks

With a variety of LAs to choose from, it is useful to keep the following points in mind when selecting an agent for nerve blockade. In general, the onset and duration of a LA are similar in nature. For example, 2-chloroprocaine has a short onset but also a relatively brief duration (Table 2-1). In contrast, bupivacaine and ropivacaine have longer durations of action but take somewhat longer to exert their effect.

The LA should be tailored to the duration of the surgical procedure and the anticipated degree of pain. For example, creation of an arteriovenous fistula is a relatively short operation with minimal postoperative pain. Therefore, selection of a short-acting agent (e.g., mepivacaine) provides excellent intraoperative conditions, without the burden of an insensate limb for 10 to 18 hours postoperatively. A rotator cuff repair involves a greater degree of postoperative pain, and therefore selection of a long-acting LA (e.g., ropivacaine) is appropriate.

Onset and duration for a given LA varies according to the nerve or plexus blocked. For example, at the brachial plexus, 0.5% ropivacaine may be expected to provide 10 to 12 hours of analgesia; the same concentration at the sciatic nerve may provide up to 24 hours of analgesia. This is likely due to differences in the local vascularity, which influences the uptake of LA.

Blocks for postoperative analgesia (often in concert with general anesthesia) do not require a high concentration of LA. Ropivacaine 0.2% is usually sufficient to provide excellent sensory analgesia but spare any motor blockade.

The toxicity of the agent should be considered. Bupivacaine provides the longest duration of the commonly used LAs but also has the worst cardiotoxic profile. However, a reduction in the dose used, seen more and more frequently with ultrasound-guided nerve blocks, may provide an equivalent

**TABLE 2-1 Choice of Local Anesthetic for Peripheral Nerve Blockade**

| ANESTHETIC | ONSET (min) | DURATION OF ANESTHESIA (h) | DURATION OF ANALGESIA (h) |
|---|---|---|---|
| 3% 2-Chloroprocaine (+$HCO_3$) | 10–15 | 1 | 2 |
| 3% 2-Chloroprocaine ($HCO_3$ + epinephrine) | 10–15 | 1.5–2 | 2–3 |
| 1.5% Mepivacaine (+ $HCO_3$) | 10–20 | 2–3 | 3–5 |
| 1.5% Mepivacaine (+ $HCO_3$ plus epinephrine) | 10–20 | 2–5 | 3–8 |
| 2% Lidocaine ($HCO_3$ + epinephrine) | 10–20 | 2–5 | 3–8 |
| 0.5% Ropivacaine | 15–30 | 4–8 | 5–12 |
| 0.75% Ropivacaine | 10–15 | 5–10 | 6–24 |
| 0.5% Bupivacaine or levobupivacaine (+ epinephrine) | 15–30 | 5–15 | 6–30 |

or greater safety profile than a larger dose of ropivacaine, the drug to which it is often compared.

Ambulatory patients who are undergoing lower limb surgery should be administered long-acting LAs with caution and with proper education regarding ambulation with assistance. Short procedures with minimal postoperative pain (most ambulatory procedures) only require a short- to intermediate-acting agent, and evidence of block resolution is often a requirement before discharge home.

Anticipated pain lasting longer than 15 to 20 hours should warrant the consideration of a perineural catheter. The appreciation that patients show for any effective block will fade quickly when it wears off in the middle of the night, leaving them unprepared, in pain, and unable to access alternative pain therapies.

## Mixing of Local Anesthetics

Mixing of LAs (e.g., lidocaine and bupivacaine) is often done in clinical practice with the intent of obtaining the faster onset of the shorter acting LAs and the longer duration of the longer acting LA. Unfortunately, when LAs are mixed, their onset, duration, and potency become much less predictable, and the end result is far from expected. For instance, work performed at our institution has shown that combining mepivacaine 1.5% with bupivacaine 0.5%, versus either drug alone for interscalene brachial plexus block, results in little clinical advantage. Onset times for all three solutions were indistinguishable, and the duration of the combined solution was significantly shorter than bupivacaine alone. Moreover, a separate experiment looking at the sequence of LAs (i.e., bupivacaine first, mepivacaine second versus mepivacaine first, bupivacaine second) showed no difference in the onset and duration between groups.

Therefore, if long duration is desired, a long-acting drug alone will provide the best conditions. In addition, mixing LAs also carries a risk of a drug error. For this reason, we rarely mix LAs; instead, we choose drugs and concentrations of single agents to achieve the desired effects.

The vast majority of nerve block goals can be met using one short/intermediate and one long-acting LA. At our institution, more than 90% of peripheral nerve blocks for surgical anesthesia are performed with one of two LAs: 1.5% mepivacaine or 0.5%–0.75% ropivacaine. Of course, there are times when other LAs are used. Chloroprocaine is used for quick knee arthroscopies, for example, when the postoperative pain is minimal and rapid return to ambulation is required. Table 2-1 shows the commonly used local anesthetics, with and without bicarbonate and/or epinephrine, and their expected onset and duration of actions. As mentioned previously, these numbers do not apply to all scenarios, all nerves, and all plexuses but can be used as a rough comparative guide to aid in decision making.

## SUGGESTED READINGS

Albright GA. Cardiac arrest following regional anesthesia with etidocaine or bupivacaine. *Anesthesiology*. 1978;51:285-287.

Auroy Y, Narchi P, Messiah A, et al. Serious complications related to regional anesthesia: results of a prospective survey in France. *Anesthesiology.* 1997;87:479-486.

Avery P, Redon D, Schaenzer G, et al. The influence of serum potassium on the cerebral and cardiac toxicity of bupivacaine and lidocaine. *Anesthesiology*. 1985;61:134-138.

Berry JS, Heindel L. Evaluation of lidocaine and tetracaine mixture in axillary brachial plexus block. *AANA J.* 1999;67:329-334.

Blanch SA, Lopez AM, Carazo J, et al. Intraneural injection during nerve stimulator-guided sciatic nerve block at the popliteal fossa. *Br J Anaesth.* 2009;102:855-861.

Braid BP, Scott DB. The systemic absorption of local analgesic drugs. *Br J Anaesth.* 1965;37:394.

Burney RG, DiFazio CA, Foster JA. Effects of pH on protein binding of lidocaine. *Anesth Analg.* 1978;57:478-480.

Butterworth JF, Strichartz GR. The molecular mechanisms by which local anesthetics produce impulse blockade: a review. *Anesthesiology.* 1990;72:711-734.

Carpenter RI, Mackey DC. Local anesthetics. In: Barash PG, Cullen BF, Stoelting RK, eds. *Clinical Anesthesia.* 2nd ed. Philadelphia, PA: Lippincott; 1992:509-541.

Casati A, Magistris L, Fanelli G, et al. Small-dose clonidine prolongs postoperative analgesia after sciatic-femoral nerve block with 0.75% ropivacaine for foot surgery. *Anesth Analg.* 2000;91:388.

Catterall WA. Cellular and molecular biology of voltage-gated sodium channels. *Physiol Rev.* 1992;72:S15-S48.

Clarkson CW, Hondeghem LM. Mechanism for bupivacaine depression of cardiac conduction: fast block of sodium channels during the action potential with slow recovery from block during diastole. *Anesthesiology.* 1985;62:396-405.

Courtney KR, Strichartz GR. Structural elements which determine local anesthetic activity. In: Strichartz GR, ed. *Handbook of Experimental Pharmacology.* Vol 81. Berlin, Germany: Springer-Verlag; 1987:53-94.

Cousins MJ, Bridenbaugh PO, eds. *Neural Blockade in Clinical Anesthesia and Management of Pain.* 3rd ed. Philadelphia, PA: Lippincott; 1995.

Cousins MJ, Mather LE. Intrathecal and epidural administration of opioids. *Anesthesiology.* 1984;61:276-310.

Covino BG. Toxicity and systemic effects of local anesthetic agents. In: Strichartz GR, ed. *Handbook of Experimental Pharmacology.* Vol 81. Berlin, Germany: Springer-Verlag; 1987:187-212.

Covino BG, Vassallo HG. *Local Anesthetics: Mechanisms of Action and Clinical Use.* New York, NY: Grune & Stratton; 1976.

De Negri P, Visconti C, DeVivo P, et al. Does clonidine added to epidural infusion of 0.2% ropivacaine enhance postoperative analgesia in adults? *Reg Anesth Pain Med.* 2000;25:39.

DiFazio CA, Rowlingson JC. Additives to local anesthetic solutions. In: Brown DL, ed. *Regional Anesthesia and Analgesia.* Philadelphia, PA: Saunders; 1996:232-239.

Gormley WP, Murray JM, Fee JPH, Bower S. Effect of the addition of alfentanil to lignocaine during axillary brachial plexus anaesthesia. *Br J Anaesth.* 1996;76:802-805.

Fibuch EE, Opper SE. Back pain following epidurally administered Nesacaine MPF. *Anesth Analg.* 1989;69:113-115.

Gadsden J, Hadzic A, Gandhi K, et al. The effect of mixing 1.5% mepivacaine and 0.5% bupivacaine on duration of analgesia and latency of block onset in ultrasound-guided interscalene block. *Anesth Analg.* 2011;112:471-6.

Garfield JM, Gugino L. Central effects of local anesthetics. In: Strichartz GR, ed. *Handbook of Experimental Pharmacology.* Vol 81. Berlin, Germany: Springer-Verlag; 1987:187-212.

Gissen AJ, Datta S, Lambert D. The chloroprocaine controversy. II. Is chloroprocaine neurotoxic? *Reg Anesth.* 1984;9:135-145.

Graf BM, Martin E, Bosnjak ZJ, et al. Stereospecific effect of bupivacaine isomers on atrioventricular conduction in the isolated perfused guinea pig heart. *Anesthesiology.* 1997;86:410-419.

Harwood TN, Butterworth JF, Colonna DM, et al. Plasma bupivacaine concentrations and effects of epinephrine after superficial cervical plexus blockade in patients undergoing carotid endarterectomy. *J Cardiothorac Vasc Anesth.* 1999;3:703-706.

Hilgier M. Alkalinization of bupivacaine for brachial plexus block. *Reg Anesth.* 1985;10:59-61.

Huang YF, Pryor ME, Mather LE, et al. Cardiovascular and central nervous system effects of intravenous levobupivacaine and bupivacaine in sheep. *Anesth Analg.* 1998;86:797-804.

Kasten GW, Martin ST. Bupivacaine cardiovascular toxicity: comparison of treatment with bretylium and lidocaine. *Anesth Analg.* 1985;64:911-916.

Moore DC. Administer oxygen first in the treatment of local anesthetic-induced convulsions. *Anesthesiology.* 1980;53:346-347.

Nath S, Haggmark S, Johansson G, et al. Differential depressant and electrophysiologic cardiotoxicity of local anesthetics: an experimental study with special reference to lidocaine and bupivacaine. *Anesth Analg.* 1986;65:1263-1270.

Ragsdale DR, McPhee JC, Scheuer T, et al. Molecular determinants of state-dependent block of $Na^+$ channels by local anesthetics. *Science.* 1994;265:1724-1728.

Raymond SA, Gissen AJ. Mechanism of differential nerve block. In: Strichartz GR, ed. *Handbook of Experimental Pharmacology.* Vol 81. Berlin, Germany: Springer-Verlag; 1987:95-164.

Reiz S, Haggmark S, Johansson G, et al. Cardiotoxicity of ropivacaine—a new amide local anesthetic agent. *Acta Anaesthesiol Scand.* 1989;33:93-98.

Ritchie JM, Greengard P. On the mode of action of local anesthetics. *Annu Rev Pharmacol.* 1966;6:405-430.

Rowlingson JC. Toxicity of local anesthetic additives. *Reg Anesth.* 1993;18:453-460.

Sage DJ, Feldman HS, Arthur GR, et al. Influence of bupivacaine and lidocaine on isolated guinea pig atria in the presence of acidosis and hypoxia. *Anesth Analg.* 1984;63:1-7.

Santos AC, Arthur GR, Lehning EJ, et al. Comparative pharmacokinetics of ropivacaine and bupivacaine in nonpregnant and pregnant ewes. *Anesth Analg.* 1997;85:87-93.

Santos AC, Arthur GR, Padderson H, et al. Systemic toxicity of ropivacaine during bovine pregnancy. *Anesthesiology.* 1994;75: 137-141.

Singelyn FJ, Gouvernuer JM, Robert A. A minimum dose of clonidine added to mepivacaine prolongs the duration of anesthesia and analgesia after axillary brachial plexus block. *Anesth Analg.* 1996;83:1046.

Stevens RA, Urmey WF, Urquhart BL, et al. Back pain after epidural anesthesia with chloroprocaine. *Anesthesiology.* 1993;78:492-497.

Strichartz GR, Ritchie JM. The action of local anesthetics on ion channels of excitable tissues. In: Strichartz GR, ed. *Handbook of Experimental Pharmacology.* Vol 81. Berlin, Germany: Springer-Verlag; 1987:21-53.

Tucker GT, Mather LE. Pharmacokinetics of local anesthetic agents. *Br J Anaesth.* 1975;47:213-214.

Wagman IH, Dejong RH, Prince DA. Effect of lidocaine on the central nervous system. *Anesthesiology.* 1967;28:155-172.

Wang BC, Hillman DE, Spiedholz NI, et al. Chronic neurologic deficits and Nesacaine-CE. An effect of the anesthetic, 2-chloro-procaine, or the antioxidant, sodium bisulfite. *Anesth Analg.* 1984;63:445-447.

Winnie AP, Tay CH, Patel KP, et al. Pharmacokinetics of local anesthetics during plexus blocks. *Anesth Analg.* 1977;56:852-861.

# 3 Equipment for Peripheral Nerve Blocks

*Ali Nima Shariat, Patrick M. Horan, Kimberly Gratenstein, Colleen McCally, and Ashton P. Frulla*

## Introduction

Over the past several decades, regional anesthesia equipment has undergone substantial technological advances. Historically, the development and consequent introduction of the portable nerve stimulator to clinical practice in the 1970s and 1980s was a critical advance in regional anesthesia, allowing the practitioner to better localize the targeted nerve. In recent years, however, the advent of ultrasound, better needles, catheter systems, and monitoring has entirely rejuvenated, if not revolutionized, the practice of regional anesthesia.

## Induction and Block Room

Regional anesthesia is ideally performed in a designated area with access to all the appropriate equipment necessary to perform blocks. Whether this area is the operating room or a separate block room, there must be adequate space, proper lighting, and equipment to ensure successful, efficient, and safe performance of peripheral nerve blocks (PNBs). Provision for proper monitoring, oxygen, equipment for emergency airway management and positive-pressure ventilation, and access to emergency drugs is of paramount importance (Figure 3-1).

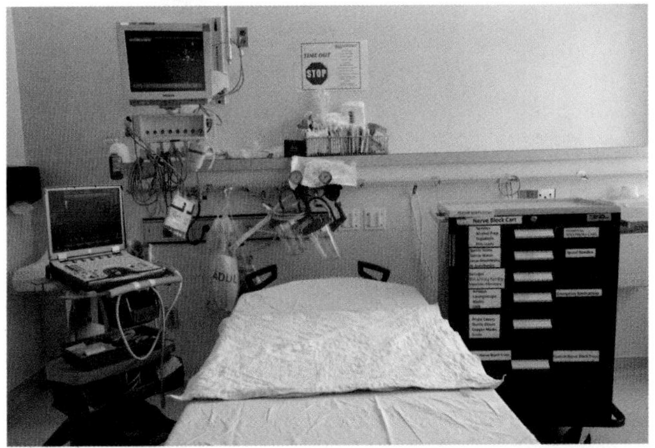


**FIGURE 3-1.** Typical block room setup. Shown are monitoring, oxygen source, suction apparatus, ultrasound machine, and nerve block cart with equipment.

### Cardiovascular and Respiratory Monitoring During Application of Regional Anesthesia

Patients receiving regional anesthesia should be monitored with the same degree of vigilance as patients receiving general anesthesia. Local anesthetic toxicity due to intravascular injection or rapid absorption into systemic circulation is a relatively uncommon but potentially life-threatening complication of regional anesthesia. Likewise, premedication, often necessary before many regional anesthesia procedures, may result in respiratory depression, hypoventilation, and hypoxia. For these reasons, patients receiving PNBs should have vascular access and be appropriately monitored. Routine cardio-respiratory monitoring should consist of pulse oximetry, noninvasive blood pressure, and electrocardiogram. Respiratory rate and mental status should also be monitored. The risk of the local anesthetic toxicity has a biphasic pattern and should be anticipated (1) during and immediately after the injection and (2) 10 to 30 minutes after the injection. Signs and symptoms of toxicity occurring during or shortly after the completion of the injection are due to an intravascular injection or channeling of local anesthetics to the systemic circulation (1–2 minutes). In the absence of an intravascular injection, the typical absorption rate of local anesthetics after injection peaks at approximately 10 to 30 minutes after performance of a PNB[1]; therefore patients should be continuously and closely monitored for at least 30 minutes for signs of local anesthetic toxicity.

**TIPS**

- Routine monitoring during administration of nerve blocks:
  - Pulse oximetry
  - Noninvasive blood pressure
  - Electrocardiogram
  - Respiratory rate
  - Mental status

## Regional Anesthesia Equipment Storage Cart

A regional anesthesia cart should have all drawers clearly labeled and be portable to enable transport to the patient's bedside. The anesthesia cart should also be well stocked with all equipment necessary to perform PNBs effectively, safely, and efficiently. Supplies such as needles and catheters of various sizes, local anesthetics, and emergency airway and resuscitation equipment should also be included (Figures 3-2,3-3, and 3-4).

Different drawers are best organized in a logical manner to ensure quick and easy access. One drawer should be designated for emergency equipment and should include laryngoscopes with an assortment of commonly used blades, styletted endotracheal tubes and airways of various sizes (Figure 3-5). Emergency drugs that should be present include atropine, ephedrine, phenylephrine, propofol, succinylcholine, and intralipid 20%. The latter can alternatively be stored in a nearby drug cart or drug-dispensing system that is immediately available and in close proximity to the block room. This way, it can be prepared within minutes in case of emergency (Figures 3-6, 3-7, and 3-8).

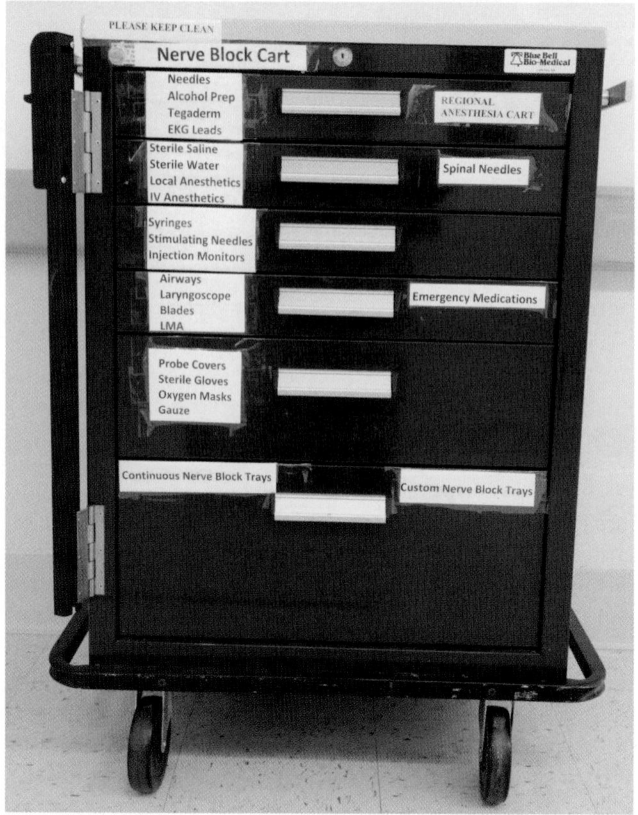


**FIGURE 3-2.** Typical nerve block cart with labels for each drawer.

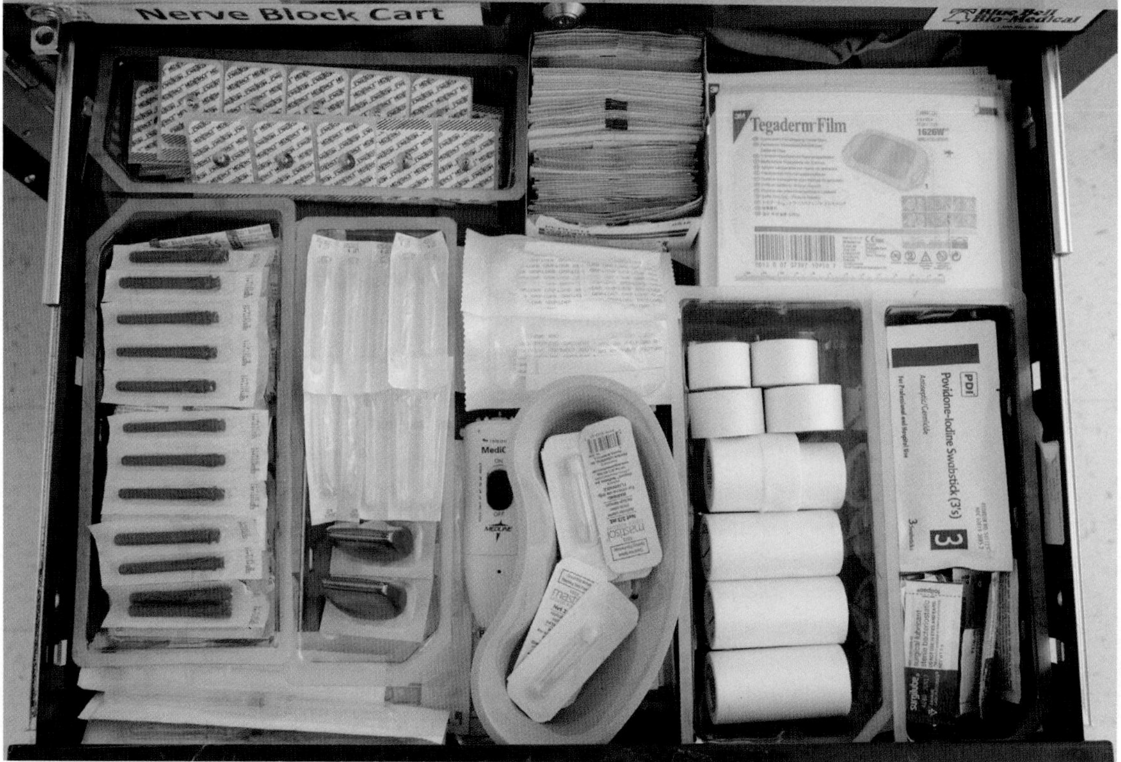


**FIGURE 3-3.** Drawer 1, including electrocardiogram leads, 18-gauge needles, skin adhesive and catheter securing systems, alcohol swabs, clear, occlusive dressing, tape, iodine swabs, and lubricating gel.

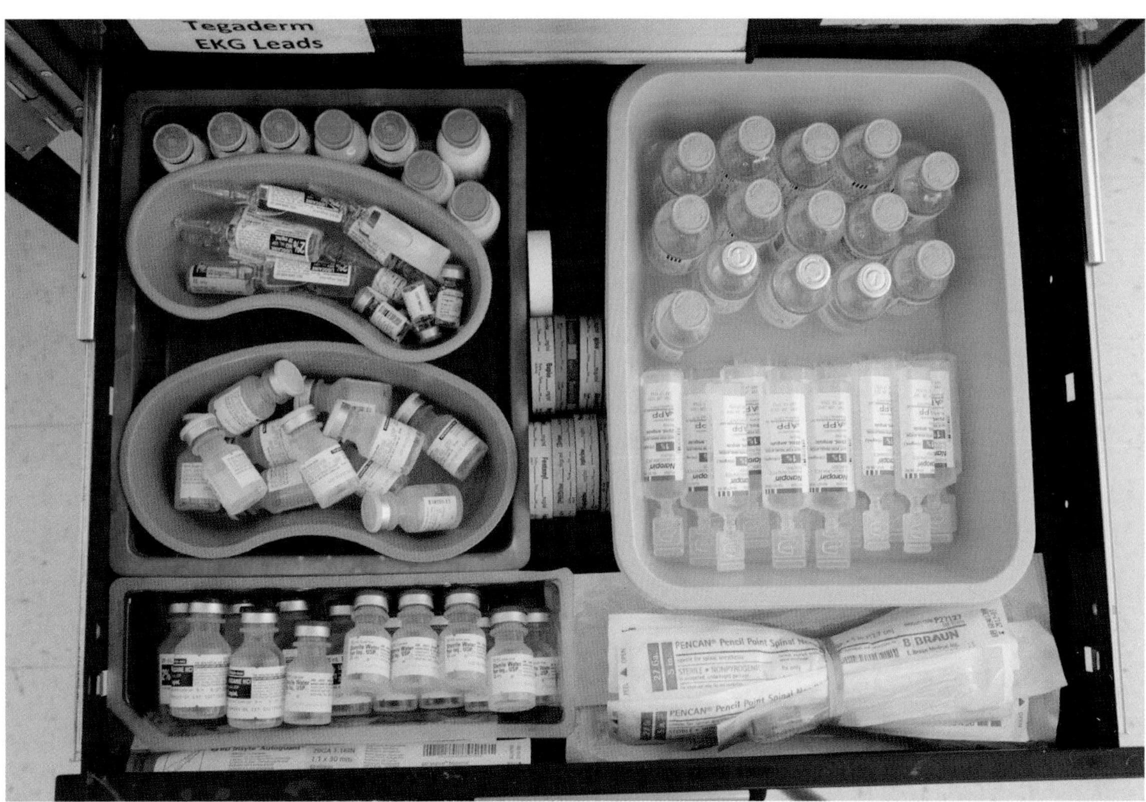


**FIGURE 3-4.** Drawer 2, including propofol, lidocaine 2%, sterile saline, and atropine, sterile saline, lidocaine 2% and sterile water, syringe labels, bupivacaine 0.5%, ropivacaine 1%, and spinal needles.

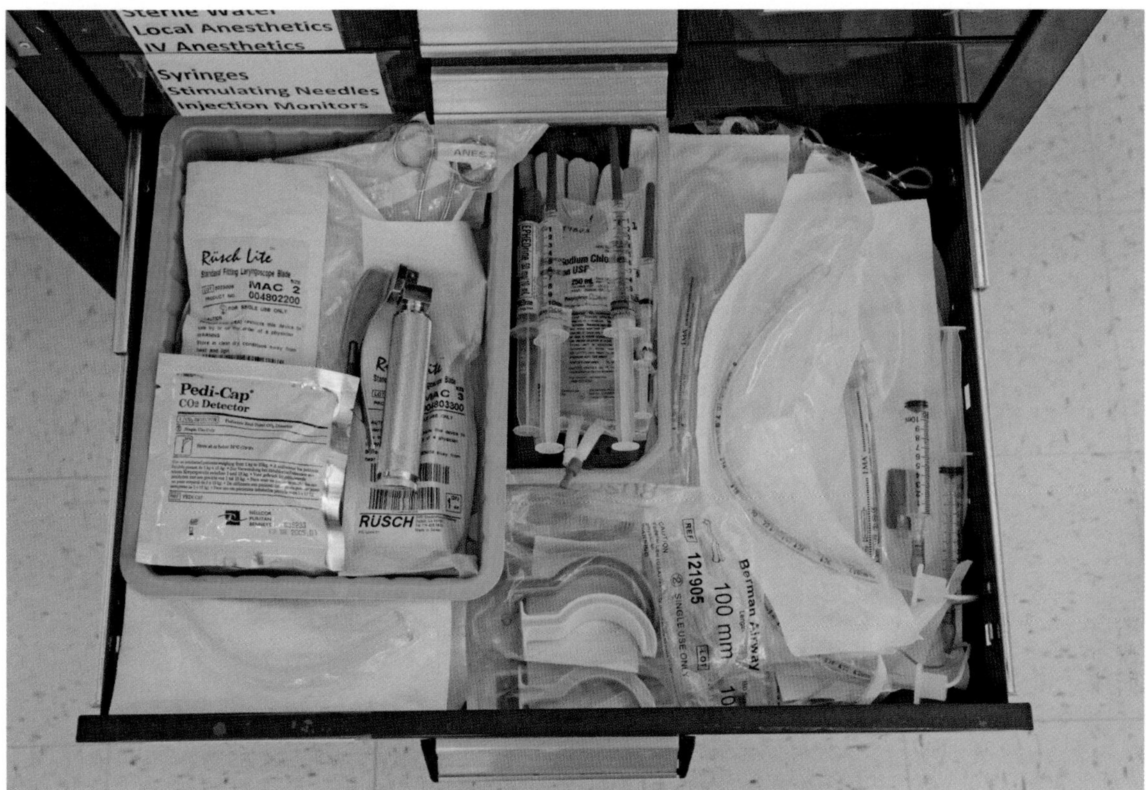


**FIGURE 3-5.** Drawer 3, including laryngoscope, assorted blades, and Magill forceps, emergency medications, stylleted endotracheal tubes, and laryngeal mask airways of assorted sizes, nasal airways, and oral airways.

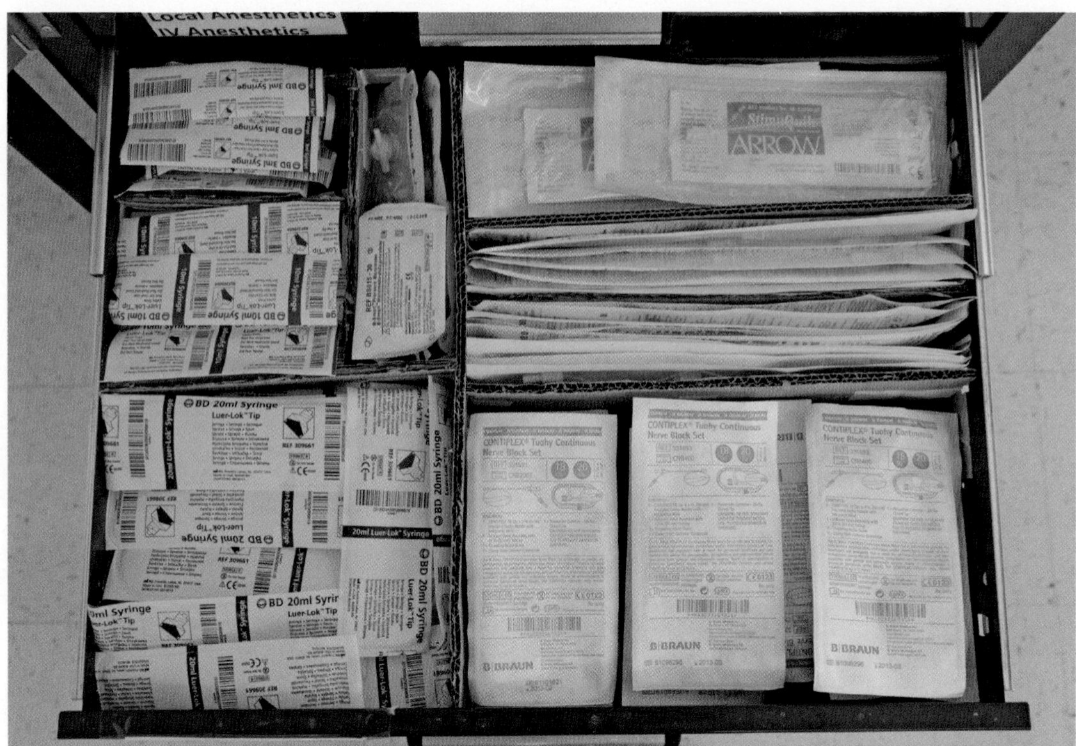


**FIGURE 3-6.** Drawer 4, including syringes of assorted sizes, pressure monitors, stimulating needles, and nonstimulating catheters.

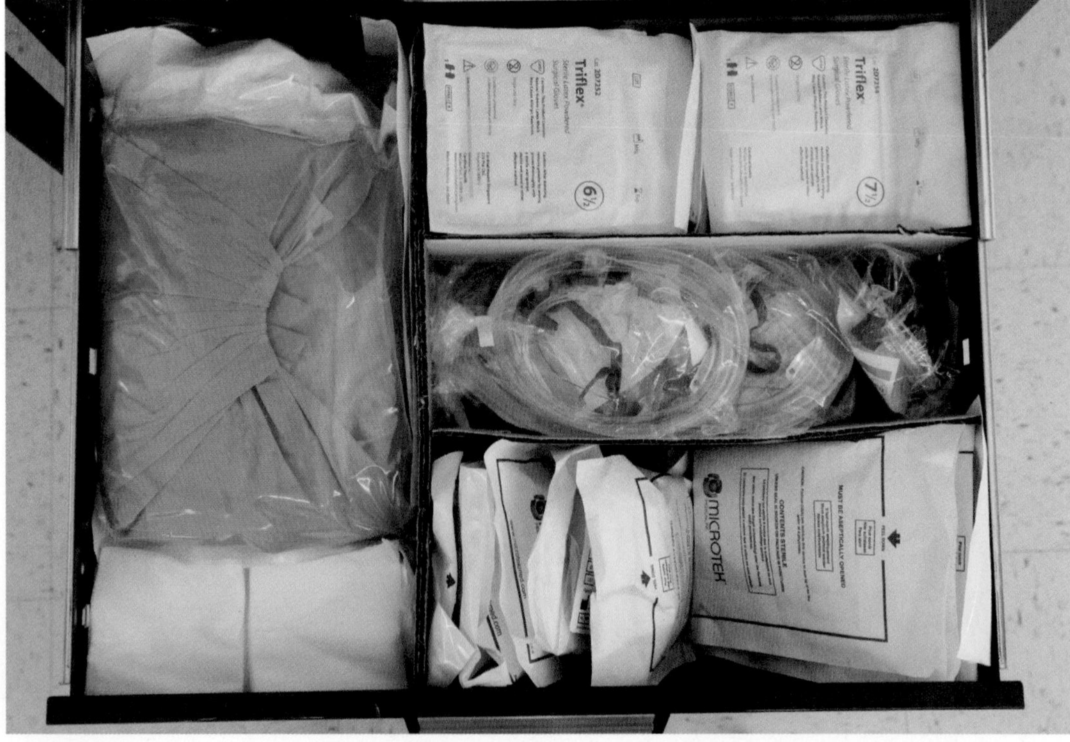


**FIGURE 3-7.** Drawer 5, including sterile drape, sponges, sterile gloves, oxygen masks, and sterile transducer coverings.

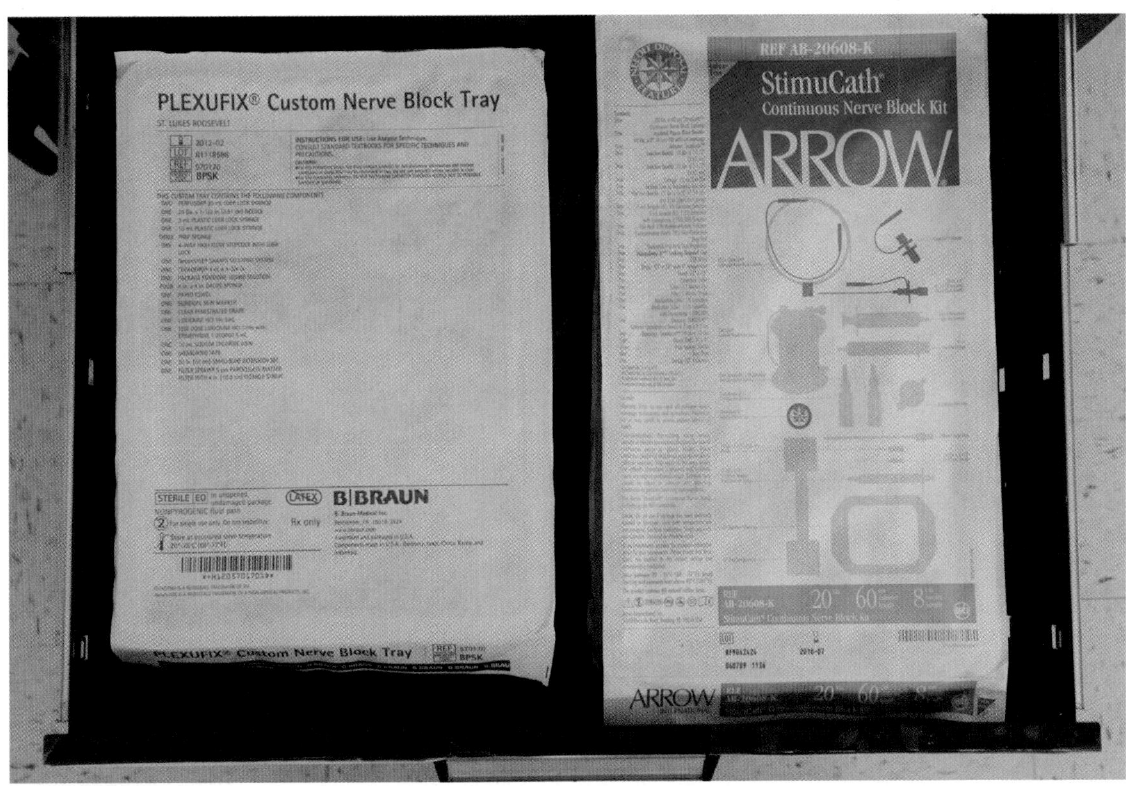


**FIGURE 3-8.** Drawer 6, including custom nerve block tray and continuous nerve block kit with stimulating catheters.

## Suggested Emergency Drugs Required During Nerve Block Procedures

See Table 3-1.

**TABLE 3-1 Suggested Emergency Drugs Required During Nerve Block Procedures**

| DRUG | SUGGESTED DOSE (70 KG ADULT) |
|---|---|
| Atropine | 0.2 mg–0.4 mg IV increments |
| Ephedrine | 5 mg–10 mg IV |
| Phenylephrine | 50 µg–200 µg IV |
| Epinephrine | 10 µg–100 µg IV |
| Midazolam | 2.0 mg–10 mg IV |
| Propofol* | 30 mg–200 mg IV |
| Muscle relaxant (succinylcholine) | Succinylcholine: 20–80 mg IV |
| Intralipid 20% | 105 mL IV bolus followed by 0.25 mL/kg/min infusion given at a rate of 400 mL over 10 min |

*A short-acting barbiturate (i.e., thiopental, Brevital) can be used instead of propofol; however, this requires dilution of the drug at the time when its prompt administration is of utmost importance. In addition, the hypnotic and sedative effects of a barbiturate may be longer lived than those of propofol. These drugs also require more intensive monitoring and airway management. The dosages recommended are for the purpose of abolishing the seizure activity.

## Treatment of Severe Local Anesthetic Toxicity

A 1998 study heralded the clinical utility of intralipid therapy in the treatment of local anesthetic toxicity. Administration of 20% intralipid solution to rats increased the lethal dose of bupivacaine by 48% when compared with untreated controls. The same study also showed increasing survival rates when used as part of a resuscitation protocol. The results were explained by the portioning of bupivacaine into the newly created lipid phase.[2] In follow-up studies, dogs that had bupivacaine-induced cardiovascular collapse were successfully resuscitated after receiving lipid infusion, demonstrating the utility of intralipid in a large animal model that more closely approximates human physiology.[3] In 2006, Rosenblatt et al published the first use of intralipids in a patient to reverse bupivacaine-induced cardiotoxicity.[4] Soon thereafter, additional case reports of successful resuscitation from local anesthetic-induced toxicity with intralipid were published[5–8] establishing intralipid infusion as an important emergency intervention in the practice of regional anesthesiology. Based on laboratory evidence and a growing body of anecdotal reports in clinical practice, it appears prudent to keep intralipid solution 20% in close proximity to locations where regional anesthesia is administered.[9]

### Peripheral Nerve Block Trays

Commercially available, specialized nerve block trays are useful for time-efficient practice of PNBs. An all-purpose tray that can be adapted to a variety of blocks may be the most practical, given the wide array of needles and catheters that may be needed for specific procedures. Appropriate needles, catheters, and other specialized equipment are simply opened and added to the generic nerve block tray as needed (Figure 3-9).

#### *Regional Nerve Block Needles*

A wide array of needles is available for performing PNBs (Figure 3-10). Choice of needle depends on the block being performed, the size of the patient, and preference of the clinician. Needles are typically classified according to tip design, length, gauge, and the presence or absence of electrical insulation or other specialized treatment of the needles (e.g., etching for better ultrasound visualization).

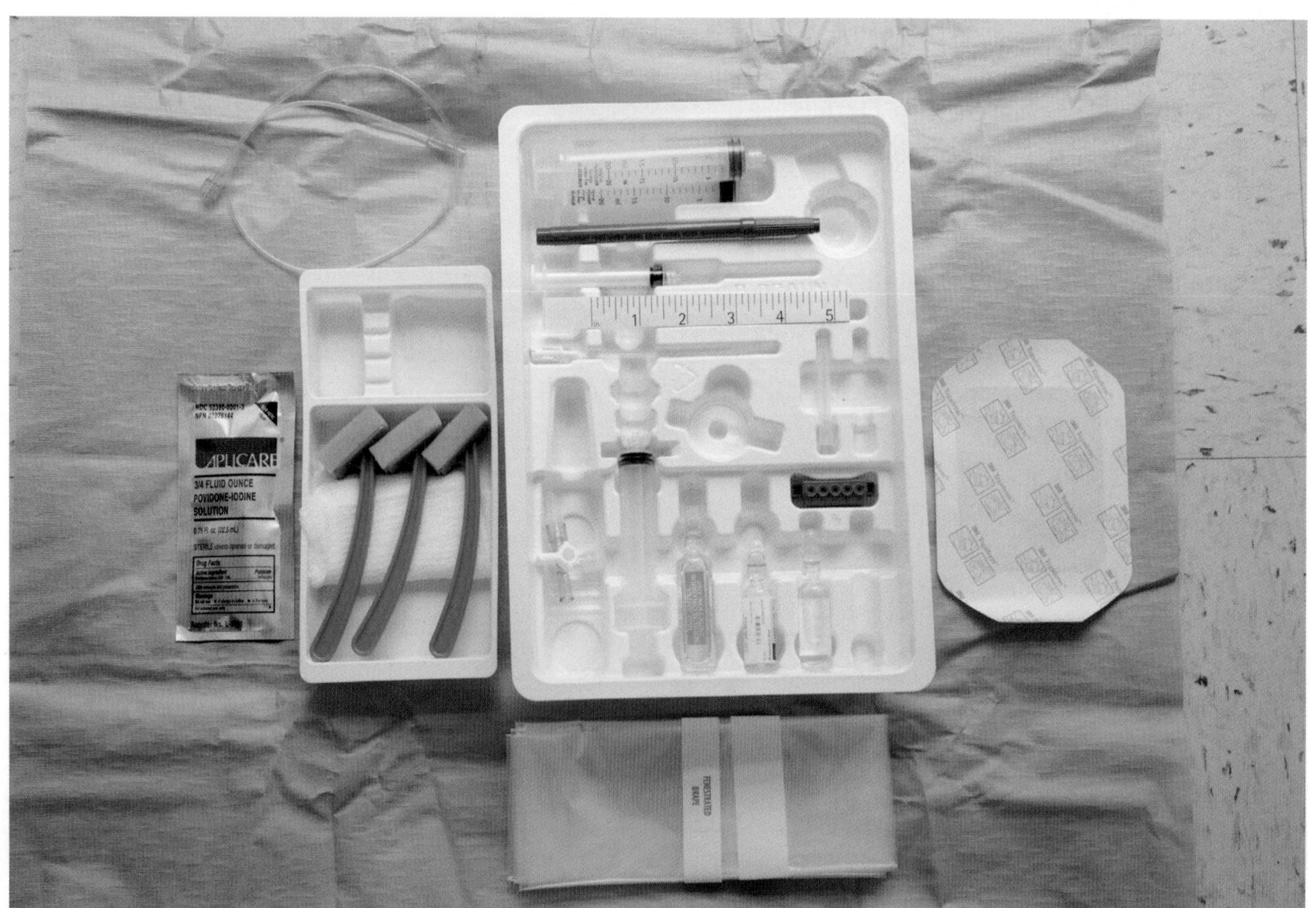


**FIGURE 3-9.** An example of a custom nerve block tray, including lidocaine 1%, lidocaine 1% with epinephrine, sterile saline, syringes, connector, and marker, prep sponges and iodine solution, sterile occlusive dressing and drape, and extension tubing.

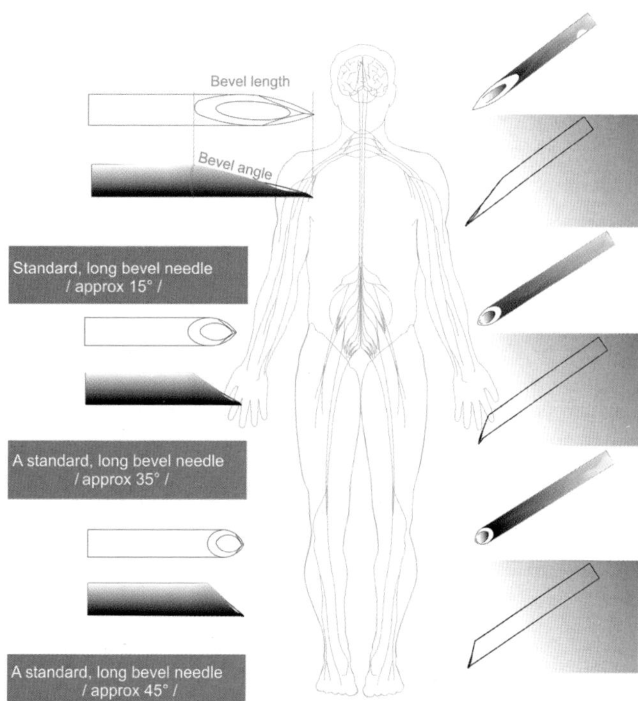


**FIGURE 3-10.** Common needle tip designs.

### *Needle Tip Design*

Direct evidence for an association between needle tip design and the incidence of nerve injury is scarce. In a rabbit sciatic nerves model, Selander demonstrated that the risk of fascicle injury was lower when a short bevel needle penetrated a nerve as opposed to a long bevel needle.[10] However, another experiment by Rice and colleagues suggested that the reverse may be true.[11] This disparity might be explained by the fact that the study of Rice et al examined the effect of needle bevel design on the severity and consequences of intrafascicular should accidental fasicular penetration occur. Therefore, although it may be more difficult to enter a nerve fascicle with a short bevel needle as compared with a long bevel needle, the short bevel needle may cause a more severe lesion should a nerve be impaled by such a needle.[12] Needle design can also have a direct effect on the anesthesiologist's ability to perceive tissue planes. Tuohy and short bevel noncutting needles provide more resistance and thus enhance the feel of the needle traversing different tissues. Long bevel cutting needles, by contrast, do not provide as much tactile information while traversing different tissues. Pencil point needles may be associated with less tissue trauma than short bevel needles when bony contact occurs during spinal anesthesia, resulting in a lower incidence of postdural puncture headache.[13] It is unclear however, whether pencil point needles have any advantage over other needle designs in practice of PNBs.

**Needle Length** The length of the needle should be selected according to the type of block being performed (Table 3-2). A short needle may not reach its target. Long needles have a greater risk of causing injury due to increased difficulty in their handling and possibility of being inserted too deeply. The needle lengths recommended in this text are based on the author's experience and are intended as a general guide. Note that the needle length is often longer by 2 to 3 cm for ultrasound-guided blocks because needles are inserted further from the target to visualize the course of the needle on the image. Needles should have depth markings on their shaft to allow monitoring for the depth of placement at all times.

**TABLE 3-2 Block Technique and Recommended Needle Length**

| BLOCK TECHNIQUE | RECOMMENDED NEEDLE LENGTH (nerve stimulator-guided blocks. For ultrasound-guided blocks, needles may be slightly longer) |
|---|---|
| Cervical plexus block | 50 mm (2 in) |
| Interscalene brachial plexus block | 25 mm (1 in) to 50 mm (2 in) |
| Infraclavicular brachial plexus block | 100 mm (4 in) |
| Axillary brachial plexus block | 25 (1 in) to 50 mm (2 in) |
| Thoracic paraverterbral block | 90 mm (3.5–4 in) |
| Lumbar paravertebral | 100 mm (4 in) |
| Lumbar plexus block | 100 mm (4 in) |
| Sciatic block: posterior approach | 100 mm (4 in) |
| Sciatic block: anterior approach | 150 mm (6 in) |
| Femoral block | 50 mm (2 in) |
| Popliteal block: posterior approach | 50 mm (2 in) |
| Popliteal block: lateral approach | 100 mm (4 in) |

**Needle Gauge** The choice of the needle gauge depends on the depth of the block and whether a continuous catheter is placed. Steinfeldt et al recently demonstrated the correlation between larger needle gauge and increasing levels of nerve damage after intentional nerve perforation in a porcine model.[14] Thus, a small gauge needle may theoretically reduce the tissue trauma and discomfort to patients, whereas a long gauge needle bends more easily, making it more difficult to control. The needles of smaller caliber however, may also be more likely to penetrate the fascicles. In addition, needles of smaller gauges have more internal resistance, making it more difficult to gauge injection resistance and aspirate blood. Needles of very small size (25 and 26 gauge) are most commonly used for superficial and field blocks. Larger gauge needles (20–22 gauge) may be used in deeper blocks to avoid bending of the shaft and to maintain better control over the needle path. When placing a continuous catheter, the needle gauge must be large enough to allow passage of the catheter. Consequently, 17-19 gauge needles are most commonly used with an 18- gauge catheter for continuous catheters.

### *Echogenic Needles*

Visualization of the needle tip is one of the more challenging aspects of performing an ultrasound-guided PNB. To facilitate the ease of needle visualization, specialized needle designs are being developed that allow greater visibility of the needle when performing ultrasound-guided PNBs. One example of such needle designs is coating with a biocompatible polymer that traps microbubbles of air, thus creating specular reflectors of air.[15] The design improves needle visibility and aids in the performance of sonographically guided biopsies.[16] Another echogenic needle design incorporates echogenic "dimples" at the tip to improve visibility.[17] Unique texturing on the needle tip also demonstrated improvement in visibility.[18] The design of echogenic needles is a continuously evolving field.

## Ultrasound Machines

Ultrasound technology allows visualization of the anatomic structures, the approaching needle, and the spread of local anesthetic.[19] Ease of use, image quality, ergonomic design, portability, and cost are all important considerations when choosing an ultrasound machine. To curtail costs, some institutions or practices purchase a single ultrasound machine to use for several purposes such as obstetrics, regional anesthesia, abdominal scanning, or echocardiography.[20] Recently, a number of newer ultrasound machine models have evolved that are portable or can be mounted on the wall, which is beneficial in a setting where there is limited space to perform a block. The ultrasound technology is continually and rapidity evolving with an increasing focus on its application in regional anesthesia.

## Sterile Technique

Strict adherence to sterile technique is of importance in the practice of regional anesthesia. Infections due to PNBs are uncommon, but potentially devastating, yet largely preventable complications. A report of a fatality due to an infectious complication of a PNB underscores the importance of sterile techniques.[21] One study found that 57% of femoral catheters demonstrated bacterial colonization, although only 3 of 208 showed signs suggestive of infection (shivering and fever) that subsided after catheter removal.[22] Another study documented 1 infectious complication of 405 axillary catheters placed,[23] reflecting the relative rarity of such events. However, several case reports reflect the severity of infections caused by indwelling catheters. One case of psoas abscess complicating a femoral catheter placement has been reported.[24] Capdevila and colleagues reported an occurrence of acute cellulitis and mediastinitis following placement of a continuous interscalene catheter that may have resulted from the refilling of local anesthetic into the elastomeric pump.[25] More recently, sepsis following interscalene catheter placement was complicated by hematoma.[26] These cases illustrate the importance of adherence to aseptic technique in all phases of needle puncture, catheter insertion and management, as well as administration of local anesthetics.

The hands of health care workers are the most common vehicles for the transfer of microorganisms from one patient to another.[27] Studies show that although soap and water may remove bacteria, only alcohol-based antiseptics provide superior disinfection, and solutions of povidone iodine and chlorhexidine possibly provide the most extended antimicrobial activity.[28] Sterile gloves should be used throughout in addition to all other measures discussed.[29] No evidence exists to prove that gowning decreases the incidence of nosocomial infection.[30] One study showed no difference between infection or colonization rates between gowning and not gowning in the pediatric intensive care unit (ICU).[31] Another study showed that use of gowns and gloves was no better than use of gloves alone in preventing rectal colonization of vancomycin-resistant enterococci in the medical ICU.[32] Therefore, although gowning during the performance of PNBs is recommended by some, there is not sufficient evidence that such practice is beneficial in decreasing the incidence of infection.[30]

Surgical masks have become commonplace when performing invasive procedures. In an experiment where volunteers were asked to speak with and without surgical masks in close proximity to agar plates, it was found that wearing a mask significantly reduced the contamination of the plates.[33] However, there is considerable debate whether their use is effective at decreasing nosocomial infection with some arguing that they represent an essential component of sterile practice[34,35] and others maintaining there is no scientific evidence to support the practice. A postal survey of 801 anesthesiologists in Great Britain found that only 41.3% routinely wore face masks while performing spinal and epidural anesthesia, whereas 50.6% did not.[36] The work of Schweizer indicates that masks may increase contamination of a sterile field possibly due to the increase in shedding skin scales.[37] These results were supported by the work of Orr et al that found a significant ($p < 0.05$) decrease in the amount of infections when masks were not worn during surgical procedures.[38] However, one case series reported four cases of meningitis due to viridans streptococci following spinal anesthesia performed by the same anesthesiologist.[39] The same causative bacteria were later cultured from the anesthesiologist's nasopharyngeal mucosa, and the anesthesiologist was noted not to wear surgical masks when performing spinal anesthesia. Another case report described two cases of bacterial meningitis following diagnostic lumbar puncture due to *Streptococcus salivarius*. The same bacteria were cultured from the oropharyngeal mucosa of the neurologist who performed the lumbar puncture.[40] At this time there is no evidence that wearing a mask can prevent infectious complications of PNBs, although some clinicians suggest this practice.[41–43]

## Transducer Covers and Gel

Sterile clear dressings or sterile ultrasound transducer covers constitute sound clinical practice and are routinely used by most clinicians. A variety of sterile ultrasound transducer covers are available. Some come in sets with sterile ultrasound gel and rubber bands to pull the transducer covers tightly over the transducers to facilitate imaging.

However, the incidence of contact dermatitis due to ultrasound gel is rare considering the frequency of its worldwide use, several case reports have emerged that have been attributed to the bacteriostatic preservatives propylene glycol and parabens.[44,45] Regardless, contact dermatitis from ultrasound gel has also been attributed to the imidazolidinyl urea.[46] Drugs such as diazepam that have propylene glycol in their solvent solutions are known to cause myotoxicity when injected intramuscularly.[47] In the 1950s, a preparation of procaine called Efocaine was introduced for its long duration of action. However, reports surfaced of neuritis and local irritation after perineural injection of Efocaine. The mechanism of action of the drug was attributed to coagulation necrosis, and it is noteworthy that the preparation of Efocaine contained 78% propylene glycol.[48] Likewise, safety of inadvertent injection of ultrasound gel during ultrasound-guided nerve blocks has been questioned. A recent study has demonstrated that the lumen of PNB needles can carry and deposit ultrasound gel in close proximity to nerves, suggesting that further studies are needed to ascertain whether the amounts of gel under consideration are enough to cause toxicity.[49]

## Injection Pressure Monitoring

Intrafascicular injections during the performance of PNBs are associated with high injection pressures during injection of the local anesthetic.[50] Such injections lead to neural damage and neurologic deficits in animal models.[51] Assessment of resistance to injection is routinely done in clinical practice to reduce a risk of an intraneural injection and constitutes a suggested routine documentation of PNB procedure.[71] Traditionally, however, anesthesiologists have relied on a subjective "syringe feel," that is, the feeling of increased resistance on injection. Recent studies have cast doubt on the ability of anesthesiologists to detect intraneural injections using this method. In fact, studies show that anesthesiologists may often inject local anesthetic at injection pressures capable of rupturing a fascicle.[52] An inline injection pressure manometer can be placed between the syringe and the injection tubing with the needle to objectively quantify and monitor the injection pressure (Figure 3-11). Injection pressures greater than 20 psi are associated with intraneural intrafascicular injection. Alternatively, an air-compression test in the syringe is used to avoid injection using pressure greater than 20 psi.[72,73] In actual clinical practice, injection with pressures <15 psi establishes a wider margin of safety in reducing the risk of an intrafascicular injection or too forceful spread of the local anesthetics.

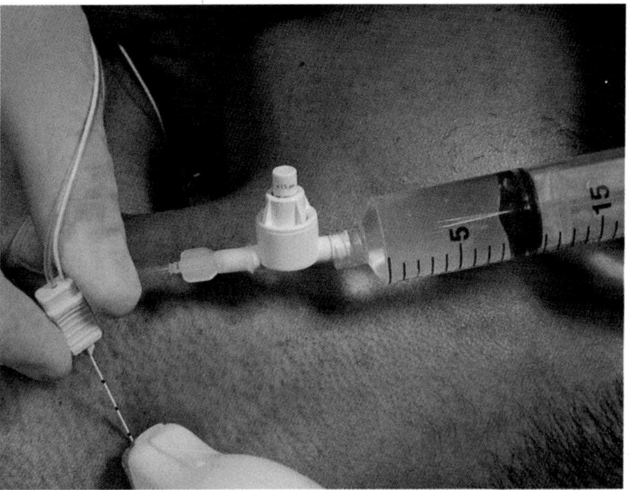

**FIGURE 3-11.** Monitoring injection pressure at the femoral nerve using an in-line injection pressure monitor (BSmart, Concert Medical USA). A color-coded piston moves during the block performance to indicate pressure during injection.

## Continuous Nerve Catheters

Sutherland was first to introduce the stimulating catheter to improve the success rates over blindly inserted catheters.[53] This was followed closely by further reports of similar techniques.[54,55] For the performance of continuous peripheral nerve catheters, a wide range of needle and catheter types are available. Two main types of catheters are the stimulating catheters, which can provide stimulation through the catheter itself, and the nonstimulating catheters, which do not allow this option. Stimulation is typically accomplished through a metal stylet or coil that conducts electricity through or around the catheter lumen. Several designs are available on the market. Although it would appear logical that the confirmation of the catheter placement using electrolocalization should result in a greater consistency of catheter placement and higher success rate, the data on any advantages of the stimulating catheters over nonstimulating catheter remain conflicting. One study in volunteers found that although there was no statistically significant difference in block success rate between stimulating and nonstimulating catheters, the stimulating catheters did provide an increase in depth of both sensory and motor block.[56] Another study found that using a stimulating catheter as opposed to a nonstimulating catheter resulted in a significant lowering of the local anesthetic volume required to block the sciatic nerve.[57]

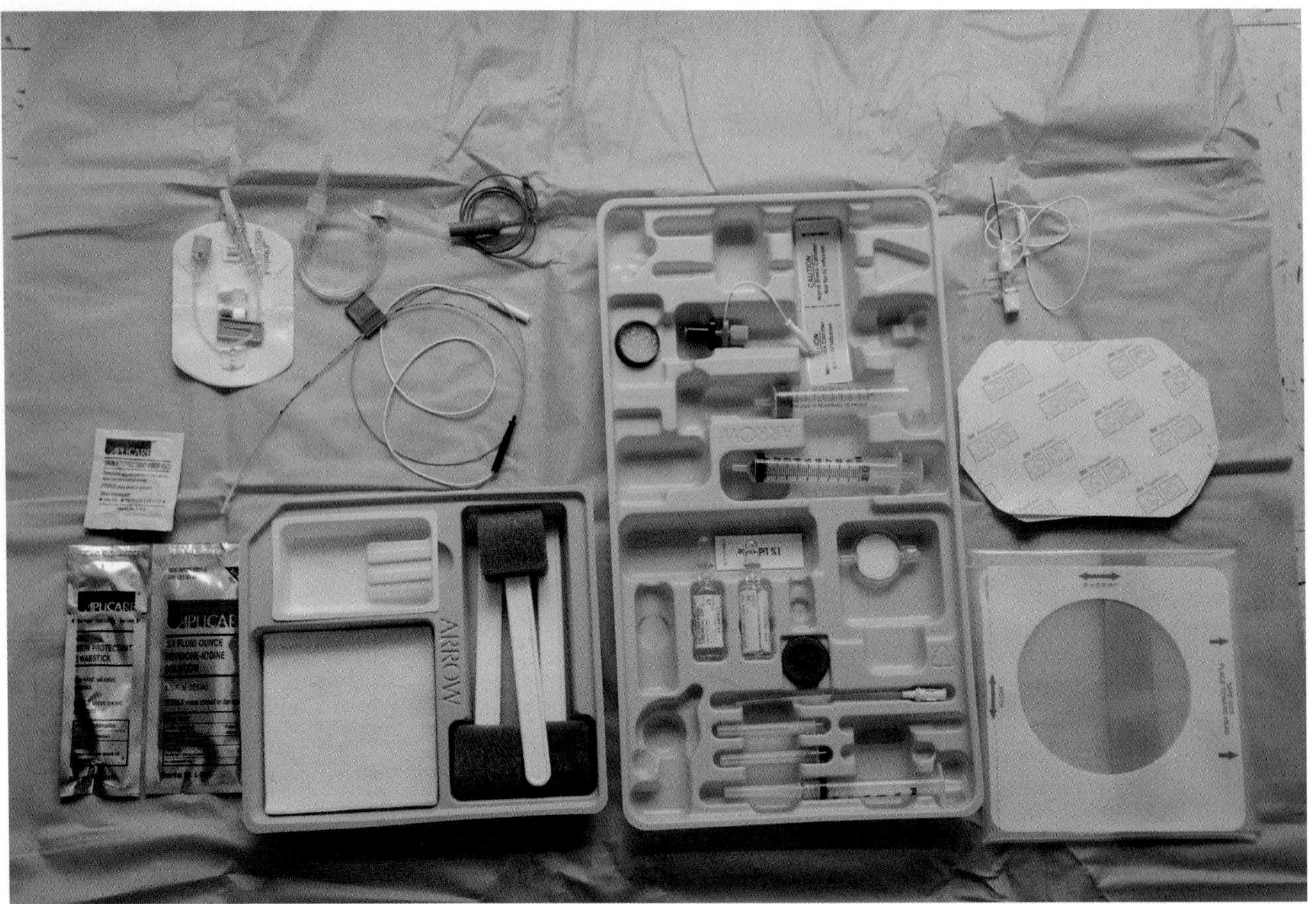

**FIGURE 3-12.** Continuous nerve block set with stimulating catheter, including lidocaine 1%, lidocaine 1% with epinephrine, needles, syringes, and gauze, sterile sponges with iodine solution, stimulating needle, securement device, stimulating catheter, sterile drape and swabstick pack, and adaptor.

Stimulating may also result in shorter onset time for sensory and motor block, a lower consumption of local anesthetics postoperatively, and less need for rescue pain medication.[58] Several other studies, however, have found no significant differences in local anesthetic required, speed of onset for motor and sensory block, visual analog scores, or opioid consumed postoperatively when comparing stimulating with nonstimulating catheters.[59–62] The most recent meta-analysis investigating 649 patients comparing stimulating and non-stimulating catheters from 11 trials showed a statistically significant benefit in analgesic effect from stimulating catheters.[63] Significantly, these studies did not use ultrasound guidance and only used nerve stimulation for localization of the nerve and confirmation of the catheter position. The position of a nonstimulating catheter can be confirmed by bolusing local anesthetic or saline through the catheter and visualizing the spread under ultrasound. If normal saline or local anesthetic is bolused through the catheter, it must be noted that should replacement of the catheter be necessary, electrical nerve stimulation will no longer be possible.[64] A nonconducting solution, such as dextrose 5% in water, may be used to ascertain the catheter tip location and preserve the ability to stimulate.[65] Any advantage of stimulating over nonstimulating catheters placed with ultrasound guidance may be even further diminished because the spread of the local anesthetic solutions injected through the catheter (as evidenced by ultrasound) is the gold standard of documenting proper catheter placement, rather than a specific motor response to nerve stimulation (Figures 3-12 and 3-13).

## Securing Perineural Catheters

Dislodgement of a catheter is relatively common and leads to ineffective analgesia and requires reinsertion of the catheter. There are a variety of methods and devices for securing indwelling continuous catheters, most of which incorporate some means of fixing the device and/or catheter to the skin via adhesive tape on one side of the device.

Some practitioners tunnel the indwelling catheters to better secure them, although there is no data documenting that tunneling a catheter decreases the incidence of dislodgement. The benefits of tunneling should be weighed against the potential for dislodging the catheter in the process of needle insertion. If the decision is made to tunnel the catheter, then application of a topical skin adhesive to the puncture site that

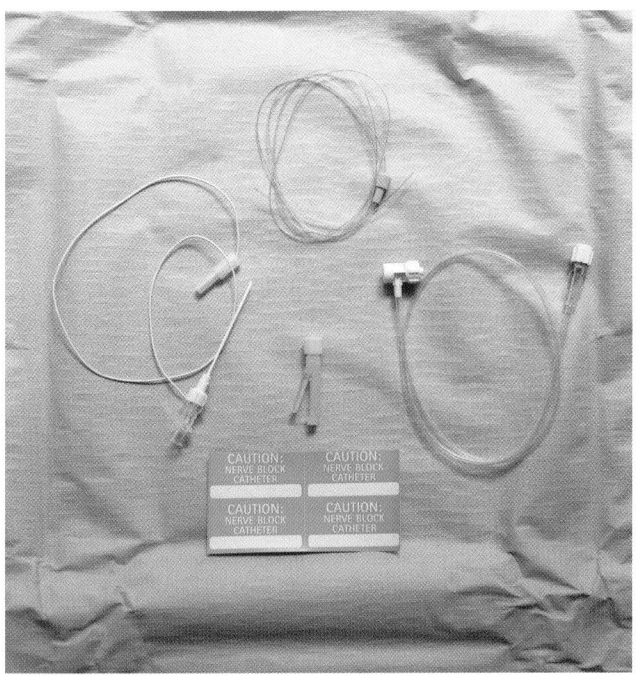


**FIGURE 3-13.** Nonstimulating catheter set, including nonstimulating catheter, extension tubing, clamp-style catheter connector, 2-inch stimulating Tuohy needle, 4-inch stimulating Tuohy needle, and label.

the catheter passes through can help secure the catheter and prevent leakage of local anesthetic. This is due to the fact that the puncture sites produced by catheters have larger diameter than the catheters themselves. The catheter should be covered with a transparent, sterile occlusive dressing to allow daily inspection of the catheter exit site. This allows for monitoring catheter migration and early signs of infection.[66]

## Infusion Pumps

Patients are increasingly being sent home with peripheral nerve catheters attached to portable infusion pumps that ensure the accurate and reliable delivery of local anesthetic. The pumps can be either elastomeric or electronic. The elastomeric pumps use a nonmechanical balloon mechanism to infuse local anesthetics and consist of an elastomeric membrane within a protective shell. The pressure generated on the fluid when the balloon is stretched is determined by the material of the elastomer (e.g., latex, silicon, or isoprene rubber) and its shape.[67] These pump sets typically contain an elastomeric pump with a fill port, a clamp, an air-eliminating filter, a variable controller, a flow rate dial, a rate-changing key, and a lockable cover. Most electronic pumps can hold 400 mL of local anesthetic, and the anesthesiologist can easily program the concentration, rate, and volume. These pumps are lightweight, typically come with carrying cases, and do not impose any limitations on mobility for the patient. One study found that the elastomeric pumps were as effective as electronic pumps in providing analgesia following ambulatory orthopedic surgery; however, the elastomeric pumps led to higher patient satisfaction scores due to fewer technical problems.[68] However, underfilling the elastomeric pump results in a faster flow rate, whereas overfilling results in a slower rate. The elastomeric pump flow rate is also affected by changes in temperature that affect the solution viscosity. Recently, the elastomeric pump was shown to have technical difficulties with 20.5% not deflating correctly after being attached to the catheter resulting in insufficient analgesia.[69] The patient should be given emergency contact information and be informed of the signs and symptoms of excessive local anesthetic absorption. Typically the catheter remains in place for 2 to 3 days postoperatively, and an anesthesiologist or another health care worker guides the patient through the removal of the catheter over the phone.

## Nerve Stimulators

The advent of nerve stimulation has been a great advance in the performance of regional anesthesia. Because the electrical properties of a nerve stimulator contribute to the performance of a successful PNB, practitioners should be familiar with the model used in their institution. Past models of electrical nerve stimulators have used a constant voltage system. However, the current, not the voltage, stimulates a nerve. Therefore, the amplitude of those nerve stimulators required constant adjustment to maintain a desirable current output. Ideally, the current output of a nerve stimulator should not change as the needle is being advanced through various resistances encountered from the tissue, needle, and connectors. Resistance is a measure of the resistance to flow of alternating current through tissue, and there is an inverse relationship between resistance and current thresholds necessary to elicit a motor response.[70] Most modern models deliver a constant current output in the presence of varied resistance. Settings that can be altered on these models include frequency, pulse-width, and current milliamperes. Nerve stimulators are described in a greater detail in Chapter 4.

## REFERENCES


1. Rettig HC, et al. The pharmacokinetics of ropivacaine after four different techniques of brachial plexus blockade. *Anaesthesia.* 2007;62(10):1008-1014.
2. Weinberg GL, et al. Pretreatment or resuscitation with a lipid infusion shifts the dose-response to bupivacaine-induced asystole in rats. *Anesthesiology.* 1998;88(4):1071-1075.
3. Weinberg G, et al. Lipid emulsion infusion rescues dogs from bupivacaine-induced cardiac toxicity. *Reg Anesth Pain Med.* 2003; 28(3):198-202.
4. Rosenblatt MA, et al. Successful use of a 20% lipid emulsion to resuscitate a patient after a presumed bupivacaine-related cardiac arrest. *Anesthesiology.* 2006;105(1):217-218.
5. Litz RJ, et al. Reversal of central nervous system and cardiac toxicity after local anesthetic intoxication by lipid emulsion injection. *Anesth Analg.* 2008;106(5):1575-1577.
6. Ludot H, et al. Successful resuscitation after ropivacaine and lidocaine-induced ventricular arrhythmia following posterior lumbar plexus block in a child. *Anesth Analg.* 2008; 106(5): 1572-1574.

7. Warren JA, et al. Intravenous lipid infusion in the successful resuscitation of local anesthetic-induced cardiovascular collapse after supraclavicular brachial plexus block. *Anesth Analg.* 2008;106(5):1578-1580.
8. Litz RJ, et al. Successful resuscitation of a patient with ropivacaine-induced asystole after axillary plexus block using lipid infusion. *Anaesthesia.* 2006;61(8):800-801.
9. Brull SJ. Lipid emulsion for the treatment of local anesthetic toxicity: patient safety implications. *Anesth Analg.* 2008; 106(5):1337-1339.
10. Selander D, Dhuner KG, Lundborg G. Peripheral nerve injury due to injection needles used for regional anesthesia. An experimental study of the acute effects of needle point trauma. *Acta Anaesthesiol Scand.* 1977;21(3):182-188.
11. Rice AS, McMahon SB. Peripheral nerve injury caused by injection needles used in regional anaesthesia: influence of bevel configuration, studied in a rat model. *Br J Anaesth.* 1992;69(5): 433-438.
12. Selander D. Peripheral nerve injury caused by injection needles. *Br J Anaesth.* 1993;71:323-325.
13. Parker RK, White PF. A microscopic analysis of cut-bevel versus pencil-point spinal needles. *Anesth Analg.* 1997;85(5):1101-1104.
14. Steinfeldt T, et al. Nerve injury by needle nerve perforation in regional anaesthesia: does size matter? *Br J Anaesth.* 2010; 104(2):245-253.
15. Gottlieb RH, et al. Coating agent permits improved visualization of biopsy needles during sonography. *AJR Am J Roentgenol.* 1998;171(5):1301-1302.
16. Bergin D, et al. Echogenic polymer coating: does it improve needle visualization in sonographically guided biopsy? *AJR Am J Roentgenol.* 2002;178(5):1188-1190.
17. Takayama W, et al. Novel echogenic needle for ultrasound-guided peripheral nerve block "Hakko type CCR" [in Japanese]. *Masui.* 2009;58(4):503-507.
18. Deam RK, et al. Investigation of a new echogenic needle for use with ultrasound peripheral nerve blocks. *Anaesth Intensive Care.* 2007;35(4):582-586.
19. Sites BD, et al. Artifacts and pitfall errors associated with ultrasound-guided regional anesthesia. Part II: a pictorial approach to understanding and avoidance. *Reg Anesth Pain Med.* 2007;32(5):419-433.
20. Wynd KP, et al. Ultrasound machine comparison: an evaluation of ergonomic design, data management, ease of use, and image quality. *Reg Anesth Pain Med.* 2009;34(4):349-356.
21. Nseir S, et al. Fatal streptococcal necrotizing fasciitis as a complication of axillary brachial plexus block. *Br J Anaesth.* 2004;92(3):427-429.
22. Cuvillon P, et al. The continuous femoral nerve block catheter for postoperative analgesia: bacterial colonization, infectious rate and adverse effects. *Anesth Analg.* 2001;93(4):1045-1049.
23. Bergman BD, et al. Neurologic complications of 405 consecutive continuous axillary catheters. *Anesth Analg.* 2003;96(1): 247-252.
24. Adam F, Jaziri S, Chauvin M. Psoas abscess complicating femoral nerve block catheter. *Anesthesiology.* 2003;99(1):230-231.
25. Capdevila X, et al. Acute neck cellulitis and mediastinitis complicating a continuous interscalene block. *Anesth Analg.* 2008; 107(4):1419-1421.
26. Clendenen SR, et al. Case report: continuous interscalene block associated with neck hematoma and postoperative sepsis. *Anesth Analg.* 2010;110(4):1236–1238.
27. Hebl JR, Neal JM. Infectious complications: a new practice advisory. *Reg Anesth Pain Med.* 2006;31(4):289-290.
28. Boyce JM, Pittet D. Guideline for Hand Hygiene in Health-Care Settings: recommendations of the Healthcare Infection Control Practices Advisory Committee and the HICPAC/SHEA/APIC/IDSA Hand Hygiene Task Force. *Infect Control Hosp Epidemiol.* 2002;23(12 Suppl):S3-S40.
29. Saloojee H, Steenhoff A. The health professional's role in preventing nosocomial infections. *Postgrad Med J.* 2001;77(903): 16-19.
30. Hebl JR. The importance and implications of aseptic techniques during regional anesthesia. *Reg Anesth Pain Med.* 2006; 31(4):311-323.
31. Pelke S, et al. Gowning does not affect colonization or infection rates in a neonatal intensive care unit. *Arch Pediatr Adolesc Med.* 1994;148(10):1016-1020.
32. Slaughter S, et al. A comparison of the effect of universal use of gloves and gowns with that of glove use alone on acquisition of vancomycin-resistant enterococci in a medical intensive care unit. *Ann Intern Med.* 1996;125(6):448–456.
33. Philips BJ, et al. Surgical face masks are effective in reducing bacterial contamination caused by dispersal from the upper airway. *Br J Anaesth.* 1992;69(4):407-498.
34. Tsen LC. The mask avenger? *Anesth Analg.* 2001;92(1): author reply 280-281.
35. Browne IM, Birnbach DJ. Unmasked mischief. *Anesth Analg.* 2001;92(1):279-281.
36. Panikkar KK, Yentis SM. Wearing of masks for obstetric regional anaesthesia. A postal survey. *Anaesthesia.* 1996;51(4):398-400.
37. Schweizer RT. Mask wiggling as a potential cause of wound contamination. *Lancet.* 1976;2(7995):1129-1130.
38. Orr NW. Is a mask necessary in the operating theatre? *Ann R Coll Surg Engl.* 1981;63(6):390-392.
39. Schneeberger PM, Janssen M, Voss A. Alpha-hemolytic streptococci: a major pathogen of iatrogenic meningitis following lumbar puncture. Case reports and a review of the literature. *Infection.* 1996;24(1):29-33.
40. de Jong J, Barrs AC. Lumbar myelography followed by meningitis. *Infect Control Hosp Epidemiol.* 1992;13(2):74-75.
41. Watanakunakorn C, Stahl C. *Streptococcus salivarius* meningitis following myelography. *Infect Control Hosp Epidemiol.* 1992; 13(8):454.
42. Aromaa U, Lahdensuu M, Cozanitis DA. Severe complications associated with epidural and spinal anaesthesias in Finland 1987–1993. A study based on patient insurance claims [see comment]. *Acta Anaesthesiol Scand.* 1997;41(4):445-452.
43. North JB, Brophy BP. Epidural abscess: a hazard of spinal epidural anaesthesia. *Aust N Z J Surg.* 1979;49(4):484-485.
44. Kessler J, Schafhalter-Zoppoth I, Gray AT, Allergic contact dermatitis caused by ultrasonic gel. *Reg Anesth Pain Med.* 2006; 31(5):480-481.
45. Eguino P, et al. Allergic contact dermatitis due to propylene glycol and parabens in an ultrasonic gel. *Contact Dermatitis.* 2003;48(5):290.
46. Ando M, et al. Allergic contact dermatitis from imidazolidinyl urea in an ultrasonic gel. *Contact Dermatitis.* 2000;42(2): 109-110.
47. Brazeau GA, Fung HL. An in vitro model to evaluate muscle damage following intramuscular injections. *Pharm Res.* 1989; 6(2):167-170.
48. Mannheimer W, Pizzolato P, Adriani J. Mode of action and effects on tissues of long-acting local anesthetics. *J Am Med Assoc.* 1954;154(1):29-32.
49. Belavy D. Regional anesthesia needles can introduce ultrasound gel into tissues. *Anesth Analg.* 2010;11(3):811-812.
50. Selander D, Sjostrand J. Longitudinal spread of intraneurally injected local anesthetics. An experimental study of the initial neural distribution following intraneural injections. *Acta Anaesthesiol Scand.* 1978;22(6):622-634.
51. Hadžić A, et al. Combination of intraneural injection and high injection pressure leads to fascicular injury and neurologic deficits in dogs. *Reg Anesth Pain Med.* 2004;29(5):417-423.
52. Theron PS, et al. An animal model of "syringe feel" during peripheral nerve block. *Reg Anesth Pain Med.* 2009;34(4):330-332.

53. Sutherland ID. Continuous sciatic nerve infusion: expanded case report describing a new approach. *Reg Anesth Pain Med.* 1998;23(5):496-501.
54. Kick O, et al. A new stimulating stylet for immediate control of catheter tip position in continuous peripheral nerve blocks. *Anesth Analg.* 1999;89(2):533-534.
55. Boezaart AP, et al. A new technique of continuous interscalene nerve block. *Can J Anaesth.* 1999;46(3):275-281.
56. Salinas FV, et al. Prospective comparison of continuous femoral nerve block with nonstimulating catheter placement versus stimulating catheter-guided perineural placement in volunteers. *Reg Anesth Pain Med.* 2004;29(3): 212-220.
57. Paqueron X, et al. A randomized, observer-blinded determination of the median effective volume of local anesthetic required to anesthetize the sciatic nerve in the popliteal fossa for stimulating and nonstimulating perineural catheters. *Reg Anesth Pain Med.* 2009;34(4):290-295.
58. Casati A, et al. Using stimulating catheters for continuous sciatic nerve block shortens onset time of surgical block and minimizes postoperative consumption of pain medication after halux valgus repair as compared with conventional nonstimulating catheters. *Anesth Analg.* 2005;101(4):1192-1197.
59. Hayek SM, et al. Continuous femoral nerve analgesia after unilateral total knee arthroplasty: stimulating versus nonstimulating catheters. *Anesth Analg.* 2006;103(6):1565-1570.
60. Morin AM, et al. Does femoral nerve catheter placement with stimulating catheters improve effective placement? A randomized, controlled, and observer-blinded trial. *Anesth Analg.* 2005; 100(5):1503-1510.
61. Jack NT, Liem EB, Vonhogen LH. Use of a stimulating catheter for total knee replacement surgery: preliminary results. *Br J Anaesth.* 2005;95(2):250-254.
62. Barrington MJ, et al. Stimulating catheters for continuous femoral nerve blockade after total knee arthroplasty: a randomized, controlled, double-blinded trial. *Anesth Analg.* 2008;106(4):1316-1321.
63. Morin AM, et al. The effect of stimulating versus nonstimulating catheter techniques for continuous regional anesthesia: a semiquantitative systematic review. *Reg Anesth Pain Med.* 2010;35(2):194-199.
64. Pham-Dang C, et al. Continuous peripheral nerve blocks with stimulating catheters. *Reg Anesth Pain Med.* 2003;28(2):83-88.
65. Tsui BC. Wagner A, Finucane B. Electrophysiologic effect of injectates on peripheral nerve stimulation. *Reg Anesth Pain Med.* 2004;29(3):189-193.
66. Boezaart AP. Perineural infusion of local anesthetics. *Anesthesiology.* 2006;104(4):872-880.
67. Grant CR, Fredrickson MJ. Regional anaesthesia elastomeric pump performance after a single use and subsequent refill: a laboratory study. *Anaesthesia.* 2009;64(7):770-775.
68. Capdevila X, et al. Patient-controlled perineural analgesia after ambulatory orthopedic surgery: a comparison of electronic versus elastomeric pumps. *Anesth Analg.* 2003;96(2):414-417.
69. Remerand F, et al. Elastomeric pump reliability in postoperative regional anesthesia: a survey of 430 consecutive devices. *Anesth Analg.* 2008;107(6):2079-2084.
70. Sauter AR, et al. Current threshold for nerve stimulation depends on electrical impedance of the tissue: a study of ultrasound-guided electrical nerve stimulation of the median nerve. *Anesth Analg.* 2009;108(4):1338-1343.
71. Gerancher JC, Viscusi ER, Liguori GA, et al. Development of standardized peripheral nerve block procedure note form. *Reg Anesth Pain Med.* 2005;30(1):67-71.
72. Tsui BC, Knezevich MP, Pillay JJ. Reduced injection pressures using a compressed air injection technique (CAIT): an in vitro study. *Reg Anesth Pain Med.* 2008;33(2):168-173.
73. Tsui BC, Li LX, Pillay JJ. Compressed air injection technique to standardize block injection pressures. *Can J Anaesth.* 2006;53(11):1098-1102.

# Electrical Nerve Stimulators and Localization of Peripheral Nerves

*Martin Simpel and Andre van Zundert*

## History of Electrical Nerve Stimulation

### Quick Facts

- 1780: Galvani[1] was the first to describe the effect of electrical neuromuscular stimulation
- 1912: Perthes[2] developed and described an electrical nerve stimulator
- 1955: Pearson[3] introduced the concept of insulated needles for nerve location
- 1962: Greenblatt and Denson[4] introduced a portable solid-state nerve stimulator with variable current output and described its use for nerve location
- 1973: Montgomery et al[5] demonstrated that noninsulated needles require significantly higher current amplitudes than the insulated needles
- 1984: Ford et al[6] reported a lack of accuracy with noninsulated needles once the needle tip passed the target nerve
- Ford et al suggested the use of nerve stimulators with a constant current source, based on the comparison of the electrical characteristics of peripheral nerve stimulators[7,8]

The use of nerve stimulation became commonplace in clinical practice only in the mid- to late 1990s. Research on the needle–nerve relationship and the effect of stimulus duration ensued.[9–11] More recently, the principles of electrical nerve stimulation were applied to surface mapping of peripheral nerves using percutaneous electrode guidance (PEG)[12–15] for confirmation and epidural catheter placement[16–18] and peripheral catheter placement.[19] This chapter discusses the electrophysiology of nerve stimulation, electrical nerve stimulators, various modes of localization of peripheral nerves, and integration of the technology into the realm of modern regional anesthesia.

## What Is Peripheral Electrical Nerve Stimulation?

Nerve stimulation is a commonly used method for localizing nerves before the injection of local anesthetic. Electrical nerve stimulation in regional anesthesia is a method of using a low-intensity (up to 5 mA) and short-duration (0.05–1 ms) electrical stimulus (at 1–2 Hz repetition rate) to obtain a defined response (muscle twitch or sensation) to locate a peripheral nerve or nerve plexus with an (insulated) needle. The goal is to inject a certain amount of local anesthetic in close proximity to the nerve to block nerve conduction and provide a sensory and motor block for surgery and/or, eventually, analgesia for pain management. The use of nerve stimulation can also help to avoid an intraneural intrafascicular injection and, consequently, nerve injury.

Electrical nerve stimulation can be used for a single-injection technique, as well as for guidance during the insertion of continuous nerve block catheters. More recently, ultrasound (US) guidance and, in particular, the so-called dual guidance technique in which both techniques (peripheral nerve stimulation [PNS] and US) are combined, has become a common practice in many institutions.

## Indications for the Use of PNS

In principle, almost all plexuses or other larger peripheral nerves can be located using PNS.[20] The goal of nerve stimulation is to place the tip of the needle (more specifically, its orifice for injection) in close proximity to the target nerve to inject the local anesthetic in the vicinity of the nerve. The motor response (twitch) to PNS is objective and reliable and independent from the patient's (subjective) response. Nerve stimulation is often helpful to confirm that the structure imaged with ultrasound (US) is actually the nerve that is sought. This is because the needle–nerve relationship may not always be visualized on US; an unexpected motor response can occur, alerting the operator that the needle tip is already in close proximity to the nerve. Likewise, the occurrence of a motor response at a current intensity of <0.3-0.2 mA can serve as an indicator of an intraneural needle placement. Although this response may not always be present even with an intraneural needle position (low sensitivity), its presence is always indicative of intraneural placement (high specificity).

The disadvantages of PNS are the need for additional equipment (nerve stimulator and insulated needles), the greater cost of insulated needles, and abnormal physiology or anatomy where it may be difficult to elicit a motor response.

## TIPS

- PNS is an adjunct to and not a substitute for knowledge of anatomy.
- Presence of neurologic disorders (e.g., polyneuropathy) can result in difficulties in obtaining a motor response. The use of a longer pulse duration (0.3 or 1.0 ms, instead of 0.1 ms), may be helpful in these cases.
- PNS is not reliable in a patient receiving muscle relaxants.
- PNS can be used in patients who have received central neuraxial blocks.

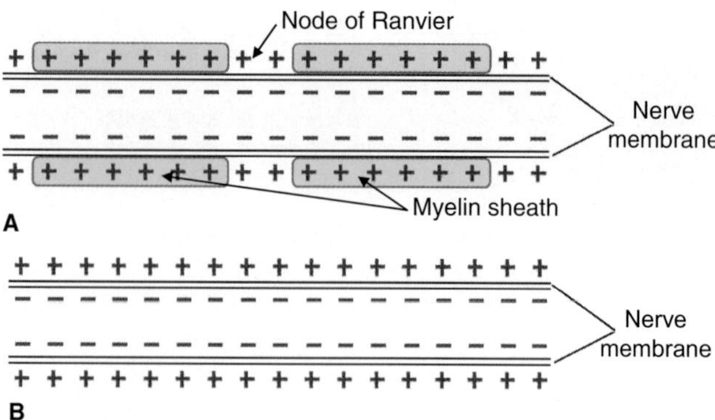


**FIGURE 4-1.** (A) Schematic anatomic and electrophysiologic structure of nerve fibers of myelinated and (B) unmyelinated nerve fibers.

# Basics of Neurophysiology and Electrophysiology

## Membrane Potential, Resting Potential, Depolarization, Action Potential, and Impulse Propagation

All living cells have a **membrane potential** (a voltage potential across their membrane, measured from the outside to the inside), which varies (depending on the species and the cell type) from about −60 mV to −100 mV. Nerve and muscle cells in mammals typically have a membrane potential (resting potential) of about −90 mV.

Only nerve and muscle cells have the capability of producing uniform electrical pulses, the so-called **action potentials** (also called spikes), which are propagated along their membranes, especially along the long extensions of nerve cells (nerve fibers, axons). A decrease in the electric potential difference (e.g., from −90 mV to −55 mV, or **depolarization**) elicits an action potential. If the depolarization exceeds a certain *threshold,* an action potential or a series of action potentials is generated by the nerve membrane (also called firing) according to the all-or-nothing rule, resulting in propagation of the action potential along the nerve fiber (axon). To **depolarize** the nerve membrane from outside the cell (extracellular stimulation), the negative **polarity** of the electrical stimulus is more effective in removing the positive charge from the outside of the membrane. This in turn decreases the potential across the membrane toward the threshold level.

There are several types of nerve fibers. Each fiber type can be distinguished anatomically by their diameter and degree of myelinization. Myelinization is formed by an insulating layer of Schwann cells wrapped around the nerve fibers. These characteristics largely determine the electrophysiologic behavior of different nerve fibers, that is, the speed of impulse propagation of action potentials and the threshold of excitability. Most commonly, the distinguishing features are motor fibers (e.g., Aα, Aβ) and pain fibers (C). The Aα motor fibers have the largest diameter and highest degree of myelinization and therefore the highest speed of impulse propagation and a relatively low threshold level to external stimulation. C-fibers (which transmit severe, dull pain) have very little to no myelinization and are of smaller diameter. Consequently, the speed of propagation in these fibers is relatively low, and the threshold levels to external stimulation, in general, are higher.

There are several other, efferent fibers, which transmit responses from various skin receptors or muscle spindles (Aδ). These are thinner than Aα fibers and have less myelinization. Some of these (afferent) sensory fibers, having a relatively low threshold level, transmit the typical tingling sensation associated with a lower level of pain sensation when electrically stimulated. Such sensation can occur during transcutaneous stimulation before a motor response is elicited.

The basic anatomic structure of myelinated Aα fibers (motor) and nonmyelinated C fibers (pain) is shown schematically in Figure 4-1. The relationship between different stimuli and the triggering of the action potential in motor and pain fibers is illustrated in Figures 4-2A, B.

## Threshold Level, Rheobase, Chronaxy

A certain minimum current intensity is necessary at a given pulse duration to reach the **threshold level** of excitation. The lowest threshold current (at infinitely long pulse durations) is called **rheobase.** The pulse duration (pulse width) at double the rheobase current is called **chronaxy.** Electrical pulses with the duration of the chronaxy are most effective (at relatively low amplitudes) to elicit action potentials. This is the reason why motor response can be elicited at such short pulse duration (e.g., 0.1 ms) at relatively low current amplitudes while avoiding the stimulation of C-type pain fibers. Typical chronaxy figures are 50 to 100 μs (Aα fibers), 170 μs (AΔ fibers), and ≥400 μs (C fibers). Figure 4-3 illustrates the relationship of the rheobase to chronaxy for motor fibers versus pain nerve fibers.

### *Impedance, Impulse Duration, and Constant Current*

The electrical circuit is formed by the nerve stimulator, the nerve block needle and its tip, the tissue characteristics of the patient, the skin, the skin electrode (grounding electrode), and the cables connecting all the elements. The resistance of this circuit is not just a simple Ohm's resistor equation because of the specific capacitances of the tissue, the electrocardiogram (ECG) electrode to skin interface, and

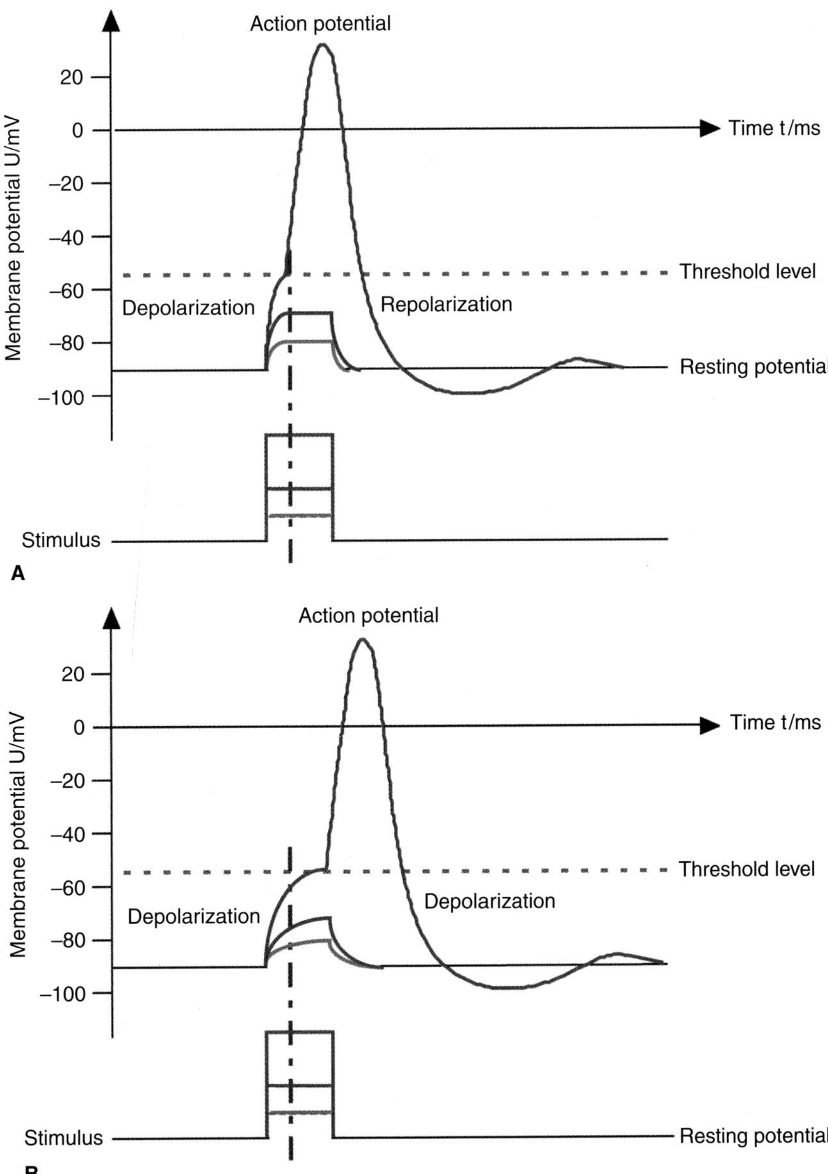


**FIGURE 4-2.** (A) Action potential, threshold level, and stimulus. Motor fibers have a short chronaxy because of the relatively low capacitance of their myelinated membrane (only the area of the nodes of Ranvier count; see Figure 4-1), therefore, it takes only a short time to depolarize the membrane up to the threshold level. (B) Pain fibers have a long chronaxy because of the higher capacitance of their nonmyelinated membrane (the entire area of the membrane counts); therefore, it takes a longer time to depolarize the membrane up to the threshold level. Short impulses (as indicated by the vertical dotted line) would not be able to depolarize the membrane to its threshold level.

the needle tip, which influence the overall resistance. The capacitance in the described circuit varies with the frequency content of the stimulation current, and it is called impedance, or a so-called *complex resistance,* which depends on the frequency content of the stimulus. In general, the shorter the impulse, the higher its frequency content, and, consequently, the lower the impedance of a circuit with a given capacitance. Conversely, a longer pulse duration has a lower frequency content. As an example, for a 0.1-ms stimulus, the main frequency content is 10 kHz plus its harmonics; whereas for a 1.0-ms impulse, the main frequency content is 1 kHz plus harmonics. In reality, the impedance of the needle tip and the electrode to skin impedance have the highest impact. The impedance of the needle tip largely depends on the geometry and insulation (conductive area). The electrode to skin impedance can vary considerably between individuals (e.g., type of skin, hydration status) and can be influenced by the quality of the ECG electrode used.

Because of the variable impedance in the circuit, created primarily by the needle tip and electrode to skin interface, a

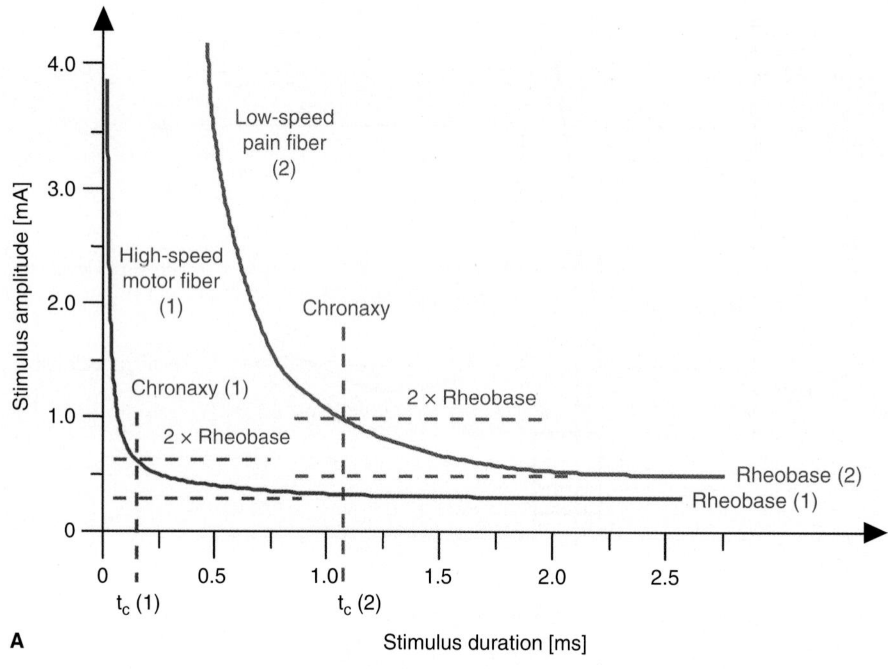


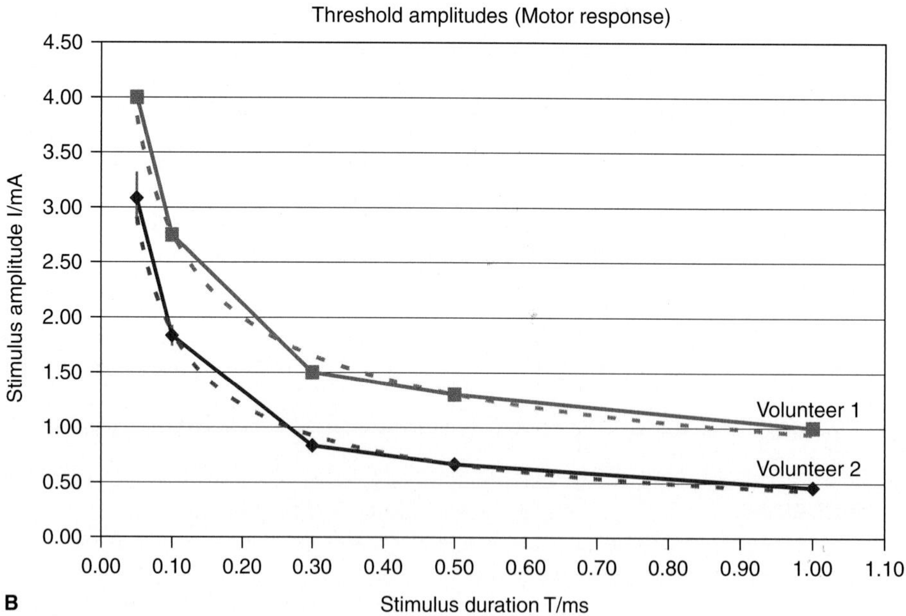


**FIGURE 4-3.** (A) Comparison of threshold curves, chronaxy, and rheobase level of motor (high speed) and pain fibers (low speed). (B) Experimental data, threshold amplitudes obtained with percutaneous stimulation (Stimuplex Pen and Stimuplex HNS 12). Stimulation obtained with percutaneous stimulation of the median nerve near the wrist looking for motor response of the thumb. (C) Experimental data, threshold amplitudes obtained with percutaneous stimulation (Stimuplex Pen and Stimuplex HNS 12). Stimulation of the median and radial nerves near the wrist and at the midforearm looking for electric paresthesia (tingling sensation) in the middle and ring finger (median nerve) or superficial pain sensation near the wrist (radial nerve), respectively.

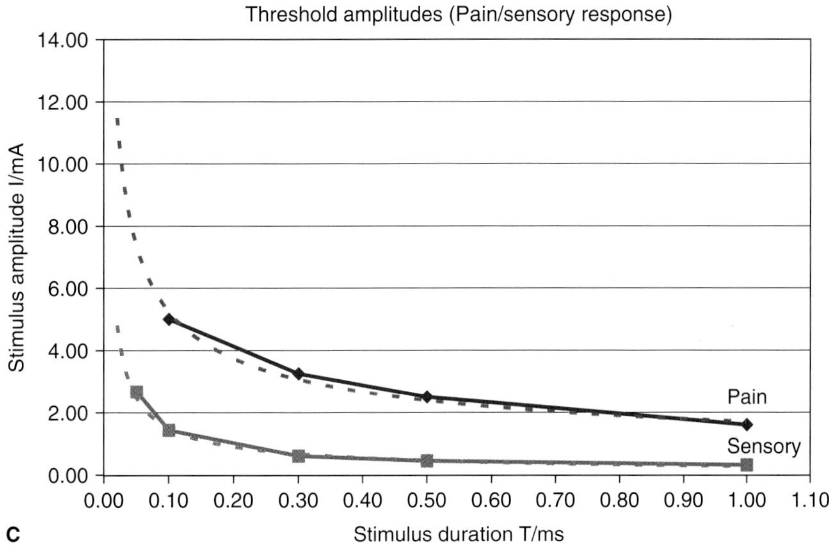


**FIGURE 4-3.** (Continued)

nerve stimulator with a constant current source and sufficient (voltage) output power is important to use to compensate for the wide range of impedances encountered clinically.

## Clinical Use of PNS

### Proper Setup and Check of the Equipment

The following are a few important aspects for successful electrolocalization of the peripheral nerves using PNS:

- Use a high-quality nerve stimulator and a high-accuracy constant current source.
- Use insulated nerve stimulation needles with a small conductive area at the tip. The smaller the conductive area, the higher the current density is at the tip, and the greater spatial discrimination in the near field.
- Use high-quality skin electrodes with a low impedance.

**TIPS**

- Some lower priced ECG electrodes can have too high of an impedance/resistance. This limits their suitability for use with nerve stimulation.
- Good quality skin electrodes have an impedance of a maximum of a few hundred ohms.
- Typically, biomedical engineers use a dummy resistor (e.g., 10 kOhm), which allows them to check that the nerve stimulator and cables are functioning properly.

- Before starting the procedure, check for the proper functioning of the nerve stimulator and the connecting cables.
- During nerve stimulator-assisted nerve localization, the negative pole (cathode) should be connected to the stimulating electrode (needle) and the positive pole (anode) to the patient's skin.
  - The design of the connectors should prevent a faulty polarity connection.
- Connect the nerve stimulation needle to the nerve stimulator (which should be turned on), and set the current amplitude and duration to the desired levels.
  - For superficial blocks, select 1.0 mA as a starting current intensity.
  - For deep blocks, select 1.5 mA as a starting current intensity.
  - Select between 0.1 and 0.3 ms of current duration for most purposes.
- For more technical details and how to operate a specific nerve stimulator, refer to the instructions for use supplied with the stimulator.

### Transcutaneous Nerve Mapping

Electrolocalization of peripheral nerves is typically accomplished by inserting a needle into the tissue and advancing the needle toward the expected location of the nerve(s) of interest. However, a nerve mapping pen can be used to locate superficial nerves (up to a maximum depth of approximately 3 cm) with transcutaneous nerve stimulation before the nerve block needle is inserted. Transcutaneous nerve mapping is particularly useful when identifying the best site for needle insertion in patients with difficult anatomy or when the landmarks prove difficult to indentify. Figure 4-4 shows three examples of commercially available nerve mapping pens.

Nerve mapping is also very useful when training anesthesia residents. It should be noted that longer stimulus duration (e.g., 1 ms) is needed to accomplish transcutaneous

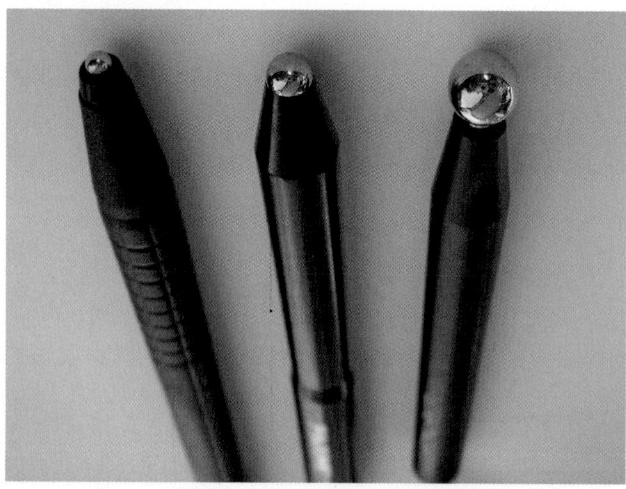

**FIGURE 4-4.** Tip configuration of several commercially available nerve mapping peripheral nerve stimulators. From left to right: Stimuplex Pen, B. Braun Melsungen (Germany); nerve mapping pen, Pajunk (Germany); NeuroMap, HDC (USA).

nerve stimulation, because the energy required to stimulate transcutaneously is larger. The electrode tip of the pen should have an atraumatic ball-shaped tip. The conductive tip diameter should not be larger than approximately 3 mm to provide sufficient current density and spatial discrimination, which may not be the case with larger tip diameters. Some nerve stimulators do not provide the required impulse duration of 1 ms or a strong enough constant current source (5 mA at minimum 12-kOhm output load) to perform nerve mapping. Therefore, it is recommended that the mapping pen and the nerve stimulator be paired, ideally by acquiring them from the same manufacturer.

The transcutaneous stimulation often results in a sensation reported by the patient as tingling, pinprick, or a slight burning sensation. The perception varies greatly among individuals. Most people tolerate transcutaneous stimulation with a nerve mapping pen very well; however, some individuals describe it as uncomfortable or even painful (depending on the stimulus amplitude and duration). However, the amount of energy delivered by nerve stimulators with a maximum output of 5 mA at 1 msec pulse duration is far too low to create any injury of the skin or the nerves. A moderate premedication is usually sufficient to make the procedure well tolerated by patients.

## Percutaneous Electrode Guidance

PEG[10,11] combines the transcutaneous nerve stimulation (nerve mapping) with nerve block needle guidance (Figure 4-5). In essence, a small aiming device is mounted and locked onto a conventional nerve block needle, which allows the conductive needle tip to make contact with the skin without scratching or penetrating the skin. Once the best response is obtained, the needle is advanced through the skin in the usual fashion and the remainder of the apparatus continues to stabilize the needle and guide it toward the target. The device also allows the operator to make indentations in the skin and tissue so the initial distance between the needle tip at the skin level and the target nerve is reduced and the nerve block needle has less distance to travel through tissue. The technique allows for prelocation of the target nerve(s) before skin puncture.

## Operating the Nerve Stimulator

The starting amplitude used for nerve stimulation depends on the local practice and the projected skin-nerve depth. For superficial nerves, amplitude of 1 mA at 0.1 (or 0.3) ms impulse duration to start is chosen in most cases. For deeper nerves, it may be necessary to increase the initial current amplitude between 1.5 and 3 mA until a muscle response is elicited at a safe distance from the nerve. Too high current intensity, however, can lead to direct muscle stimulation or discomfort for the patient, both of which are undesirable.

Once the sought-after muscle response is obtained, the current intensity amplitude is gradually reduced and the needle is advanced further slowly. The needle must be advanced slowly to avoid too rapid advancement between the stimuli. Advancement of the needle and current reduction are continued until the desired motor response is achieved with a current of 0.2–0.5 mA at 0.1 ms stimulus duration. The threshold level and duration of the stimulus are interdependent; in general, a short pulse duration is a better discriminator of the distance between the needle and the nerve.[20] When the motor twitch is lost during needle advancement, the stimulus intensity first should be increased to regain the muscle twitch rather than move the needle blindly. Once a proper motor response is obtained with a current of 0.2–0.5 mA (most nerve blocks), the needle is positioned correctly for an injection of local anesthetic. A small test dose

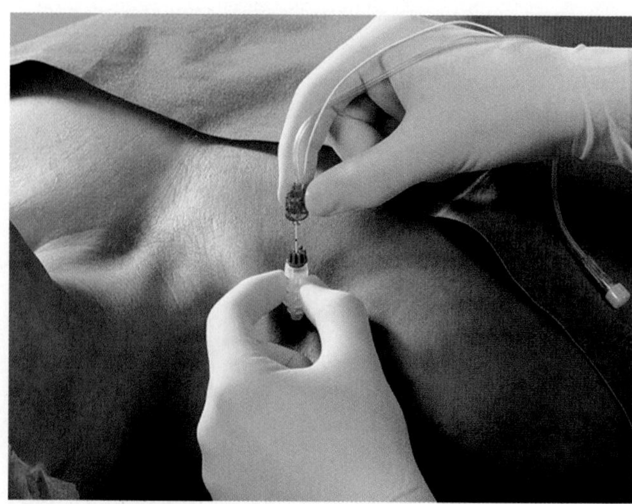

**FIGURE 4-5.** Percutaneous electrode guidance technique using Stimuplex Guide (B. Braun Melsungen, Germany) during a vertical infraclavicular block procedure.

of local anesthetic is injected, which abolishes the muscle twitch. Then the total amount of local anesthetic appropriate for the desired nerve block is injected. Of note, the highly conductive injectate (e.g., local anesthetic or normal saline solution) short-circuits the current to the surrounding tissue, effectively abolishing the motor response. In such situations, increasing the amplitude may not bring back the muscle twitch. Tsui and Kropelin[21] demonstrated that injection of dextrose 5% in water (D5W) (which has a low conductivity) does not lead to loss of the muscle twitch if the needle position is not changed.

It should be remembered that the absence of the motor response with a stimulating current even up to 1.5 mA does not rule out an intraneural needle placement (low sensitivity). However, the presence of a motor response with a low-intensity current (<0.2–0.3 mA) occurs only with intraneural and, possibly, intrafascicular needle placement. For this reason, if the motor response is still present at <0.2–0.3 mA (0.1 ms), the needle should be slightly withdrawn to avoid the risk of intrafascicular injection. Figure 4-6A–C illustrates the principle of the needle to nerve approach and its relation to the stimulation.

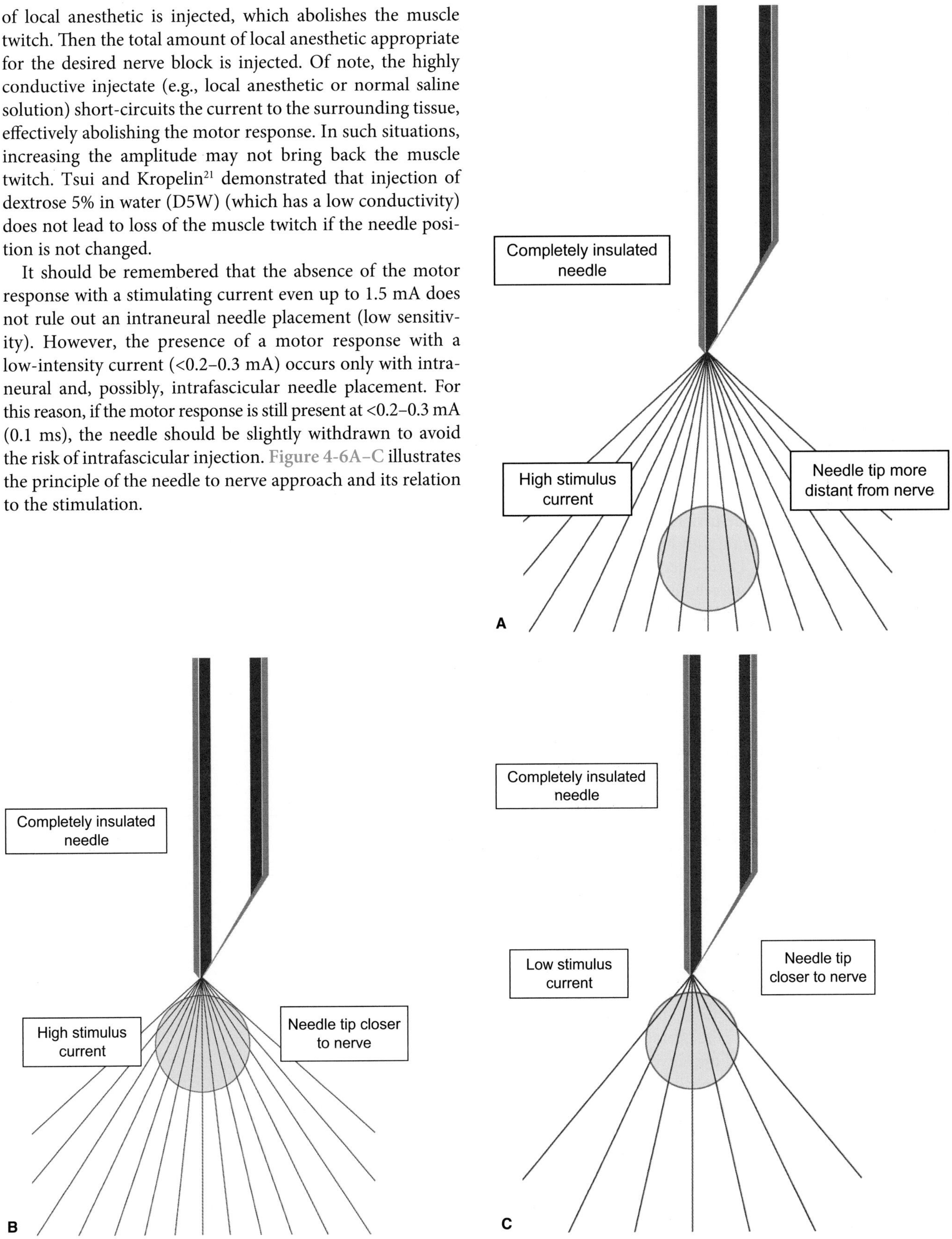

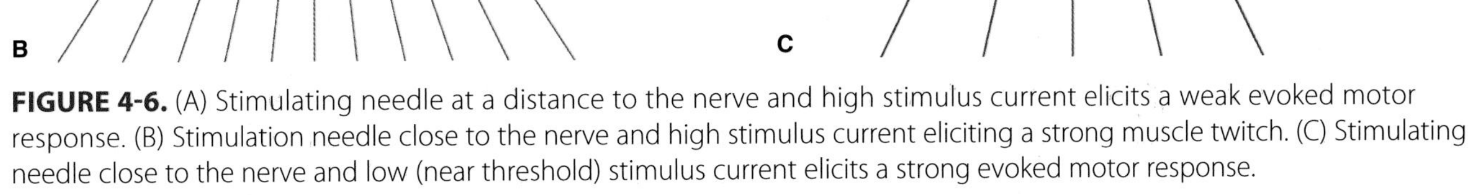


**FIGURE 4-6.** (A) Stimulating needle at a distance to the nerve and high stimulus current elicits a weak evoked motor response. (B) Stimulation needle close to the nerve and high stimulus current eliciting a strong muscle twitch. (C) Stimulating needle close to the nerve and low (near threshold) stimulus current elicits a strong evoked motor response.

To avoid or minimize discomfort for the patient during the nerve location procedure, it is recommended that a too high stimulating current be avoided. The needle should not be advanced too fast because it can increase the risk of injuries and the evoked motor response may be missed.

## The Role of Impedance Measurement

Measurement of the impedance can provide additional information if the electrical circuit is optimal. Theoretically, impedance can identify an intraneural or intravascular placement of the needle tip. Tsui and colleagues[22] reported that the electrical impedance nearly doubles (12.1–23.2 kOhm), which is significant, when the needle is advanced from an extraneural to intraneural position in a porcine sciatic nerve. Likewise, injection of a small amount of (D5W), which has a high impedance, results in a significantly higher increase of impedance in the perineural tissue than it does within the intravascular space.[23] Thus measurement of the impedance before and after dextrose injection can potentially detect intravascular placement of the needle tip, thus identifying the placement before the injection of local anesthetic. In this report, the perineural baseline impedance [25.3 (±2.0) kOhm] was significantly higher than the intravascular [17.2 (±1.8) kOhm]. Upon injection of 3 mL of D5W, the perineural impedance increased by 22.1 (±6.7) kOhm to reach a peak of 50.2 (±7.6) kOhm and remained almost constant at about 42 kOhm during the 30-second injection time. By contrast, intravascular impedance increased only by 2.5 (±0.9) kOhm, which is significantly less compared with the perineural needle position. At the present time, however, more data are needed before these findings can be incorporated as an additional safely monitoring method in clinical practice.

## Sequential Electrical Nerve Stimulation

Current nerve stimulation uses stimuli of identical duration (typically 0.1 ms), usually at 1 or 2 Hz repetition frequency. A common problem during nerve stimulation is that the evoked motor response is often lost while moving the needle to optimize its position. In such cases, it its recommended that the operator either increase the stimulus amplitude (mA) or increase the impulse duration (ms), the latter of which may not be possible. Alternatively, the operator can take a couple of steps, depending on type of the nerve stimulator used. The SENSe (sequential electrical nerve stimulation) technique incorporates an additional stimulus with a longer pulse duration after two regular impulses at 0.1 msec duration, creating a 3 Hz stimulation frequency.[24] The third longer impulse delivers more charge than the first two and therefore has a longer reach into the tissue. Consequently, an evoked motor response often is elicited at 1 Hz, even when the needle is distant from the nerve. Once the needle tip is positioned closer to the nerve, muscle twitches are seen at 3 Hz. The advantage of the SENSe is that a motor response (at 1/second) is maintained even when the motor response previously elicited by the first two impulses is lost due to slight needle movement. This feature helps prevent the operator from moving the needle "blindly."[24]

Figure 4-7 shows examples of the particular SENSe impulse patterns at different stimulus amplitudes. Eventually the

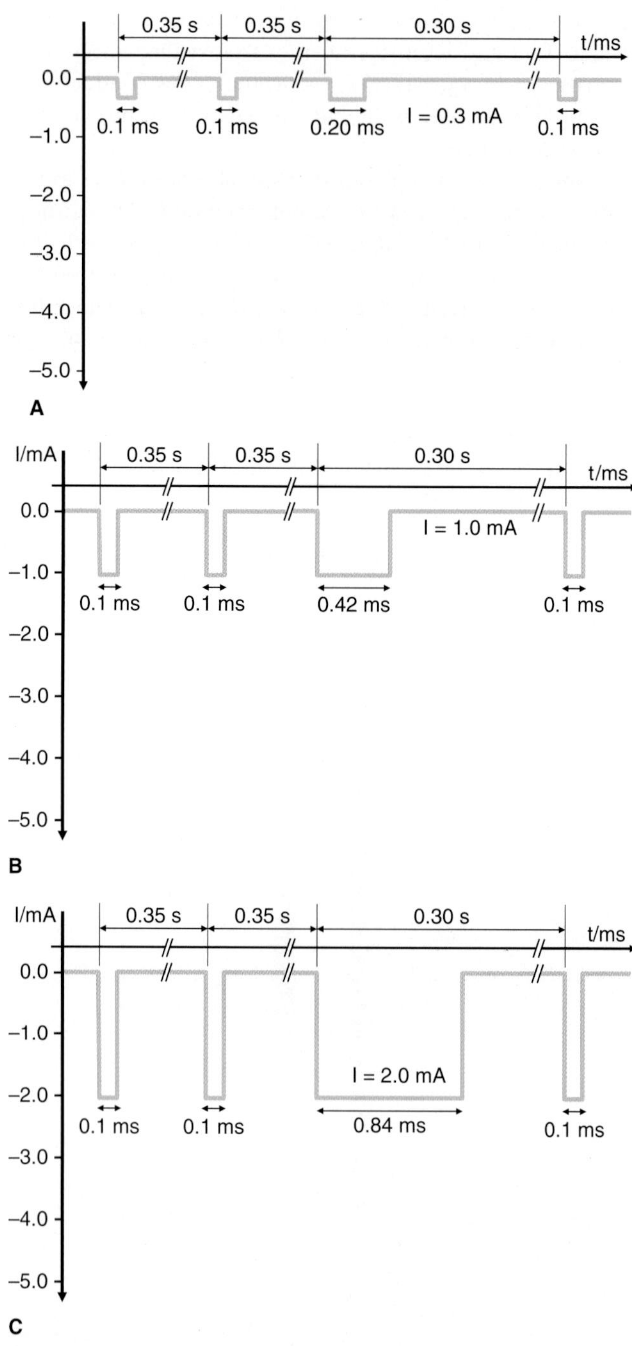


**FIGURE 4-7.** Sequential electrical nerve stimulation (SENSe) impulse pattern of the Stimuplex HNS 12 nerve stimulator (B. Braun Melsungen, Germany) depending on the actual stimulus amplitude. The impulse duration of the third impulse decreases with the stimulus amplitude below 2.5 mA from 1.0 ms to a minimum of 0.2 ms compared with the constant impulse duration of 0.1 ms of the first two impulses. (A) Impulse pattern at 0.3 mA (threshold level). (B) Impulse pattern at 1.0 mA. (C) Impulse pattern at 2.0 mA.

**TABLE 4-1 Common Problems during Electrolocalization of Nerves and Corrective Actions**

| PROBLEM | SOLUTION |
|---|---|
| Nerve stimulator does not work at all. | Check and replace battery; refer to stimulator operator's manual. |
| Nerve stimulator suddenly stops working. | Check and replace battery. |
| No motor response is achieved despite the appropriate needle placement. | Check connectors, skin electrode, cables, and stimulation needle for an interrupted circuit or too high impedance. |
| | Check and make sure that current is flowing. |
| | Check the setting of amplitude (mA) and impulse duration. |
| | Check stimulator setting (some stimulators have a test mode or pause mode, which prevents current delivery. |
| | Double-check for puncture site. Consider surface mapping because the target nerve might be at a different site than expected due to some anatomic abnormalities. |
| Motor response disappears and cannot be regained even after increasing stimulus amplitude or/and duration. | Check for the causes listed previously. Can be caused by injection of local anesthetic. |

target threshold amplitude remains the same as usual (about 0.3 mA) but at 3 stimuli per second. With the SENSe technique, a motor response at only 1/second indicates that the needle is not yet placed correctly.

### Troubleshooting During Nerve Stimulation

Table 4-1 lists the most common problems encountered during electrolocalization of the peripheral nerves and the corrective action.

## Characteristics of the Modern Equipment for Nerve Stimulator Guided Peripheral Nerve Blocks

### Most Important Features of Nerve Stimulators[20,25]

*Electrical Features*

- An adjustable constant current source with an operating range of 10 kOhm, minimally, output load (impedance) and ideally at ≥15 kOhm.
- A precisely adjustable stimulus amplitude (0–5 mA): An analog control dial is preferred over up/down keys.
- A large and easy-to-read digital display of actual current flowing to maintain precise control of the stimulus.
- A selectable pulse duration (width), at least between 0.1 ms and 1.0 ms, to allow the operator to selectively stimulate motor fibers (0.1 ms) and to stimulate sensory fibers as well (1.0 ms).
- A stimulus frequency between 1 and 3 Hz (meaning 1–3 pulses per second) because the use of a too low frequency can lead to "blind" advancement of the needle in between stimuli. Use of a too high frequency will lead to superimposing of muscle twitches, which makes the detection of twitches more difficult.
- A monophasic rectangular output pulse to provide reproducible stimuli.
- Configurable start-up parameters so the machine will comply with the hospital protocol and to avoid mistakes when multiple users are working with the same device.
- A display of the circuit impedance (kOhm) is recommended to allow the operator to check the integrity of the electrical circuit and to detect a potential intraneural or intravascular placement of the needle tip.
- An automatic self-check process of the internal functioning of the unit with a warning message if something is wrong.
- An optional remote control (handheld remote control or foot pedal).

*Safety Features*

- Easy and intuitive use
- A large and easy-to-read display
- Limited current range (0–5 mA) because a too high amplitude may be uncomfortable to the patient
- A display of all relevant parameters such as Amplitude (mA) [alternatively stimulus charge (nC)], stimulus duration (ms), stimulus frequency (Hz), impedance (kOhm), and battery status
- Clear identification of output polarity (negative polarity at the needle)
- Meaningful instructions for use, with lists of operating ranges and allowed tolerances

- Battery operation of the nerve stimulator, as opposed to electrical operation, provides intrinsic safety: no risk of serious electric shock or burns caused by a short circuit to main supply of electricity
- The maximum energy delivered by a nerve stimulator with 5 mA and 95 V output signal at 1 ms impulse duration is only 0.475 mWs (see Section 7.3).
- Combined units for *peripheral* (for PNB) and *transcutaneous* (for muscle relaxation measurement) electrical nerve stimulation are not to be used because the transcutaneous function produces an unwanted high energy charge

Alarms/warnings:

- Open circuit/disconnection alarm (optical and acoustical)
- Warning/indication if impedance is too high; that is, the desired current is not delivered
- The display of actual impedance appears to be useful and recommendable
- Near threshold amplitude indication or alarm
- Low battery alarm
- Internal malfunction alarm

Table 4-2 provides a comparison of the most important features of commonly used nerve stimulators.

## Stimulating Needles

### *Needle*

A modern stimulating needle should have the following characteristics:

- A fully insulated needle hub and shaft to avoid current leakage
- The conductive electrode area should be able to accomplish higher current density at the tip for precise nerve location
- Depth markings for easy identification and documentation of the needle insertion depth

Figures 4-8A and B show a comparison of the electrical characteristics of noninsulated and insulated needles with uncoated bevel (Figure 4-8A) and fully coated needles with a pinpoint electrode (Figure 4-8B). Even though a noninsulated needle provides for discrimination (change in threshold amplitude) while approaching the nerve, there is virtually no ability to discriminate once the needle tip has passed the nerve. The discrimination near the nerve is more precise in needles with a pinpoint electrode tip (Figure 4-8B) compared with needles with an uncoated bevel (Figure 4-8A).

### *Connectors*

Connectors and cables should be fully insulated and include a safety connector to prevent current leakage as well as the risk of electric charge if the needle is not connected to the stimulator. Extension tubing with a Luer lock connector should be present for immobile needle techniques.

### *Visualization of the Needle Under Ultrasound Imaging*

Because US imaging is more in use (in particular with the use of the "dual guidance" technique), the importance of good visualization of the nerve block needle is becoming an additional important feature. The visibility (distinct reflection signal) of the needle tip certainly is the most important aspect because this is the part of the needle that is placed in the target area next to the nerve. However, in particular when using the in-plane approach, the visibility of the needle shaft is of interest as well because it helps to align the needle properly with the US beam and to visualize its entire length up to the target nerve.

## Stimulating Catheters

In principle, stimulating catheters function like insulated needles. The catheter body is made from insulating plastic material and usually contains a metallic wire inside, which conducts the current to its exposed tip electrode. Such stimulating catheters are usually placed using a continuous nerve block needle, which is placed by first using nerve stimulation as described and acts as an introducer needle for the catheter. Once this needle is placed close to the nerve or plexus to be blocked, the stimulating catheter is introduced through it and the nerve stimulator is connected to the catheter. Stimulation through the catheter should reconfirm that the catheter tip is positioned in close proximity to the target nerve(s). However, it must be noted that the threshold currents with stimulating catheters may be considerably higher. Injection of local anesthetic or saline (which is frequently used to widen the space for threading the catheter more easily) should be avoided because this may increase the threshold current considerably and can even prevent a motor response. D5W can be used to avoid losing a motor response.[21] Since the ultimate test for the properly positioned catheter is the distribution of the local anesthetic, rather than evoked motor response, the role of the catheter stimulating with US-guided blocks is not clear.

## Recommendations for Best Practice

- Adequate knowledge of anatomy
- Correct patient positioning
- Proper technique and equipment

Standard nerve stimulator settings for peripheral nerve blocks:

- Stimulus duration: 0.1 ms for mixed nerves
- Amplitude range: 0–5 mA or 0–1 mA (sufficient for superficial nerves)
- Stimulus frequency: 2 or 3 Hz, or SENSe

Nerve stimulator check:

- Check battery status
- Check that all connections are placed properly (cable, needle, skin electrode)

## TABLE 4-2 Comparison of Most Relevant Features of Modern Nerve Stimulators

| Feature / Product/company | Stimuplex HNS 12 (w/ SENSe) B. Braun | Stimuplex HNS 11 (replaced by HNS 12) B. Braun | Stimuplex DIG RC B. Braun | Multistim Sensor Pajunk | Multistim Vario Pajunk | Multistim Plex Pajunk | Plexygon Vygon | Polystim II Polymedic | Tracer III Life-Tech | NeuroTrace III / NMS 300 HDC/Xavant technology |
|---|---|---|---|---|---|---|---|---|---|---|
| **Amplitude setting** | Digital dial, 1 or 2 turns for full scale | Analog dial | Analog dial | Digital dial | Up/down keys | Up/down keys | Digital dial up/down keys | Analog dial | Analog dial | Up/down keys |
| **Display size [WxH, mm] / type** | 62 × 41 graphic LCD | 50 × 20 standard LCD | 21 × 8 red LED | 47 × 36 custom LCD | 47 × 18 custom LCD | 47 × 18 custom LCD | 47.5 × 33.5 custom LCD | 50 × 20 standard LCD | 50 × 20 custom LCD | 41 × 22 graphic LCD |
| **Current range [mA]** | 0–1<br>0–5 | 0–1<br>0–5 | 0.2–5 | 0–6<br>0–60<br>(for nerve mapping only, max. 1 kOhm) | 0–6<br>0–60<br>(for TENS only, max. 1.3 kOhm) | 0–6 | 0–6 (at 0.05 ms)<br>0–5 (at 0.15 ms)<br>0–4 (at 0.3 ms) | 0–1<br>0–5 | 0.05–5<br>0.05–1.5<br>(w/ foot pedal) | 0.1–5<br>0–20 (nerve mapping)<br>0–80 (TENS) |
| **Max. output voltage [V]** | 95 | 61 | 32 | 65 | 80 | 80 | 48 | 72 | 60 | 400<br>(for TENS) |
| **Max. output load (impedance) nominal/max.** | 12/17 kOhm (5 mA)<br>90 kOhm (1 mA) | 12/12 kOhm (mA)<br>60 kOhm (mA) | 6/6 kOhm (5 mA)<br>30 kOhm (mA) | 12/13 kOhm (5 mA)<br>65 kOhm (1 mA) | 12/15 kOhm (5 mA)<br>80 kOhm (1 mA) | 12/15 kOhm (5 mA)<br>80 kOhm (1 mA) | 9/9 kOhm (5 mA)<br>48 kOhm (1 mA) | 10/13 (5 mA)<br>72 kOhm (1 mA) | 12/11 kOhm (5 mA) | 80 kOhm (5 mA)<br>(for TENS) |
| **Impulse duration [ms]** | 0.05, 0.1, 0.3, 0.5, 1.0 | 0.1, 0.3, 1.0 | 0.1 | 0.05, 0.1, 0.2, 0.3, 0.5, 1.0 | 0.1, 0.3, 0.5, 1.0 | 0.1 | 0.05, 0.15, 0.3 | 0.1, 0.3, 1.0 | 0.05, 0.1, 0.3, 0.5, 1.0 | 0.04–0.200 |
| **Stimulus frequency [Hz]** | 1, 2,<br>3 (SENSe) | 1, 2 | 1, 2 | 1, 2 | 1, 2,<br>TOF, 50 Hz, 100 Hz | 1, 2 | 1, 2, 4 | 1, 2, 3, 4, 5 | 1, 2 | 1, 2<br>TOF, DB, 50 Hz, 100 Hz |
| **Display of patient current** | YES | YES<br>activated by key | NO | YES | YES<br>activated by key | NO | YES | YES | NO | NO |
| **Display of set current** | YES<br>if patient current is lower | YES<br>activated by key | YES<br>flashes if patient current is lower | YES<br>if PAUSE key is pressed, or dial is turned | YES<br>activated by key | YES<br>(permanent) | YES<br>if dial is turnd | YES<br>activated by key | YES | YES; no indication if patient current deviates from displayed value |
| **Display of impulse duration (ms)** | YES | YES<br>key LED | - | YES | YES | - | YES | YES<br>key LED | YES | NO |
| **Display of impedance** | 0–90 kOhm | NO | NO | NO | NO | NO | NO | NO | NO | NO |
| **Display of charge (nC)** | Optional, in addition to display of mA | NO | NO | NO | NO | NO | Alternative to mA | NO | NO | NO |
| **Alarm signals** | Special alarm and warning sounds; LED (red/yellow/green), display of respective text messages | Change of beep tone and LED stops flashing when no current, display icon | No tone and no yellow LED flash if no current; blinking display if current is lower than set | Change of beep tone if no current, display icon | Change of beep tone, display symbol, LED stops flashing if no current | Change of beep tone, display symbol, LED stops flashing if no current | Constant tone if open circuit, flashing display if current is lower than set | Click tone changes, LED stops flashing when current is lower than set | Flashing display and chirp sounds on open circuit | Chirp tone and display symbol for open circuit; no indication if current is lower than set |
| **Threshold amplitude warning** | Acoustic, LED yellow and display of text message | NO | NO | NO | NO | NO | NO | NO | NO | NO |
| **Menu for setup and features** | YES, full text menu, 26 languages | NO | NO | NO<br>(setup w/o menu) | NO | NO | NO | NO | NO | YES, limited text |
| **Percutaneous nerve mapping** | YES<br>stimuplex pen | YES<br>stimuplex pen | NO | YES<br>Pen + bipolar probe | NO | NO | NO | NO | NO | YES<br>NeuroMap pen |
| **Remote control** | Handheld RC | NO | Hand held RC | NO | NO | NO | NO | NO | Foot pedal RC | NO |
| **Power consumption at 5 mA output [mA]** | 3.6 | 3.6<br>(key LEDs off) | 6.0 | 4.8 | 4.2 | 5.0 | 15.5 | 11.8<br>(key LEDs off) | No data | 5.7 |
| **Size H x W x D [mm]** | 157 × 81 × 35 | 145 × 80 × 39 | 126 × 77 × 38 | 120 × 65 × 22 | 121 × 65 × 22 | 122 × 65 × 22 | 200 × 94 × 40 | 245 × 80 × 39 | 153 × 83 × 57 | 125 × 80 × 37 |
| **Weight w/ battery [g]** | 277 | 266 | 210 | 167 | 168 | 169 | 251 | 247 | 275 | 235 |

**Note:** Nerve stimulator models, features, and availability, July 2008.

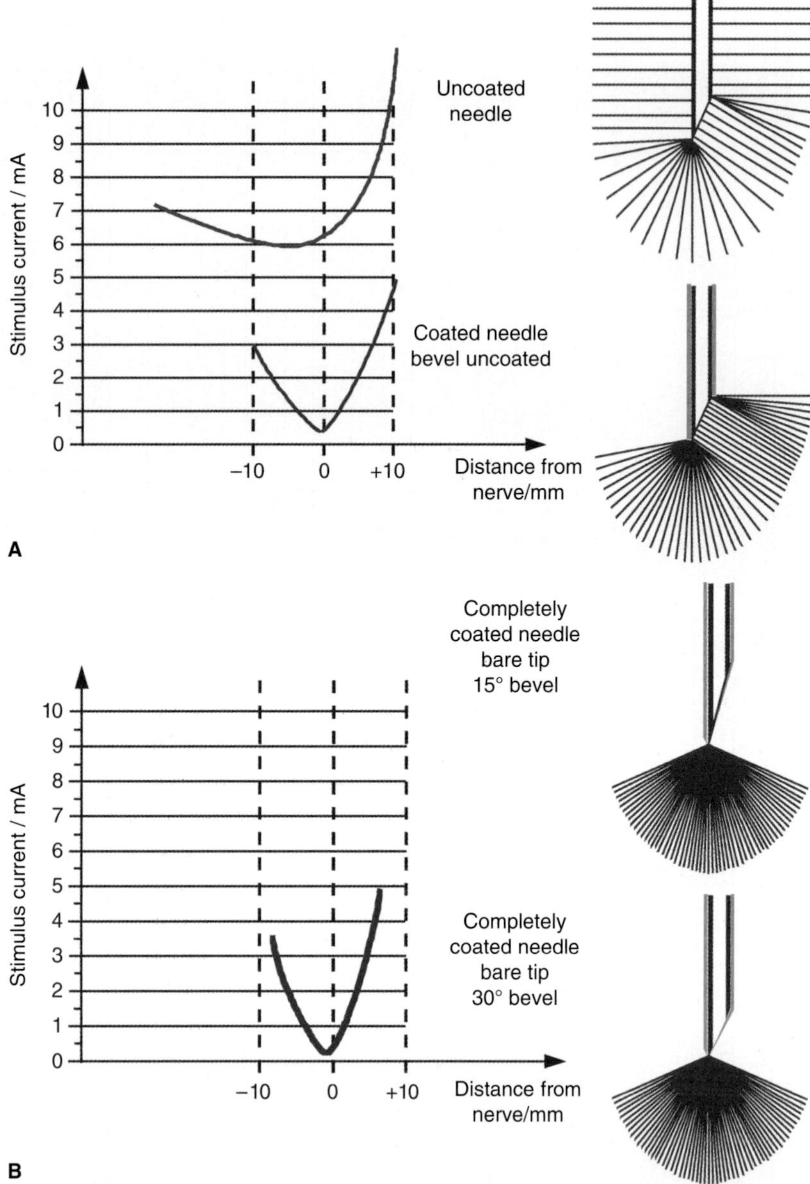


**FIGURE 4-8.** (A) Threshold amplitude achieved with an uncoated needle and a coated needle with an uncoated bevel. (B) Threshold amplitude achieved with a fully coated needle and a pinpoint electrode.

- Check the entire nerve stimulator function using a test resistor (this automatically checks connectors and cable as well)

Needles:

- Use fully insulated nerve block needles, Figure 4-8.
- Use the appropriate gauge size and length (avoid too long needles; see Table 4-3)

End point of nerve stimulation:

- Threshold current 0.2 to 0.3 mA (at 0.1 ms)
- Higher threshold current (≥0.5 mA) means the needle tip is too far from the nerve end point and block failure becomes more likely
- Lower threshold current (≤0.2 mA) signals a risk of intraneural/fascicular injection, and consequently, the risk for neural damage increases

To avoid discomfort for the patient and take precautions for safety:

- Use a low-intensity current nerve stimulation
- Limit the stimulus energy by limiting the initial stimulus current amplitude: 1 mA (superficial blocks), 2 mA (deeper blocks), maximum 5 mA (e.g., psoas compartment and deep sciatic blocks), and the stimulus duration; do not use long stimulus duration (1 ms) if it is not needed

**TABLE 4-3 Stimulation Needle Sizes Recommended for Various Nerve Blocks**

| | SINGLE-SHOT TECHNIQUE | | CATHETER TECHNIQUE (INTRODUCER NEEDLE) | |
|---|---|---|---|---|
| **NERVE BLOCK** | **LENGTH (mm)** | **SIZE, OD (mm/G)** | **LENGTH (mm)** | **SIZE, OD (mm/G)** |
| Anterior interscalene | 25–50 | 0.5-0.7/25-22 | 33–55 | 1.1-1.3/20-18 |
| Posterior interscalene | 80–100 | 0.7/22 | 80–110 | 1.3/18 |
| Vertical infraclavicular (VIB) | 50 | 0.7/22 | 50–55 | 1.3/18 |
| Axillary blockade | 35–50 | 0.5-0.7/25-22 | 40–55 | 1.3/18 |
| Suprascapular | 35–50 | 0.5-0.7/25-22 | 40–55 | 1.3/18 |
| Psoas compartment | 80–120 | 0.7-0.8/22-21 | 80–150 | 1.3/18 |
| Femoral nerve | 50 | 0.7/22 | 50–55 | 1.3/18 |
| Saphenous nerve | 50–80 | 0.7/22 | 55–80 | 1.3/18 |
| Obturator | 80 | 0.7/22 | 80 | 1.3/18 |
| Parasacral sciatic | 80–120 | 0.7-0.8/22-21 | 80–110 | 1.3/18 |
| Transgluteal sciatic | 80–100 | 0.7-0.8 / 22 - 21 | 80–110 | 1.3/18 |
| Anterior sciatic | 100–150 | 0.7-0.9/22-20 | 100–150 | 1.3/18 |
| Subtrochanteric sciatic | 80–100 | 0.7-0.8/22-21 | 80–110 | 1.3/18 |
| Lateral distal sciatic | 50–80 | 0.7/22 | 55–80 | 1.3/18 |
| Popliteal sciatic | 50 | 0.7/22 | 55 | 1.3/18 |

Note: The nerve location needle sizes given here are only estimates. Depending on the patient's size a slightly shorter or longer size of needle may be needed. Some manufacturers also offer smaller needle sizes for pediatric use.

Caution: Never use needles with a longer length than actually needed because the risk of complications may increase when inserting the needle too deep.

- Do not inject at exceedingly high pressure or if the threshold current is <0.2–0.3 mA (0.1 ms) to avoid a intraneural/fascicular injection and subsequent neurologic damage
- Apply appropriate anesthesia technique (e.g., infiltration of puncture site, light sedation)

## Appendix: Glossary of Physical Parameters

### Voltage, Potential, Current, Resistance/Impedance

**Voltage (U)** is the difference in electrical potential between two points carrying different amounts of positive and negative charge. It is measured in volts (V) or millivolts (mV). Voltage can be compared with the filled level of a water tank, which determines the pressure at the bottom outlet (Figure 4-9A). In modern nerve stimulators using constant current sources, voltage is adapted automatically and cannot nor needs to be influenced by the user.

**Current (I)** is the measure of the flow of a positive or negative charge. It is expressed in amperes (A) or milliamperes (mA). Current can be compared with the flow of water.

A total charge (**Q**) applied to a nerve equals the product of the intensity (I) of the applied current and the duration (t) of the square pulse of the current: $Q = I \times t$.

The minimum current intensity (I) required to produce an action potential can be expressed by the relationship

$$I_{Threshold} = \frac{I_{Rheobase}}{1 - e^{-t/c}}$$

where, t = pulse duration, c = time constant of nerve membrane related to chronaxy.

The **electrical resistance R** limits the flow of current at a given voltage (see Ohm's law) and is measured in ohms (Ω) or kilo Ohms (kΩ).

If there is capacitance in addition to Ohm's resistance involved (which is the case for any tissue), the resistance becomes a so-called complex resistance, or **impedance.** The main difference between the two is that the value of the impedance depends on the frequency of the applied voltage/current, which is not the case for an Ohm's resistor. In clinical practice, this means the impedance of the tissue is higher for low frequencies (i.e., a long pulse duration) and lower for higher frequencies (i.e., a short impulse duration). Consequently, a constant current source (which delivers longer duration impulses, e.g., 1 ms versus 0.1 ms) needs to have a stronger output stage (higher output voltage) to compensate for the higher tissue impedance involved and to deliver the desired current. However, the basic principles of Ohm's law remain the same.

## Ohm's Law

**Ohm's law** describes the relationship between voltage, resistance, and current according to the equation:

$$\mathbf{U\ [V] = R\ [\Omega] \cdot I\ [A]}$$

or conversely,

$$\mathbf{I\ [A] = U\ [V]/R\ [\Omega]}$$

This means that at a given voltage, current changes with resistance. If a constant current must be achieved (as needed for nerve stimulation), the voltage has to adapt to the varying resistance of the entire electrical circuit. For nerve localization in particular, the voltage must adapt to the resistance of the needle tip, the electrode to skin interface, and the tissue layers. A constant current source does this automatically. Ohm's law and the functional principle of a constant current source are illustrated in Figures 4-9A–C.

## Coulomb's Law, Electric Field, Current Density, and Charge

According to **Coulomb's law,** the strength of the **electric field** and, therefore, the corresponding **current density** (J) in relation to the distance from the current source is given by:

$$\mathbf{J(r) = k \cdot I_0/r^2}$$

$$(k = \text{constant},\ I_0 = \text{initial current})$$

This means the current (or charge) that reaches the nerve decreases by a factor of 4 if the distance to the nerve is doubled, or conversely, it increases by a factor of 4 if the distance is divided in half (ideal conditions assumed).

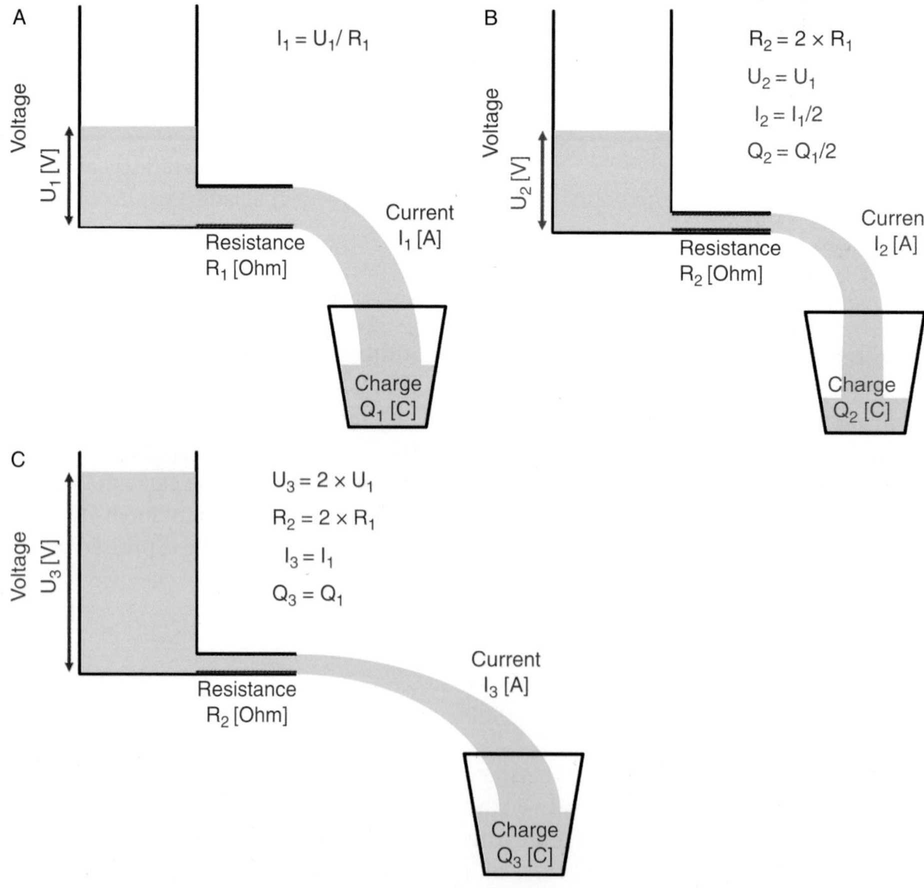


**FIGURE 4-9.** Ohm's law and principle of a constant current source. Functional principle of a constant current source. (A) Low resistance $R_1$ requires voltage $U_1$ to achieve desired current $I_1$. (B) High resistance $R_2 = 2 \times R_1$ causes current I to decrease to $I_2 = I_1/2$ if voltage U remains constant ($U_2 = U_1$). (C) Constant current source automatically increases output voltage to $U_3 = 2 \times U_1$ to comPNSate for the higher resistance $R_2$ and, therefore, current I increases to the desired level of $I_3 = I_1$.

The **charge Q** is the product of current multiplied by time and is given in ampere seconds (As) or coulomb (C). As an example, rechargeable batteries often have an indication of Ah or mAh as the measure of their capacitance of charge (kilo = 1000 or $10^3$; milli = 0.001 or $10^{-3}$; micro = 0.000001 or $10^{-6}$; nano = 0.000000001 or $10^{-9}$).

## Energy of Electrical Impulses Delivered by Nerve Stimulators and Related Temperature Effects

According to a worst-case scenario calculation, the temperature increase caused by a stimulus of 5 mA current and 1 ms duration, at a maximum output voltage of 95 V, would be <0.5 C, if all the energy were concentrated within a small volume of only 1 $mm^3$ and no temperature dissipation into the surrounding tissue occurred. This calculation can be applied for the tip of a nerve stimulation needle.

The maximum energy (E) of the electrical impulse delivered by a common nerve stimulator would be:

$$E \leq U \times I \times t = 95\ V\ 5\ mA \times 1\ ms$$
$$= 0.475\ mWs = 0.475\ mJ.$$

The caloric equivalent for water is $c_w = 4.19\ J\ g^{-1}\ K^{-1}$

One stimulus creates a temperature difference $\Delta T$ within 1 $mm^3$ of tissue around the tip of a nerve stimulation needle. For the calculation that follows, it is assumed that tissue contains a minimum of 50% water and the mass (M) of 1 $mm^3$ of tissue is 1 mg.

$$\Delta T \leq 2 \times E/(M \times c_w) = 2 \times 0.475 \times 10^{-3}\ J/(10^{-3}\ g \times 4.19\ g/K)$$
$$= 0.45\ K$$

That is, the maximum temperature increase in this worst-case scenario calculation is <0.5 C. In practice, this means the temperature effect of normal nerve stimulation on the tissue can be neglected.

## REFERENCES


1. Keithley J. *The Story of Electrical and Magnetic Measurements.* New York: IEEE; 1999.
2. von Perthes G. Überleitungsanästhesie unter Zuhilfenahme elektrischer Reizung. *Münch med Wochenschr.* 1912;47: 2545-2548.
3. Pearson RB. Nerve block in rehabilitation: a technique of needle localization. *Arch Phys Med Rehabil.* 1955;26:631-633.
4. Greenblatt GM, Denson JS. Needle nerve stimulator locator. Nerve blocks with a new instrument for locating nerves. *Anesth Analg.* 1962;41:599-602.
5. Montgomery SJ, Raj PP, Nettles D, Jenkins MT. The use of the nerve stimulator with standard unsheathed needles in nerve blockade. *Anesth Analg.* 1973;52:827-831.
6. Ford DJ, Pither C, Raj PP. Comparison of insulated and uninsulated needles for locating peripheral nerves with a peripheral nerve stimulator. *Anesth Analg.* 1984;63:925-928.
7. Ford DJ, Pither CE, Raj PP. Electrical characteristics of peripheral nerve stimulators: Implications for nerve localization. *Reg Anesth.* 1984;9:73-77.
8. Pither CE, Ford DJ, Raj PP. The use of peripheral nerve stimulators for regional anesthesia, a review of experimental characteristics, technique, and clinical applications. *Reg Anesth.* 1985;10:49-58.
9. Kaiser H, Neuburger M. How close is close enough—how close is safe enough. *Reg Anesth Pain Med.* 2002;27(2):227-228.
10. Neuburger M, Rotzinger M, Kaiser H. Electric nerve stimulation in relation to impulse strength. A quantitative study of the distance of the electrode point to the nerve. *Acta Anaesthesiol Scand.* 2007;51(7):942-948.
11. Hadžić A, Vloka JD, Claudio RE, Thys DM, Santos AC. Electrical nerve localization: effects of cutaneous electrode placement and duration of the stimulus on motor response. *Anesthesiology.* 2004;100:1526-1530.
12. Bosenberg AT, Raw R, Boezaart AP. Surface mapping of peripheral nerves in children with a nerve stimulator. *Paediatr Anaesth.* 2002;12:398-403.
13. Urmey WF, Grossi P. Percutaneous electrode guidance. A non-invasive technique for prelocation of peripheral nerves to facilitate peripheral plexus or nerve block. *Reg Anesth Pain Med.* 2002;27:261-267.
14. Urmey WF, Grossi P. Percutaneous electrode guidance and subcutaneous stimulating electrode guidance. Modifications of the original technique. *Reg Anesth Pain Med.* 2003;28:253-255.
15. Capdevilla X, Lopez S, Bernard N, et al. Percutaneous electrode guidance using the insulated needle for prelocation of peripheral nerves during axillary plexus blocks. *Reg Anesth Pain Med.* 2004;29:206-211.
16. Tsui BC, Gupta S, Finucane B. Confirmation of epidural catheter placement using nerve stimulation. *Can J Anesth.* 1998;45:640-644.
17. Tsui BC, Guenther C, Emery D, Finucane B. Determining epidural catheter location using nerve stimulation with radiological confirmation. *Reg Anesth Pain Med.* 2000;25:306-309.
18. Tsui BC, Seal R, Koller J, Entwistle L, Haugen R, Kearney R. Thoracic epidural analgesia via the caudal approach in pediatric patients undergoing fundoplication using nerve stimulation guidance. *Anesth Analg.* 2001;93:1152-1155.
19. Boezaart AP, de Beer JF, du Toit C. van Rooyen K. A new technique of continuous interscalene nerve block. *Can J Anesth.* 1999;46:275-281.
20. Kaiser H. Periphere elektrische Nervenstimulation. In: Niesel HC, Van Aken H, eds. *Regionalanästhesie, Lokalanästhesie, Regionale Schmerztherapie.* 2nd ed. Stuttgart, Germany: Thieme; 2002.
21. Tsui BC, Kropelin B. The electrophysiological effect of dextrose 5% in water on single-shot peripheral nerve stimulation. *Anesth Analg.* 2005;100:1837-1839.
22. Tsui BC. Electrical impedance to distinguish intraneural from extraneural needle placement in porcine nerves during direct exposure and ultrasound guidance. *Anesthesiology.* 2008;109:479-483.
23. Tsui BC, Chin JH. Electrical impedance to warn of intravascular needle placement. Abstract ASRA 2007. *Reg Anesth Pain Med.* 2007;32:A-51.
24. Urmey WF, Grossi P. Use of sequential electrical nerve stimuli (SENS) for location of the sciatic nerve and lumbar plexus. *Reg Anesth Pain Med.* 2006;31(5):463-469.
25. Jochum D, Iohom G, Diarra DP, Loughnane F, Dupré LJ, Bouaziz H. An objective assessment of nerve stimulators used for peripheral nerve blockade. *Anaesthesia.* 2006, 61:557-564.

# 5 Monitoring and Documentation

*Jeff Gadsden*

## Introduction

The incidence of complications from general anesthesia has diminished substantially in recent decades, largely due to advances in respiratory monitoring.[1] The use of objective monitors such as pulse oximetry and capnography allows anesthesiologists to quickly identify changing physiologic parameters and intervene rapidly and appropriately.

In contrast, the practice of regional anesthesia has traditionally suffered from a lack of similar objective monitors that aid the practitioner in preventing injury. Practitioners of peripheral nerve blocks were made to rely on subjective end points to gauge the potential risk to the patient. This is changing, however, with the introduction and adoption of standardized methods by which to safely perform peripheral nerve blocks with the minimal possible risk to the patient. For example, instead of relying on feeling "clicks," "pops," and "scratches" to identify needle tip position, the anesthesiologist can now directly observe it using ultrasonography. It follows that advancements such as this may help in reducing the three most feared complications of peripheral nerve blockade: nerve injury, local anesthetic toxicity, and inadvertent damage to adjacent structures ("needle misadventure").

Objective monitoring, and the rationale for its use, is discussed in the first part of this chapter. The later section focuses on documentation of nerve block procedures, which is a natural accompaniment to the use of these empirical monitors. The proper documentation of *how* a nerve block was performed has obvious medicolegal implications and aids the future practitioner in choosing the best nerve block regimen for that particular patient.

## SECTION I: MONITORING

### What Are the Available Monitors?

Monitors, as used in the medical sense, are devices that assess a specific physiologic state and warn the clinician of impending harm. The monitors discussed in this chapter include nerve stimulation, ultrasonography, and the monitoring of injection pressure. Each of these has its own distinct set of both advantages and limitations. For this reason, these three technologies are best used in a complementary fashion (Figure 5-1), to minimize the potential for patient injury, rather than just relying on the information provided by one monitor alone. The combination of all three monitors is likely to produce the safest possible environment in which to perform a peripheral nerve block.

A fourth monitor that many clinicians use regularly is the use of epinephrine in the local anesthetic. Good evidence supports this practice as a means of improving safety during peripheral nerve blocks, particularly in patients receiving higher doses of local anesthetic. First, it acts as a marker of intravascular absorption. About 10 to 15 μg of epinephrine injected intravenously reliably increases the systolic blood pressure >15 mm Hg, even in sedated or beta-blocked individuals (whereas a heart rate increase is not reliable in sedated patients).[2,3] The recognition of this increase permits the clinician to halt the injection promptly and increase his or her vigilance for signs of systemic toxicity. Second, epinephrine truncates the peak plasma level of local anesthetic,

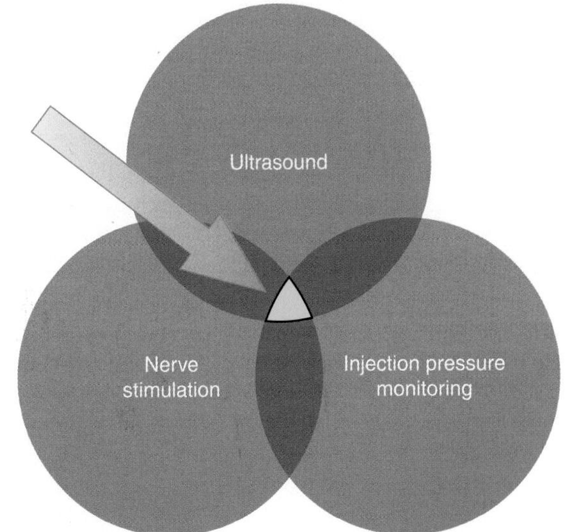


**FIGURE 5-1.** Three modes of monitoring peripheral nerve blocks for patient injury. The overlapping area of all three (yellow area) represents the safest means of performing a block.

resulting in a lower risk for systemic toxicity.[4,5] Concerns regarding the effects of epinephrine on nutritive vessel vasoconstriction and nerve ischemia have been unsubstantiated. In contrast, concentrations of 2.5 μg/mL have been associated with an increase in nerve blood flow, likely due to the predominance of the beta effect of the drug.[6] Therefore, when added to local anesthetics, epinephrine can enhance safety during administration of larger doses of local anesthetics.

##  Nerve Stimulation

Neurostimulation has largely replaced paresthesia as the primary means of nerve localization in the 1980s and has only recently been challenged by ultrasound guidance. Its effectiveness as a method of nerve localization has been challenged since the publication of a series of studies showing that, despite intimate needle–nerve contact as witnessed by ultrasonography, a motor response may be absent.[7] In some instances, a current intensity as high as >1.5 mA may be necessary to elicit motor response with needle placement within epineurium of the nerve.[8] There are probably multiple factors that contribute to the explanation of this phenomenon, including the nonuniform distribution of motor and sensory fibers in the compound nerve and the unpredictable pattern of current dispersion in the tissue depending on tissue conductances and impedances.

Although this has led some clinicians to de-value nerve stimulation in an era of ultrasound-guided blocks, a growing body of evidence suggests that the presence of a motor response at a very low current (i.e., <0.2 mA) is associated with an intraneural needle tip placement (Table 5-1). In a 2005 trial, Voelckel et al conducted percutaneous sciatic nerve blocks in pigs and demonstrated that when local anesthetic was injected at currents between 0.3 and 0.5 mA, the resulting nerve tissue showed no signs of an inflammatory process, whereas injections at <0.2 mA resulted in lymphocytic and granulocytic infiltration in 50% of the nerves.[9] Tsai et al performed a similar study investigating the effect of distance to the nerve on current required; although a range of currents were recorded for a variety of distances, the only instances in which the motor response

**TABLE 5-1 Studies of Intensity of the Current (mA) and Needle Tip Location**

| STUDY | SUBJECTS | METHODS | RESULTS |
|---|---|---|---|
| Voelckel et al[9] | Pigs ($n$ = 10) | • Posterior sciatic nerve blocks performed bilaterally<br>• Two groups<br>  ◦ Accepted twitch at 0.3–0.5 mA<br>  ◦ Only accepted twitch at <0.2 mA<br>• 6 h postinjection, sciatic nerves harvested for histologic analysis | • Normal, healthy appearance of nerves in "high-current" group<br>• 50% of nerves in "low-current" group showed evidence of lymphocyte and polymorphic granulocyte sub-, peri-, and intraneurally<br>• One specimen in "low current" group showed gross disruption of perineurium and multiple nerve fibers |
| Tsai et al[10] | Pigs ($n$ = 20) | • General anesthesia<br>• Sciatic nerves exposed bilaterally<br>• Current applied with needle at various distances from 2 cm away to intraneural<br>• Two blinded observers agreed on minimal current required to obtain hoof twitch<br>• 40 attempts at each distance | • Sciatic nerve twitches only obtainable 0.1 cm or closer<br>• Wide range of currents required to elicit motor response<br>• Only when intraneural did a motor response result from current <0.2 mA |
| Bigeleisen et al[11] | Patients for hand/wrist surgery ($n$ = 55) | • Supraclavicular block<br>• Minimum current recorded<br>  ◦ With needle outside nerve trunk (but contacting nerve)<br>  ◦ inside trunk<br>• Intraneural position sonographically confirmed with 5 mL injection of local anesthetic | • Median minimal current threshold outside nerve was 0.60 mA ± 0.37 mA<br>• Median minimal current threshold outside nerve was 0.30 mA ± 0.19 mA<br>• No twitch observed at any time when needle placed outside nerve and current <0.2 mA |

was obtained at <0.2 mA was when the needle tip was intraneural.[10]

More recently, a study was conducted on 55 patients scheduled for upper limb surgery who received ultrasound-guided supraclavicular brachial plexus blocks. The authors set out to determine the minimum current threshold for motor response both inside and outside the first trunk encountered.[11] They discovered that the median minimum stimulation threshold was 0.60 mA outside the nerve and 0.3 mA inside the nerve. Interestingly, stimulation currents of ≤0.2 mA were not observed outside the nerve, whereas 36% of patients experienced a twitch at currents <0.2 mA while the needle was intraneural.

Taken together, these data suggest that although the sensitivity of a "low-current" twitch for intraneural placement is not high, the specificity is. Put another way, the needle tip can be in the nerve and not elicit a motor response at very low currents; however, if a twitch *is* elicited at <0.2 mA, it is certain that the tip is intraneural.

Most regional anesthesiologists agree that injection of local anesthetic into the nerve may be a risk factor for injury and that extra-neural deposition minimizes the potential for an intrafascicular injection.[12] Ultrasonography is good, but not perfect, at delineating the exact position of the needle tip. In our attempts to get "close, but not too close" to the nerve so we might have the best block result, needles occasionally but inevitably cross the epineurium into the substance of the nerve. This event in and of itself may be of minimal consequence.[13] However, injection into a fascicle carries a high risk of injury.[14] It is for this reason that a reliable electrical monitor of needle tip position is a useful safety instrument. If a motor twitch is elicited at currents <0.2 mA, our approach is to gently withdraw the needle until the motor response disappears and then attempt to reelicit the twitch at the more appropriate (0.3–0.5 mA) current.

Overall, nerve stimulation adds little to the cost of a nerve block procedure, in terms of time, clinician effort, or dollars. It also serves as a useful functional confirmation of the anatomic image shown on the ultrasound screen (e.g. "Is that the median or ulnar nerve?"). In our practice, nerve stimulator is routinely used in conjunction with ultrasound guidance as an invaluable monitor of the needle tip position with respect to the nerve, based on the association of low currents with intraneural placement. In addition, an unexpected motor response during ultrasound-guided blocks may alert the operator of the needle-nerve relationship that was missed on ultrasound.

## Ultrasonography

The use of ultrasound guidance to assist in nerve block placement has become very popular, for a number of reasons. First, ultrasound allows visualization of the needle in real time and therefore quickly and accurately guide the needle toward the target. Multiple injection techniques that were difficult, or indeed dangerous, to do in the era of nerve stimulation alone are now easy to perform because the nerves can be seen and injectate carefully deposited at various points around them. Also, because a motor response is not technically required, blocks can now be performed in amputees who do not have a limb to twitch. Not surprisingly, ultrasound has the potential to improve the safety of peripheral nerve blocks for a number of reasons.

First, adjacent structures of importance can be seen and avoided. The resurgence in popularity of the supraclavicular block is a testament to this. Before ultrasound, the highly effective block was relatively unpopular as a means of anesthetizing the brachial plexus, for fear of causing a pneumothorax, despite the paucity of data regarding its actual incidence. However, now that the brachial plexus and, more importantly, the rib, pleura, and subclavian artery can all be seen at the supraclavicular level, this block has become common in clinical practice. However, recent reports of pneumothoraces serve as a reminder that while ultrasound may reduce the incidence of complications of nerve blocks, it is unlikely to entirely prevent when used as a sole monitor.[15,16] Similarly, there are reports of intravascular and intraneural needle placement witnessed (and despite the use of) ultrasound, highlighting the need to use care with this technology that is, in the end, a tool that is not failsafe.[17–19]

A useful adjunct to the visualization of structures on the ultrasound screen is the ability to measure the distance from skin to target using electronic calipers (Figure 5-2). This, coupled with needles that have depth markings etched on the side of the nerve block needles, confers a great safety advantage by warning the clinician of a "stop distance," or a depth beyond which he or she should stop, reassess the needle visualization, and perhaps withdraw and begin again.

Another important advantage that ultrasound can confer is the ability to see the local anesthetic distribution on the screen image (Figure 5-3). If corresponding tissue expansion is not seen when injection begins, then the needle tip is *not* where it is thought to be, and the clinician should immediately halt injection and relocate the tip of the needle. This is particularly worrisome in vascular areas because the lack of spread can signal the intravascular needle placement. However, ultrasound has been used successfully to diagnose an intra-arterial needle tip placement when an echogenic "blush" was noted in the lumen of the artery, allowing for rapid cessation of the block technique and avoidance of what surely would have been systemic toxicity.[20,21]

Similarly, ultrasound may also be able to reduce the likelihood of systemic toxicity by allowing clinicians to use less local anesthetic. Several authors have published large reductions in the volume required to affect an equivalent block to standard nerve stimulation techniques. For example, Casati et al demonstrated a significant reduction in volume required to produce an effective three-in-one block (22 mL vs. 41 mL).[22] Sandhu et al showed in a feasibility study that infraclavicular block was possible using ultrasound with

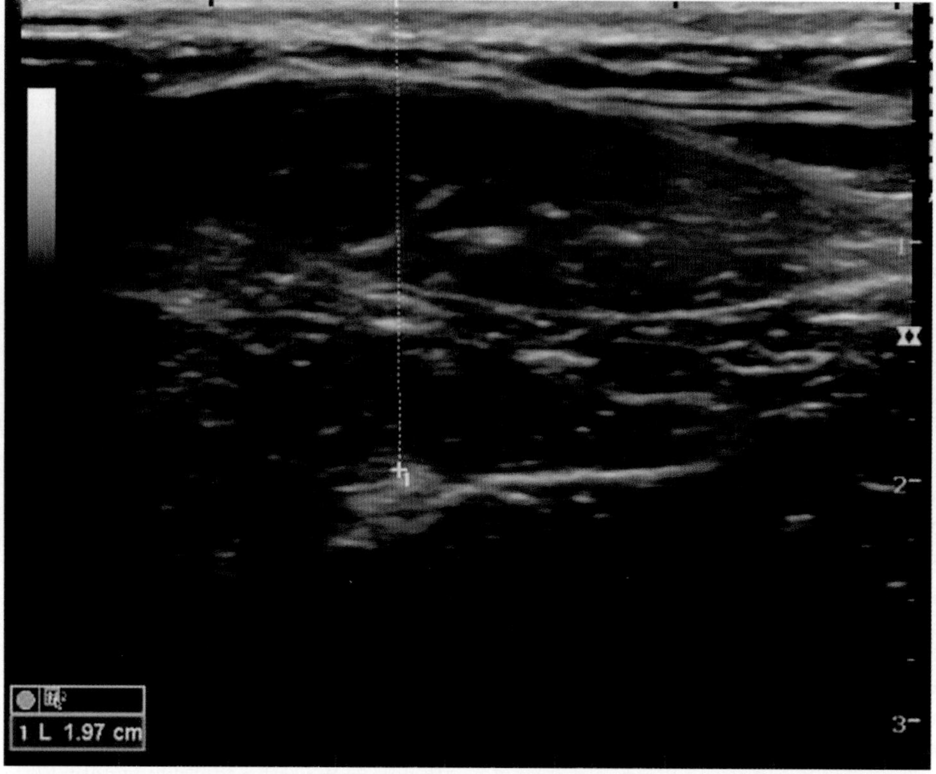


**FIGURE 5-2.** An example of ultrasound being used to determine the depth of a structure of interest.

volumes typically half of what were used with nerve stimulation alone (16.1 ± 1.9 mL).[23] Riazi et al published a study in 2008 showing that ultrasound guidance allowed for a substantial reduction of volume for interscalene block used for postoperative pain while still providing a quality block (5 mL vs. 20 mL).[24] Interestingly, this low dose also resulted in less diaphragmatic impairment related to phrenic nerve paresis.

The utility of ultrasound in prevention of nerve injury during peripheral nerve blockade is likely over-estimated. The problem is threefold: First, observing the needle tip in relation to the nerve is user dependent, and one can often be fooled by poor technique or simply unfavorable echogenic characteristics of the tissue–needle interface; second, the current resolution available is not adequate to distinguish

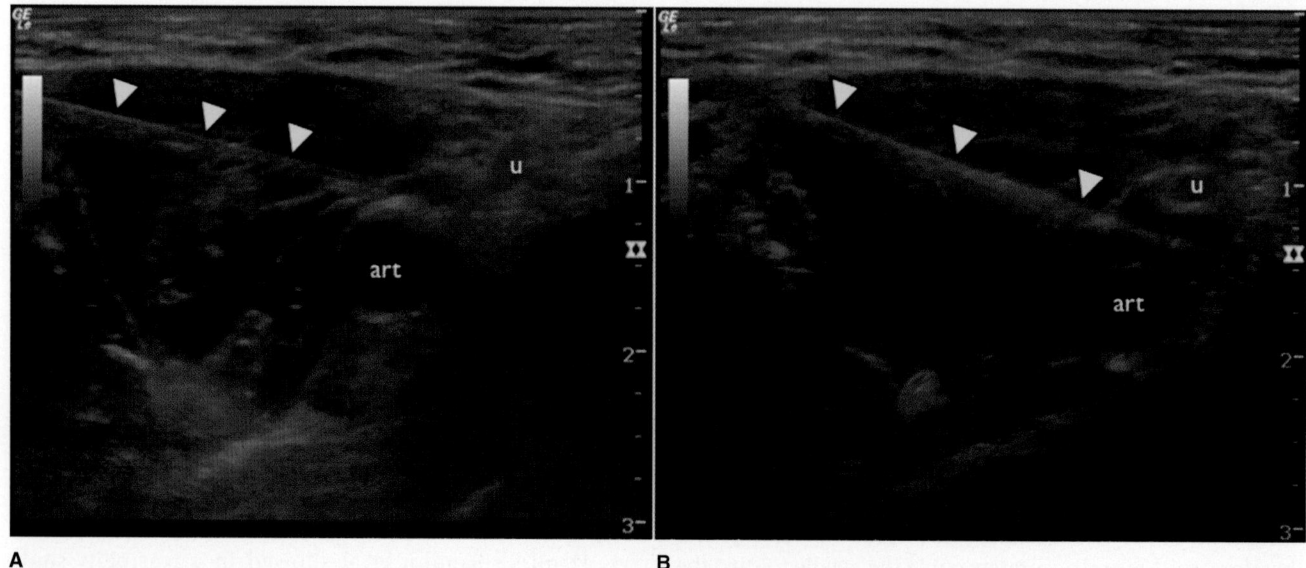


**FIGURE 5-3.** Axillary block with axillary artery (art), ulnar nerve (u), needle (arrowheads), (A) before and (B) after injection of small amount of local anesthetic, showing spread of injectate between artery and nerve.

between an intra- versus extrafascicular needle tip location. This difference is crucial because evidence is mounting that an intraneural (but extrafascicular) injection is likely not associated with injury, whereas injection inside the fascicles themselves produces clinical and histologic damage.[14,25] Lastly, once injection has begun, even a minuscule amount of local anesthetic can produce damage if intrafascicular.[26] Relying on the visual confirmation of tissue expansion may result in damage before expansion is detected on the screen. It is, in other words, probably too late.

## Injection Pressure Monitoring

How, then, can the clinician distinguish the intrafascicular versus the extrafascicular needle tip placement, if ultrasound guidance is insufficient? An additional modality to ultrasound and nerve stimulation is monitoring of injection pressures. In a study of intraneural injections in dog sciatic nerves, a slow injection of lidocaine while the needle tip was intrafascicular was associated with an immediate and substantial rise in the pressure of the syringe-tubing-needle system (>20 psi), followed by return of the pressure tracing to normal (i.e., <5 psi) levels. In contrast, those nerves that underwent extrafascicular injection showed no high pressure whatsoever.[14] Moreover, those limbs in which the nerves were exposed to high-injection pressures all experienced clinical signs of neuropathy (muscle wasting, weakness) as well as histologic evidence (inflammation, disruption of the nerve architecture). The implication is that injection into a low compliance compartment, such as within the tough, durable perineurium, is likely to result in generation of high pressures that can either directly damage delicate nerve fibers or rupture the fascicle itself, leading to nerve injury.

The use of "hand feel" to avoid high injection pressure is unfortunately not reliable. Studies of experienced practitioners blinded to the injection pressure and asked to perform a mock injection using standard equipment reveals wide variations in applied pressure, some grossly exceeding the established thresholds for safety.[27] Similarly, anesthesiologists perform poorly when asked to distinguish between intraneural injection and injection into other tissues such as muscle or tendon in an animal model.[28] It is therefore important to use an objective and quantifiable method of gauging injection pressure.

Although the practice of injection pressure monitoring during peripheral nerve blocks is relatively young, monitoring options do exist. Tsui et al described a method of "compressed air injection technique" where 10 mL of air was drawn into the syringe along with the local anesthetic.[29] Holding the syringe upright, it is then possible to avoid exceeding a maximum threshold of 1 atmosphere (or approximately 15 psi) by only allowing the gas portion of the syringe contents to compress to half of its original volume, or 5 mL. This makes use of Boyle's law, which states that pressure times volume must be constant. A pressure <15 psi is probably a safe threshold for initiating injection during peripheral nerve blocks.

Another option is disposable pressure manometers specifically manufactured for this purpose. These devices bridge the syringe and needle tubing, and via a spring-loaded piston, allow the clinician to gauge the pressure in the system continuously. On the shaft of the piston are markings delineating three different pressure thresholds: <15 psi, 15 to 20 psi, and >20 psi (Figure 5-4). An advantage of this method is

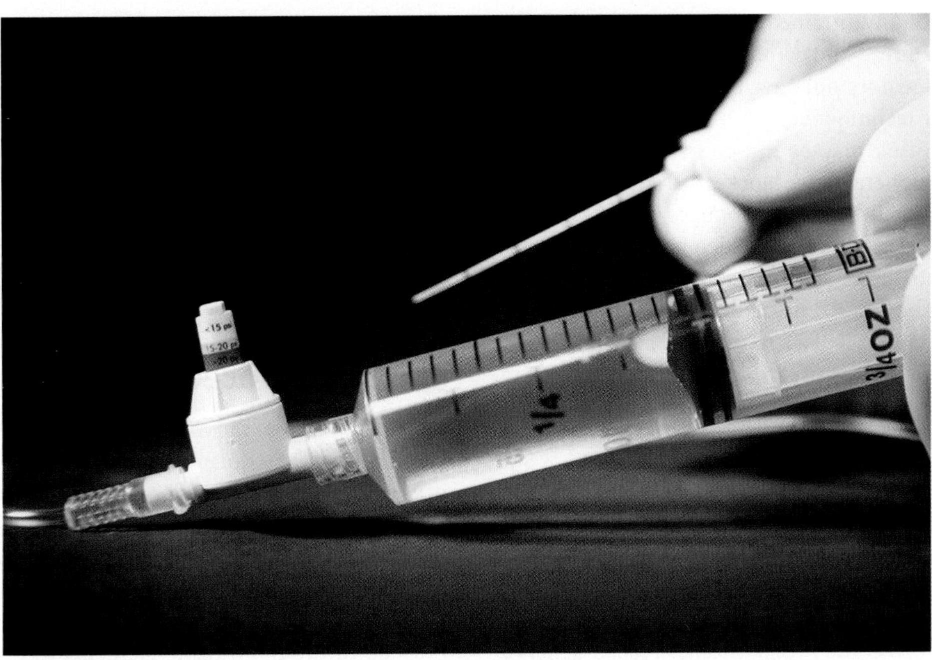


**FIGURE 5-4.** Inline pressure manometer with graded markings on the side (B-smart, Concert Medical, Needham, MA).

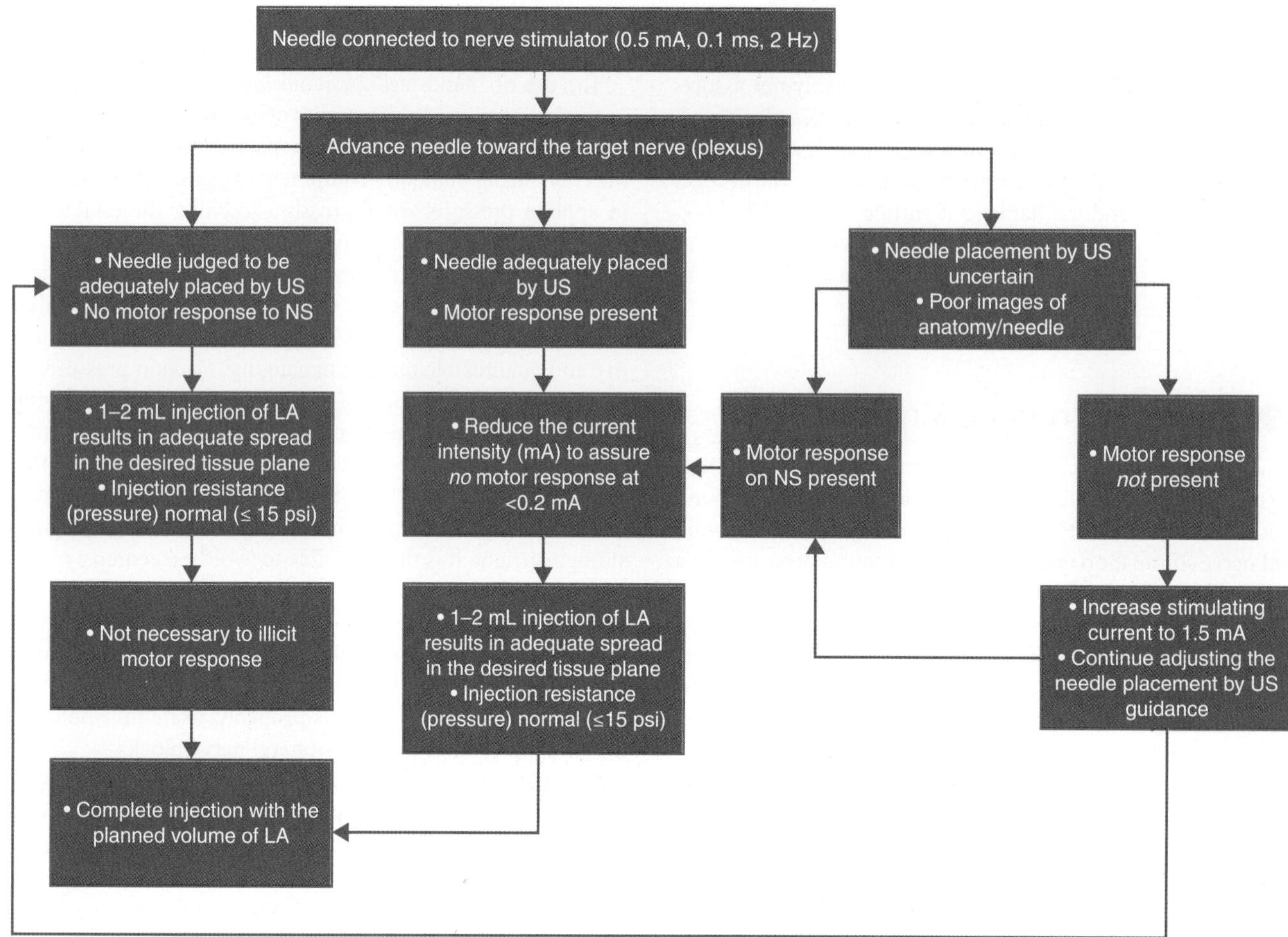


**FIGURE 5-5.** Flowchart depicting the order of correctly documenting nerve block procedures: combining ultrasound (US), nerve stimulation (NS), and injection pressure monitoring.

the ease with which an untrained assistant who is performing the injection can read and communicate the pressures. In addition, the syringe does not have to be held upright, as in the compressed air technique.

Pressure monitoring may be a useful safety monitor for other aspects of peripheral nerve blocks. In a study of patients receiving lumbar plexus blocks randomized to low (<15 psi) versus high (>20 psi) pressures, Gadsden et al demonstrated that 60% of patients in the high-pressure group experienced a bilateral epidural block.[30] Furthermore, 50% in the same group reported an epidural block in the thoracic distribution. No patient in the low-pressure group experienced bilateral or epidural blockade. This has now become an important adjunct to lumbar plexus blockade in our institution, to avoid this potentially dangerous complication.

## Summary

Regional anesthesia has been making a transition from art to science as more rigorous and precise means of locating nerves are developed. The same process should be expected for monitoring peripheral blockade. The use of neurostimulation, ultrasonography, and injection pressure monitoring together provides a complementary package of objective data that can guide clinicians to perform the safest blocks possible. The flowchart in Figure 5-5 outlines how these monitors can be combined.

# SECTION II: DOCUMENTATION

## Block Procedure Notes

Documentation of nerve block procedures has, by and large, lagged behind the documentation of general anesthesia, and it is often relegated to a few scribbled lines in the corner of the anesthetic record. Increasing pressure from legal, billing, and regulatory sources has provoked an effort to improve the documentation for peripheral nerve blocks. A sample of a peripheral nerve block documentation form that incorporates all of the monitoring elements discussed in this book (ultrasound, nerve stimulation, and injection pressure monitoring) and can be adopted to individual practice is shown

## PERIPHERAL NERVE BLOCK PROCEDURE NOTE

| Patient Name: | | | | | |
|---|---|---|---|---|---|
| Medical Record #: | | | | | |
| Age: | | ASA: | | Allergies: | |

**Consents:** ☐ Surgery ☐ Anesthesia
**Indication:** ☐ Analgesia ☐ Surgical Anesthesia
☐ Block requested by Dr. ____________

☐ Laterality Check (Time Out): ( : )
☐ Initials _______

**Site of Surgery**:
☐ Left ☐ Right

**Surgery**: ______________________________

**Block(s) Performed**: ______________________________

**Date:** ___/___/_____ **Procedure Start Time** ( : ) **End Time** ( : )

**Vital Signs:** BP: ___/___ HR: _____ ☐ $O_2$ Saturation _____ %
☐ Awake ☐ Sedated ☐ Anesthetized

**Premedication:** Midazolam …… (mcg) Fentanyl …… (mcg) Alfentayl …… (mcg) Sufentanyl ……. (mcg)

**Asepsis:** ☐ Povid-iodine ☐ Sterile Gloves ☐ Block Tray ☐ Other ……………………………..

**Patient Position:** ☐ Supine ☐ Prone ☐ LLD ☐ RLD ☐ Sitting

**ASA Monitoring:** ☐ BP ☐ EKG ☐ $O_2$ Sat ☐ Supplemental $O_2$ ☐ Resuscitation equipment

**Technique:** ☐ Single Injection ☐ Catheter (depth at skin ……… cm.)

**Needle:** ☐ 2" 22 G ☐ 4" 21 G ☐ 18 G Tuohy ☐ Other: ………………………….

**Skin Anesthesia:** ……… mL of ☐Lidocaine ☐ Other: ………………………., with ☐ 25 G needle.

**Monitoring:** ☐ Ultrasound ☐ Nerve Stimulation ☐ Injection Resistance (Pressure)
→ *Transducer*: ☐ *Curved* ☐ *Linear*, ☐ *In Plane* ☐ *Out of Plane*

| Motor response (specify) | Minimal current (mA) before injection | Ultrasound image quality | Local Anesthetic | Conc. (%) | Volume (mL) | Epinephrine/ Additives |
|---|---|---|---|---|---|---|
| | | ☐ Clear | ☐ Bupivacaine | | | ☐ 1/___00,000 |
| | | | ☐ Ropivacaine | | | |
| | | | ☐ Mepivacaine | | | ☐ Other: ………………………… |
| | | ☐ Poor | ☐ Lidocaine | | | |
| | | | ☐ 2-CP | | | |

**Catheter Infusion:** Rate ……… (mL/hr) PCA ……… (mL/hr) ☐ ……… mL (Q 30 mins) ☐ ……… mL (Q1hr)

Blood Aspirated? ☐ No ☐ Yes
Intravenous test using epinephrine? ☐ Negative ☐ Positive
Pain on injection? ☐ No ☐ Yes
Resistance on injection? ☐ Normal (<15 psi) ☐ High ( >15 psi)
Notes ……………………………………………………………………………………

**Events:** ☐ Uneventful ☐ Other ……………………………………

**Block Success:** ☐ Complete ☐ Partial ☐ Failed ☐ Aborted ☐ A full evaluation pending

**Post Procedure Condition:** BP: ___/___ HR: _____ ☐ $O_2$ Saturation _____ % ☐ Awake ☐ Comfortable

☐ **MD SIGNATURE:** ______________________________

**FIGURE 5-6.** Example of a procedure note.

in Figure 5-6. This form has a number of features that should be considered by institutions attempting to formulate their own procedure note. These include the following:

| USEFUL FEATURES OF A PERIPHERAL NERVE BLOCK PROCEDURE NOTE | EXAMPLE |
|---|---|
| Elements that guide the practitioner to meet a given standard of care. | A space to indicate the use of epinephrine in the local anesthetic solution; if none was used, why not? |
| A compromise between efficiency and ability to individualize. | Information is recorded using both checkboxes and blank line spaces. |
| Documentation to safeguard against common medicolegal challenges. | Practitioner must indicate patient's level of consciousness. |
| Documentation of compliance with regulatory agencies (e.g., The Joint Commission). | Checkboxes to indicate laterality. |
| Elements to facilitate successful billing. | Language required by many insurance companies indicating block specifically requested by surgeon. |
| Documentation of clinicians involved and in what capacity. | Was the attending the individual performing the block, or was he or she medically directing a resident? |

Another useful aspect of peripheral nerve block documentation is the recording of an ultrasound image or video clip, to be stored either as a hard copy in the patient's chart or as an electronic copy in a database. This is not only good practice from a medicolegal point of view but is a required step that must be taken if the clinician wishes to bill for the use of ultrasound guidance. Any hard copies should have a patient identification sticker attached, the date recorded, and any pertinent findings highlighted with a marker, such as local anesthetic spreading around nerve circumferentially (Figure 5-6).

## Informed Consent

Documentation of informed consent is another issue that is of importance to regional anesthesiologists. Practice patterns vary widely on this issue, and specific written consent for nerve block procedures is often not obtained. However, the written documentation of this process can be important for a number of reasons:

- Patients are often distracted and anxious on the day of surgery (when many consents are obtained), and they may not remember the details of a discussion with their anesthesiologist. Studies have shown that a written record of the informed consent process improves patient recall of risks and benefits.[31]
- A written consent establishes that a discussion of risks and benefits occurred between the patient and the physician.
- A specific document for regional anesthesia can be tailored to include all the common and serious risks. This allows the physician to explain them to the patient as a matter of routine and reduce the chance of omitting important risks.

| SUGGESTIONS FOR IMPROVING THE CONSENT PROCESS |
|---|
| Be brief. A simple, short explanation helps recall of the risks and benefits more than lengthy paragraphs. |
| Include serious and common risks but also the benefits and expected results of the proposed regional anesthetic procedure. It is difficult for patients to make an informed choice if only risks are discussed. |
| Use the consent process as a means to educate the patient at the same time. |
| Offer a copy of the form to the patient. This has been shown to aid in recall of consent-related information. |

The following tips can be used to maximize the consent process:

A specific regional anesthesia consent form should be included as well. This will not be applicable to all institutions but can be modified to suit the needs of each individual department.

## REFERENCES


1. Buhre W, Rossaint R. Perioperative management and monitoring in anaesthesia. *Lancet*. 2003;362:1839-1846.
2. Guinard JP, Mulroy MF, Carpenter RL, Knopes KD. Test doses: optimal epinephrine content with and without acute beta-adrenergic blockade. *Anesthesiology*. 1990;73:386-392
3. Tanaka M, Sato M, Kimura T, Nishikawa T. The efficacy of simulated intravascular test dose in sedated patients. *Anesth Analg*. 2001;93:1612-1617.
4. Karmakar MK, Ho AM, Law BK, Wong AS, Shafer SL, Gin T. Arterial and venous pharmacokinetics of ropivacaine with and without epinephrine after thoracic paravertebral block. *Anesthesiology*. 2005;103:704-711.
5. Van Obbergh LJ, Roelants FA, Veyckemans F, Verbeeck RK. In children, the addition of epinephrine modifies the pharmacokinetics of ropivacaine injected caudally. *Can J Anaesth*. 2003;50:593-598.
6. Neal JM. Effects of epinephrine in local anesthetics on the central and peripheral nervous systems: neurotoxicity and neural blood flow. *Reg Anesth Pain Med*. 2003;28:124-134.

7. Perlas A, Niazi A, McCartney C, Chan V, Xu D, Abbas S. The sensitivity of motor response to nerve stimulation and paresthesia for nerve localization as evaluated by ultrasound. *Reg Anesth Pain Med.* 2006;31:445-450.
8. Chan VW, Brull R, McCartney CJ, Xu D, Abbas S, Shannon P. An ultrasonographic and histological study of intraneural injection and electrical stimulation in pigs. *Anesth Analg.* 2007;104:1281-1284.
9. Voelckel WG, Klima G, Krismer AC, et al. Signs of inflammation after sciatic nerve block in pigs. *Anesth Analg.* 2005;101:1844-1846.
10. Tsai TP, Vuckovic I, Dilberovic F, et al. Intensity of the stimulating current may not be a reliable indicator of intraneural needle placement. *Reg Anesth Pain Med.* 2008;33:207-210.
11. Bigeleisen PE, Moayeri N, Groen GJ. Extraneural versus intraneural stimulation thresholds during ultrasound-guided supraclavicular block. *Anesthesiology.* 2009;110:1235-1243.
12. Hogan QH. Pathophysiology of peripheral nerve injury during regional anesthesia. *Reg Anesth Pain Med.* 2008;33:435-441.
13. Sala-Blanch X, Ribalta T, Rivas E, et al. Structural injury to the human sciatic nerve after intraneural needle insertion. *Reg Anesth Pain Med.* 2009;34:201-205.
14. Hadžić A, Dilberovic F, Shah S, et al. Combination of intraneural injection and high injection pressure leads to fascicular injury and neurologic deficits in dogs. *Reg Anesth Pain Med.* 2004;29:417-423.
15. Koscielniak-Nielsen ZJ, Rasmussen H, Hesselbjerg L. Pneumothorax after an ultrasound-guided lateral sagittal infraclavicular block. *Acta Anaesthesiol Scand.* 2008;52:1176-1177.
16. Bryan NA, Swenson JD, Greis PE, Burks RT. Indwelling interscalene catheter use in an outpatient setting for shoulder surgery: technique, efficacy, and complications. *J Shoulder Elbow Surg.* 2007;16:388-395.
17. Russon K, Blanco R. Accidental intraneural injection into the musculocutaneous nerve visualized with ultrasound. *Anesth Analg.* 2007;105:1504-1505.
18. Schafhalter-Zoppoth I, Zeitz ID, Gray AT. Inadvertent femoral nerve impalement and intraneural injection visualized by ultrasound. *Anesth Analg.* 2004;99:627-628.
19. Loubert C, Williams SR, Helie F, Arcand G. Complication during ultrasound-guided regional block: accidental intravascular injection of local anesthetic. *Anesthesiology.* 2008;108:759-760.
20. VadeBoncouer TR, Weinberg GL, Oswald S, Angelov F. Early detection of intravascular injection during ultrasound-guided supraclavicular brachial plexus block. *Reg Anesth Pain Med.* 2008;33:278-279.
21. Martinez Navas A, DE LA Tabla González RO. Ultrasound-guided technique allowed early detection of intravascular injection during an infraclavicular brachial plexus block. *Acta Anaesthesiol Scand.* 2009;53:968-970.
22. Casati A, Baciarello M, Di Cianni S, et al. Effects of ultrasound guidance on the minimum effective anaesthetic volume required to block the femoral nerve. *Br J Anaesth.* 2007;98:823-827.
23. Sandhu NS, Bahniwal CS, Capan LM. Feasibility of an infraclavicular block with a reduced volume of lidocaine with sonographic guidance. *J Ultrasound Med.* 2006;25:51-56
24. Riazi S, Carmichael N, Awad I, Holtby RM, McCartney CJ. Effect of local anaesthetic volume (20 vs 5 ml) on the efficacy and respiratory consequences of ultrasound-guided interscalene brachial plexus block. *Br J Anaesth.* 2008;101:549-556.
25. Bigeleisen PE. Nerve puncture and apparent intraneural injection during ultrasound-guided axillary block does not invariably result in neurologic injury. *Anesthesiology.* 2006;105:779-783.
26. Selander D, Dhuner KG, Lundborg G. Peripheral nerve injury due to injection needles used for regional anesthesia. An experimental study of the acute effects of needle point trauma. *Acta Anaesthesiol Scand.* 1977;21:182-188.
27. Claudio R, Hadžić A, Shih H, et al. Injection pressures by anesthesiologists during simulated peripheral nerve block. *Reg Anesth Pain Med.* 2004;29:201-205.
28. Theron PS, Mackay Z, Gonzalez JG, Donaldson N, Blanco R. An animal model of "syringe feel" during peripheral nerve block. *Reg Anesth Pain Med.* 2009;34:330-332.
29. Tsui BC, Knezevich MP, Pillay JJ. Reduced injection pressures using a compressed air injection technique (CAIT): an in vitro study. *Reg Anesth Pain Med.* 2008;33:168-173.
30. Gadsden JC, Lindenmuth DM, Hadžić A, Xu D, Somasundarum L, Flisinski KA. Lumbar plexus block using high-pressure injection leads to contralateral and epidural spread. *Anesthesiology.* 2008;109:683-688.
31. Gerancher JC, Grice SC, Dewan DM, Eisenach J. An evaluation of informed consent prior to epidural analgesia for labor and delivery. *Int J Obstet Anesth.* 2000;9:168-173.

# 6 Indications for Peripheral Nerve Blocks

*Jeff Gadsden*

## Introduction

During the past 20 years, increasing knowledge in functional regional anesthesia anatomy, coupled with new technologies for locating peripheral nerves, has resulted in expansion of regional anesthesia techniques. This phenomenon served to provide the clinician with a wide variety of techniques from which to choose. Nevertheless, many nerve block techniques are quite similar and result in a similar, if not exact, distribution of anesthesia. The proper choice of the nerve block for a particular surgical procedure and/or patient, however, is far more important than deliberation on the minutia of various technical techniques. In this chapter, a rational selection of the nerve block techniques is approached in three sections. In the first section, indications for common nerve blocks are listed with a short summary of the advantages and disadvantages of each technique selected. In the second section, specific protocols for intraoperative anesthesia and postoperative analgesia for the common surgical procedures are suggested as practiced by anesthesiologists affiliated with the St. Luke's and Roosevelt Hospitals in New York. This cookbook approach was chosen to allow clinicians to duplicate the results that we have found, via trial and error, to work best in our own practice. The last section is a more comprehensive compendium of published medical literature on the indications for peripheral nerve blocks.

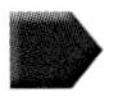

## Section I: Advantages and Disadvantages of Specific Nerve Blocks

### Upper Limb Blocks

With the advent of ultrasound guidance for nerve blocks, the choice of which brachial plexus block to perform has become less relevant because the block can be extended by needle repositioning into the desired area. For example, the interscalene approach was not recommended in the past for procedures on the hand or elbow because it was believed that local anesthetic would not sufficiently cover the inferior trunk of the brachial plexus. However, this barrier can be overcome with the use of a low-interscalene approach or by using sonographic guidance to target all three trunks. Multiple injections at different levels of the brachial plexus through a single-needle insertion site can make the interscalene brachial plexus applicable for most upper limb procedures. Regardless, the common approaches to brachial plexus block are sufficiently different in their anesthetic coverage to deserve knowledgeable consideration when making a decision about which block to use. In addition to the anesthetic coverage, the block selection should also take into consideration other factors, such as patient comfort, preexisting respiratory dysfunction, and practitioner experience. Table 6-1 lists common nerve block procedures and their indications.

### Lower Limb Blocks

Achieving quality anesthesia or analgesia of the lower limb is more challenging than with an upper extremity. This is because its innervation stems from two major plexuses, the lumbar and the sacral. The lumbar plexus is formed by the roots of L1-L4 and gives rise to the femoral, obturator, and lateral femoral cutaneous nerves, among others. The sacral plexus originates from L4-S3, and its principal branch is the sciatic nerve. Most of the indications for lower limb blockade involve joint surgery on either the hip or the knee. Because both joints are supplied by elements of each plexus, complete anesthesia often requires at least two nerve blocks. Consequently, many clinicians choose to perform just one block for the purpose of *analgesia*. Table 6-2 lists some common lower limb blocks and their advantages and disadvantages.

## Section II: Protocols

A variety of different methods are available to provide intraoperative and postoperative analgesia for surgery on the extremity. Any anesthetic or analgesic plan is based on patient and surgical factors as well as practical considerations such as the practitioner's skill level, availability of a block room, availability of skilled assistants, and departmental and hospital policies. The protocols for most common major orthopedic procedures outlined in this section were refined through trial and error and are the actual methods used in our daily practice.

**TABLE 6-1 Common Upper Limb Blocks**

| PERIPHERAL NERVE BLOCK | INDICATIONS | ADVANTAGES | DISADVANTAGES |
|---|---|---|---|
| Interscalene brachial plexus block | • Shoulder surgery<br>• Any surgery on the arm and humerus<br>• Manipulation of a frozen shoulder | • Also results in anesthesia of supraclavicular nerves<br>• Superficial, easy to perform, and comfortable for patient | • Hemidiaphragmatic paralysis<br>• Unless certain of inferior trunk blockade (by using US or a low-interscalene approach), not recommended for elbow, forearm, hand surgery |
| Supraclavicular brachial plexus block | • Any surgery of the arm distal to the shoulder | • Anesthesia of all portions of the arm distal to shoulder<br>• Fast onset. Simple to perform with US guidance<br>• Superficial/comfortable to the patient<br>• Requires relatively small amount of LA (20–25 mL) | • Potential for pneumothorax (may be less with ultrasound guidance) |
| Infraclavicular brachial plexus block | • Any surgery of the arm distal to the axilla | • Provides anesthesia to the entire arm distal to axilla<br>• Good choice for catheter placement because pectoralis muscles "hold" catheter in place | • Deeper block<br>• Greater discomfort during block placement<br>• Requires more expertise |
| Axillary brachial plexus block | • Any surgery on the elbow or below | • No risk of pneumothorax, neuraxial block, or phrenic nerve blockade | • Hematoma resulting in post-block local discomfort and/or discoloration relatively common (with trans-arterial technique)<br>• Site of injection can be tender postoperatively |
| Distal blocks of the median, ulnar, and radial nerves (at elbow, forearm) | • Hand surgery | • Avoids motor block of biceps and triceps, allowing patient greater postoperative function while maintaining analgesia of hand<br>• Reduction in dose and volume of LA, compared with other proximal brachial plexus block approaches | • Procedures on lateral forearm/wrist require separate blockade of either lateral cutaneous nerve of forearm or its parent nerve, musculocutaneous nerve<br>• Tourniquet on arm/forearm may not be tolerated for long periods; requires separate sedation/analgesia |

LA, local anesthesia; US, ultrasound.

The choice of the block combination for postoperative pain is based on several factors. The orthopedic surgeons at St. Luke's-Roosevelt Hospital prefer a regimen of twice-daily dosing of low molecular weight heparin (LMWH) for thromboprophylaxis, which makes the use of an indwelling epidural catheter for postoperative pain impractical or unsuitable. Similarly, although we recognize there is some controversy regarding the use of lumbar plexus catheters in the same setting, by and large, we treat them as neuraxial catheters and remove them before the first dose of LMWH. Other perineural catheters are routinely placed and maintained even in patients who are treated with anticoagulants.

In recent years, we have made an effort to minimize the use of parenteral opioids for postoperative pain if possible. In particular, patients admitted to the ward with a perineural catheter and intravenous patient-controlled opioid analgesia can find it confusing to have two buttons to press, and therefore they do not use the catheter effectively, leading to inadequate analgesia. For this reason, we strive to make use of a multimodal regimen instead, consisting of acetaminophen, a nonsteroidal anti-inflammatory drug, and an oral opioid.

For lower limb surgery, such as total knee replacement, clinicians often debate whether the sciatic nerve and/or obturator blocks should be routinely used in addition to the femoral (or lumbar plexus) block. We do not routinely do this but rather assess the patient after the femoral/lumbar plexus blockade is performed. In our practice, in the majority of patients, postoperative pain is adequately managed (visual analog scale [VAS] ≤3) by continuous femoral nerve block alone. A small proportion of patients (about 20%) may require

**TABLE 6-2 Common Lower Limb Blocks**

| PERIPHERAL NERVE BLOCK | INDICATIONS | ADVANTAGES | DISADVANTAGES |
|---|---|---|---|
| Lumbar plexus block | • Surgical anesthesia for knee arthroscopy<br>• Superficial procedures of the anterior thigh<br>• Patella tendon repair<br>• Quadriceps tendon repair<br>• Postoperative analgesia for hip or knee arthroplasty | • Block of obturator nerve (supplies both hip and knee joints)<br>• Covers lateral femoral cutaneous nerve, site of incision for hip replacement<br>• Can be combined easily with spinal anesthesia with patients in lateral position | • Risk of bilateral & epidural spread<br>• Higher risk of toxicity due to absorption of LA injected in the muscles<br>• Deep block: care with anticoagulated patient<br>• Other reported complications include peritoneal puncture, renal subcapsular hematoma<br>• Risk of hypotension due to high/epidural/spinal anesthesia<br>• Cardiac arrests reported |
| Femoral nerve block | • Knee arthroscopy<br>• Superficial procedures of the anterior thigh<br>• Quadriceps tendon repair<br>• Patella fracture ORIF<br>• Postoperative analgesia for hip or knee arthroplasty | • Superficial, simple to perform<br>• Can be used in anticoagulated patient | • Incomplete analgesia for hip or knee surgery (sciatic, obturator, LFCN)<br>• Lumbar plexus provides better coverage for knee and hip |
| Posterior (transgluteal or subgluteal) sciatic block | • Anesthesia for procedures on the knee (combined with femoral)<br>• Lower limb surgery below the knee (i.e., foot and ankle)<br>• Supplementary analgesia for procedures about the knee | • Reliable landmarks makes location easy to find<br>• Provides motor block of hamstrings, if desired<br>• Little risk of vascular puncture | • Relatively deep blocks<br>• Can be uncomfortable for patients, requiring significant premedication<br>• Requires semiprone/prone position<br>• Requires advanced skill to visualize by US<br>• Posterior cutaneous nerve of thigh not blocked |
| Anterior sciatic block | • Anesthesia for procedures on the lower limb below the knee (i.e., foot and ankle)<br>• Supplementary analgesia for procedures about the knee | • No need for lateral/prone position for block placement<br>• Convenient to combine with femoral block | • Risk of femoral vessel puncture<br>• Deep block; uncomfortable for patients<br>• May require multiple attempts to localize the nerve |
| Popliteal sciatic nerve block | • Surgical anesthesia for procedures on the foot and ankle<br>• Lesser saphenous nerve stripping<br>• Supplementary analgesia for procedures about the knee | • Can be done in supine, oblique, and prone position<br>• Posterior approach simple to perform<br>• Not uncomfortable for patients; intertendinous approach does not require needle insertion through muscle | • Does not provide anesthesia for Tourniquet; calf Tourniquet must be used, except for short procedures. |

LA, local anesthetic; LFCN, lateral femoral cutaneous nerve; ORIF, open reduction and internal fixation; US, ultrasound.

a sciatic nerve block for adequate pain control. Although often debated and taught in various regional courses, the usefulness of the obturator block in our practice is questionable at best. Consequently, we do not use obturator blocks in patients having knee arthroplasty.

The timing of block placement is institution dependent, and it relies on the presence of various factors, such as availability of the designated block personnel, operating room flow, ancillary staff, and a separate block area. Single-injection nerve blocks for surgery are performed either in the holding area or

**TABLE 6-3 Common Surgical Procedures and Analgesic Options**

| SURGICAL PROCEDURE | PRE/INTRAOPERATIVE ANESTHESIA | POSTOPERATIVE ANALGESIA |
|---|---|---|
| Rotator cuff repair | 1. Midazolam 2 mg IV, alfentanil 250–500 μg IV as premedication<br>2. Interscalene block<br>• 20–25 mL ropivacaine 0.5% or<br>• 15–20 mL of bupivacaine 0.5% with epinephrine 1:300,000*<br>3. Propofol sedation 25–50 μg/kg/min | 1. Ketorolac 30 mg IV<br>2. Intravenous Acetaminophen 1 gm loading dose, then 1 gm q 6 Hrs<br>3. Instruct to take ibuprofen 400 mg q6h at home |
| Total shoulder replacement | 1. Midazolam 2 mg IV, alfentanil 250–500 μg IV as premedication<br>2. Interscalene catheter<br>• 20–25 mL ropivacaine 0.5%<br>• If catheter not used, 15–25 mL of bupivacaine 0.5% with epinephrine 1:300,000*<br>3. Propofol sedation 25–50 μg/kg/min | 1. Ketorolac 15 mg IV q6h × 24 h<br>2. Intravenous Acetaminophen 1 gm loading dose, then 1 gm q 6 Hrs<br>3. Ibuprofen 400 mg q6h × 48 h at home<br>4. Catheter settings:<br>• Ropivacaine 0.2%<br>• 5 mL/h plus 5 mL bolus q15–30 min<br>• If sent home with catheter, instruct patient to remove at 48–72 h |
| Elbow replacement | 1. Midazolam 4 mg IV, alfentanil 250–500 μg IV as premedication<br>2. Infraclavicular or supraclavicular catheter<br>• 20–25 mL ropivacaine 0.5%<br>• If catheter not used, supraclavicular block with 15–20 mL of bupivacaine 0.5% with epinephrine 1:300,000*<br>3. Propofol sedation 25–50 μg/kg/min | 1. Ketorolac 15 mg IV q6h while in hospital<br>2. Intravenous Acetaminophen 1 gm loading dose, then 1 gm q 6 Hrs<br>3. Ibuprofen 400 mg q6h × 48 h at home<br>4. Catheter settings:<br>• Ropivacaine 0.2%<br>• 5 mL/h plus 5 mL bolus q15–30 min |
| Creation of AV fistula | 1. Midazolam 2 mg IV, alfentanil 250–500 μg IV (premedication)<br>2. Supraclavicular block<br>• 20–25 mL mepivacaine 1.5%<br>3. Propofol sedation 25–50 μg/kg/min | Tylenol 3 (acetaminophen 300 mg/codeine 30 mg) or oxycodone 5–10 mg for breakthrough pain |
| Total hip replacement | 1. In holding area:<br>• Intravenous Acetaminophen 1 gm loading dose, then 1 gm q 6 Hrs<br>• Celecoxib 400 mg PO<br>• Gabapentin 600 mg PO<br>2. Move to operating room<br>3. Position in lateral position with operative side up<br>4. Mark skin for lumbar plexus block before sterile prep<br>5. Midazolam 2–4 mg, alfentanil 500 μg<br>6. Perform single-injection spinal anesthesia (or combined spinal-epidural)<br>• 12.5–15 mg of bupivacaine 0.5% (isobaric)<br>7. Propofol sedation 25–50 μg/kg/min | 1. Ketorolac 15 mg IV q6h × 24 h<br>2. Intravenous Acetaminophen 1 gm loading dose, then 1 gm q 6 Hrs<br>3. OxyContin 10 mg PO q12h<br>4. Oxycodone 5 mg q4h PRN for breakthrough |

(Continued)

**TABLE 6-3 Common Surgical Procedures and Analgesic Options (*Continued*)**

| SURGICAL PROCEDURE | PRE/INTRAOPERATIVE ANESTHESIA | POSTOPERATIVE ANALGESIA |
|---|---|---|
| Total knee replacement | 1. In holding area:<br>• Intravenous Acetaminophen 1 gm loading dose, then 1 gm q 6 Hrs<br>• Celecoxib 400 mg PO<br>• Gabapentin 600 mg PO<br>2. Move to operating room<br>3. Midazolam 2–4 mg, alfentanil 500 μg<br>4. Perform single-injection spinal (or combined spinal-epidural)<br>• 12.5–15 mg of bupivacaine 0.5% (isobaric)<br>5. Propofol sedation 25–50 μg/kg/min | 1. In postanesthetic care unit, perform femoral nerve catheter:<br>• Inject 15–20 mL 0.2% ropivacaine via needle or catheter as initial bolus<br>2. Catheter settings:<br>• Ropivacaine 0.2%<br>• 5 mL/h plus 5 mL bolus q1h<br>3. Following catheter placement and bolusing, evaluate pain (especially posterior knee pain). If present and VAS >3, perform sciatic nerve block via either popliteal approach or subgluteal approach using 15 mL of ropivacaine 0.2%<br>4. Ketorolac 15 mg IV q6h × 24 h<br>5. Intravenous Acetaminophen 1 gm loading dose, then 1 gm q 6Hrs<br>6. OxyContin 10 mg PO q12h2) oxycodone 5 mg q4h PRN for breakthrough pain |
| Anterior cruciate ligament repair | 1. Midazolam 2–4 mg, alfentanil 500 μg<br>2. Perform single-injection spinal (or combined spinal-epidural)<br>• 12.5–15 mg of bupivacaine 0.5% (isobaric)<br>3. Femoral nerve block (0.5% bupivacaine with 1:300,000 epinephrine 15 mL)* or<br>4. Femoral nerve catheter:<br>• Inject 15 mL 0.2% ropivacaine via needle or catheter as initial bolus<br>5. Propofol sedation 25–50 μg/kg/min | 1. Ketorolac 30 mg IV<br>2. Intravenous Acetaminophen 1 gm loading dose, then 1 gm q 6 Hrs<br>3. Instruct to take ibuprofen 400 mg q6h at home<br>4. Home femoral nerve catheter settings:<br>• Ropivacaine 0.2%<br>• 5 mL/h plus 5 mL bolus q1h<br>• Instruct patient to remove catheter at 36–48 h postoperative |
| Below-knee amputation | 1. Midazolam 2–4 mg, alfentanil 500 μg<br>2. Perform single-injection femoral nerve block<br>• 15–20 mL of ropivacaine<br>3. 0. 5% bupivacaine with 1:300,000 epinephrine 15 mL)*<br>4. Perform sciatic nerve catheter (may be done anteriorly or posteriorly, depending on habitus and ability of patient to cooperate):<br>• Inject 15–20 mL 0.5% ropivacaine via needle or catheter as initial bolus<br>5. Propofol sedation 25–50 μg/kg/min | 1. Catheter settings:<br>• Ropivacaine 0.2%<br>• 5 mL/h plus 5 mL bolus q1h<br>2. Intravenous Acetaminophen 1 gm loading dose, then 1 gm q 6 Hrs<br>3. OxyContin 10 mg PO q12h<br>4. Oxycodone 5 mg q4h PRN for breakthrough |
| ORIF ankle fracture | 1. Midazolam 2 mg IV, alfentanil 500–1000 μg IV as premedication<br>2. Position patient supine or oblique<br>3. Lateral popliteal block<br>• 20–30 mL ropivacaine 0.5%<br>4. Supplementary saphenous block (e.g., ultrasound-guided at adductor canal)<br>• 10 mL lidocaine 2%. Propofol sedation 25–50 μg/kg/min | 1. Ketorolac 15 mg IV q6h × 24 h<br>2. Intravenous Acetaminophen 1 gm loading dose, then 1 gm q 6 Hrs<br>3. OxyContin 10 mg PO q12h<br>4. Oxycodone 5 mg q4h PRN for breakthrough |

*Bupivacaine is increasingly used in our practice when longer duration of analgesia is desired. With ultrasound guidance, the doses and volumes required for successful block can be substantially reduced, thus reducing the risk for severe systemic toxicity.
AV, arteriovenous; ORIF, open reduction and internal fixation; VAS, visual analog scale.

operating room immediately prior to the surgical procedure. Catheters for upper limb surgery are usually placed in a similar manner if the technique is used for surgical anesthesia as well. In contrast, most of our lower limb nerve blocks or catheters are placed in the postanesthesia care unit *before* the resolution of the neuraxial block. Although the practice of performing blocks in anesthetized patients (in this case in the presence of spinal anesthesia), we believe that when modern monitoring is used (combination of ultrasound, nerve stimulation, and injection pressure monitoring), it is irrelevant whether the blocks are performed in anesthetized or nonanesthetized patients.

Finally, we do not routinely combine general anesthesia with regional anesthesia, although this is a widely used practice elsewhere. Our regional anesthetics are often used as the primary anesthesia modality, rather then solely for the purpose of postoperative analgesia. Instead of general anesthesia, we typically use sedation with propofol and/or intravenous midazolam titrated to light sleep and spontaneous breathing with supplemental oxygen via a facemask. Table 6-3 lists some common surgical procedures, peripheral nerve blocks that are suitable for anesthesia and analgesia, as well as other common analgesic options.

## Section III: Compendium of the Literature

The previous two sections described some of the most common indications for peripheral nerve blocks in our practice. However, the usefulness of peripheral nerve blocks is much greater than the few common ones discussed here. For the sake of completeness, the compendium of indications for peripheral nerve blocks reported in medical literature is listed in the accompanying chart. Readers should use their own discretion when determining whether any indications would fit the realm of their own clinical practice.

### I. INDICATIONS FOR CERVICAL PLEXUS BLOCK

Vocal cord surgery - medialization thyroplasty[1]
Cervicogenic headache[2]
Carotid endarterectomy[3]
Zenker diverticulum excision in a patient with ankylosing spondylitis[4]
Drainage of dental abscess in adults with difficult airways[5]
Drainage of submandibular and submental abscesses[6]
Minimally invasive parathyroidectomy[7]
Carotid body tumor excision in a patient with Eisenmenger syndrome[8]
Postoperative analgesia after clavicle surgery[9]
Thyroid surgery under general anesthesia[10]
Management of neuropathic cancer pain[11]

### II. INDICATIONS FOR INTERSCALENE BRACHIAL PLEXUS BLOCK

Reduction of shoulder dislocation[12]
Treatment of shoulder adhesive capsulitis[13]
Post-thoracotomy shoulder pain[14]
Open shoulder surgery[15]
Ambulatory shoulder surgery[16]
Venodilatation in the creation of upper extremity arteriovenous fistulae[17]
Outpatient rotator cuff surgery[18]

### III. INDICATIONS FOR SUPRACLAVICULAR BRACHIAL PLEXUS BLOCK

Emergency department patients with fractures, dislocations, or abscesses of the upper extremities[19]
Sole anesthetic technique for children undergoing closed reduction of arm fractures[20]
Surgery on upper extremities[21]
Upper limb surgery[22,23]

### IV. INDICATIONS FOR INFRACLAVICULAR BRACHIAL PLEXUS BLOCK

Elective hand surgery[24-28]
Forearm surgeries[26,27]
Wrist surgery[26,28]
Forearm and hand surgeries in children[29,30]
Arteriovenous fistula at the lateral aspect of the distal forearm[31]
Complex regional pain syndrome type I[32]
Blockade in dermatomes C5-T1[33]
Analgesia or anesthesia of all five nerves distal to the elbow[34]
Emergency upper limb surgery[35]

(Continued)

## V. INDICATIONS FOR AXILLARY BLOCK

Ambulatory surgery at or below the elbow[36-38]
Elective hand surgery[39-43]
Emergency surgery of the upper arm[44]
Forearm surgery[41]
Creation of an arteriovenous fistula at the lateral aspect of the distal forearm[31]
Postoperative pain control and rigorous physiotherapy (children/continuous)[45]
Routine surgery and reimplantation of fingers, hand, or forearm[46]
Distal upper extremity surgery[47]
Fracture of the distal radius[48]
Double corrective osteotomy of the humerus[49]
Pain relief and sympatholysis in patients suffering from CRPS[50]
Ulnar nerve transposition surgery[51]
Treatment of severe limb ischemia after arterial catheterization in neonates and premature infants[52]
Preexisting ulnar neuropathy in patients undergoing ulnar nerve transposition[53]
Improve circulation in peripheral microvascular interventions[54]
Immobilization of the upper extremities at groin flap coverage[55]
Manipulation of forearm fractures in children[56]

## VI. INDICATIONS FOR WRIST BLOCK

Flexor and extensor tenolysis depends on postoperative hand rehabilitation[57]
Pain free active early mobilization after hand surgery[58]
Ambulatory endoscopic carpal tunnel release[59-62]
Treatment of palmar hyperhidrosis with botulinum toxin type A (BTX A) injections[63,64]
Exploring complex wounds of the hand[65]
Repair of hand injuries[66]
Common problems of the hands and fingers (fractures, lacerations, and infections requiring drainage)[67]
Functional treatment after operations at gliding structures (tendons) or periarticular structures[68]
Management of finger ulcers in scleroderma[69]
Control of vasospasm following trauma and microvascular surgery[70]
Sympathetic blockade following replantation and revascularization of the digits[71]

## VII. INDICATIONS FOR DIGITAL BLOCK

Digital injuries[72,73]
Excision of a mucous cyst of the index finger[74]
Injuries to the fingers and to the palmar aspect of the thumb[75]
Raynaud disease[76]
Immediate pain-free mobilization after tenolysis or tenosynovectomy in zone II[77]

## VIII. INDICATIONS FOR THORACIC PARAVERTEBRAL BLOCK

Pain relief for thoracotomy[78–80]
Major breast surgery[81–83]
Implantable cardioverter defibrillator and laser lead extraction[84]
Right lobe hepatectomy[85]
Postoperative analgesia after robotic-assisted coronary artery bypass graft[86]
Open cholecystectomy[87]
Abdominoplasty[88]
Submuscular breast augmentation[89]
Radiofrequency ablation of a metastatic carcinoid liver lesion[90]
Single-injection/continuous block technique for major renal surgery in children[91,92]
Thymectomy performed with a bilateral thoracoscopic approach[93]
Video-assisted thoracic surgery procedures[94]
Percutaneous transhepatic biliary drainage[95]
Thoracoabdominal esophageal surgery[96]
Conventional on-pump cardiac surgery[97]

*(Continued)*

Multiple rib fracture[98,99]
Minimally invasive direct coronary artery bypass surgery[100]
Pleuritic pain[101]
Esophagogastrectomy[102]

## IX. INDICATIONS FOR THORACOLUMBAR PARAVERTEBRAL BLOCK

Outpatient lithotripsy[103]
Inguinal hernia repair[104]
Ventral hernia repair[105]
Hip arthroscopy[106]
Femoral-popliteal bypass in high-risk patient[107]
Labor analgesia[108,109]

## X. INDICATIONS FOR LUMBAR PLEXUS BLOCK

Urologic surgeries (with flank incision)[110]
Open reduction internal fixation of hip fracture[111–113]
Pain management after total hip or knee arthroplasty114
Hip arthroplasty[115,116]
Continuous block for analgesia after total hip arthroplasty[114,116–119]
Anesthesia and analgesia of proximal part of lower limb[120]
Percutaneous renal procedures[121]
Analgesia for labor[122]
Treatment for flexor spasticity of hip[123]
Infrainguinal artery bypass graft surgery[124]
Femoral-popliteal bypass in high-risk patients[107]
Knee arthroplasty[125]
Lower limb surgery in children[126]
Surgery in the hip region (children)[127]

## XI. INDICATIONS FOR SCIATIC NERVE BLOCK

Minor knee surgery[128]
Outpatient knee arthroscopy and knee arthroplasty[129–131]
Foot surgery[132]
Leg amputation[133]
Femoral-popliteal bypass in high-risk patients[107]
Intractable stump pain[134]
Bilateral lower limb amputation[135]
Hallux valgus repair[136]
Saphenous vein stripping[137]

## XII. INDICATIONS FOR FEMORAL NERVE BLOCK

Outpatient knee arthroscopy[130,131]
Knee arthroplasty[129,138]
Total knee replacement[139–141]
Anterior cruciate ligament reconstruction[142]
Analgesia in emergency department for diaphyseal or distal femoral fractures[143]
Major knee surgery[144]
Leg amputation[133]
Patellar realignment surgery[145]
Awake off pump coronary artery bypass grafting (CABG)[146,147]
Fractured femur in children[148]
Saphenous vein stripping[137]
Preclinical administration for severe knee trauma[149]

(*Continued*)

## XIII. INDICATIONS FOR OTHER LOWER LIMB NERVE BLOCKS

*Medial or Lateral Cutaneous Antebrachial Nerve Block*
Insertion or revision of a forearm Gortex arteriovenous fistula[150]

*Lateral Femoral Cutaneous Nerve*
Skin split grafting[151,152]
Muscle biopsy for determination of susceptibility to malignant hyperthermia[153]
Osteosynthesis of femur neck fracture[154]
Meralgia paresthetica[155,156]
Combined block of femoral, sciatic, obturator nerves, and the lateral cutaneous nerve for above-knee amputation[157]

*Posterior Cutaneous Nerve of the Thigh*
Short saphenous vein stripping[158]

*Saphenous Nerve Block*
Postmeniscectomy pain relief: analgesic method for arthroscopic interventions[159]
Foot and ankle surgery (in association with popliteal nerve block)160
Lower leg and ankle[161]

*Ankle Block*
Foot surgery[160,162,163]
Mid- and forefoot surgery[164,165]

## XIV. INDICATIONS FOR INTRAVENOUS REGIONAL ANESTHESIA

Outpatient hand surgery[166]
Cases involving the hand, forearm, foot, and lower leg that last ≥60 min[167]
Limb surgery in the ambulatory patient[168]
Complex regional pain syndrome (CRPS) type 1[169–171]
Upper extremity fractures and dislocations[172]
Treatment of children's upper extremity fractures in the emergency department[173]
Ambulatory management of fractures in children[174]
Pain relief in the treatment of patients with palmar hyperhidrosis with brevetoxin (BTX)-A[175,176]
Treating distal radius fractures in adults[177]
Management of complex regional pain syndrome (CRPS) of the knee[178]
Management of forearm injuries (i.e., forearm, wrist, or hand)[179]

## REFERENCES


1. Suresh S, Templeton L. Superficial cervical plexus block for vocal cord surgery in an awake pediatric patient. *Anesth Analg.* 2004;98:1656-1657.
2. Goldberg ME, Schwartzman RJ, Domsky R, Sabia M, Torjman MC. Deep cervical plexus block for the treatment of cervicogenic headache. *Pain Physician.* 2008;11:849-854.
3. Stoneham MD, Knighton JD. Regional anaesthesia for carotid endarterectomy. *Br J Anaesth.* 1999;82:910-919.
4. Naja ZM, Al-Tannir MA, Zeidan A, et al. Bilateral guided cervical block for Zenker diverticulum excision in a patient with ankylosing spondylitis. *J Anesth.* 2009;23:143-146.
5. Ling KU, Hasan MS, Ha KO, Wang CY. Superficial cervical plexus block combined with auriculotemporal nerve block for drainage of dental abscess in adults with difficult airways. *Anaesth Intensive Care.* 2009;37:124-126.
6. Shteif M, Lesmes D, Hartman G, Ruffino S, Laster Z. The use of the superficial cervical plexus block in the drainage of submandibular and submental abscesses—an alternative for general anesthesia. *J Oral Maxillofac Surg.* 2008;66:2642-2645.
7. Pintaric TS, Hocevar M, Jereb S, Casati A, Jankovic VN. A prospective, randomized comparison between combined (deep and superficial) and superficial cervical plexus block with levobupivacaine for minimally invasive parathyroidectomy. *Anesth Analg.* 2007;105:1160-1163; table of contents.
8. Jones HG, Stoneham MD. Continuous cervical plexus block for carotid body tumour excision in a patient with Eisenmenger's syndrome. *Anaesthesia.* 2006;61:1214-1218.
9. Choi DS, Atchabahian A, Brown AR. Cervical plexus block provides postoperative analgesia after clavicle surgery. *Anesth Analg.* 2005;100:1542-1543.
10. Aunac S, Carlier M, Singelyn F, De Kock M. The analgesic efficacy of bilateral combined superficial and deep cervical plexus block administered before thyroid surgery under general anesthesia. *Anesth Analg.* 2002;95:746-750.
11. Nadig M, Ekatodramis G, Borgeat A. Continuous brachial plexus block at the cervical level using a posterior approach in the management of neuropathic cancer pain. *Reg Anesth Pain Med.* 2002;27:446; author reply 446-447.
12. Christiansen TG, Nielsen R. Reduction of shoulder dislocations under interscalene brachial blockade. *Arch Orthop Trauma Surg.* 1988;107:176-177.
13. Roubal PJ, Dobritt D, Placzek JD. Glenohumeral gliding manipulation following interscalene brachial plexus block in patients with adhesive capsulitis. *J Orthop Sports Phys Ther.* 1996;24:66-77.
14. Barak M, Iaroshevski D, Poppa E, Ben-Nun A, Katz Y. Low-volume interscalene brachial plexus block for post-thoracotomy shoulder pain. *J Cardiothorac Vasc Anesth.* 2007;21:554-557.

15. Casati A, Borghi B, Fanelli G, et al. Interscalene brachial plexus anesthesia and analgesia for open shoulder surgery: a randomized, double-blinded comparison between levobupivacaine and ropivacaine. *Anesth Analg.* 2003;96:253-259.
16. Faryniarz D, Morelli C, Coleman S, et al. Interscalene block anesthesia at an ambulatory surgery center performing predominantly regional anesthesia: a prospective study of one hundred thirty-three patients undergoing shoulder surgery. *J Shoulder Elbow Surg.* 2006;15:686-690.
17. Hingorani AP, Ascher E, Gupta P, et al. Regional anesthesia: preferred technique for venodilatation in the creation of upper extremity arteriovenous fistulae. *Vascular.* 2006;14:23-26.
18. Hadzic A, Williams BA, Karaca PE, et al. For outpatient rotator cuff surgery, nerve block anesthesia provides superior same-day recovery over general anesthesia. *Anesthesiology.* 2005;102:1001-1007.
19. Stone MB, Price DD, Wang R. Ultrasound-guided supraclavicular block for the treatment of upper extremity fractures, dislocations, and abscesses in the ED. *Am J Emerg Med.* 2007;25:472-475.
20. Harmon D, Frizelle HP. Supraclavicular block for day-case anaesthesia at altitude. *Anaesthesia.* 2001;56:197.
21. Ortells-Polo MA, Garcia-Guiral M, Garcia-Amigueti FJ, Carral-Olondris JN, Garcia-Godino T, Aguiar-Mojarro JA. Brachial plexus anesthesia: results of a modified perivascular supraclavicular technique [in Spanish]. *Rev Esp Anestesiol Reanim.* 1996;43:94-98.
22. Rigal MC, Esteve E, Alran R, Pech C. Brachial plexus block anesthesia in the upper limb surgery [author's translation]. *Anesth Analg (Paris).* 1979;36:231-234.
23. Thompson AM, Newman RJ, Semple JC. Brachial plexus anaesthesia for upper limb surgery: a review of eight years' experience. *J Hand Surg Br.* 1988;13:195-198.
24. Dhir S, Ganapathy S. Comparative evaluation of ultrasound-guided continuous infraclavicular brachial plexus block with stimulating catheter and traditional technique: a prospective-randomized trial. *Acta Anaesthesiol Scand.* 2008;52:1158-1166.
25. Morimoto M, Popovic J, Kim JT, Kiamzon H, Rosenberg AD. Case series: Septa can influence local anesthetic spread during infraclavicular brachial plexus blocks. *Can J Anaesth.* 2007;54:1006-1010.
26. Gurkan Y, Hosten T, Solak M, Toker K. Lateral sagittal infraclavicular block: clinical experience in 380 patients. *Acta Anaesthesiol Scand.* 2008;52:262-266.
27. Dingemans E, Williams SR, Arcand G, et al. Neurostimulation in ultrasound-guided infraclavicular block: a prospective randomized trial. *Anesth Analg.* 2007;104:1275-1280.
28. Hadžić A, Arliss J, Kerimoglu B, et al. A comparison of infraclavicular nerve block versus general anesthesia for hand and wrist day-case surgeries. *Anesthesiology.* 2004;101:127-132.
29. De Jose Maria B, Banus E, Navarro Egea M, Serrano S, Perello M, Mabrok M. Ultrasound-guided supraclavicular vs infraclavicular brachial plexus blocks in children. *Paediatr Anaesth.* 2008;18:838-844.
30. Ponde VC. Continuous infraclavicular brachial plexus block: a modified technique to better secure catheter position in infants and children. *Anesth Analg.* 2008;106:94-96; table of contents.
31. Niemi TT, Salmela L, Aromaa U, Poyhia R, Rosenberg PH. Single-injection brachial plexus anesthesia for arteriovenous fistula surgery of the forearm: a comparison of infraclavicular coracoid and axillary approach. *Reg Anesth Pain Med.* 2007;32:55-59.
32. Day M, Pasupuleti R, Jacobs S. Infraclavicular brachial plexus block and infusion for treatment of long-standing complex regional syndrome type 1: a case report. *Pain Physician.* 2004;7:265-268.
33. Rettig HC, Gielen MJ, Boersma E, Klein J. A comparison of the vertical infraclavicular and axillary approaches for brachial plexus anaesthesia. *Acta Anaesthesiol Scand.* 2005;49:1501-1508.
34. Sauter AR, Dodgson MS, Stubhaug A, Halstensen AM, Klaastad O. Electrical nerve stimulation or ultrasound guidance for lateral sagittal infraclavicular blocks: a randomized, controlled, observer-blinded, comparative study. *Anesth Analg.* 2008;106:1910-1915.
35. Minville V, Fourcade O, Bourdet B, et al. The optimal motor response for infraclavicular brachial plexus block. *Anesth Analg.* 2007;104:448-451.
36. Rodriguez J, Taboada M, Oliveira J, Ulloa B, Bascuas B, Alvarez J. Radial plus musculocutaneous nerve stimulation for axillary block is inferior to triple nerve stimulation with 2% mepivacaine. *J Clin Anesth.* 2008;20:253-256.
37. Kang SB, Rumball KM, Ettinger RS. Continuous axillary brachial plexus analgesia in a patient with severe hemophilia. *J Clin Anesth.* 2003;15:38-40.
38. Brown AR. Anaesthesia for procedures of the hand and elbow. *Best Pract Res Clin Anaesthesiol.* 2002;16:227-246.
39. Chan VW, Perlas A, McCartney CJ, Brull R, Xu D, Abbas S. Ultrasound guidance improves success rate of axillary brachial plexus block. *Can J Anaesth.* 2007;54:176-182.
40. Andersson A, Akeson J, Dahlin LB. Efficacy and safety of axillary brachial plexus block for operations on the hand. *Scand J Plast Reconstr Surg Hand Surg.* 2006;40:225-229.
41. Freitag M, Zbieranek K, Gottschalk A, et al. Comparative study of different concentrations of prilocaine and ropivacaine for intraoperative axillary brachial plexus block. *Eur J Anaesthesiol.* 2006;23:481-486.
42. Schwemmer U, Schleppers A, Markus C, Kredel M, Kirschner S, Roewer N. Operative management in axillary brachial plexus blocks: comparison of ultrasound and nerve stimulation [in German]. *Anaesthesist.* 2006;55:451-456.
43. Kefalianakis F, Spohner F. Ultrasound-guided blockade of axillary plexus brachialis for hand surgery [in German]. *Handchir Mikrochir Plast Chir.* 2005;37:344-348.
44. Fuzier R, Fourcade O, Pianezza A, Gilbert ML, Bounes V, Olivier M. A comparison between double-injection axillary brachial plexus block and midhumeral block for emergency upper limb surgery. *Anesth Analg.* 2006;102:1856-1858.
45. Theroux MC, Dixit D, Brislin R, Como-Fluero S, Sacks K. Axillary catheter for brachial plexus analgesia in children for postoperative pain control and rigorous physiotherapy—a simple and effective procedure. *Paediatr Anaesth.* 2007;17:302-303.
46. Kjelstrup T. Transarterial block as an addition to a conventional catheter technique improves the axillary block. *Acta Anaesthesiol Scand.* 2006;50:112-116.
47. Lim WS, Gammack JK, Van Niekerk J, Dangour AD. Omega 3 fatty acid for the prevention of dementia. *Cochrane Database Syst Rev.* 2006:CD005379.
48. Woods RK, Thien FC, Abramson MJ. Dietary marine fatty acids (fish oil) for asthma in adults and children. *Cochrane Database Syst Rev.* 2002:CD001283.
49. Bullmann V, Waurick R, Rodl R, et al. Corrective osteotomy of the humerus using perivascular axillary anesthesia according to Weber in a patient suffering from McCune-Albright syndrome [in German]. *Anaesthesist.* 2005;54:889-894.
50. Gradl G, Beyer A, Azad S, Schurmann M. Evaluation of sympathicolysis after continuous brachial plexus analgesia using laser Doppler flowmetry in patients suffering from CRPS I [in German]. *Anasthesiol Intensivmed Notfallmed Schmerzther.* 2005;40:345-349.
51. Liu HT, Yu YS, Liu CK, et al. Delayed recovery of radial nerve function after axillary block in a patient receiving ipsilateral ulnar nerve transposition surgery. *Acta Anaesthesiol Taiwan.* 2005;43:49-53.

52. Breschan C, Kraschl R, Jost R, Marhofer P, Likar R. Axillary brachial plexus block for treatment of severe forearm ischemia after arterial cannulation in an extremely low birth-weight infant. *Paediatr Anaesth.* 2004;14:681-684.
53. Hebl JR, Horlocker TT, Sorenson EJ, Schroeder DR. Regional anesthesia does not increase the risk of postoperative neuropathy in patients undergoing ulnar nerve transposition. *Anesth Analg.* 2001;93:1606-1611.
54. van den Berg B, Berger A, van den Berg E, Zenz M, Brehmeier G, Tizian C. Continuous plexus anesthesia to improve circulation in peripheral microvascular interventions [in German]. *Handchir Mikrochir Plast Chir.* 1983;15:101-104.
55. Bekler H, Beyzadeoglu T, Mercan A. Groin flap immobilization by axillary brachial plexus block anesthesia. *Tech Hand Up Extrem Surg.* 2008;12:68-70.
56. Kriwanek KL, Wan J, Beaty JH, Pershad J. Axillary block for analgesia during manipulation of forearm fractures in the pediatric emergency department: a prospective randomized comparative trial. *J Pediatr Orthop.* 2006;26:737-740.
57. Jablecki J, Syrko M. The application of nerve block in early post-operative rehabilitation after tenolysis of the flexor tendon. *Ortop Traumatol Rehabil.* 2005;7:646-650.
58. Broekhuysen CL, Fechner MR, Kerkkamp HE. The use of a selective peripheral median nerve block for pain-free early active motion after hand surgery. *J Hand Surg Am.* 2006;31:857-859.
59. Macaire P, Choquet O, Jochum D, Travers V, Capdevila X. Nerve blocks at the wrist for carpal tunnel release revisited: the use of sensory-nerve and motor-nerve stimulation techniques. *Reg Anesth Pain Med.* 2005;30:536-540.
60. Gebhard RE, Al-Samsam T, Greger J, Khan A, Chelly JE. Distal nerve blocks at the wrist for outpatient carpal tunnel surgery offer intraoperative cardiovascular stability and reduce discharge time. *Anesth Analg.* 2002;95:351-355.
61. Delaunay L, Chelly JE. Blocks at the wrist provide effective anesthesia for carpal tunnel release. *Can J Anaesth.* 2001;48:656-660.
62. Derkash RS, Weaver JK, Berkeley ME, Dawson D. Office carpal tunnel release with wrist block and wrist tourniquet. *Orthopedics.* 1996;19:589-590.
63. Siebert T, Sinkgraven R, Fuchslocher M, Rzany B. Efficacy, side effects and patient satisfaction with wrist conduction block anaesthesia prior to the treatment of palmar hyperhidrosis with botulinum toxin type A [in German]. *J Dtsch Dermatol Ges.* 2003;1:876-883.
64. Campanati A, Lagalla G, Penna L, Gesuita R, Offidani A. Local neural block at the wrist for treatment of palmar hyperhidrosis with botulinum toxin: technical improvements. *J Am Acad Dermatol.* 2004;51:345-348.
65. Thompson WL, Malchow RJ. Peripheral nerve blocks and anesthesia of the hand. *Mil Med.* 2002;167:478-482.
66. Ferrera PC, Chandler R. Anesthesia in the emergency setting: Part I. Hand and foot injuries. *Am Fam Physician.* 1994;50:569-573.
67. Leversee JH, Bergman JJ. Wrist and digital nerve blocks. *J Fam Pract.* 1981;13:415-421.
68. Braun C, Henneberger G, Racenberg E. Techniques of continuous nerve block at the level of the wrist [in French]. *Ann Chir Main Memb Super.* 1992;11:141-145.
69. Ward WA, Van Moore A. Management of finger ulcers in scleroderma. *J Hand Surg Am.* 1995;20:868-872.
70. Phelps DB, Rutherford RB, Boswick JA Jr. Control of vasospasm following trauma and microvascular surgery. *J Hand Surg Am.* 1979;4:109-117.
71. Taras JS, Behrman MJ. Continuous peripheral nerve block in replantation and revascularization. *J Reconstr Microsurg.* 1998;14:17-21.
72. Hart RG, Fernandas FA, Kutz JE. Transthecal digital block: an underutilized technique in the ED. *Am J Emerg Med.* 2005;23:340-342.
73. Keramidas EG, Rodopoulou SG, Tsoutsos D, Miller G, Ioannovich J. Comparison of transthecal digital block and traditional digital block for anesthesia of the finger. *Plast Reconstr Surg.* 2004;114:1131-1134; discussion 1135-1136.
74. Harness NG. Digital block anesthesia. *J Hand Surg Am.* 2009;34:142-145.
75. Kollersbeck C, Walcher T, Gradl G, Genelin F. Clinical experiences and dosage pattern in subcutaneous single-injection digital block technique [in German]. *Handchir Mikrochir Plast Chir.* 2004;36:64-66.
76. Freedman RR, Mayes MD, Sabharwal SC. Digital nerve blockade in Raynaud's disease. *Circulation.* 1989;80:1923-1924.
77. Kirchhoff R, Jensen PB, Nielsen NS, Boeckstyns ME. Repeated digital nerve block for pain control after tenolysis. *Scand J Plast Reconstr Surg Hand Surg.* 2000;34:257-258.
78. Daly DJ, Myles PS. Update on the role of paravertebral blocks for thoracic surgery: are they worth it? *Curr Opin Anaesthesiol.* 2009;22:38-43.
79. Davies RG, Myles PS, Graham JM. A comparison of the analgesic efficacy and side-effects of paravertebral vs epidural blockade for thoracotomy—a systematic review and meta-analysis of randomized trials. *Br J Anaesth.* 2006;96:418-426.
80. Joshi GP, Bonnet F, Shah R, et al. A systematic review of randomized trials evaluating regional techniques for postthoracotomy analgesia. *Anesth Analg.* 2008;107:1026-1040.
81. Boezaart AP, Raw RM. Continuous thoracic paravertebral block for major breast surgery. *Reg Anesth Pain Med.* 2006;31:470-476.
82. Pusch F, Freitag H, Weinstabl C, Obwegeser R, Huber E, Wildling E. Single-injection paravertebral block compared to general anaesthesia in breast surgery. *Acta Anaesthesiol Scand.* 1999;43:770-774.
83. Coveney E, Weltz CR, Greengrass R, et al. Use of paravertebral block anesthesia in the surgical management of breast cancer: experience in 156 cases. *Ann Surg.* 1998;227:496-501.
84. Tsai T, Rodriguez-Diaz C, Deschner B, Thomas K, Wasnick JD. Thoracic paravertebral block for implantable cardioverter-defibrillator and laser lead extraction. *J Clin Anesth.* 2008;20:379-382.
85. Moussa AA. Opioid saving strategy: bilateral single-site thoracic paravertebral block in right lobe donor hepatectomy. *Middle East J Anesthesiol.* 2008;19:789-801.
86. Mehta Y, Arora D, Sharma KK, Mishra Y, Wasir H, Trehan N. Comparison of continuous thoracic epidural and paravertebral block for postoperative analgesia after robotic-assisted coronary artery bypass surgery. *Ann Card Anaesth.* 2008;11:91-96.
87. Serpetinis I, Bassiakou E, Xanthos T, Baltatzi L, Kouta A. Paravertebral block for open cholecystectomy in patients with cardiopulmonary pathology. *Acta Anaesthesiol Scand.* 2008;52:872-873.
88. Rudkin GE, Gardiner SE, Cooter RD. Bilateral thoracic paravertebral block for abdominoplasty. *J Clin Anesth.* 2008;20:54-56.
89. Cooter RD, Rudkin GE, Gardiner SE. Day case breast augmentation under paravertebral blockade: a prospective study of 100 consecutive patients. *Aesthetic Plast Surg.* 2007;31:666-673.
90. Culp WC, Payne MN, Montgomery ML. Thoracic paravertebral block for analgesia following liver mass radiofrequency ablation. *Br J Radiol.* 2008;81:e23-e25.
91. Berta E, Spanhel J, Smakal O, Smolka V, Gabrhelik T, Lonnqvist PA. Single injection paravertebral block for renal surgery in children. *Paediatr Anaesth.* 2008;18:593-597.

92. Lonnqvist PA, Olsson GL. Paravertebral vs epidural block in children. Effects on postoperative morphine requirement after renal surgery. *Acta Anaesthesiol Scand.* 1994;38:346-349.
93. Lopez-Berlanga JL, Garutti I, Martinez-Campos E, Pineiro P, Salvatierra D. Bilateral paravertebral block anesthesia for thymectomy by video-assisted thoracoscopy in patients with myasthenia gravis [in Spanish]. *Rev Esp Anestesiol Reanim.* 2006;53:571-574.
94. Kaya FN, Turker G, Basagan-Mogol E, Goren S, Bayram S, Gebitekin C. Preoperative multiple-injection thoracic paravertebral blocks reduce postoperative pain and analgesic requirements after video-assisted thoracic surgery. *J Cardiothorac Vasc Anesth.* 2006;20:639-643.
95. Culp WC Jr, Culp WC. Thoracic paravertebral block for percutaneous transhepatic biliary drainage. *J Vasc Interv Radiol.* 2005;16:1397-1400.
96. Kelly FE, Murdoch JA, Sanders DJ, Berrisford RG. Continuous paravertebral block for thoraco-abdominal oesophageal surgery. *Anaesthesia.* 2005;60:98-99.
97. Canto M, Sanchez MJ, Casas MA, Bataller ML. Bilateral paravertebral blockade for conventional cardiac surgery. *Anaesthesia.* 2003;58:365-e70.
98. Karmakar MK, Ho AM. Acute pain management of patients with multiple fractured ribs. *J Trauma.* 2003;54:615-625.
99. Karmakar MK, Critchley LA, Ho AM, Gin T, Lee TW, Yim AP. Continuous thoracic paravertebral infusion of bupivacaine for pain management in patients with multiple fractured ribs. *Chest.* 2003;123:424-431.
100. Dhole S, Mehta Y, Saxena H, Juneja R, Trehan N. Comparison of continuous thoracic epidural and paravertebral blocks for postoperative analgesia after minimally invasive direct coronary artery bypass surgery. *J Cardiothorac Vasc Anesth.* 2001;15:288-292.
101. Paniagua P, Catala E, Villar Landeira JM. Successful management of pleuritic pain with thoracic paravertebral block. *Reg Anesth Pain Med.* 2000;25:651-653.
102. Sabanathan S, Shah R, Tsiamis A, Richardson J. Oesophagogastrectomy in the elderly high risk patients: role of effective regional analgesia and early mobilisation. *J Cardiovasc Surg (Torino).* 1999;40:153-156.
103. Jamieson BD, Mariano ER. Thoracic and lumbar paravertebral blocks for outpatient lithotripsy. *J Clin Anesth.* 2007;19:149-151.
104. Weltz CR, Klein SM, Arbo JE, Greengrass RA. Paravertebral block anesthesia for inguinal hernia repair. *World J Surg.* 2003;27:425-429.
105. Naja Z, Ziade MF, Lonnqvist PA. Bilateral paravertebral somatic nerve block for ventral hernia repair. *Eur J Anaesthesiol.* 2002;19:197-202.
106. Lee EM, Murphy KP, Ben-David B. Postoperative analgesia for hip arthroscopy: combined L1 and L2 paravertebral blocks. *J Clin Anesth.* 2008;20:462-465.
107. Basagan-Mogol E, Turker G, Yilmaz M, Goren S. Combination of a psoas compartment, sciatic nerve, and T12-L1 paravertebral blocks for femoropopliteal bypass surgery in a high-risk patient. *J Cardiothorac Vasc Anesth.* 2008;22:337-339.
108. Nair V, Henry R. Bilateral paravertebral block: a satisfactory alternative for labour analgesia. *Can J Anaesth.* 2001;48:179-184.
109. Suelto MD, Shaw DB. Labor analgesia with paravertebral lumbar sympathetic block. *Reg Anesth Pain Med.* 1999;24:179-181.
110. Akin S, Aribogan A, Turunc T, Aridogan A. Lumbar plexus blockade with ropivacaine for postoperative pain management in elderly patients undergoing urologic surgeries. *Urol Int.* 2005;75:345-349.
111. Asao Y, Higuchi T, Tsubaki N, Shimoda Y. Combined paravertebral lumbar plexus and parasacral sciatic nerve block for reduction of hip fracture in four patients with severe heart failure [in Japanese]. *Masui.* 2005;54:648-652.
112. Ho AM, Karmakar MK. Combined paravertebral lumbar plexus and parasacral sciatic nerve block for reduction of hip fracture in a patient with severe aortic stenosis. *Can J Anaesth.* 2002;49:946-950.
113. Morimoto M, Kim JT, Popovic J, Jain S, Bekker A. Ultrasound-guided lumbar plexus block for open reduction and internal fixation of hip fracture. *Pain Pract.* 2006;6:124-126.
114. Bogoch ER, Henke M, Mackenzie T, Olschewski E, Mahomed NN. Lumbar paravertebral nerve block in the management of pain after total hip and knee arthroplasty: a randomized controlled clinical trial. *J Arthroplasty.* 2002;17:398-401.
115. Stevens RD, Van Gessel E, Flory N, Fournier R, Gamulin Z. Lumbar plexus block reduces pain and blood loss associated with total hip arthroplasty. *Anesthesiology.* 2000;93:115-121.
116. Siddiqui ZI, Cepeda MS, Denman W, Schumann R, Carr DB. Continuous lumbar plexus block provides improved analgesia with fewer side effects compared with systemic opioids after hip arthroplasty: a randomized controlled trial. *Reg Anesth Pain Med.* 2007;32:393-398.
117. Marino J, Russo J, Kenny M, Herenstein R, Livote E, Chelly JE. Continuous lumbar plexus block for postoperative pain control after total hip arthroplasty. A randomized controlled trial. *J Bone Joint Surg Am.* 2009;91:29-37.
118. Capdevila X, Macaire P, Dadure C, et al. Continuous psoas compartment block for postoperative analgesia after total hip arthroplasty: new landmarks, technical guidelines, and clinical evaluation. *Anesth Analg.* 2002;94:1606-1613.
119. Ilfeld BM, Ball ST, Gearen PF, et al. Ambulatory continuous posterior lumbar plexus nerve blocks after hip arthroplasty: a dual-center, randomized, triple-masked, placebo-controlled trial. *Anesthesiology.* 2008;109:491-501.
120. Zetlaoui PJ. Block of the lumbar plexus [in French]. *Cah Anesthesiol.* 1994;42:771-780.
121. Mongan PD, Strong WE, Menk EJ. Anesthesia for percutaneous renal procedures. *Reg Anesth.* 1991;16:296-298.
122. Meguiar RV, Wheeler AS. Lumbar sympathetic block with bupivacaine: analgesia for labor. *Anesth Analg.* 1978;57:486-492.
123. Meelhuysen FE, Halpern D, Quast J. Treatment of flexor spasticity of hip by paravertebral lumbar spinal nerve block. *Arch Phys Med Rehabil.* 1968;49:717-722.
124. Asakura Y, Kandatsu N, Kato N, Sato Y, Fujiwara Y, Komatsu T. Ultra-sound guided sciatic nerve block combined with lumbar plexus block for infra-inguinal artery bypass graft surgery. *Acta Anaesthesiol Scand.* 2008;52:721-722.
125. Campbell A, McCormick M, McKinlay K, Scott NB. Epidural vs. lumbar plexus infusions following total knee arthroplasty: randomized controlled trial. *Eur J Anaesthesiol.* 2008;25:502-507.
126. Mello SS, Saraiva RA, Marques RS, Gasparini JR, Assis CN, Goncalves MH. Posterior lumbar plexus block in children: a new anatomical landmark. *Reg Anesth Pain Med.* 2007;32:522-527.
127. Dalens B, Tanguy A, Vanneuville G. Lumbar plexus block in children: a comparison of two procedures in 50 patients. *Anesth Analg.* 1988;67:750-758.
128. Ota J, Sakura S, Hara K, Saito Y. Ultrasound-guided anterior approach to sciatic nerve block: a comparison with the posterior approach. *Anesth Analg.* 2009;108:660-665.
129. del Fresno Caniaveras J, Campos A, Galiana M, Navarro-Martinez JA, Company R. Postoperative analgesia in knee arthroplasty using an anterior sciatic nerve block and a femoral nerve block [in Spanish]. *Rev Esp Anestesiol Reanim.* 2008;55:548-551.
130. Montes FR, Zarate E, Grueso R, et al. Comparison of spinal anesthesia with combined sciatic-femoral nerve block for outpatient knee arthroscopy. *J Clin Anesth.* 2008;20:415-420.
131. Casati A, Cappelleri G, Fanelli G, et al. Regional anaesthesia for outpatient knee arthroscopy: a randomized clinical comparison of two different anaesthetic techniques. *Acta Anaesthesiol Scand.* 2000;44:543-547.

132. Taboada Muniz M, Rodriguez J, Bermudez M, et al. Low volume and high concentration of local anesthetic is more efficacious than high volume and low concentration in Labat's sciatic nerve block: a prospective, randomized comparison. *Anesth Analg.* 2008;107:2085-2088.
133. Raith C, Kolblinger C, Walch H. Combined transgluteal ischial and femoral nerve block: retrospective data on 65 risk patients with leg amputation [in German]. *Anaesthesist.* 2008;57:555-561.
134. Fischler AH, Gross JB. Ultrasound-guided sciatic neuroma block for treatment of intractable stump pain. *J Clin Anesth.* 2007;19:626-628.
135. van Geffen GJ, Scheuer M, Muller A, Garderniers J, Gielen M. Ultrasound-guided bilateral continuous sciatic nerve blocks with stimulating catheters for postoperative pain relief after bilateral lower limb amputations. *Anaesthesia.* 2006;61:1204-1207.
136. Casati A, Fanelli G, Danelli G, et al. Stimulating or conventional perineural catheters after hallux valgus repair: a double-blind, pharmaco-economic evaluation. *Acta Anaesthesiol Scand.* 2006;50:1284-1289.
137. Serri S. Venous surgery of the lower limb: value of nerve blocks [in French]. *Cah Anesthesiol.* 1996;44:441-445.
138. Brodner G, Buerkle H, Van Aken H, et al. Postoperative analgesia after knee surgery: a comparison of three different concentrations of ropivacaine for continuous femoral nerve blockade. *Anesth Analg.* 2007;105:256-262.
139. Allen HW, Liu SS, Ware PD, Nairn CS, Owens BD. Peripheral nerve blocks improve analgesia after total knee replacement surgery. *Anesth Analg.* 1998;87:93-97.
140. Ng HP, Cheong KF, Lim A, Lim J, Puhaindran ME. Intraoperative single-shot "3-in-1" femoral nerve block with ropivacaine 0.25%, ropivacaine 0.5% or bupivacaine 0.25% provides comparable 48-hr analgesia after unilateral total knee replacement. *Can J Anaesth.* 2001;48:1102-1108.
141. Good RP, Snedden MH, Schieber FC, Polachek A. Effects of a preoperative femoral nerve block on pain management and rehabilitation after total knee arthroplasty. *Am J Orthop.* 2007;36:554-557.
142. Iskandar H, Benard A, Ruel-Raymond J, Cochard G, Manaud B. Femoral block provides superior analgesia compared with intra-articular ropivacaine after anterior cruciate ligament reconstruction. *Reg Anesth Pain Med.* 2003;28:29-32.
143. Mutty CE, Jensen EJ, Manka MA Jr, Anders MJ, Bone LB. Femoral nerve block for diaphyseal and distal femoral fractures in the emergency department. Surgical technique. *J Bone Joint Surg Am.* 2008;90 Suppl:218-226.
144. Fowler SJ, Symons J, Sabato S, Myles PS. Epidural analgesia compared with peripheral nerve blockade after major knee surgery: a systematic review and meta-analysis of randomized trials. *Br J Anaesth.* 2008;100:154-164.
145. Luhmann SJ, Schootman M, Schoenecker PL, Gordon JE, Schrock C. Use of femoral nerve blocks in adolescents undergoing patellar realignment surgery. *Am J Orthop.* 2008;37:39-43.
146. Noiseux N, Prieto I, Bracco D, Basile F, Hemmerling T. Coronary artery bypass grafting in the awake patient combining high thoracic epidural and femoral nerve block: first series of 15 patients. *Br J Anaesth.* 2008;100:184-189.
147. Hemmerling TM, Noiseux N, Basile F, Noel MF, Prieto I. Awake cardiac surgery using a novel anesthetic technique. *Can J Anaesth.* 2005;52:1088-1092.
148. Stewart B, Tudur Smith C, Teebay L, Cunliffe M, Low B. Emergency department use of a continuous femoral nerve block for pain relief for fractured femur in children. *Emerg Med J.* 2007;24:113-114.
149. Barker R, Schiferer A, Gore C, et al. Femoral nerve blockade administered preclinically for pain relief in severe knee trauma is more feasible and effective than intravenous metamizole: a randomized controlled trial. *J Trauma.* 2008;64:1535-1538.
150. Viscomi CM, Reese J, Rathmell JP. Medial and lateral antebrachial cutaneous nerve blocks: an easily learned regional anesthetic for forearm arteriovenous fistula surgery. *Reg Anesth.* 1996;21:2-5.
151. Cook JL, Cook J. The lateral femoral cutaneous nerve block. *Dermatol Surg.* 2000;26:81-83.
152. Wardrop PJ, Nishikawa H. Lateral cutaneous nerve of the thigh blockade as primary anaesthesia for harvesting skin grafts. *Br J Plast Surg.* 1995;48:597-600.
153. Maccani RM, Wedel DJ, Melton A, Gronert GA. Femoral and lateral femoral cutaneous nerve block for muscle biopsies in children. *Paediatr Anaesth.* 1995;5:223-227.
154. Hotta K, Sata N, Suzuki H, Takeuchi M, Seo N. Ultrasound-guided combined femoral nerve and lateral femoral cutaneous nerve blocks for femur neck fracture surgery—case report [in Japanese]. *Masui.* 2008;57:892-894.
155. Tumber PS, Bhatia A, Chan VW. Ultrasound-guided lateral femoral cutaneous nerve block for meralgia paresthetica. *Anesth Analg.* 2008;106:1021-1022.
156. Hurdle MF, Weingarten TN, Crisostomo RA, Psimos C, Smith J. Ultrasound-guided blockade of the lateral femoral cutaneous nerve: technical description and review of 10 cases. *Arch Phys Med Rehabil.* 2007;88:1362-1364.
157. Hirabayashi Y, Hotta K, Suzuki H, Igarashi T, Saitoh K, Seo N. Combined block of femoral, sciatic, obturator nerves and lateral cutaneous nerve block with ropivacaine for leg amputation above the knee [in Japanese]. *Masui.* 2002;51:1013-1035.
158. Vloka JD, Hadžić A, Mulcare R, Lesser JB, Koorn R, Thys DM. Combined popliteal and posterior cutaneous nerve of the thigh blocks for short saphenous vein stripping in outpatients: an alternative to spinal anesthesia. *J Clin Anesth.* 1997;9:618-622.
159. Akkaya T, Ersan O, Ozkan D, et al. Saphenous nerve block is an effective regional technique for post-meniscectomy pain. *Knee Surg Sports Traumatol Arthrosc.* 2008;16:855-858.
160. Singelyn FJ. Single-injection applications for foot and ankle surgery. *Best Pract Res Clin Anaesthesiol.* 2002;16:247-254.
161. van der Wal M, Lang SA, Yip RW. Transsartorial approach for saphenous nerve block. *Can J Anaesth.* 1993;40:542-546.
162. Reilley TE, Gerhardt MA. Anesthesia for foot and ankle surgery. *Clin Podiatr Med Surg.* 2002;19:125-147, vii.
163. Sarrafian SK, Ibrahim IN, Breihan JH. Ankle-foot peripheral nerve block for mid and forefoot surgery. *Foot Ankle.* 1983;4:86-90.
164. Rudkin GE, Rudkin AK, Dracopoulos GC. Bilateral ankle blocks: a prospective audit. *ANZ J Surg.* 2005;75:39-42.
165. Rudkin GE, Rudkin AK, Dracopoulos GC. Ankle block success rate: a prospective analysis of 1,000 patients. *Can J Anaesth.* 2005;52:209-210.
166. Reuben SS, Steinberg RB, Maciolek H, Manikantan P. An evaluation of the analgesic efficacy of intravenous regional anesthesia with lidocaine and ketorolac using a forearm versus upper arm tourniquet. *Anesth Analg.* 2002;95: 457-460.
167. Johnson CN. Intravenous regional anesthesia: new approaches to an old technique. *CRNA.* 2000;11:57-61.
168. Estebe JP. Locoregional intravenous anesthesia [in French]. *Ann Fr Anesth Reanim.* 1999;18:663-673.
169. Bernateck M, Rolke R, Birklein F, Treede RD, Fink M, Karst M. Successful intravenous regional block with low-dose tumor necrosis factor-alpha antibody infliximab for treatment of complex regional pain syndrome 1. *Anesth Analg.* 2007;105:1148-1151.

170. Toda K, Muneshige H, Asou T. Intravenous regional block with lidocaine for treatment of complex regional pain syndrome. *Clin J Pain.* 2006;22:222-224.
171. Lake AP. Intravenous regional sympathetic block: past, present and future? *Pain Res Manag.* 2004;9:35-37.
172. Bolte RG, Stevens PM, Scott SM, Schunk JE. Mini-dose Bier block intravenous regional anesthesia in the emergency department treatment of pediatric upper-extremity injuries. *J Pediatr Orthop.* 1994;14:534-537.
173. Barnes CL, Blasier RD, Dodge BM. Intravenous regional anesthesia: a safe and cost-effective outpatient anesthetic for upper extremity fracture treatment in children. *J Pediatr Orthop.* 1991;11:717-720.
174. McCarty EC, Mencio GA, Green NE. Anesthesia and analgesia for the ambulatory management of fractures in children. *J Am Acad Orthop Surg.* 1999;7:81-91.
175. Blaheta HJ, Vollert B, Zuder D, Rassner G. Intravenous regional anesthesia (Bier's block) for botulinum toxin therapy of palmar hyperhidrosis is safe and effective. *Dermatol Surg.* 2002;28:666-671.
176. Blaheta HJ, Deusch H, Rassner G, Vollert B. Intravenous regional anesthesia (Bier's block) is superior to a peripheral nerve block for painless treatment of plantar hyperhidrosis with botulinum toxin. *J Am Acad Dermatol.* 2003;48:302-304.
177. Handoll HH, Madhok R, Dodds C. Anaesthesia for treating distal radial fracture in adults. *Cochrane Database Syst Rev.* 2002:CD003320.
178. Reuben SS, Sklar J. Intravenous regional anesthesia with clonidine in the management of complex regional pain syndrome of the knee. *J Clin Anesth.* 2002;14:87-91.
179. Mohr B. Safety and effectiveness of intravenous regional anesthesia (Bier block) for outpatient management of forearm trauma. *CJEM.* 2006;8:247-250.

# 7 Continuous Peripheral Nerve Blocks in Outpatients

*Brian M. Ilfeld, Elizabeth M. Renehan, and F. Kayser Enneking*

## Introduction

- Single-injection nerve blocks provide up to 16 hours of postoperative analgesia.
- Portable infusion pumps allow outpatients to receive continuous nerve blocks.

More than 40% of ambulatory patients experience moderate to severe postoperative pain at home following orthopedic procedures.[1] Up to 16 hours of analgesia may be provided by single-injection peripheral nerve blocks with long-acting local anesthetics. However, following block resolution, ambulatory patients must usually rely on oral opioids to control pain. Unfortunately, opioids are associated with undesirable side effects, such as pruritus, nausea and vomiting, sedation, and constipation. To improve postoperative analgesia following ambulatory surgery, there has been an increasing interest in providing "perineural local anesthetic infusions," also called, "continuous peripheral nerve blocks," to outpatients. This technique involves the percutaneous insertion of a catheter directly adjacent to the peripheral nerve(s) supplying the surgical site. Local anesthetic is then infused via the catheter providing potent, site-specific analgesia. Outpatients may theoretically experience the same level of analgesia previously afforded only to those remaining hospitalized by combining the perineural catheter with a portable infusion pump.

In 1946, Ansbro first described continuous regional blockade using a cork to stabilize a needle placed adjacent to the brachial plexus divisions to provide a "continuous" supraclavicular block.[2] However, for decades patients were required to remain hospitalized because the available pumps used to infuse local anesthetic were large, heavy, and technically sophisticated. It was not until 52 years later that Rawal described outpatient perineural infusion using a percutaneous catheter and a small lightweight, portable infusion pump.[3]

## Advantages and Evidence

- Significant decreases in postoperative pain and opioid side effects are possible.
- Earlier home discharge is possible for a select subset of hospitalized patients.

Following Rawal's article, case reports or series of ambulatory perineural infusion were described via catheters in various anatomic locations, including paravertebral,[4] interscalene,[5–7] intersternocleidomastoid,[8] infraclavicular,[6] axillary,[9] psoas compartment,[9,10] femoral,[9,11] fascia iliaca,[5] sciatic/Labat,[9,10] sciatic/popliteal,[6,12] and tibial nerve.[6] Ambulatory continuous peripheral nerve blocks in pediatric patients have also been reported in patients as young as 8 years of age.[13] However, Klein et al provided the first prospective evidence *quantifying* infusion benefits in 2000.[14]

This randomized, double-masked, placebo-controlled investigation by Klein et al involved subjects undergoing open rotator cuff repair who received an interscalene block and perineural catheter preoperatively, and they were randomized to receive either perineural ropivacaine 0.2% or normal saline postoperatively (10 mL/h). Patients receiving perineural placebo averaged a 3 on a visual analog pain scale of 0 to 10, compared with a 1 for subjects receiving ropivacaine. Although a portable pump was used, patients remained hospitalized during local anesthetic infusion <24 hours, and catheters were removed by investigators prior to home discharge. Patients had access to intravenous morphine via patient-controlled opioid analgesia because the investigators "felt compelled to provide more than oral analgesics," since patients remained hospitalized.[14] As a result, patients receiving normal saline theoretically received a greater degree of analgesia than that available to ambulatory patients who must rely on oral instead of intravenous opioids. Consequently, although these data suggested perineural infusion may improve postoperative analgesia following hospital discharge, the extent of improvement for patients actually *at home* remained unknown.

Data involving perineural infusion in outpatients were subsequently provided in four randomized double-masked, placebo-controlled studies.[15–18] Patients receiving perineural local anesthetic achieved both clinically and statistically significant lower resting and breakthrough pain scores compared with those using exclusively oral opioids for analgesia (Figure 7-1). In addition, they required dramatically fewer oral analgesics to achieve their improved level of analgesia (Figure 7-1). Preoperatively, subjects scheduled for moderately painful procedures had a perineural catheter placed: an infraclavicular catheter for hand/forearm procedures,[15] a popliteal catheter for foot/ankle surgeries,[16,18] or an interscalene

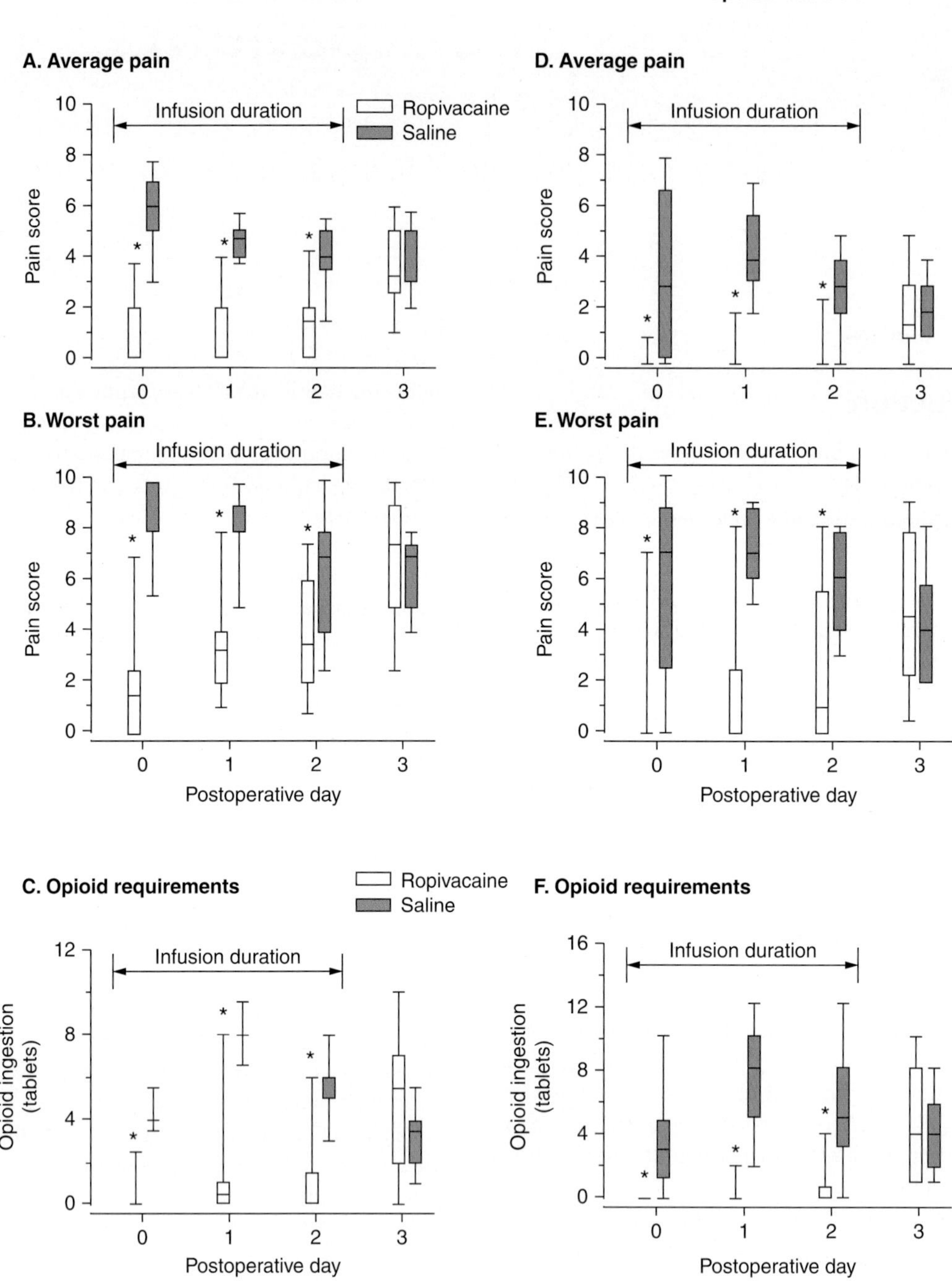


**FIGURE 7-1.** Effects of interscalene and sciatic/popliteal perineural infusion of either ropivacaine or placebo on average pain at rest (panels A and D), worst pain overall (panels B and E), and opiate use (panels C and F) following moderately painful shoulder or lower extremity surgery (scale: 0–10). Each opiate tablet consisted of oxycodone, 5 mg. *Note*: The infusion was discontinued after postoperative day 2 as indicated by the horizontal lines. Data are expressed as median (horizontal bar) with 25th–75th (box) and 10th–90th (whiskers) percentiles for patients randomly assigned to receive either 0.2% ropivacaine or 0.9% saline placebo. For tightly clustered data (e.g., panel A, postoperative days 0 and 1, ropivacaine group), the median approximated the 10th and 25th percentile values. In this case, the median is zero and only the 75th and 90th percentiles are clearly noted; $p < 0.05$: *, compared with saline for a given postoperative day. Reproduced with permission.[16,17]

catheter for shoulder procedures.[17] Postoperatively, patients received either perineural local anesthetic or normal saline and were followed at home for up to 60 hours. All patients were instructed to use a bolus from their infusion pump for breakthrough pain and oral analgesics if this maneuver failed. In patients with an interscalene catheter following shoulder surgery, the local anesthetic infusion provided analgesia so complete that 80% of patients receiving ropivacaine required one or fewer opioid tablets per day during their infusion, and they reported average resting pain <1.5 on a scale of 0–10.[17] This compares with all patients receiving placebo requiring four or more opioid tablets per day, beginning the evening of surgery, and reporting average resting pain scores between 3 and 4. For breakthrough pain, the differences between treatment groups were even more pronounced in all of these four placebo-controlled studies (Figure 7-1).

Additional benefits related to improved analgesia were experienced by patients who received perineural local anesthetic. Of patients receiving perineural ropivacaine, 0 to 30% reported insomnia due to pain, compared with 60 to 70% of patients receiving placebo.[15–17] Additionally, awakenings from sleep because of pain averaged 0.0 to 0.2 times on the first postoperative night, compared with 2.0 to 2.3 times for patients using only oral opioids.[15–17] Using fewer opioid tablets was associated with a lower rate of nausea, vomiting, pruritus, and sedation.[15–18] Satisfaction with postoperative analgesia was both clinically and statistically higher for patients receiving local anesthetic.[15–18] Finally, patients with popliteal local anesthetic infusion rated their "quality of recovery" (0–100; 100 = highest) an average of 96 compared with 83 for patients receiving placebo.[18] Whether these demonstrated benefits result in an improvement in patients' health-related quality-of-life remains unexamined.[19] Also uninvestigated to date is the relative superiority of one location over another for similar procedures (e.g., axillary vs. infraclavicular for hand surgery).

The possible advantages of using outpatient perineural infusion to allow earlier discharge of patients who require potent analgesia has only recently been explored. Individual benefits of a shorter hospitalization may include a decrease in nosocomial infection,[20,21] harmful medical errors,[22,23] and increases in health-related quality-of-life.[19] Societal benefits include a potentially enormous cost savings.[24–26] Using ambulatory perineural infusion, patients have been discharged home directly from the recovery room following total elbow (unpublished data, Ilfeld et al, 2004) and shoulder replacement,[27] and on the first postoperative day following total hip (unpublished data, Ilfeld et al, 2004) and knee replacement.[28] Additional data are required to define the appropriate subset of patients and assess the benefits and incidence of complications associated with this practice.

## Patient Selection

- Outpatient infusion is often limited to patients expected to have moderate pain.
- Appropriate patient selection is crucial for safe outpatient infusion.

Many investigators have limited the use of ambulatory infusion to patients who are expected to have *moderate or severe* postoperative pain >24 hours that is not easily managed with oral opioids. This practice is in an attempt to balance the potential benefits of this technique with the potential risks,[29,30] financial cost, and patient inconvenience of carrying an infusion pump and up to 600 mL of local anesthetic.[27] However, outpatient infusion may be used following *mildly* painful procedures—defined here as usually well-managed with oral opioids—to decrease opioid requirements and opioid-related side effects.[3,31] Appropriate patient selection is crucial for safe outpatient infusion because not all patients desire, or are capable of accepting, the extra responsibility that comes with the catheter and pump system. Because some degree of postoperative cognitive dysfunction is common following surgery,[32] patients are often required to have a "caretaker" during infusion.[15–17,33–36] Whether a caretaker is necessary for one night or for the entire duration of infusion remains unresolved.[37] If removal of the catheter is expected to occur at home, then a caretaker willing to perform this procedure must be available at the infusion conclusion if the patient is unwilling or unable to do this themselves (e.g., psoas compartment catheter).

In medically unsupervised outpatients, complications may take longer to identify or be more difficult to manage than for hospitalized patients. Therefore, hepatic or renal insufficiency have been relative contraindications to outpatient infusion in an effort to avoid local anesthetic toxicity.[38] For infusions that may effect the phrenic nerve and ipsilateral diaphragm function (e.g., interscalene or cervical paravertebral catheters), patients with heart or lung disease are often excluded because continuous interscalene local anesthetic infusions have been shown to cause frequent ipsilateral diaphragm paralysis.[39] Conservative application of this technique is warranted until additional investigation of hospitalized medically supervised patients documents its safety,[40,41] although the effect on overall pulmonary function may be minimal for relatively healthy patients.[42]

## Selection of Insertion Technique

- The optimal equipment and insertion techniques have yet to be determined.
- A "test dose" of local anesthetic and epinephrine via the catheter is mandatory.
- Securing the catheter adequately is of paramount concern.

In a substantial number of cases—as high as 40% in some reports[43]—inaccurate catheter placement may occur.[17,44,45] This issue is of critical importance for outpatients because catheter replacement is not an option after leaving the medical facility. Many techniques and types of equipment have been described for catheter insertion. Using one common technique, the initial local anesthetic bolus is given via the needle, followed by catheter placement. However, using this method, it is possible to provide a successful surgical block but inaccurate catheter placement.[17] For ambulatory patients, the inadequate perineural infusion often will not be detected until after surgical block resolution following home discharge.[17] Using another technique, investigators have first inserted the catheter and then administered a bolus of local anesthetic via the catheter, with a reported failure rate of 1 to 8%.[46,47]

In an attempt to further improve catheter-placement success rates, "stimulating" catheters have been developed that deliver current to the catheter tip.[48] This design provides feedback on the positional relationship of the catheter tip to the target nerve prior to local anesthetic dosing.[33,34] To date, there are no studies comparing stimulating and nonstimulating catheters. However, there is limited evidence that passing current via the catheter may improve the accuracy of catheter placement.[49] The optimal placement techniques and equipment for ambulatory perineural infusion have yet to be determined and require further investigation.[50] A local anesthetic and epinephrine "test dose" should be injected via the catheter in an effort to identify intrathecal,[51] epidural,[52] or intravascular[53] placement before infusion initiation, regardless of the equipment/technique used.

## Local Anesthetic and Adjuvant Selection

- Most outpatient infusions reported involved ropivacaine or bupivacaine.
- No adjuvant added to local anesthetic has been demonstrated to be of benefit.

Although perineural infusions of levobupivacaine[54] and shorter-acting agents have been reported,[55–57] most publications have involved ropivacaine 0.2% or bupivacaine 0.125 to 0.25%. Currently, there is insufficient information to determine if there is an optimal local anesthetic (or concentration) for ambulatory infusions.[31,54,58] The optimal concentration and infusion rate for a particular catheter site in relationship to the degree of motor block has not been established either.

## Patient-Controlled Regional Analgesia

- Providing patients the ability to self-administer bolus doses maximizes benefits
- The optimal basal rate, bolus volume, and lockout time have not been determined
- Commonly used: basal 4–8 mL/h, bolus 2–5 mL, and lockout time 20–60 minutes

Available inpatient and outpatient data suggest that following procedures producing moderate to severe pain, providing patients with the ability to self-administer local anesthetic doses (patient-controlled regional analgesia) increases perioperative benefits and/or decreases local anesthetic consumption.[33,34,36,59–61] However, no information is available to base recommendations on the optimal basal rate, bolus volume, or lockout period, other than for interscalene catheters.[33] Until recommendations based on prospectively collected data are published, practitioners should be aware that investigators have reported successful analgesia using the following with long-acting local anesthetics: basal rate of 4 to 8 mL/h, bolus volume of 2 to 5 mL, and lockout duration of 20 to 60 minutes. Practitioners should be aware that the maximum safe doses for the long-acting local anesthetics remain unknown. However, multiple investigations involving patients free of renal or hepatic disease have reported blood concentrations within acceptable limits following up to 5 days of perineural infusion with similar dosing schedules.[38,62–64] Extrapolating from data involving patients receiving epidural bupivacaine infusion, a maximum infusion rate of 0.5 mg/kg per hour of bupivacaine may be considered.[38]

Following ambulatory shoulder surgery with an interscalene catheter, infusion duration may be increased and similar baseline analgesia may be provided by decreasing the basal rate from 8 to 4 mL/h when patients supplement their block with large bolus doses (6 mL).[33] However, patients experience an increase in breakthrough pain incidence and intensity, sleep disturbances, and a decrease in satisfaction with their analgesia. Therefore, if ambulatory patients do not return for additional local anesthetic, practitioners are left with the dilemma of superior analgesia for a shorter duration versus a lesser degree of analgesia for a longer period of time. Of note, the infusion duration may be increased by progressively decreasing the basal infusion rate with a reprogrammable infusion pump, thus theoretically maximizing postoperative analgesia.[7]

The publications that investigated the optimal dosing regimen for outpatients involved surgical procedures producing moderate postoperative pain. For procedures inducing *mild* postoperative pain, it is possible—even probable—that adequate analgesia would be adequately treated with a bolus-only dosing regimen.[31] There is also the possibility that stimulating catheters may be placed, on average, closer to the target nerve/plexus compared with nonstimulating devices.[49] If so, then the optimal dosing regimens, basal rates, and bolus doses may vary among different catheter types. Unfortunately, there are currently insufficient published data to draw any conclusions.

## Equipment

- There is no one perfect infusion pump for all applications.
- A multitude of factors must be taken into account when choosing a pump.

Multiple small portable infusion pumps are currently available (Table 7-1; Figures 7-2 and 7-3), each with benefits

**TABLE 7-1 Infusion Pump Distributors**

| PUMP (REFERENCE) | DISTRIBUTOR | CITY | STATE |
|---|---|---|---|
| 6060 MT[69] | Baxter Healthcare | Deerfield | IL |
| Accufuser[65] and Accufuser Plus XL[66,67,69] | McKinley Medical | Wheat Ridge | CO |
| ambIT LPM[69] and ambIT PCA[69] | Sorenson Medical | West Jordan | UT |
| AutoMed 3200[69] and AutoMed 3400[67] | Algos, LC | Salt Lake City | UT |
| BlockIt (WalkMed)[66] | McKinley Medical | Wheat Ridge | CO |
| CADD-Legacy PCA[66] and CADD-Prism PCS[66] | Smiths Medical | St. Paul | MN |
| C-Bloc[65] | I-Flow Corporation | Lake Forest | CA |
| Infusor LV5[67] | Baxter Healthcare | Deerfield | IL |
| Ipump[69] | Baxter Healthcare | Deerfield | IL |
| Microject PCA[65,66] and Microject PCEA[67] | Sorenson Medical | West Jordan | UT |
| On-Q C-Bloc with OnDemand[69] | I-Flow Corporation | Lake Forest | CA |
| Pain Care 3200[67] | Breg, Inc. | Vista | CA |
| Pain Pump I[65] | Stryker Instruments | Kalamazoo | MI |
| Sgarlato[65] | Sgarlato Labs | Los Gatos | CA |

Reproduced with permission.[79]

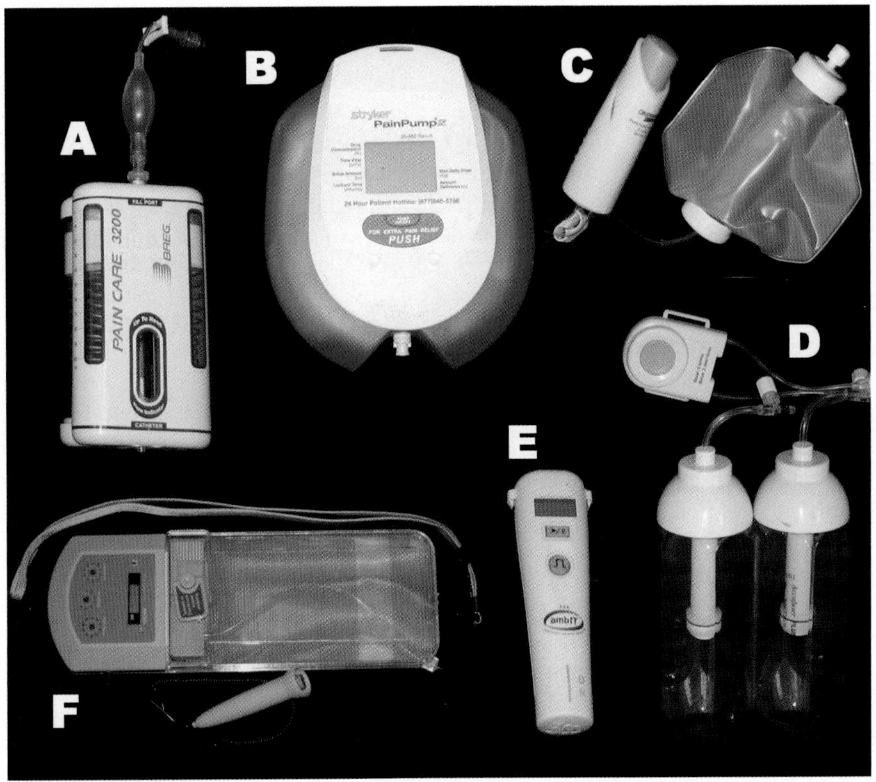


**FIGURE 7-2.** Examples of portable *disposable* basal- and bolus-capable infusion pumps. (A) Pain Care 3200, (B) Pain Pump II, (C) On-Q C-Bloc with OnDemand, (D) Accufuser Plus XL, (E) ambIT PCA, (F) AutoMed 3200. Distributor information and pump attributes are included in the appendix and Table 7-2. Note that the ambIT PCA is produced as a disposable model as well as a more expensive reusable unit and therefore appears in both Figures 7-2 and 7-3.

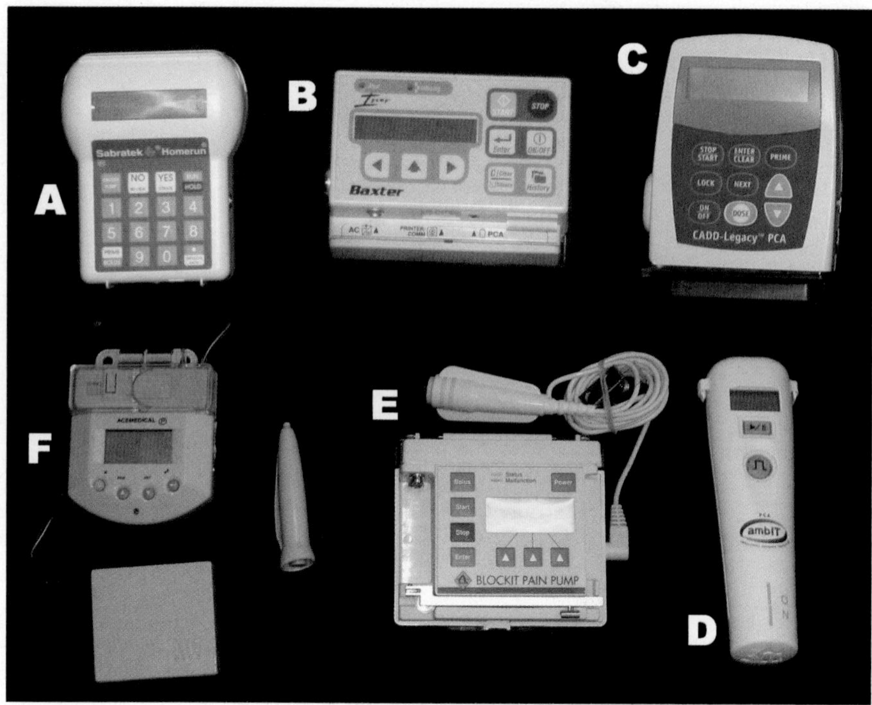


**FIGURE 7-3.** Examples of portable *reusable* basal- *and* bolus-capable infusion pumps. (A) 6060 MT, (B) Ipump PMS, (C) CADD-Legacy PCA, (D) ambIT PCA, (E) BlockIt, (F) AutoMed 3400. Distributor information and pump attributes are included in the appendix and Table 7-2. Note that the ambIT PCA is produced as a disposable model as well as a more expensive reusable unit, and therefore appears in both Figures 7-2 and 7-3.

and limitations (Table 7-2). Many factors must be taken into account when determining the optimal device for a given clinical situation. The provided list of infusion devices includes those for which performance data are available from independent sources and is not meant to be an exhaustive list of available units.

## Bolus-Dose Capability

Various pumps allow for both patient-controlled local anesthetic boluses and a basal infusion (Table 7–2); others allow for only one of these.[65–69] Bolus-dose capability (also termed patient-controlled regional analgesia, or PCRA) offers two significant benefits over continuous infusions alone. First, higher doses of oral opiates are often required for breakthrough pain without patient-controlled bolus doses.[34,68] Second, for outpatients using a limited local anesthetic reservoir, PCRA allows a provider to minimize the basal rate and, in turn, allows maximum infusion duration and minimal motor block[7] yet also permits bolus dosing for breakthrough pain[34] and physical therapy.[27,33,36,70] Compared with continuous infusions alone, equivalent or superior analgesia with a lower rate of local anesthetic consumption may be provided by using patient-controlled local anesthetic.[34,59–61]

## Disposability and Cost

Reusable electronic infusion pumps are generally more expensive than the available single-use/disposable models (Table 7–2). However, reusable pumps that use relatively inexpensive disposable "cassettes" for each new patient (usually about US$10) may be more cost effective for practitioners who use these devices repeatedly (Table 7–2). But a reusable unit requires the patient to return the infusion pump by either the mail service or revisiting the surgical center.[33,34,36]

## Patient Instructions

- A prescription for oral opioids should be filled by patients following discharge.
- Oral and written instructions, including health care provider contact numbers, should be provided.

Following a single-injection nerve block for ambulatory surgery, discharge with an insensate extremity results in minimal complications.[71] However, whether or not patients should weight-bear with a continuous peripheral nerve block remains unexamined. Therefore, conservative management may be optimal, and some investigators have recommended that patients avoid using their surgical limb for weightbearing.[8,16,36] A prescription for oral analgesics should be provided to all patients, and the importance of filling the prescription immediately after leaving the surgical center should be emphasized. If patients wait to fill the prescription until after they have determined if oral analgesics are required, a period of inadequate analgesia may result.

**TABLE 7-2 Infusion Pump Attributes**

| PUMP MODEL (REFERENCES) | WEIGHTT[1] (g) | RESERVOIR VOLUME (max mL) | BASAL INFUSION (mL/h) | BOLUS DOSE (mL) | BOLUS LOCKOUT (min–h) | RETAIL PRICE (U.S. $) | POWER SOURCE |
|---|---|---|---|---|---|---|---|
| **Programmable, Reusable Models** | | | | | | | |
| 6060 MT[69] | 525 | IV bag[2] | 0.1–50.0 | 0–50 | 0–60 | 3995 | Electronic |
| ambIT PCA[69] | 133 | IV bag[2] | 0–20 | 0– 0 | 5–24 | 500–800[3] | Electronic |
| AutoMed 3400[67] | 325 | IV bag[2] | 0–50 | 0–50 | 0–60 | 675 | Electronic |
| BlockIt (WalkMed)[66] | 323 | IV bag[2] | 0–30 | 0–30 | 0–24 | 1750–2300 | Electronic |
| CADD-Legacy PCA[66] | 372 | IV bag[2] | 0–50 | 0–9.9 | 5–24 | 3595 | Electronic |
| CADD-Prism PCS[66] | 547 | IV bag[2] | 0–30 | 0–9.9 | 5–24 | 4125 | Electronic |
| Ipump PMS[69] | 415 | IV bag[2] | 0–19.9[4] | 0–9.9 | 1–6 | 4295 | Electronic |
| Microject PCA[5,65,66] | 198 | IV bag[2] | 0–9.9 | 0–2 | 6–1 | N/A[5] | Electronic |
| Microject PCEA[5,67] | 198 | IV bag[2] | 0–29 | 0–10 | 10–120 | N/A[5] | Electronic |
| **Programmable, Disposable Models** | | | | | | | |
| ambIT LPM[69] | 133 | IV bag[2] | 0–20 | 0–20 | 5–24 | 250–350[3] | Electronic |
| AutoMed 3200[69] | 350 | 250 | 0–10 | 0–5 | 2–60 | 255 | Electronic |
| **Nonprogrammable, Disposable, Basal- *and* Bolus-Capable Models** | | | | | | | |
| Accufuser Plus XL[66,67,69] | 109 | 550 | 5, 8, or 10[6] | 2 | 15, 60 min | 260 | Elastomeric |
| Pain Care 3200[67] | 290 | 200 | 5.7–2.9[6,7] | 4–6[6,7] | 40–1.3[6,7] | 175 | Spring |
| On-Q C-Bloc with OnDemand[69] | 135 | 400[8] | 5 | 5 | 60 min[6] | 250–500 | Elastomeric |
| **Nonprogrammable, Disposable, Basal- *or* Bolus-Only Models** | | | | | | | |
| Accufuser[65] | 95 | 275 | 2, 4, 5, 8, 10[6] | N/A | N/A | 150–225 | Elastomeric |
| C-Bloc[65] | 65 | 400 | 5 or 10[6] | N/A | N/A | 395[3] | Elastomeric |
| Infusor LV5[67] | 65 | 275 | 2, 5, 7, 10[6] | N/A | N/A | 55 | Elastomeric |
| Pain Pump I[65] | 104 | 120 | 0.8, 2.1, 4.2[6] | N/A | N/A | 150[3] | Vacuum |
| Sgarlato[65] | 225 | 200 | 0.5, 1, 2, 4[6] | N/A | N/A | 225[3] | Spring |

Reproduced with permission.[79]

N/A, not applicable.

1. Including batteries and disposable cassette in electronic pumps; and excluding infusate for all pumps.
2. Local anesthetic reservoir is an external syringe or IV-style bag of any size.
3. Approximate price for Florida (USA): other regions may vary.
4. If a bolus dose is not provided, the maximum basal rate is 90 mL/h.
5. The Microject pumps may be reused because disposable cassettes are used with the mechanical pump, but the pumps themselves are less expensive than some "disposable" pumps and may thus be considered disposable, if desired. Not available in the United States.
6. Fixed during manufacture.
7. Basal infusion rate described as "4 mL/h continuous flow" on product packaging and marketing materials. However, product information contained within the instruction manual specifies that the rate is 5.7 mL/h at the beginning of the infusion, and steadily declines to 2.9 mL/h by reservoir exhaustion. Bolus dose is variable and lockout increases as infusion progresses.[67]
8. On-Q C-Block with OnDemand may be "overfilled" to 500 mL, decreasing the basal rate for a portion of the infusion but allowing for a longer infusion duration.[69]

**Florida Surgical Center**
AT SHANDS HOSPITAL AT THE UNIVERSITY OF FLORIDA

PATIENT LABEL

## Progress Note for Ambulatory Perineural Local Anesthetic Infusion

Surgery Date_____/_____/200__ Surgeon:_______________________ Home phone: ( _______ ) ________ - ____________

Procedure:_______________________________________________ Other phone: ( _______ ) ________ - ____________

Post-op in PACU
- ☐ Catheter w/ neg. aspiration & ____ mL of ______________ w/ ____ μg epinephrine/mL to catheter w/ neg. aspiration q2 mL
- ☐ No heart rate or sensory changes within 3 minutes
- ☐ Verbal and written instructions given to patient/care-taker & all questions answered, MD phone #s provided
- ☐ Pump tubing secured to catheter, pump programmed & infusion begun

Notes:

_______________________ Physician Signature

POD #0 ____:____
- ☐ Patient or patient's caretaker contacted by phone
- ☐ Symptoms of local anesthetic toxicity, catheter migration and infection denied
- ☐ Appropriate sensory/motor function of affected extremity acknowledged
- ☐ Surgical pain under control
- ☐ Patient would like to have catheter remain in situ at this time
- ☐ All questions answered

Notes:

_______________________ Physician Signature

POD #1 ____:____
- ☐ Patient or patient's caretaker contacted by phone
- ☐ Symptoms of local anesthetic toxicity, catheter migration and infection denied
- ☐ Appropriate sensory/motor function of affected extremity acknowledged
- ☐ Surgical pain under control
- ☐ Patient would like to have catheter remain in situ at this time
- ☐ All questions answered

Notes:

_______________________ Physician Signature

POD #2 ____:____
- ☐ Patient or patient's caretaker contacted by phone
- ☐ Symptoms of local anesthetic toxicity, catheter migration and infection denied
- ☐ Appropriate sensory/motor function of affected extremity acknowledged
- ☐ Surgical pain under control
- ☐ Patient would like to have catheter remain in situ at this time
- ☐ Catheter removed by patient's caretaker with MD on phone, tip reported to be blue/silver
- ☐ All questions answered

Notes:

_______________________ Physician Signature

POD #3 ____:____
- ☐ Patient or patient's caretaker contacted by phone
- ☐ Symptoms of local anesthetic toxicity, catheter migration and infection denied
- ☐ Appropriate sensory/motor function of affected extremity acknowledged
- ☐ Surgical pain under control
- ☐ Patient would like to have catheter remain in situ at this time
- ☐ Catheter removed by patient's caretaker with MD on phone, tip reported to be blue/silver
- ☐ All questions answered

Notes:

_______________________ Physician Signature

POD #4 ____:____
- ☐ Patient or patient's caretaker contacted by phone
- ☐ Symptoms of local anesthetic toxicity, catheter migration and infection denied
- ☐ Appropriate sensory/motor function of affected extremity acknowledged
- ☐ Surgical pain under control
- ☐ Patient would like to have catheter remain in situ at this time
- ☐ Catheter removed by patient's caretaker with MD on phone, tip reported to be blue/silver
- ☐ All questions answered

Notes:

_______________________ Physician Signature

**FIGURE 7-4.** An example of a progress note that may be used to record telephone contacts with ambulatory patients. Reproduced with permission.[79]

Most investigators educate both the patient and his or her caretaker at the same time before discharge because most patients have some degree of postoperative cognitive dysfunction. Both verbal and written instructions should be provided, along with contact numbers for health care providers who are available throughout the infusion duration.[6,15,31,72] In addition to standard outpatient instructions, topics reviewed often include expectations regarding surgical block resolution, infusion pump instructions, breakthrough pain treatment, catheter site care, limb protection, and the plan for catheter removal. Forewarning that pain in the operative limb is anticipated following surgical block resolution and fluid leakage at the catheter site is common—and what to do if these are experienced—often proves helpful. Signs and symptoms of possible catheter- and local anesthetic-related complications include, but are not limited to, pulmonary compromise,[40,41] nerve injury,[73] site infection,[74] and local anesthetic toxicity.[53] Although there are case reports of *initially* misplaced catheters, *migration* following a documented correct placement has not been described but remains a theoretical risk.[51–53,75,76] Possible complications of an unidentified *initially* misplaced catheter or of a catheter *migration* include intravascular or interpleural catheterization resulting in local anesthetic toxicity, intramuscular catheterization resulting in myonecrosis, and epidural/intrathecal catheterization when using interscalene, intersternocleidomastoid, paravertebral, or psoas compartment catheters. As is standard of care for inpatients, health care providers may want to consider documenting each patient contact (Figure 7-4).

Catheter removal may be achieved with various techniques: Patients may be discharged with written instructions,[12] a health care provider may perform this procedure,[77] or patients' caretakers (or occasionally the patients themselves) may remove the catheters with instructions given by a provider over the telephone.[15–17,33,34,36] Although one technique has not been demonstrated to be superior to the others, one survey revealed that with instructions given by phone, 98% of patients felt comfortable removing their catheter at home.[78] Of note, only 4% would have preferred to return for a health care provider to remove the catheter, and 43% responded they would have felt comfortable with exclusively written instructions.[78] Nonsterile gloves may be provided for patients having their catheters removed at home.[15–17]

## REFERENCES


1. Rawal N, Hylander J, Nydahl PA, Olofsson I, Gupta A. Survey of postoperative analgesia following ambulatory surgery. *Acta Anaesthesiol Scand.* 1997;41:1017-1022.
2. Ansbro FP. A method of continuous brachial plexus block. *Am J Surg.* 1946;71:716-722.
3. Rawal N, Axelsson K, Hylander J, et al. Postoperative patient-controlled local anesthetic administration at home. *Anesth Analg.* 1998;86:86-89.
4. Buckenmaier CC III, Klein SM, Nielsen KC, Steele SM. Continuous paravertebral catheter and outpatient infusion for breast surgery. *Anesth Analg.* 2003;97:715-717.
5. Ganapathy S, Amendola A, Lichfield R, Fowler PJ, Ling E. Elastomeric pumps for ambulatory patient controlled regional analgesia. *Can J Anaesth.* 2000;47:897-902.
6. Macaire P, Gaertner E, Capdevila X. Continuous post-operative regional analgesia at home. *Minerva Anesthesiol.* 2001;67:109-116.
7. Ilfeld BM, Enneking FK. A portable mechanical pump providing over four days of patient-controlled analgesia by perineural infusion at home. *Reg Anesth Pain Med.* 2002;27:100-104.
8. Corda DM, Enneking FK. A unique approach to postoperative analgesia for ambulatory surgery. *J Clin Anesth.* 2000;12:595-599.
9. Grant SA, Nielsen KC, Greengrass RA, Steele SM, Klein SM. Continuous peripheral nerve block for ambulatory surgery. *Reg Anesth Pain Med.* 2001;26:209-214.
10. Klein SM, Greengrass RA, Grant SA, Higgins LD, Nielsen KC, Steele SM. Ambulatory surgery for multi-ligament knee reconstruction with continuous dual catheter peripheral nerve blockade. *Can J Anaesth.* 2001;48:375-378.
11. Chelly JE, Gebhard R, Coupe K, Greger J, Khan A. Local anesthetic delivered via a femoral catheter by patient-controlled analgesia pump for pain relief after an anterior cruciate ligament outpatient procedure. *Am J Anesthesiol.* 2001;28:192-194.
12. Klein SM, Greengrass RA, Gleason DH, Nunley JA, Steele SM. Major ambulatory surgery with continuous regional anesthesia and a disposable infusion pump. *Anesthesiology.* 1999;91:563-565.
13. Ilfeld BM, Smith DW, Enneking FK. Continuous regional analgesia following ambulatory pediatric orthopedic surgery. *Am J Orthop.* 2004;33:405-408.
14. Klein SM, Grant SA, Greengrass RA, et al. Interscalene brachial plexus block with a continuous catheter insertion system and a disposable infusion pump. *Anesth Analg.* 2000;91:1473-1478.
15. Ilfeld BM, Morey TE, Enneking FK. Continuous infraclavicular brachial plexus block for postoperative pain control at home: a randomized, double-blinded, placebo-controlled study. *Anesthesiology.* 2002;96:1297-1304.
16. Ilfeld BM, Morey TE, Wang RD, Enneking FK. Continuous popliteal sciatic nerve block for postoperative pain control at home: a randomized, double-blinded, placebo-controlled study. *Anesthesiology.* 2002;97:959-965.
17. Ilfeld BM, Morey TE, Wright TW, Chidgey LK, Enneking FK. Continuous interscalene brachial plexus block for postoperative pain control at home: a randomized, double-blinded, placebo-controlled study. *Anesth Analg.* 2003;96:1089-1095.
18. White PF, Issioui T, Skrivanek GD, Early JS, Wakefield C. The use of a continuous popliteal sciatic nerve block after surgery involving the foot and ankle: does it improve the quality of recovery? *Anesth Analg.* 2003;97:1303-1309.
19. Wu CL, Naqibuddin M, Rowlingson AJ, Lietman SA, Jermyn RM, Fleisher LA. The effect of pain on health-related quality of life in the immediate postoperative period. *Anesth Analg.* 2003;97:1078-1085.
20. Public health focus: surveillance, prevention, and control of nosocomial infections. *MMWR CDC Surveill Summ.* 1992;41:783-787.
21. Wenzel RP, Edmond MB. The impact of hospital-acquired bloodstream infections. *Emerg Infect Dis.* 2001;7:174-177.
22. Relman AS. The institute of medicine report on the quality of health care. *N Engl J Med.* 2001;345:702-703.
23. Leape LL. Institute of Medicine medical error figures are not exaggerated. *JAMA.* 2000;284:95-97.
24. Mushinski M. Average charges for hip replacement surgeries: United States, 1997. *Stat Bull Metrop Insur Co.* 1999;80:32-40.
25. Mushinski M. Average charges for a total knee replacement: United States, 1994. *Stat Bull Metrop Insur Co.* 1996;77:24-30.
26. Weinstein J. *The Dartmouth Atlas of Musculoskeletal Health Care.* Chicago, IL: AHA Press; 2000:72-78.

27. Ilfeld BM, Wright TW, Enneking FK, et al. Effect of interscalene perineural local anesthetic infusion on postoperative physical therapy following total shoulder replacement. *Reg Anesth Pain Med.* 2004;29:A18.
28. Ilfeld BM, Gearen PF, Enneking FK, et al. Effect of femoral perineural local anesthetic infusion on postoperative functional ability following total knee arthroplasty. *Anesthesiology.* 2004;101:A945.
29. Ekatodramis G, Macaire P, Borgeat A. Prolonged Horner syndrome due to neck hematoma after continuous interscalene block. *Anesthesiology.* 2001;95:801-803.
30. Ribeiro FC, Georgousis H, Bertram R, Scheiber G. Plexus irritation caused by interscalene brachial plexus catheter for shoulder surgery. *Anesth Analg.* 1996;82:870-872.
31. Rawal N, Allvin R, Axelsson K, et al. Patient-controlled regional analgesia (PCRA) at home: controlled comparison between bupivacaine and ropivacaine brachial plexus analgesia. *Anesthesiology.* 2002;96:1290-1296.
32. Johnson T, Monk T, Rasmussen LS, et al. Postoperative cognitive dysfunction in middle-aged patients. *Anesthesiology.* 2002;96:1351-1357.
33. Ilfeld BM, Morey TE, Wright TW, Chidgey LK, Enneking FK. Interscalene perineural ropivacaine infusion: a comparison of two dosing regimens for postoperative analgesia. *Reg Anesth Pain Med.* 2004;29:9-16.
34. Ilfeld BM, Morey TE, Enneking FK. Infraclavicular perineural local anesthetic infusion: a comparison of three dosing regimens for postoperative analgesia. *Anesthesiology.* 2004;100:395-402.
35. Ilfeld BM, Morey TE, Enneking FK. Continuous infraclavicular perineural infusion with clonidine and ropivacaine compared with ropivacaine alone: a randomized, double-blinded, controlled study. *Anesth Analg.* 2003;97:706-712.
36. Ilfeld BM, Thannikary LJ, Morey TE, Vander Griend RA, Enneking FK. Popliteal sciatic perineural local anesthetic infusion: a comparison of three dosing regimens for postoperative analgesia. *Anesthesiology.* 2004;101:970-977.
37. Klein SM, Steele SM, Nielsen KC, et al. The difficulties of ambulatory interscalene and intra-articular infusions for rotator cuff surgery: a preliminary report. *Can J Anaesth.* 2003;50:265-269.
38. Denson DD, Raj PP, Saldahna F, et al. Continuous perineural infusion of bupivacaine for prolonged analgesia: pharmacokinetic considerations. *Int J Clin Pharmacol Ther Toxicol.* 1983;21:591-597.
39. Pere P. The effect of continuous interscalene brachial plexus block with 0.125% bupivacaine plus fentanyl on diaphragmatic motility and ventilatory function. *Reg Anesth.* 1993;18:93-97.
40. Smith MP, Tetzlaff JE, Brems JJ. Asymptomatic profound oxyhemoglobin desaturation following interscalene block in a geriatric patient. *Reg Anesth Pain Med.* 1998;23:210-213.
41. Sardesai AM, Chakrabarti AJ, Denny NM. Lower lobe collapse during continuous interscalene brachial plexus local anesthesia at home. *Reg Anesth Pain Med.* 2004;29:65-68.
42. Borgeat A, Perschak H, Bird P, Hodler J, Gerber C. Patient-controlled interscalene analgesia with ropivacaine 0.2% versus patient-controlled intravenous analgesia after major shoulder surgery: effects on diaphragmatic and respiratory function. *Anesthesiology.* 2000;92:102-108.
43. Salinas FV. Location, location, location: Continuous peripheral nerve blocks and stimulating catheters. *Reg Anesth Pain Med.* 2003;28:79-82.
44. Coleman MM, Chan VW. Continuous interscalene brachial plexus block. *Can J Anaesth.* 1999;46:209-214.
45. Ganapathy S, Wasserman RA, Watson JT, et al. Modified continuous femoral three-in-one block for postoperative pain after total knee arthroplasty. *Anesth Analg.* 1999;89:1197-1202.
46. Borgeat A, Dullenkopf A, Ekatodramis G, Nagy L. Evaluation of the lateral modified approach for continuous interscalene block after shoulder surgery. *Anesthesiology.* 2003;99:436-442.
47. Borgeat A, Blumenthal S, Karovic D, Delbos A, Vienne P. Clinical evaluation of a modified posterior anatomical approach to performing the popliteal block. *Reg Anesth Pain Med.* 2004;29:290-296.
48. Boezaart AP, de Beer JF, du Toit C, van Rooyen K. A new technique of continuous interscalene nerve block. *Can J Anaesth.* 1999;46:275-281.
49. Salinas FV, Neal JM, Sueda LA, Kopacz DJ, Liu SS. Prospective comparison of continuous femoral nerve block with nonstimulating catheter placement versus stimulating catheter-guided perineural placement in volunteers. *Reg Anesth Pain Med.* 2004;29:212-220.
50. Chelly JE, Williams BA. Continuous perineural infusions at home: narrowing the focus. *Reg Anesth Pain Med.* 2004;29:1-3.
51. Litz RJ, Vicent O, Wiessner D, Heller AR. Misplacement of a psoas compartment catheter in the subarachnoid space. *Reg Anesth Pain Med.* 2004;29:60-64.
52. Cook LB. Unsuspected extradural catheterization in an interscalene block. *Br J Anaesth.* 1991;67:473-475.
53. Tuominen MK, Pere P, Rosenberg PH. Unintentional arterial catheterization and bupivacaine toxicity associated with continuous interscalene brachial plexus block. *Anesthesiology.* 1991;75:356-358.
54. Casati A, Borghi B, Fanelli G, et al. Interscalene brachial plexus anesthesia and analgesia for open shoulder surgery: a randomized, double-blinded comparison between levobupivacaine and ropivacaine. *Anesth Analg.* 2003;96:253-259.
55. Buettner J, Klose R, Hoppe U, Wresch P. Serum levels of mepivacaine-HCl during continuous axillary brachial plexus block. *Reg Anesth.* 1989;14:124-127.
56. Wajima Z, Shitara T, Nakajima Y, et al. Comparison of continuous brachial plexus infusion of butorphanol, mepivacaine and mepivacaine-butorphanol mixtures for postoperative analgesia. *Br J Anaesth.* 1995;75:548-551.
57. Bergman BD, Hebl JR, Kent J, Horlocker TT. Neurologic complications of 405 consecutive continuous axillary catheters. *Anesth Analg.* 2003;96:247-252.
58. Borgeat A, Kalberer F, Jacob H, Ruetsch YA, Gerber C. Patient-controlled interscalene analgesia with ropivacaine 0.2% versus bupivacaine 0.15% after major open shoulder surgery: the effects on hand motor function. *Anesth Analg.* 2001;92:218-223.
59. Singelyn FJ, Gouverneur JM: Extended "three-in-one" block after total knee arthroplasty: continuous versus patient-controlled techniques. *Anesth Analg.* 2000;91:176-180.
60. Singelyn FJ, Seguy S, Gouverneur JM. Interscalene brachial plexus analgesia after open shoulder surgery: continuous versus patient-controlled infusion. *Anesth Analg.* 1999;89:1216-1220.
61. Singelyn FJ, Vanderelst PE, Gouverneur JM: Extended femoral nerve sheath block after total hip arthroplasty: continuous versus patient-controlled techniques. *Anesth Analg.* 2001;92:455-459.
62. Ekatodramis G, Borgeat A, Huledal G, Jeppsson L, Westman L, Sjovall J. Continuous interscalene analgesia with ropivacaine 2 mg/ml after major shoulder surgery. *Anesthesiology.* 2003;98:143-150.
63. Kaloul I, Guay J, Cote C, Halwagi A, Varin F. Ropivacaine plasma concentrations are similar during continuous lumbar plexus blockade using the anterior three-in-one and the posterior psoas compartment techniques. *Can J Anaesth.* 2004;51:52-56.
64. Anker-Moller E, Spangsberg N, Dahl JB, Christensen EF, Schultz P, Carlsson P. Continuous blockade of the lumbar plexus after knee surgery: a comparison of the plasma concentrations and analgesic effect of bupivacaine 0.250% and 0.125%. *Acta Anaesthesiol Scand.* 1990;34:468-472.

65. Ilfeld BM, Morey TE, Enneking FK. The delivery rate accuracy of portable infusion pumps used for continuous regional analgesia. *Anesth Analg.* 2002;95:1331-1336.
66. Ilfeld BM, Morey TE, Enneking FK. Delivery rate accuracy of portable, bolus-capable infusion pumps used for patient-controlled continuous regional analgesia. *Reg Anesth Pain Med.* 2003;28:17-23.
67. Ilfeld BM, Morey TE, Enneking FK. Portable infusion pumps used for continuous regional analgesia: delivery rate accuracy and consistency. *Reg Anesth Pain Med.* 2003;28:424-432.
68. Ilfeld BM, Morey TE. Use of term "patient-controlled" may be confusing in study of elastometric pump. *Anesth Analg.* 2003;97:916-917.
69. Ilfeld BM, Morey TE, Enneking FK. New portable infusion pumps: real advantages or just more of the same in a different package? *Reg Anesth Pain Med.* 2004;29:371-376.
70. Ilfeld BM, Gearen PF, Enneking FK, et al. Effect of femoral perineural local anesthetic infusion on postoperative functional ability following total knee arthroplasty. *Anesthesiology.* 2004;101:A945.
71. Klein SM, Nielsen KC, Greengrass RA, Warner DS, Martin A, Steele SM. Ambulatory discharge after long-acting peripheral nerve blockade: 2382 blocks with ropivacaine. *Anesth Analg.* 2002;94:65-70.
72. Grant SA, Nielsen KC. Continuous peripheral nerve catheters for ambulatory anesthesia. *Curr Anesthesiol Reports.* 2000;2:304-307.
73. Borgeat A, Ekatodramis G, Kalberer F, Benz C. Acute and nonacute complications associated with interscalene block and shoulder surgery: a prospective study. *Anesthesiology.* 2001;95:875-880.
74. Cuvillon P, Ripart J, Lalourcey L, et al. The continuous femoral nerve block catheter for postoperative analgesia: bacterial colonization, infectious rate and adverse effects. *Anesth Analg.* 2001;93:1045-1049.
75. Souron V, Reiland Y, De Traverse A, Delaunay L, Lafosse L. Interpleural migration of an interscalene catheter. *Anesth Analg.* 2003;97:1200-1201.
76. Hogan Q, Dotson R, Erickson S, Kettler R, Hogan K. Local anesthetic myotoxicity: a case and review. *Anesthesiology.* 1994;80:942-947.
77. Chelly JE, Greger J, Gebhard R. Ambulatory continuous perineural infusion: are we ready? [letter]. *Anesthesiology.* 2000;93:581-582.
78. Ilfeld BM, Esener DE, Morey TE, Enneking FK. Ambulatory perineural infusion: the patients' perspective. *Reg Anesth Pain Med.* 2003;28:418-423.
79. Ilfeld BM, Enneking FK. Continuous nerve blocks at home: a review. *Anesth Analg.* 2005;100:1822–1833.

# 8 Regional Anesthesia in the Anticoagulated Patient

*Honorio T. Benzon*

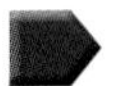

## Intraspinal Hematoma

The incidence of intraspinal hematoma is approximately 0.1 per 100,000 patients per year.[1] It is more likely to occur in anticoagulated or thrombocytopenic patients, patients with neoplastic disease, or in those with liver disease or alcoholism.[2] The incidence of neurologic dysfunction resulting from hemorrhagic complications associated with neuraxial blockade is estimated to be <1 in 150,000 epidural procedures and <1 in 220,000 with spinal anesthetics. The risk of formation of intraspinal hematoma after administration of neuraxial injections is increased in patients who received anticoagulant therapy or have a coagulation disorder, technical difficulties in the performance of the neuraxial procedures due to anatomic abnormalities of the spine, and multiple or bloody punctures. The American Society of Regional Anesthesia and Pain Medicine (ASRA) issued recommended guidelines for the safe performance of neuraxial blocks in patients who are on anticoagulants.[3,4] The third edition of the ASRA guidelines was published in 2010.

## Antiplatelet Therapy

Antiplatelet medications inhibit platelet cyclo-oxygenase and prevent the synthesis of thromboxane A2. Thromboxane A2 is a potent vasoconstrictor and facilitates secondary platelet aggregation and release reactions. An adequate, although potentially fragile, clot may form.[5] Platelet function in patients receiving antiplatelet medications should be assumed to be decreased for 1 week after treatment with aspirin and 1 to 3 days with nonsteroidal anti-inflammatory drugs (NSAIDs). New platelets are produced every day, and these new platelets partly explain the relative safety of performing neuraxial procedures in these patients.

Although Vandermeulen et al[6] implicated antiplatelet therapy in 3 of the 61 cases of spinal hematoma occurring after spinal or epidural anesthesia, the results of several large studies demonstrated the relative safety of neuraxial blockade in combination with antiplatelet therapy. The Collaborative Low-Dose Aspirin Study in Pregnancy Group[7] included 1422 high-risk obstetric patients who were administered 60 mg aspirin daily and underwent epidural anesthesia without any neurologic sequelae. The studies of Horlocker et al,[8,9] of approximately 1000 patients in each study, showed no spinal hematomas, although blood was noted during needle or catheter placement in 22% of the patients. A later study in patients who were on NSAIDs and underwent epidural steroid injections did not develop the signs and symptoms of intraspinal hematoma.[10] A review of the case reports of intraspinal hematoma in patients on aspirin and NSAIDs showed complicating factors that included concomitant heparin administration, epidural venous angioma, and technical difficulty when performing the procedure.[11]

The thienopyridine drugs, ticlopidine and clopidogrel, prevent platelet aggregation by inhibiting adenosine diphosphate (ADP) receptor-mediated platelet activation. Ticlopidine is rarely used because it causes neutropenia, thrombocytopenic purpura, and hypercholesterolemia. Clopidogrel is preferred because of its increased safety profile and proven efficacy. The maximal inhibition of ADP-induced platelet aggregation with clopidogrel occurs 3 to 5 days after the initiation of a standard dose (75 mg), but within 4 to 6 hours after the administration of a large loading dose of 300 to 600 mg.[12] There is a case report of spinal hematoma in a patient on ticlopidine[13] and a case of quadriplegia in a patient on clopidogrel, diclofenac, and possibly aspirin.[14]

Neuraxial blocks can be safely performed on patients taking aspirin or NSAIDs.[4] It is safe to perform neuraxial blocks on patients taking cyclo-oxygenase (COX)-2 inhibitors. For the thienopyridine drugs, it is recommended that clopidogrel be discontinued for 7 days and ticlopidine for 10 to 14 days before a neuraxial injection. It is possible for epidural catheters to be removed or neuraxial injections to be performed 5 days, and not 7 days, after clopidogrel is discontinued.[15] If a neuraxial injection is to be performed in a patient on clopidogrel before 7 days of discontinuation, a P2Y12 assay, a new assay of residual antiplatelet activity, can be performed; <10% activity probably means that a neuraxial block is safe.[16]

Here is a summary of current recommendations:

1. Neuraxial blocks can be performed on patients taking aspirin or NSAIDs.[4]
2. It is safe to perform neuraxial blocks on patients taking COX-2 inhibitors.

3. For the thienopyridine drugs, the ASRA recommendation is that clopidogrel be discontinued for 7 days and ticlopidine for 10 to 14 days before a neuraxial injection.
4. Epidural catheters can be removed safely and neuraxial injections can be performed 5 days (not 7 days, as once advised) after clopidogrel is discontinued.[15]
5. If a neuraxial injection is to be performed in a patient on clopidogrel before 7 days of discontinuation, a P2Y12 assay, a new assay of residual antiplatelet activity, is performed; <10% activity probably means that a neuraxial block is safe.[16]

## Oral Anticoagulants

Warfarin exerts its anticoagulant effect by interfering with the synthesis of the vitamin K–dependent clotting factors (VII, IX, X, and thrombin).[17] It also inhibits the anticoagulants protein C and S. Factor VII and protein C have short half-lives (6–8 hours), and the prolongation of the international normalized ratio (INR) during the early phase of warfarin therapy is the result of the competing effects of reduced factor VII and protein C.[18] Adequate anticoagulation is not achieved until the levels of biologically active factors II (half-life of 50 hours) and X are sufficiently depressed, that is, 4 to 6 days.

Few data exist regarding the risk of spinal hematoma in patients with indwelling spinal or epidural catheters who are subsequently anticoagulated with warfarin. Horlocker et al[19] and Wu and Perkins[20] found no neuraxial hemorrhagic complications in patients who received postoperative epidural analgesia in conjunction with low-dose warfarin after total knee arthroplasty. Because intraspinal hematomas have occurred after removal of the catheter,[6] some have recommended that the same laboratory values apply to placement and removal of an epidural catheter.[21] The current ASRA guidelines recommends an INR value of ≤1.4 as acceptable for the performance of neuraxial blocks.[4] The value was based on studies that showed excellent perioperative hemostasis when the INR value was ≤1.5. The concurrent use of other medications, such as aspirin, NSAIDs, and heparins that affect the clotting mechanism, increases the risk of bleeding complications without affecting the INR.

A controversy exists regarding whether or not the epidural catheter can be removed on postoperative day 1, or 12–14 hours after warfarin is started, when the INR is >1.4. In the absence of other risk factors for increased bleeding, the catheter can probably be removed. The factor VII activity should be determined if risk factors such as low platelets, advanced age, kidney failure, or intake of other anticoagulants are present.[18]

Warfarin is metabolized primarily by the CYP2C9 enzyme of the cytochrome P450 system. Mutations in the gene coding for the cytochrome P450 2C9 hepatic microsomal enzyme affect the elimination clearance of warfarin by impairing the patient's ability to metabolize S-warfarin. Other genetic factors affecting the warfarin dose–response relationship include polymorphisms of the vitamin K oxide reductase (VKOR) enzyme. Mutations in the gene encoding for isoforms of the protein that can lead to enzymes with varied sensitivities to warfarin is rare, and the American College of Chest Physicians (ACCP) advises against pharmacokinetic-based initial dosing of warfarin at this time.[17]

## Intravenous Heparin

Heparin is a complex polysaccharide that exerts its anticoagulant effect by binding to antithrombin III. The conformational change in antithrombin accelerates its ability to inactivate thrombin, factor Xa, and factor IXa. The anticoagulant effect of subcutaneous heparin takes 1 to 2 hours, but the effect of intravenous heparin is immediate. Heparin has a half-life of 1.5 to 2 hours. The activated partial thromboplastin time (aPTT) is used to monitor the effect of heparin; therapeutic anticoagulation is achieved with a prolongation of the aPTT to >1.5 times the baseline value.

There were no spinal hematomas in >4000 patients who underwent lower extremity vascular surgery under continuous spinal or epidural anesthesia.[22] In this study, patients with preexisting coagulation disorders were excluded, heparinization occurred at least 60 minutes after catheter placement, the level of anticoagulation was carefully monitored, and the indwelling catheters were removed at a time when heparin activity was low. Ruff and Dougherty[23] noted the occurrence of spinal hematomas in patients who underwent lumbar puncture with subsequent heparinization. The presence of blood during the procedure, concomitant aspirin therapy, and heparinization within 1 hour were identified as risk factors for the development of a spinal hematoma.

When intraoperative anticoagulation is planned, neuraxial technique should be avoided in patients with coexisting coagulopathies. The following considerations are in order:

1. There should be at least a 1-hour delay between needle placement and heparin administration.
2. The catheter should be removed 1 hour before subsequent heparin administration and 2 to 4 hours after the last heparin dose.[4]
3. The partial thromboplastin time or activated clotting time should be monitored to avoid excessive heparin effect.

## Subcutaneous Heparin

The therapeutic basis of low-dose subcutaneous heparin (5000 units every 8–12 hours) is heparin-mediated inhibition of activated factor X. Following intramuscular or subcutaneous injection of 5000 units of heparin, maximum anticoagulation effect is observed in 40 to 50 minutes and returns to baseline within 4 to 6 hours. The aPTT may remain in the normal range and often is not monitored. However, wide variations in individual patient responses to subcutaneous heparin have been reported. Neuraxial techniques are not contraindicated during subcutaneous (mini-dose) prophylaxis. Some have suggested that the risk of bleeding can be further reduced by delay of the heparin administration until after the block.[4]

The 2008 ACCP guidelines have suggested a more frequent dosing of subcutaneous heparin to three times a day.[24] Case reports show an increased risk for bleeding in patients receiving thrice-daily subcutaneous heparin.[25] In view of this increased bleeding and in the absence of prospective studies that looked into the implications of neuraxial injections in this setting, the third edition of the ASRA guidelines will advise that patients not receive thrice-daily heparin when receiving epidural infusions.

## Low Molecular Weight Heparin

The anticoagulant effect of low molecular weight heparin (LMWH) is similar to unfractionated heparin, that is, activation of antithrombin and acceleration of its interaction with thrombin and factor Xa.[26] LMWH has a greater activity against factor Xa; unfractionated heparin has equivalent activity against thrombin and factor Xa. The plasma half-life of the LMWH ranges from 2 to 4 hours after an intravenous injection and 3 to 6 hours after a subcutaneous injection. Its half-life is two to four times that of standard heparin. The recovery of anti-factor Xa activity after a subcutaneous injection of LMWH approaches 100%. This characteristic makes laboratory monitoring unnecessary, except in patients with renal insufficiency or those with body weight <50 kg or >80 kg.

The summary of recommendations for patients receiving LMWH and neuraxial anesthesia are as follows[4]:

1. The administration of other anticoagulant medications with LMWHs may increase the risk of spinal hematoma.
2. The presence of blood during needle placement and catheter placement does not necessitate postponement of surgery. However, the initiation of LMWH therapy should be delayed for 24 hours postoperatively.
3. The first dose of LMWH prophylaxis should be given no earlier than 24 hours postoperatively and only in the presence of adequate hemostasis.
4. In patients who are on LMWH, needle/catheter placement (or catheter removal) should be performed at least 12 hours after the last prophylactic dose of enoxaparin or 24 hours after higher doses of enoxaparin (1 mg/kg every 12 hours), and 24 hours after dalteparin (120 U/kg every 12 hours or 200 U/kg every 12 hours) or tinzaparin (175 U/kg daily).
5. The LMWH can be administered 2 hours after the epidural catheter is removed.
6. Monitoring of anti-Xa level is not recommended.

## Thrombolytic Therapy

Thrombolytic agents actively dissolve fibrin clots that have already formed, secondary to the action of plasmin. Plasminogen activators, such as streptokinase and urokinase, dissolve thrombus and affect circulating plasminogen leading to decreased levels of both plasminogen and fibrin. Clot lysis leads to elevation of fibrin degradation products, which have an anticoagulant effect by inhibiting platelet aggregation. Fibrinogen and plasminogen are maximally depressed at 5 hours after thrombolytic therapy and remain significantly depressed at 27 hours.[4,27]

Although epidural or spinal needle and catheter placement with subsequent heparinization appears relatively safe, the risk of spinal hematoma in patients who receive thrombolytic therapy is less well-defined. Cases of spinal hematoma in patients who received neuraxial injections and thrombolytic agents were reported recently in the medical literature.

Fibrinolytic and thrombolytic agents pose a unique problem when performing neuraxial anesthesia. The time frame for avoidance of these drugs and puncture of noncompressible vessels is 10 days. Except in highly unusual circumstances, patients who received fibrinolytic or thrombolytic drugs should be cautioned against receiving spinal or epidural anesthesia.[4,27] There are no available data to clearly determine the length of time after discontinuation of these drugs for the safe performance of a neuraxial technique. There is no definitive recommendation on the timing of removal of neuraxial catheters in patients who unexpectedly receive fibrinolytic or thrombolytic therapy. Measurement of fibrinogen levels may be helpful in guiding a decision about removal of the catheter.

## Herbal Therapy

Herbal preparations do have some effect on platelet aggregation. For example, garlic inhibits platelet aggregation and its effect on hemostasis appears to last 7 days. Ginkgo biloba inhibits platelet-activating factor and its effect lasts 36 hours. These effects last 24 hours with the use of ginseng.[4] The effects of dietary supplements on platelet function and coagulation are not well described, and outcomes are difficult to predict.[28] In spite of these characteristics, herbal preparations appear to present no added significant risk in the development of spinal hematoma in patients having epidural or spinal anesthesia. At this time, there appears to be no specific concerns as to the timing of neuraxial block in relationship to the dosing of herbal therapy, postoperative monitoring, or the timing of neuraxial catheter removal.[4]

## Fondaparinux

Fondaparinux is a synthetic anticoagulant that produces its antithrombotic effect through selective inhibition of factor Xa.[29] The drug exhibits consistency in its anticoagulant effect because it is chemically synthesized and its bioavailability is 100%. Rapidly absorbed, it reaches maximum concentration within 1.7 hours of administration. Its half-life is 17 to 21 hours, allowing once-daily dosing.[30] The actual risk of spinal hematoma with fondaparinux is unknown. The daily dosing makes safe catheter removal harder to predict. The ASRA[4] recommends against the use of fondaparinux in the presence of an indwelling epidural catheter. These recommendations were based on the sustained and irreversible antithrombotic effect of fondaparinux, early postoperative dosing (6 hours after surgery), and the spinal hematoma reported during initial clinical trials. Performance of neuraxial techniques should occur under the conditions used in clinical trials (single needle pass, atraumatic needle placement, and avoidance of indwelling neuraxial catheters).[4]

A 2007 study showed no complications in patients who had neuraxial injections or deep peripheral nerve blocks.[31] In this study, the catheters were removed 36 hours after the last dose of fondaparinux and dosing was delayed for 12 hours after the catheter was removed. In a review article, Rosencher et al[32] recommended that catheter removal should be delayed at least 36 hours (equivalent to two half-lives) and that the subsequent injection should be timed to at least 7 hours after the removal of the catheter.

## Thrombin Inhibitors

Recombinant hirudin derivatives, such as desirudin (Revasc), lepirudin (Refludan), and bivalirudin (Angiomax), inhibit both free and clot-bound thrombin.[4] Argatroban, although an L-arginine derivative, is also a thrombin inhibitor. These drugs are used in the treatment of heparin-induced thrombocytopenia and as an adjunct when angioplasty is performed.[33] Their anticoagulant effect is present for 1 to 3 hours after intravenous administration and is monitored by the aPTT. There is no pharmacologic reversal to the effect of these drugs. Desirudin is used as thromboprophylaxis after total hip replacement.[34] There are no published reports of spinal hematoma related to neuraxial anesthesia in patients who have received a thrombin inhibitor, probably because of the hesitancy of clinicians to perform neuraxial injections in patients taking the drugs, which is probably related to their unfamiliarity with the drugs. The most recent ASRA guidelines recommend against the performance of neuraxial techniques in patients who received thrombin inhibitors.

## Newer Anticoagulants

### Dabigatran Etexilate

Dabigatran is an oral direct thrombin inhibitor. Its bioavailability is only 5%, peak plasma levels occur at 2 hours, and its half-life is 8 hours after a single dose but up to 17 hours after multiple doses. The drug is approved for clinical use in Europe. Studies showed dabigatran (150 or 220 mg daily) to be less effective than enoxaparin (30 mg twice daily) when used for thromboprophylaxis after total joint surgery.[35,36] A 48-hour interval is recommended before a neuraxial injection.

### Rivaroxaban

Rivaroxaban is an oral factor Xa inhibitor approved for use in Europe and Canada. It is awaiting approval by the Food and Drug Administration (FDA) in the United States. It has an 80% bioavailability; its peak effect occurs after 1 hour; the duration of effect is 12 hours; and it has a half-life of 9 to 13 hours. Clinical studies comparing rivaroxaban, at doses of 5 to 40 mg, to enoxaparin showed similar or superior efficacy.[37–40] There were no reports of spinal hematoma in these studies. Apparently, a 24-hour interval (2 × half-life) was observed between the rivaroxaban dose and epidural catheter placement or removal; subsequent dosing of the drug was 6 hours after removal of the catheter (personal communication with the company). The drug offers several salutary characteristics including efficacy and simplicity with once-daily oral dosing.

### Prasugrel

Prasugrel is an oral anticoagulant approved for use by the FDA in July 2009. Its mechanism of action is similar to clopidogrel; that is, it acts as a noncompetitive antagonist of P2Y12, inhibiting the ability of platelet ADP to induce aggregation for the life of the platelet.[41] Prasugrel and clopidogrel are prodrugs; however, prasugrel has a quicker onset of action, a longer duration (the effect of 60 mg is 1–1.5 hours compared with 6 hours with 300 mg clopidogrel); it is 10 times more potent; and less prone to drug–drug interactions and variability in patient response than clopidogrel.[41,42] A 7–10 day interval is recommended before a neuraxial injection. Other novel antiplatelet drugs are in development, including ticagrelor and cangrelor, which are under study for use in patients with acute coronary syndromes.[43]

## Anticoagulation and Peripheral Nerve Blocks

Spontaneous hematomas have been reported in patients who took anticoagulants. Abdominal wall hematomas, intracranial hemorrhage, psoas hematoma, and intrahepatic hemorrhage

**TABLE 8-1 Summary of Guidelines on Anticoagulants and Neuraxial Blocks***

I. Antiplatelet medications
  1. Aspirin, NSAIDs, COX-2 inhibitors
     Surgery: May continue
     Pain Clinic: ASA preferably stopped 2–3 d in thoracic/cervical epidurals
  2. Thienopyridine derivatives
     a. Clopidogrel (Plavix): discontinue for 7 d
     b. Ticlopidine (Ticlid): discontinue for 14 d
     Do not perform a neuraxial block in patients on more than one antiplatelet drug.
     If a neuraxial or deep plexus block has to be performed in patients whose clopidogrel was discontinued <7 d, then a P2Y12 assay should be performed.
  3. GPIIB/IIIA inhibitors: Time to normal platelet aggregation
     a. Abciximab (ReoPro) = 48 h
     b. Eptifibatide (Integrilin) = 8 h
     c. Tirofiban (Aggrastat) = 8 h

II. Warfarin
   Check INR; discontinue 4–5 d
   INR ≤1.4 before neuraxial block or epidural catheter removal

III. Heparin
  1. Subcutaneous heparin (5000 U SC q12h)
     Subcutaneous heparin is not a contraindication against a neuraxial block
     Neuraxial block should preferably be performed before SC heparin is given
     Risk of decreased platelet count with SC heparin therapy >5 d
  2. Intravenous heparin
     Neuraxial block: 2–4 h after the last intravenous heparin dose
     Wait ≥1 h after neuraxial block before giving intravenous heparin

IV. Low molecular weight heparin (LMWH)
   No concomitant antiplatelet medication, heparin, or dextran
   Time interval between placement/removal of catheter after last dose
     a. Enoxaparin (Lovenox) 0.5 mg/kg BID (prophylactic dose): 12 h
     b. 24-h interval:
        Enoxaparin (Lovenox), 1 mg/kg BID (therapeutic dose)
        Enoxaparin (Lovenox), 1.5 mg/kg QD
        Dalteparin (Fragmin), 120 U/kg BID, 200 U/kg QD
        Tinzaparin (Innohep), 175 U/kg QD
   LMWH Postop: LMWH should not be started until after 24 h postsurgery.
   LMWH should not be given until ≥2 h after epidural catheter removal.

V. Specific Xa inhibitor: Fondaparinux (Arixtra)
   ASRA: If neuraxial procedure *has to be performed*, recommend single needle, atraumatic placement, avoid indwelling catheter.
   EXPERT Study (reference 31): Epidural placement or catheter removal: 36 h after.
   Fondaparinux (half-lives); subsequent dose 12 h after catheter removal.

VI. Fibrinolytic/Thrombolytic drugs (Streptokinase, alteplase [TPA])
   Recommended interval: 10 d (ASRA: no definite recommendation).
   No data on safety interval for performance of neuraxial procedure.

(*Continued*)

**TABLE 8-1 Summary of Guidelines on Anticoagulants and Neuraxial Blocks* (*Continued*)**

VII. Thrombin Inhibitors
Desirudin (Revasc)
Lepirudin (Refludan)
Bivalirudin (Angiomax)
Argatroban (Acova)
Anticoagulant effect lasts 3 h; monitored by aPTT
ASRA: no recommendation because of paucity of data

VII. Herbal therapy
Mechanism of anticoagulant effect and time to normal hemostasis:
Garlic: inhibits platelet aggregation, increased fibrinolysis; 7 d
Ginkgo: inhibits platelet-activating factor; 36 h
Ginseng: increased PT and PTT; 24 hs
ASRA: Neuraxial block not contraindicated for single herbal medication use

Note: The guidelines are the same for the placement and removal of epidural catheters.

*Modified from Benzon HT. Anticoagulants and neuraxial injections. In: Benzon HT, Raja S, Molloy RE, Liu SS, Fishman FM, eds. *Essentials of Pain Medicine and Regional Anesthesia.* New York: Elsevier/Churchill Livingstone; 2005:708-720. Copyright Elsevier 2005.

have occurred after LMWH.[44-47] Major hemorrhagic complications occur in 1.9 to 6.5% of patients on enoxaparin.[48] The increased bleeding that occurs after vascular or cardiac procedures and regional nerve blocks in these patients can result in an expanding hematoma with resultant ischemia of the nerve.

There has been no prospective study on peripheral nerve blocks in the presence of anticoagulants. However, there have been several case reports of hematomas when peripheral blocks are performed in patients who are on these drugs. The hematomas occurred in patients with abnormal and normal coagulation status, and in patients who were given LMWH, ticlopidine and clopidogrel, warfarin, heparin, or a combination of the drugs.[49-55] In most cases, however, recovery of neurologic deficits occurred within a year.

The diagnosis of bleeding after peripheral nerve block in patients on anticoagulants include pain (flank, paravertebral, or in the groin with psoas bleeding), tenderness in the area, fall in hemoglobin/hematocrit, fall in blood pressure, and sensory and motor deficits. Although definite diagnosis is made by computed tomography, ultrasound can be a diagnostic aid, and its increasing use will make this modality a useful tool for the diagnosis and subsequent monitoring of peripheral hematomas. Treatment of peripheral hematomas usually includes surgical consult, blood transfusion as necessary, and watchful waiting versus surgical drainage.

The most recent ASRA guidelines recommended that the same guidelines on neuraxial injections apply to deep plexus or peripheral nerve blocks. Some clinicians may find this to be too restrictive and apply the same guidelines only to deep plexus and noncompressible blocks (e.g., lumbar plexus block, deep cervical plexus blocks) or to blocks near vascular areas, such as celiac plexus blocks or superior hypogastric plexus blocks. If peripheral nerve blocks are performed in the presence of anticoagulants, the anesthesiologist must discuss the risks and benefits of the block with the patient and the surgeon, and follow the patient very closely after the block.

## Guidelines of Various Societies

Guidelines on use of regional anesthesia in the presence of anticoagulants have been published by a number of societies throughout the world to better fit them to the realm of the local practices. By necessity, there are similarities and differences among them. A good example is the new ASRA guidelines[56] and the Belgian and German guidelines.[57,58] The guidelines of the three organizations are similar with regard to antiplatelet medications, unfractionated heparin, and thrombolytic agents. With regard to LMWH, the ASRA guidelines are more conservative, partly due to the differences in the dosing of the drug. For fondaparinux, the German guidelines allow an indwelling epidural catheter, whereas the ASRA and the Belgian guidelines recommend against it. The Belgian and German guidelines allow neuraxial injections in patients on direct thrombin inhibitors; the ASRA guidelines do not. Finally, some of the newer anticoagulants have been approved for use in Europe and are awaiting approval in the United States so the guidelines for these drugs are forthcoming.

## Summary

Adherence to the discussed guidelines should lead to a lesser risk of hemorrhagic complications after regional anesthesia, including spinal hematomas. Likewise, implementation of the guidelines leads to improved vigilance and better care of patients on anticoagulants in whom nerve blocks are performed or entertained. Consensus guidelines, however, should be viewed only as recommendations; specific decisions on nerve blocks in patients on anticoagulants should be individualized. Adequate monitoring, follow-up, and timely treatment should be implemented in patients on anticoagulants who are receiving neuraxial or peripheral nerve blocks (see algorithms on the following pages).

## DECISION MAKING ALGORITHM IN THE SELECTION OF NEURAXIAL OR PERIPHERAL NERVE BLOCKADE

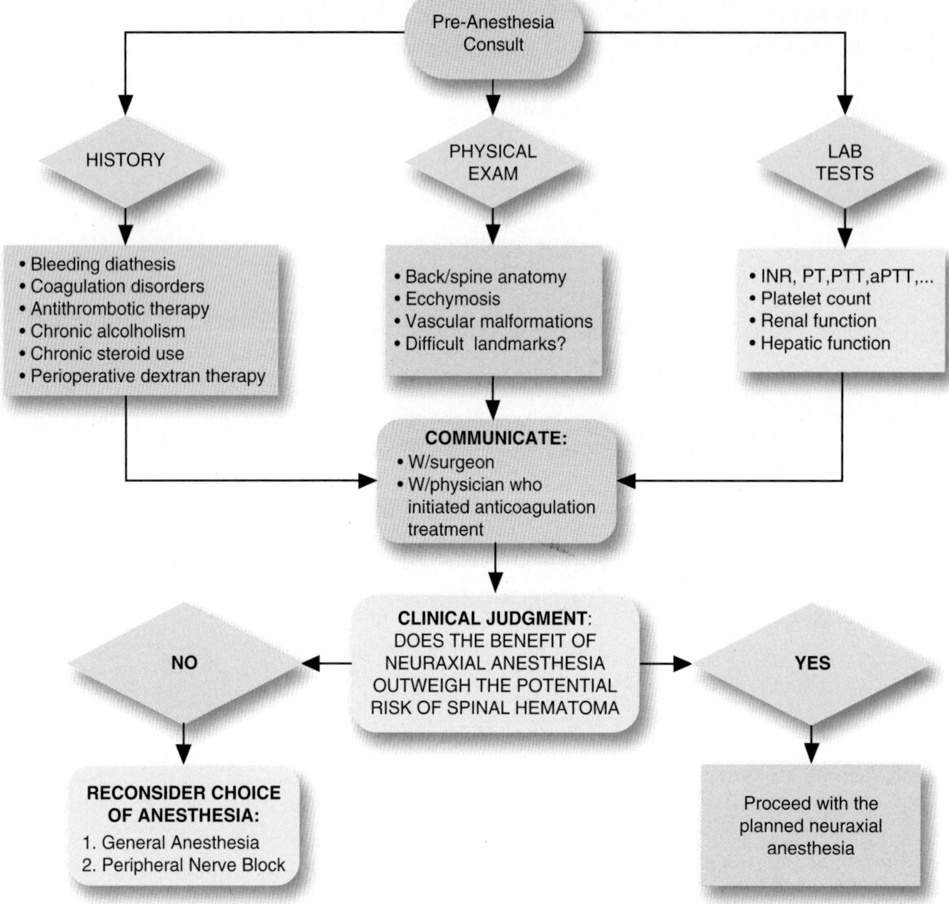


## FOLLOW-UP OF PATIENTS WHO ARE AT RISK FOR SPINAL OR PERIPHERAL HEMATOMA

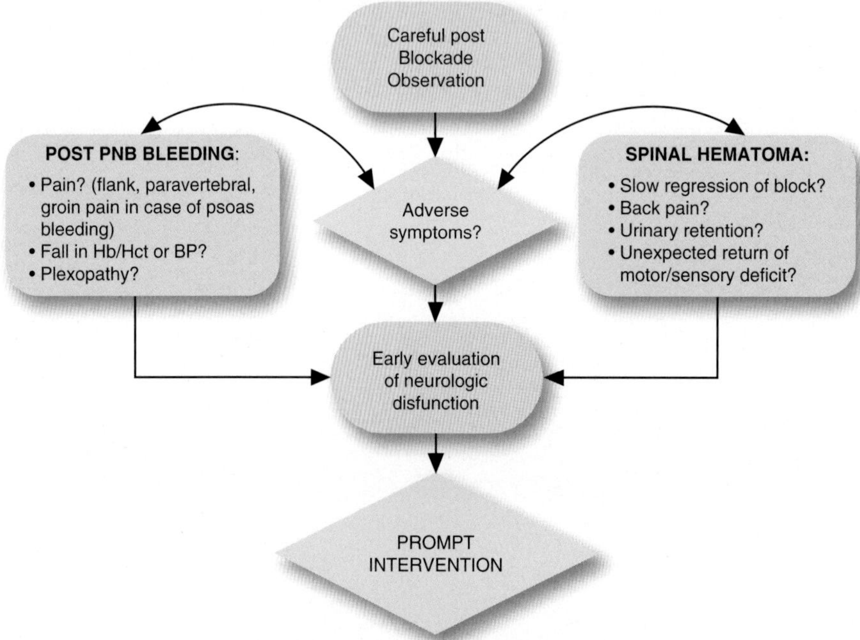

## ANTICOAGULANTS: MECHANISM OF ACTION AND RECOMMENDED GUIDELINES FOR PRACTICE OF NEURAXIAL ANESTHESIA

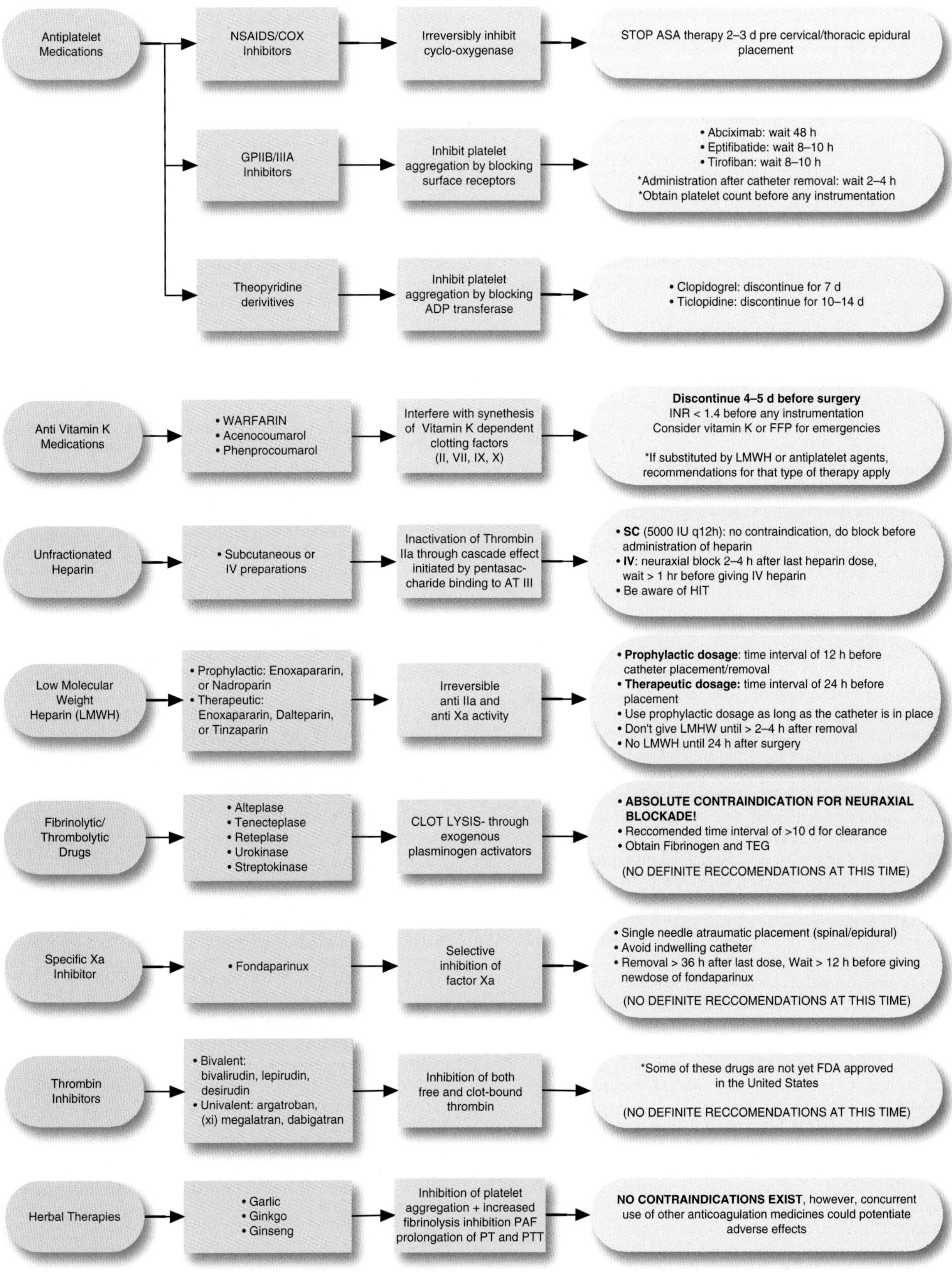

## REFERENCES


1. Hejazi N, Thaper PY, Hassler W. Nine cases of nontraumatic spinal epidural hematoma. *Neurol Med Chir.* 1998;38:718-723.
2. Mattle H, Sieb JP, Rohner M, Mumenthaler M. Nontraumatic spinal epidural and subdural hematomas. *Neurology.* 1987;37:1351-1356.
3. Heit JA, Horlocker TT, eds. Neuraxial anesthesia and anticoagulation. *Reg Anesth Pain Med.* 1998;23:S129-193.
4. Horlocker TT, Wedel DJ, Benzon HT, et al. Regional anesthesia in the anticoagulated patient: defining the risks (The second ASRA Consensus Conference on Neuraxial Anesthesia and Anticoagulation). *Reg Anesth Pain Med.* 2003;28:172-197.
5. Benzon HT, Brunner EA, Vaisrub N. Bleeding time and nerve blocks after aspirin. *Reg Anesth.* 1984;9:86-90.
6. Vandermeulen EP, Van Aken H, Vermylen J. Anticoagulants and spinal-epidural anesthesia. *Anesth Analg.* 1994;79:1165-1177.
7. CLASP (Collaborative Low-Dose Aspirin Study in Pregnancy) Collaborative Group. CLASP: a randomized trial of low-dose aspirin for the prevention and treatment of pre-eclampsia among 9364 pregnant women. *Lancet.* 1994;343:619-629.
8. Horlocker TT, Wedel DJ, Offord KP. Does preoperative antiplatelet therapy increase the risk of hemorrhagic complications associated with regional anesthesia? *Anesth Analg.* 1990;70:631-634.
9. Horlocker TT, Wedel DJ, Schroeder DR, et al. Preoperative antiplatelet therapy does not increase the risk of spinal hematoma associated with regional anesthesia. *Anesth Analg.* 1995;80:303-309.
10. Horlocker TT, Bajwa ZH, Ashraft Z, et al. Risk assessment of hemorrhagic complications associated with nonsteroidal antiinflammatory medications in ambulatory pain clinic patients undergoing epidural steroid injection. *Anesth Analg.* 2002;95:1691-1697.
11. Benzon HT, Wong HY, Siddiqui T, Ondra S. Caution in performing epidural injections in patients on several antiplatelet drugs. *Anesthesiology.* 1999;91:1558-1559.
12. Helft G, Osende JI, Worthley SG, et al. Acute antithrombotic effect of a front-loaded regimen of clopidogrel in patients with atherosclerosis on aspirin. *Arterioscler Thromb Vasc Biol.* 2000;29:2316-2321.
13. Mayumi T, Dohi S. Spinal subarachnoid hematoma after lumbar puncture in a patient receiving antiplatelet therapy. *Anesth Analg.* 1983;62:777-779.
14. Benzon HT, Wong HY, Siddiqui T, Ondra S. Caution in performing epidural injections in patients on several antiplatelet drugs. *Anesthesiology.* 1999;91:1558-1559.
15. Broad L, Lee T, Conroy M, et al. Successful management of patients with a drug-eluting coronary stent presenting for elective, non-cardiac surgery. *Br J Anaesth.* 2007;98:19-22.
16. Benzon HT, Fragen R, Benzon HA, Savage J, Robinson J, Puri L. Clopidogrel and neuraxial block: the role of the PFA II and P2Y12 assays. *Reg Anesth Pain Med.* 2010;35:115.
17. Ansell J, Hirsh J, Hylek E, Jacobson A, Crowther M, Palareti G. Pharmacology and management of the vitamin K antagonists. *Chest.* 2008;133:160S-190S.
18. Benzon HT, Benzon HA, Kirby-Nolan M, Avram MJ, Nader A. Factor VII levels and risk factors for increased international normalized ratio in the early phase of warfarin therapy. *Anesthesiology.* 2010;112:298-304.
19. Horlocker TT, Wedel DJ, Schlichting JL. Postoperative epidural analgesia and oral anticoagulant therapy. *Anesth Analg.* 1994;79:89-93.
20. Wu CL, Perkins FM. Oral anticoagulant prophylaxis and epidural catheter removal. *Reg Anesth.* 1996;21:517-524.
21. Horlocker TT. When to remove a spinal or epidural catheter in an anticoagulated patient. *Reg Anesth.* 1993;18:264-265.
22. Rao TL, El-Etr AA. Anticoagulation following placement of epidural and subarachnoid catheters: an evaluation of neurologic sequelae. *Anesthesiology.* 1981;55:618-620.
23. Ruff DL, Dougherty JH. Complications of anticoagulation followed by anticoagulation. *Stroke.* 1981;12:879-881.
24. Geerts WH, Bergqvist D, Pineo GF, et al. Prevention of venous thromboembolism. American College of Chest Physicians Evidence-Based Clinical Practice Guidelines (8th Edition). *Chest.* 2008;133:381S-453S.
25. King CS, Holley AB, Jackson JL, et al. Twice versus three times daily heparin dosing for thromboembolism prophylaxis in the general population: a metaanalysis. *Chest.* 2007;131:507-516.
26. Horlocker TT, Heit JA. Low molecular weight heparin: biochemistry, pharmacology, perioperative prophylaxis regimens, and guidelines for regional anesthetic management. *Anesth Analg.* 1997;85:874-885.
27. Rosenquist RW, Brown DL. Neuraxial bleeding: fibrinolytics/thrombolytics. *Reg Anesth Pain Med.* 1998;23S:152-156.
28. Basila D, Yuan CS. Effects of dietary supplements on coagulation and platelet function. *Thromb Res.* 2005;117:49-53.
29. Bauer KA. Fondaparinux: basic properties and efficacy and safety in venous thromboembolism prophylaxis. *Am J Orthop.* 2002;31:4-10.
30. Turpie AG, Gallus AS, Hoek JA. Pentasaccharide investigators. A synthetic pentasaccharide for the prevention of deep-vein thrombosis after total hip replacement. *N Engl J Med.* 2001;344:619-625.
31. Singelyn FJ, Verheyen CC, Piovella F, Van Aken HK, Rosenceher N. EXPERT Study Investigators. The safety and efficacy of extended thromboprophylaxis with fondaparinux after major orthopedic surgery of the lower limb with or without a neuraxial or deep peripheral nerve catheter: the EXPERT Study. *Anesth Analg.* 2007;105:1540-1547.
32. Rosencher N, Bonnet MP, Sessler DI. Selected new antithrombotic agents and neuraxial anesthesia for major orthopedic surgery: management strategies. *Anaesthesia.* 2007;62:1154-1160.
33. Greinacher A, Lubenow N. Recombinant hirudin in clinical practice: focus on lepirudin. *Circulation.* 2001;103:1479-1484.
34. Ericksson BI, Wille-Jorgensen P, Kalebo P, et al. A comparison of recombinant hirudin with a low-molecular-weight heparin to prevent thromboembolic complications after total hip replacement. *N Engl J Med.* 1997;337:1329-1335.
35. Ericksson BI, Dahl OE, Rosencher N, et al. RE-MODEL Study Group: Oral dabigatran etexilate vs. subcutaneous enoxaparin for the prevention of venous thromboembolism after total knee replacement: the RE-MODEL randomized trial. *J Thromb Haemost.* 2007;5:2178-2185.
36. The RE-MOBILIZE Writing Committee. Oral thrombin inhibitor dabigatran etexilate versus North American enoxaparin regimen for prevention of venous thromboembolism after knee arthroplasty surgery. *J Arthroplasty.* 2009;24:1-9.
37. Ericksson BI, Borris LC, Dahl OE, et al; ODIXa-HIP Study Investigators. A once-daily, oral, direct factor Xa inhibitor, rivaroxaban (BAY 59-7939), for thromboprophylaxis after total hip replacement. *Circulation.* 2006;114:2374-2381.
38. Eriksson BI, Borris LC, Friedman RJ, et al; RECORD1 Study group. Rivaroxaban versus enoxaparin for thromboprophylaxis after hip arthroplasty. *N Engl J Med.* 2008;358:2765-2775.
39. Lassen MR, Ageno W, Borris LC, et al; RECORD3 Investigators. Rivaroxaban versus enoxaparin for thromboprophylaxis after total knee arthroplasty. *N Eng J Med.* 2008;358:2776-2786.
40. Kakkar AK, Brenner B, Dahl O, et al. RECORD2 Investigators. Extended duration rivaroxaban versus short-term enoxaparin for the prevention of venous thromboembolism after total hip arthroplasty: a double-blind, randomized controlled trial. *Lancet.* 2008;372:31-39.
41. Reinhart KM, White CM, Baker WL. *Pharmacotherapy.* 2009;29:1441-1451.
42. Bhatt DL. Prasugrel in clinical practice. *N Engl J Med.* 2009;361:940-942.

43. Shalito I, Kopyleva O, Serebruany V. Novel antiplatelet agents in development: prasugrel, ticagrelor, and cangrelor and beyond. *Am J Ther.* 2009;16:451-458.
44. Antonelli D, Fares L, Anene C. Enoxaparin associated with huge abdominal wall hematomas: a report of two cases. *Am Surgeon.* 2000;66:797-800.
45. Dickinson LD, Miller L, Patel CP, Gupta SK. Enoxaparin increases the incidence of postoperative intracranial hemorrhage when initiated preoperatively for deep vein thrombosis prophylaxis with brain tumors. *Neurosurgery.* 1998;43:1074-1081.
46. Ho KJ, Gawley SD, Young MR. Psoas hematoma and femoral neuropathy associated with enoxaparin therapy. *Int J Clin Pract.* 2003;57:553-554.
47. Houde JP, Steinberg G. Intrahepatic hemorrhage after use of low-molecular-weight heparin for total hip arthroplasty. *J Arthroplasty.* 1999;14:372-374.
48. Noble S, Spencer CM. Enoxaparin: a review of its clinical potential in the management of coronary artery disease. *Drugs.* 1998;56:259-272.
49. Klein SM, D'Ercole F, Greengrass RA, Warner DS. Enoxaparin associated with psoas hematoma and lumbar plexopathy after lumbar plexus block. *Anesthesiology.* 1997;87:1576-1579.
50. Weller RS, Gerancher JC, Crews JC, Wade KL. Extensive retroperitoneal hematoma without neurologic deficit in two patients who underwent lumbar plexus block and were later anticoagulated. *Anesthesiology.* 2003;98:581-583.
51. Maier C, Gleim M, Weiss T, et al. Severe bleeding following lumbar sympathetic blockade in two patients under medication with irreversible platelet aggregation inhibitors. *Anesthesiology.* 2002;97:740-743.
52. Nielsen CH. Bleeding after intercostal nerve block in a patient anticoagulated with heparin. *Anesthesiology.* 1989;71:162-164.
53. Aida S, Takahashi H, Shimoji K. Renal subcapsular hematoma after lumbar plexus block. *Anesthesiology.* 1996;84:452-455.
54. Mishio M, Matsumoto T, Okuda Y, Kitayama T. Delayed severe airway obstruction due to hematoma following stellate ganglion block. *Reg Anesth Pain Med.* 1998;23:516-519.
55. Maier C, Gleim M, Weiss T, Stachetzki U, Nicolas V, Zenz M. Severe bleeding following lumbar sympathetic block in two patients under medication with irreversible platelet aggregation inhibitors. *Anesthesiology.* 2002;97:740-743.
56. Horlocker TT, Wedel DJ, Rowlingson JC, et al. Regional anesthesia in the patient receiving antithrombotic or thrombolytic therapy: American Society of Regional Anesthesia and Pain Medicine evidence-based guidelines (third edition). *Reg Anesth Pain Med.* 2010;35:64-101.
57. The Belgian Association for Regional Anesthesia Working Party on Anticoagulants and Central Nerve Blocks: Vandermeulen E, Singelyn F, Vercauteren M, Brichant JF, Icks BE, Gautier P. Belgian guidelines concerning central neural blockade in patients with drug-induced alteration of coagulation: an update. *Acta Anaesth Belg.* 2005;56:139-146.
58. Gogarten W, Van Aken H, Buttner J, Reiss H, Wulf H, Burkle H. Regional anesthesia and thromboembolism prophylaxis/anticoagulation—revised recommendations of the German Society of Anaesthesiology and Intensive Care Medicine. *Anaesth Intensive Med.* 2007;48:S109-S124.

# 9 Toxicity of Local Anesthetics

Steven Dewaele, and Alan C. Santos

##  Introduction

Systemic toxicity of local anesthetics can occur after administration of an excessive dose, with rapid absorption, or because of an accidental intravenous injection. The management of local anesthetic toxicity can be challenging, and in the case of cardiac toxicity, prolonged resuscitation efforts may be necessary.[1,2] Therefore, understanding the circumstances that can lead to systemic toxicity of local anesthetics and being prepared for treatment is essential to optimize the patient outcome.

Systemic toxicity is typically manifested as central nervous system (CNS) toxicity (tinnitus, disorientation, and ultimately, seizures) or cardiovascular toxicity (hypotension, dysrhythmias, and cardiac arrest).[3] The dose capable of causing CNS symptoms is typically lower than the dose and concentration result in cardiovascular toxicity. This is because the CNS is more susceptible to local anesthetic toxicity than the cardiovascular system. However, bupivacaine toxicity may not adhere to this sequence, and cardiac toxicity may precede the neurologic symptoms.[4] Although less common, cardiovascular toxicity is more serious and more difficult to treat than CNS toxicity.

Other reported, but much less common, adverse effects of certain local anesthetics include allergic reactions,[5] methemoglobinemia,[6] and bronchospasm.[7] Direct neural[8] and local tissue toxicity[9] have been reported also; however, discussion about these topics is beyond the scope of this chapter.

##  Signs and Symptoms of Systemic Local Anesthetic Toxicity

The earliest signs of systemic toxicity are usually caused by blockade of inhibitory pathways in the cerebral cortex.[10] This allows for disinhibition of facilitator neurons resulting in excitatory cell preponderance and unopposed (generally enhanced) excitatory nerve activity. As a result, initial subjective symptoms of CNS toxicity include signs of excitation, such as lightheadedness and dizziness, difficulty focusing, tinnitus, confusion, and circumoral numbness.[11,12] Likewise, the objective signs of local anesthetic toxicity are excitatory, for example, shivering, myoclonia, tremors, and sudden muscular contractions.[13] As the local anesthetic level rises, tonic-clonic convulsions occur. Symptoms of CNS excitation typically are followed by signs of CNS depression: Seizure activity ceases rapidly and ultimately is succeeded by respiratory depression and respiratory arrest. In the concomitant presence of other CNS depressant drugs (e.g., premedication), CNS depression can develop without the preceding excitatory phase.

The CNS toxicity is directly correlated with local anesthetic potency.[14–17] However, there is an inverse relationship between the toxicity of local anesthetics and the rate at which the agents are injected: Increasing speed of injection will decrease the blood-level threshold for symptoms to appear.

All local anesthetics can induce cardiac dysrhythmias,[18,19] and all, except cocaine, are myocardium depressants.[20–25] Local anesthetic–induced arrhythmias can manifest as conduction delays (from prolonged PR interval to complete heart block, sinus arrest, and asystole) to ventricular dysrhythmias (from simple ventricular ectopy to torsades de pointes and fibrillation). The negative inotropic action of local anesthetics is exerted in a dose-dependent fashion and consists of depressed myocardial contractility and a decrease in cardiac output. Dysrhythmias due to local anesthetic overdose may be recalcitrant to traditional therapies; the reduced myocardial contractility and low output state further complicate the treatment.

The sequence of cardiovascular events is ordinarily as follows: Low blood levels of local anesthetic usually generate a small increase in cardiac output, blood pressure, and heart rate, which is most likely due to a boost in sympathetic activity and direct vasoconstriction. As the blood level of local anesthetic rises, hypotension ensues as a result of peripheral vasodilation due to relaxation of the vascular smooth muscles. Further rise of local anesthetic blood levels leads to severe hypotension, resulting from the combination of reduced peripheral vascular resistance, reduced cardiac output, and/or malignant arrhythmias. Eventually, extreme hemodynamic instability may lead to cardiac arrest.

Acid–base status plays an important role in the setting of local anesthetic toxicity.[26] Acidosis and hypercarbia amplify the CNS effects of local anesthetic overdose and exacerbate cardiotoxicity. Hypercarbia enhances cerebral blood flow; consequently, more local anesthetic is made accessible to the cerebral circulation. Diffusion of carbon dioxide across the nerve membrane can cause intracellular acidosis, and as such, it is promoting the conversion of the local anesthetic into the cationic, or active, form. Because it is impossible for the cationic form to travel across the nerve membrane, ionic trapping occurs, worsening the CNS toxicity of the local anesthetic. Hypercarbia and/or acidosis also reduce the binding of local anesthetics by plasma proteins,[27] and as a result, the fraction of free drug readily available for diffusion expands.

## Prevention

Prevention of toxicity is key to safer practice, and it starts with making sure that the work environment is optimized for performing regional anesthesia.[28] The logistics for treating an emergency, including equipment for airway management and treating cardiac arrest, must be readily available and functioning.

A judicious selection of the type, dose, and concentration of the local anesthetic, and the regional anesthesia technique, is important. As a rule, the optimal dose and concentration is the lowest one that achieves the aimed for effect. The effects of pretreatment with a benzodiazepine is often debated but almost routinely used in our practice. Benzodiazepines lower the probability of seizures[29–32] but can mask early signs of toxicity.[33] A sedated patient is theoretically less able to keep the physician updated on the subjective symptoms of light toxicity, and severe toxicity can establish itself without a recognizable toxic prodrome. This concern remains only theoretical; many symptoms of limited, mild CNS toxicity can be prevented by routine premedication with benzodiazepines in addition to making the PNB procedure more pleasant to patients.

Therefore, the presence of premedication or general anesthesia is not perceived to increase the risk of local anesthetic toxicity. Considerable research has been invested into the subject of the ideal test for detecting intravenous injection and to what constitutes the ideal test dose. Epinephrine (5–15 μg) is still widely in use as a marker of intravascular injection. End points with an acceptable sensitivity are defined by an increase in heart rate >10 bpm, increase in systolic blood pressure by >15 mm Hg,[34] or a 25% decrease in lead II T-wave amplitude.[35] However, elderly patients are less responsive to beta stimulation[36] as are those on beta-blocking agents. Low cardiac output can prolong drug circulation and delay the clinical effect of the beta mimetic, and therefore, the sensitivity of the test. Accordingly, the interpretation of the test result is not always as straightforward as one would wish. The significant proportion of false negative test results warrants a reevaluation of the routine use of this test as a sole determinant to detect inadvertent intravenous injection.

Regardless of whether epinephrine is used as a marker of an intravascular injection, it is of utmost importance to use slow, incremental injections of local anesthetic, with frequent aspirations (every 3–5 mL) between injections while monitoring the patient for signs of toxicity.[37] A slow rate of injection of divided doses at distinct intervals can decrease the possibility of summating intravascular injections. With a rapid injection the seizures may occur at higher blood level because there is no time for distribution of the drug as compared to a slow infusion where the seizure occurs at a lower drug level because of the distribution. It is prudent to decrease the local anesthetic dosage in elderly or debilitated patients and in any patient with diminished cardiac output. However, there are no firm recommendations on the degree of dose reduction.

## Treatment

Early recognition of the toxicity and early discontinuation of the administration is of crucial importance.[38] The administration of local anesthetics should be stopped immediately. The airway should be maintained at all times, and supplemental oxygen is provided while ensuring that the monitoring equipment is functional and properly applied. Neurologic parameters and cardiovascular status should be assessed until the patient is completely asymptomatic and stable.[39]

Administration of a benzodiazepine to offset or ameliorate excitatory neurological symptoms or a potential tonic-clonic seizure is indicated.[40] Early treatment of convulsions is particularly meaningful because convulsions can result in metabolic acidosis, thus aggravating the toxicity. Seizures should be controlled at all times. Based on the recent data in animal studies,[41–43] as well as mounting case reports,[44–53] starting an infusion of lipid emulsion (intralipid), especially in those cases where symptoms of cardiac toxicity are present, should be contemplated early.[54] Importantly, there is a mounting consensus that infusion of intralipids may be initiated early, to also *prevent*, rather then treat cardiac arrest. If available, arrangements for transfer to an operating room where cardiopulmonary bypass can be instituted should also be contemplated in situations where the response to early treatment is not favorable.[55–58]

Malignant arrhythmias and asystole are managed using standard cardiopulmonary resuscitation protocols,[59,60] acknowledging that a prolonged effort may be needed to increase the chance of resuscitation. The rationale of this approach is to maintain the circulation until the local anesthetic is redistributed or metabolized below the level associated with cardiovascular toxicity, at which time spontaneous circulation should resume. Because the contractile depression is a core factor underlying severe cardiotoxicity, it would be intuitive to believe that the use of sympathomimetics should be helpful. Nonetheless, epinephrine can induce dysrhythmia or it can exacerbate the ongoing arrhythmia associated with local anesthetic overdose.[61,62] Consequently, in the setting of local anesthetic toxicity, vasopressin may be more appropriate to maintain the blood pressure, support coronary perfusion, and facilitate local anesthetic metabolism.[63] The appropriateness of phosphodiesterase inhibitors administration is not corroborated by published research results. Although these inhibitors can promote hemodynamics, there is no evidence of a better outcome. As potent vasodilators, phosphodiesterase inhibitors do no support blood pressure,[64] and they have been associated with ventricular arrhythmias.[65]

The current advanced cardiac life support algorithm emphasizes amiodarone as the mainstay drug for treatment of arrhythmias.[66,67] Also, for ventricular arrhythmias prompted by local anesthetic overdose, current data favor amiodarone. Published studies of using lidocaine to treat arrhythmias reveal conflicting results, but it is logical to think that treating local anesthetic–induced arrhythmias with just another local anesthetic antiarrhythmic is likely to add to the cardiotoxicity. The use of bretylium is no longer endorsed. Occurrence of Torsades des Pointes with bupivacaine toxicity may require overdrive pacing if that rhythm predominates.

Calcium channel blockers and phenytoin are contraindicated because their coadministration with local anesthetics may increase the risk of mortality.[68,69] Recovery from local anesthetic–induced cardiac arrest can take enduring resuscitation efforts for more than an hour. Propofol is not an adequate alternative for treatment with intralipid, although judicious administration to control seizures when used in small divided doses is appropriate.[70,71] Administration of the lipid emulsion has become an important addition to the treatment of severe local anesthetic toxicity.[72] Because it is still an innovative therapy, future laboratory and clinical experiences are needed for a better understanding of the mechanisms and further refinement of the treatment protocols.[73]

## Allergic Reactions

The amino-esters, such as chloroprocaine, are all derivatives of the allergen paraaminobenzoic acid (PABA). Accordingly, the local anesthetics belonging to the ester group may cause positive skin reactions, ranging from toxic eruptions in situ to generalized rash or urticaria.[74] Previous study results indicate an incidence of 30%, but no subject developed anaphylaxis. However, true allergic reactions to the local anesthetics of the amino-amide group are extremely rare. By and large, preparations of amide anesthetics do not cause allergic reactions, unless they contain the preservative methylparaben, which is in its chemical structure virtually the same as PABA.[75] For patients who reported an allergy to amino-amides, one can safely use a preservative-free amide anesthetic unless a well-documented allergology reports point to an unambiguous allergy. Anaphylaxis due to local anesthetics remains a rare event, even within the ester group. It should be considered if the patient starts wheezing or develops respiratory distress instantly following injection. However, many symptoms can be explained by a variety of other causes including anxiety, hyperventilation, toxic effects of the drug, vasovagal reactions, reactions to epinephrine, or contamination with latex.

Management of local anesthetic triggered allergic reactions does not differ from the treatment algorithms for other more common allergic reactions. Intravenous lidocaine can result in paradoxical airway narrowing and bronchospasm in patients with asthma. The mechanism of this reaction is not well understood. Apparently, it is not explained by an exacerbation of the asthmatic condition itself or by some anaphylactoid cascade activated by lidocaine or its preservatives.

A unique side effect of some local anesthetics is methemoglobinemia.[76,77] It has been associated with the topical, epidural, and intravenous administration of prilocaine. Hepatic metabolism of prilocaine produces orthotoluidine, which converts hemoglobin into methemoglobin. The doses needed to effectuate diminished oxygen saturation levels that are clinically significant, however, are typically above what is used in the clinical practice of regional anesthesia. Regardless, because of this theoretical possibility, in some countries, the use of prilocaine in regional anesthesia is banned. The condition of methemoglobinemia caused by prilocaine is spontaneously self-limiting and reversible. Reversal can be accelerated with the administration of methylene blue intravenously (1 mg/kg).

## Summary

**Prevention**

- Always maintain a high degree of suspicion.
- Monitor electrocardiogram, blood pressure, and arterial oxygen saturation.
- When feasible, communicate with the patient.
- Be conservative with local anesthetic (LA) dose in patients with advanced age, poor cardiac function, conduction abnormalities, or abnormally low plasma protein concentration.
- Gently aspirate every 3–5 mL.
- Inject slowly (<20 mL/min), and avoid forceful high-pressure injections.
- Use a pharmacologic marker (e.g., epinephrine 5 μg/mL of LA) with high-volume blocks.
- Monitor the patient after high-dose blocks for 30 minutes.
- Be prepared: A plan for managing systemic local anesthetic toxicity should be established in facilities where local anesthetics are used.
- Current recommendations are to have 20% lipid emulsion stocked close to sites where local anesthetics are used.
- Consider infusing lipid emulsion early to help prevent cardiac toxicity.

**Detection of Systemic LA Toxicity**

- Maintain a high degree of suspicion.
- The single most important step in treating local anesthetic toxicity is to consider its diagnosis.
- CNS symptoms are often subtle or absent.
- Cardiovascular signs (e.g., hypertension, hypotension, tachycardia, or bradycardia) may be the first signs of local anesthetic toxicity.
- CNS excitation (agitation, confusion, twitching, seizure), depression (drowsiness, obtundation, coma, or apnea), or nonspecific neurologic symptoms (metallic taste, circumoral paresthesias, diplopia, tinnitus, dizziness) are typical of LA toxicity.

- Ventricular ectopy, multiform ventricular tachycardia, and ventricular fibrillation are hallmarks of cardiac toxicity of LA.
- Progressive hypotension and bradycardia, leading to asystole, are the hallmark of severe cardiovascular toxicity.

**Treatment of Systemic LA Toxicity**

- Get help and call for 20% lipid emulsion.
- Perform airway management. Hyperventilate with 100% oxygen.
- Abolish the seizures.
- Perform cardiopulmonary resuscitation
- Epinephrine–controversial; may have to use higher doses then recommended in ACLS.
- Consider using vasopressin to support circulation
- Alert the nearest facility having cardiopulmonary bypass capability.
- Perform lipid emulsion treatment (for a 70-kg adult patient):
  - Bolus 1.5 mL/kg intravenously over 1 minute (about 100 mL)
  - Continuous infusion 0.25 mL/kg per minute (about 500 mL over 30 minutes)
  - Repeat bolus every 5 minutes for persistent cardiovascular collapse.
  - Double the infusion rate if blood pressure returns but remains low.
  - Continue infusion for a minimum of 30 minutes.

## DIAGNOSIS AND TREATMENT OF LOCAL ANESTHETIC TOXICITY

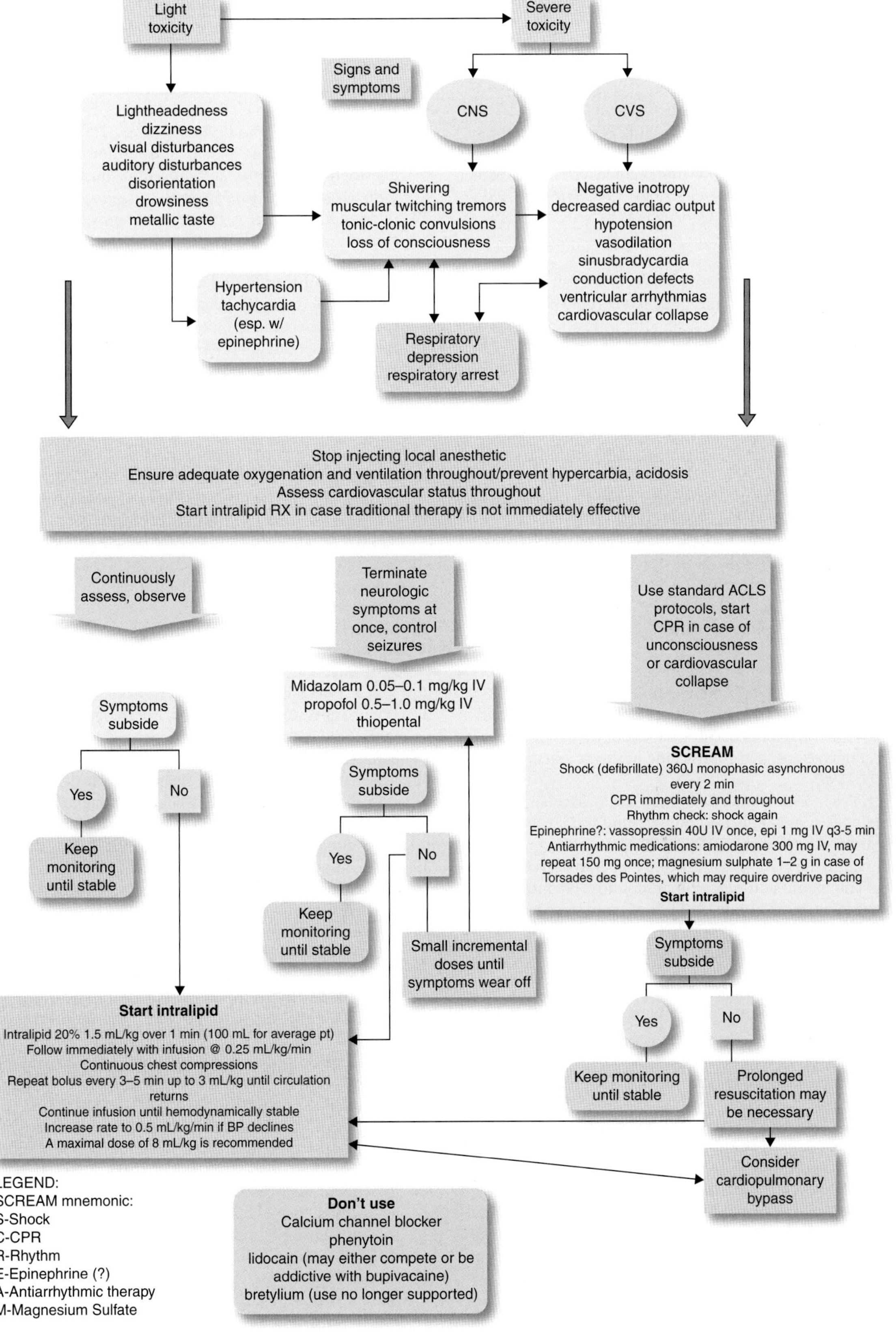

## REFERENCES


1. Weinberg GL. Current concepts in resuscitation of patients with local anesthetic cardiac toxicity. *Reg Anesth Pain Med.* 2002;27:568-575.
2. Long WB, Rosenblum S, Grady IP. Successful resuscitation of bupivacaine-induced cardiac arrest using cardiopulmonary bypass. *Anesth Analg.* 1989;69:403-406.
3. Feldman HS. Toxicity of local anesthetic agents. In: Rice SA, Fish KJ, eds. *Anesthetic Toxicity.* New York, NY: Raven Press; 1994.
4. Albright GA. Cardiac arrest following regional anesthesia with etidocaine or bupivacaine. *Anesthesiology.* 1979;51(4):285-287.
5. Boren E, Teuber S, Naguwa S, Gershwin M. A critical review of local anesthetic sensitivity. *Clin Rev Allergy Immunol.* 2007;32(1):119-127.
6. Guay J. Methemoglobinemia related to local anesthetics: a summary of 242 episodes. *Anest Analg.* 2009;108(3):837-845.
7. Burches B, Warner D. Bronchospasm after intravenous lidocaine. *Anesth Analg.* 2008;107(4):1260-1262.
8. Kalichman MW. Physiologic mechanisms by which local anesthetics may cause injury to nerve and spinal cord. *Reg Anesth.* 1993;18(6 Suppl):448-452.
9. Sadove S, Kolodny S. Local anesthetic agents in combination with vasoconstrictors part I, epinephrine. *Acta Anaesth Scand.* 1961;5(1):13-19.
10. Scott DB. Toxic effects of local anaesthetic agents on the central nervous system. *Br J Anaesth.* 1986;58:732-735.
11. Scott DB. Evaluation of the toxicity of local anaesthetic agents in man. *Br J Anaesth.* 1975;47:56-61.
12. Mather LE, Tucker GT, Murphy TM, Stanton-Hicks MD, Bonica JJ. Cardiovascular and subjective central nervous system effects of long-acting local anaesthetics in man. *Anaesth Intensive Care.* 1979;7:215-221.
13. Scott DB. Evaluation of clinical tolerance of local anaesthetic agents. *Br J Anaesth.* 1975;47 Suppl:328-331.
14. Rutten AJ, Nancarrow C, Mather LE, et al. Hemodynamic and central nervous system effects of intravenous bolus doses of lidocaine, bupivacaine, and ropivacaine in sheep. *Anesth Analg.* 1989;69:291-299.
15. Huang YF, Pryor ME, Mather LE, et al. Cardiovascular and central nervous system effects of bupivacaine and levobupivacaine in sheep. *Anesth Analg.* 1998;86:797-804.
16. Feldman HS, Arthur GR, Covino BG. Comparative systemic toxicity of convulsant and supraconvulsant doses of intravenous ropivacaine, bupivacaine, and lidocaine in the conscious dog. *Anesth Analg.* 1989;69:794-801.
17. Liu P, Feldman H, Giasi R, Patterson M, Covino B. Comparative CNS toxicity of lidocaine, etidocaine, bupivacaine, and tetracaine in awake dogs following rapid administration. *Anesth Analg.* 1983;62:375-379.
18. Reiz S, Nath S. Cardiotoxicity of local anaesthetic agents. *Br J Anaesth.* 1986;58:736-746.
19. Hogan Q. Local anesthetic toxicity: an update. *Reg Anesth.* 1996;21(6S):43-50.
20. Feldman HS, Covino BM, Sage DJ. Direct chronotropic and inotropic effects of local anesthetic agents in isolated guinea pig atria. *Reg Anesth.* 1982;7:149-156.
21. Lynch C. Depression of myocardial contractility in vitro by bupivacaine, etidocaine, and lidocaine. *Anesth Analg.* 1986;65:551-559.
22. Block A, Covino B. Effect of local anesthetic agents on cardiac conduction and contractility. *Reg Anesth.* 1982;6:55-61.
23. Stewart D, Rogers W, Mahaffrey J, Witherspoon S, Woods E. Effect of local anesthetics on the cardiovascular system in the dog. *Anesthesiology.* 1963;24:620-624.
24. Tanz RD, Heskett T, Loehning RW, Fairfax CA. Comparative cardiotoxicity of bupivacaine and lidocaine in the isolated perfused mammalian heart. *Anesth Analg.* 1984;63:549-556.
25. Pitkanen M, Feldman HS, Authur GR, Covino BG. Chronotropic and inotropic effects of ropivacaine, bupivacaine, and lidocaine in the spontaneously beating and electrically paced isolated, perfused rabbit heart. *Reg Anesth Pain Med.* 1992;17:183-192.
26. Englesson S. The influence of acid-base changes on central nervous system toxicity of local anaesthetic agents. I. An experimental study in cats. *Acta Anaesth Scand.* 1974;18:79-87.
27. Burney R, DiFazio C, Foster J. Effects of pH on protein binding of lidocaine. *Anesth Analg.* 1978; 57:478-480.
28. Mulroy M. Systemic toxicity and cardiotoxicity from local anesthetics: incidence and preventive measures. *Reg Anesth Pain Med.* 2002;27(6):556-561.
29. de Jong RH, Heavner JE. Diazepam prevents local anesthetic seizures. *Anesthesiology.* 1971;34:523-531.
30. de Jong RH, Heavner JE. Diazepam prevents and aborts lidocaine convulsions in monkeys. *Anesthesiology.* 1974;41:226-230.
31. de Jong RH, Bonin JD. Benzodiazepines protect mice from local anesthetic convulsions and deaths. *Anesth Analg.* 1981;60:385-389.
32. Ausinsch B, Malagodi MH, Munson ES. Diazepam in the prophylaxis of lignocaine seizures. *Br J Anaesth.* 1976;48:309-313.
33. Liguori G, Chimento GF, Borow L, Figgie M. Possible bupivacaine toxicity after intraarticular injection for postarthroscopic analgesia of the knee: implications of the surgical procedure. *Anesth Analg.* 2002; 94:1010-1013.
34. Kahn RL, Quinn TJ. Blood pressure, not heart rate, as a marker of intravascular injection of epinephrine in an epidural test dose. *Reg Anesth.* 1991;16:292-295.
35. Tanaka M, Nishikawa T. A comparative study of hemodynamic and T-wave criteria for detecting intravascular injection of the test dose (epinephrine) in sevoflurane-anesthetized adults. *Anesth Analg.* 1999;89:32-36.
36. Schoenwald PK, Whalley DG, Schluchter MD, Gottlieb A, Ryckman JV, Bedocs NM. The hemodynamic responses to an intravenous test dose in vascular surgical patients. *Anesth Analg.* 1995;80:864-868.
37. Weinberg G. Current concepts in resuscitation of patients with local anesthetic cardiac toxicity. *Reg Anesth Pain Med.* 2002;27(6):568-575.
38. Feldman HS, Arthur GR, Pitkanen M, Hurley R, Doucette AM, Covino BG. Treatment of acute systemic toxicity after the rapid intravenous injection of ropivacaine and bupivacaine in the conscious dog. *Anesth Analg.* 1991;73:373-384.
39. Association of Anaesthetists of Great Britain and Ireland. *Guidelines for the Management of Severe Local Anaesthetic Toxicity.* London, UK: AAGBI, 2007.
40. Crews JC, Rothman TE. Seizure after levobupivacaine for interscalene brachial plexus block. *Anesth Analg.* 2003; 96:1188-1190.
41. Weinberg G, VadeBoncouer T, Ramaraju G, Garcia- Amaro M, Cwik M. Pretreatment or resuscitation with a lipid infusion shifts the dose-response to bupivacaine-induced asystole in rats. *Anaesthesiology.* 1998;88:1071-1075.
42. Weinberg G, Ripper R, Feinstein D, Hoffman W. Lipid emulsion infusion rescues dogs from bupivacaine induced cardiac toxicity. *Reg Anesth Pain Med.* 2003; 8:198-202.
43. Weinberg G, Di Gregorio G, Ripper R, et al. Resuscitation with lipid versus epinephrine in a rat model of bupivacaine overdose. *Anesthesiology.* 2008;108:907-913.
44. Rosenblatt M, Abel M, Fischer G, Itzkovich C, Eisenkraft J. Successful use of a 20% lipid emulsion to resuscitate a patient after a presumed bupivacaine related cardiac arrest. *Anaesthesiology.* 2006;105:217-218.
45. Litz R, Popp M, Stehr S, Koch T. Successful resuscitation of a patient with ropivacaine-induced asystole after axillary plexus block using lipid infusion. *Anaesthesia.* 2006;61:800-801.
46. McCutchen T, Gerancher J. Early Intralipid may have prevented bupivacaine associated cardiac arrest. *Reg Anaesth Pain Med.* 2008;33:178-180.

47. Foxall G, McCahon R, Lamb J, Hardman J, Bedforth N. Levobupivacaine-induced seizures and cardiovascular collapse treated with Intralipid. *Anaesthesia.* 2007;62:516–518.
48. Whiteside J. Reversal of local anaesthetic induced CNS toxicity with lipid emulsion. *Anaesthesia.* 2008;63:203–204.
49. Spence A. Lipid reversal of central nervous system symptoms of bupivacaine toxicity. *Anaesthesiology.* 2007;107:516–517.
50. Litz R, Roessel T, Heller A, Stehr S. Reversal of central nervous system and cardiac toxicity following local anaesthetic intoxication by lipid emulsion injection. *Anesth Analg.* 2008;106:1575–1577.
51. Zimmer C, Piepenbrink K, Riest G, Peters J. Cardiotoxic and neurotoxic effects after accidental intravascular bupivacaine administration. Therapy with lidocaine propofol and lipid emulsion. *Anaesthesist.* 2007;56(5):449-453.
52. Ludot H, Tharin JY, Belouadah M, Mazoit JX, Malinovsky JM. Successful resuscitation after ropivacaine and lidocaine-induced ventricular arrhythmia following posterior lumbar plexus block in a child. *Anesth Analg.* 2008;106(5):1572-1574.
53. Warren JA, Thoma RB, Georgescu A, Shah SJ. Intravenous lipid infusion in the successful resuscitation of local anesthetic-induced cardiovascular collapse after supraclavicular brachial plexus block. *Anesth Analg.* 2008;106(5):1578-1580.
54. Picard J, Meek T. Lipid emulsion to treat overdose of local anaesthetic: the gift of the glob. *Anaesthesia.* 2006;61:107–109.
55. Tsai MH, Tseng CK, Wong KC. Successful resuscitation of a bupivacaine-induced cardiac arrest using cardiopulmonary bypass and mitral valve replacement. *J Cardiothorac Anesth.* 1987;1:454-456.
56. Long WB, Rosenblum S, Grady IP. Successful resuscitation of bupivacaine-induced cardiac arrest using cardiopulmonary bypass. *Anesth Analg.* 1989;69:403-406.
57. Freedman MD, Gal J, Freed CR. Extracorporeal pump assistance—novel treatment for acute lidocaine poisoning. *Eur J Clin Pharmacol.* 1982;22:129-135.
58. Soltesz EG, van Pelt F, Byrne JG. Emergent cardiopulmonary bypass for bupivacaine cardiotoxicity. *J Cardiothorac Anesth.* 2003;17:357-358.
59. Chazalon P, Tourtier JP, Villevieille T, et al. Ropivacaine-induced cardiac arrest after peripheral nerve block: successful resuscitation. *Anesthesiology.* 2003;99:1449–1451.
60. Huet O, Eyrolle LJ, Mazoit JX, Ozier YM. Cardiac arrest and plasma concentration after injection of ropivacaine for posterior lumbar plexus blockade. *Anesthesiology.* 2003;99:1451–1453.
61. Heavner JE, Pitkanen MT, Shi B, Rosenberg PH. Resuscitation from bupivacaine-induced asystole in rats: comparison of different cardioactive drugs. *Anesth Analg.* 1995;80:1134-1139.
62. Bernards CM, Carpenter RL, Kenter ME, Brown DL, Rupp SM, Thompson GE. Effect of epinephrine on central nervous system and cardiovascular system toxicity of bupivacaine in pigs. *Anesthesiology.* 1989;71:711-717.
63. Krismer AC, Hogan QH, Wenzel V, et al. The efficacy of epinephrine or vasopressin for resuscitation during epidural anesthesia. *Anesth Analg.* 2001;93:734-742.
64. Arnold JM. The role of phosphodiesterase inhibitors in heart failure. *Pharmacol Ther.* 1993;57:161-161.
65. DiBianco R, Shabetai R, Kostuk W, Moran J, Schlant RC, Wright R. A comparison of oral milrinone, digoxin, and their combination in the treatment of patients with chronic heart failure. *N Engl J Med.* 1989;320:677-683.
66. Nolan JP, Deakin CD, Soar J, Böttiger BW, Smith G. European Resuscitation Council Guidelines for Resuscitation 2005 Section 4. Adult advanced life support. *Resuscitation.* 2005;67S1:S39-S86.
67. 2005 American Heart Association Guidelines for Cardiopulmonary Resuscitation and Emergency Cardiovascular Care: Part 7.3: Management of Symptomatic Bradycardia and Tachycardia. *Circulation.* 2005;112:IV-67-IV-77.
68. Tallman RD Jr, Rosenblatt RM, Weaver JM, Wang YL. Verapamil increases the toxicity of local anesthetics. *J Clin Pharmacol.* 1988;28:317-321.
69. Simon L, Kariya N, Pelle-Lancien E, Mazoit JX. Bupivacaine-induced QRS prolongation is enhanced by lidocaine and by phenytoin in rabbit hearts. *Anesth Analg.* 2002; 94:203-207.
70. Heavner JE, Arthur J, Zou J, McDaniel K, Tyman-Szram B, Rosenberg PH. Comparison of propofol with thiopentone for treatment of bupivacaine-induced seizures in rats. *Br J Anaesth.* 1993;71:715-719.
71. Momota Y, Artru AA, Powers KM, Mautz DS, Ueda Y. Posttreatment with propofol terminates lidocaine induced epileptiform electroencephalogram activity in rabbits: effects on cerebrospinal fluid dynamics. *Anesth Analg.* 1998;87:900-906.
72. Weinberg GL. Lipid infusion therapy: translation to clinical practice. *Anesth Analg.* 2008;106(5):1340-1342.
73. Cave G, Harvey M. Intravenous lipid emulsion as antidote beyond local anesthetic toxicity: a systematic review. *Acad Emerg Med.* 2009;16(9):815-824.
74. Aldrete JA, Johnson DA. Evaluation of intracutaneous testing for investigation of allergy to local anesthetic agents. *Anesth Analg.* 1970;49:173-183.
75. Cashman AL, Warshaw EM. Parabens: a review of epidemiology, structure, allergenicity, and hormonal properties. *Dermatitis.* 2005;16(2):57-66.
76. Lund PC, Cwik JC. Propitocaine (Citanest) and methemoglobinemia. *Anesthesiology.* 1965; 26:569-571.
77. Scott DB, Owen JA, Richmond J. Methemoglobinemia due to prilocaine. *Lancet.* 1964;284:728-729.

# 10 Neurologic Complications of Peripheral Nerve Blocks

*Jeff Gadsden*

Nerve injury following peripheral nerve blockade (PNB) is a potentially devastating complication that can result in permanent disability.[1] Data from a recent review of published studies suggest that the incidence of neurologic symptoms following PNB varies depending on the anatomic location, ranging from 0.03% for supraclavicular blocks to 0.3% for femoral blocks to up to 3% for interscalene blocks.[2] Fortunately, the vast majority of these neuropathies appear to be temporary rather than permanent neuropathy and resolve over weeks to months.

The exact etiology of neurologic injury related to PNB remains unclear in many instances. Suggested etiologies include mechanical trauma from the needle, nerve edema and/or hematoma, pressure effects of the local anesthetic injectate, and neurotoxicity of the injected solutions (both local anesthetics and adjuvants, e.g., epinephrine).[3] Confounding factors that may play a role in nerve injury include preexisting neuropathies (e.g., diabetes mellitus), surgical manipulation, prolonged tourniquet pressure, or compression from postoperative casting.[4]

It is well-established that direct injection into peripheral nerves (i.e., accidentally during intramuscular administration) can result in nerve injury.[5] This is one of the reasons why intraneural injections are avoided during peripheral nerve blockade. More recent data however, suggest that intraneural injections are not always associated with nerve injury. This chapter summarizes the clinically relevant considerations regarding the etiology of nerve injury during peripheral nerve blockade.

## Histology and Histopathology of Peripheral Nerves

Knowledge of the functional histology of nerves is essential to understanding the consequences of intraneural injection. Nerves are made up of fascicles supported and enveloped by perineurium and a loose collection of collagen fibers termed the *epineurium*. The epineurium is easy permeable and carries the nutritive vessels of larger nerves. Each fascicle is made up of bundles of nerve fibers (axons) and their associated Schwann cells held together by a tough squamous epithelial sheath called the *perineurium*, which acts as a semipermeable barrier to local anesthetics. The nerve fibers are supported within the perineurium by a delicate connective tissue matrix called the *endoneurium*, which contains capillaries that arise from the larger epineurial vessels. Figure 10-1 features normal anatomy of a mixed peripheral nerve and relationship of the epineurium and perineurium.

Peripheral nerve lesions can be classified in terms of their degree of functional disruption.[6] *Neurapraxia* refers to a mild insult in which the axons and connective tissue structures supporting them remain intact. This type of injury is often associated with focal demyelination and generally reversible over the course of weeks to several months. Axonal interruption with conservation of the neural connective tissues is termed *axonotmesis*. Regeneration at a rate of 1 to 2 mm/day occurs, and recovery is generally favorable although not always complete. *Neurotmesis* represents complete fascicular interruption, including the axons and the connective tissue supporting tissues. Because the nerve is severed, recovery

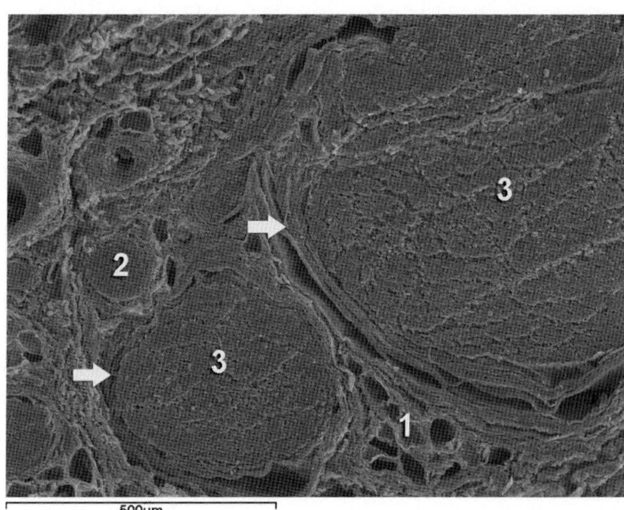


**FIGURE 10-1.** Anatomy of the peripheral nerve as seen on an electron microscopy image. 1-Epineurium, 2-Fascicle, 3-Fascicular bundles (several fascicles bound together), Arrows-perineurium.

depends on surgical reapproximation of the two stumps. Even with prompt surgical intervention, recovery is often poor. It is important to note that most nerve injuries are mixed, with different fascicles exhibiting characteristics of these three different injury types.

## The Problem, or Is It?

Selander *et al* provided evidence of the deleterious effects of intraneural injection over 30 years ago[7] Indeed, the objective during peripheral nerve blockade has been to deposit local anesthetic in the vicinity, but not within, the substance of the nerve. This tacit convention has been challenged in recent years with the publication of a series of reports suggesting that intraneural needle placement, and indeed injection of local anesthetic, may not necessarily result in detectable clinical injury. In 2004 Sala-Blanch *et al* described two cases of placement of a catheter within the epineurium of the sciatic nerve, confirmed by computerized tomographic imaging.[8] Both patients demonstrated clinically efficacious blocks without postoperative neurologic deficit. The advent of ultrasound guidance for nerve blocks has likely led to an increase in the recognition of inadvertent intraneural injections. Accidental femoral[9] and musculocutaneous[10] intraneural injections have been described, as evidenced by nerve swelling on the ultrasound image, both without lasting neurologic effect.

In 2006, Bigeleisen published a series of axillary brachial plexus blocks performed on 22 patients undergoing thumb surgery.[11] Using ultrasound guidance, the authors deliberately placed the needle intraneurally and injected 2 to 3 mL of local anesthetic, which resulted in 72 intraneural injections as evidenced by nerve swelling. Despite the common occurrence of paresthesia or dysesthesia (66 times), none of the patients developed an overt neurologic deficit up to 6 months postoperatively.

Similarly, Robards *et al* studied 24 patients receiving sciatic nerve blocks in the popliteal fossa using both nerve stimulation and ultrasound guidance.[12] The end point for needle advancement was a motor response using a current intensity of 0.2 to 0.5 mA, or an apparent intraneural needle tip location, whichever came first. These investigators found that the motor response could only be obtained upon entry of the needle into the nerve in 83.3% of patients; in the remaining 16.7%, a motor response with a stimulating current of 1.5 mA could not be obtained, even when the needle tip was intraneural. There was no postoperative neurologic dysfunction.

Taken together, these studies suggest that an intraneural needle placement with resultant injection of the local anesthetic within internal epineurium does not lead to an imminent neurologic injury. The data by Robards *et al*, suggest that many nerve blocks without the benefit of ultrasound visualization, have likely resulted in intraneural (intra-epineural) injections. The reason why nerve injury is infrequent is that the vast majority of these injections do not occur within fascicles.

## Extrafascicular versus Intrafascicular Injections

A needle placed within a peripheral nerve can be in one of two locations: within the loose epineurial matrix that surrounds the fascicles or inside a fascicle itself. It is well-established that injection of even very small amounts of local anesthetic within the fascicle can lead to widespread axonal degeneration and permanent neural damage in animals, whereas extrafascicular injection does not disrupt the normal nerve architecture.[7,13] Part of this can be explained mechanically because the perineurium, a tough multilayer epithelial sheath, is not easily distensible to compensate to an increase in intrafascicular pressure. Intrafascicular pressure rises on injection and can remain higher than the capillary perfusion pressure longer than the duration of the injection itself, predisposing to neural ischemia and inflammation.[14] Furthermore, pressure curves derived from intrafascicular versus extrafascicular injections in canine sciatic nerves show that a pattern of very high initial injection pressures followed by a sharp drop to baseline is associated with poor outcome and severe neural histologic damage, and may suggest fascicular rupture.[15] In contrast, injections into the compliant epineurial space appear to be associated with a minimal rise in pressure, which can be explained by its loose and accommodating stromal architecture.

The risk of an intrafascicular injection differs from site to site in the peripheral nervous system, and it correlates with the cross-sectional fascicle-epineurium ratio. For example, the sciatic nerve at the popliteal fossa contains more non-neural tissue than fascicles in its cross-sectional area, which corresponds with its low incidence of post-PNB neuropathy.[16] By contrast, the brachial plexus at the level of the trunks contains much more neural than connective tissue; a needle entering the nerve here is more likely to encounter a fascicle on its trajectory that may contribute to the disproportionately higher rate of postoperative neuropathy following PNB with interscalene blocks.[17] As peripheral nerves move away from the neuraxis, the ratio of connective tissue to neural tissue within the nerve tends to increase. The brachial plexus elements below the clavicle have a ratio of connective tissue to neural tissue of approximately 2:1, whereas the more proximal trunks and divisions have a ratio of 1:1.[18]

## Mechanisms of Nerve Injury Following Intraneural Injection

Once the perineurium is breached, the spectrum of subsequent injury is wide and multifactorial.

## Needle Trauma

The mechanical disruption of the perineurial sheath may result in injury to the axons and/or the leakage/herniation of endoneural contents.[19] However, the composition of the injectate may play a larger role in the outcome of intrafascicular injection. For example, normal saline injected into fascicles did not cause any damage in one study, suggesting that mere puncture of the perineurium does not necessarily result in clinically overt injury.[13] In contrast, nerve puncture with intravenous cannulae or electroneurography needles has been shown to result in lasting neurologic deficit.[20–22] A variety of cellular changes accompany needle trauma, including alterations in membrane channel expression, activation of signal transduction, neuropeptide production, and an overall increase in excitability at the dorsal horn.[23,24] The effect of the needle size on the likelihood and severity of the injury is controversial, however, smaller needles (24 gauge) may lead to less nerve injury than larger needles (19 gauge).[25]

Despite the concern over fascicular puncture, due to their compact nature, fascicles are more likely to escape the advancing needle, rather than be penetrated under normal PNB conditions. Early work by Selander *et al* in rabbits demonstrated that needle tip characteristics influenced the likelihood of fascicular penetration.[26] This study demonstrated that long-bevel (12–15°) needles were more likely to puncture the fascicle than short-bevel (45°) needles, and resulted in the author advocating for their use during PNB. A more recent study compared blunt (30°) versus sharp (15°) needles by passing these needles through a cadaveric sciatic nerve and examining the nerve microscopically afterward for signs of fascicular damage.[27] Although a total of 134 fascicles were identified as being in contact with the needle tracks, only 4 fascicles were damaged, all of which belonged to the sharp-tip group. These data suggest that a needle passing through a fascicle is more likely only to encounter epineurium and may in fact displace the tough fascicles away from the needle path. Although blunt needles are less likely to enter the fascicle, once penetrated, blunt needles appear to cause a greater degree of injury compared with sharp needles, especially if the sharp needles are oriented with the bevel in the same direction as the nerve fibers (i.e., not cutting transversely across the fibers).[28] Regardless of which needle type or size enters the nerve, a needle insertion into nerve and consequent injection invariably leads to inflammation and cellular infiltration regardless of whether a clinical injury occurs.

## Toxicity of Local Anesthetics and Additives

Although all local anesthetics are potentially neurotoxic,[29] the mechanism remains unclear. Proposed mechanisms include increases in intracellular calcium concentration, disturbance in mitochondrial function, interference with membrane phospholipids, and cell apoptosis.[30–33] The perineurium and blood vessel endothelium serve as a barrier to entry into the fascicle. However, even local anesthetics placed within the epineurium have been shown to cause altered perineural permeability and fascicular edema, leading to compression of the fascicle and reduced neural blood flow.[13,34] This effect appears to be dose dependent.

Intraneural administration of local anesthetics exposes the axons to higher concentrations of drug than extraneural application. One study comparing the extraneural, extrafascicular, and intrafascicular administration of ropivacaine 0.75% showed that histologic damage was least severe extraneurally and most severe intrafascicularly.[35] However, even when injected inside the epineurium, others have shown ropivacaine 0.75% to have no adverse effect on functional recovery.[36] Ester local anesthetics such as tetracaine and chloroprocaine were shown in some studies to cause a greater degree of injury than those of the amide group, but recent data have challenged those conclusions.[34,37] What is well known is that the injection of local anesthetics into the fascicle results in widespread and immediate axonal injury.[14]

Local anesthetics alone are also capable of decreasing neural blood flow. Lidocaine 2% reduces neural blood flow in rat sciatic nerves by 20–40%, and this difference persists after washout of the local anesthetic solution.[38,39] Increasing concentrations of lidocaine appear to reduce neural blood flow further; the reverse is true for bupivacaine. Altering the concentration of tetracaine appears to have no effect on neural blood flow. Various concentrations of levobupivacaine and ropivacaine have been found to reduce rat sciatic nerve blood flow significantly.[40]

Epinephrine is a common adjuvant used to prolong the duration of blockade and to warn of intravascular injection/absorption. At concentrations of 5 μg/mL and 10 μg/mL, epinephrine reduces neural blood flow by 20% and 35%, respectively.[39] In contrast, at lower concentrations (2.5 μg/mL), neural blood flow increases by 20% transiently before returning to baseline, suggesting that at lower concentrations the β-adrenergic effects predominate. The effects of combining lidocaine and epinephrine are additive: A solution of 2% lidocaine plus 5 μg/mL of epinephrine reduced neural blood flow by 80%.[38]

The clinical significance of the effects of various local anesthetics and additives is unknown. The experimental data must be weighed within the context of clinical practice; countless of nerve blocks of blocks are performed in daily practice using a combination of local anesthetic and epinephrine with no neurologic consequences. This reinforces the hypothesis that nerve injury is multifactorial, and one theoretical aspect may be insufficient to cause injury consistently.

# Prevention of Peripheral Nerve Injury

Several techniques have been advocated to enhance safety during the performance of PNBs. The merits of each technique in preventing nerve injury are addressed individually.

## Pain on Injection

Pain on injection has traditionally been taught as a reliable and effective means to guard against intraneural injection because intraneural injections are thought to be exquisitely painful. However, there are multiple problems with this logic. First, pain is notoriously difficult to evaluate in terms of intensity and quality. Consequently, differentiating between a benign, commonly present discomfort during injection of local anesthetic (pressure paresthesia) and that of intrafascicular injection can be elusive. Second, various patient conditions (e.g., diabetes mellitus, peripheral neuropathy) and premedication may interfere with pain perception. Third, there appears to be little evidence that pain on injection is either sensitive or specific. Fanelli et al conducted a prospective study of nearly 4000 patients receiving multiple-injection PNBs and found that the overall rate of neurologic complications was 1.7%, independent of whether the patient reported a paresthesia or not.[41] In other words, it does not appear to matter whether the patient reports a paresthesia or not—they have an equal likelihood of postoperative neuropathy. Bigeleisen's report of 72 intraneural injections was associated with 66 reports of paresthesia or dysesthesia, yet none of the patients had neurologic complications, suggesting the symptom itself has a low specificity for complications.[11] Fourth, the nature of nerve injury might preclude its use as a useful monitor: By the time a patient registers pain, communicates it to the anesthesiologist, and the injection is halted, the damage is likely to have been done. Because a fraction of a milliliter is sufficient to cause irreversible fascicular damage, the patient's subjective symptom may be too late.[7,15] Finally, there are situations in which performing PNBs in an asleep/heavily sedated/blocked patient might be the safest approach, for example, pediatric cases, mentally incompetent patients, the traumatically injured, patients needing rescue or repeat blocks, and so on. The use of more objective monitors, as listed here, may provide increased confidence that an intrafascicular injection can be avoided when compared with a subjective patient symptom.

## Electrical Nerve Stimulation

Electrical stimulation is a means to locate nerves but also may be used to rule out an intraneural (intrafascicular) location of the needle. Voelckel et al demonstrated that sciatic blocks in pigs performed with a motor response at <0.2 mA resulted in inflammatory nerve changes in 50% of the specimens, compared with none when the motor response was achieved at 0.3 to 0.5 mA.[42] Others have investigated the relationship between current intensity and needle-nerve distance in pigs and found that, although the relationship is unpredictable outside the epineurium, a motor response at a current intensity of <0.3 mA occurs only with intraneural needle placement.[43,44] These findings have been substantiated in a clinical study of patients undergoing ultrasound-guided supraclavicular block, in which minimal threshold currents were recorded at "extraneural" and "intraneural" positions.[45] The investigators found that no motor response could be elicited at a current of ≤0.2 mA unless the needle tip was intraneural.

These studies suggest that, although neurostimulation techniques may not be a highly sensitive method of detecting intraneural needle tip position (i.e., high current intensities may still be required to elicit motor responses even with intra-epineural needle placement), neurostimulation has a high specificity for identifying intraneural needle tip placement (i.e., motor response at ≤0.2 mA obtained only with intraneural needle tip location) Based on the cumulative experimental and clinical data, using *no* motor response at <0.2–0.3 mA as a cutoff for safe practice before injecting local anesthetic makes clinical sense as a routine monitoring method for most nerve blocks.

## Ultrasonography

Ultrasound guidance is theoretically an attractive means of preventing intraneural injection due to real-time imaging of the needle and nerve. Indeed, nerve swelling visualized on the sonographic image appears to represent true histologic intraneural injection as evaluated by the presence of India ink staining within the epineurium.[44,46] However, the clinical implications of this are also unclear because nerve swelling and even histologic changes associated with nerve injury appear not to result in detectable neurologic deficit in pigs, although there may be subtle changes that cannot be assessed by the evaluators.[47]

Ultrasound guidance may not be a substantially effective means of preventing nerve injury. The reliability of ultrasound to keep the needle tip extraneural depends largely on the skill of the operator and the imaging characteristics of the needle and tissue. Several case reports of accidental nerve (and vascular) puncture despite the use of ultrasound guidance highlight the fact that ultrasound monitoring is not a fail-proof method of avoiding neurologic (and other mechanical) complications.[9,10,48] Furthermore, at the present time the resolution of the sonographic image is such that it would be impossible to tell if the needle tip was intrafascicular or extrafascicular, which is the critical anatomic differentiation to make to avoid nerve injury. Finally, as is the case with paresthesia, by the time the nerve is seen swelling on the image, the damage may have already been done if the injection is made with the needle tip inside the fascicle.

## Injection Pressure Monitoring

The crux of the intraneural injection problem thus far appears to lie in the avoidance of penetrating the perineurium and entering the fascicle. The presence of a high opening injection pressure (>20 psi) in a canine model is a very sensitive (if not highly specific) sign of intrafascicular needle tip placement, whereas extrafascicular needle tip placement is associated with low (<10 psi) pressures.[15] Another dog study showed that some, but not all, intraneural injections resulted in high (>20 psi) pressures, whereas high pressures were absent during extraneural injection.[49] More importantly, high pressure injection was associated with neurologic deficits and severe axonal damage after the block, in contrast to normal neurologic and histologic findings following any low-pressure injection (extra or intraneural). Indeed, PNBs associated with high injection pressure, despite a lack of paresthesia, have been reported to result in permanent neurologic injury.[50] Although objective injection pressure monitoring and documentation has not yet been universally adopted, assessment of resistance to injection is a standard clinical practice. Unfortunately, clinical data on the role of injection pressure monitoring may never become available as it would be unethical to randomize patients to receive a high versus low pressure nerve block injection. However, the available clinical and experimental evidence points that injection pressure is useful in detecting needle-nerve contact (Table 10-1).

Given this, safe practice should include the objective assessment of the resistance to injection with most single injection peripheral nerve blocks. An assessment of injection resistance is often assessed using a "syringe-hand-feel" technique. However, it has been well documented (in at least two models) that practitioners are unable to gauge injection pressure by using a syringe-hand-feel subjective technique.[51,52] Therefore, if monitoring of resistance to injection is to have clinical merit, objective monitoring of injection pressure should be used to standardize the injection force. This may be achieved by use of commercially available inline devices or with the use of a "compressed air injection technique."[53] One shortcoming of injection pressure monitoring is that injection pressure is highly sensitive but lacks specificity. In other words, absence of high injection pressure appears to effectively rule out an intrafascicular injection. However, high injection pressure also can be caused by PNB needle obstruction, attempted injection into a tendon, or tissue compression caused by the ultrasound transducer.

## Future Directions

The regional anesthesia community is witnessing the beginning of a paradigm shift in the thinking surrounding intraneural injection during PNB. Clearly they can be performed safely in certain patients. The question is: Should they?

**TABLE 10-1**

| KEY LABORATORY DATA | KEY FINDINGS |
|---|---|
| *Selander D et al.* Acta Anaesthesiol Scand. 1978;22:622-34. | Intrafascicular injections in a rabbit sciatic nerve model result in high injection pressure (≥11 psi) and back-tracking of LA proximally towards centroneuraxis |
| *Kapur E et al.* Acta Anaesthesiol Scand. 2007;51:101-7. | Perineural and extrafascicular intraneural injections resulted in low injection pressure (<5 psi). Intraneural intrafascicular injection resulted in ≥25 psi. |
| *Hadzic A et al.* Reg Anesth Pain Med. 2004;29:417-23. | Perineural and extrafascicular intraneural injections resulted in low injection pressure (<5 psi). Intraneural intrafascicular injection resulted in ≥20 psi and neurologic deficit. |
| *Steinfeld T et al.* Anesth Analg 2011;113:417-20. | Needle-nerve contact with forced needle advancement [0.15 N/mm2 (21 psi)] in pigs led to severe structural nerve injury. |
| *Orebaugh SL et al.* Abstracts of ASRA Annual Meeting, Las Vegas, May 2011 | Injection into fascicles in fresh cadavers resulted in high injection pressures (≥38 psi) |
| **KEY CLINICAL OBSERVATIONS** | |
| *Robards C et al.* Anesth Analg. 2009;109:673-7. | Intraneural injections (as seen by ultrasound) resulted in combination of 1. Pain on injection, 2. Low current (< 0.3 mA) nerve stimulation and 3. High injection pressures (>20 psi) |
| *Bigeleisen P et al.* Anesthesiology. 2009;110:1235-43. | Intraneural injections (as seen by ultrasound) resulted in combination of 1. Pain on injection, 2. Low current (< 0.3 mA) nerve stimulation and 3. High resistance to injection |
| *Gadsden J et al.* Anesthesiology. 2008;109:683-8. | High injection pressures during lumbar plexus block resulted in epidural spread of block in all patients |
| *de Leeuw MA et al.* Anesth Analg. 2011 Mar;112:719-24. | Slow injection speed (pressure) did not result in significant hemodynamic changes after psoas compartment block, indicating the lack of epidural spread with slow injection (low pressure/force) |

Even intranueral extrafascicular injection of local anesthetic often results in histologic evidence of inflammation in animal experiments. However, intraneural extrafascicular injection in patients often does not result in symptoms. The risk may be different in patients who have preexisting or subclinical neuropathy. It is important to note that the studies demonstrating safe intraneural injections in humans deliberately excluded patients with preexisting neuropathy.

Deliberate injection of local anesthetic into peripheral nerves and plexuses is controversial with regards to its safety and clinical advantages. Such injections in distal nerves may be more forgiving, owing to their increased ratio of nonneural tissue to neural tissue. In particular, injuries to the sciatic nerve at the popliteal fossa appear to be uncommon following intraneural injection or intraneural catheter placement.[54,55] In fact, it has been noted that intraneural injection of local anesthetic in the popliteal sciatic nerve leads to a rapid onset of sensory and motor blockade, without complications.[55] Some practitioners now routinely attempt to place the needle tip within the epineurium at this location, in an attempt to hasten onset, improve block success, and decrease the total amount of local anesthetic required. However, this practice should be done only with a combination of objective monitoring because the need to remain extrafascicular is paramount.

One of the challenges is to elucidate the precise factors that provide for a safe intraneural injection, whether anatomic (popliteal sciatic versus subgluteal), technological (injection pressure monitoring, improved resolution of ultrasound imaging), educational (improved training), or otherwise. More clinical research is needed to clarify the safety of intraneural injection in various nerves such as the femoral nerve, and distal nerves of the upper and lower limbs. This should be undertaken with care and with proper safeguards to prevent penetration of the perineurium. Lastly, intraneural injection may allow for reduction in the volume and/or concentration of local anesthetic required for effective nerve block.[54] This is a worthwhile avenue to explore, both in terms of the implications for nerve injury and for reducing the potential for systemic local anesthetic toxicity. A combination of monitoring to decrease the risk of an intrafascicular injection during peripheral nerve blocks is demonstrated in Figure 10-2 as well as in Chapter 5.

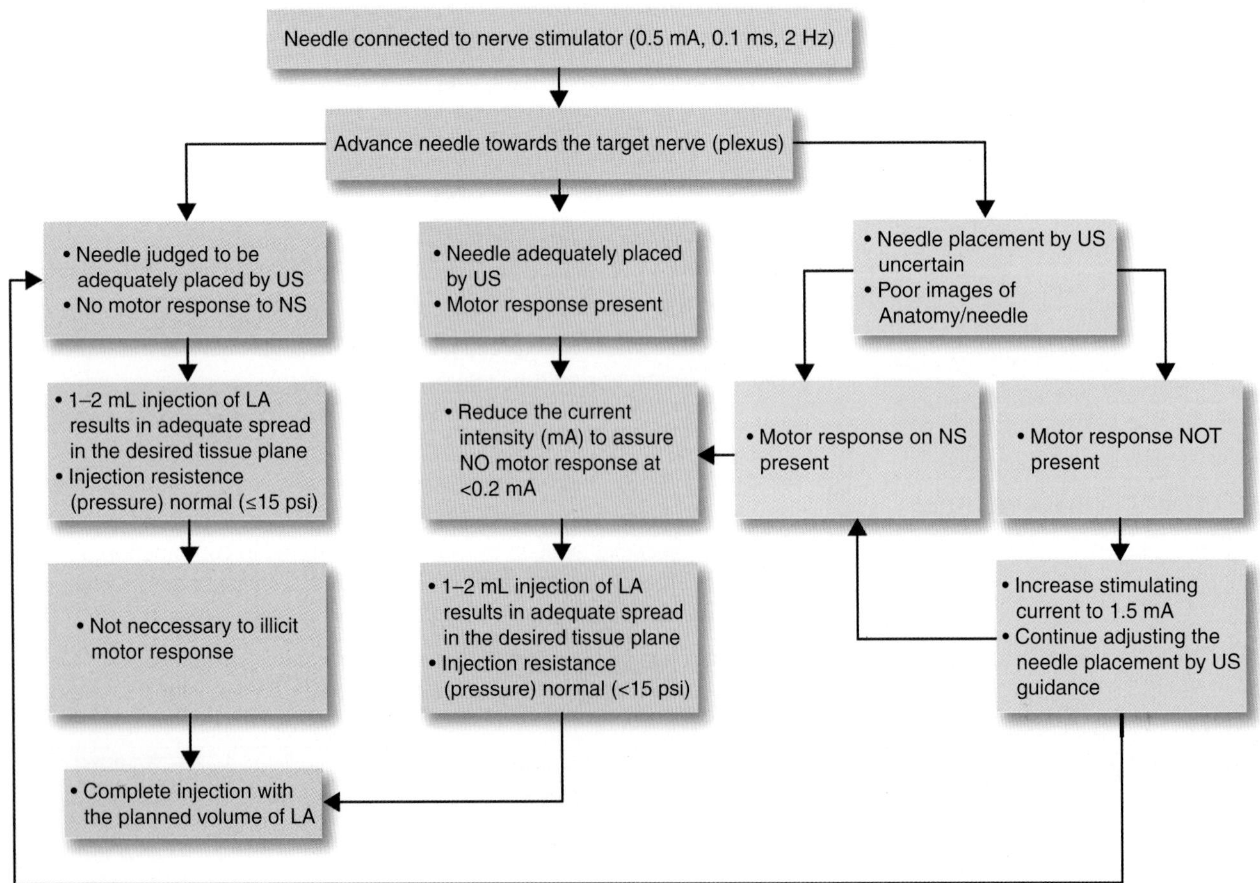


**FIGURE 10-2.**

## Practical Management of Postoperative Neuropathy

Despite the best precautions, a postoperative sensory or motor deficit that outlasts the expected duration of the PNB may occur. It is important to note that the vast majority of neuropathies resolve spontaneously, and patient reassurance is vital.[36] Processes that are either evolving (i.e. compartment syndrome) or are reparable (i.e. surgical transection of a nerve) should be ruled out. Here are a few principles to bear in mind when managing a postoperative neuropathy:

1. Good communication is essential, both from a patient care and medicolegal standpoint.
2. Approximately 95% of postoperative sensory changes will resolve within 4–6 weeks, and most of these will occur during the first week. 99% of sensory changes will resolve within the first year.
3. Early diagnosis of postoperative peripheral nerve injury can be challenging due to:
   - residual sedation and/or PNB
   - pain that limits the examination
   - casts, dressings, splints, slings
   - movement restrictions
   - patient expectations regarding block—"I didn't know how long it was supposed to last"
4. Neuropathies can also be caused by prolonged tourniquets, casting, excessive intraoperative traction, or a misplaced surgical clip. Early involvement of the surgical team is prudent.
5. In general, the presence of motor deficits is an ominous sign, and a referral to a neurologist and/or neurosurgeon is indicated.
6. Neuropathies that are evolving, and those that are severe/complete should be seen immediately by a neurologist and/or neurosurgeon.

Referral for electrophysiologic testing may be indicated when the symptoms are not purely sensory, or when the neuropathy is severe and/or long-lasting. Studies performed usually consist of the following:

1. Electromyography. This is undertaken to determine which muscle units are affected by a denervation lesion. Small needle electrodes are placed in various muscles and the pattern of electrical activity both at rest and with contraction is analyzed. The results can help to localize a lesion, and, depending on the pattern, suggest a time frame for the injury.
2. Nerve conduction studies. In these tests, a device similar to the peripheral nerve stimulator used by anesthesiologists to monitor the degree of neuromuscular blockade is attached over various nerves in the affected area. A characteristic waveform is generated following stimulation of the nerve, which may allow the neurologist to pinpoint a conduction block.

The optimal timing of these tests depends on the indication. An exam within 2–3 days of the onset of injury may give information regarding the completeness of the lesion (and therefore prognosis), as well as clues about the duration of the lesion, which often has medicolegal ramifications, particularly if the lesion is deemed to predate the nerve block or surgical procedure. As such, this can be seen as a "baseline" exam. More information is obtained at approximately 4 weeks post-injury, when the electrophysiologic changes have had an opportunity to evolve more fully.

A practical algorithm for the management of postoperative neuropathy is shown in Figure 10-3.

# PRACTICAL APPROACH TO MANAGEMENT OF A PATIENT WITH NEUROLOGIC DEFICIT AFTER PERIPHERAL NERVE BLOCK

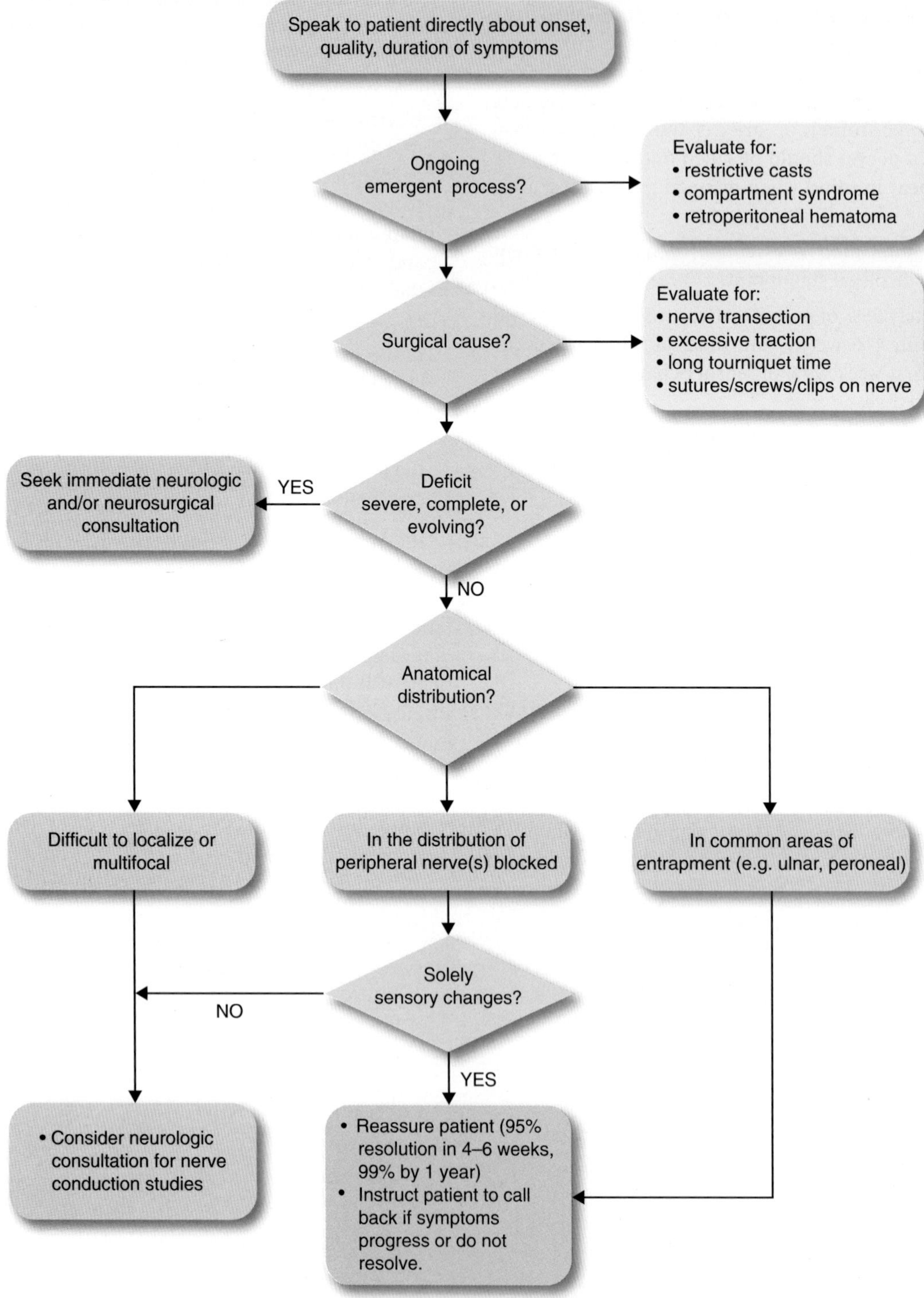


**FIGURE 10-3.**

## REFERENCES


1. Borgeat A, Blumenthal S. Nerve injury and regional anaesthesia. *Curr Opin Anaesthesiol.* 2004;17(5):417-421.
2. Brull R, McCartney CJL, Chan VWS, El-Beheiry H. Neurological complications after regional anesthesia: contemporary estimates of risk. *Anesth Analg.* 2007;104(4):965-974.
3. Hogan QH. Pathophysiology of peripheral nerve injury during regional anesthesia. *Reg Anesth Pain Med.* 2008;33(5):435-441.
4. Sorenson EJ. Neurological injuries associated with regional anesthesia. *Reg Anesth Pain Med.* 2008;33(5):442-448.
5. Clark K, Williams PE, Willis W, McGavran WL. Injection injury of the sciatic nerve. *Clin Neurosurg.* 1970;17:111-125.
6. Seddon HJ. Three types of nerve injury. *Brain.* 1943;66(4): 237-288.
7. Selander D, Brattsand R, Lundborg G, Nordborg C, Olsson Y. Local anesthetics: importance of mode of application, concentration and adrenaline for the appearance of nerve lesions. An experimental study of axonal degeneration and barrier damage after intrafascicular injection or topical application of bupivacaine (Marcain). *Acta Anaesthesiol Scand.* 1979;23(2):127-136.
8. Sala-Blanch X, Pomés J, Matute P, et al. Intraneural injection during anterior approach for sciatic nerve block. *Anesthesiology.* 2004;101(4):1027-1030.
9. Schafhalter-Zoppoth I, Zeitz ID, Gray AT. Inadvertent femoral nerve impalement and intraneural injection visualized by ultrasound. *Anesth Analg.* 2004;99(2):627-628.
10. Russon K, Blanco R. Accidental intraneural injection into the musculocutaneous nerve visualized with ultrasound. *Anesth Analg.* 2007;105(5):1504-1505.
11. Bigeleisen PE. Nerve puncture and apparent intraneural injection during ultrasound-guided axillary block does not invariably result in neurologic injury. *Anesthesiology.* 2006;105(4):779-783.
12. Robards C, Hadzic A, Somasundaram L, et al. Intraneural injection with low-current stimulation during popliteal sciatic nerve block. *Anesth Analg.* 2009;109(2):673-677.
13. Gentili F, Hudson AR, Hunter D, Kline DG. Nerve injection injury with local anesthetic agents: a light and electron microscopic, fluorescent microscopic, and horseradish peroxidase study. *Neurosurgery.* 1980;6(3):263-272.
14. Selander D, Sjöstrand J. Longitudinal spread of intraneurally injected local anesthetics. An experimental study of the initial neural distribution following intraneural injections. *Acta Anaesthesiol Scand.* 1978;22(6):622-634.
15. Hadzic A, Dilberovic F, Shah S, et al. Combination of intraneural injection and high injection pressure leads to fascicular injury and neurologic deficits in dogs. *Reg Anesth Pain Med.* 2004;29(5):417-423.
16. Moayeri N, Groen GJ. Differences in quantitative architecture of sciatic nerve may explain differences in potential vulnerability to nerve injury, onset time, and minimum effective anesthetic volume. *Anesthesiology.* 2009;111(5):1128-1134.
17. Liu SS, Zayas VM, Gordon MA, et al. A prospective, randomized, controlled trial comparing ultrasound versus nerve stimulator guidance for interscalene block for ambulatory shoulder surgery for postoperative neurological symptoms. *Anesth Analg.* 2009;109(1):265-271.
18. Moayeri N, Bigeleisen PE, Groen GJ. Quantitative architecture of the brachial plexus and surrounding compartments, and their possible significance for plexus blocks. *Anesthesiology.* 2008;108(2):299-304.
19. Sugimoto Y, Takayama S, Horiuchi Y, Toyama Y. An experimental study on the perineurial window. *J Peripher Nerv Syst.* 2002;7(2):104-111.
20. Fredrickson MJ. Case report: Neurological deficit associated with intraneural needle placement without injection. *Can J Anaesth.* 2009;56(12):935-938.
21. Inglis JT, Leeper JB, Wilson LR, Gandevia SC, Burke D. The development of conduction block in single human axons following a focal nerve injury. *J Physiol (Lond).* 1998;513(Pt 1): 127-133.
22. Eckberg DL, Wallin BG, Fagius J, Lundberg L, Torebjörk HE. Prospective study of symptoms after human microneurography. *Acta Physiol Scand.* 1989;137(4):567-569.
23. Hogan Q. Animal pain models. *Reg Anesth Pain Med.* 2002;27(4):385-401.
24. Gold MS. Spinal nerve ligation: what to blame for the pain and why. *Pain.* 2000;84(2-3):117-120.
25. Steinfeldt T, Nimphius W, Werner T, et al. Nerve injury by needle nerve perforation in regional anaesthesia: does size matter? *Br J Anaesth.* 2010;104(2):245-253.
26. Selander D, Dhunér KG, Lundborg G. Peripheral nerve injury due to injection needles used for regional anesthesia. An experimental study of the acute effects of needle point trauma. *Acta Anaesthesiol Scand.* 1977;21(3):182-188.
27. Sala-Blanch X, Ribalta T, Rivas E, et al. Structural injury to the human sciatic nerve after intraneural needle insertion. *Reg Anesth Pain Med.* 2009;34(3):201-205.
28. Rice AS, McMahon SB. Peripheral nerve injury caused by injection needles used in regional anaesthesia: influence of bevel configuration, studied in a rat model. *Br J Anaesth.* 1992;69(5):433-438.
29. Lambert LA, Lambert DH, Strichartz GR. Irreversible conduction block in isolated nerve by high concentrations of local anesthetics. *Anesthesiology.* 1994;80(5):1082-1093.
30. Kitagawa N, Oda M, Totoki T. Possible mechanism of irreversible nerve injury caused by local anesthetics: detergent properties of local anesthetics and membrane disruption. *Anesthesiology.* 2004;100(4):962-967.
31. Johnson ME, Saenz JA, DaSilva AD, Uhl CB, Gores GJ. Effect of local anesthetic on neuronal cytoplasmic calcium and plasma membrane lysis (necrosis) in a cell culture model. *Anesthesiology.* 2002;97(6):1466-1476.
32. Floridi A, Di Padova M, Barbieri R, Arcuri E. Effect of local anesthetic ropivacaine on isolated rat liver mitochondria. *Biochem Pharmacol.* 1999;58(6):1009-1016.
33. Sturrock JE, Nunn JF. Cytotoxic effects of procaine, lignocaine and bupivacaine. *Br J Anaesth.* 1979;51(4):273-281.
34. Myers RR, Kalichman MW, Reisner LS, Powell HC. Neurotoxicity of local anesthetics: altered perineurial permeability, edema, and nerve fiber injury. *Anesthesiology.* 1986;64(1):29-35.
35. Whitlock EL, Brenner MJ, Fox IK, et al. Ropivacaine-induced peripheral nerve injection injury in the rodent model. *Anesth Analg.* 2010;111(1):214-220.
36. Iohom G, Lan GB, Diarra DP, et al. Long-term evaluation of motor function following intraneural injection of ropivacaine using walking track analysis in rats. *Br J Anaesth.* 2005;94(4):524-529.
37. Kalichman MW, Moorhouse DF, Powell HC, Myers RR. Relative neural toxicity of local anesthetics. *J Neuropathol Exp Neurol.* 1993;52(3):234-240.
38. Myers RR, Heckman HM. Effects of local anesthesia on nerve blood flow: studies using lidocaine with and without epinephrine. *Anesthesiology.* 1989;71(5):757-762.
39. Partridge BL. The effects of local anesthetics and epinephrine on rat sciatic nerve blood flow. *Anesthesiology.* 1991;75(2):243-250.
40. Bouaziz H, Iohom G, Estèbe J, Campana WM, Myers RR. Effects of levobupivacaine and ropivacaine on rat sciatic nerve blood flow. *Br J Anaesth.* 2005;95(5):696-700.
41. Fanelli G, Casati A, Garancini P, Torri G. Nerve stimulator and multiple injection technique for upper and lower limb blockade: failure rate, patient acceptance, and neurologic complications. Study Group on Regional Anesthesia. *Anesth Analg.* 1999;88(4):847-852.
42. Voelckel WG, Klima G, Krismer AC, et al. Signs of inflammation after sciatic nerve block in pigs. *Anesth Analg.* 2005;101(6):1844-1846.

43. Tsai TP, Vuckovic I, Dilberovic F, et al. Intensity of the stimulating current may not be a reliable indicator of intraneural needle placement. *Reg Anesth Pain Med.* 2008;33(3):207-210.
44. Chan VWS, Brull R, McCartney CJL, et al. An ultrasonographic and histological study of intraneural injection and electrical stimulation in pigs. *Anesth Analg.* 2007;104(5):1281-1284.
45. Bigeleisen PE, Moayeri N, Groen GJ. Extraneural versus intraneural stimulation thresholds during ultrasound-guided supraclavicular block. *Anesthesiology.* 2009;110(6):1235-1243.
46. Altermatt FR, Cummings TJ, Auten KM, et al. Ultrasonographic appearance of intraneural injections in the porcine model. *Reg Anesth Pain Med.* 2010;35(2):203-206.
47. Lupu CM, Kiehl T, Chan VWS, et al. Nerve expansion seen on ultrasound predicts histologic but not functional nerve injury after intraneural injection in pigs. *Reg Anesth Pain Med.* 2010;35(2):132-139.
48. Loubert C, Williams SR, Hélie F, Arcand G. Complication during ultrasound-guided regional block: accidental intravascular injection of local anesthetic. *Anesthesiology.* 2008;108(4):759-760.
49. Kapur E, Vuckovic I, Dilberovic F, et al. Neurologic and histologic outcome after intraneural injections of lidocaine in canine sciatic nerves. *Acta Anaesthesiol Scand.* 2007;51(1):101-107.
50. Shah S, Hadzic A, Vloka JD, et al. Neurologic complication after anterior sciatic nerve block. *Anesth Analg.* 2005;100(5):1515-1517.
51. Claudio R, Hadzic A, Shih H, et al. Injection pressures by anesthesiologists during simulated peripheral nerve block. *Reg Anesth Pain Med.* 2004;29(3):201-205.
52. Theron PS, Mackay Z, Gonzalez JG, Donaldson N, Blanco R. An animal model of "syringe feel" during peripheral nerve block. *Reg Anesth Pain Med.* 2009;34(4):330-332.
53. Tsui BCH, Knezevich MP, Pillay JJ. Reduced injection pressures using a compressed air injection technique (CAIT): an in vitro study. *Reg Anesth Pain Med.* 2008;33(2):168-173.
54. Rodríguez J, Taboada M, Blanco M, et al. Intraneural catheterization of the sciatic nerve in humans: a pilot study. *Reg Anesth Pain Med.* 2008;33(4):285-290.
55. Sala Blanch X, López AM, Carazo J, et al. Intraneural injection during nerve stimulator-guided sciatic nerve block at the popliteal fossa. *Br J Anaesth.* 2009;102(6):855-861.

SECTION 2

# Nerve Stimulator and Surface-Based Nerve Block Techniques

# 11 Cervical Plexus Block

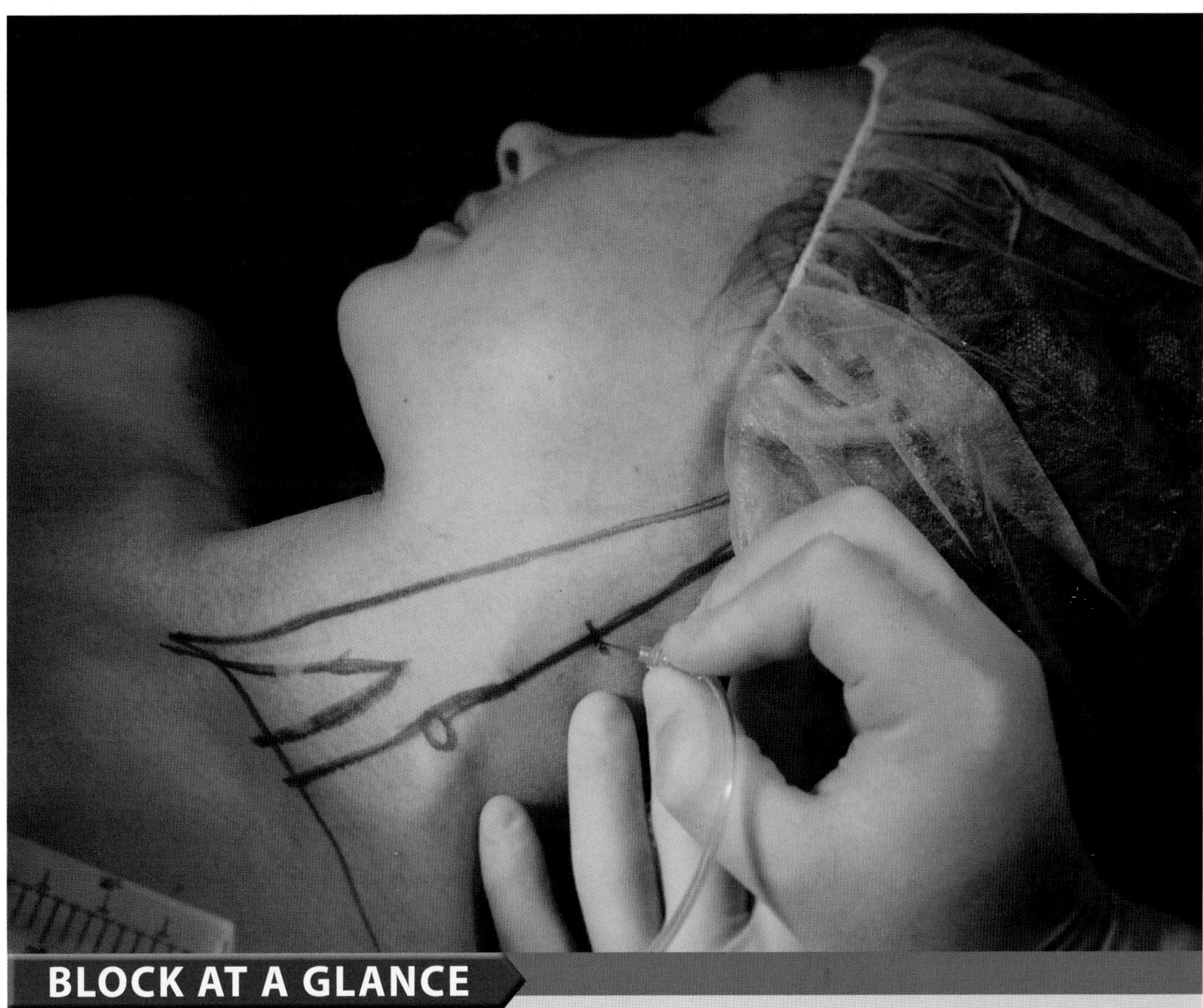

## BLOCK AT A GLANCE

- Indications: carotid endarterectomy, superficial neck surgery
- Landmarks: mastoid process, sternocleidomastoid muscle, C6 transverse process
- Equipment, *superficial:* 1½-in, 25-gauge needle
- Equipment, *deep:* 2-in, 22-gauge, short bevel needle connected to a syringe via a flexible tubing
- Local anesthetic: 15–20 mL

**FIGURE 11-1.** Needle insertion for superficial cervical plexus block. The needle is inserted behind the posterior border of the sternocleidomastoid muscle.

## General Considerations

Cervical plexus block can be performed using two different methods. One is a deep cervical plexus block, which is essentially a paravertebral block of the C2-4 spinal nerves (roots) as they emerge from the foramina of their respective vertebrae. The other method is a superficial cervical plexus block, which is a subcutaneous blockade of the distinct nerves of the anterolateral neck. The most common clinical uses for this block are carotid endarterectomy and excision of cervical lymph nodes. The cervical plexus is anesthetized also when a large volume of local anesthetic is used for an interscalene brachial plexus block. This is because local anesthetic invariably escapes the interscalane groove and layers out underneath the deep cervical fascia where the branches of the cervical plexus are located.

The sensory distribution for the deep and superficial blocks is similar for neck surgery, so there is a trend toward favoring the superficial approach. This is because of the potentially greater risk for complications associated with the deep block, such as vertebral artery puncture, systemic toxicity, nerve root injury, and neuraxial spread of local anesthetic.

## Functional Anatomy

The cervical plexus is formed by the anterior rami of the four upper cervical nerves. The plexus lies just lateral to the tips of the transverse processes in the plane just behind the sternocleidomastoid muscle, giving off both cutaneous and muscular branches. There are four cutaneous branches, all of which are innervated by roots C2-4. These emerge from the posterior border of the sternocleidomastoid muscle at approximately its midpoint, and they supply the skin of the anterolateral neck (Figures 11-2 and 11-3). The second, third, and fourth cervical nerves typically send a branch each to the spinal accessory nerve or directly into the deep surface of the trapezius to supply sensory fibers to this muscle. In addition, the fourth cervical nerve may send a branch downward to join the fifth cervical nerve and participates in formation of the brachial plexus. The

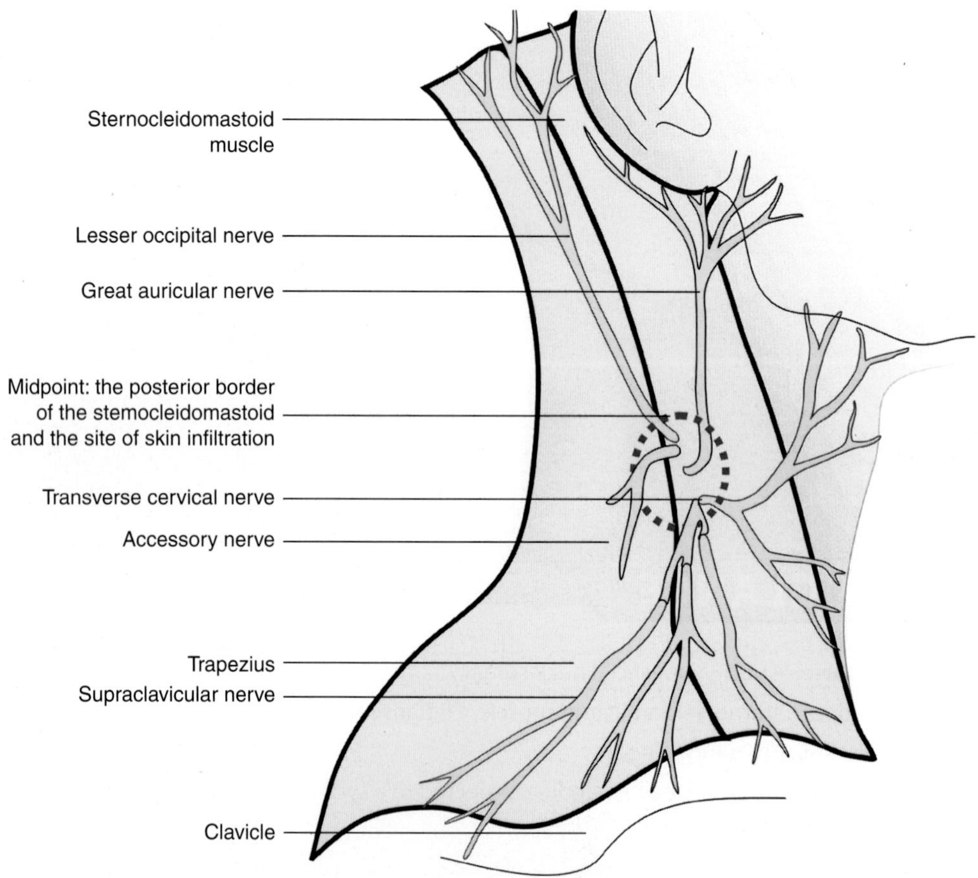


**FIGURE 11-2.** The superficial cervical plexus and its terminal nerves. Anatomy of the superficial cervical plexus and its branches are shown emerging behind the posterior border of the sternocleidomastoid muscle.

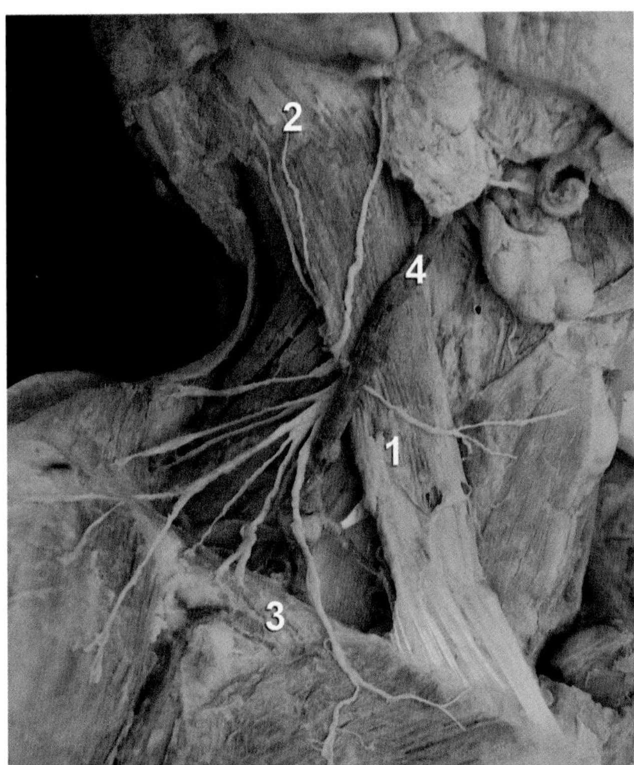


**FIGURE 11-3.** Anatomy of the superficial cervical plexus. ❶ Sternocleidomastoid muscle ❷ mastoid process ❸ clavicle ❹ external jugular vein.

| TABLE 11-1 | Cervical Plexus Branches |
|---|---|
| *Cutaneous branches* | • Lesser occipital nerve (C2, 3)<br>• Greater auricular nerve (C2, 3)<br>• Transverse cervical nerve (C3, 4)<br>• Supraclavicular nerve (C3, 4) |
| *Muscular branches* | • Ansa cervicalis (C1-3)<br>• Branches to posterolateral neck musculature |

motor component of the cervical plexus consists of the looped ansa cervicalis (C1-C3), from which the nerves to the anterior neck muscles originate, and various branches from individual roots to posterolateral neck musculature (Figure 11-4). The C1 spinal nerve (the suboccipital nerve) is strictly a motor nerve, and is not blocked with either technique. One other significant muscle innervated by roots of the cervical plexus includes the diaphragm (phrenic nerve, C3,4,5) (Table 11-1).

## Distribution of Blockade

Cutaneous innervation of both the deep and the superficial cervical plexus blocks includes the skin of the anterolateral neck and the ante- and retroauricular areas (Figure 11-5).

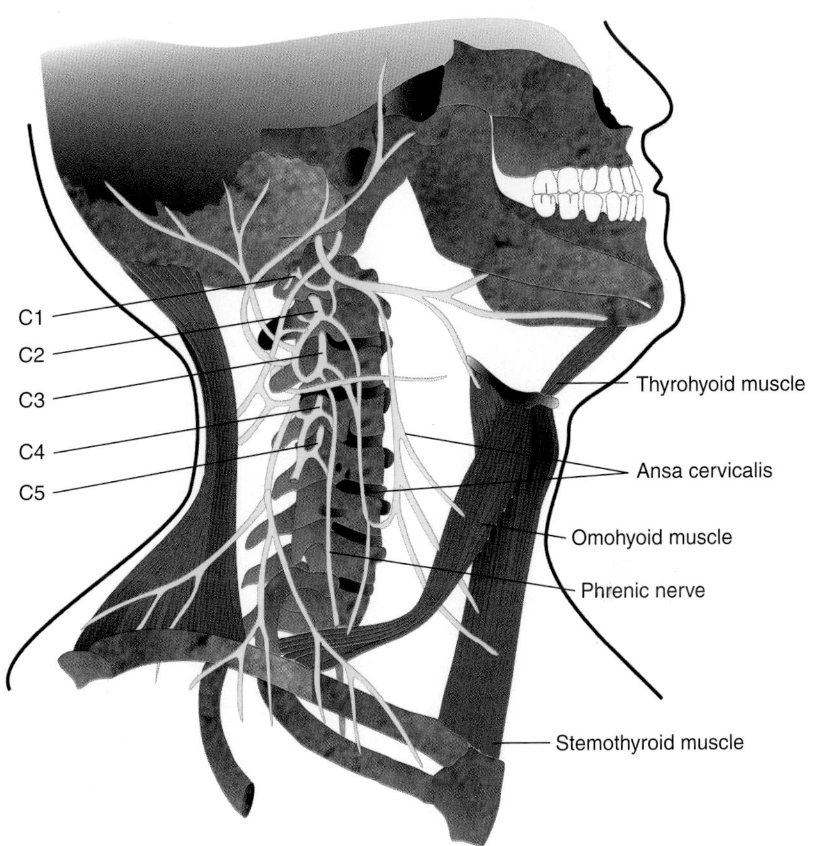


**FIGURE 11-4.** The roots origin of the cervical plexus.

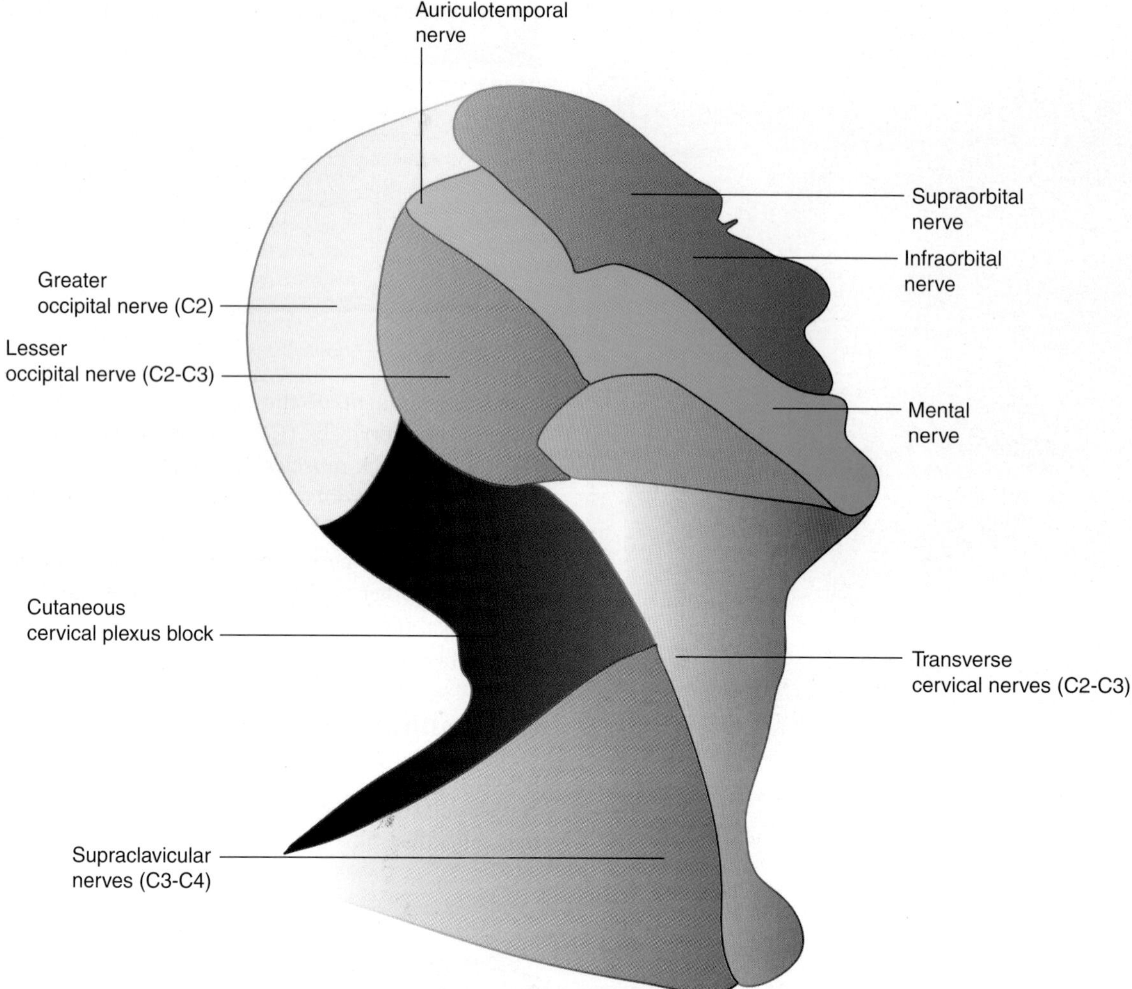


**FIGURE 11-5.** Sensory innervation of the lateral aspect of the head and neck and contribution of the superficial cervical plexus.

In addition, the deep cervical block anesthetizes three of the four strap muscles of the neck, geniohyoid, the prevertebral muscles, sternocleidomastoid, levator scapulae, the scalenes, trapezius, and the diaphragm (via blockade of the phrenic nerve).

## Superficial Cervical Plexus Block

### Equipment

A standard regional anesthesia tray is prepared with the following equipment:

- Sterile towels and gauze packs
- A 20-mL syringe with local anesthetic, attached to a 1½-in, 25-gauge needle, typically via a flexible tubing
- Sterile gloves, marking pen

### Landmarks and Patient Positioning

The patient is in a supine or semi-sitting position with the head facing away from the side to be blocked. These are the primary landmarks (Figure 11-6) for performing this block:

1. Mastoid process
2. Clavicular head of the sternocleidomastoid
3. The midpoint of the posterior border of the sternocleidomastoid (this is aided by identifying the first two landmarks)

#### *Maneuvers to Facilitate Landmark Identification*

The sternocleidomastoid muscle can be better differentiated from the deeper neck structures by asking the patient to raise their head off the table.

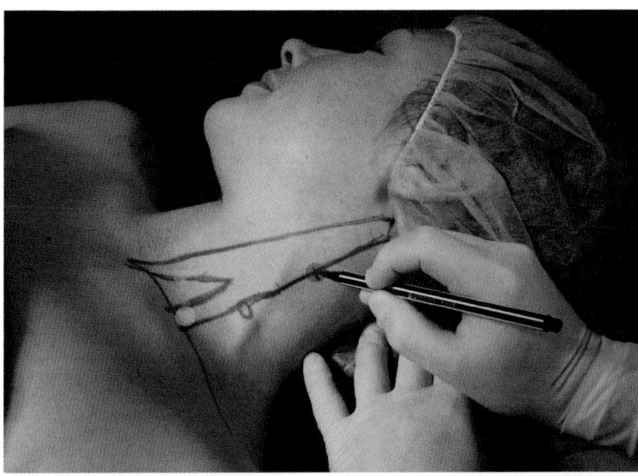

**FIGURE 11-6.** Surface landmarks for superficial cervical plexus block. White dot: insertion of the clavicular head of the sternocleidomastoid muscle. Blue dot: Mastoid process. Uncolored circle: Transverse process of C6 vertebrate. Red dot: Needle insertion site at the midpoint between C6 and mastoid process behind the posterior border of the sternocleidomastoid muscle.

## TIP

- The proportions of the shoulder girdle, size of the neck, prominence of the muscles, and other areas vary among patients. When in doubt, always perform a "reality check" and estimate the two bony landmarks, the clavicle and the mastoid process.

## Technique

After cleaning the skin with an antiseptic solution, the needle is inserted along the posterior border of the sternocleidomastoid, and three injections of 5 mL of local anesthetic are injected behind the posterior border of the sternocleidomastoid muscle subcutaneously, perpendicularly, cephalad, and caudad in a "fan" fashion (Figure 11-7).

## GOAL

The goal of the injection is to infiltrate the local anesthetic subcutaneously but deep to the cervical fascia and behind the sternocleidomastoid muscle. Deep needle insertion (i.e., >1–2 cm) should be avoided to minimize the risk of subarachnoid or vertebral artery injection.

## Block Dynamics and Perioperative Management

A superficial cervical plexus block is associated with minor patient discomfort. Small doses of midazolam 1 to 2 mg for sedation and alfentanil 250 to 500 μg for analgesia just before needle insertion should result in a comfortable, cooperative patient during block injection. The onset time for this block is 10 to 15 minutes. Excessive sedation should be avoided before and during head and neck procedures because airway management, when necessary, can prove difficult because access to the head and neck is shared with the surgeon. Due to the complex arrangement of the sensory innervation of the neck and the cross-coverage from the contralateral side, the anesthesia achieved with a cervical plexus block is rarely complete. Although this should not discourage the use of the cervical block, the surgeon must be willing to supplement the block with a local anesthetic if necessary.

## TIPS

- A subcutaneous midline injection of local anesthetic extending from the thyroid cartilage distally to the suprasternal notch will block the branches crossing from the opposite side. This injection can be considered a "field" block. It is useful for preventing pain from surgical skin retractors on the medial aspect of the neck.
- Carotid surgery requires blockade of the glossopharyngeal nerve branches. The surgeon can accomplish this intraoperatively by injecting local anesthetic inside the carotid artery sheath.

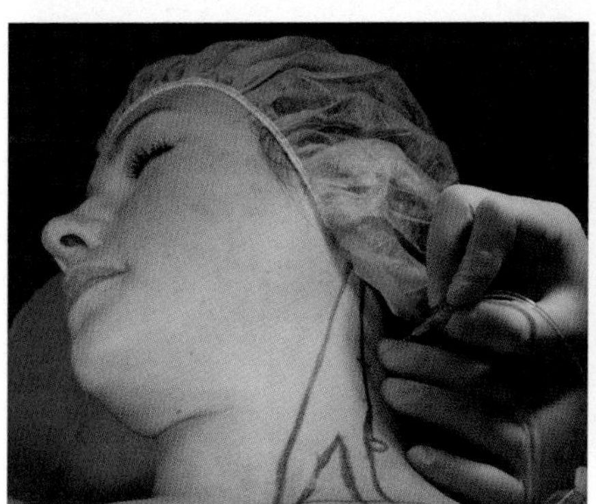

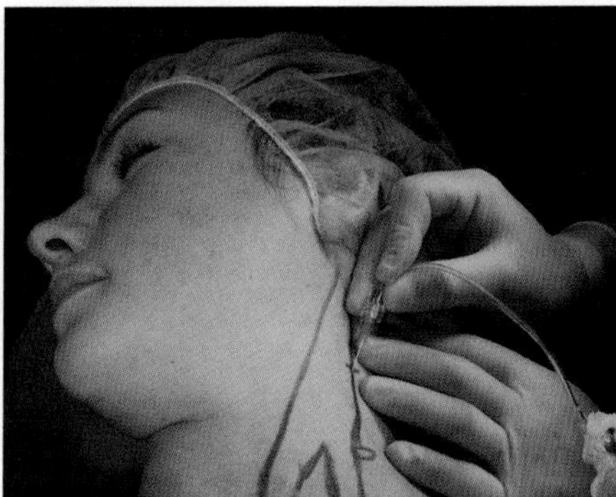

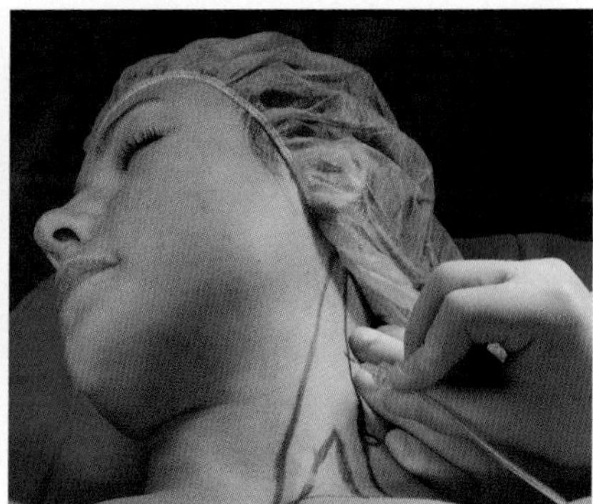

**FIGURE 11-7.** Injection of local anesthetic for superficial cervical plexus. The injection is made fan-wise behind the posterior border of the sternocleidomastoid muscle at a depth of approximately 1 cm in average-size patients.

## Deep Cervical Plexus Block

### Equipment

A standard regional anesthesia tray is prepared with the following equipment:

- Sterile towels and gauze packs
- A 20-mL syringe with local anesthetic, attached via tubing to 1½ to 2 in, 22-gauge short bevel needle
- A 3-mL syringe plus 25-gauge needle with local anesthetic for skin infiltration
- Sterile gloves, marking pen, ruler

### Landmarks and Patient Positioning

The patient is in the same position as for the superficial cervical plexus block. The three landmarks for a deep cervical plexus block are similar to those for the superficial cervical plexus block:

1. Mastoid process
2. Chassaignac tubercle (transverse process of C6) (Figure 11-8)
3. Posterior border of the sternocleidomastoid muscle (Figure 11-9)

To estimate the line of needle insertion overlying the transverse processes, the mastoid process and the transverse process of C6 are identified and marked. The latter is easily palpated behind the clavicular head of the sternocleidomastoid muscle just below the level of the cricoid cartilage.

Next, a line is drawn connecting the mastoid process to the C6 transverse process. The palpating hand is best positioned just behind the posterior border of the sternocleidomastoid muscle. Once this line is drawn, the insertion sites over C2 through C4 are labeled as follows: C2: 2 cm caudad to the mastoid process, C3: 4 cm caudad to the mastoid process, and C4: 6 cm caudad to the mastoid process (Figure 11-10).

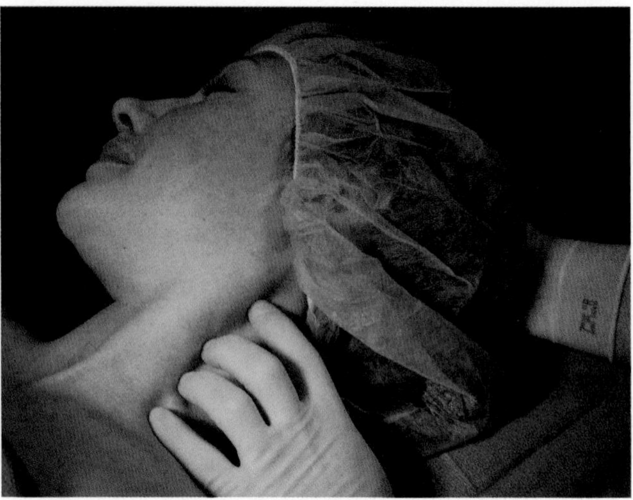

**FIGURE 11-9.** Palpation technique to determine the posterior border of the sternocleidomastoid muscle. With the head of the patient rotated away from the palpation side, the patient is asked to lift his or her head off of the bed to accentuate the sternocleidomastoid muscle.

#### *Maneuvers to Facilitate Landmark Identification*

The sternocleidomastoid muscle can be accentuated by asking the patient to raise his or her head off of the table.

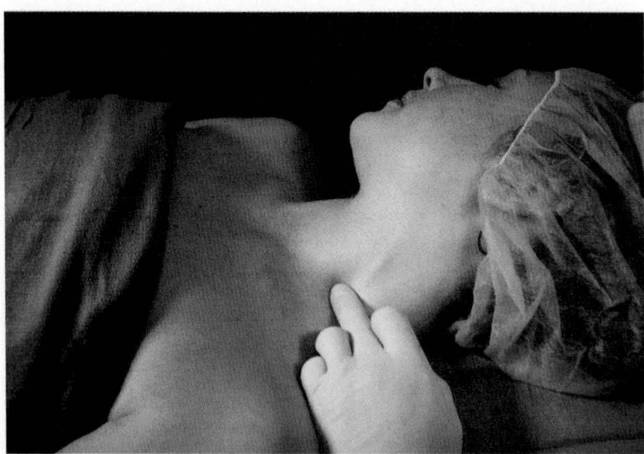

**FIGURE 11-8.** Palpation technique to determine location of the transverse process of C6. The head is rotated away from the palpated side while the palpated fingers explore for the most lateral bony prominence, often in the vicinity of the external jugular vein.

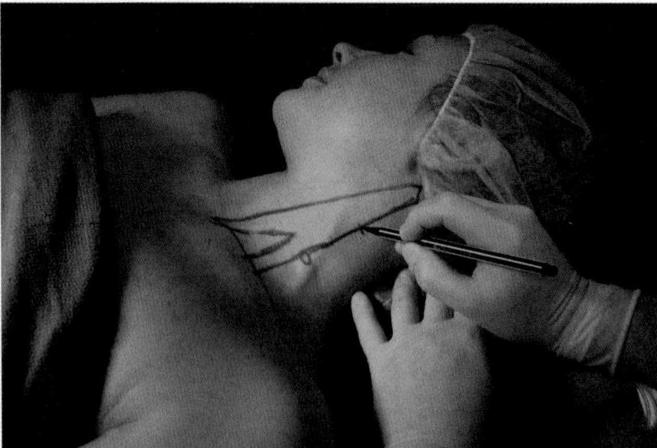

**FIGURE 11-10.** The landmarks for the deep cervical plexus block. White circle indicates the transverse process of C6 The pen is outlining the transverse process of C4.

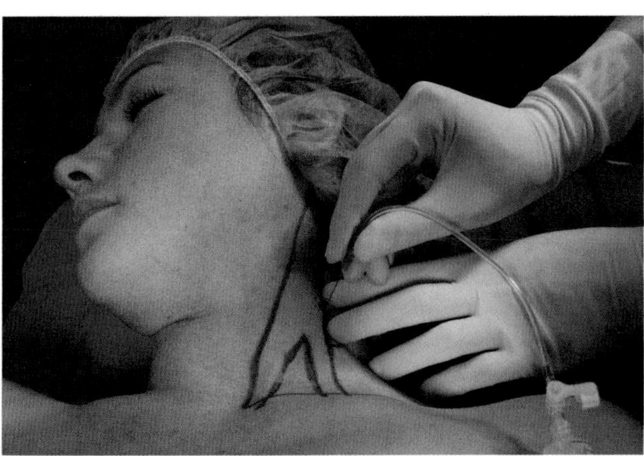

**FIGURE 11-11.** Needle insertion for the deep cervical plexus block. The needle is inserted between fingers palpating individual transverse processes.

## Technique

After cleaning the skin with an antiseptic solution, local anesthetic is infiltrated subcutaneously along the line estimating the position of the transverse processes. The local anesthetic is infiltrated over the entire length of the line, rather than at the projected insertion sites. This allows reinsertion of the needle slightly caudally or cranially when the transverse process is not contacted, without the need to infiltrate the skin at a new insertion site.

A needle is connected via flexible tubing to a syringe containing local anesthetic. The needle is inserted between the palpating fingers and advanced at an angle perpendicular to the skin plane (Figure 11-11). The needle should never be oriented cephalad. A slightly caudal orientation of the needle is important to prevent inadvertent insertion of the needle toward the cervical spinal cord. The needle is advanced slowly until the transverse process is contacted. At this point, the needle is withdrawn 1 to 2 mm and firmly stabilized, and 4 to 5 mL of local anesthetic is injected after a negative aspiration test for blood. The needle is removed, and the entire procedure is repeated at consecutive levels.

### TIPS

- The transverse processes are typically contacted at a depth of 1–2 cm in most patients. This distance can be further shortened by exerting pressure on the skin during needle advancement.
- The needle should never be advanced beyond 2.5 cm to avoid the risk of cervical cord injury or carotid or vertebral artery puncture.

### GOAL

- Contact with the posterior tubercle of the transverse process.
- Slightly withdraw the needle after the contact and before making an injection.

## Troubleshooting Deep Cervical Plexus Blocks

When insertion of the needle does not result in contact with the transverse process within 2 cm, the following maneuvers are used:

1. While avoiding skin movement, keep the palpating hand in the same position and the skin between the fingers stretched.
2. Withdraw the needle to the skin, redirect it 15° inferiorly, and repeat the procedure.
3. Withdraw the needle to the skin, reinsert it 1 cm caudal, and repeat the procedure.

### TIPS

- When these maneuvers fail to result in contact with the transverse process, the needle should be withdrawn and the landmarks reassessed.
- Redirecting the needle cephalad in an attempt to contact the transverse process should be avoided because it carries a risk of cervical cord injury when the needle is advanced too deeply.

## Block Dynamics and Perioperative Management

Premedication is useful for patient comfort; however, excessive sedation should be avoided. During neck surgery, airway management can be difficult because the anesthesiologist must share access to the head and neck with the surgeon. Surgeries like carotid endarterectomy require the patient to be fully conscious, oriented, and cooperative during the entire procedure. In addition, excessive sedation and the consequent lack of patient cooperation can result in restlessness and create difficulty for the surgeon. The onset time for this block is 10 to 20 minutes. The first sign is decreased sensation in the area of distribution of the respective components of the cervical plexus. Complications of cervical plexus blocks and strategies to avoid them are listed in Table 11-2.

**TABLE 11-2 Complications and How to Avoid Them**

| | |
|---|---|
| *Infection* | • Low risk.<br>• A strict aseptic technique should be used. |
| *Hematoma* | • Avoid multiple needle insertions, particularly in patients on anticoagulant therapy.<br>• Keep a 5-min steady pressure on the site if a blood vessel is inadvertently punctured. |
| *Phrenic nerve blockade* | • Phrenic nerve blockade (diaphragmatic paresis) is expected with a deep cervical plexus block<br>• A bilateral deep cervical block may be contraindicated in patients with symptomatic respiratory disease<br>• Blockade of the phrenic nerve does not occur following a superficial cervical plexus block. |
| *Local anesthetic toxicity* | • Central nervous system toxicity is the most common complication of the cervical plexus block.<br>• This complication occurs because of the rich vascularity of the neck (vertebral and carotid artery vessels); the toxicity usually results from the inadvertent intravascular injection rather than absorption of local anesthetic.<br>• Frequent aspiration for blood should be performed during the injection. |
| *Nerve injury* | • Local anesthetic should never be injected against excessive resistance (pressure) or when the patient complains of severe pain on injection. |
| *Spinal anesthesia* | • This complication may occur with injection of a large volume of local anesthetic inside the dural sleeve surrounding the nerves of the cervical plexus.<br>• Avoidance of high volumes and high pressure during injection are the best measures to avoid this complication.<br>• It should be noted that negative results from an aspiration test for cerebrospinal fluid do not rule out the possibility of intrathecal spread of local anesthetic. |

# DEEP CERVICAL PLEXUS BLOCK

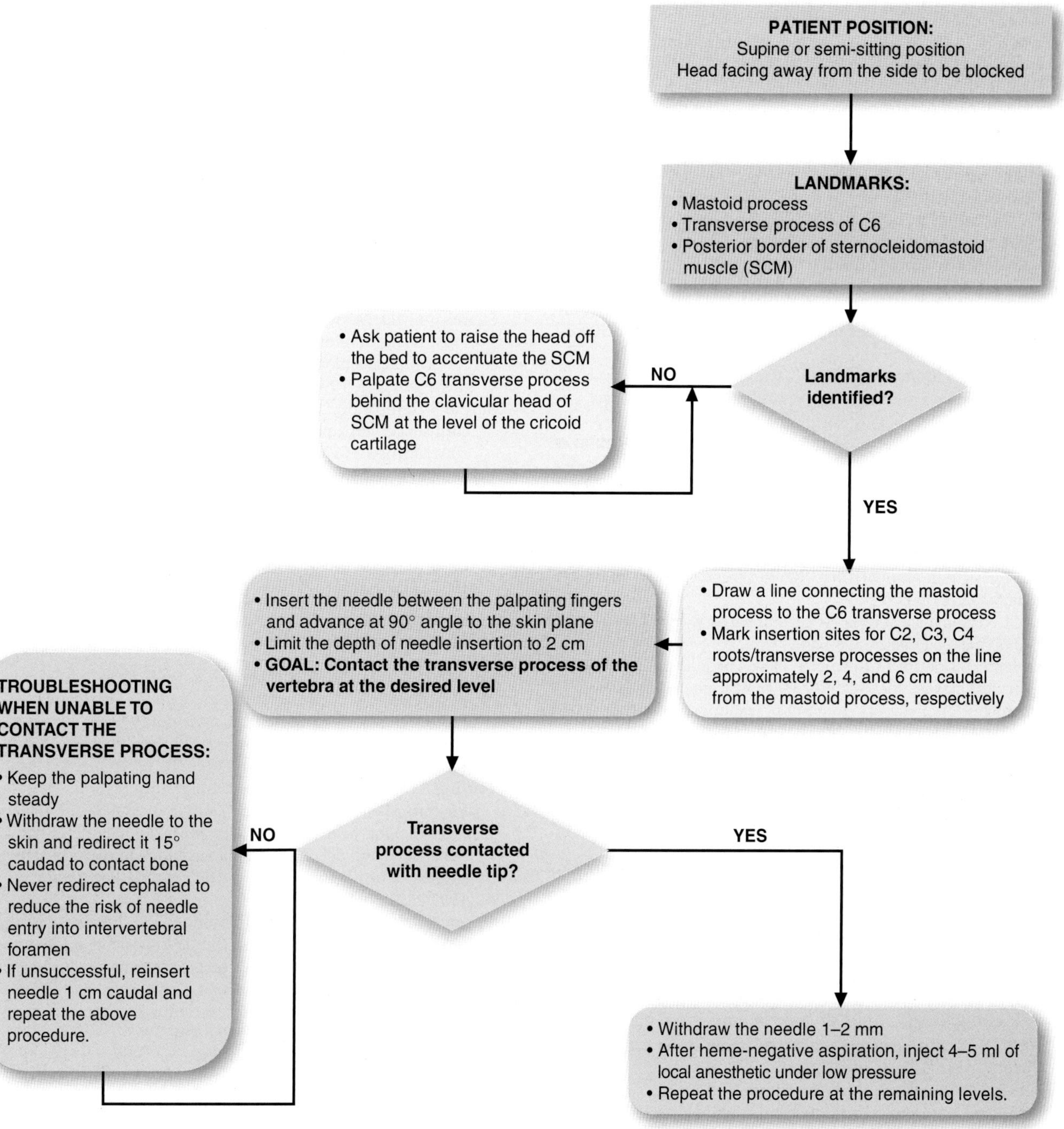

## SUGGESTED READING

### Superficial Cervical Plexus Block

Aunac S, Carlier M, Singelyn F, De Kock M. The analgesic efficacy of bilateral combined superficial and deep cervical plexus block administered before thyroid surgery under general anesthesia. *Anesth Analg.* 2002;95:746-750.

Brogly N, Wattier JM, Andrieu G, et al. Gabapentin attenuates late but not early postoperative pain after thyroidectomy with superficial cervical plexus block. *Anesth Analg.* 2008;107:1720-1725.

Choi DS, Atchabahian A, Brown AR. Cervical plexus block provides postoperative analgesia after clavicle surgery. *Anesth Analg.* 2005;100:1542-1543.

de Sousa AA, Filho MA, Faglione W Jr, Carvalho GT. Superficial vs combined cervical plexus block for carotid endarterectomy: a prospective, randomized study. *Surg Neurol.* 2005;63 Suppl 1:S22-25.

D'Honneur G, Motamed C, Tual L, Combes X. Respiratory distress after a deep cervical plexus block. *Anesthesiology.* 2005;102:1070.

Dieudonne N, Gomola A, Bonnichon P, Ozier YM. Prevention of postoperative pain after thyroid surgery: a double-blind randomized study of bilateral superficial cervical plexus blocks. *Anesth Analg.* 2001;92:1538-1542.

Eti Z, Irmak P, Gulluoglu BM, Manukyan MN, Gogus FY. Does bilateral superficial cervical plexus block decrease analgesic requirement after thyroid surgery? *Anesth Analg.* 2006;102:1174-1176.

Guay J. Regional anesthesia for carotid surgery. *Curr Opin Anaesthesiol.* 2008;21:638-644.

Herbland A, Cantini O, Reynier P, et al. The bilateral superficial cervical plexus block with 0.75% ropivacaine administered before or after surgery does not prevent postoperative pain after total thyroidectomy. *Reg Anesth Pain Med.* 2006;31:34-39.

Heyer EJ, Gold MI, Kirby EW, et al. A study of cognitive dysfunction in patients having carotid endarterectomy performed with regional anesthesia. *Anesth Analg.* 2008;107:636-642.

Jankovic D, Wells C, eds. *Regional Nerve Blocks.* 2nd ed. Berlin, Germany: Blackwell Scientific Publications; 2001.

Junca A, Marret E, Goursot G, Mazoit X, Bonnet F. A comparison of ropivacaine and bupivacaine for cervical plexus block. *Anesth Analg.* 2001;92:720-724.

Kim YK, Hwang GS, Huh IY, et al. Altered autonomic cardiovascular regulation after combined deep and superficial cervical plexus blockade for carotid endarterectomy. *Anesth Analg.* 2006;103:533-539.

Kwok AO, Silbert BS, Allen KJ, Bray PJ, Vidovich J. Bilateral vocal cord palsy during carotid endarterectomy under cervical plexus block. *Anesth Analg.* 2006;102:376-377.

Luchetti M, Canella M, Zoppi M, Massei R. Comparison of regional anesthesia versus combined regional and general anesthesia for elective carotid endarterectomy: a small exploratory study. *Reg Anesth Pain Med.* 2008;33:340-345.

Masters RD, Castresana EJ, Castresana MR. Superficial and deep cervical plexus block: technical considerations. *AANA J.* 1995;63:235-243.

Mulroy M. *Regional Anesthesia: An Illustrated Procedural Guide.* 3rd ed. Philadelphia, PA: Lippincott, Williams & Wilkins; 2002.

Murphy T. Somatic blockade of head and neck. In: Cousins MJ, Bridenbaugh PO, eds. *Neuronal Blockade in Clinical Anesthesia and Management of Pain.* Philadelphia, PA: Lippincott-Raven; 1988:489-514.

Nash L, Nicholson HD, Zhang M. Does the investing layer of the deep cervical fascia exist? *Anesthesiology.* 2005;103:962-968.

Pandit JJ, Bree S, Dillon P, Elcock D, McLaren ID, Crider B. A comparison of superficial versus combined (superficial and deep) cervical plexus block for carotid endarterectomy: a prospective, randomized study. *Anesth Analg.* 2000;91:781-786.

Pintaric TS, Hocevar M, Jereb S, Casati A, Jankovic VN. A prospective, randomized comparison between combined (deep and superficial) and superficial cervical plexus block with levobupivacaine for minimally invasive parathyroidectomy. *Anesth Analg.* 2007;105:1160-1163.

Schneemilch CE, Bachmann H, Ulrich A, Elwert R, Halloul Z, Hachenberg T. Clonidine decreases stress response in patients undergoing carotid endarterectomy under regional anesthesia: a prospective, randomized, double-blinded, placebo-controlled study. *Anesth Analg.* 2006;103:297-302.

Stoneham MD, Doyle AR, Knighton JD, Dorje P, Stanley JC. Prospective, randomized comparison of deep or superficial cervical plexus block for carotid endarterectomy surgery. *Anesthesiology.* 1998;89:907-912.

Suresh S, Templeton L. Superficial cervical plexus block for vocal cord surgery in an awake pediatric patient. *Anesth Analg.* 2004;98:1656-1657.

Umbrain VJ, van Gorp VL, Schmedding E, et al. Ropivacaine 3.75 mg/ml, 5 mg/ml, or 7.5 mg/ml for cervical plexus block during carotid endarterectomy. *Reg Anesth Pain Med.* 2004;29:312-316.

Winnie AP, Ramamurthy S, Durrani Z, Radonjic R. Interscalene cervical plexus block: a single-injection technic. *Anesth Analg.* 1975;54:370-375.

### Deep Cervical Plexus Block

Benzon HT, Raja SN, Borsook D, Molloy RE, Strichartz G. *Essentials of Pain Medicine and Regional Anesthesia.* Philadelphia, PA: Churchill Livingstone; 1999.

Brown D. *Atlas of Regional Anesthesia.* Philadelphia, PA: Saunders; 1992.

Carling A, Simmonds M. Complications from regional anaesthesia for carotid endarterectomy. *Br J Anaesth.* 2000;84:797-800.

Davies MJ, Silbert BS, Scott DA, Cook RJ, Mooney PH, Blyth C. Superficial and deep cervical plexus block for carotid artery surgery: a prospective study of 1000 blocks. *Reg Anesth.* 1997;22:442-446.

Emery G, Handley G, Davies MJ, Mooney PH. Incidence of phrenic nerve block and hypercapnia in patients undergoing carotid endarterectomy under cervical plexus block. *Anaesth Intensive Care.* 1998;26:377-381.

Johnson TR. Transient ischaemic attack during deep cervical plexus block. *Br J Anaesth.* 1999;83:965-967.

Kulkarni RS, Braverman LE, Patwardhan NA. Bilateral cervical plexus block for thyroidectomy and parathyroidectomy in healthy and high risk patients. *J Endocrinol Invest.* 1996;19:714-718.

Lo Gerfo P, Ditkoff BA, Chabot J, Feind C. Thyroid surgery using monitored anesthesia care: an alternative to general anesthesia. *Thyroid.* 1994;4:437-439.

Stoneham MD, Wakefield TW. Acute respiratory distress after deep cervical plexus block. *J Cardiothorac Vasc Anesth.* 1998;12:197-198.

Weiss A, Isselhorst C, Gahlen J, et al. Acute respiratory failure after deep cervical plexus block for carotid endarterectomy as a result of bilateral recurrent laryngeal nerve paralysis. *Acta Anaesthesiol Scand.* 2005;49:715-719.

# 12 Interscalene Brachial Plexus Block

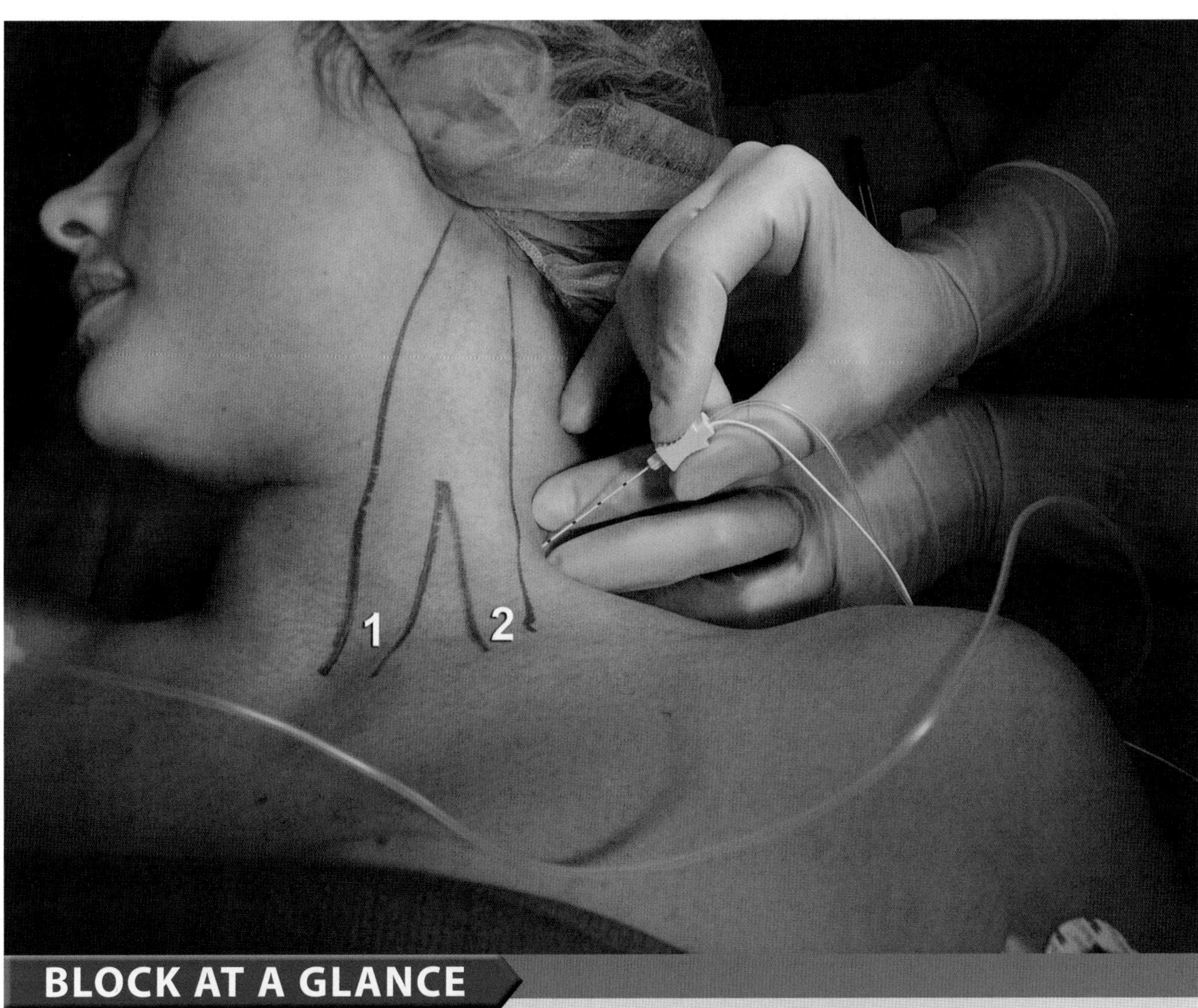


## BLOCK AT A GLANCE

- Indications: shoulder, arm, and elbow surgery
- Landmarks: the clavicular head of the sternocleidomastoid muscle, clavicle, external jugular vein
- Nerve stimulation: twitch of the pectoralis, deltoid, arm, forearm, or hand muscles at 0.2–0.5 mA
- Local anesthetic: 25–35 mL
- Complexity level: intermediate

**FIGURE 12-1.** Needle insertion for interscalene brachial plexus block. The needle is inserted between palpating fingers that are positioned in the scalene groove (between anterior and middle scalene muscles). 1 = sternal head of the sternocleidomastoid muscle. 2 = clavicular head of the sternocleidomastoid muscle.

## General Considerations

An interscalene block relies on the spread of a relatively large volume of local anesthetic within the interscalene groove to accomplish blockade of the brachial plexus. In our practice, we almost always use a low interscalene block technique, which consists of inserting the needle more caudally than in the commonly described procedure performed at the level of the cricoid cartilage. Our reasoning is that at the lower neck, the interscalene groove is more shallow and easier to identify, and the distribution of anesthesia is also adequate for elbow and forearm surgery. In addition, the needle insertion is more lateral, which makes puncture of the carotid artery less likely and performance of the block easier to master by trainees. Low approach to interscalene block is used in shoulder, arm, and forearm surgery. In our practice, the most common indications for this procedure are shoulder and humerus surgery and the insertion of an arteriovenous graft for hemodialysis.

## Functional Anatomy

The brachial plexus supplies innervation to the upper limb and consists of a branching network of nerves derived from the anterior rami of the lower four cervical and the first thoracic spinal nerves. Starting from their origin and descending distally, the components of the plexus are named roots, trunks, divisions, cords, and, finally, terminal branches. The five roots of the cervical and the first thoracic spinal nerves (anterior rami) give rise to three trunks (superior, middle, and inferior) that emerge between the medial and anterior scalene muscles to lie on the floor of the posterior triangle of the neck (Figure 12-2). The roots of the plexus lie deep to the prevertebral fascia, whereas the trunks are covered by its lateral extension, the axillary sheath. Each trunk divides into an anterior and a posterior division behind the clavicle, at the apex of the axilla (Figure 12-3). The divisions combine to produce the three cords, which are named lateral, median, and posterior according to their relationship to

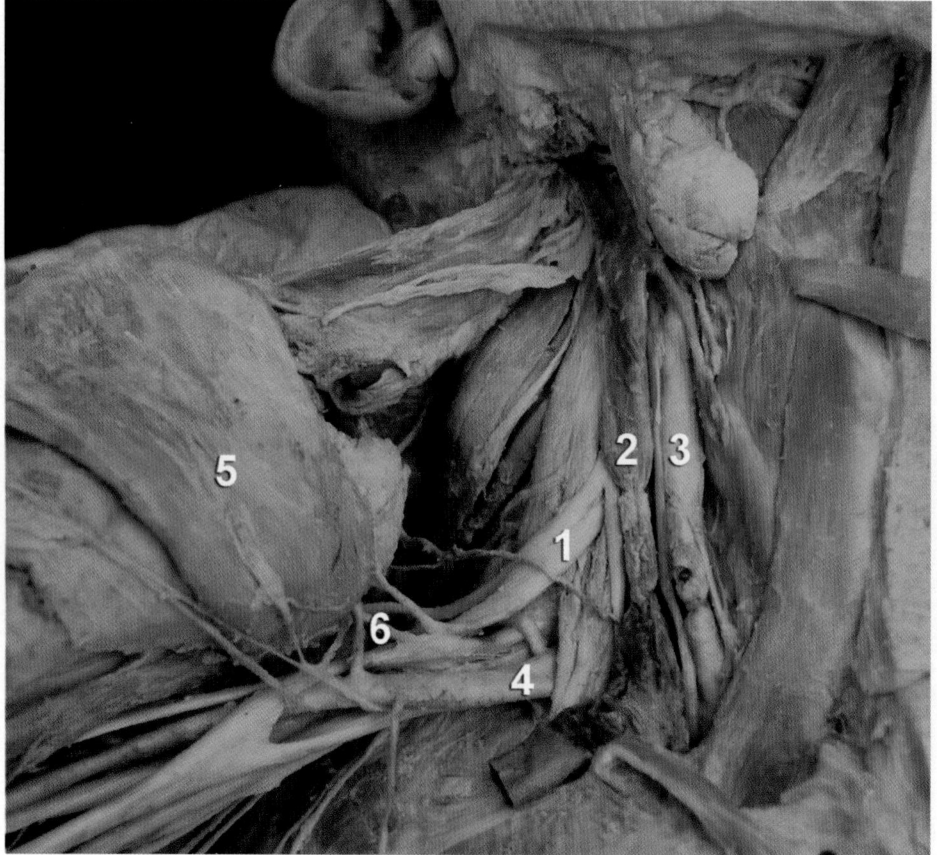


**FIGURE 12-2.** Anatomy of the brachial plexus. The sternocleidomastoid muscle is removed and the brachial plexus ❶ is seen emerging between the scalene muscles. ❷ internal jugular vein. ❸ carotid artery. ❹ subclavian artery. ❺ Retracted pectoralis muscle. ❻ medial and lateral pectoral nerves. The number "1" also indicates the approximate level at which the block is performed where the roots of the muscles are emerging between the scalene muscles.

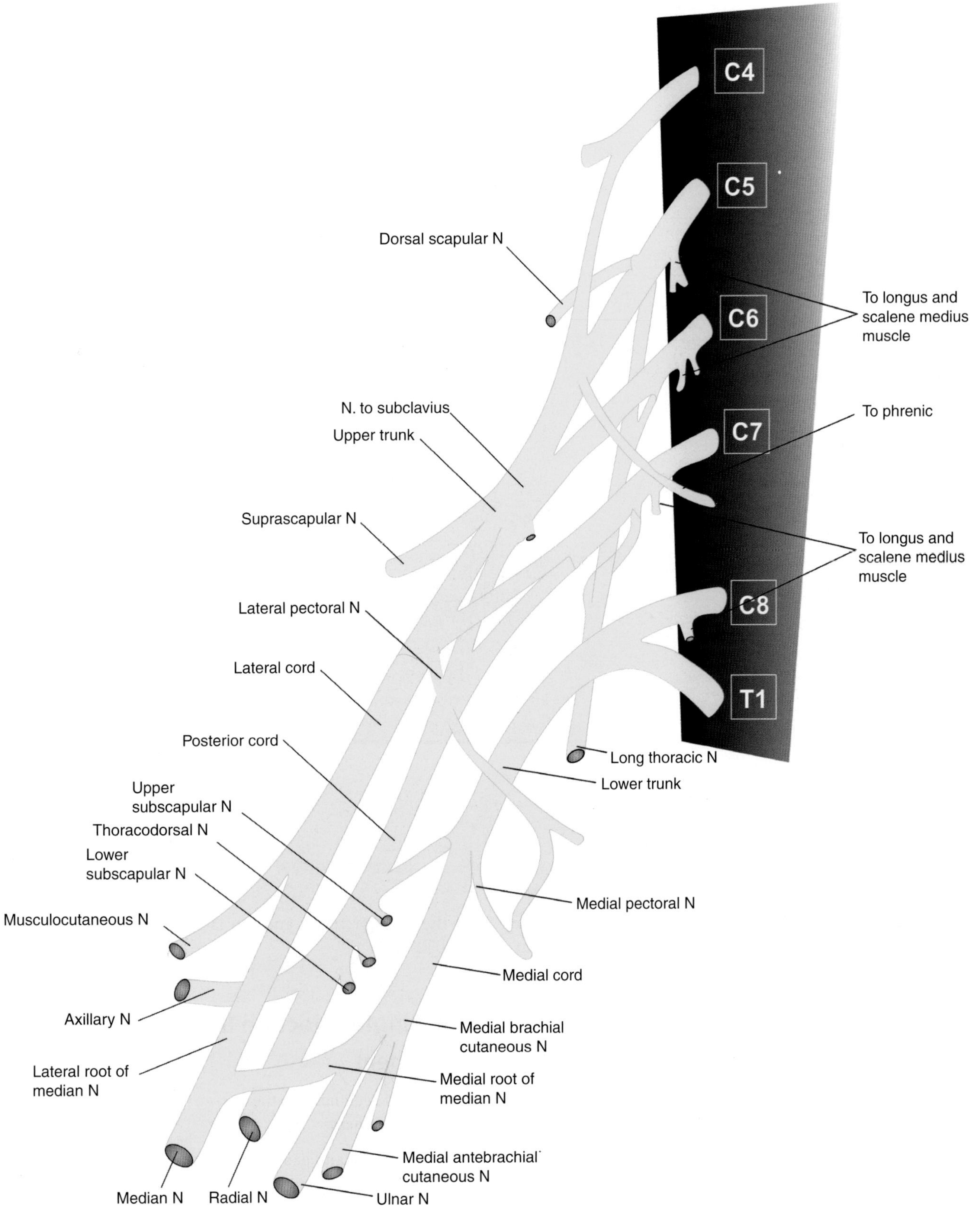


**FIGURE 12-3.** Functional organization of the brachial plexus and formation of the terminal nerves.

**TABLE 12-1 Distribution of the Brachial Plexus**

| NERVE(S) | SPINAL SEGMENT(S) | DISTRIBUTION |
|---|---|---|
| Nerves to subclavius | C5,C6 | Subclavius muscle |
| Dorsal scapular nerve | C5 | Rhomboid muscles and levator scapulae muscle |
| Long thoracic nerve | C5 through C7 | Serratus anterior muscle |
| Suprascapular nerve | C5, C6 | Supraspinatus and infraspinatus muscles |
| Pectoralis nerve (medial and lateral) | C5 through T1 | Pectoralis muscles |
| Subscapular nerves | C5, C6 | Subscapularis and teres major muscles |
| Thoracodorsal nerve | C6 through C8 | Latissimus dorsi muscle |
| Axillary nerve | C5 and C6 | Deltoid and teres minor muscles; skin of shoulder |
| Radial nerve | C5 through T1 | Extensor muscles of the arm and forearm (triceps brachii, extensor carpi radialis, extensor carpi ulnaris), supinator, anconeus, and brachioradialis muscles; digital extensors and abductor pollicis longus muscle; skin over posterolateral surface of the arm, forearm, and hand |
| Musculocutaneous nerve | C5 through C7 | Flexor muscles of the arm (biceps brachii, brachialis, coracobrachialis); skin over lateral surface of the forearm |
| Median nerve | C6 through T1 | Flexor muscles of the forearm (flexor carpi radialis, palmaris longus); pronator quadratus and pronator teres muscles; digital flexors (through the palmar interosseous nerve); skin over anterolateral surface of the hand |
| Ulnar nerve | C8, T1 | Flexor carpi ulnaris muscle, adductor pollicis muscle, the hypothenar muscles and small digital muscles; skin over medial surface of the hand |

the axillary artery. From this point on, individual nerves are formed as these neuronal elements descend distally (Figure 12-3 and Table 12-1).

## Distribution of Blockade

The interscalene approach to brachial plexus blockade results in anesthesia of the shoulder, arm, and elbow (Figure 12-4). Note that the skin over and medial to the acromion is supplied by the supraclavicular nerve, which is a branch of the cervical plexus. Supraclavicular nerves are usually blocked with the brachial plexus when an interscalene block is performed. This is because the local anesthetic invariably spills over from the interscalene space into the prevertebral fascia and blocks the branches of the cervical plexus. The classic interscalene block is not recommended for hand surgery due to potential sparing of the inferior trunk and the lack of blockade of the C8 and T1 roots.

## Single-Injection Interscalene Block

### Equipment

A standard regional anesthesia tray is prepared with the following equipment:

- Sterile towels and gauze packs
- 2 × 20-mL syringes containing local anesthetic
- A 3-mL syringe and 25-gauge needle with local anesthetic for skin infiltration
- A 3.5-cm, 22-gauge, short-bevel insulated stimulating needle
- Peripheral nerve stimulator
- Sterile gloves; marking pen

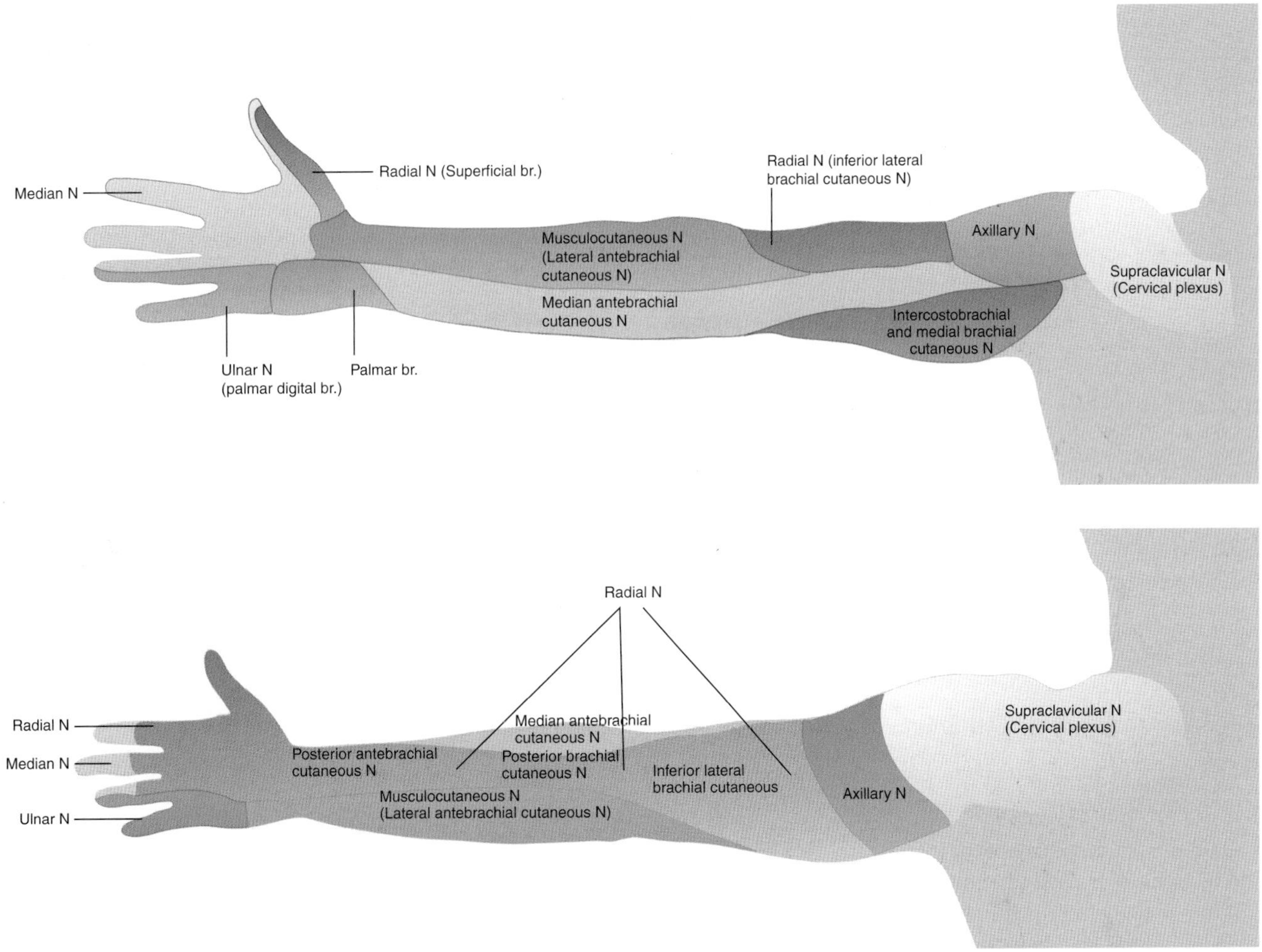

**FIGURE 12-4.** Sensory distribution of the brachial plexus. The innervation is shown for didactic purposes; the exact extent of anesthesia with interscalane block varies considerably and often spares the hand.

## Landmarks and Patient Positioning

The patient is in a supine or semi-sitting position with the head facing away from the side to be blocked (Figure 12-5). The arm should rest comfortably on the bed, abdomen, or arm-board to allow detection of responses to nerve stimulation. Removal of a cast (when present) can help to detect motor response, although removal is not essential because the responses to nerve stimulation are usually mixed (stimulation of trunks and divisions rather than specific nerves) and proximal motor response is adequate (e.g., deltoid, pectoralis).

These are the primary landmarks for performing this block:

1. The clavicle
2. Posterior border of the clavicular head of the sterno-cleidomastoid muscle
3. External jugular vein (usually crosses the interscalene groove at the level of the trunks)

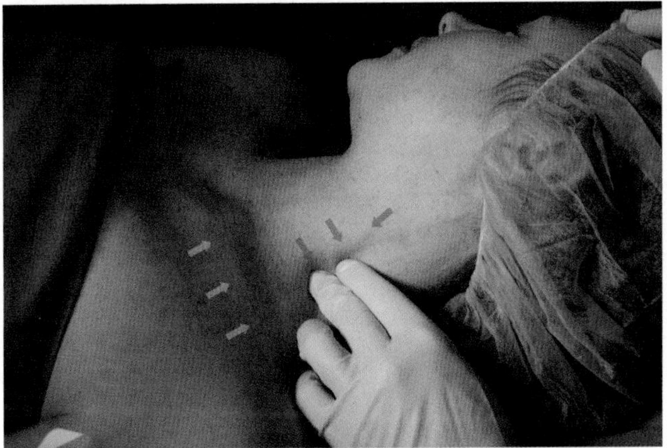

**FIGURE 12-5.** Landmarks for the interscalene brachial plexus. White arrows: clavicle. Red arrows: posterior border of the sternocleidomastoid muscle. Blue arrow: external jugular vein. The palpating fingers are positioned lateral and posterior to the clavicular head of the sternocleidomastoid muscle in the space between anterior and middle scalene muscles. The scalene groove is often palpated just in front or behind the external jugular vein.

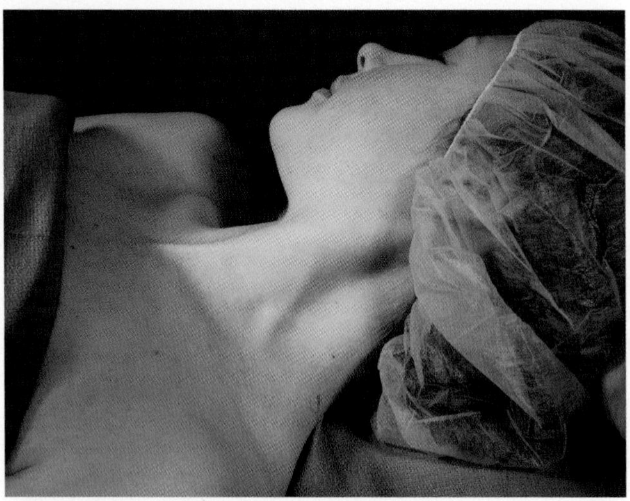

**FIGURE 12-6.** Maneuver to extenuate the posterior border of the sternocleidomastoid muscle and external jugular vein by asking the patient to lift her head off of the table while looking away from the side to be blocked.

### *Maneuvers to Facilitate Landmark Identification*

Identification of the interscalene groove can be made easier by performing the following steps:

- Ask the patient to reach for the ipsilateral knee with the limb to be blocked or passively pull the patient's wrist inferiorly. This maneuver flattens the skin of the neck and helps identify both the scalene muscles and the external jugular vein.
- The sternocleidomastoid muscle can be accentuated by asking the patient to raise the head off the table (Figure 12-6).
- The external jugular vein can be accentuated by asking the patient to perform a brief Valsalva maneuver.
- While palpating the interscalene groove, ask the patient to sniff forcefully. Sniffing tenses the scalene muscles, and the fingers of the palpating hand often fall into the interscalene groove.

The described landmarks should routinely be marked on the patient's skin prior to performing the block.

**TIP**

- The proportions of the shoulder girdle, size of the neck, prominence of the muscles, and other anatomic features vary among patients. When in doubt, always perform a "reality check" and estimate three bony landmarks: the sternal notch, clavicle, and mastoid process. This helps identify the sternocleidomastoid muscle and its relations.

## Technique

After cleaning the skin with an antiseptic solution, 1 to 3 mL of local anesthetic is infiltrated subcutaneously at the determined needle insertion site.

**TIP**

- During skin infiltration, care should be taken to infiltrate local anesthetic into the subcutaneous tissue plane *only* because the brachial plexus is very shallow at this location. A deeper needle insertion can result in deposition of local anesthetic into the plexus; this can result in nerve injury and/or make attempts at obtaining a motor response unsuccessful.

The fingers of the palpating hand should be gently but firmly pressed between the anterior and middle scalene muscles to shorten the skin-brachial plexus distance. The skin over the neck can be very mobile, and care should be taken to stabilize the fingers as well as to stretch the skin gently between the two fingers to ensure accuracy in needle advancement and redirection. The palpating hand should not be allowed to move during the entire block procedure to allow for precise redirection of the needle when necessary.

**GOAL**

The goal is stimulation of the brachial plexus with a current intensity of 0.2–0.5 mA (0.1 ms). The following motor responses result in a similar success rate:

- Pectoralis muscle
- Deltoid muscle
- Triceps muscles
- Biceps muscle
- Any twitch of the hand or forearm

The needle is inserted 3–4 cm (approximately 2 fingerbreadths) above the clavicle and advanced at an angle almost perpendicular to the skin plane (Figure 12-7).

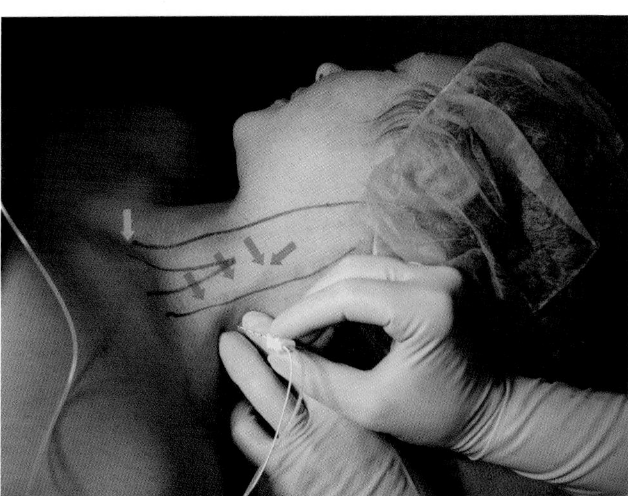

**FIGURE 12-7.** Needle insertion for interscalene brachial plexus block. The needle is inserted between fingers positioned in the interscalene groove with a slight caudad orientation to decrease the chance of entrance in the cervical spinal cord. White arrow: insertion of the sternal head of the sternocleidomastoid muscle. Red arrows: posterior border of the sternocleidomastoid muscle. Blue arrow: external jugular vein. The insertion point for the block is often immediately posterior to the external jugular vein.

The needle must never be oriented cephalad; a slight caudal orientation reduces a chance for an inadvertent insertion of the needle into the cervical spinal cord. The nerve stimulator should be initially set to deliver 0.8 to 1.0 mA (2 Hz, 0.1 ms). The needle is advanced slowly until stimulation of the brachial plexus is obtained. This typically occurs at a depth of 1 to 2 cm in most all patients. Once appropriate twitches of the brachial plexus are elicited, 25 to 35 mL of local anesthetic are injected slowly with intermittent aspiration to rule out intravascular injection.

This "low-interscalene" approach differs from the classic description of the interscalene block, which uses the cricoid cartilage as a landmark. The principal advantage to the low approach is that the brachial plexus is more compact at the lower levels, and reliable coverage of the upper, middle, and lower trunks can be achieved with a single injection (Figure 12-8). In contrast, the classic approach may spare the lower trunk, which limits its use for forearm and elbow surgery.

When insertion of the needle does not result in upper extremity muscle stimulation, the following maneuvers can be used (Figure 12-9):

1. Keep the palpating hand in the same position and the skin between the fingers stretched.
2. Withdraw the needle to the skin level, redirect it 15° posteriorly, and repeat the needle advancement.
3. Withdraw the needle to the skin level, redirect it 15° anteriorly, and repeat the needle insertion.

## TIPS

- The needle should never be advanced beyond 2.5 cm to avoid the risk of mechanical complications (cervical cord injury, pneumothorax, vascular puncture).
- *Never inject* when resistance (high pressure) on injection of local anesthetic is met. High resistance to injection (>15 psi) may indicate an intrafascicular needle placement. Instead, withdraw and/or rotate the needle slightly and reattempt the injection to assure absence of resistance.
- Stimulation of the brachial plexus with a higher stimulating current (e.g., >1.0 mA) results in an exaggerated response and unnecessary discomfort for the patient. In addition, an unpredictably strong response often causes dislodgment of the needle and a withdrawal reaction by the patient.
- Local anesthetic should not be injected when a motor response is obtained at a current intensity <0.2 mA because this is associated with intraneural needle placement.
- Intraneural injection of the trunks can lead not only to nerve injury but also retrograde backflow of local anesthetic toward neuraxial space, resulting in total spinal anesthesia.
- Care should always be taken to avoid attributing diaphragmatic and trapezius twitches to stimulation of the brachial plexus. Misinterpretation of these twitches is one of the most common causes of block failure.
- When in doubt, palpate the muscle that appears to be twitching to ensure the proper response.

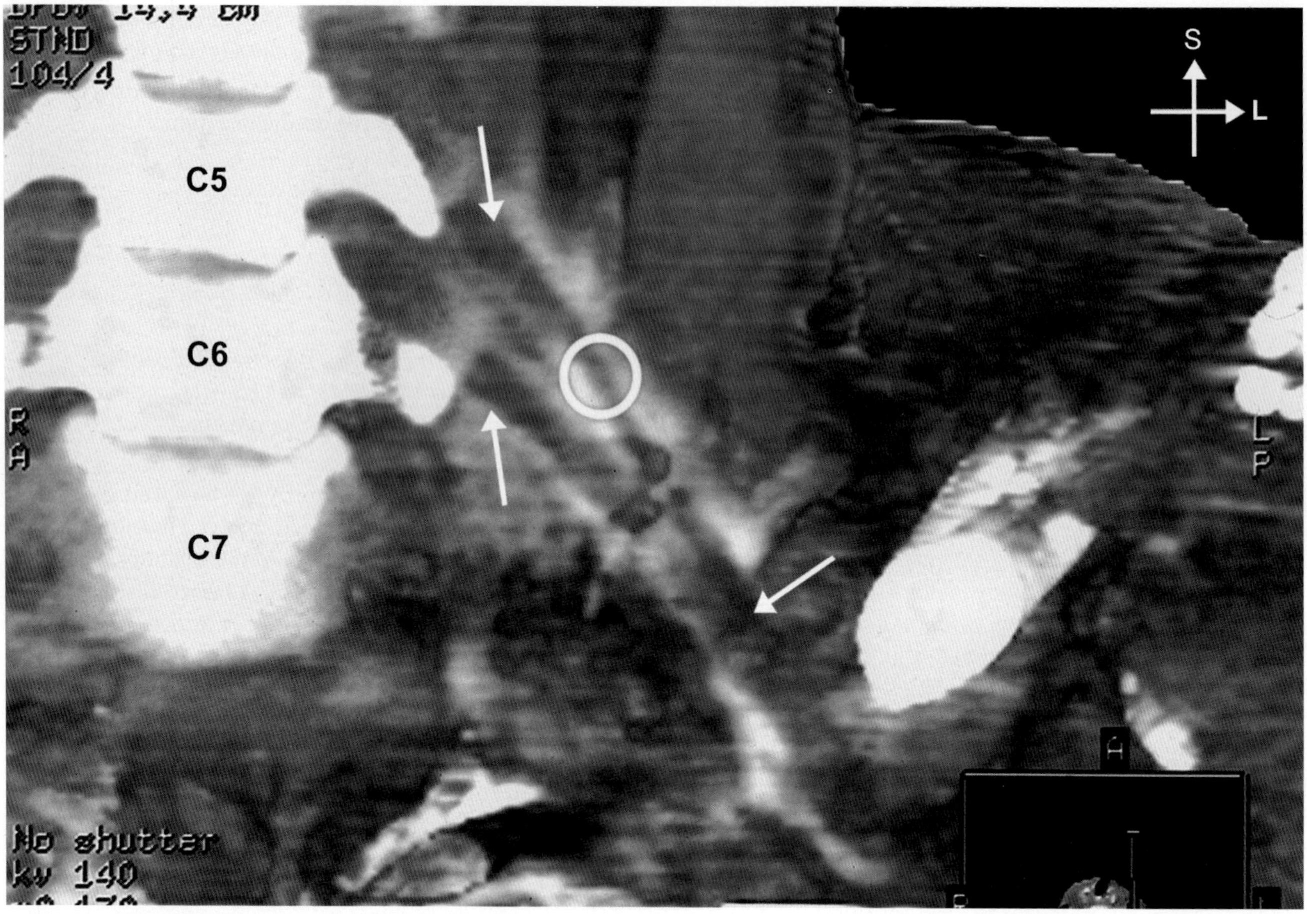

**FIGURE 12-8.** Distribution of the mixture of local anesthetic and a radiopaque contrast after an interscalene brachial plexus injection. The arrows and the circle indicate "negative" contrast image of the roots of the brachial plexus.

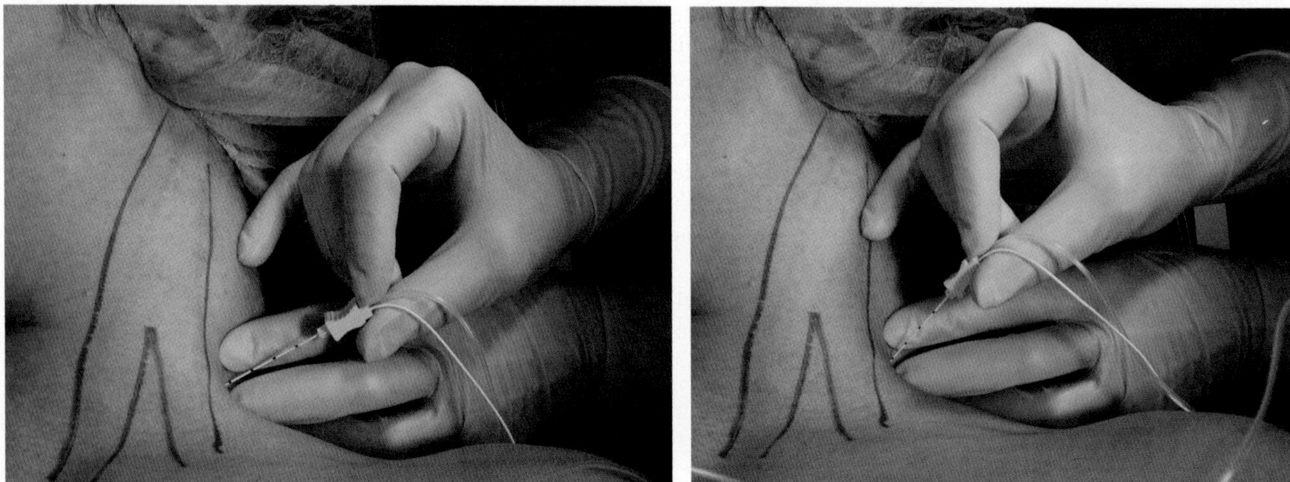

**FIGURE 12-9.** Maneuvers to obtain a motor response of the brachial plexus during electric nerve localization. When the motor response is not obtained on the initial needle pass, the needle is redirected anteriorly or posteriorly to the original insertion plane as shown in the figure.

## Troubleshooting

**TABLE 12-2 Common Problems During Nerve Localization and the Corrective Action**

| RESPONSE OBTAINED | INTERPRETATION | PROBLEM | ACTION |
|---|---|---|---|
| Local twitch of the neck muscles | Direct stimulation of the anterior scalene or sternocleidomastoid muscle | Needle pass is in the wrong plane | Withdraw the needle to the skin level and reinsert it slightly anteriorly or posteriorly |
| Needle contacts bone at 1- to 2-cm depth; no twitches are seen | Needle stopped by the transverse process (or first rib) | Needle is inserted too posteriorly; the needle is contacting the anterior tubercles of the transverse process | Withdraw the needle to the skin level and reinsert it 15° anteriorly |
| Twitches of the diaphragm | Results from stimulation of the phrenic nerve | Needle is inserted too anteriorly | Withdraw the needle and reinsert it 15° posteriorly |
| Arterial blood noticed in the tubing | Puncture of the carotid artery (most common) | Needle insertion and angulation are too anterior | Withdraw the needle and keep a steady pressure for 2-3 min; reinsert it 1-2 cm posteriorly |
| Pectoralis muscle twitch | Brachial plexus stimulation (C4 through C5) | None | Accept and inject local anesthetic |
| Twitch of the scapula | Twitch of the serratus anterior muscle; stimulation of the thoracodorsal nerve | Needle position is posterior and deep to the brachial plexus | Withdraw the needle to the skin level and reinsert it anteriorly |
| Trapezius muscle twitches | Accessory nerve stimulation | Needle is posterior to the brachial plexus | Withdraw the needle and reinsert it anteriorly |
| Twitch of pectorals, deltoid, triceps, biceps, forearm, and hand muscles | Stimulation of the brachial plexus | None | Accept and inject local anesthetic |

**TIPS**

- Always assess the risk-benefit ratio of using large volumes and concentrations of long-acting local anesthetic for interscalene brachial plexus block.
- Smaller volumes and concentrations can be used successfully (e.g., 15–20 mL). However failure rate may be somewhat higher because the spread of local anesthetic can be seen as is the case with ultrasound guidance.

## Block Dynamics and Perioperative Management

When stimulation with a low-intensity current and slow needle advancement are used, interscalene brachial plexus block is associated with minor patient discomfort. Excessive sedation is not only unnecessary but also potentially disadvantageous because patient cooperation during landmark assessment and block performance is beneficial. The administration of benzodiazepines also may decrease the tone of the scalene and sternocleidomastoid muscles, making their recognition more difficult. We typically use small doses of midazolam (e.g., 1–2 mg) and/or short acting opioid (e.g., alfentanyl 250-500 mcg), so that the patient is comfortable and cooperative during nerve localization.

The onset time of this block is relatively short. The first sign of the blockade is typically a loss of coordination of the shoulder and arm muscles. This sign is seen sooner than the onset of a sensory blockade or a temperature change and, when observed within 1 to 2 minutes after injection, is highly predictive of a successful brachial plexus blockade. In patients undergoing shoulder arthroscopic procedures, it is important to note that the arthroscopic portals are often inserted outside the cutaneous distribution of the interscalene block. Local infiltration at the site of the incision by the surgeon is all that is needed because the entire shoulder joint and deep tissues are anesthetized with the interscalene block alone.

Education of the patient regarding block effects and side effects is important with interscalene block. Patients should be instructed to take prescribed oral analgesics and use ice packs before the block resolves. This regimen is of particular importance with ambulatory patients who may experience significant pain after discharge if they are unprepared.

## TIPS

- Due to blockade of neighboring neural structures, many patients develop a hoarse voice (recurrent laryngeal nerve), mild ipsilateral ptosis and miosis, and nasal congestion (Horner syndrome: sympathetic chain) following an interscalene block. A proper explanation and reassurance are all that such patients need.
- Interscalene block inevitably results in ipsilateral diaphragmatic paralysis (a phrenic nerve block). The significance of this is debated, and avoidance of this block is suggested in patients with severe chronic respiratory disease, especially restrictive lung diseases. Patients with chronic obstructive pulmonary disease often already have diaphragms that are flattened and inefficient, and the subsequent paresis is thought to have a limited effect on these individuals.
- We avoid the use of this block only in patients whose breathing involves the use of accessory respiratory muscles.
- Appropriate intravenous sedation, communication with the patient, lifting drapes off the patient's face, and shielding the ears from noise are all necessary ingredients for success with interscalene blocks in patients undergoing shoulder surgery.

## Continuous Interscalene Block

A continuous interscalene block is a more advanced regional anesthesia technique, and adequate experience with the single-injection technique is necessary. Paradoxically, although a single-injection interscalene block is one of the easiest intermediate techniques to perform and master, placement of the catheter can be one of the more technically challenging procedures. This is because the shallow position of the brachial plexus does not allow for an easy needle stabilization during catheter advancement and catheters can easily get dislodged during needle withdrawal. Otherwise, the technique is similar to the single-injection procedure, apart from a slight difference in the angle of the needle. This procedure provides excellent analgesia in patients following shoulder, arm, and elbow surgery.

### Equipment

A standard regional anesthesia tray is prepared with the following equipment:

- Sterile towels and gauze packs
- 2 × 20-mL syringes containing local anesthetic
- Sterile gloves, marking pen, and surface electrode
- A 3-mL syringe and 25-gauge needle with local anesthetic for skin infiltration
- Peripheral nerve stimulator
- Catheter kit (including a 4- to 5-cm large-gauge stimulating needle and catheter)

Kits come in two varieties based on catheter construction: nonstimulating (conventional) and stimulating catheters. During the placement of a conventional nonstimulating catheter, the stimulating needle is first advanced until appropriate twitches are obtained. Then, 5 to 10 mL of local anesthetic or other injectate (e.g., dextrose 5% in water) can be injected to "open up" a space for the catheter to advance freely without resistance. The catheter is then inserted through the needle approximately 3 to 5 cm beyond the tip of the needle. The needle is withdrawn, the catheter is secured, and the remaining local anesthetic is injected via the catheter. Stimulating catheters are insulated and have a filament or core that transmits current to a bare metal tip. After obtaining twitches with the needle, the catheter is advanced with the nerve stimulator connected until the anesthesiologist is satisfied with the quality of the motor response. If the twitch is lost, the catheter may be withdrawn until it reappears, and the catheter is readvanced. This method requires no conducting solution to be injected through the needle (i.e., local anesthetic, saline) before catheter advancement, or difficulty obtaining a motor response will result.

### Landmarks and Patient Positioning

The patient is in the same position as for the single-injection technique. However, it is imperative that the anesthesiologist assume an ergonomic position to allow maneuvering during catheter insertion. It is often easiest for the clinician to stand at the head of the bed to avoid inserting the needle at an awkward angle because it is desirable to advance the catheter in an inferolateral direction (i.e., the same direction as the plexus). It is also important that all equipment, including the catheter, be immediately available and prepared in advance because small movements of the needle that might occur while trying to prepare the catheter can result in dislodging the needle from its position in the brachial plexus sheath.

The landmarks for a continuous interscalene brachial plexus block are similar to those for the single-shot technique:

1. Clavicle
2. Posterior border of the clavicular head of the sternocleidomastoid muscle
3. External jugular vein

## Technique

The subcutaneous tissue at the projected site of needle insertion is anesthetized with local anesthetic. The block needle is attached to a nerve stimulator (1.0 mA, 2 Hz, 0.1 ms). With this technique, the palpating hand must firmly stabilize the skin to facilitate needle insertion and insertion of the catheter. A 3- to 5-cm block needle is inserted in the interscalene groove, with a more pronounced caudal angle than the single-shot technique, and advanced until the brachial plexus twitch is elicited at 0.2 to 0.5 mA. Precautions should be taken to avoid inserting the needle through the external jugular vein because this invariably results in prolonged oozing from the site of puncture. This can be avoided by retracting the external jugular vein and inserting the needle slightly in *front* of or *posteriorly* to the external jugular vein. Paying meticulous attention to the position of the needle, the catheter is inserted no more than 3 to 5 cm beyond the tip of the needle (Figure 12-10).

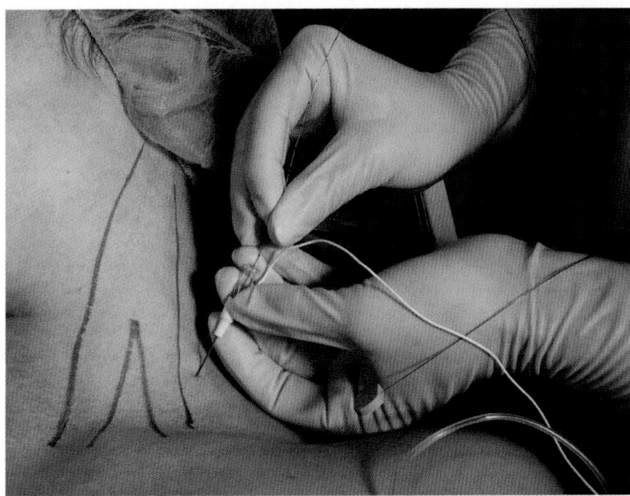

**FIGURE 12-10.** Insertion of a catheter into the interscalene space. Insertion of the catheter often requires lowering of the needle angle to facilitate catheter passage. Catheters are typically inserted 3–5 cm past the needle tip to prevent inadvertent removal.

### TIPS

- The most challenging aspect of this technique is stabilization of the needle for catheter insertion after the brachial plexus is localized.
- When the needle encounters the brachial plexus at a very shallow location, it is helpful to have an assistant advance the catheter in a sterile fashion to ensure that the needle does not move from its original position.
- In patients with less than ideal landmarks, it may be prudent to first use a single-shot needle to localize the brachial plexus and to determine the needle insertion point and proper angulation before inserting a large-gauge continuous block needle.

The catheter is secured using an adhesive skin preparation such as benzoin, followed by application of a clear dressing. Several securing devices are also commercially available. The infusion port should be clearly marked "continuous nerve block," and the catheter should be carefully checked for intravascular placement before administering a bolus or infusion of local anesthetics.

## Management of the Continuous Infusion

Continuous infusion is initiated after an initial bolus of dilute local anesthetic is administered through the needle or catheter. For this purpose, we routinely use 0.2% ropivacaine 15 to 20 mL. Diluted bupivacaine or levobupivacaine are suitable also but can result in greater motor blockade. Other adjuvants (clonidine, epinephrine, or opioids) do not appear to be of benefit in continuous nerve blocks. The infusion is maintained at 5 mL/h when a dose of patient-controlled regional analgesia (PCRA) (5 mL every 30-60 minutes) is planned. Additional catheter management directions are also discussed in Chapter 7.

Inpatients should be seen and instructed on the use of PCRA at least once a day. During each visit, the insertion site should be checked for erythema and swelling and the extent of motor and sensory blockade documented. The infusion and PCRA dose should be adjusted accordingly. When the patient complains of breakthrough pain, the extent of the blockade should be checked first. A bolus of dilute local anesthetic (e.g., 10–15 mL of 0.2% ropivacaine) can be injected to reactivate the catheter. Increasing the infusion rate alone never results in improvement in analgesia. When the bolus fails to result in blockade after 30 minutes, the catheter should be considered to have migrated and should be removed. Alternatively, where equipment and expertise is available, the position of the catheter can be confirmed ultrasonographically by documenting the location of an injection bolus through the catheter. Every patient receiving a continuous nerve block infusion should be prescribed an immediately available alternative pain management protocol because incomplete analgesia and catheter dislodgment can occur. Complications of interscalane brachial plexus blocks and means of their prevention are listed in Table 12-3.

## TIPS

- Breakthrough pain in patients undergoing continuous infusion is always managed by administering a bolus of local anesthetic. Increasing the rate of infusion alone is rarely adequate.
- For patients on the ward, a small bolus (e.g. 5 mL) of a shorter acting, higher concentration epinephrine-containing local anesthetic (e.g., 1% mepivacaine or lidocaine with 1:300,000 epinephrine) can be used to test the position of the catheter; failure to obtain a sensory block indicates catheter migration.

**TABLE 12-3 Complications and How to Avoid Them**

| | |
|---|---|
| *Infection* | • A strict aseptic technique is used. |
| *Hematoma* | • Avoid insertion of the needle through the external jugular vein.<br>• Avoid multiple needle insertions, particularly in patients undergoing anticoagulant treatment.<br>• Use a single-injection needle to localize the brachial plexus in patients with difficult anatomy. |
| *Vascular puncture* | • Apply a steady pressure of for 5 min if the carotid artery is punctured (uncommon). |
| *Local anesthetic toxicity* | • Systemic toxicity most commonly occurs during or shortly after the injection of local anesthetic; it is most commonly caused by inadvertent intravascular injection or channeling of forcefully injected local anesthetic into small veins or lymphatic channels that were cut during needle manipulation.<br>• Large volumes of long-acting anesthetic should be avoided in older and frail patients.<br>• Careful, frequent aspiration should be performed during the injection.<br>• Avoid fast, forceful injection of local anesthetic. |
| *Nerve injury* | • Never inject local anesthetic when excessive pressure (>15 psi) is required to initiate the injection.<br>• Local anesthetic injection should be stopped when the patient complains of severe pain or exhibits a withdrawal reaction on injection. |
| *Total spinal anesthesia* | • When stimulation is obtained with a current intensity of <0.2 mA, the needle should be pulled back to achieve the same response with a current >0.2 mA before injecting local anesthetic to avoid injection into the dural sleeves and consequent epidural or spinal spread. |
| *Horner syndrome* | • The occurrence of ipsilateral ptosis, hyperemia of the conjunctiva, and nasal congestion is common and depends on the site of injection (it is less common with the low interscalene approach) and the total volume of local anesthetic injected.<br>• The patient should be instructed about the occurrence of this syndrome and reassured about its benign nature. |
| *Diaphragmatic paralysis* | • Invariably present; avoid interscalene blockade or the use of a large volume of local anesthetic in patients who have severe chronic respiratory disease and use accessory respiratory muscles during breathing at rest. |

# INTERSCALENE BRACHIAL PLEXUS BLOCK: DECISION MAKING ALGORITHM

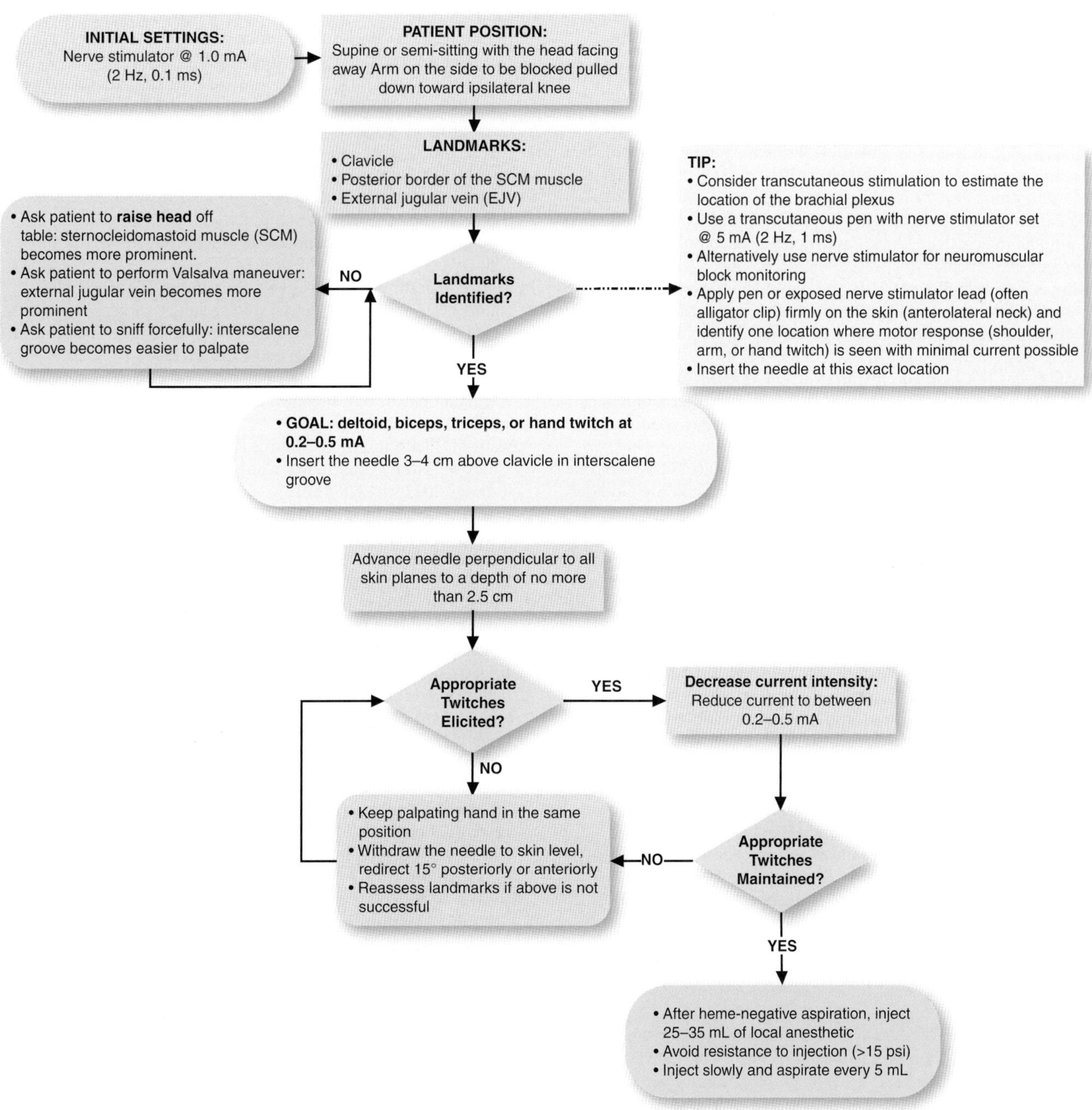

## SUGGESTED READINGS


Adam F, Menigaux C, Sessler DI, Chauvin M. A single preoperative dose of gabapentin (800 milligrams) does not augment postoperative analgesia in patients given interscalene brachial plexus blocks for arthroscopic shoulder surgery. *Anesth Analg.* 2006;103:1278-1282.

Agostoni M, Marchesi M, Fanelli G, Reineke R. Analgesic brachial plexus block for reduction of shoulder dislocation. *Reg Anesth.* 1996;21:373.

Aguirre J, Ekatodramis G, Ruland P, Borgeat A: Interscalene block should she a block for shoulder and proximal humerus sugery, and nothing else. *J Clin Anesth* 2010;22.

Alemanno F, Capozzoli G, Egarter-Vigl E, Gottin L, Alberto B. The middle interscalene block: cadaver study and clinical assessment. *Reg Anesth Pain Med.* 2006;31:563-568.

Altintas F, Gumus F, Kaya G, et al. Interscalene brachial plexus block with bupivacaine and ropivacaine in patients with chronic renal failure: diaphragmatic excursion and pulmonary function changes. *Anesth Analg.* 2005;100:1166-1171.

Arcas-Bellas JJ, Cassinello F, Cercos B, del Valle M, Leal V, Alvarez-Rementeria R. Delayed quadriparesis after an interscalene brachial plexus block and general anesthesia: a differential diagnosis. *Anesth Analg.* 2009;109:1341-1343.

Barak M, Iaroshevski D, Poppa E, Ben-Nun A, Katz Y. Low-volume interscalene brachial plexus block for post-thoracotomy shoulder pain. *J Cardiothorac Vasc Anesth.* 2007;21:554-557.

Baskan S, Taspinar V, Ozdogan L, Gulsoy KY, Erk G, Dikmen B, Gogus N: Comparison of 0.25% levobupivacaine and 0.25% bupivacaine for posterior approach interscalene brachial plexus block. *J Anesth* 2010;24:38-42.

Baskan S, Taspinar V, Ozdogan L, et al. Comparison of 0.25% levobupivacaine and 0.25% bupivacaine for posterior approach interscalene brachial plexus block. *J Anesth.* 2010;24:38-42.

Beaudet V, Williams SR, Tetreault P, Perrault MA. Perioperative interscalene block versus intra-articular injection of local anesthetics for postoperative analgesia in shoulder surgery. *Reg Anesth Pain Med.* 2008;33:134-138.

Benumof JL. Permanent loss of cervical spinal cord function associated with interscalene block performed under general anesthesia. *Anesthesiology.* 2000;93:1541-1544.

Bittar DA. Attempted interscalene block procedures. *Anesthesiology.* 2001;95:1303-1304.

Blumenthal S, Jutzi H, Borgeat A. Is the interscalene brachial plexus block the best approach? *Anesth Analg.* 2006;102: 652-653; author reply 653.

Blumenthal S, Nadig M, Borgeat A. Pectoralis major motor for interscalene block: what to do with it? *Reg Anesth Pain Med.* 2003;28:155.

Bollini CA, Urmey WF, Vascello L, Cacheiro F. Relationship between evoked motor response and sensory paresthesia in interscalene brachial plexus block. *Reg Anesth Pain Med.* 2003;28:384-388.

Borgeat A, Ekatodramis G, Blumenthal S. Interscalene brachial plexus anesthesia with ropivacaine 5 mg/mL and bupivacaine 5 mg/mL: effects on electrocardiogram. *Reg Anesth Pain Med.* 2004;29:557-563.

Borgeat A, Ekatodramis G, Gaertner E. Performing an interscalene block during general anesthesia must be the exception. *Anesthesiology.* 2001;95:1302-1303.

Borgeat A, Ekatodramis G, Kalberer F, Benz C. Acute and nonacute complications associated with interscalene block and shoulder surgery: a prospective study. *Anesthesiology.* 2001;95:875-880.

Borgeat A, Kalberer F, Jacob H, Ruetsch YA, Gerber C. Patient-controlled interscalene analgesia with ropivacaine 0.2% versus bupivacaine 0.15% after major open shoulder surgery: the effects on hand motor function. *Anesth Analg.* 2001;92:218-223.

Brown DL, Bridenbaugh LD. The upper extremity: somatic block. In: Cousins MJ, Bridenbaugh PO, eds. *Neuronal Blockade in Clinical Anesthesia and Management of Pain.* Philadelphia, PA: Lippincott-Raven; 1988:345-371.

Brull R, McCartney CJ, Chan VW, El-Beheiry H. Neurological complications after regional anesthesia: contemporary estimates of risk. *Anesth Analg.* 2007;104:965-974.

Brull R, Wijayatilake DS, Perlas A, et al. Practice patterns related to block selection, nerve localization and risk disclosure: a survey of the American Society of Regional Anesthesia and Pain Medicine. *Reg Anesth Pain Med.* 2008;33:395-403.

Candido KD, Sukhani R, Doty R Jr, et al. Neurologic sequelae after interscalene brachial plexus block for shoulder/upper arm surgery: the association of patient, anesthetic, and surgical factors to the incidence and clinical course. *Anesth Analg.* 2005;100:1489-1495.

Casati A, Borghi B, Fanelli G, et al. Interscalene brachial plexus anesthesia and analgesia for open shoulder surgery: a randomized, double-blinded comparison between levobupivacaine and ropivacaine. *Anesth Analg.* 2003;96:253-259.

Casati A, Chelly JE. Neurological complications after interscalene brachial plexus blockade: what to make of it? *Anesthesiology.* 2002;97:279-280.

Casutt M, Ekatodramis G, Maurer K, Borgeat A. Projected complex sensations after interscalene brachial plexus block. *Anesth Analg.* 2002;94:1270-1271.

Chelly JE, Greger J, Gebhard R, Casati A. How to prevent catastrophic complications when performing interscalene blocks. *Anesthesiology.* 2001;95:1302.

Choquet O, Jochum D, Estebe JP, Dupre LJ, Capdevila X. Motor response following paresthesia during interscalene block: methodological problems may lead to inappropriate conclusions. *Anesthesiology.* 2003;98:587-588.

Christ S, Rindfleisch F, Friederich P. Superficial cervical plexus neuropathy after single-injection interscalene brachial plexus block. *Anesth Analg.* 2009;109:2008-2011.

Cohen JM, Gray AT: Functional deficits after intraneural injection during interscalene block. *Reg Anesth Pain Med* 2010;35:397-399.

Coleman MM, Peng P. Pectorialis major in interscalene brachial plexus blockade. *Reg Anesth Pain Med.* 1999;24:190-191.

Crews JC, Rothman TE. Seizure after levobupivacaine for interscalene brachial plexus block. *Anesth Analg.* 2003;96: 1188-1190.

Culebras X, Van Gessel E, Hoffmeyer P, Gamulin Z. Clonidine combined with a long acting local anesthetic does not prolong postoperative analgesia after brachial plexus block but does induce hemodynamic changes. *Anesth Analg.* 2001;92: 199-204.

Delaunay L, Souron V, Lafosse L, Marret E, Toussaint B. Analgesia after arthroscopic rotator cuff repair: subacromial versus interscalene continuous infusion of ropivacaine. *Reg Anesth Pain Med.* 2005;30:117-122.

Devera HV, Furukawa KT, Scavone JA, Matson M, Tumber S. Interscalene blocks in anesthetized pediatric patients. *Reg Anesth Pain Med.* 2009;34:603-604.

Ekatodramis G, Borgeat A. The "interscalene triangular swelling": an early sign for successful interscalene brachial plexus block. *Reg Anesth Pain Med.* 2000;25:662-663.

Eroglu A, Uzunlar H, Sener M, Akinturk Y, Erciyes N. A clinical comparison of equal concentration and volume of ropivacaine and bupivacaine for interscalene brachial plexus anesthesia and analgesia in shoulder surgery. *Reg Anesth Pain Med.* 2004;29:539-543.

Faryniarz D, Morelli C, Coleman S, et al. Interscalene block anesthesia at an ambulatory surgery center performing predominantly regional anesthesia: a prospective study of one hundred thirty-three patients undergoing shoulder surgery. *J Shoulder Elbow Surg.* 2006;15:686-690.

Gadsden JC, Tsai T, Iwata T, Somasundarum L, Robards C, Hadžić A. Low interscalene block provides reliable anesthesia for surgery at or about the elbow. *J Clin Anesth.* 2009;21:98-102.

Ganesh A. Interscalene brachial plexus block-anatomic considerations. *Reg Anesth Pain Med.* 2009;34:525.

Hadžić A, Vloka JD, Claudio RE, Hadžić N, Thys DM, Santos AC. Electrical nerve localization: effects of cutaneous electrode placement and duration of the stimulus on motor response. *Anesthesiology.* 2004;100:1526-1530.

Hadžić A, Vloka JD, Kuroda MM, Koorn R, Birnbach DJ. The practice of peripheral nerve blocks in the United States: a national survey [p2e comments]. *Reg Anesth Pain Med.* 1998;23:241-246.

Hadžić A, Williams BA, Karaca PE, et al. For outpatient rotator cuff surgery, nerve block anesthesia provides superior same-day recovery over general anesthesia. *Anesthesiology.* 2005;102: 1001-1007.

Harrop-Griffiths W, Denny N. Is a deltoid twitch a satisfactory endpoint for all interscalene blocks? *Reg Anesth Pain Med.* 2001;26:182-183.

Hermanns H, Braun S, Werdehausen R, Werner A, Lipfert P, Stevens MF. Skin temperature after interscalene brachial plexus blockade. *Reg Anesth Pain Med.* 2007;32:481-487.

Hingorani AP, Ascher E, Gupta P, et al. Regional anesthesia: preferred technique for venodilatation in the creation of upper extremity arteriovenous fistulae. *Vascular.* 2006;14:23-26.

Homer JR, Davies JM, Amundsen LB. Persistent hiccups after attempted interscalene brachial plexus block. *Reg Anesth Pain Med.* 2005;30:574-576.

Ilfeld BM, Wright TW, Enneking FK, et al. Total shoulder arthroplasty as an outpatient procedure using ambulatory perineural local anesthetic infusion: a pilot feasibility study. *Anesth Analg.* 2005;101:1319-1322.

Iskandar H, Benard A, Ruel-Raymond J, Cochard G, Manaud B. The analgesic effect of interscalene block using clonidine as an analgesic for shoulder arthroscopy. *Anesth Analg.* 2003;96: 260-262.

Iskandar H, Wakim N, Benard A, et al. The effects of interscalene brachial plexus block on humeral arterial blood flow: a Doppler ultrasound study. *Anesth Analg.* 2005;101: 279-281.

Jafari S, Kalstein AI, Nasrullah HM, Hedayatnia M, Yarmush JM, SchianodiCola J. A randomized, prospective, double-blind trial comparing 3% chloroprocaine followed by 0.5% bupivacaine to 2% lidocaine followed by 0.5% bupivacaine for interscalene brachial plexus block. *Anesth Analg.* 2008;107:1746-1750.

Karaca P, Hadžić A, Yufa M, et al. Painful paresthesiae are infrequent during brachial plexus localization using low-current peripheral nerve stimulation. *Reg Anesth Pain Med.* 2003;28:380-383.

Kempen PM, O'Donnell J, Lawler R, Mantha V. Acute respiratory insufficiency during interscalene plexus block. *Anesth Analg.* 2000;90:1415-1416.

Klein SM, Nielsen KC, Martin A, et al. Interscalene brachial plexus block with continuous intraarticular infusion of ropivacaine. *Anesth Analg.* 2001;93:601-605.

Klein SM, Pietrobon R, Nielsen KC, Warner DS, Greengrass RA, Steele SM. Peripheral nerve blockade with long-acting local anesthetics: a survey of the Society for Ambulatory Anesthesia. *Anesth Analg.* 2002;94: 71-76.

Koorn R, Tenhundfeld Fear KM, Miller C, Boezaart A. The use of cervical paravertebral block as the sole anesthetic for shoulder surgery in a morbid patient: a case report. *Reg Anesth Pain Med.* 2004;29:227-229.

Krone SC, Chan VW, Regan J, et al. Analgesic effects of low-dose ropivacaine for interscalene brachial plexus block for outpatient shoulder surgery—a dose-finding study. *Reg Anesth Pain Med.* 2001;26:439-443.

Langen KE, Candido KD, King M, Marra G, Winnie AP. The effect of motor activity on the onset and progression of brachial plexus block with bupivacaine: a randomized prospective study in patients undergoing arthroscopic shoulder surgery. *Anesth Analg.* 2008;106:659-663.

Lierz P, Gustorff B, Felleiter P. Pain therapy with interscalene local anesthetic. *Anesth Analg.* 2001;93:1624.

Liguori GA, Zayas VM, YaDeau JT, et al. Nerve localization techniques for interscalene brachial plexus blockade: a prospective, randomized comparison of mechanical paresthesia versus electrical stimulation. *Anesth Analg.* 2006;103:761-767.

Long TR, Wass CT, Burkle CM. Perioperative interscalene blockade: an overview of its history and current clinical use. *J Clin Anesth.* 2002;14:546-556.

Marhofer P, Harrop-Griffiths W, Willschke H, Kirchmair L. Fifteen years of ultrasound guidance in regional anaesthesia: Part 2—recent developments in block techniques. *Br J Anaesth.* 2010;104:673-683.

Maurer K, Ekatodramis G, Rentsch K, Borgeat A. Interscalene and infraclavicular block for bilateral distal radius fracture. *Anesth Analg.* 2002;94:450-452.

Moayeri N, Bigeleisen PE, Groen GJ. Quantitative architecture of the brachial plexus and surrounding compartments, and their possible significance for plexus blocks. *Anesthesiology.* 2008;108:299-304.

Nadig M, Blumenthal S, Ekatodramis G, Borgeat A. Interscalene brachial plexus anesthesia and analgesia for open shoulder surgery: what about pharmacokinetics? *Anesth Analg.* 2003;97: 605-606.

Naik VN, Perlas A, Chandra DB, Chung DY, Chan VW. An assessment tool for brachial plexus regional anesthesia performance: establishing construct validity and reliability. *Reg Anesth Pain Med.* 2007;32:41-45.

Neal JM, McDonald SB, Larkin KL, Polissar NL. Suprascapular nerve block prolongs analgesia after nonarthroscopic shoulder surgery but does not improve outcome. *Anesth Analg.* 2003;96:982-986.

Orebaugh SL, Williams BA, Vallejo M, Kentor ML. Adverse outcomes associated with stimulator-based peripheral nerve blocks with versus without ultrasound visualization. *Reg Anesth Pain Med.* 2009;34:251-255.

Paqueron X, Gentili ME, Willer JC, Coriat P, Riou B. Time sequence of sensory changes after upper extremity block: swelling sensation is an early and accurate predictor of success. *Anesthesiology.* 2004;101:162-168.

Patel V, Hadzic A, Gadsden J, Gandhi K: An electrocardiopraph artifact caused by peripheral nerve stimulation during an interscalene brachial plexus nerve block. *Reg Anesth Pain Med* 2010; 35:118-9.

Raj PP. *Textbook of Regional Anesthesia.* London, UK: Churchill Livingstone; 2002.

Reuben SS. Interscalene block superior to general anesthesia. *Anesthesiology.* 2006;104:207.

Robaux S, Bouaziz H, Boisseau N, Raucoules-Aime M, Laxenaire MC. Persistent phrenic nerve paralysis following interscalene brachial plexus block. *Anesthesiology.* 2001;95:1519-1521.

Rose M, Ness TJ. Hypoxia following interscalene block. *Reg Anesth Pain Med.* 2002;27:94-96.

Sardesai AM, Patel R, Denny NM, et al. Interscalene brachial plexus block: can the risk of entering the spinal canal be reduced? A study of needle angles in volunteers undergoing magnetic resonance imaging. *Anesthesiology.* 2006;105:9-13.

Sciard D, Matuszczak M, Gebhard R, Kocieniewska D. Interscalene block-, sedation-, lateral positioning-, and hydralazine-induced hypotension: is it really prudent? *Anesthesiology.* 2002;97:280-281.

Sia S, Sarro F, Lepri A, Bartoli M. The effect of exogenous epinephrine on the incidence of hypotensive/bradycardic events during shoulder surgery in the sitting position during interscalene block. *Anesth Analg.* 2003;97:583-588.

Silverstein WB, Saiyed MU, Brown AR. Interscalene block with a nerve stimulator: a deltoid motor response is a satisfactory endpoint for successful block. *Reg Anesth Pain Med.* 2000;25: 356-359.

Singelyn FJ. Difficult insertion of interscalene brachial plexus catheter. *Anesth Analg.* 2001;92:1074.

Singelyn FJ, Lhotel L, Fabre B. Pain relief after arthroscopic shoulder surgery: a comparison of intraarticular analgesia, suprascapular nerve block, and interscalene brachial plexus block. *Anesth Analg.* 2004;99:589-592.

Sukhani R, Candido KD. Interscalene brachial plexus block: shoulder paresthesia versus deltoid motor response: revisiting the anatomy to settle the controversy. *Anesth Analg.* 2002;95:1818; author reply 1818-1819.

Tonidandel WL, Mayfield JB. Successful interscalene block with a nerve stimulator may also result after a pectoralis major motor response. *Reg Anesth Pain Med.* 2002;27:491-493.

Urmey WF. Interscalene block: the truth about twitches. *Reg Anesth Pain Med.* 2000;25:340-342.

Urmey WF. Is a deltoid twitch a satisfactory endpoint for all interscalene blocks? *Reg Anesth Pain Med.* 2001;26:183.

Urmey WF, Stanton J. Inability to consistently elicit a motor response following sensory paresthesia during interscalene block administration. *Anesthesiology.* 2002;96:552-554.

Walton JS, Folk JW, Friedman RJ, Dorman BH. Complete brachial plexus palsy after total shoulder arthroplasty done with interscalene block anesthesia. *Reg Anesth Pain Med.* 2000;25:318-321.

Weber SC, Parise CA, Jain R. Interscalene block superior to general anesthesia: a discussion of the conclusions regarding these two anesthesia techniques. *Anesthesiology.* 2006;104:208.

Whitaker EE, Edelman AL, Wilkens JH, Richman JM: Severe hypotension after interscalene block for outpatient shoulder surgery: a case report. *J Clin Anesth* 2010;22:132-134.

White JL. Catastrophic complications of interscalene nerve block. *Anesthesiology.* 2001;95:1301.

Winnie AP. Interscalene brachial plexus block. *Anesth Analg.* 1970;49:455-466.

Winnie AP. *Plexus Anesthesia, Perivascular Techniques of Brachial Plexus Block.* 2nd ed. Philadelphia, PA: Saunders; 1990.

Wong GY, Brown DL, Miller GM, Cahill DR. Defining the cross-sectional anatomy important to interscalene brachial plexus block with magnetic resonance imaging. *Reg Anesth Pain Med.* 1998;23:77-80.

Wurm WH, Concepcion M, Sternlicht A, et al. Preoperative interscalene block for elective shoulder surgery: loss of benefit over early postoperative block after patient discharge to home. *Anesth Analg.* 2003;97:1620-1626.

### Continuous Interscalene Brachial Plexus Block

Blumenthal S, Nadig M, Borgeat A. The analgesic effect of interscalene block using clonidine as an analgesic for shoulder arthroscopy: where is the catheter? *Anesth Analg.* 2003;97:928.

Borgeat A, Aguirre J, Curt A. Case scenario: neurologic complication after continuous interscalene block. *Anesthesiology.* 2010;112:742-745.

Borgeat A, Dullenkopf A, Ekatodramis G, Nagy L. Evaluation of the lateral modified approach for continuous interscalene block after shoulder surgery. *Anesthesiology.* 2003;99:436-442.

Borgeat A, Perschak H, Bird P, Hodler J, Gerber C. Patient-controlled interscalene analgesia with ropivacaine 0.2% versus patient-controlled intravenous analgesia after major shoulder surgery: effects on diaphragmatic and respiratory function. *Anesthesiology.* 2000;92:102-108.

Borgeat A, Aguirre J, Curt A: Case scenario: neurologic complication after continuous interscalene block. Anesthesiology 2010; 112: 742-5.

Capdevila X, Dadure C, Bringuier S, et al. Effect of patient-controlled perineural analgesia on rehabilitation and pain after ambulatory orthopedic surgery: a multicenter randomized trial. *Anesthesiology*. 2006;105:566-573.

Capdevila X, Jaber S, Pesonen P, Borgeat A, Eledjam JJ. Acute neck cellulitis and mediastinitis complicating a continuous interscalene block. *Anesth Analg.* 2008;107:1419-1421.

Chelly JE, Casati A, Fanelli G. *Continuous Peripheral Nerve Block Techniques: An Illustrated Guide.* London, UK: Mosby International; 2001.

Clendenen SR, Robards CB, Wang RD, Greengrass RA. Case report: continuous interscalene block associated with neck hematoma and postoperative sepsis. *Anesth Analg.* 2010;110:1236-1238.

Clendenen SR, Robards CB, Wang RD, Greengrass RA: Case report: continuous interscalene block associated with neck hematoma and postoperative sepsis. *Anesth Analg* 2010;110: 1236-1238.

Coleman MM, Chan VW. Continuous interscalene brachial plexus block. *Can J Anaesth.* 1999;46:209-214.

Despond O, Kohut GN. Broken interscalene brachial plexus catheter: surgical removal or not? *Anesth Analg.* 2010;110:643-644.

Dooley J, Fingerman M, Melton S, Klein SM: Contralateral local anesthetic spread from an outpatient interscalene catheter. *Can J Anaesth* 2010;10:936-939.

Ekatodramis G, Borgeat A, Huledal G, Jeppsson L, Westman L, Sjovall J. Continuous interscalene analgesia with ropivacaine 2 mg/ml after major shoulder surgery. *Anesthesiology.* 2003;98: 143-150.

Ekatodramis G, Macaire P, Borgeat A. Prolonged Horner syndrome due to neck hematoma after continuous interscalene block. *Anesthesiology*. 2001;95:801-803.

Faust A, Fournier R, Hagon O, Hoffmeyer P, Gamulin Z. Partial sensory and motor deficit of ipsilateral lower limb after continuous interscalene brachial plexus block. *Anesth Analg.* 2006;102:288-290.

Fredrickson MJ, Abeyeskera A, Price DJ, Wong AC: Patient-initiated mandatory boluses for ambulatory continuous interscalene analgesia: an effective strategy for optimizing analgesia and minimizing side-effects. *Br J Anaesth* 2011; 106:239-245.

Fredrickson MJ, Ball CM, Dalgleish AJ. Successful continuous interscalene analgesia for ambulatory shoulder surgery in a private practice setting. *Reg Anesth Pain Med.* 2008;33:122-128.

Fredrickson MJ, Ball CM, Dalgeish AJ: Analgesic effectiveness of a continuous versus single-injection intersclane block for minor arthroscopic shoulder surgery. *Reg Anesth Pain Med* 2010;35:28-33.

Fredrickson MJ, Ball CM, Dalgleish AJ: A prospective randomized comparison of ultrasound guidance versus neurotimulation for interscalene catheter placement. *Reg Anesth Pain Med* 2009;34: 590-594.

Hofmann-Kiefer K, Eiser T, Chappell D, Leuschner S, Conzen P, Schwender D. Does patient-controlled continuous interscalene block improve early functional rehabilitation after open shoulder surgery? *Anesth Analg.* 2008;106:991-996.

Horlocker TT, O'Driscoll SW, Dinapoli RP. Recurring brachial plexus neuropathy in a diabetic patient after shoulder surgery and continuous interscalene block. *Anesth Analg.* 2000;91:688-690.

Horlocker TT, Weiss WT, Olson CA. Whodunnit: the mysterious case of mediastinitis after continuous interscalene block. *Anesth Analg.* 2008;107:1095-1097.

Ilfeld BM, Enneking FK. A portable mechanical pump providing over four days of patient-controlled analgesia by perineural infusion at home. *Reg Anesth Pain Med.* 2002;27:100-104.

Ilfeld BM, Morey TE, Thannikary LJ, Wright TW, Enneking FK. Clonidine added to a continuous interscalene ropivacaine perineural infusion to improve postoperative analgesia: a randomized, double-blind, controlled study. *Anesth Analg.* 2005;100:1172-1178.

Ilfeld BM, Morey TE, Wright TW, Chidgey LK, Enneking FK. Continuous interscalene brachial plexus block for postoperative pain control at home: a randomized, double-blinded, placebo-controlled study. *Anesth Analg.* 2003;96:1089-1095.

Ilfeld BM, Morey TE, Wright TW, Chidgey LK, Enneking FK. Interscalene perineural ropivacaine infusion:a comparison of two dosing regimens for postoperative analgesia. *Reg Anesth Pain Med.* 2004;29:9-16.

Ilfeld BM, Vandenborne K, Duncan PW, et al. Ambulatory continuous interscalene nerve blocks decrease the time to discharge readiness after total shoulder arthroplasty: a randomized, triple-masked, placebo-controlled study. *Anesthesiology.* 2006;105:999-1007.

Ilfeld BM, Wright TW, Enneking FK, Morey TE. Joint range of motion after total shoulder arthroplasty with and without a continuous interscalene nerve block: a retrospective, case-control study. *Reg Anesth Pain Med.* 2005;30:429-433.

Klein SM, Grant SA, Greengrass RA, et al. Interscalene brachial plexus block with a continuous catheter insertion system and a disposable infusion pump. *Anesth Analg.* 2000;91:1473-1478.

Le LT, Loland VJ, Mariano ER, et al. Effects of local anesthetic concentration and dose on continuous interscalene nerve blocks: a dual-center, randomized, observer-masked, controlled study. *Reg Anesth Pain Med.* 2008;33:518-525.

Lehtipalo S, Koskinen LO, Johansson G, Kolmodin J, Biber B. Continuous interscalene brachial plexus block for postoperative analgesia following shoulder surgery. *Acta Anaesthesiol Scand.* 1999;43:258-264.

Macfarlane AJ, Brull R. Continuous interscalene block for open shoulder surgery. *Anesth Analg.* 2008;107:726.

Maurer K, Ekatodramis G, Hodler J, Rentsch K, Perschak H, Borgeat A. Bilateral continuous interscalene block of brachial plexus for analgesia after bilateral shoulder arthroplasty. *Anesthesiology*. 2002;96:762-764.

Pere P, Pitkanen M, Rosenberg PH, et al. Effect of continuous interscalene brachial plexus block on diaphragm motion and on ventilatory function. *Acta Anaesthesiol Scand.* 1992; 36:53-57.

Rawal N, Allvin R, Axelsson K, et al. Patient-controlled regional analgesia (PCRA) at home: controlled comparison between bupivacaine and ropivacaine brachial plexus analgesia. *Anesthesiology*. 2002;96:1290-1296.

Sandefo I, Bernard JM, Elstraete V, et al. Patient-controlled interscalene analgesia after shoulder surgery: catheter insertion by the posterior approach. *Anesth Analg.* 2005;100:1496-1498.

Sardesai AM, Chakrabarti AJ, Denny NM. Lower lobe collapse during continuous interscalene brachial plexus local anesthesia at home. *Reg Anesth Pain Med.* 2004;29:65-68.

Singelyn FJ, Seguy S, Gouverneur JM. Interscalene brachial plexus analgesia after open shoulder surgery: continuous versus patient-controlled infusion. *Anesth Analg.* 1999;89: 1216-1220.

Souron V, Reiland Y, Delaunay L. Pleural effusion and chest pain after continuous interscalene brachial plexus block. *Reg Anesth Pain Med.* 2003;28:535-538.

Souron V, Reiland Y, De Traverse A, Delaunay L, Lafosse L. Interpleural migration of an interscalene catheter. *Anesth Analg.* 2003;97:1200-1201.

Stevens MF, Werdehausen R, Golla E, et al. Does interscalene catheter placement with stimulating catheters improve postoperative pain or functional outcome after shoulder surgery? A prospective, randomized and double-blinded trial. *Anesth Analg.* 2007;104:442-447.

Vranken JH, van der Vegt MH, Zuurmond WW, Pijl AJ, Dzoljic M. Continuous brachial plexus block at the cervical level using a posterior approach in the management of neuropathic cancer pain. *Reg Anesth Pain Med.* 2001;26:572-575.

Wiegel M, Gottschaldt U, Hennebach R, Hirschberg T, Reske A. Complications and adverse effects associated with continuous peripheral nerve blocks in orthopedic patients. *Anesth Analg.* 2007;104:1578-1582.

# 13 Supraclavicular Brachial Plexus Block

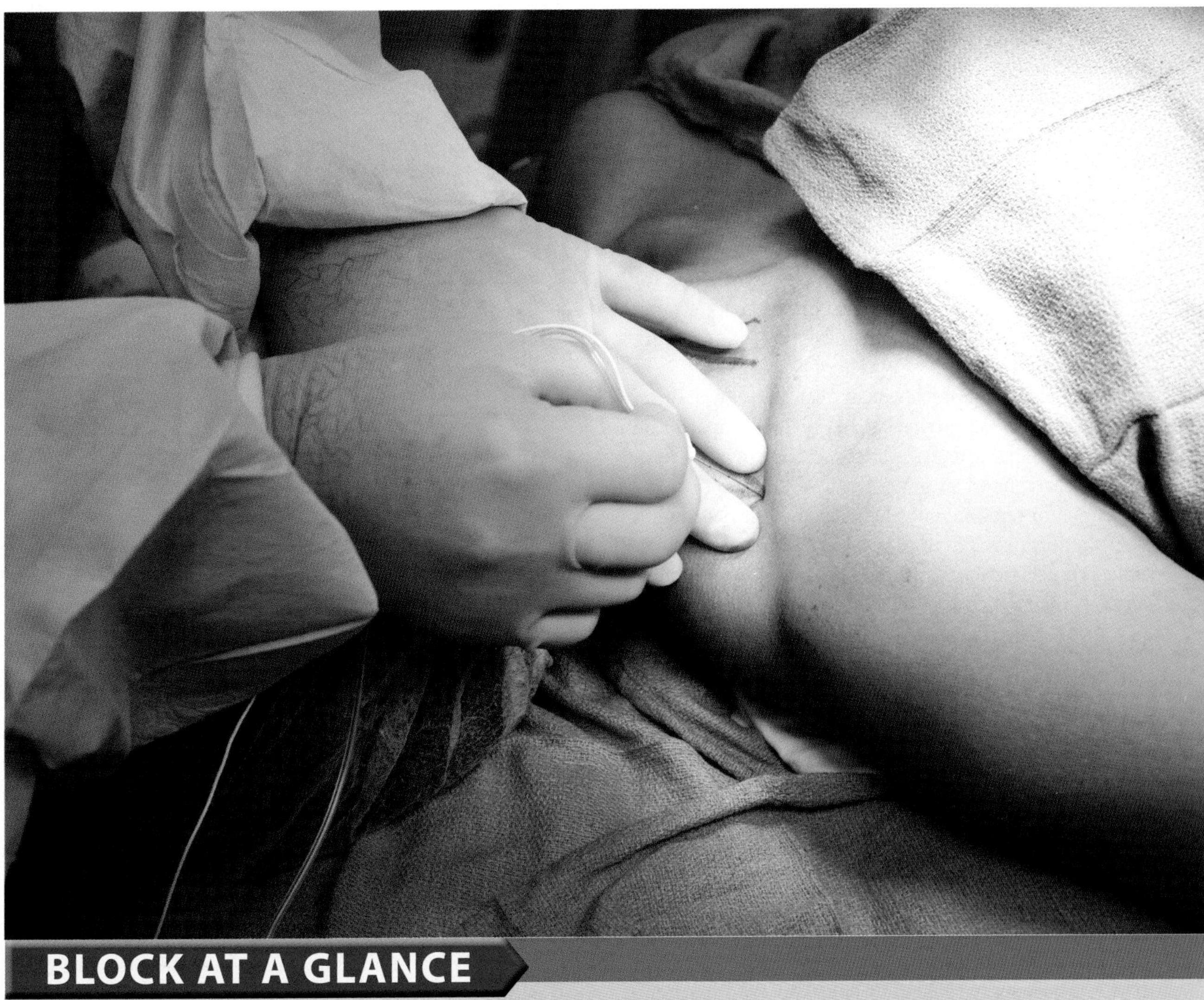

## BLOCK AT A GLANCE

- Indications: upper extremity surgery (arm, elbow, forearm, wrist, hand)
- Landmarks: the clavicular head of the sternocleidomastoid muscle
- Equipment:
  - A 5-cm, 22-gauge, short-bevel insulated needle
  - Peripheral nerve stimulator
- Local anesthetic: 25–35 mL

**FIGURE 13-1.** Insertion of the needle in the supraclavicular brachial plexus block. The needle is inserted lateral to the insertion of the clavicular head of the sternocleidomastoid muscle.

# Supraclavicular Block

## General Considerations

The supraclavicular approach to the brachial plexus characteristically is associated with a rapid onset of anesthesia and a high success rate. The first percutaneous supraclavicular block was performed by Kulenkampff in Germany in 1911, reportedly on himself. A few months after, Hirschel described a method of brachial plexus with an axillary approach. In 1928, Kulenkampff and Persky published their experiences with a thousand blocks without apparent major complications.

Kulenkampff's technique required the patient to be in the sitting position. The needle insertion was above the midpoint of the clavicle in the direction of the spinous process of T2 or T3. Unfortunately, this medial orientation of the needle was associated with a risk of pneumothorax, which eventually became the reason for the supraclavicular block to fall into disfavor in many centers. Since then, many modifications to the original technique were proposed to decrease the risk for pneumothorax. The technique described in this chapter takes into account the location of the dome of the pleura to reduce the risk for pneumothorax.

The advantages of a supraclavicular technique over other brachial plexus block approaches are its rapid onset and complete and predictable anesthesia for entire upper extremity and particularly, hand surgery. The introduction of ultrasound guidance to regional anesthesia in the last decade has resulted in significant renewed interest in the clinical application of the supraclavicular block, as well as a greater understanding of its mechanics.

## Functional Anatomy

The supraclavicular block is often called the "spinal anesthesia of the upper extremity" because of its ubiquitous application for upper extremity surgery. The reasons for its high success rate are in its anatomic characteristics. The block is performed at the level of the distal trunks and origin of the divisions, where the brachial plexus is confined to its smallest surface area (Figure 13-2A). The three trunks carry the entire sensory, motor, and sympathetic innervation of the upper extremity, with the exception of the uppermost part of the medial side of the arm (T2). The densely packed divisions, in contrast, carry a similar amount of innervation in a slightly larger surface area, but there is a larger surface of absorption. Another important anatomic feature of the supraclavicular block is the presence of the subclavian artery in front of the lower trunk and its divisions (Figure 13-2B). To increase the chance of blocking C8-T1 dermatomes it may be beneficial to insert the needle in the proximity of the lower trunk and make it the focal point of injection.

The sternocleidomastoid muscle inserts on the medial third of the clavicle, the trapezius inserts on the lateral third, and the neurovascular bundle passes underneath the middle third, which includes the midpoint of the clavicle. During a supraclavicular block, the pleura potentially can be breached either at the pleural dome (more likely) or through the first intercostal space.

A practical knowledge of the anatomical position of the pleura is important to decrease the risk of pneumothorax. The pleural dome is contained within the concavity of the first rib. Because the first rib crosses under the junction between the medial and middle thirds of the clavicle (Figure 13-3), its path coincides with the insertion of the sternocleidomastoid muscle, which inserts on the medial third of the clavicle. Therefore, the lateral insertion of the sternocleidomastoid muscle on the clavicle can be used as a landmark for the location of the first rib and of the lateral edge of the dome of the pleura. The first intercostal space, in contrast, is for the most part infraclavicular, and consequently it should not be reached during a supraclavicular block.

### TIPS

- With the shoulder pulled down, the entire brachial plexus is located above the clavicle, making it unnecessary to insert the needle below the clavicle.
- The first intercostal space is located below the clavicle for the most part; therefore, it is unlikely to be breached during a supraclavicular block that is performed *above* the clavicle, as its name implies.
- The dome of the pleura is contained within the concavity of the first rib. The crossing of the first rib under the clavicle coincides with the lateral insertion of the sternocleidomastoid into the clavicle; therefore, keeping the needle lateral to this sagittal plane should decrease the risk for pneumothorax.

## Distribution of Blockade

The supraclavicular block results in anesthesia of dermatomes C5 through T1, making it suitable for anesthesia or analgesia of the entire upper extremity distal to the shoulder, including the upper arm and elbow as well as the forearm, wrist, and hand.

## Equipment

- Antiseptic solution
- Two 20-mL syringes with desired local anesthetic solution
- A 3-mL syringe and a 27-gauge needle with local anesthetic for skin infiltration
- A 5-cm, 22-gauge, short bevel, insulated needle
- Peripheral nerve stimulator
- Marking pen and gloves

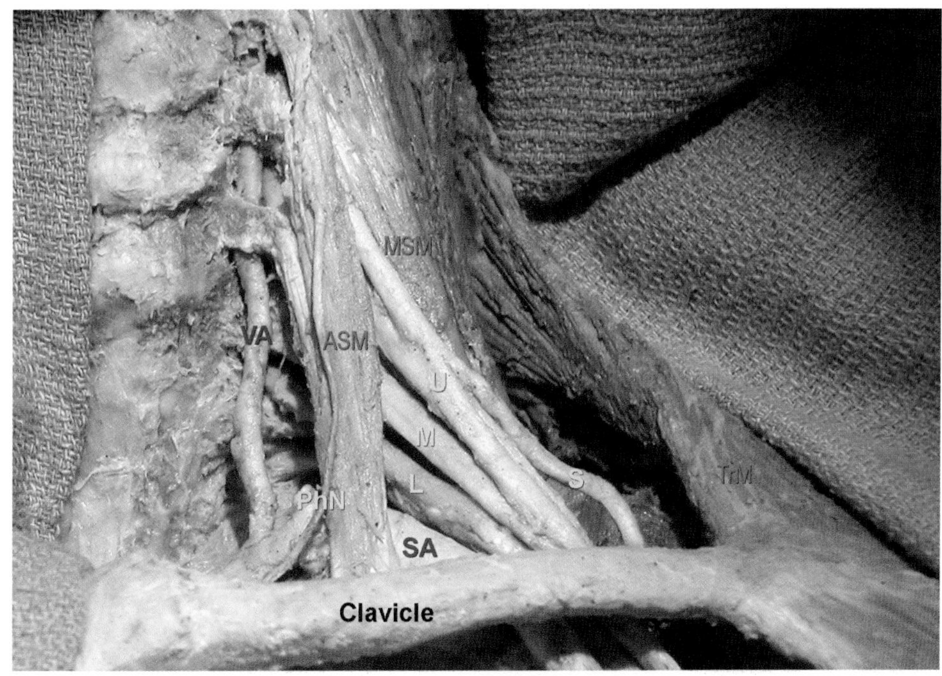


A

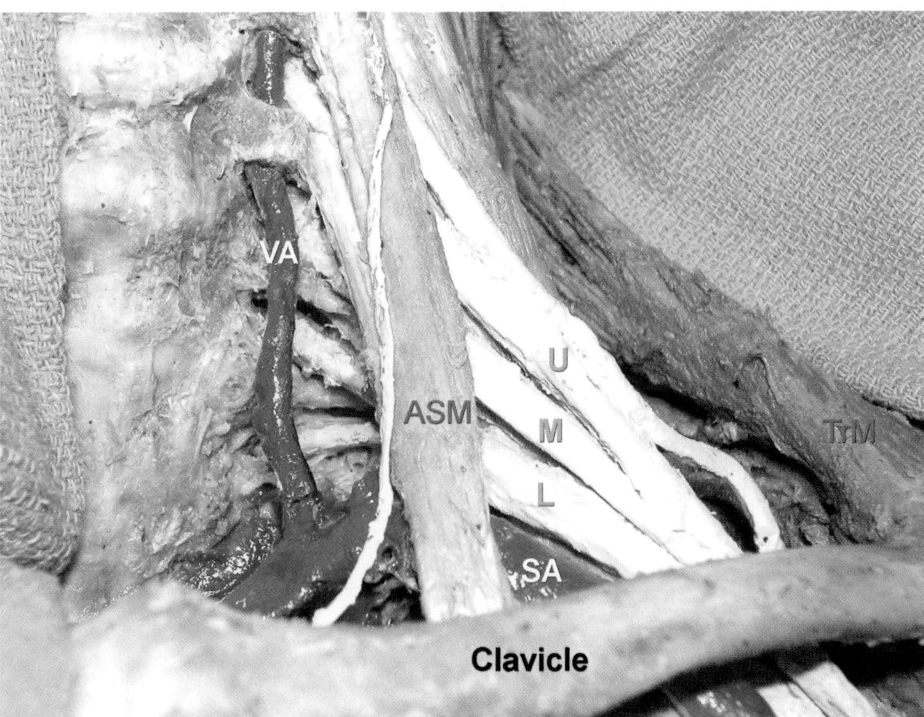


B

**FIGURE 13-2.** (A) Anatomy of brachial plexus about the clavicle. Shown are upper (U), middle (M), and lower (L) roots of the brachial plexus emerging between anterior (ASM) and middle (MSM) scalene muscles. Phrenic nerve (PhN) is shown descending on the anterior-medial surface of the anterior scalene muscle. Other shown anatomic details of importance are vertebral artery (VA), suprascapular nerve (S), trapezius muscle (TrM), and subclavian artery (SA). Note the intimate relationship of the brachial plexus trunks to the subclavian artery as they both pass underneath the clavicle. (B) Relationship of the arterial vasculature and the brachial plexus at the level above the clavicle.

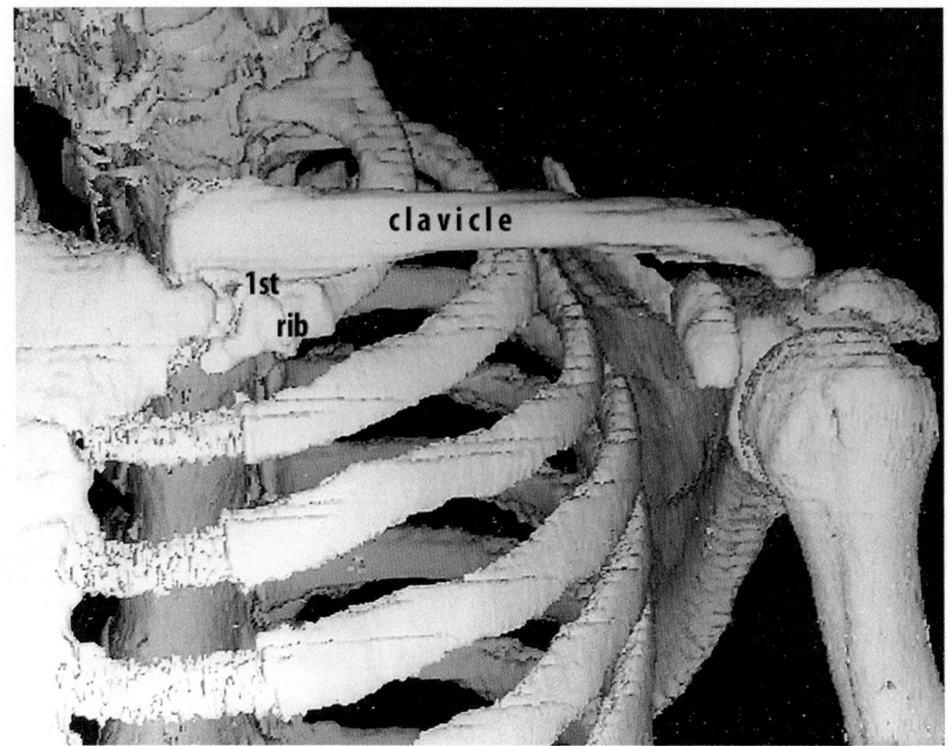


**FIGURE 13-3.** Radiocontrast image of the mixture of local anesthetic and radiopaque solution injected in the supraclavicular brachial plexus. The contrast is shown descending from the lower aspect of the clavicle toward the axillary fossa.

## Landmarks and Patient Positioning

The patient is placed in a semi-sitting position with the head rotated away from the site to be blocked and the shoulder pulled down. The arm rests comfortably on the side while the wrist, if possible, is supinated (Figure 13-4). The main landmarks for this block are the lateral insertion of the sternocleidomastoid muscle onto the clavicle and the clavicle itself.

Light premedication (e.g., midazolam 1 mg and fentanyl 50 μg IV repeated as necessary) is beneficial for patient comfort.

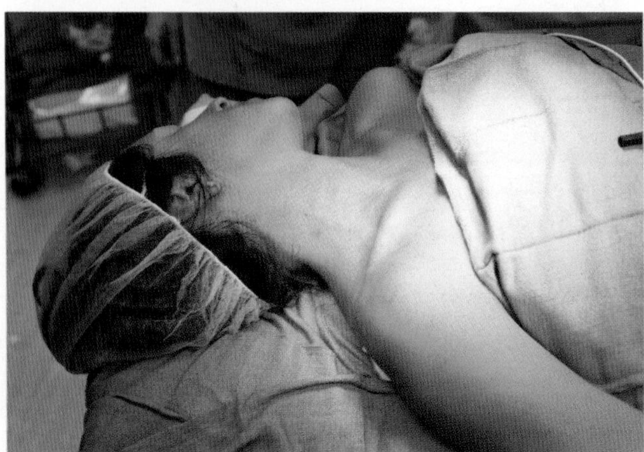

**FIGURE 13-4.** Patient position for the supraclavicular brachial plexus block.

## Maneuvers to Facilitate Landmarks Identification

To facilitate the recognition of the sternocleidomastoid muscle, the patient can be asked to elevate the head off the pillow, as shown in Figure 13-5. Once the sternocleidomastoid is identified, a mark is placed on the clavicle at its lateral insertion, as shown in Figure 13-6.

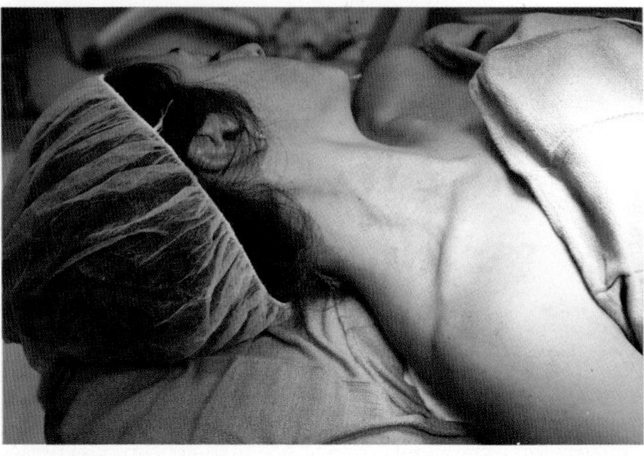

**FIGURE 13-5.** Sternocleidomastoid muscle can be accentuated by asking the patient to lift the head off of the table while glazing away from the side to be blocked.

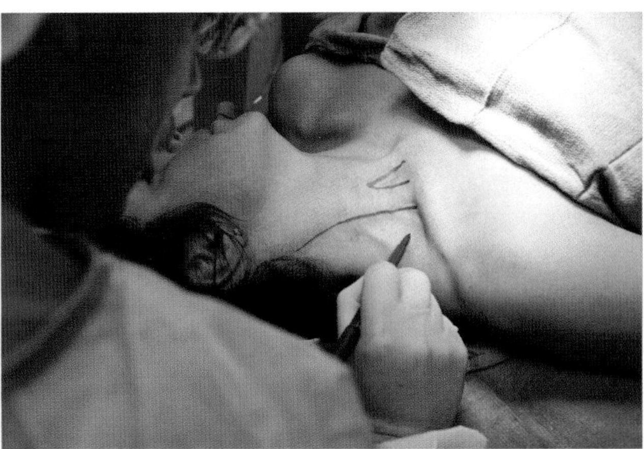

**FIGURE 13-6.** Outlining landmarks for supraclavicular brachial plexus block. Shown are the palpated contours of the sternal and clavicular heads of the sternocleidomastoid muscle.

## TIPS

- The lateral insertion of the sternocleidomastoid to the clavicle determines the most lateral boundary of the pleural dome.
- This point establishes a parasagittal plane, medial to which the needle should not cross to avoid placement of the needle toward the pleural dome.

## Technique

After identifying the lateral insertion of the sternocleidomastoid muscle on the clavicle, the operator locates the plexus by palpation, which in adults is found at about 2.5 cm lateral to the sternocleidomastoid. Once the plexus is found, the point of needle insertion is located immediately cephalad to the palpating finger, as shown in Figure 13-7.

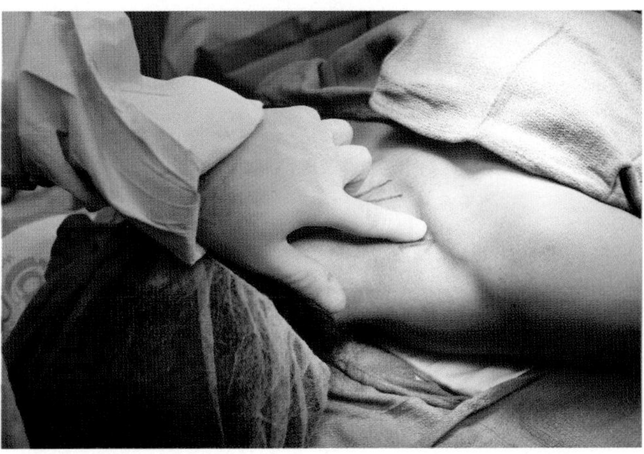

**FIGURE 13-7.** Insertion point for the supraclavicular brachial plexus block is outlined approximately 1–2 cm lateral to the insertion of the clavicular head of the sternocleidomastoid muscle.

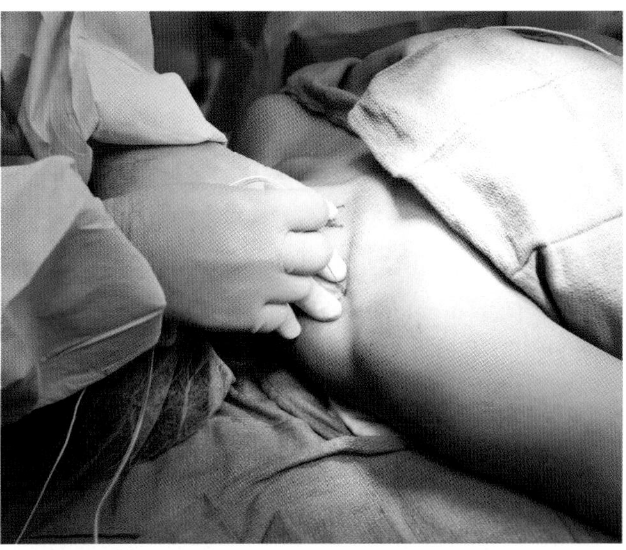

**FIGURE 13-8.** Insertion of the needle for the supraclavicular brachial plexus block.

The nerve stimulator is connected to the stimulating needle and set to deliver a 0.8 to 1.0 mA current at 1 Hz frequency and 0.1 ms of pulse duration.

The needle is inserted first in an anteroposterior direction, almost perpendicularly to the skin with a slight caudal orientation, as shown in Figure 13-1. The needle is slowly advanced until the upper trunk is identified by a muscle twitch of the shoulder muscles or up to 1 cm, if there is no response. At this point, the orientation of the needle is changed to advance it now caudally under the palpating finger, with a slight posterior angle, as shown in Figure 13-8. This strategy directs the needle from the vicinity of the upper trunk (shoulder twitch) to the front of the medial trunk (biceps, triceps, pectoralis twitch) on its way to the lower trunk (fingers twitch).

## GOAL

The goal of this block is to bring the tip of the needle in the proximity of the lower trunk, which is manifested by a twitch of the fingers in either flexion or extension.

Once the elicited motor response of the fingers is obtained at 0.5 mA, the injection is carried out after gentle aspiration. Injecting in the proximity of the lower trunk (motor response of the fingers) is the most important factor in accomplishing a successful supraclavicular brachial plexus block.

For surgical anesthesia, we commonly select 25 to 35 mL of 1.5% mepivacaine with 1:300,000 epinephrine, for a 3- to

4-hour duration of anesthesia and a variable, but usually short, duration of analgesia. We use a similar volume of 3% 2-chloroprocaine for a duration of 60 to 90 minutes of anesthesia for shorter cases. For analgesia, 20 mL of 0.2% ropivacaine with 1:300,000 epinephrine as an intravascular marker can be selected.

## Troubleshooting Maneuvers

- If the plexus is not found by palpation at 2.5 cm from the lateral insertion of the sternocleidomastoid:
  - Verify that the lateral insertion of the sternocleidomastoid on the clavicle is marked correctly. This insertion is usually vertical into the clavicle, and if an outward curve is noted, it is most likely part of the omohyoid muscle.
  - Palpate a few mm more medial or lateral than 2.5 cm.
- If the needle in its first perpendicular insertion does not make contact with the upper trunk:
  - Verify that the nerve stimulator connections and settings are correct.
- Failure to elicit a muscle twitch from the middle and lower trunks after eliciting a twitch from the upper trunk:
  - This usually means that the orientation plane of the needle, which is advancing caudally, does not match the frontal orientation plane of the trunks. Bring the needle back to the vicinity of the upper trunk (shoulder twitch) and increase the posterior orientation of the needle a few degrees.

## Contraindications

Supraclavicular block should not be done bilaterally because of the potential risk of respiratory compromise secondary to pneumothorax or phrenic nerve block. Although this recommendation seems logical, there is no evidence in the literature that bilateral supraclavicular block is actually contraindicated. Although phrenic nerve palsy may occur after approximately 50% of supraclavicular blocks, very few patients are symptomatic.

Regardless, performing the block in patients with chronic respiratory problems, especially those using accessory respiratory muscles, is a decision that must be made on a case-by-case basis because any choice of anesthesia, including general anesthesia, will have important implications in these patients.

### TIPS

- The risk of an intrafascicular injection can be minimized by using low injection pressures and overall meticulous technique.
- The injection is performed slowly with frequent aspirations while carefully observing the patient and the monitors for any change or sign of trouble.
- If pain or undue pressure is felt at any point during injection, the needle should be withdrawn 1 to 2 mm before a new attempt to inject is made.

# NERVE STIMULATOR-GUIDED SUPRACLAVICULAR BRACHIAL PLEXUS BLOCK: DECISION-MAKING ALGORITHM

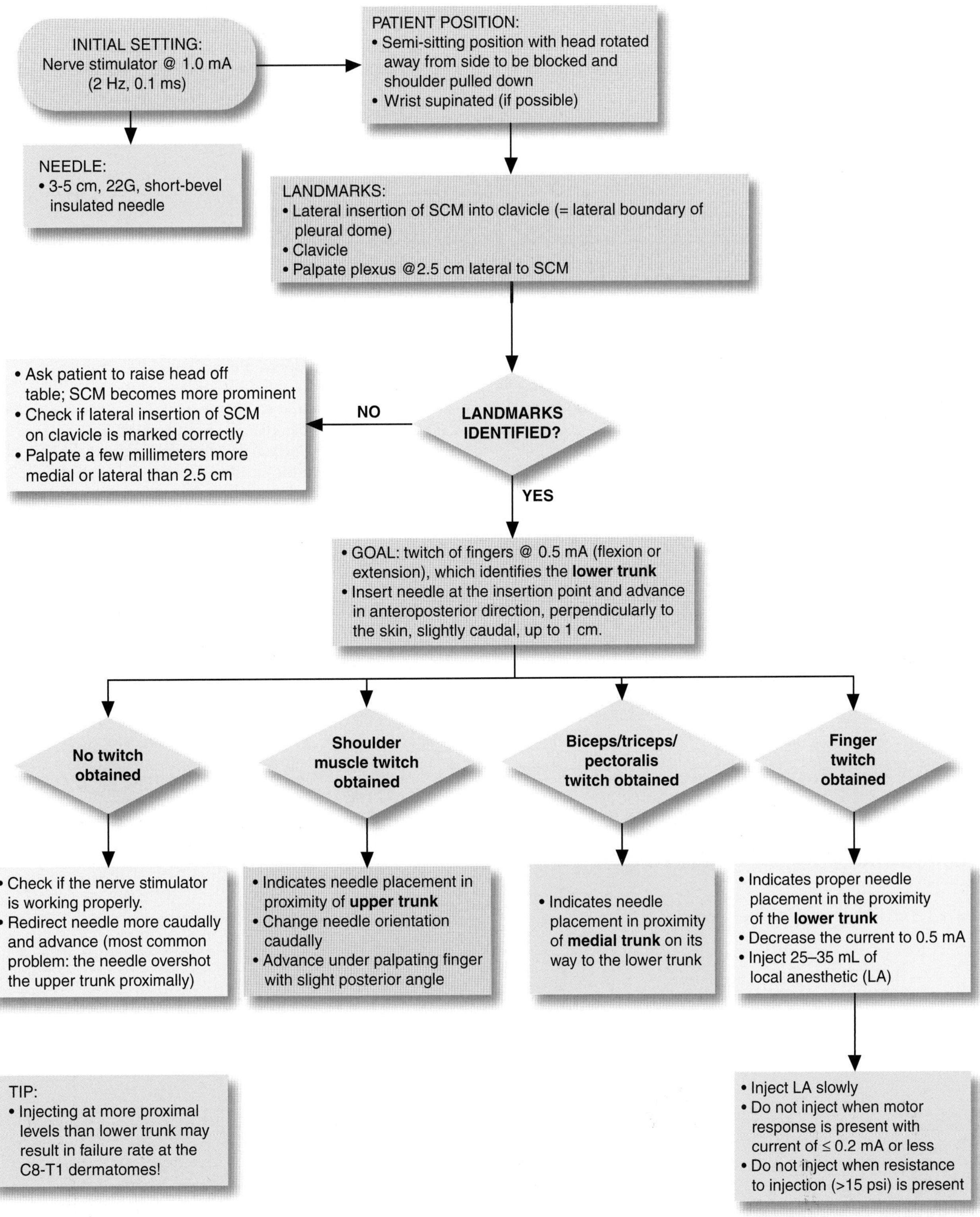

## SUGGESTED READING


Accardo N, Adriani J. Brachial plexus block: a simplified technique using the axillary route. *South Med J*. 1949;42:920.

Brand L, Papper E. A comparison of supraclavicular and axillary techniques for brachial plexus blocks. *Anesthesiology*. 1961;22:226-229.

Brown DL, Cahill D, Bridenbaugh D. Supraclavicular nerve block: anatomic analysis of a method to prevent pneumothorax. *Anesth Analg*. 1993;76:530-534.

Burnham P. Regional anesthesia of the great nerves of the upper arm. *Anesthesiology*. 1958;19:281-284.

De Jong R. Axillary block of the brachial plexus. *Anesthesiology*. 1961;22:215-225.

Franco C, Domashevich V, Voronov G, et al. The supraclavicular block with a nerve stimulator: to decrease or not to decrease, that is the question. *Anesth Analg*. 2004;98:1167-1171.

Franco C, Vieira Z. 1,001 subclavian perivascular brachial plexus blocks: success with a nerve stimulator. *Reg Anesth Pain Med*. 2000;25:41-46.

Franco CD. The subclavian perivascular block. *Tech Reg Anesth Pain Manage*. 1999;3:212-216.

Greengrass R, Steele S, Moretti G, et al. Peripheral nerve blocks. In: Raj P, ed. *Textbook of Regional Anesthesia*. New York, NY: Churchill Livingstone; 2002:325-377.

Harley N, Gjessing J. A critical assessment of supraclavicular brachial plexus block. *Anesthesia*. 1969;24:564-570.

Kulenkampff D, Persky M. Brachial plexus anesthesia. Its indications, technique and dangers. *Ann Surg*. 1928;87:883-891.

Labat G. *Regional Anesthesia—Its Techniques and Clinical Application*. Philadelphia, PA: Saunders; 1922.

Lanz E, Theiss D, Jankovic D. The extent of blockade following various techniques of brachial plexus block. *Anesth Analg*. 1983;62:55-58.

Moore D. Supraclavicular approach for block of the brachial plexus. In: Moore D, ed. *Regional Block. A Handbook for Use in the Clinical Practice of Medicine and Surgery*. 4th ed. Springfield, IL: Charles C Thomas; 1981:221-242.

Murphey D. Brachial plexus block anesthesia: an improved technique. *Ann Surg*. 1944;119:935-943.

Neal J, Moore J, Kopacz D, et al. Quantitative analysis of respiratory, motor, and sensory function after supraclavicular block. *Anesth Analg*. 1998;86:1239-1244.

Neal JM, Gerancher JC, Hebl JR, et al. Upper extremity regional anesthesia: essentials of our current understanding. *Reg Anesth Pain Med*. 2009;34:134-70.

Patrick J. The technique of brachial plexus block anesthesia. *Br J Surg*.1940;27:734-739.

Urmey W. Upper extremity blocks. In: Brown D, ed. *Regional Anesthesia and Analgesia*. Philadelphia, PA: Saunders; 1996:254-278.

Winnie A. *Plexus Anesthesia. Perivascular Techniques of Brachial Plexus Block*. Philadelphia, PA: Saunders; 1993.

Winnie A, Collins V. The subclavian perivascular technique of brachial plexus anesthesia. *Anesthesiology*. 1964;25:353-363.

# 14 Infraclavicular Brachial Plexus Block

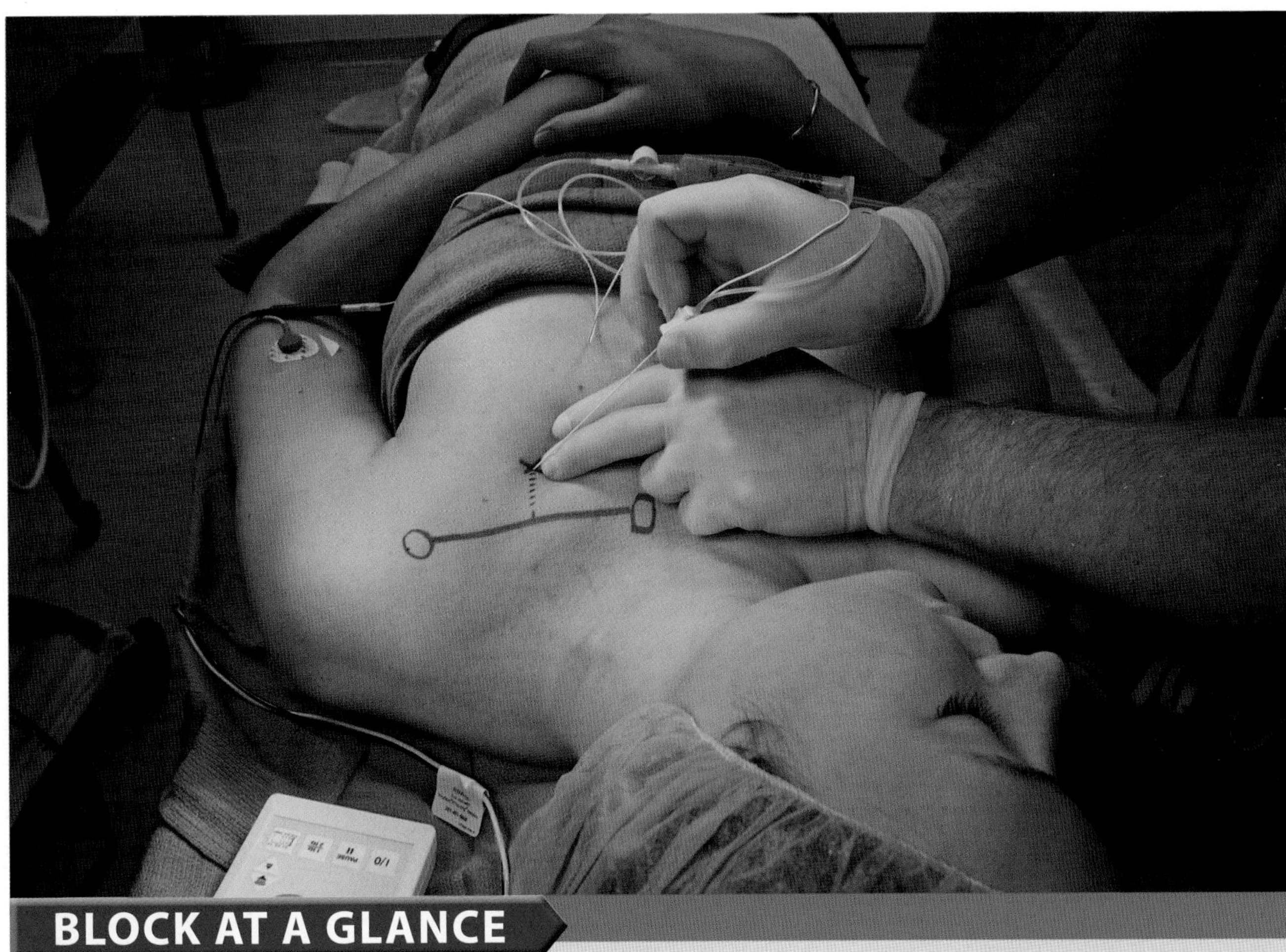

## BLOCK AT A GLANCE

- Indications: elbow, forearm, hand surgery
- Landmarks: medial clavicular head, coracoid process
- Nerve stimulation: hand twitch at 0.2–0.5 mA
- Local anesthetic: 25–35 mL

**FIGURE 14-1.** Patient position and needle insertion for infraclavicular brachial plexus block.

## General Considerations

The infraclavicular block is a method of accomplishing brachial plexus anesthesia below the level of the clavicle. Experience with basic brachial plexus techniques and understanding of the anatomy of the infraclavicular fossa and axilla is necessary for its safe and efficient implementation. This block is well suited for hand, wrist, elbow, and distal arm surgery. It also provides excellent analgesia for an arm tourniquet. Infraclavicular block is functionally similar to supraclavicular block, therefore the two techniques are often used interchangeably, depending on whether the patient's anatomy is more conducive to one or the other.

### Functional Anatomy

The infraclavicular block is performed below the clavicle, where the axillary vessels and the cords of the brachial plexus lie deep to the pectoralis muscles, just inferior and slightly medial to the coracoid process. The boundaries of the space are the pectoralis minor and major muscles anteriorly, ribs medially, clavicle and the coracoid process superiorly, and humerus laterally. The connective tissue sheath surrounding the plexus also contains the axillary artery and vein. Axillary and musculocutaneous nerves may leave the common tissue sheath at or before the coracoid process in 50% of patients (Table 14-1 and Figure 14-2). Consequently, deltoid and biceps twitches should not be accepted as reliable signs of infraclavicular brachial plexus identification.

| TABLE 14-1 | Distribution of the Branches of the Brachial Plexus |
|---|---|
| ***Chest*** | • Medial and lateral pectoral nerves (motor to pectoralis muscles) |
| ***Shoulder*** | • Subscapular nerves (motor to subscapularis and teres major)<br>• Axillary |
| ***Arm, forearm, shoulder, hand*** | • Musculocutaneous<br>• Medial cutaneous nerve of the arm<br>• Medial cutaneous nerve of the forearm<br>• Median<br>• Ulnar<br>• Radial |

The important anatomic structures are exposed in Figure 14-3.

### Distribution of Anesthesia/Analgesia

The typical distribution of anesthesia following an infraclavicular brachial plexus block includes the hand, wrist, forearm, elbow, and distal arm (Figure 14-4). The skin of the axilla and proximal medial arm (unshaded areas) are not anesthetized (intercostobrachial nerve).

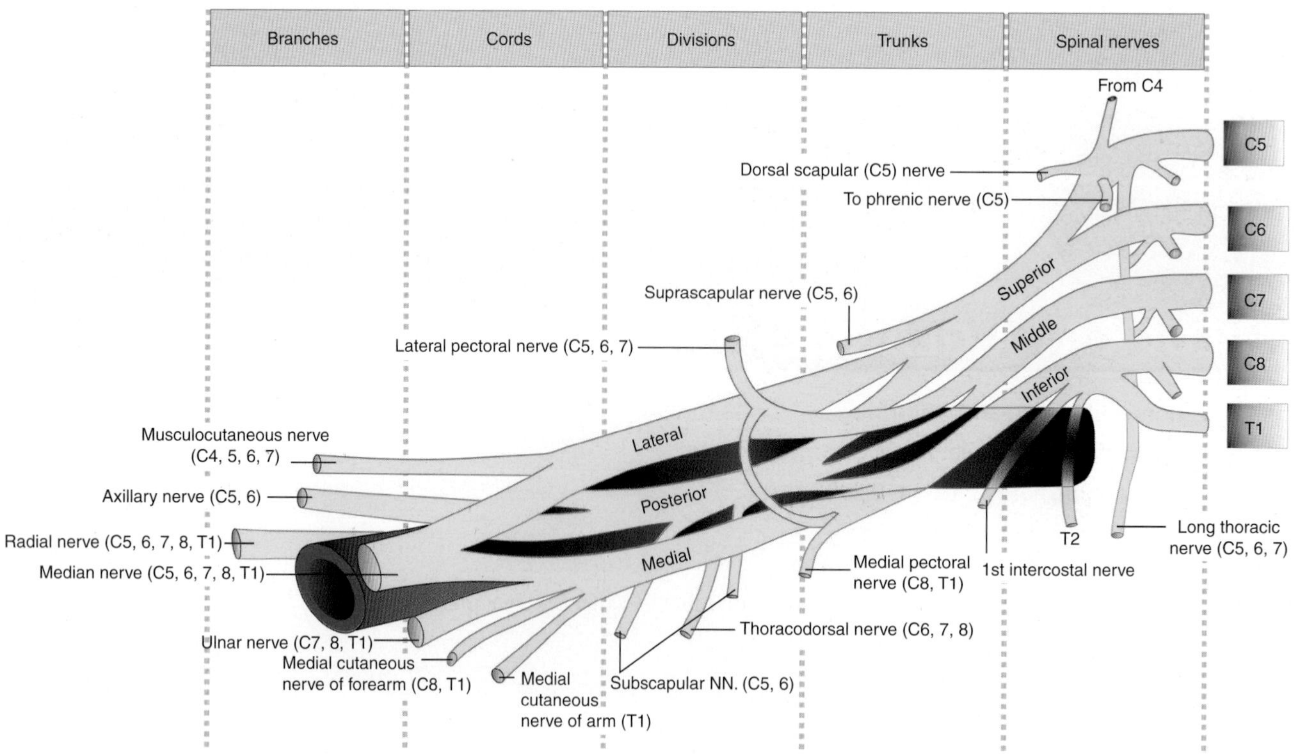


**FIGURE 14-2.** Functional organization of the brachial plexus into trunks, divisions, and cords.

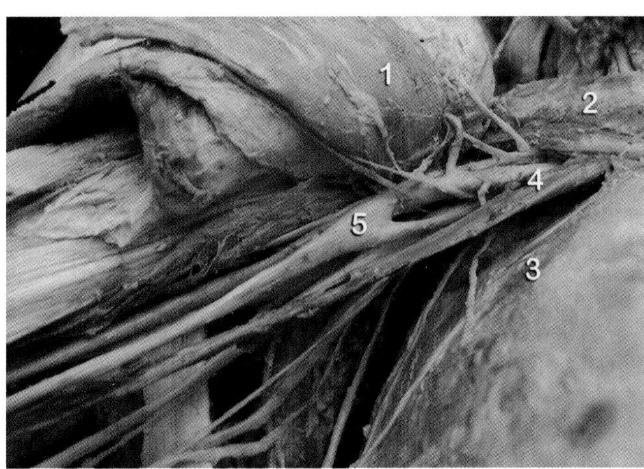


**FIGURE 14-3.** Anatomy of the infraclavicular fossa. Shown are retracted pectoralis muscles (1), clavicle (2), chest wall (3), axillary (subclavian) artery and vein (4) and brachial plexus "wrapped" around the artery (5).

## Single-Injection Infraclavicular Block

### Equipment

A standard regional anesthesia tray is prepared with the following equipment:

- Sterile towels and gauze packs
- 2 × 20-mL syringes containing local anesthetic
- 3 mL syringe + 25-gauge needle with local anesthetic for skin infiltration
- 10-cm, 21-gauge short-bevel insulated stimulating needle
- Peripheral nerve stimulator
- Sterile gloves; marking pen

### Landmarks and Patient Positioning

The patient is in the supine position with the head facing away from the side to be blocked. The anesthesiologist also stands opposite the side to be blocked to assume an ergonomic position during the block performance. It may be beneficial to keep the patient's arm abducted and flexed at

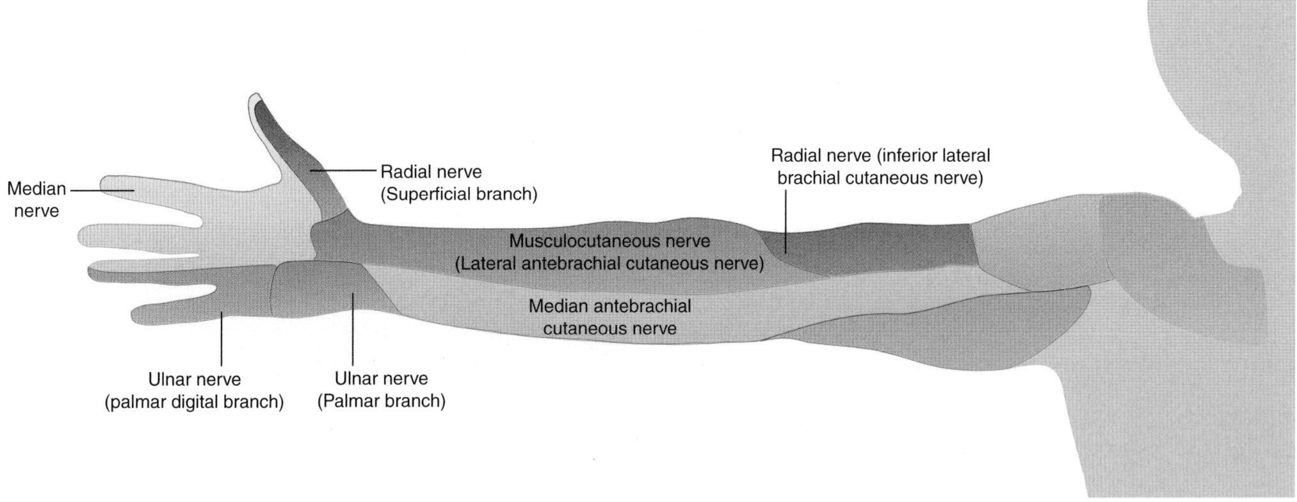


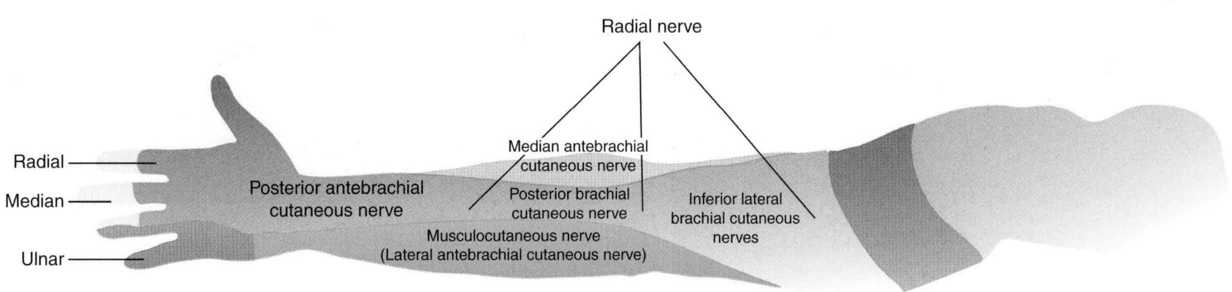


**FIGURE 14-4.** Distribution of sensory blockade with infraclavicular brachial plexus block.

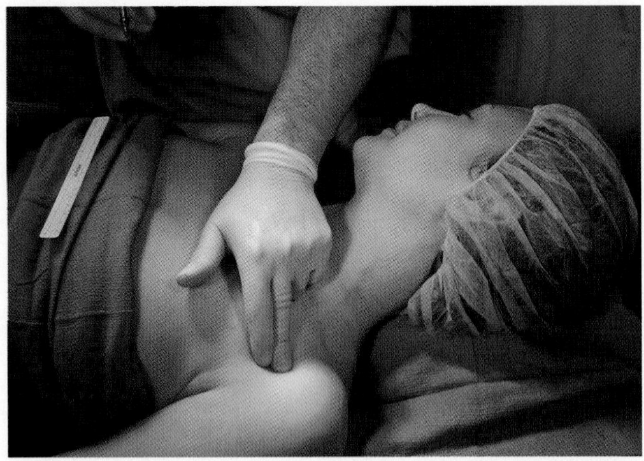

**FIGURE 14-5.** Technique of palpation of the coracoid process.

the elbow to keep the relationship of the landmarks to the brachial plexus constant. After a certain level of comfort with the technique is reached, the arm can be in any position during the block performance. The arm should be supported at the wrist to allow a clear, unobstructed view and interpretation of twitches of the hand.

The following landmarks are useful in estimating the site for an infraclavicular block:

1. Coracoid process (Figure 14-5)
2. Medial clavicular head (Figure 14-6)
3. Midpoint of line connecting landmarks 1 and 2.

The needle insertion site is marked approximately 3 cm caudal to the midpoint of landmark 3 (Figure 14-7).

An X-ray film demonstrates the relevant anatomy (Figure 14-8):

1. Coracoid process
2. Clavicle
3. Humerus
4. Scapula
5. Rib cage.

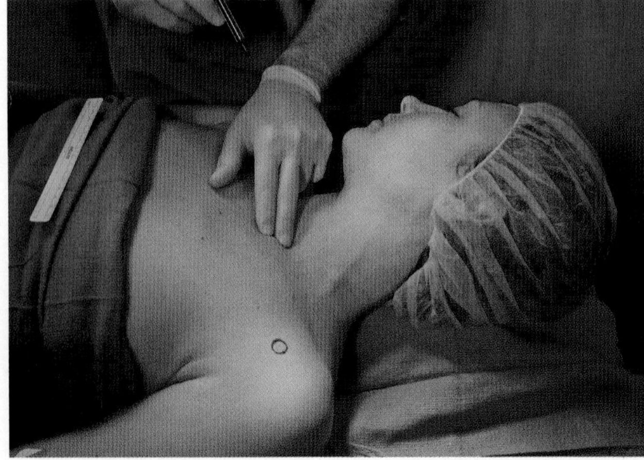

**FIGURE 14-6.** Palpation of the medial head of the clavicle. The circle outlines the coracoid process.

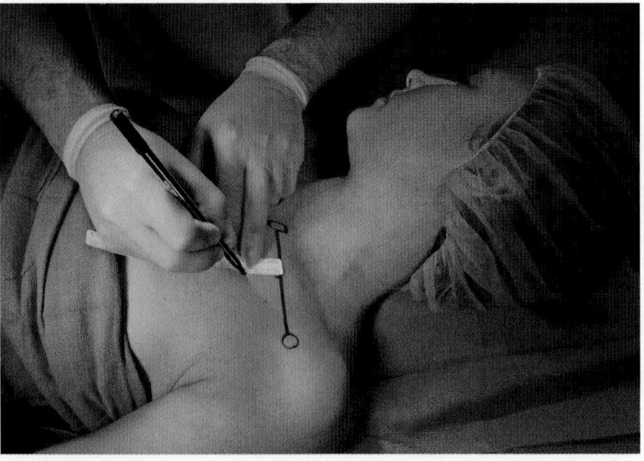

**FIGURE 14-7.** Needle insertion point for infraclavicular brachial plexus block. The medial and lateral circles outline the sternal head of the clavicle and coracoid process, respectively.

## TIPS

- The coracoid process can be identified by palpating the bony prominence just medial to the shoulder while the arm is elevated and lowered.
- As the arm is lowered, the coracoid process meets the fingers of the palpating hand.

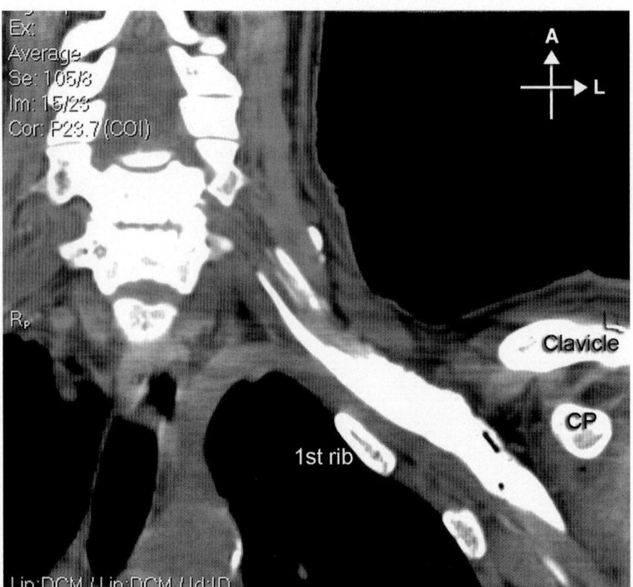


**FIGURE 14-8.** Osseous prominences of significance to infraclavicular brachial plexus block and relationship to the chest wall. Shown also is distribution of the local anesthetic underneath the clavicle after injection of the contrast-containing local anesthetic.

## Technique

The needle insertion site is infiltrated with local anesthetic using a 25-gauge needle. Local anesthetic should also be infiltrated deeper into the pectoralis muscle to decrease discomfort during needle insertion through the muscle layers.

A 10-cm, 21-gauge insulated needle, attached to a nerve stimulator, is inserted at a 45° angle to the skin and advanced parallel to the line connecting the medial clavicular head with the coracoid process (Fig. 14-1). The nerve stimulator is initially set to deliver 1.5 mA. A local twitch of the pectoralis muscle is typically elicited as the needle is advanced beyond the subcutaneous tissue. Once these twitches disappear, the needle advancement should be slow and methodical while the patient is observed for motor responses of the brachial plexus.

### TIPS

- When the pectoralis muscle twitch is absent despite an appropriately deep needle insertion, the landmarks should be checked because the needle has most likely been inserted too cranially (underneath the clavicle).
- Twitches from the biceps or deltoid muscles should not be accepted because the musculocutaneous or axillary nerve may exit the brachial plexus sheath before the coracoid process. Injection of local anesthetic outside the sheath would result in a weak block of slow onset.
- Hand stabilization and precision are crucial in this block because the tissue sheath separating the brachial plexus from the pectoralis minor muscle is thin at this location. Small movements of the needle may result in injection of local anesthetic outside the sheath and within the muscle.
- After the twitches of the pectoralis muscle cease, the stimulating current should be lowered to <1.0 mA to decrease patient discomfort. The needle is then slowly advanced or withdrawn until hand twitches are obtained at 0.2 to 0.5 mA.
- The success rate with this block decreases when local anesthetic is injected after obtaining stimulation with a current intensity >0.5 mA.

### GOAL

The goal is to achieve a hand twitch (ideally finger extension) using a current of 0.2 to 0.5 mA.

When insertion of the needle does not result in brachial plexus stimulation, the following maneuvers should be undertaken:

1. Keep the palpating hand in the same position, with the palpating finger firmly seated in the pectoralis and the skin between the fingers stretched (Figure 14-9A).
2. Withdraw the needle to skin level, redirect it 10° cephalad, and repeat the procedure (Figure 14-9B).
3. Withdraw the needle from the skin, redirect it 10° caudal, and repeat the procedure (Figure 14-9C).

If these maneuvers fail to result in a motor response, withdraw the needle and reassess the landmarks. Assure that the nerve stimulator is properly connected and delivering the set stimulus. Insert the needle 2 cm laterally and repeat the preceding steps.

## Troubleshooting

Table 14-2 lists some common responses to nerve stimulation and the course of action needed to obtain the proper response.

## Block Dynamics and Perioperative Management

Adequate sedation and analgesia are crucial during nerve localization to ensure patient comfort and to facilitate the interpretation of responses to nerve stimulation. For instance, midazolam 2 to 6 mg intravenously (IV) can be used to achieve sedation. Because the needle passage through the pectoralis muscle is moderately painful, a short-acting narcotic (e.g., alfentanil 250–750 μg) is added just before needle insertion. A typical onset time for this block is 15 to 20 minutes, depending on the local anesthetic chosen. Waiting beyond 20 minutes will not result in further enhancement of the blockade. The first sign of an impending successful blockade is loss of muscle coordination within minutes after the injection. This loss can be easily tested by asking the patient to touch the nose, paying close attention that they do not injure an eye. The loss of motor coordination typically occurs before sensory blockade can be documented. In case of inadequate skin anesthesia, despite the apparently timely onset of the blockade, local infiltration by the surgeon at the site of the incision is often all that is needed to allow the surgery to proceed.

## Continuous Infraclavicular Block

A continuous infraclavicular block is an advanced regional anesthesia technique, and adequate experience with the single-injection technique is necessary for its safe,

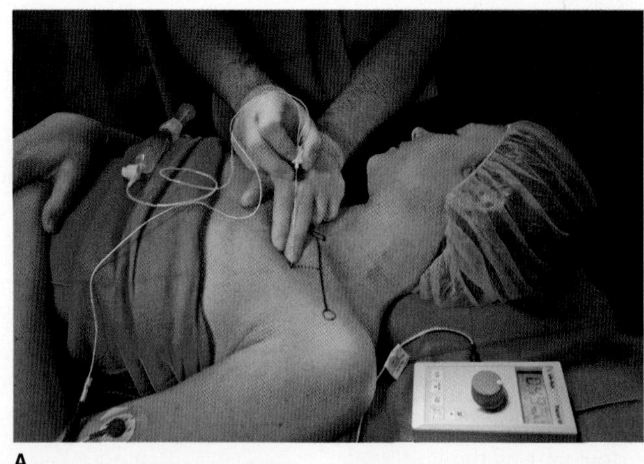

A

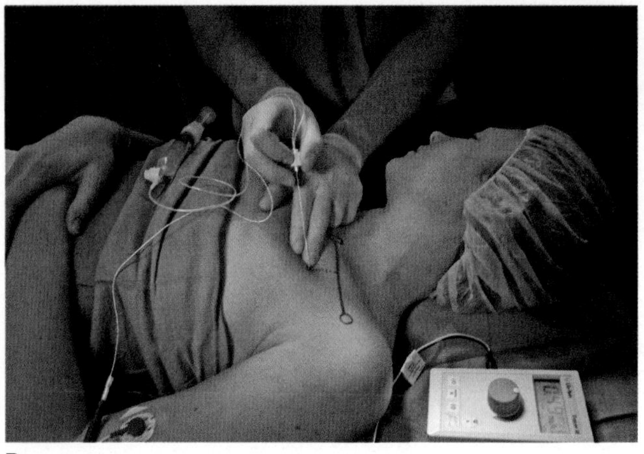

B

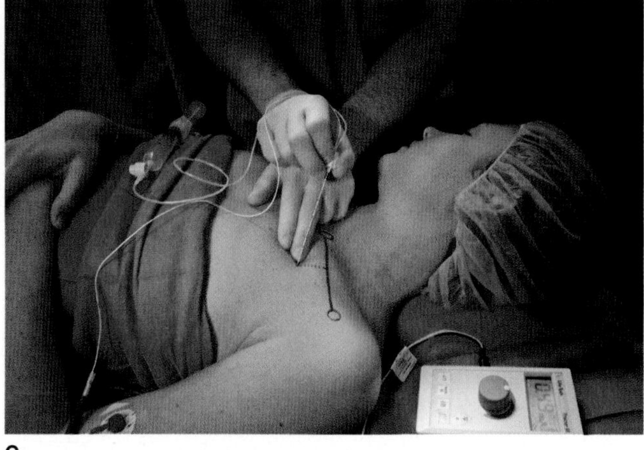

C

**FIGURE 14-9.** (A) Maneuvers to obtain motor response when it is not obtained on the first needle pass. The needle is withdrawn back to the skin and reinserted (B) cephalad or (C) caudad to obtain the motor response of the hand.

**TABLE 14-2 Common Problems During Nerve Localizations and Corrective Actions**

| STIMULATION | MOTOR RESPONSE | EXPLANATION | ACTION |
|---|---|---|---|
| Pectoralis muscle, direct muscle stimulation | Arm adduction | Too shallow a placement of needle | Continue advancing the needle |
| Subscapularis muscle | Local twitch resembling latissimus twitch | Too deep a placement of needle | Withdraw the needle to skin level and reinsert in another direction (superior or inferior) |
| Axillary nerve | Deltoid muscle | Needle placed too inferiorly | Withdraw the needle to skin level and reinsert with a superior orientation |
| Musculocutaneous nerve | Biceps twitch | Needle placed too superiorly | Withdraw the needle to skin level and reinsert with a light caudal orientation |

successful implementation. The use of a catheter significantly increases the utility of an infraclavicular block. The brachial plexus is encountered at a relatively deep location, which decreases the chance of inadvertent catheter dislodgment. Additionally, the catheter insertion site is easily approached for maintenance and inspection. This technique can be used for surgery on the hand, wrist, elbow, or distal arm and for surgery at the same anatomic location requiring prolonged postoperative pain management, repeated procedures (e.g., debridement) or a sympathetic block.

## Equipment

A standard regional anesthesia tray is prepared with the following equipment:

- Sterile towels and gauze packs
- Two 20-mL syringes containing local anesthetic
- Sterile gloves, marking pen, and surface electrode
- 3-mL syringe + 25-gauge needle with local anesthetic for skin infiltration
- Peripheral nerve stimulator
- Catheter kit (including a 17-18 cm gauge stimulating needle and catheter)

The block technique is very similar to that in the single-injection block. The brachial plexus localization is begun with a current of 1.5 mA, similarly to the single-injection technique. Once the motor response of the hand is obtained with a current of 0.5 mA, 5 to 10 mL of local anesthetic is injected and the catheter is inserted approximately 3 to 5 cm is beyond the tip of the needle. When the stimulating catheter is used, solution of dextrose in water (D5W) is used instead to allow electrolocation through the catheter. The needle is then withdrawn, the catheter secured, and the remaining volume of the planned dose of the local injected via the catheter. When a stimulating catheter is used, the catheter is manipulated with the nerve stimulator connected until the desired motor response is obtained with <1.0 mA.

## Landmarks and Patient Positioning

The patient is in the same position as for the single-injection technique (Fig. 14-1). However, the anesthesiologist must be in an ergonomic position to allow for maneuvering during catheter insertion. It is also important that all the equipment, including the catheter, be immediately available and prepared in advance because small movements of the needle while trying to prepare the catheter may result in dislodging the needle from its position in the brachial plexus sheath.

### *Maneuvers to Facilitate Landmark Identification*

The landmarks are the same as for the single-injection technique:

1. Medial clavicular head
2. Coracoid process
3. Midpoint of line connecting landmarks 1 and 2.

Elevating and raising the arm while palpating for the bony prominence of the coracoid process determines the exact location of the coracoid process. The point of needle insertion is labeled 3 cm caudal to the midpoint between the medial clavicular head and the coracoid process.

**TIPS**

- Inserting the needle too medially should be carefully avoided, as well as advancing the needle at too steep an angle, which carries a risk of pneumothorax.
- With proper technique, the risk of pneumothorax is almost negligible.

## Technique

The skin and subcutaneous tissue at the projected site of needle insertion is anesthetized with local anesthetic. Local infiltration of the skin, subcutaneous tissue, and the pectoralis muscles makes the procedure more comfortable for the patient. The block needle is then attached to the nerve stimulator (1.5 mA, 2 Hz). The fingers of the palpating hand should be firmly positioned on the pectoralis muscle and the needle inserted at a 45° angle to the horizontal plane and approximately parallel to the medial clavicular head–coracoid process line (Figure 14-10). As the needle is

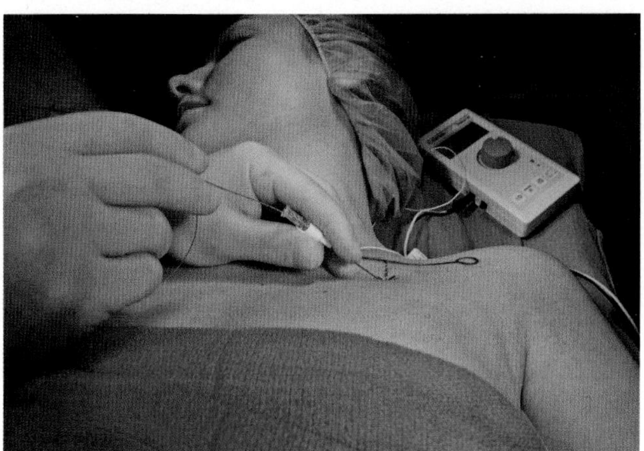

**FIGURE 14-10.** Needle position and catheter insertion in continuous infraclavicular block.

advanced beyond the subcutaneous tissue, direct stimulation of the pectoralis muscle is obtained as the needle passes through the muscle. Stimulation of the brachial plexus is encountered after the pectoralis muscle twitches cease. The desired response is that of the posterior cord, indicated by extension of the wrist and fingers at a current of 0.2 to 0.5 mA. The catheter tip should be advanced no more than 5 cm beyond the needle tip. To prevent it from being dislodged, the needle is carefully withdrawn as the catheter is simultaneously advanced. The most important aspect of this technique is stabilization of the needle for catheter insertion after the brachial plexus is localized.

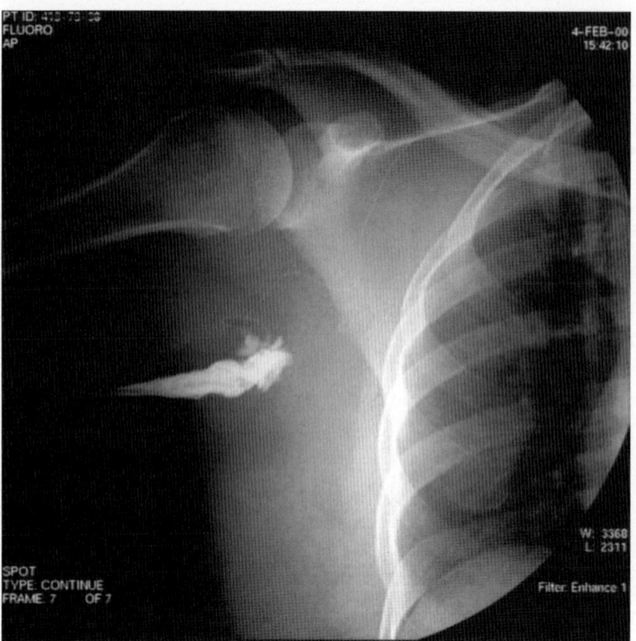


**FIGURE 14-11.** Disposition of radiopaque dye in the brachial plexus sheath after the injection of 2 mL through an infraclavicular catheter. The dye is seen descending into the axillary brachial plexus sheath, a testimony to the continuous nature of the brachial plexus sheath.

## TIPS

- This block should be reconsidered in patients with coagulopathy because the combination of a large-diameter needle and the immediate vicinity of the large vessels in the infraclavicular are (subclavian/axillary artery and vein) carries a risk of hematoma should these vessels be accidentally punctured during needle advancement.
- The stimulating characteristics of larger gauge Tuohy-style needles vary from those of small gauge single-injection needles. A slight needle rotation or angle change can make a significant difference in the ability to stimulate.

The catheter is checked for inadvertent intravascular placement and secured to the chest using an adhesive skin preparation such as benzoin, followed by application of a clear dressing. The infusion port should be clearly marked "continuous nerve block."

## Management of the Continuous Infusion

The catheter is activated by injecting a bolus of local anesthetic (20–25 mL) followed by an infusion at 5 mL/h and patient-controlled regional analgesia (PCRA) dose of 5 mL/h (Figure 14-11). For continuous infusion, we typically use 0.2% ropivacaine. Other adjuvants do not appear to be of benefit in continuous nerve blocks, such as clonidine, epinephrine, or opioids.

Patients should be seen and instructed on the use of PCRA at least once a day. During each visit, the insertion site should be checked for erythema and swelling and the extent of motor and sensory blockade documented. The infusion regimen should then be adjusted accordingly. When the patient complains of breakthrough pain, the extent of the sensory block should be checked first. A bolus of dilute local anesthetic (e.g., 10–15 mL of 0.2% ropivacaine) can be injected to reactivate the catheter. Increasing the infusion rate alone never results in improvement of analgesia. When the bolus fails to result in blockade after 30 minutes, the catheter should be considered to have migrated and should be removed. As with all continuous nerve block infusion, patients must be prescribed an immediately available alternative pain management protocol because incomplete analgesia and catheter dislodgment can occur. Table 14-3 lists possible complications with infraclavicular block and methods to reduce the risk of the complications.

## TIPS

- Breakthrough pain in patients undergoing continuous infusion is always managed by administering a bolus of local anesthetic. Increasing the rate of infusion alone is never adequate.
- For patients on the ward, a bolus of a short-acting higher concentration epinephrine-containing local anesthetic (e.g., 1% mepivacaine or lidocaine) is good to test the position of the catheter.

**TABLE 14-3 Complications and How to Avoid Them**

| | |
|---|---|
| ***Hematoma*** | • Avoid multiple needle insertions through the pectoralis muscle.<br>• Apply firm pressure over the site of needle insertion after needle withdrawal.<br>• Consider advantages and risks when planning continuous infraclavicular block in patients with abnormal coagulation. |
| ***Systemic toxicity*** | • Consider risks and benefits of using long-acting local anesthetics for each and every patient and/or surgical indication.<br>• Inject local anesthetic with frequent aspiration to rule out intravascular injection while carefully assessing the patient for signs of local anesthetic toxicity.<br>• Inject local anesthetic slowly and avoid rapid, forceful injection to reduce the risk of systemic toxicity. |
| ***Nerve injury*** | • Make sure the nerve stimulator is fully functional and connected properly.<br>• Use nerve stimulation to confirm the needle position. This technique requires deep needle insertion, and the use of paresthesia is not acceptable.<br>• Advance the needle slowly when the twitches of the pectoralis muscle cease.<br>• Do not inject against high pressures (>15 psi). Instead, withdraw the needle, check its patency by flushing it, and repeat the procedure.<br>• Stop injecting immediately when the patient complains of pain on injection. |
| ***Pneumothorax*** | • This is an often feared but uncommon complication.<br>• Attention should be paid to the site and angle of needle insertion to ensure the needle is in a plane away from the chest wall. |

## INFRACLAVICULAR BRACHIAL PLEXUS BLOCK: DECISION-MAKING ALGORITHM

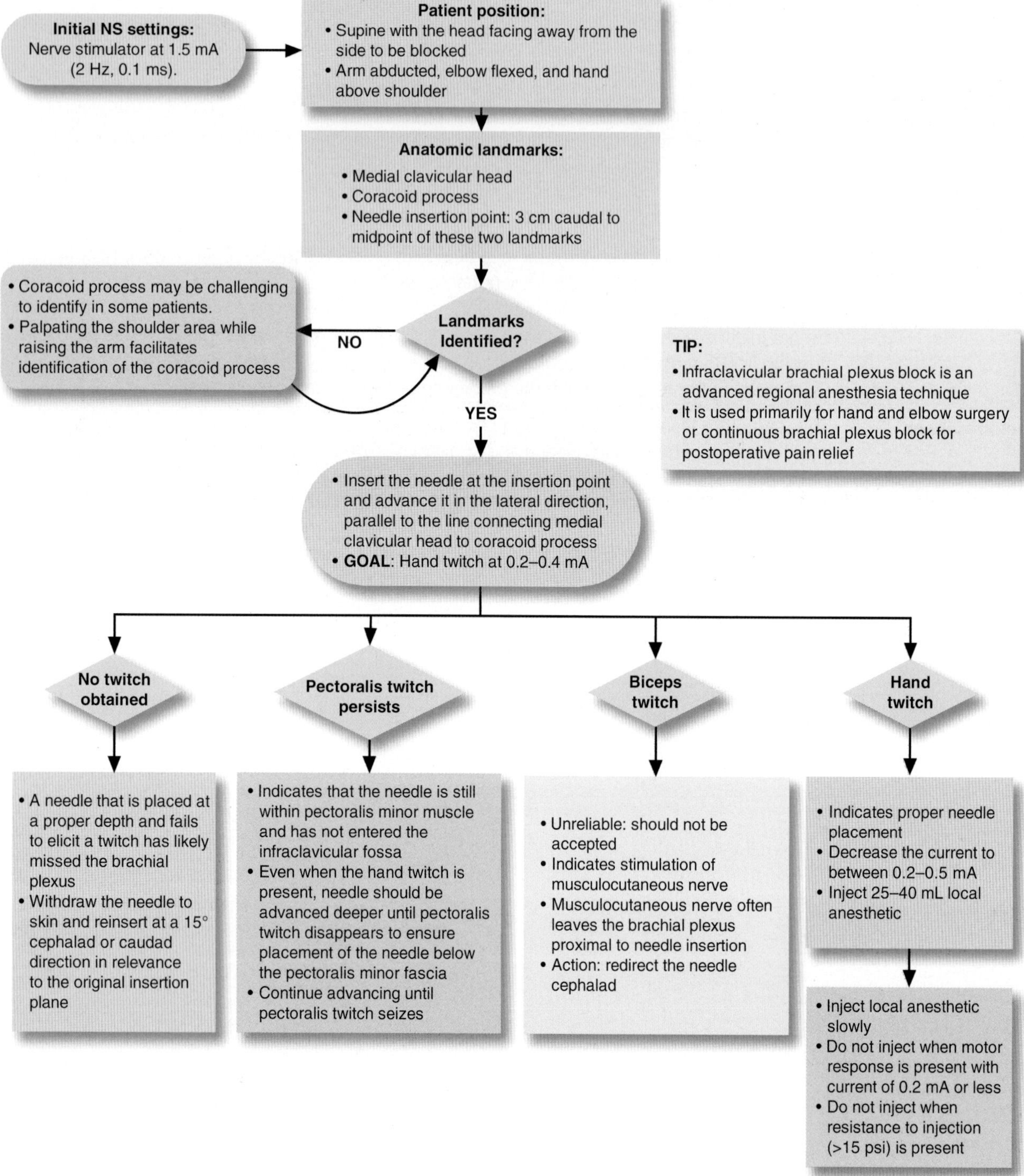

## SUGGESTED READING


Bloc S, et al. Single-stimulation, low-volume infraclavicular plexus block: influence of the evoked distal motor response on success rate. *Reg Anesth Pain Med.* 2006;31(5):433-437.

Bloc S, et al. Spread of injectate associated with radial or median nerve-type motor response during infraclavicular brachial-plexus block: an ultrasound evaluation. *Reg Anesth Pain Med.* 2007;32(2):130-135.

Blumenthal S, Nadig M, Borgeat A. Combined infraclavicular plexus block with suprascapular nerve block for humeral head surgery in a patient with respiratory failure: is an alternative approach really the best option for the lungs? *Anesthesiology.* 2004;100(1):190.

Borene SC, Edwards JN, Boezaart AP. At the cords, the pinkie towards: interpreting infraclavicular motor responses to neurostimulation. *Reg Anesth Pain Med.* 2004;29(2):125-129.

Borgeat A, Ekatodramis G, Dumont C. An evaluation of the infraclavicular block via a modified approach of the Raj technique. *Anesth Analg.* 2001;93(2):436-441.

Brown DL, Bridenbaugh LD. The upper extremity. Somatic block. In: Cousins MJ, Bridenbaugh PO, eds. *Neuronal Blockade in Clinical Anesthesia and Management of Pain.* Philadelphia, PA: Lippincott-Raven; 1988:345-371.

Chelly JE, Casati A, Fanelli G. *Continuous Peripheral Nerve Block Technique: An Illustrated Guide.* London, UK; Mosby International; 2001.

Chin KJ, et al. Continuous infraclavicular plexus blockade. *Anesth Analg.* 2009;109(4):1347–1348; author reply 1348-1349.

Comlekci M, et al. An approach to infraclavicular brachial plexus block: the highest point of the shoulder as a reference. *Anesth Analg.* 2006;103(6):1634-1635.

Cornish PB, Nowitz M. A magnetic resonance imaging analysis of the infraclavicular region: can brachial plexus depth be estimated before needle insertion? *Anesth Analg.* 2005;100(4):1184-1188.

Crews JC, Gerancher JC, Weller RS. Pneumothorax after coracoid infraclavicular brachial plexus block. *Anesth Analg.* 2007;105(1):275-277.

Dadure C, et al. Continuous infraclavicular brachial plexus block for acute pain management in children. *Anesth Analg.* 2003;97(3):691-693.

Day M, Pasupuleti R, Jacobs S. Infraclavicular brachial plexus block and infusion for treatment of long-standing complex regional syndrome type 1: a case report. *Pain Physician.* 2004;7(2):265-268.

Deleuze A, et al. A comparison of a single-stimulation lateral infraclavicular plexus block with a triple-stimulation axillary block. *Reg Anesth Pain Med.* 2003;28(2):89-94.

Desroches J. The infraclavicular brachial plexus block by the coracoid approach is clinically effective: an observational study of 150 patients. *Can J Anaesth.* 2003;50(3):253-257.

Dullenkopf A, et al. Diaphragmatic excursion and respiratory function after the modified Raj technique of the infraclavicular plexus block. *Reg Anesth Pain Med.* 2004;29(2):110-114.

Fuzier R, et al. The infraclavicular block is a useful technique for emergency upper extremity analgesia. *Can J Anaesth.* 2004;51(2):191-192.

Gaertner E, et al. Infraclavicular plexus block: multiple injection versus single injection. *Reg Anesth Pain Med.* 2002;27(6):590-594.

Greher M, et al. Ultrasonographic assessment of topographic anatomy in volunteers suggests a modification of the infraclavicular vertical brachial plexus block. *Br J Anaesth.* 2002;88(5):632-636.

Groen GJ, et al. At the cords, the pinkie towards: interpreting infraclavicular motor responses to neurostimulation. *Reg Anesth Pain Med.* 2004;29:505-507.

Hadžić A, et al. The practice of peripheral nerve blocks in the United States: a national survey. *Reg Anesth Pain Med.* 1998;23(3):241-246.

Hadžić A, et al. A comparison of infraclavicular nerve block versus general anesthesia for hand and wrist day-case surgeries. *Anesthesiology.* 2004;101(1):127-132.

Ilfeld BM. Single- versus multiple-stimulation infraclavicular blocks. *Reg Anesth Pain Med.* 2003;28(2):149-150.

Ilfeld BM, Enneking FK. Brachial plexus infraclavicular block success rate and appropriate endpoints. *Anesth Analg.* 2002;95(3):784.

Ilfeld BM, et al. The effects of local anesthetic concentration and dose on continuous infraclavicular nerve blocks: a multicenter, randomized, observer-masked, controlled study. *Anesth Analg.* 2009;108(1):345-350.

Ilfeld BM, Morey TE, Enneking FK. Continuous infraclavicular brachial plexus block for postoperative pain control at home: a randomized, double-blinded, placebo-controlled study. *Anesthesiology.* 2002;96(6):1297-1304.

Ilfeld BM, Morey TE, Enneking FK. Continuous infraclavicular perineural infusion with clonidine and ropivacaine compared with ropivacaine alone: a randomized, double-blinded, controlled study. *Anesth Analg.* 2003;97(3):706-712.

Ilfeld BM, Morey TE, Enneking FK. Infraclavicular perineural local anesthetic infusion: a comparison of three dosing regimens for postoperative analgesia. *Anesthesiology.* 2004;100(2):395-402.

Ilfeld BM, et al. Total elbow arthroplasty as an outpatient procedure using a continuous infraclavicular nerve block at home: a prospective case report. *Reg Anesth Pain Med.* 2006;31(2): 172-176.

Jandard C, et al. Infraclavicular block with lateral approach and nerve stimulation: extent of anesthesia and adverse effects. *Reg Anesth Pain Med.* 2002;27(1):37-42.

Klaastad O, et al. Magnetic resonance imaging demonstrates lack of precision in needle placement by the infraclavicular brachial plexus block described by Raj et al. *Anesth Analg.* 1999;88(3):593-598.

Klaastad O, et al. A magnetic resonance imaging study of modifications to the infraclavicular brachial plexus block. *Anesth Analg.* 2000;91(4):929-933.

Klaastad O, et al. A novel infraclavicular brachial plexus block: the lateral and sagittal technique, developed by magnetic resonance imaging studies. *Anesth Analg.* 2004;98(1):252-256.

Klaastad O, et al. The vertical infraclavicular brachial plexus block: a simulation study using magnetic resonance imaging. *Anesth Analg.* 2005;101(1):273-278.

Klaastad O, et al. Lateral sagittal infraclavicular block (LSIB). *Reg Anesth Pain Med.* 2006;31(1):86; author reply 86-87.

Koscielniak-Nielsen ZJ, et al. Clinical evaluation of the lateral sagittal infraclavicular block developed by MRI studies. *Reg Anesth Pain Med.* 2005;30(4):329-334.

Koscielniak-Nielsen ZJ, et al. Infraclavicular block causes less discomfort than axillary block in ambulatory patients. *Acta Anaesthesiol Scand.* 2005;49(7):1030-1034.

Koscielniak-Nielsen ZJ, Rotbøll Nielsen P, Risby Mortensen C. A comparison of coracoid and axillary approaches to the brachial plexus. *Acta Anaesthesiol Scand.* 2000;44(3):274-279.

Lecamwasam H, et al. Stimulation of the posterior cord predicts successful infraclavicular block. *Anesth Analg.* 2006;102(5): 1564-1568.

Macleod DB, et al. Identification of coracoid process for infraclavicular blocks. *Reg Anesth Pain Med.* 2003;28(5):485.

Martinez J, et al. Combined infraclavicular plexus block with suprascapular nerve block for humeral head surgery in a patient with respiratory failure: an alternative approach. *Anesthesiology.* 2003;98(3):784-785.

Maurer K, et al. Interscalene and infraclavicular block for bilateral distal radius fracture. *Anesth Analg.* 2002;94(2):450-452.

Minville V, et al. Hyperbaric oxygen therapy and pain management in a child with continuous infraclavicular brachial plexus block. *Anesth Analg.* 2004;99(6):1878.

Minville V, et al. A modified coracoid approach to infraclavicular brachial plexus blocks using a double-stimulation technique in 300 patients. *Anesth Analg.* 2005;100(1):263-265.
Minville V, et al. Infraclavicular brachial plexus block versus humeral approach: comparison of anesthetic time and efficacy. *Anesth Analg.* 2005;101(4):1198-1201.
Minville V, et al. Resident versus staff anesthesiologist performance: coracoid approach to infraclavicular brachial plexus blocks using a double-stimulation technique. *Reg Anesth Pain Med.* 2005;30(3):233-237.
Minville V, et al. Infraclavicular brachial plexus block versus humeral block in trauma patients: a comparison of patient comfort. *Anesth Analg.* 2006;102(3):912-915.
Minville V, et al. The optimal motor response for infraclavicular brachial plexus block. *Anesth Analg.* 2007;104(2):448-451.
Moayeri N, Bigeleisen PE, Groen GJ. Quantitative architecture of the brachial plexus and surrounding compartments, and their possible significance for plexus blocks. *Anesthesiology.* 2008;108(2):299-304.
Morimoto M, et al. Case series: Septa can influence local anesthetic spread during infraclavicular brachial plexus blocks. *Can J Anaesth.* 2007;54(12):1006-1010.
Niemi TT, et al. Single-injection brachial plexus anesthesia for arteriovenous fistula surgery of the forearm: a comparison of infraclavicular coracoid and axillary approach. *Reg Anesth Pain Med.* 2007;32(1):55-59.
Pandin P, et al. Somatosensory evoked potentials as an objective assessment of the sensory median nerve blockade after infraclavicular block. *Can J Anaesth.* 2006;53(1):67-72.
Ponde VC. Continuous infraclavicular brachial plexus block: a modified technique to better secure catheter position in infants and children. *Anesth Analg.* 2008;106(1):94-96.
Porter JM, McCartney CJ, Chan VW. Needle placement and injection posterior to the axillary artery may predict successful infraclavicular brachial plexus block: a report of three cases. *Can J Anaesth.* 2005;52(1):69-73.
Raj PP. Infraclavicular approaches to brachial plexus anesthesia. *Reg Anesth Pain Manage.* 1997;1:169-177.
Raj PP, Pai U, Rawal N. Techniques of regional anesthesia in adults. In: Raj PP, ed. *Clinical Practice of Regional Anesthesia.* New York, NY: Churchill Livingstone; 1991:276-300.
Raphael DT, et al. Frontal slab composite magnetic resonance neurography of the brachial plexus: implications for infraclavicular block approaches. *Anesthesiology.* 2005;103(6):1218-1224.
Renes S, et al. A simplified approach to vertical infraclavicular brachial plexus blockade using hand-held Doppler. *Anesth Analg.* 2008;106(3):1012-1014.
Rettig HC, et al. Vertical infraclavicular block of the brachial plexus: effects on hemidiaphragmatic movement and ventilatory function. *Reg Anesth Pain Med.* 2005;30(6):529-535.
Rodriguez J, et al. Infraclavicular brachial plexus block effects on respiratory function and extent of the block. *Reg Anesth Pain Med.* 1998;23(6):564-568.
Rodriguez J, Barcena M, Alvarez J. Restricted infraclavicular distribution of the local anesthetic solution after infraclavicular brachial plexus block. *Reg Anesth Pain Med.* 2003;28(1):33-36.
Rodriguez J, Barcena M, Alvarez J. Shoulder dislocation after infraclavicular coracoid block. *Reg Anesth Pain Med.* 2003;28(4): 351-353.
Rodriguez J, et al. A comparison of single versus multiple injections on the extent of anesthesia with coracoid infraclavicular brachial plexus block. *Anesth Analg.* 2004;99(4):1225-1230; table of contents.
Rodriguez J, et al. Median versus musculocutaneous nerve response with single-injection infraclavicular coracoid block. *Reg Anesth Pain Med.* 2004;29(6):534-538; discussion 520-523.
Sala-Blanch X, et al. Interpreting infraclavicular motor responses to neurostimulation of the brachial plexus: from anatomic complexity to clinical evaluation simplicity. *Reg Anesth Pain Med.* 2004;29(6):618-620.
Sauter AR, et al. Use of magnetic resonance imaging to define the anatomical location closest to all three cords of the infraclavicular brachial plexus. *Anesth Analg.* 2006;103(6):1574-1576.
Sedeek KA, Goujard E. The lateral sagittal infraclavicular block in children. *Anesth Analg.* 2007; 105(1):295-297.
Tran de, QH, Charghi R, Finlayson RJ. The "double bubble" sign for successful infraclavicular brachial plexus blockade. *Anesth Analg.* 2006;103(4):1048-1049.
Tran QD, et al. Retained and cut stimulating infraclavicular catheter. *Can J Anaesth.* 2005;52(9):998-999.
Whiffler K. Coracoid block—a safe and easy technique. *Br J Anaesth.* 1981;53(8):845-848.
Wilson JL, et al. Infraclavicular brachial plexus block: parasagittal anatomy important to the coracoid technique. *Anesth Analg.* 1998;87(4):870-873.
Zimmermann P, et al. Vertical infraclavicular brachial plexus block in a child with cystic fibrosis. *Anesth Analg.* 2002;95(6):1825-1826.

# 15 Axillary Brachial Plexus Block

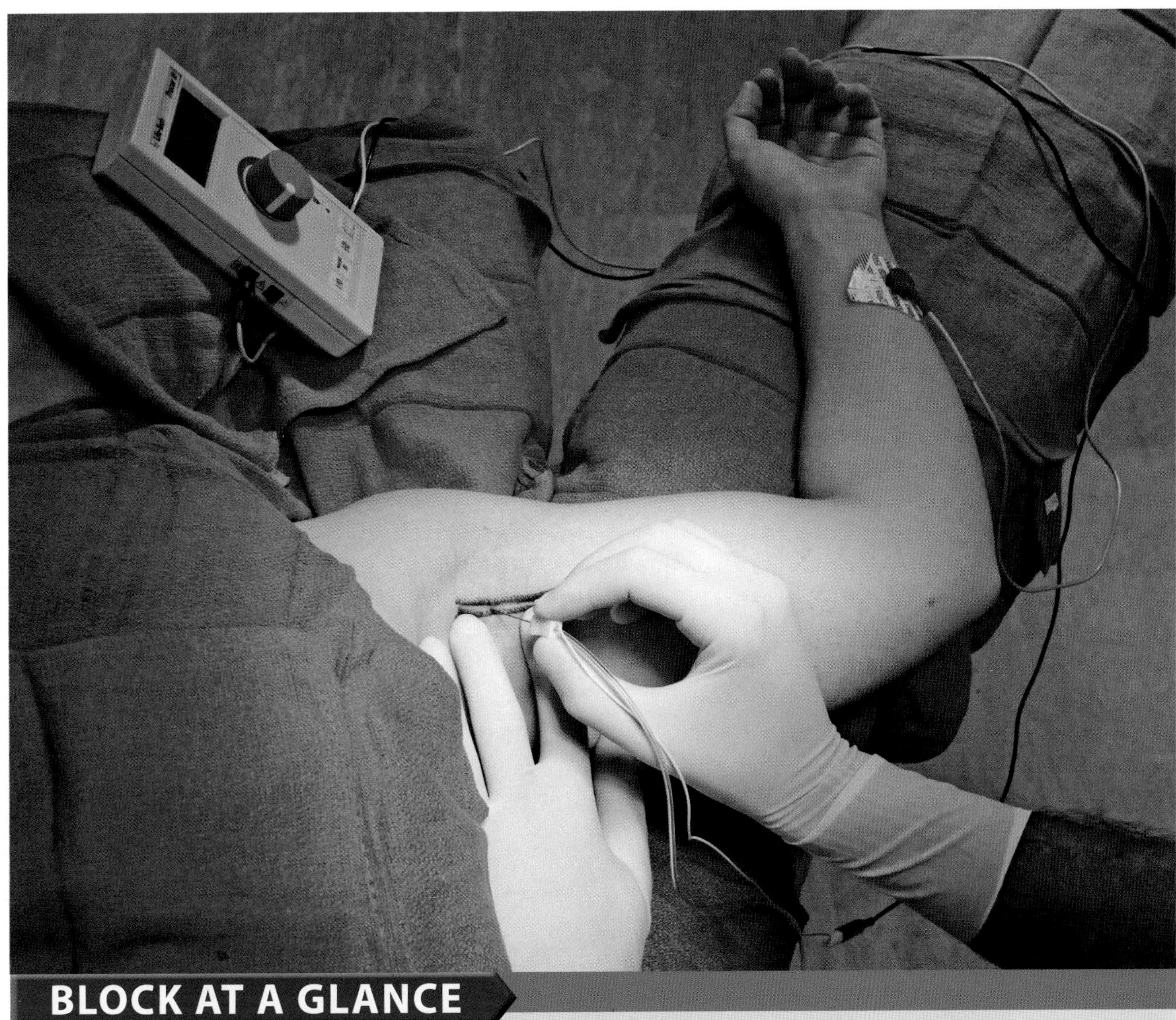

## BLOCK AT A GLANCE

- Indications: forearm and hand surgery
- Landmarks: axillary artery pulse
- Any of the following three end points: nerve stimulation, hand twitch at 0.3-0.5 mA current; hand paresthesia; arterial blood on aspiration (axillary artery)
- Local anesthetic: 20–30 mL

**FIGURE 15-1.** The needle is inserted toward the axillary artery (line) until either motor response of the hand or arterial blood on aspiration is obtained.

## General Considerations

The axillary brachial plexus block was first described by Halsted in 1884 at the Roosevelt Hospital in New York City. The axillary brachial plexus block is one of the most commonly used regional anesthesia techniques. The proximity of the terminal nerves of the brachial plexus to the axillary artery makes identification of the landmarks consistent (axillary artery) equally for both the nerve stimulator and surface-based ultrasound-guided techniques. The axillary block is an excellent choice of anesthesia technique for elbow, forearm, and hand surgery.

## Functional Anatomy

By the time the brachial plexus passes behind the lower border of the pectoralis minor muscle in the axilla, the cords quickly begin to form the principal terminal nerves of the brachial plexus, namely, the median, ulnar, radial, and musculocutaneous nerves (Figure 15-2). The arrangement of the individual nerves and their relationship to the axillary artery is important in axillary blockade (Figure 15-3). With the arm abducted at 90° and the axillary arterial pulsation as a point of reference, the nerves are located as follows: The median nerve is positioned superficially and immediately above the pulse; the ulnar nerve is found superficial slightly deeper than the median nerve; the radial nerve is located behind the pulse. The musculocutaneous nerve can be found 1 to 3 cm deeper and above the pulse, often outside the brachial plexus sheath as it moves distally away from the axillary fossa (Figure 14-2).

### Musculocutaneous Nerve

The musculocutaneous nerve is a terminal branch of the *lateral* cord. It pierces the coracobrachialis muscle to descend between the biceps and brachialis muscles, giving innervation to both. The nerve continues distally as the lateral cutaneous nerve of the forearm, which emerges from the deep fascia between the biceps and brachioradialis to emerge superficially at the level of the cubital fossa. From here on, the nerve supplies cutaneous sensory branches to the lateral aspect of the forearm.

### Median Nerve

The median nerve derives its origin from both the lateral and medial cords. It provides motor branches to the flexors of the hand and wrist, and sensation to the palmar surface of the first, second, third digits and the lateral half of the fourth digit. Interestingly, the median and ulnar nerves both traverse the entire length of the arm without giving off branches above the elbow joint.

### Ulnar Nerve

The ulnar nerve is a terminal branch of the medial cord. Together with the medial cutaneous nerve of the forearm, it

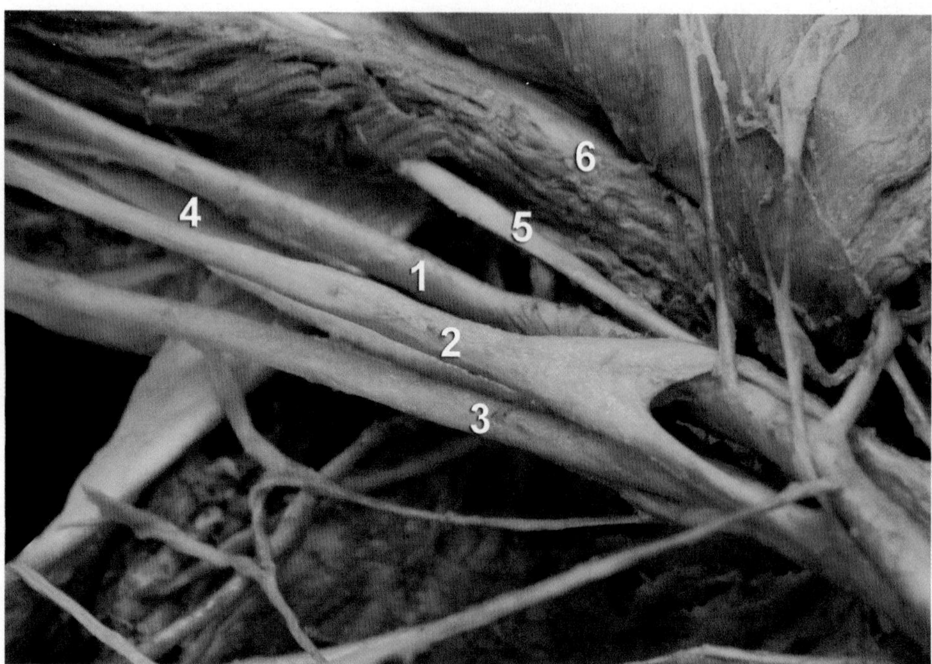


**FIGURE 15-2.** Anatomy of the brachial plexus in the axilla. ❶ axillary artery. ❷ median nerve. ❸ ulnar nerve. ❹ radial nerve. ❺ musculocutaneous nerve as it enters the coracobrachialis muscle. ❻ coracoid brachialis muscle. Pectoralis muscles are show retracted laterally (right upper corner).

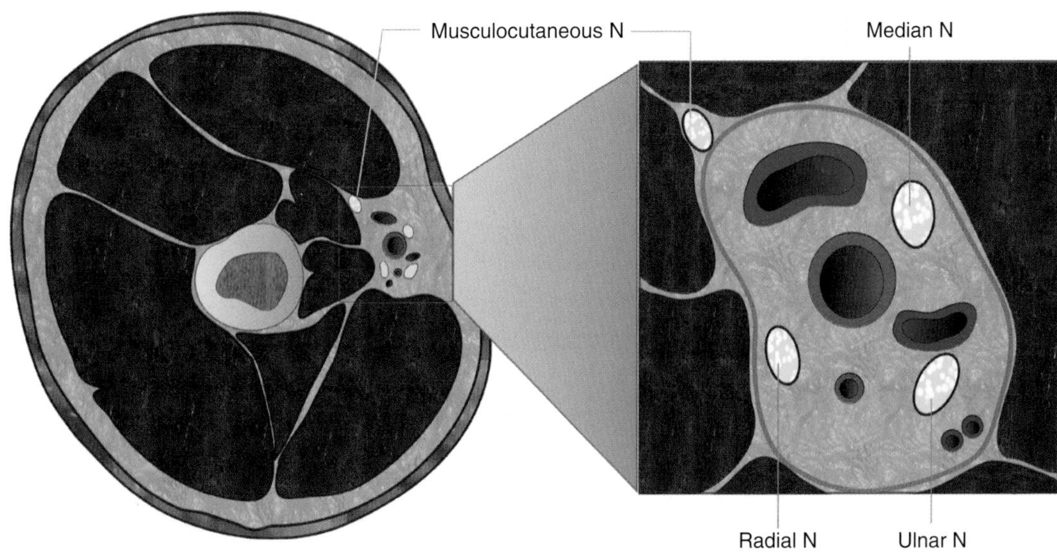


**FIGURE 15-3.** Spatial organization of the brachial plexus in the axilla. Note that the musculocutaneous nerve is outside of the axillary plexus sheath.

initially lies medial to the brachial artery but leaves the artery at midarm to pass behind the medial epicondyle to enter the forearm. The ulnar nerve has articular branches to the elbow joint and muscular branches to the hand and forearm. The nerve provides sensory innervation to the fourth and fifth digits.

### Radial Nerve

The radial nerve, a terminal branch of the posterior cord, leaves the axilla by passing below the teres major and between the humerus and the long head of the triceps. The radial nerve supplies branches to the triceps, brachioradialis, and extensor radialis longus muscles. Cutaneous branches innervate the lateral aspect of the arm and the posterior aspect of the forearm and hand.

## Distribution of Blockade

Axillary brachial plexus block provides anesthesia to the elbow, forearm, and hand (Figure 15-4).

## Equipment

A standard regional anesthesia tray is prepared with the following equipment:

- Sterile towels and gauze packs
- 2 × 20-mL syringes containing local anesthetic
- A 3-mL syringe + 25-gauge needle with local anesthetic for skin infiltration
- A 3–5 cm 22-gauge short-bevel insulated stimulating needle
- Peripheral nerve stimulator
- Sterile gloves, marking pen

## Landmarks and Patient Positioning

The patient is placed in the supine position with the head facing away from the side to be blocked. The arm is abducted to form an approximately 90° angle in the elbow joint (Figure 15-5).

**TIPS**

- Excessive abduction in the shoulder joint should be avoided because it makes palpation of the axillary artery pulse difficult.
- Excessive abduction can also result in stretching and "fixing" of the brachial plexus. Such stretching of the plexus components can increase its vulnerability during needle advancement. This is because the stretching predisposes the nerves in the axilla to penetration, as opposed to "rolling" away from the advancing needle.

Surface landmarks for the axillary brachial plexus block include the following:

1. Pulse of the axillary artery
2. Coracobrachialis muscle
3. Pectoralis major muscle

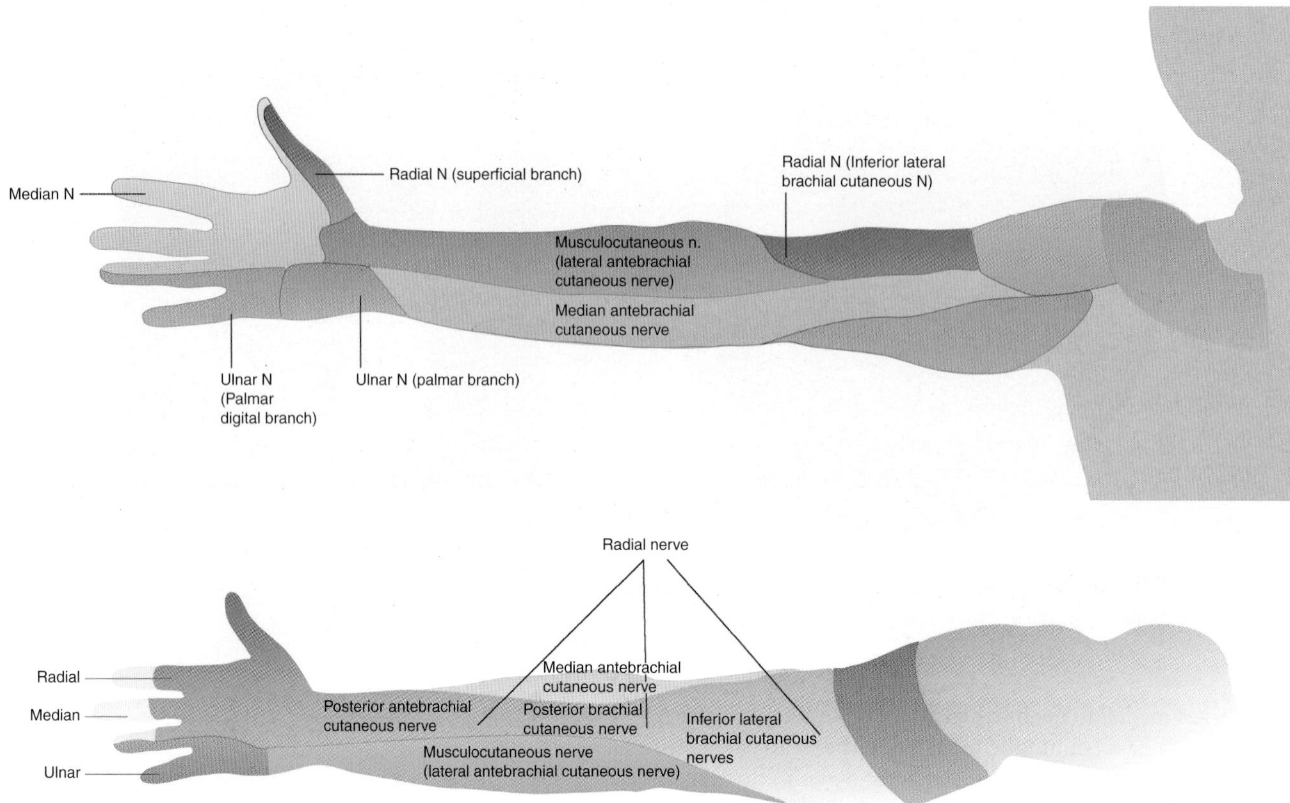


**FIGURE 15-4.** Cutaneous distribution of anesthesia after axillary brachial plexus block. Axillary block results in anesthesia in the labeled areas.

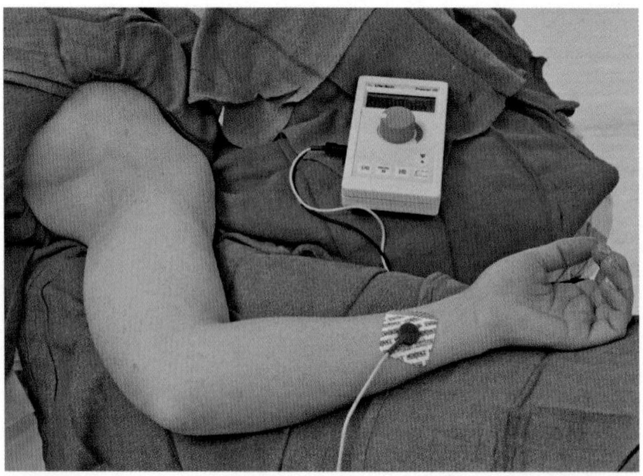

**FIGURE 15-5.** Patient position for the axillary brachial plexus block.

## TIPS

- In some patients, palpation of the axillary artery is difficult, a common scenario in young muscular men.
- When identification of the axillary artery proves difficult, the location of the brachial plexus can be estimated by percutaneous nerve stimulation (surface mapping). The nerve stimulator is set to deliver 4 to 5 mA, and a blunt probe or an "alligator" clip is firmly applied over the skin in front of the palpating fingers until twitches of the brachial plexus are elicited. At this point, the probe is replaced by a needle directed toward the estimated direction of the brachial plexus sheath.

## Technique

After thorough skin preparation, the pulse of the axillary artery is palpated high in the axilla, Figure 15-6. Once the pulse is felt, the artery is fixed between the index and the middle fingers and firmly pressed against the humerus to prevent "rolling" of the axillary artery during block performance. At this point, movement of the palpating hand and the patient's arm should be minimized

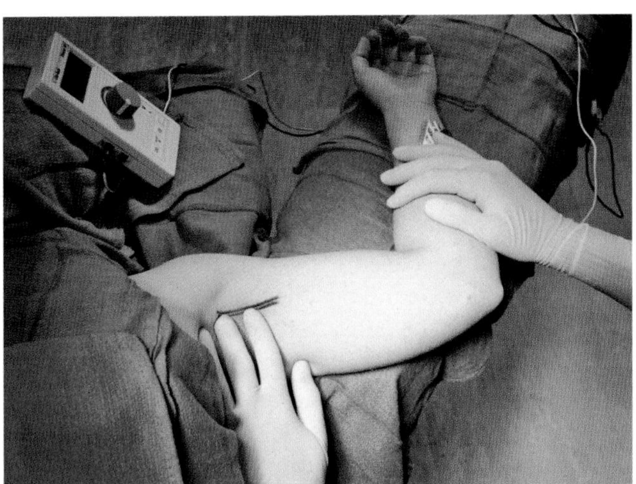

**FIGURE 15-6.** Palpation of the axillary artery.

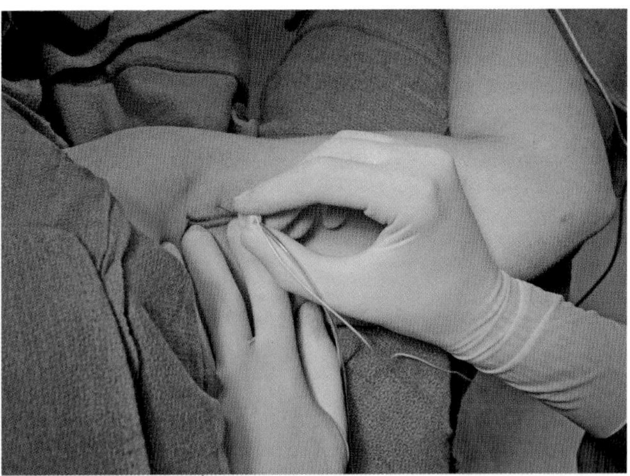

**FIGURE 15-7.** Insertion of the needle slightly above the axillary artery to block the medialis nerve.

because the axillary artery is highly movable in the adipose tissue of the axillary fossa. The anesthesiologist should assume a sitting position by the patient's side to avoid strain and unwanted hand movement during block performance. The index and middle fingers of the palpating hand should be pressed firmly against the arm, straddling the pulse of the axillary artery immediately distal to the insertion of the pectoralis major muscle (Figure 15-6). This maneuver shortens the distance between the needle insertion site and the brachial plexus block by compressing the subcutaneous tissue. It also helps in stabilizing the position of the artery and needle during performance of the block. The palpating hand should not be moved during the entire procedure to allow for precise redirection of the angle of needle insertion when necessary. Local anesthetic is infiltrated subcutaneously at the determined needle insertion site. Axillary brachial plexus blocks can also be accomplished using multiple injections after electrolocation of each nerve. Several studies have documented faster onset and better success rate compared with the single-injection technique. Multiple injections are possible due to the shallow and relatively predictable location of the nerves. With this technique, the mental image of the position the nerves in relationship to the artery should be kept in mind, Figure 15-3.

A needle connected to the nerve stimulator (0.5–1.0 mA, 2 Hz, 0.1-0.3 ms) is inserted at an angle of 45° cephalad (Figure 15-7).

Once through the skin, the needle is slowly advanced directly below the pulse until stimulation of the brachial plexus is obtained. Typically, this occurs at a depth of 1 to 2 cm in most patients. The needle should be advanced gently until a radial nerve twitch (extension of wrist and/or fingers) is obtained, and 10 to 15 mL of local anesthetic is deposited after negative aspiration.

The needle is then withdrawn completely and reinserted above the artery without moving the palpating hand (Figure 15-8). Advancing slowly, the median nerve should be encountered within 1 to 2 cm, resulting in finger flexion. The needle is then advanced slightly deeper until the ulnar twitch reappears. At this point, a further 5 to-10 mL of local anesthetic is deposited after negative aspiration.

Finally, through the same insertion site, the needle is brought back to the skin, redirected up into the bulk of the coracobrachialis, and advanced slowly. Once the needle tip is in proximity to the musculocutaneous nerve, the local coracobrachialis twitch will disappear and a more

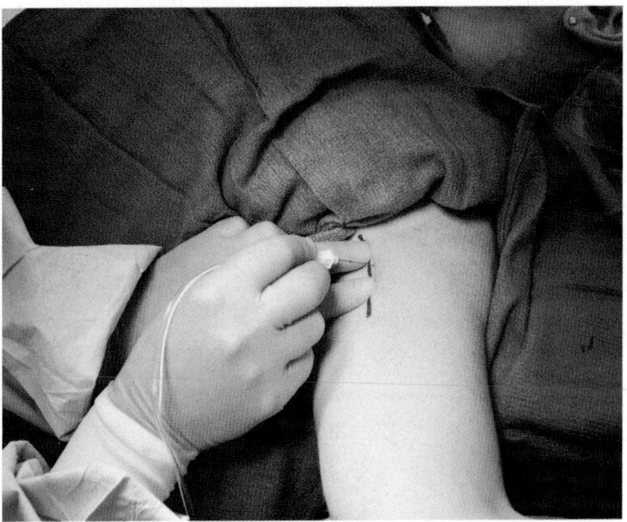

**FIGURE 15-8.** To block the musculocutaneous nerve, the needle is inserted above the axillary artery and directed upward to localize the musculocutaneous nerve.

vigorous biceps brachii twitch will materialize. The last 5 to 8 mL of local anesthetic should be administered here. Occasionally, no biceps twitch will be obtained, in which case it is sufficient to deposit the local anesthetic in the substance of the coracobrachialis muscle itself for coverage of the musculocutaneous nerve.

### TIPS

- It has been suggested that the axillary brachial plexus sheath contains septa preventing local anesthetic from reaching all nerves contained within the sheath.
- Although the clinical significance of these septa remains controversial, it makes sense to inject local anesthetic in divided doses at several locations within the sheath (e.g., at each nerve).
- Twitches of every nerve are not always obtained, especially after the administration of 1 to 2 aliquots of local anesthetic, but injecting on two distinct motor responses is more likely to result in complete plexus blockade than administration at a single location.

### GOAL

The goal for the axillary brachial plexus block is injection of the local anesthetic around the axillary artery as median, ulnar and radial nerve are all located within the neurovascular sheath. A separate injection is needed to block the musculocutaneous nerve.

When insertion of the needle does not result in nerve stimulation, the following maneuvers should be made:

1. Keep the palpating hand in the same position and the patient's skin between the fingers stretched.
2. Withdraw the needle completely, reassess the location of the arterial pulsation, and choose a new insertion site 1–2 cm more distal to the initial location.

### TIPS

- To reduce the risk of vascular puncture, the axillary artery is carefully palpated/identified, and the operator's hand is kept stable with the artery straddled between the fingers.
- Should the needle enter the artery (bright red blood noticed in tubing), the operator should best proceed with the transarterial technique instead of using nerve stimulation.
- The needle is advanced further until the aspiration is negative for blood. This indicates that the needle tip is now outside of the artery and positioned posterior to the artery.
- With intermittent aspiration, two thirds of the local anesthetic can be deposited here.
- The needle is then withdrawn back through the artery to again obtain the blood flow.
- When the needle reenters the artery (blood flow on aspiration) and exits anterior to the vessel, the remaining one third of the local anesthetic is injected at this superficial location.

## Troubleshooting

Some common responses to nerve stimulation and the course of action to obtain the proper response are shown in Table 15-1.

## Block Dynamics and Perioperative Management

An axillary brachial plexus block is associated with relatively minor patient discomfort at the time of placement. However, some patients complain of the sensation of soreness in the axillary region after the block resolution, which may be related the intramuscular needle insertion or hematoma formation from inadvertent vascular puncture. Intravenous midazolam 1 to 2 mg with alfentanil 250 to 500 μg at the time of needle insertion should produce a comfortable, cooperative patient during nerve localization. The onset time for this block ranges between 15 and 25 minutes. The first sign of the blockade is loss of coordination of the arm and forearm muscles. This sign is usually seen sooner than the onset of a sensory or temperature change. When this sign is observed shortly after injection, it is highly predictive of an oncoming successful brachial plexus blockade.

**TABLE 15-1 Some Common Responses to Nerve Stimulation and the Course of Action for Proper Response**

| RESPONSE OBTAINED | INTERPRETATION | PROBLEM | ACTION |
|---|---|---|---|
| Local twitch of the arm muscles | Direct stimulation of the biceps or triceps muscles | Needle is inserted in a direction that is too superior or too inferior, respectively | Withdraw needle and redirect it accordingly |
| The needle contacts bone at a 2- to 3-cm depth; no twitches are seen | Needle stopped by the humerus | Brachial plexus was missed - the needle is inserted too deeply | Withdraw needle to skin level and reinsert it at an angle 15–30° anteriorly or posteriorly |
| Twitches of the hand | Stimulation of the medial, radial, or ulnar nerve | Correct needle position | Accept, and inject local anesthetic |
| Arterial blood noticed in the tubing | Puncture of the axillary artery | Needle entered the lumen of the axillary artery | Proceed with the "trans-arterial" technique: Inject two-thirds of the local anesthetic posterior to the artery, and one-third anterior to the artery |
| Paresthesia: no motor response | Contact of the needle with the brachial plexus branches | Possible equipment malfunction (stimulator, needle, electrode); contact with sensory part of nerve only | Carefully assess the distribution of the paresthesia and, if typical, inject local anesthetic |

## Complications and How to Avoid Them

**TABLE 15-2 Complications of Axillary Block and Techniques to Avoid Them**

| | |
|---|---|
| ***Infection*** | • An aseptic technique is used. |
| ***Hematoma*** | • Avoid multiple needle insertions, particularly in patients on anticoagulant therapy. |
| ***Vascular puncture*** | • A steady pressure at the site of needle insertion for 3–5 min should be maintained if the axillary artery is punctured. |
| ***Local anesthetic toxicity*** | • Systemic toxicity occurs most commonly during or shortly after the injection of local anesthetic. The most common cause is inadvertent intravascular injection.<br>• Careful reconsideration of the use of large volumes of long-acting anesthetic in frail and elderly patients is needed.<br>• Careful, frequent aspiration should be performed during the injection.<br>• Avoid fast, forceful injection of local anesthetic. |
| ***Nerve injury*** | • Never inject local anesthetic when abnormal resistance (high injection pressure) is encountered on injection.<br>• Local anesthetic should never be injected when a patient complains of severe pain or exhibits a withdrawal reaction suggestive of severe discomfort on injection.<br>• When stimulation is obtained with a current intensity of <0.2-0.3 mA, the needle should be withdrawn slightly to obtain the same response with the current ≥0.2mA. |

# AXILLARY BRACHIAL PLEXUS BLOCK

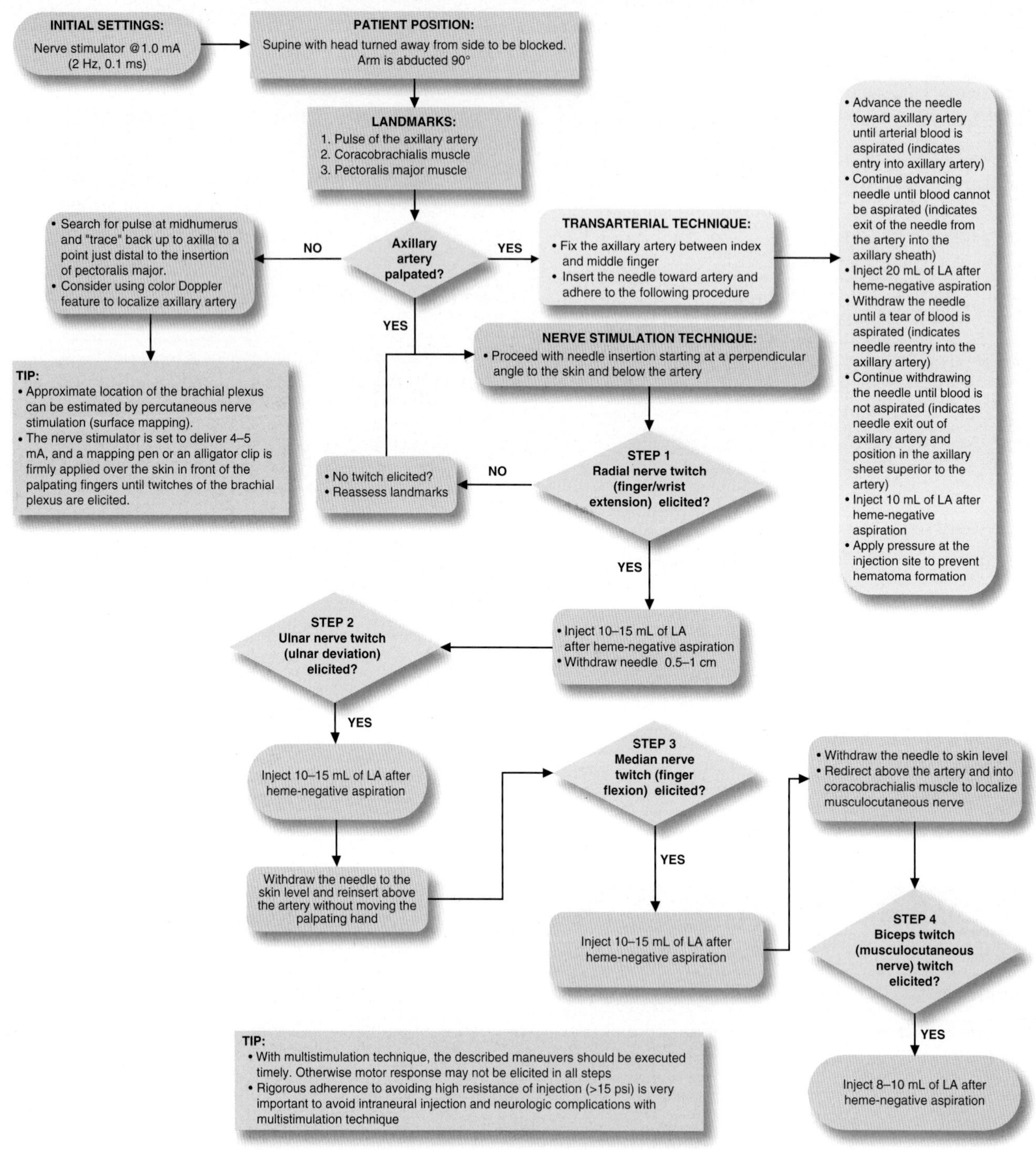

## SUGGESTED READING


Ababou A, Marzouk N, Mosadiq A, Sbihi A. The effects of arm position on onset and duration of axillary brachial plexus block. *Anesth Analg.* 2007;104:980-981.

Andersson A, Akeson J, Dahlin LB. Efficacy and safety of axillary brachial plexus block for operations on the hand. *Scand J Plast Reconstr Surg Hand Surg.* 2006;40:225-229.

Bekler H, Beyzadeoglu T, Mercan A. Groin flap immobilization by axillary brachial plexus block anesthesia. *Tech Hand Up Extrem Surg.* 2008;12:68-70.

Benhamou D. Axillary plexus block using multiple nerve stimulation: a European view. *Reg Anesth Pain Med.* 2001;26:495-498.

Bergman BD, Hebl JR, Kent J, Horlocker TT. Neurologic complications of 405 consecutive continuous axillary catheters. *Anesth Analg.* 2003;96:247-252.

Bertini L, Palmisani S, Mancini S, Martini O, Ioculano R, Arcioni R. Does local anesthetic dilution influence the clinical effectiveness of multiple-injection axillary brachial plexus block?: a prospective, double-blind, randomized clinical trial in patients undergoing upper limb surgery. *Reg Anesth Pain Med.* 2009;34:408-413.

Bhat R. Transient vascular insufficiency after axillary brachial plexus block in a child. *Anesth Analg.* 2004;98:1284-1285.

Bouaziz H, Narchi P, Mercier FJ, et al. Comparison between conventional axillary block and a new approach at the midhumeral level. *Anesth Analg.* 1997;84:1058-1062.

Breschan C, Kraschl R, Jost R, Marhofer P, Likar R. Axillary brachial plexus block for treatment of severe forearm ischemia after arterial cannulation in an extremely low birth-weight infant. *Paediatr Anaesth.* 2004;14:681-684.

Brown AR. Anaesthesia for procedures of the hand and elbow. *Best Pract Res Clin Anaesthesiol.* 2002;16:227-246.

Brull R, McCartney CJ, Chan VW, et al. Effect of transarterial axillary block versus general anesthesia on paresthesiae 1 year after hand surgery. *Anesthesiology.* 2005;103:1104-1105.

Bullmann V, Waurick R, Rodl R, et al. Corrective osteotomy of the humerus using perivascular axillary anesthesia according to Weber in a patient suffering from McCune-Albright syndrome [in German]. *Anaesthesist.* 2005;54:889-894.

Candido KD, Winnie AP, Ghaleb AH, Fattouh MW, Franco CD. Buprenorphine added to the local anesthetic for axillary brachial plexus block prolongs postoperative analgesia. *Reg Anesth Pain Med.* 2002;27:162-167.

Capdevila X, Lopez S, Bernard N, et al. Percutaneous electrode guidance using the insulated needle for prelocation of peripheral nerves during axillary plexus blocks. *Reg Anesth Pain Med.* 2004;29:206-211.

Carles M, Pulcini A, Macchi P, Duflos P, Raucoules-Aime M, Grimaud D. An evaluation of the brachial plexus block at the humeral canal using a neurostimulator (1417 patients): the efficacy, safety, and predictive criteria of failure. *Anesth Analg.* 2001;92:194-198.

Chan VW, Perlas A, McCartney CJ, Brull R, Xu D, Abbas S. Ultrasound guidance improves success rate of axillary brachial plexus block. *Can J Anaesth.* 2007;54:176-182.

Choyce A, Chan VW, Middleton WJ, Knight PR, Peng P, McCartney CJ. What is the relationship between paresthesia and nerve stimulation for axillary brachial plexus block? *Reg Anesth Pain Med.* 2001;26:100-104.

Cockings E. Axillary block complicated by hematoma and radial nerve injury. *Reg Anesth Pain Med.* 2000;25:103.

Cordell CL, Schubkegel T, Light TR, Ahmad F. Lipid infusion rescue for bupivacaine-induced cardiac arrest after axillary block. *J Hand Surg Am.* 2010;35:144-146.

Crews JC, Weller RS, Moss J, James RL. Levobupivacaine for axillary brachial plexus block: a pharmacokinetic and clinical comparison in patients with normal renal function or renal disease. *Anesth Analg* 2002;95:219-223.

De Jong RH. Axillary block of the brachial plexus. *Anesthesiology.* 1961;22:215-225.

Deleuze A, Gentili ME, Marret E, Lamonerie L, Bonnet F. A comparison of a single-stimulation lateral infraclavicular plexus block with a triple-stimulation axillary block. *Reg Anesth Pain Med.* 2003;28:89-94.

Dhir S, Tureanu L, Stewart SA. Axillary brachial plexus block complicated by cervical disc protrusion and radial nerve injury. *Acta Anaesthesiol Scand.* 2009;53:411.

Dogru K, Duygulu F, Yildiz K, Kotanoglu MS, Madenoglu H, Boyaci A. Hemodynamic and blockade effects of high/low epinephrine doses during axillary brachial plexus blockade with lidocaine 1.5%: A randomized, double-blinded study. *Reg Anesth Pain Med.* 2003;28:401-405.

Ekatodramis G, Hutter B, Borgeat A. Efficacy of ropivacaine in continuous axillary brachial plexus block. *Reg Anesth Pain Med.* 2000;25:664-665.

El Saied AH, Steyn MP, Ansermino JM. Clonidine prolongs the effect of ropivacaine for axillary brachial plexus blockade. *Can J Anaesth.* 2000;47:962-967.

Erlacher W, Schuschnig C, Koinig H, et al. Clonidine as adjuvant for mepivacaine, ropivacaine and bupivacaine in axillary, perivascular brachial plexus block. *Can J Anaesth.* 2001;48:522-525.

Ertug Z, Yegin A, Ertem S, et al. Comparison of two different techniques for brachial plexus block: infraclavicular versus axillary technique. *Acta Anaesthesiol Scand.* 2005;49:1035-1039.

Finucane BT, Yilling F. Safety of supplementing axillary brachial plexus blocks. *Anesthesiology.* 1989;70:401-403.

Freitag M, Zbieranek K, Gottschalk A, et al. Comparative study of different concentrations of prilocaine and ropivacaine for intraoperative axillary brachial plexus block. *Eur J Anaesthesiol.* 2006;23:481-486.

Fuzier R, Fourcade O, Pianezza A, Gilbert ML, Bounes V, Olivier M. A comparison between double-injection axillary brachial plexus block and midhumeral block for emergency upper limb surgery. *Anesth Analg* 2006;102:1856-1858.

Gianesello L, Pavoni V, Coppini R, et al. Comfort and satisfaction during axillary brachial plexus block in trauma patients: comparison of techniques. *J Clin Anesth.* 2010;22:7-12.

Gonzalez-Suarez S, Pacheco M, Roige J, Puig MM. Comparative study of ropivacaine 0.5% and levobupivacaine 0.33% in axillary brachial plexus block. *Reg Anesth Pain Med.* 2009;34:414–419.

Gradl G, Beyer A, Azad S, Schurmann M. Evaluation of sympathicolysis after continuous brachial plexus analgesia using laser Doppler flowmetry in patients suffering from CRPS I [in German]. *Anasthesiol Intensivmed Notfallmed Schmerzther.* 2005;40:345-349.

Grant CR, Coventry DM. A more logical sequence of nerve location when performing multiple-injection axillary block. *Reg Anesth Pain Med.* 2006;31:483-484.

Gunduz A, Bilir A, Gulec S. Magnesium added to prilocaine prolongs the duration of axillary plexus block. *Reg Anesth Pain Med.* 2006;31:233-236.

Hadžić A, Vloka JD, Kuroda MM, Koorn R, Birnbach DJ. The practice of peripheral nerve blocks in the United States: a national survey [p2e comments]. *Reg Anesth Pain Med.* 1998;23:241-246,

Handoll HH, Koscielniak-Nielsen ZJ. Single, double or multiple injection techniques for axillary brachial plexus block for hand, wrist or forearm surgery. *Cochrane Database Syst Rev.* 2006:CD003842.

Hanouz JL, Grandin W, Lesage A, Oriot G, Bonnieux D, Gerard JL. Multiple injection axillary brachial plexus block: influence of obesity on failure rate and incidence of acute complications. *Anesth Analg.* 2010;111:230-233.

Hebl JR, Horlocker TT, Sorenson EJ, Schroeder DR. Regional anesthesia does not increase the risk of postoperative neuropathy in patients undergoing ulnar nerve transposition. *Anesth Analg.* 2001;93:1606-1611.

Hebl JR, Kopp SL, Schroeder DR, Horlocker TT. Neurologic complications after neuraxial anesthesia or analgesia in patients with preexisting peripheral sensorimotor neuropathy or diabetic polyneuropathy. *Anesth Analg.* 2006;103:1294-1299.

Hepp M, King R. Transarterial technique is significantly slower than the peripheral nerve stimulator technique in achieving successful block. *Reg Anesth Pain Med.* 2000;25:660-661.

Horlocker TT, Kufner RP, Bishop AT, Maxson PM, Schroeder DR. The risk of persistent paresthesia is not increased with repeated axillary block. *Anesth Analg.* 1999;88:382-387.

Jankowski CJ, Keegan MT, Bolton CF, Harrison BA. Neuropathy following axillary brachial plexus block: is it the tourniquet? *Anesthesiology.* 2003;99:1230-1232.

Kaabachi O, Ouezini R, Koubaa W, Ghrab B, Zargouni A, Ben Abdelaziz A. Tramadol as an adjuvant to lidocaine for axillary brachial plexus block. *Anesth Analg.* 2009;108:367-370.

Kang SB, Rumball KM, Ettinger RS. Continuous axillary brachial plexus analgesia in a patient with severe hemophilia. *J Clin Anesth.* 2003;15:38-40.

Karakaya D, Buyukgoz F, Baris S, Guldogus F, Tur A. Addition of fentanyl to bupivacaine prolongs anesthesia and analgesia in axillary brachial plexus block. *Reg Anesth Pain Med.* 2001;26:434-438.

Kefalianakis F, Spohner F. Ultrasound-guided blockade of axillary plexus brachialis for hand surgery [in German]. *Handchir Mikrochir Plast Chir.* 2005;37:344-348.

Kjelstrup T. Transarterial block as an addition to a conventional catheter technique improves the axillary block. *Acta Anaesthesiol Scand.* 2006;50:112-116.

Klaastad O, Smedby O, Thompson GE, et al. Distribution of local anesthetic in axillary brachial plexus block: a clinical and magnetic resonance imaging study. *Anesthesiology.* 2002;96:1315-1324.

Koscielniak-Nielsen Z. Axillary block by double-, triple-, or quadruple-nerve stimulation. *Reg Anesth Pain Med* 2002;27:442-443.

Koscielniak-Nielsen ZJ. Multiple injections in axillary block: where and how many? *Reg Anesth Pain Med.* 2006;31:192-195.

Koscielniak-Nielsen ZJ, Rassmussen H, Jepsen K. Effect of impulse duration on patients' perception of electrical stimulation and block effectiveness during axillary block in unsedated ambulatory patients. *Reg Anesth Pain Med.* 2001;26:428-433.

Koscielniak-Nielsen ZJ, Rasmussen H, Nielsen PT. Patients' perception of pain during axillary and humeral blocks using multiple nerve stimulations. *Reg Anesth Pain Med.* 2004;29:328-332.

Kriwanek KL, Wan J, Beaty JH, Pershad J. Axillary block for analgesia during manipulation of forearm fractures in the pediatric emergency department: a prospective randomized comparative trial. *J Pediatr Orthop.* 2006;26:737-740.

Lanz E, Theiss D, Jankovic D. The extent of blockade following various techniques of brachial plexus block. *Anesth Analg.* 1983;62:55-58.

Lavoie J, Martin R, Tetrault JP, Cote DJ, Colas MJ. Axillary plexus block using a peripheral nerve stimulator: single or multiple injections. *Can J Anaesth.* 1992;39:583-586.

Lim WS, Gammack JK, Van Niekerk J, Dangour AD. Omega 3 fatty acid for the prevention of dementia. *Cochrane Database Syst Rev.* 2006:CD005379.

Lipman ZJ, Isaacson SA. Potentially concerning reason why adding methylprednisolone to local anesthetic may increase the duration of axillary block. *Reg Anesth Pain Med.* 2005;30:114.

Liu HT, Yu YS, Liu CK, et al. Delayed recovery of radial nerve function after axillary block in a patient receiving ipsilateral ulnar nerve transposition surgery. *Acta Anaesthesiol Taiwan.* 2005;43:49-53.

March X, Pardina B, Torres-Bahi S, Navarro M, del Mar Garcia M, Villalonga A. A comparison of a triple-injection axillary brachial plexus block with the humeral approach. *Reg Anesth Pain Med.* 2003;28:504-508.

McCartney CJ, Brull R, Chan VW, et al. Early but no long-term benefit of regional compared with general anesthesia for ambulatory hand surgery. *Anesthesiology.* 2004;101:461-467.

McCartney CJ, Duggan E, Apatu E. Should we add clonidine to local anesthetic for peripheral nerve blockade? A qualitative systematic review of the literature. *Reg Anesth Pain Med.* 2007;32:330-338.

Mezzatesta JP, Scott DA, Schweitzer SA, Selander DE. Continuous axillary brachial plexus block for postoperative pain relief. Intermittent bolus versus continuous infusion. *Reg Anesth.* 1997;22:357-362.

Moon JK. Dissociation of paresthesia, motor response, and success of axillary block—another factor besides needle proximity. *Reg Anesth Pain Med.* 2002;27:332-333.

Moorthy SS, Dill DW. Tremor of the forearm during performance of axillary brachial plexus block. *Reg Anesth Pain Med.* 2004;29:510.

Movafegh A, Nouralishahi B, Sadeghi M, Nabavian O. An ultra-low dose of naloxone added to lidocaine or lidocaine-fentanyl mixture prolongs axillary brachial plexus blockade. *Anesth Analg.* 2009;109:1679-1683.

Niemi TT, Salmela L, Aromaa U, Poyhia R, Rosenberg PH. Single-injection brachial plexus anesthesia for arteriovenous fistula surgery of the forearm: a comparison of infraclavicular coracoid and axillary approach. *Reg Anesth Pain Med.* 2007;32:55-59.

Partridge BL, Katz J, Benirschke K. Functional anatomy of the brachial plexus sheath: implications for anesthesia. *Anesthesiology.* 1987;66:743-747.

Perlas A, Niazi A, McCartney C, Chan V, Xu D, Abbas S. The sensitivity of motor response to nerve stimulation and paresthesia for nerve localization as evaluated by ultrasound. *Reg Anesth Pain Med.* 2006;31:445-450.

Popping DM, Elia N, Marret E, Wenk M, Tramer MR. Clonidine as an adjuvant to local anesthetics for peripheral nerve and plexus blocks: a meta-analysis of randomized trials. *Anesthesiology.* 2009;111:406-415.

Reuben SS, Pristas R, Dixon D, Faruqi S, Madabhushi L, Wenner S. The incidence of complex regional pain syndrome after fasciectomy for Dupuytren's contracture: a prospective observational study of four anesthetic techniques. *Anesth Analg.* 2006;102:499-503.

Reuben SS, Steinberg RB. Continuous shoulder analgesia via an indwelling axillary brachial plexus catheter. *J Clin Anesth.* 2000;12:472-475.

Rodriguez J, Taboada M, Del Rio S, Barcena M, Alvarez J. A comparison of four stimulation patterns in axillary block. *Reg Anesth Pain Med.* 2005;30:324-348.

Rodriguez J, Taboada M, Oliveira J, Ulloa B, Bascuas B, Alvarez J. Radial plus musculocutaneous nerve stimulation for axillary block is inferior to triple nerve stimulation with 2% mepivacaine. *J Clin Anesth.* 2008;20:253-256.

Rodriguez J, Taboada M, Valino C, Barcena M, Alvarez J. A comparison of stimulation patterns in axillary block: part 2. *Reg Anesth Pain Med.* 2006;31:202-205.

Salonen MH, Haasio J, Bachmann M, Xu M, Rosenberg PH. Evaluation of efficacy and plasma concentrations of ropivacaine in continuous axillary brachial plexus block: high dose for surgical anesthesia and low dose for postoperative analgesia. *Reg Anesth Pain Med.* 2000;25:47-51.

Schroeder LE, Horlocker TT, Schroeder DR. The efficacy of axillary block for surgical procedures about the elbow. *Anesth Analg.* 1996;83:747-751.

Schwemmer U, Schleppers A, Markus C, Kredel M, Kirschner S, Roewer N. Operative management in axillary brachial plexus blocks: comparison of ultrasound and nerve stimulation [in German]. *Anaesthesist.* 2006;55:451-456.

Selander D. Catheter technique in axillary plexus block. Presentation of a new method. *Acta Anaesthesiol Scand.* 1977;21:324-329.

Selander D. Axillary plexus block: paresthetic or perivascular. *Anesthesiology.* 1987;66:726-728.

Serradell A, Herrero R, Villanueva JA, Santos JA, Moncho JM, Masdeu J. Comparison of three different volumes of mepivacaine in axillary plexus block using multiple nerve stimulation. *Br J Anaesth.* 2003;91:519-524.

Sia S. Peripheral nerve stimulation and axillary brachial plexus block. *Reg Anesth Pain Med.* 2002;27:327; author reply 327-328.

Sia S. A comparison of injection at the ulnar and the radial nerve in axillary block using triple stimulation. *Reg Anesth Pain Med.* 2006;31:514-518.

Sia S, Bartoli M. Selective ulnar nerve localization is not essential for axillary brachial plexus block using a multiple nerve stimulation technique. *Reg Anesth Pain Med.* 2001;26:12-16.

Sia S, Lepri A, Magherini M, Doni L, Di Marco P, Gritti G. A comparison of proximal and distal radial nerve motor responses in axillary block using triple stimulation. *Reg Anesth Pain Med.* 2005;30:458-463.

Sia S, Lepri A, Marchi M. Axillary block by "selective" injections at the nerves involved in surgery using a peripheral nerve stimulator: a comparison with a "standard" triple-injection technique. *Reg Anesth Pain Med.* 2010;35:22-27.

Sia S, Lepri A, Ponzecchi P. Axillary brachial plexus block using peripheral nerve stimulator: a comparison between double- and triple-injection techniques. *Reg Anesth Pain Med.* 2001;26:499-503.

Stan T, Goodman EJ, Bravo-Fernandez C, Holbrook CR. Adding methylprednisolone to local anesthetic increases the duration of axillary block. *Reg Anesth Pain Med.* 2004;29:380-381.

Stan TC, Krantz MA, Solomon DL, Poulos JG, Chaouki K. The incidence of neurovascular complications following axillary brachial plexus block using a transarterial approach. A prospective study of 1,000 consecutive patients. *Reg Anesth.* 1995;20:486-492.

Theroux MC, Dixit D, Brislin R, Como-Fluero S, Sacks K. Axillary catheter for brachial plexus analgesia in children for postoperative pain control and rigorous physiotherapy—a simple and effective procedure. *Paediatr Anaesth.* 2007;17:302-303.

Thompson GE. Some historical perspectives on axillary plexus block. *Reg Anesth Pain Med.* 2002;27:333.

Thompson GE, Rorie DK. Functional anatomy of the brachial plexus sheaths. *Anesthesiology.* 1983;59:117-122.

van den Berg B, Berger A, van den Berg E, Zenz M, Brehmeier G, Tizian C. Continuous plexus anesthesia to improve circulation in peripheral microvascular interventions [in German]. *Handchir Mikrochir Plast Chir.* 1983;15:101-104.

Wang LK, Chen HP, Chang PJ, Kang FC, Tsai YC. Axillary brachial plexus block with patient controlled analgesia for complex regional pain syndrome type I: a case report. *Reg Anesth Pain Med.* 2001;26:68-71.

Winnie A. Perivascular techniques of brachial plexus blocks. In: *Plexus Anesthesia.* Vol 1. Edinburgh, UK: Churchill-Livingstone; 1984.

Winnie AP, Radonjic R, Akkineni SR, Durrani Z. Factors influencing distribution of local anesthetic injected into the brachial plexus sheath. *Anesth Analg.* 1979;58:225-234.

Woods RK, Thien FC, Abramson MJ. Dietary marine fatty acids (fish oil) for asthma in adults and children. *Cochrane Database Syst Rev.* 2002:CD001283.

Zeidan AM. Unilateral tremor of the upper and lower limb after an axillary brachial plexus block. *Reg Anesth Pain Med.* 2005;30:308.

# 16 Wrist Block

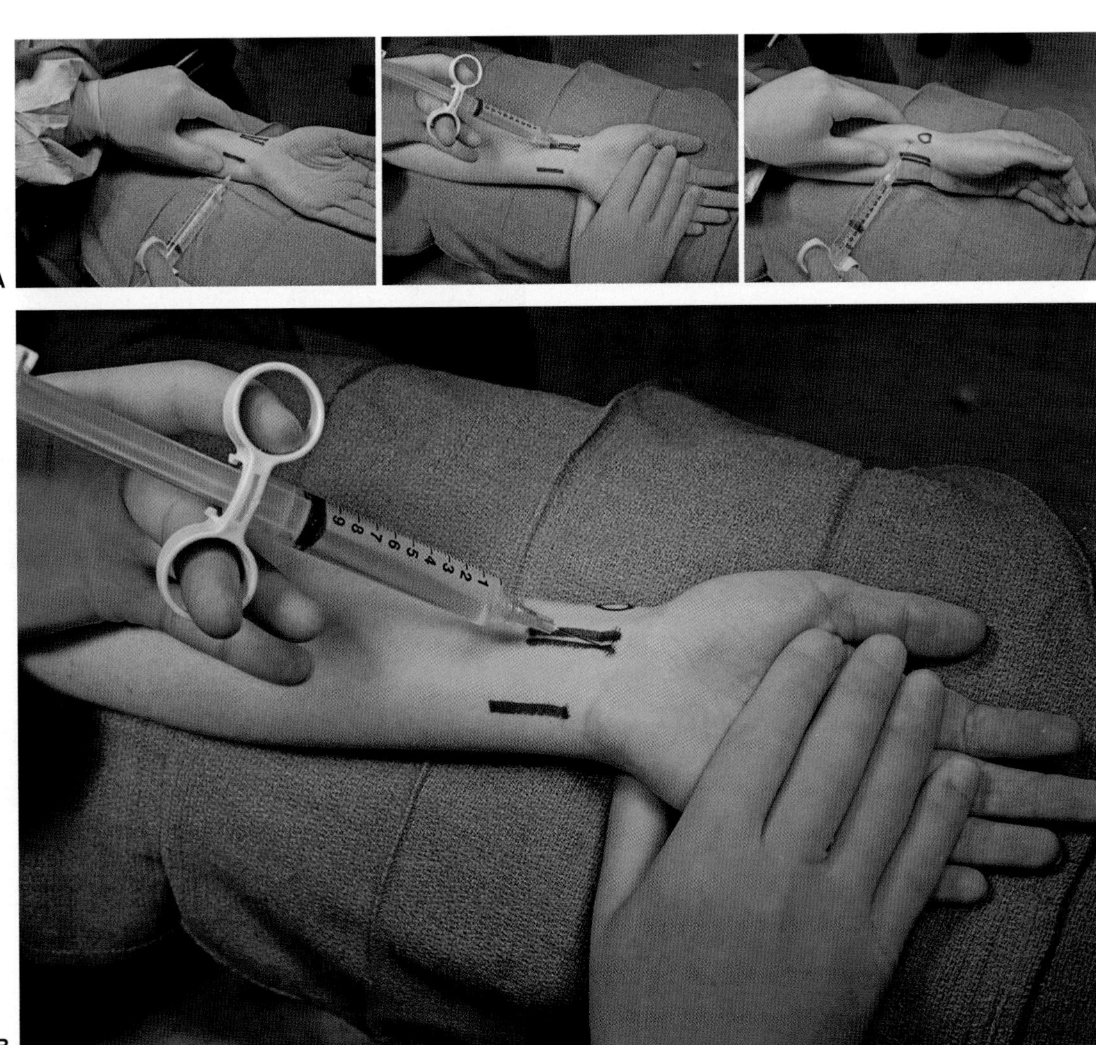

## BLOCK AT A GLANCE

- Indications: surgery on the hand and fingers
- Nerves: radial, ulnar, median
- Local anesthetic: 5 mL for median and ulnar nerve, 10 mL for radial nerve
- Never use an epinephrine-containing local anesthetic

**FIGURE 16-1.** (A) Technique to accomplish a wrist block. (B) Median nerve block. Needle is inserted medial or lateral to the flexor palmaris longus tendon and carefully advanced to avoid paresthesia. Then 5 mL of local anesthetic is injected.

## General Considerations

A wrist block consists of anesthetizing the terminal branches of the ulnar, median, and radial nerves at the level of the wrist. It is an infiltration technique that is simple to perform, essentially devoid of systemic complications, and highly effective for a variety of procedures on the hand and fingers. The relative simplicity, low risk of complications, and high efficacy of the procedure mandates this block to be a standard part of the armamentarium of an anesthesiologist. Several different techniques of wrist blockade and their modifications are in clinical use; in this chapter, however, we describe the one most commonly used at our institution. Wrist blocks are used often for carpal tunnel and hand and finger surgery.

## Functional Anatomy

Innervation of the hand is shared by the ulnar, median, and radial nerves (Figure 16-2 and 16-3). The ulnar nerve provides sensory innervation to the skin of the fifth digit and the medial half of the fourth digit, and to the corresponding area of the palm. The same area is covered on the corresponding dorsal side of the hand. Motor branches innervate the three hypothenar muscles, the medial two lumbrical muscles, the palmaris brevis muscle, all the interossei, and the adductor pollicis muscle. The median nerve traverses the carpal tunnel and terminates as digital and recurrent branches. The digital branches supply the skin of the lateral three and a half digits and the corresponding area of the palm. Motor branches supply the two lateral lumbricals and the three thenar muscles (recurrent median branch).

Although there is significant variability in the innervation of the ring and middle fingers, the skin on the anterior surface of the thumb is always supplied by the median nerve and that of the 5th finger by the ulnar nerve. The palmar digital branches of the median and ulnar nerves also innervate the nail beds of the respective digits.

The radial nerve lies on the anterior aspect of the radial side of the forearm. About 7 cm above the wrist, the nerve deviates from the artery and emerges from the deep fascia, dividing into medial and lateral branches to supply sensation to the dorsum of the thumb and the dorsum of the hand (the first three and one-half digits as far as the distal interphalangeal joint).

## Distribution of Blockade

Blocking the ulnar, median, and radial nerves results in anesthesia of the entire hand. The nerve contribution to innervation of the hand varies considerably; Figure 16-3 shows the most common arrangement.

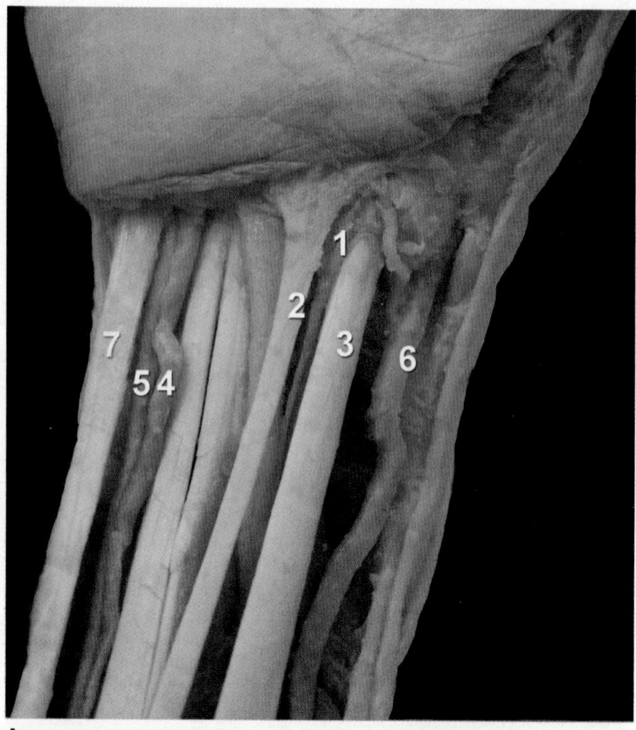


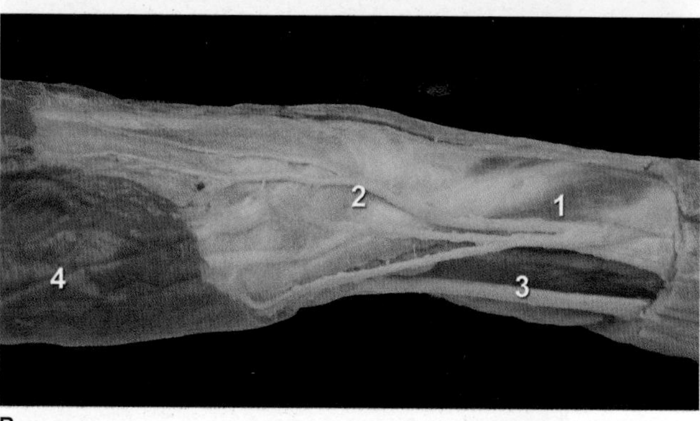


**FIGURE 16-2.** (A) Anatomy of the right wrist. 1 median nerve. 2 flexor palmaris longus. 3 flexor carpi radialis. 4 ulnar artery. 5 Ulnar nerve. 6 radial artery 7 flexor carpi ulnaris. (B) Anatomy of the right superficial radial nerve. 1 superficial radial nerve. 2 radial styloid. 3 flexor carpi radialis tendon. 4 thumb.

## Equipment

A standard regional anesthesia tray is prepared with the following equipment:

- Sterile towels and gauze packs
- Two 10-mL syringes containing local anesthetic
- A 1.5-inch, 25-gauge needle

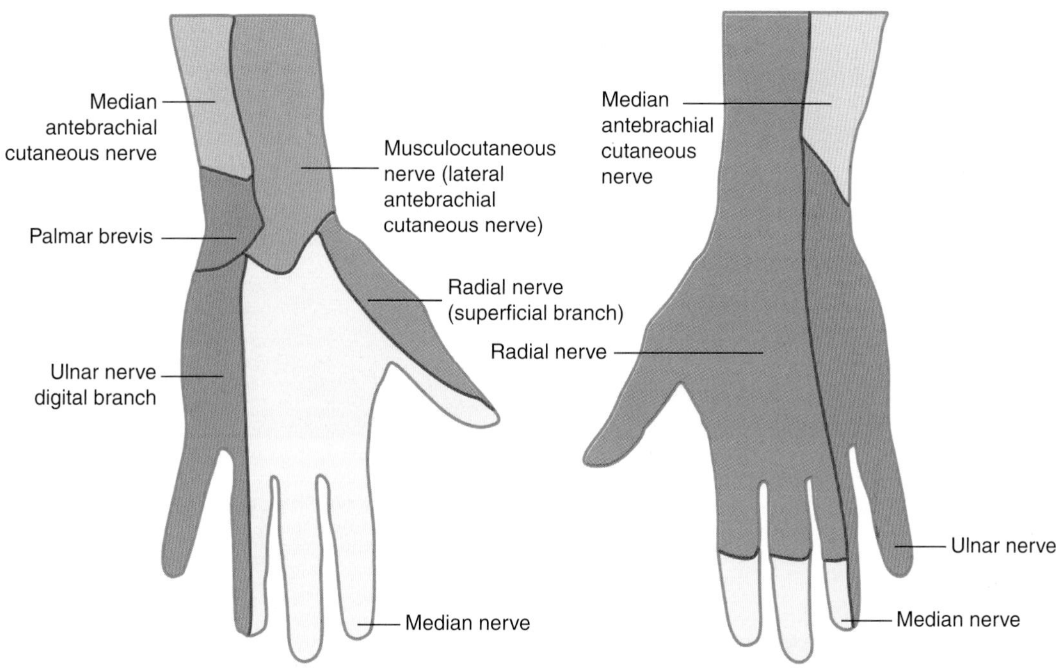


**FIGURE 16-3.** Cutaneous innervation of the left hand.

## Landmarks and Patient Positioning

The patient is positioned supine, with the arm in abduction. The wrist is best kept in slight extension.

### Maneuvers to Facilitate Landmark Identification

The superficial branch of the radial nerve emerges from between the tendon of the brachioradialis and the radius just proximal to the easily palpable styloid process of the radius (circle) (Figure 16-4). Then it divides into the medial and lateral branches, which continue subcutaneously on the dorsum of the thumb and hand. Several of the branches pass superficially over the anatomic "snuffbox."

The median nerve is located between the tendons of the flexor palmaris longus (white arrow) and the flexor carpi radialis (red arrow) (Figure 16-5A and B). The flexor palmaris longus tendon is usually the more prominent of the two, and it can be accentuated by asking the patient to oppose the thumb and 5th finger while flexing the wrist (Figure 16-6); the median nerve passes just lateral to it. The ulnar nerve passes between the ulnar artery and tendon of the flexor carpi ulnaris (Figure 16-7). The tendon of flexor carpi ulnaris is superficial to the ulnar nerve.

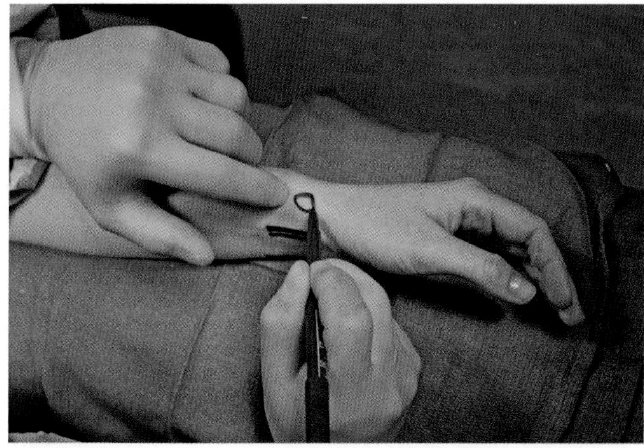

**FIGURE 16-4.** Palpation of the radial styloid. The superficial radial nerve is blocked by an injection just proximal to the styloid.

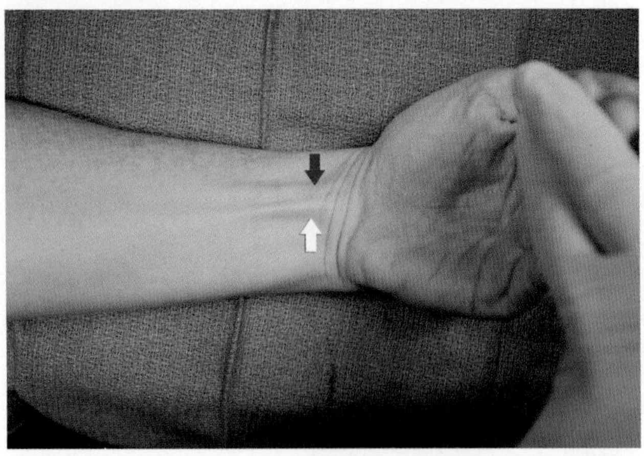
A

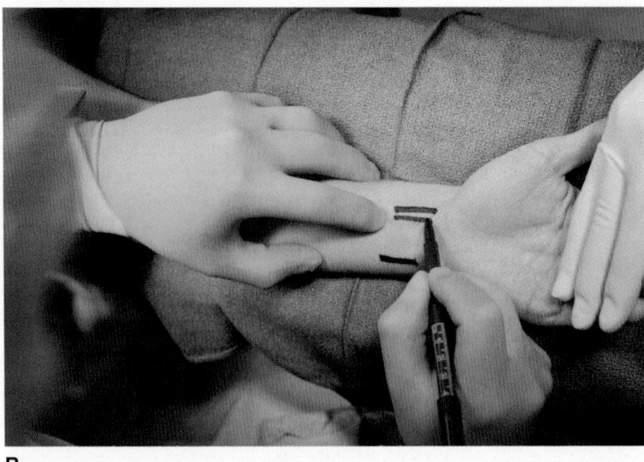
B

**FIGURE 16-5.** A maneuver to accentuate the tendons of the flexors of the wrist. (A) Shown are flexor palmaris longus (white arrow) and flexor carpi radialis (red arrow) tendons. (B) Outlining flexor palmaris longus tendon.

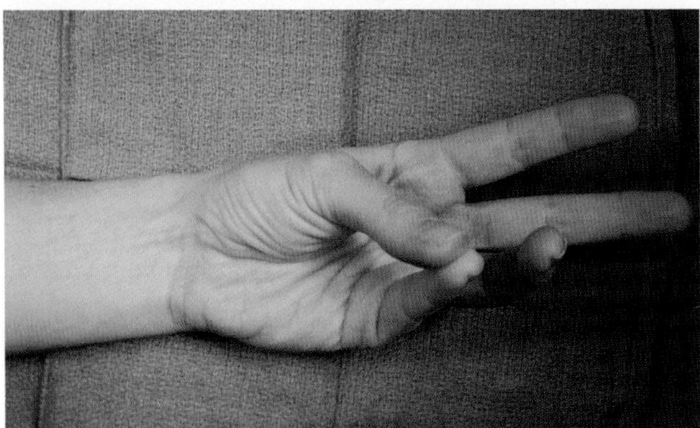

**FIGURE 16-6.** The flexor palmaris longus tendon can be accentuated by asking the patient to oppose the thumb and fifth finger while flexing the wrist.

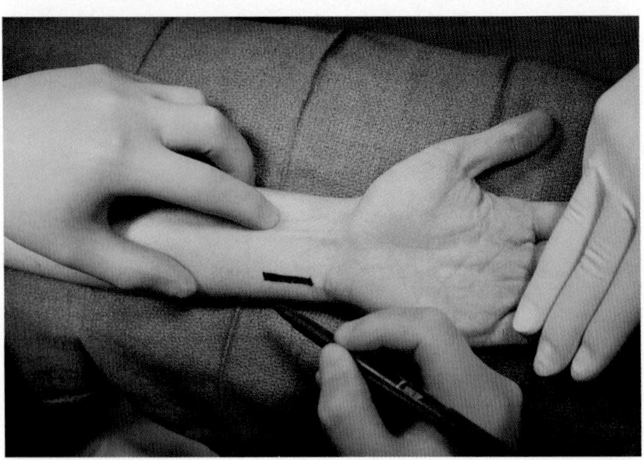

**FIGURE 16-7.** Outlining flexor carpi ulnaris tendon.

**TIP**

- The position of the radial nerve in relationship to the radial artery often is confusing to trainees. The illustration in Figure 16-8 clarifies the course of the radial nerve branches at the wrist.

## Technique

The entire surface of the wrist and palm should be disinfected.

### Block of the Ulnar Nerve

The ulnar nerve is anesthetized by inserting the needle under the tendon of the flexor carpi ulnaris muscle close to its distal attachment just above the styloid process of the ulna. The needle is advanced 5 to 10 mm to just past the tendon of the flexor carpi ulnaris (Figure 16-9A). After negative aspiration, 3 to 5 mL of local anesthetic solution is injected. A subcutaneous injection of 2 to 3 mL of local anesthesia just above the tendon of the flexor carpi ulnaris is advisable for blocking the cutaneous branches of the ulnar nerve, which often extend to the hypothenar area.

### Block of the Median Nerve

The median nerve is blocked by inserting the needle between the tendons of the flexor palmaris longus and flexor carpi radialis (Figure 16-9B). The needle is inserted until it pierces the deep fascia, and 3 to 5 mL of local anesthetic is injected.

**FIGURE 16-8.** Common arrangement of superficial branches of the radial nerve.

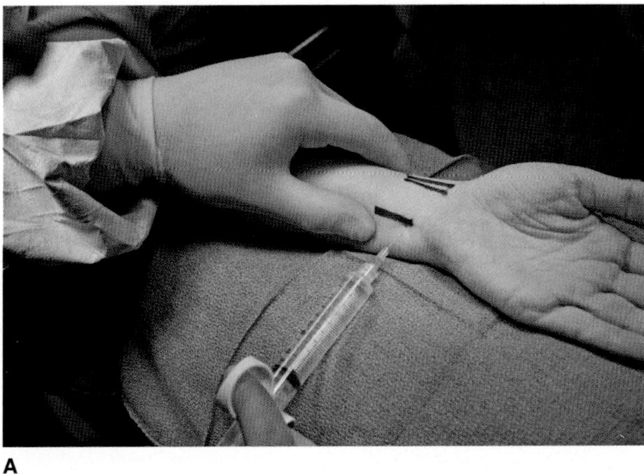

A

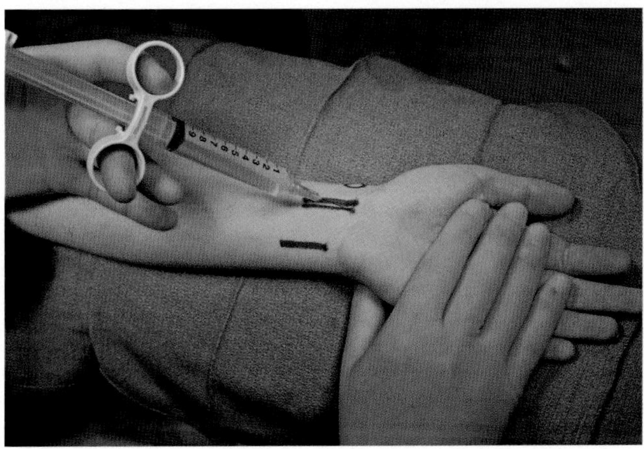

B

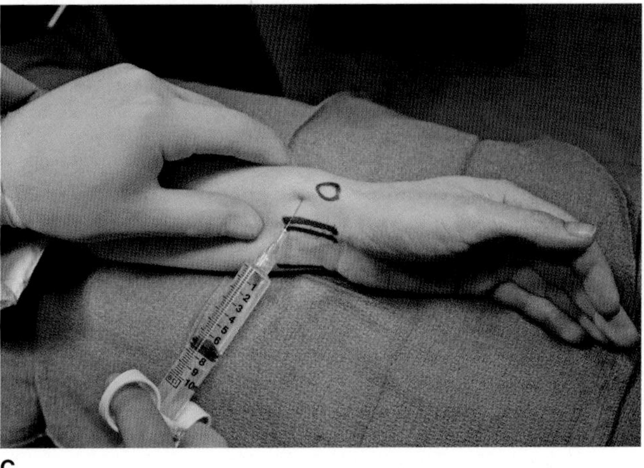

C

**FIGURE 16-9.** (A) Ulnar nerve block. The needle is inserted just medial to and underneath the flexor carpi ulnaris tendon to inject local anesthetic in the immediate proximity of the ulnar artery. (B) Median nerve block. The needle is inserted medial or lateral to the flexor palmaris longus tendon and carefully advanced to avoid paresthesia. Then 5 mL of local anesthetic is injected. (C) Radial nerve block. The superficial branches of the radial nerve are blocked by a subcutaneous injection of local anesthetic in a circular fashion. The injection is made proximal to the radial styloid head (circle).

Although piercing of the deep fascia has been described to result in a fascial "click," it is more reliable to simply insert the needle until it contacts the bone. The needle is withdrawn 2 to 3 mm, and the local anesthetic is injected.

### Block of the Radial Nerve

The radial nerve block is essentially a "field block" and requires more extensive infiltration because of its less predictable anatomic location and division into multiple smaller cutaneous branches. Five milliliters of local anesthetic should be injected subcutaneously just proximal to the radial styloid, aiming medially. Then the infiltration is extended laterally, using an additional 5 mL of local anesthetic (Figure 16-9C).

### TIPS

- A "fan" technique is recommended to increase the success rate of the median nerve block. After the initial injection, the needle is withdrawn back to skin level, redirected 30° laterally, and advanced again to contact the bone. After pulling back the needle 1 to 2 mm from the bone, an additional 2 mL of local anesthetic is injected. A similar procedure is repeated with medial redirection of the needle.
- Paresthesia in the median nerve distribution warrants a 1- to 2-mm withdrawal of the needle, followed by a slow measured injection of the local anesthetic. If paresthesia worsens or persists, the needle should be removed and reinserted.

## Block Dynamics and Perioperative Management

The wrist block technique is associated with moderate patient discomfort because multiple insertions and subcutaneous injections are required. Appropriate sedation and analgesia (midazolam 2–4 mg and alfentanil 250–500 μg) are useful to ensure the patient's comfort. A typical onset time for a wrist block is 10 to 15 minutes, depending on the concentration and volume of local anesthetic used. Sensory anesthesia of the skin develops faster than the motor block. Placement of an Esmarch bandage or a tourniquet at the level of the wrist is well tolerated and does not require additional blockade.

## Complications and How to Avoid Them

Complications following a wrist block are typically limited to residual paresthesias due to inadvertent intraneural injection. Systemic toxicity is rare because of the distal location of the blockade and the relatively small volumes of local anesthetics (Table 16-1).

**TABLE 16-1 Complications of Wrist Block and Techniques to Avoid Them**

| | |
|---|---|
| ***Infection*** | • Should be very rare with the use of an aseptic technique. |
| ***Hematoma*** | • Avoid multiple needle insertions.<br>• Use a 25-gauge needle and avoid puncturing superficial veins. |
| ***Vascular complications*** | • Do not use epinephrine for wrist and finger blocks. |
| ***Nerve injury*** | • Do not inject when the patient complains of pain or high pressure is detected on injection. |
| ***Other*** | • Instruct the patient on care of the insensate hand. |

# WRIST BLOCK

**Patient position:**

Supine, arm abducted with the wrist kept in slight extension

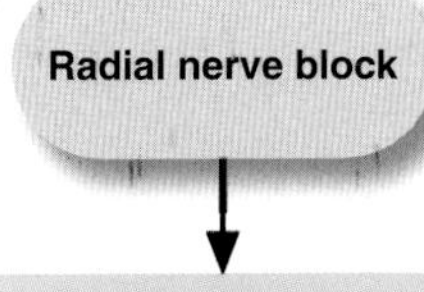


**Anatomic landmark:**
- The radial styloid

→

- Inject 5 mL of LA subcutaneously immediately proximal to radial styloid aiming first medially over the wrist crease.

→

Extend the infiltration by injecting an additional 5 mL of LA laterally, on the dorsal aspect of the wrist.

---

**Ulnar nerve block**

Anatomic landmarks:
- The ulnar styloid
- Tendon of flexor carpi ulnaris
- Pulse of ulnar artery

→

- Advance needle 0.5–1 cm past the tendon of flexor carpi ulnaris in the vicinity of ulnar artery pulse
- After negative aspiration, 3–5 mL of LA is injected.

→

Inject another 2–3 mL of LA subcutaneously just above tendon of flexor carpi ulnaris to block the cutaneous branches of the nerve.

---

**Median nerve block**

Anatomic landmarks:
- Tendon of flexor palmaris longus
- Tendon of flexor carpi radialis

→

- Insert needle in between the two landmarks until it contacts bone
- Withdraw the needle 2–3 mm after bone contact
- Inject 3–5 mL of LA

→

- If paresthesia occurs, withdraw needle 1- to 2-mm followed by slow measured injection of LA.

## SUGGESTED READINGS

Brown DL, Bridenbaugh LD. The upper extremity: somatic block. In: Cousins MJ, Bridenbaugh PO, eds. *Neuronal Blockade in Clinical Anesthesia and Management of Pain.* Philadelphia, PA: Lippincott-Raven, 1988;345-371.

Delaunay L, Chelly JE. Blocks at the wrist provide effective anesthesia for carpal tunnel release. *Can J Anaesth.* 2001;48:656-660.

Derkash RS, Weaver JK, Berkeley ME, Dawson D. Office carpal tunnel release with wrist block and wrist tourniquet. *Orthopedics.* 1996;19:589-590.

Gebhard RE, Al-Samsam T, Greger J, Khan A, Chelly JE. Distal nerve blocks at the wrist for outpatient carpal tunnel surgery offer intraoperative cardiovascular stability and reduce discharge time. *Anesth Analg.* 2002;95:351-355.

Hahn MB, McQuillan PM, Sheplock GJ. *Regional Anesthesia: An Atlas of Anatomy and Techniques.* St. Louis, MO: Mosby; 1996.

McCahon R, Bedforth N. Peripheral nerve block at the elbow and wrist. *Contin Ed Anaesth Crit Care Pain.* 2007;7:42-44.

Mulroy MF. *Regional Anesthesia: An Illustrated Procedural Guide.* 3rd ed. Philadelphia, PA: Lippincott; 2002.

Ramamurthy S, Hickey R. Anesthesia. In: Green DP, Hotchkiss RN, eds. *Operative Hand Surgery.* New York, NY: Churchill Livingstone, 1993;25-52.

# 17 Cutaneous Nerve Blocks of the Upper Extremity

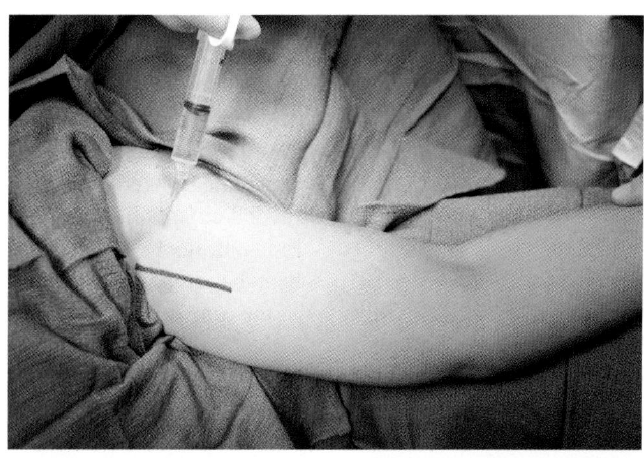

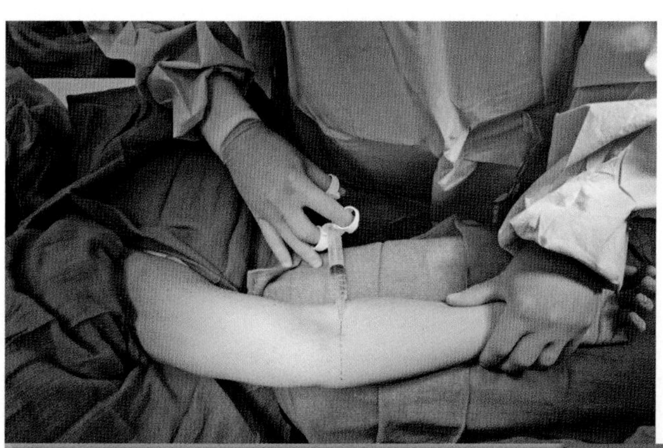

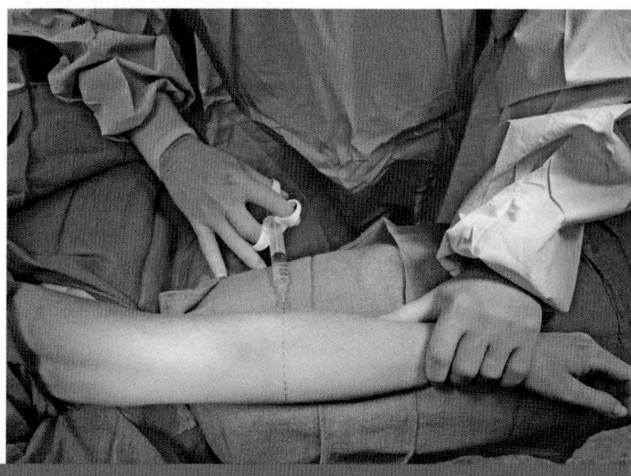

## BLOCK AT A GLANCE

- Indications: mostly used as a supplement to major blocks of the upper extremity
- Local anesthetic: 5–10 mL

**FIGURE 17-1.** Techniques to block the cutaneous nerves of the upper extremity.

##  General Considerations

Cutaneous nerve blocks of the upper extremity are used mainly as a supplement to brachial plexus blocks. These blocks are simple to learn and perform. They are essentially devoid of complications and can be useful as complements to major conduction blocks of the upper extremity. Their judicious use can be used for superficial surgery or to help salvage an incomplete brachial plexus block. The techniques discussed in this chapter focus primarily on the blocks that are most useful clinically: blocks of the intercostobrachial nerve and the medial and lateral cutaneous nerves of the forearm, Figure 17-1.

##  Functional Anatomy

Cutaneous nerve blockade is achieved by the injection of local anesthetic into the subcutaneous layers above the muscle fascia. The subcutaneous tissue contains a variable amount of fat, superficial nerves, and vessels. Deeper, there is a tough membranous layer, the deep fascia of the upper extremity, which encloses the muscles of the arm and forearm. Numerous superficial nerves and vessels penetrate the deep fascia.

The cutaneous innervation of the upper extremity originates from the superficial cervical plexus, the brachial plexus, and the intercostal nerves (Table 17-1; Figure 17-2A and B). Familiarity with their relevant anatomy is important to avoid sparing of cutaneous anesthesia during a nerve block procedure. For example, a brachial plexus block does not anesthetize the intercostobrachial nerve, a branch of T2 that is responsible for sensation of the skin of the proximal medial arm. Failure to supplement this may result in discomfort at skin incision during upper extremity surgery. Similarly, a single-injection axillary brachial plexus block typically does not cover the musculocutaneous nerve (and its terminal branch, the lateral cutaneous nerve of the forearm). A cutaneous block of this terminal branch is a more distal alternative to a musculocutaneous nerve block that provides the same sensory anesthesia.

##  Intercostobrachial Nerve Block

### Anatomy

The intercostobrachial nerve is the lateral cutaneous branch of the ventral primary ramus of T2. It provides innervation to the skin of the axilla and the medial aspect of the proximal arm. The intercostobrachial nerve communicates with the medial cutaneous nerve of the arm, which is a branch of the brachial plexus (Figure 17-3). Both nerves are anesthetized by subcutaneous infiltration of the skin of the medial aspect of the arm.

### Indications

Blocks of these nerves are typically combined with brachial plexus block to achieve more complete anesthesia of the upper arm.

### Technique

A 1.5-in, 25-gauge needle is inserted at the level of the axillary fossa (Figure 17-4A). The entire width of the medial aspect of the arm is infiltrated with local anesthetic to raise a subcutaneous wheal of anesthesia.

**TABLE 17-1 Origin of the Cutaneous Nerves of the Upper Extremity**

| SUPERFICIAL CERVICAL PLEXUS | BRACHIAL PLEXUS | INTERCOSTAL NERVES |
|---|---|---|
| Supraclavicular nerves | Superior lateral cutaneous nerve of arm | Intercostobrachial nerve (T2 and occasionally T3) |
| | Posterior cutaneous nerve of the arm | |
| | Posterior cutaneous nerve of the forearm | |
| | Medial cutaneous nerve of the forearm | |
| | Lateral cutaneous nerve of the forearm (musculocutaneous nerve) | |
| | Superficial radial nerve | |
| | Dorsal cutaneous branch of the ulnar nerve | |
| | Palmar cutaneous branch of the median nerve | |

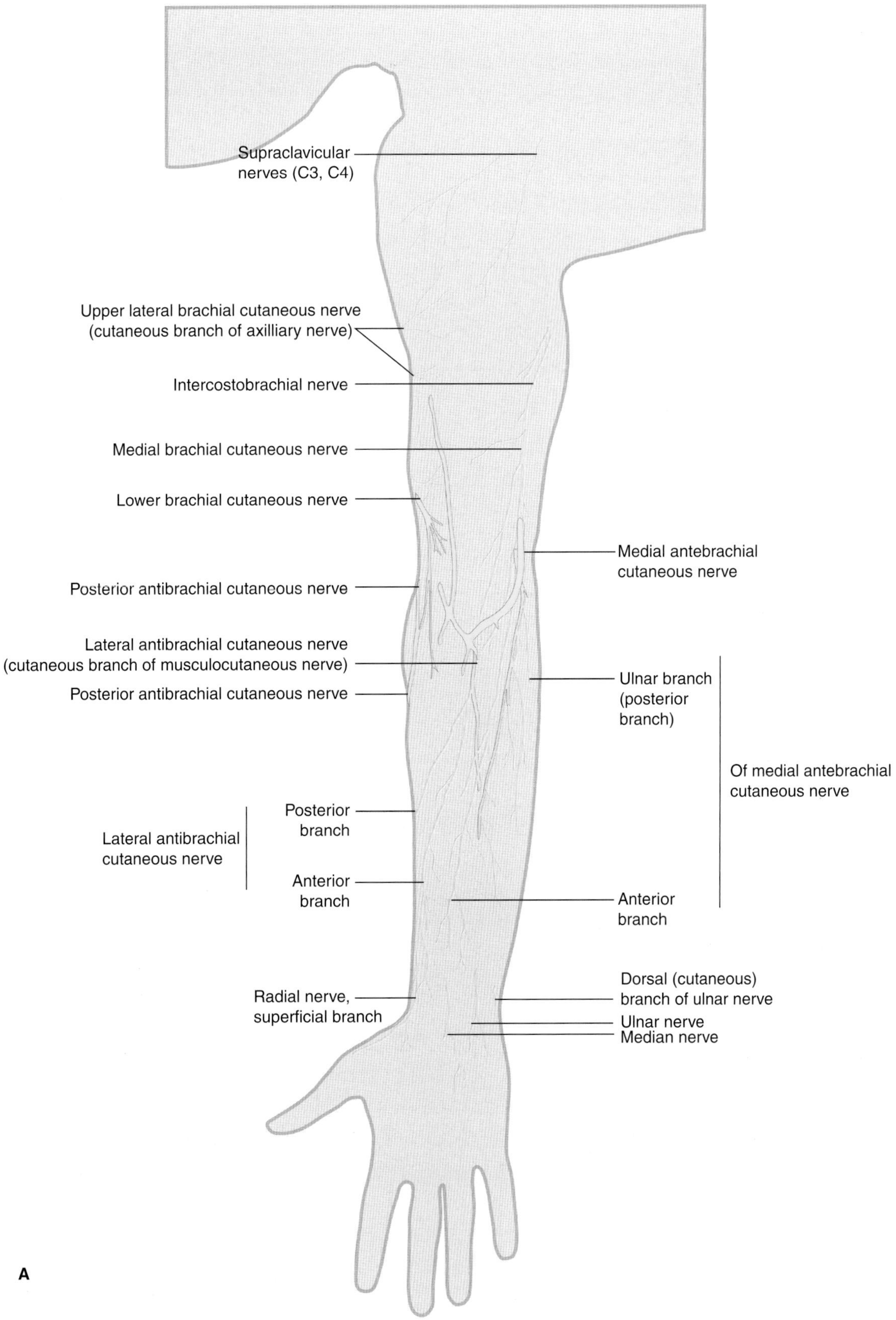

**FIGURE 17-2.** (A) Cutaneous innervation of the upper extremity (front).

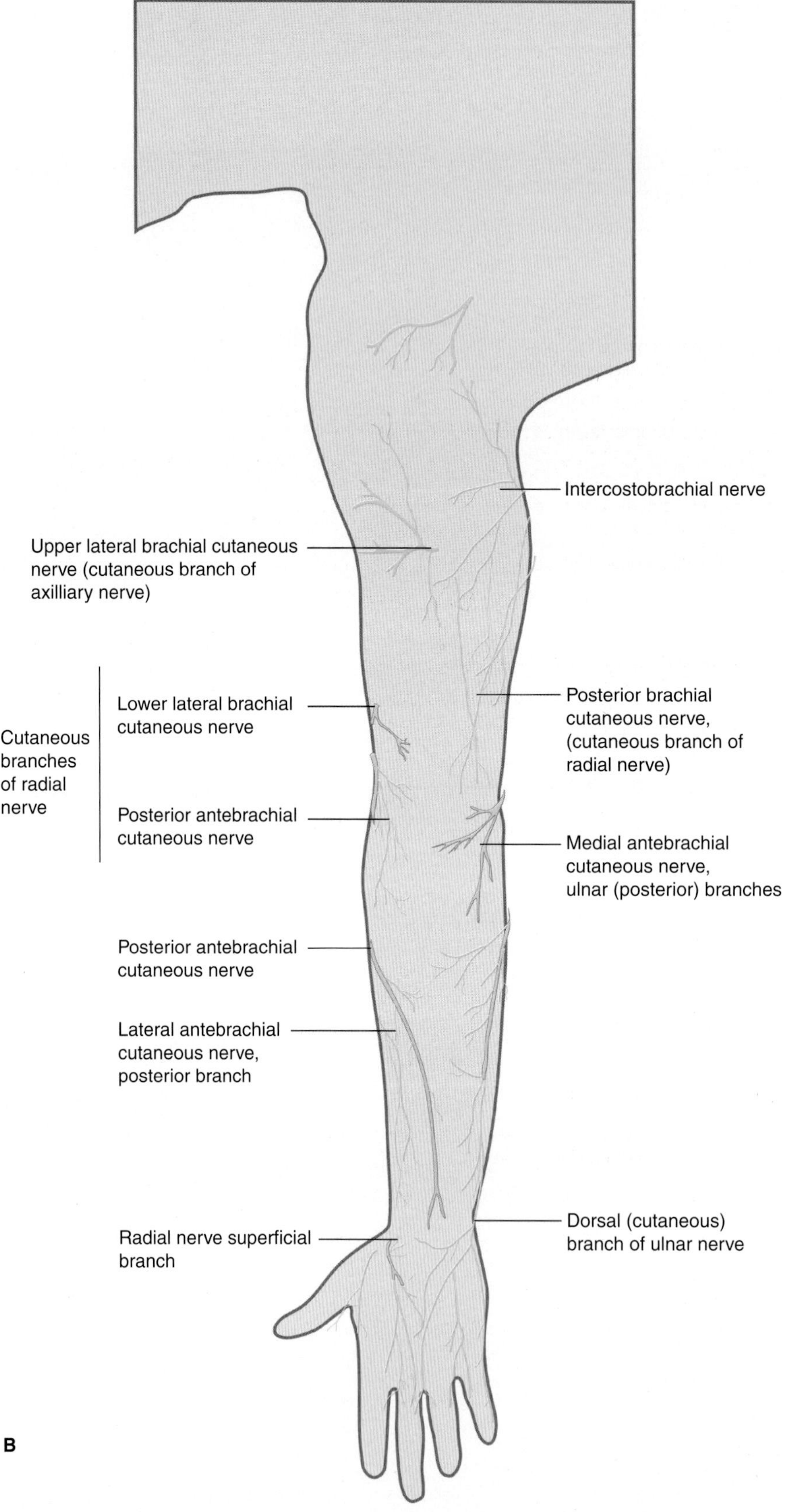


**FIGURE. 17-2.** (B) Cutaneous innervation of the upper extremity (back).

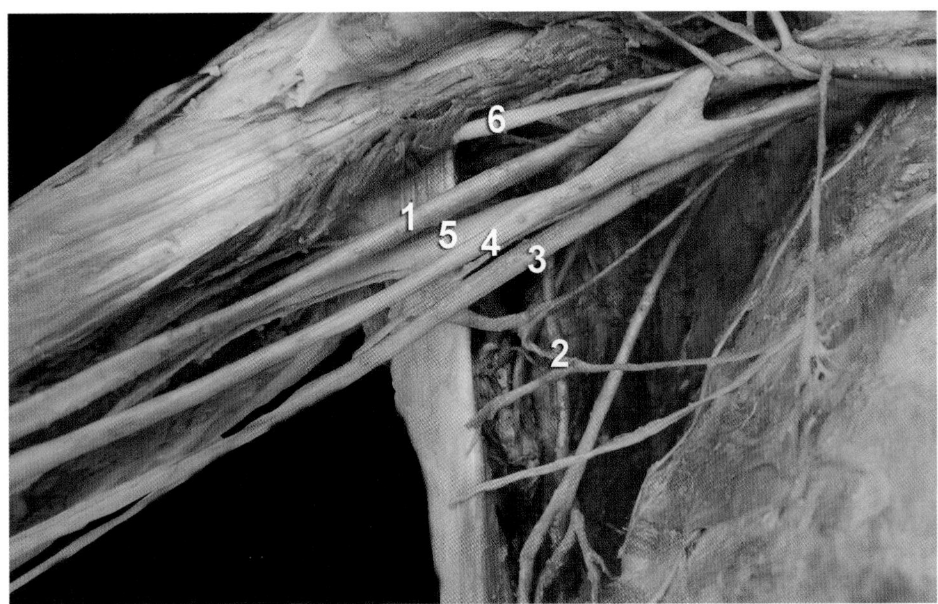


**FIGURE 17-3.** Anatomy of the terminal nerves of the upper extremity at the level of the axillary fossa. ❶ axillary artery. ❷ intercostobrachial nerve. ❸ ulnar nerve. ❹ median nerve. ❺ radial nerve. ❻ musculocutaneous nerve.

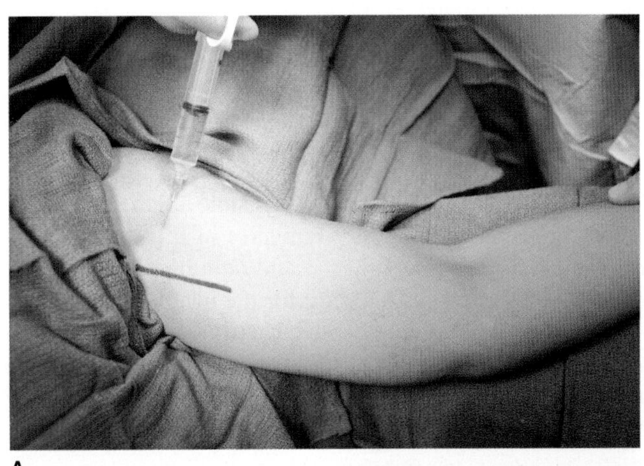

A

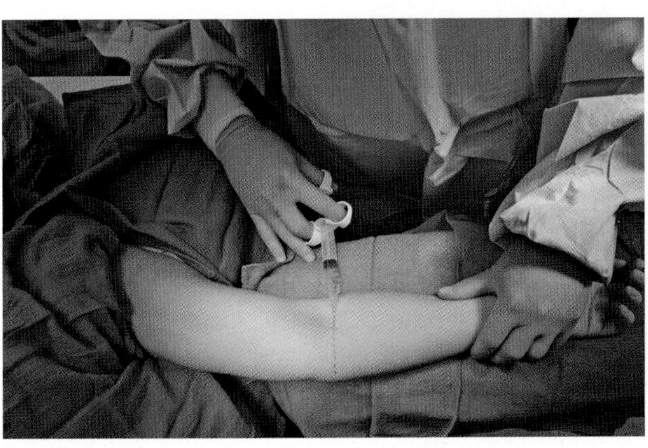

B

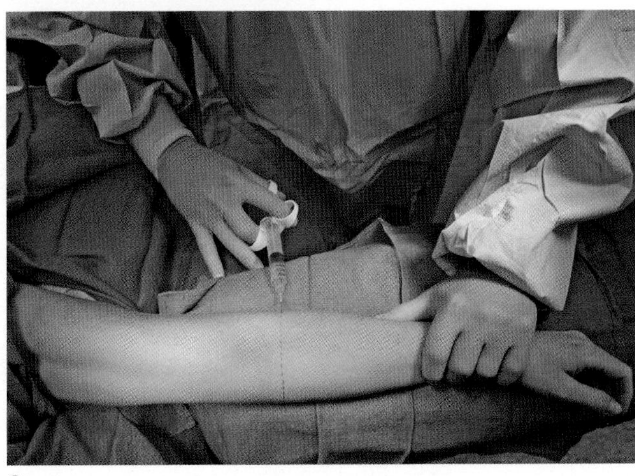

C

**FIGURE 17-4.** (A) Block of the intercostobrachial nerve. (B) Block of the medial cutaneous nerve of the forearm. (C) Block of the lateral cutaneous nerve of the forearm.

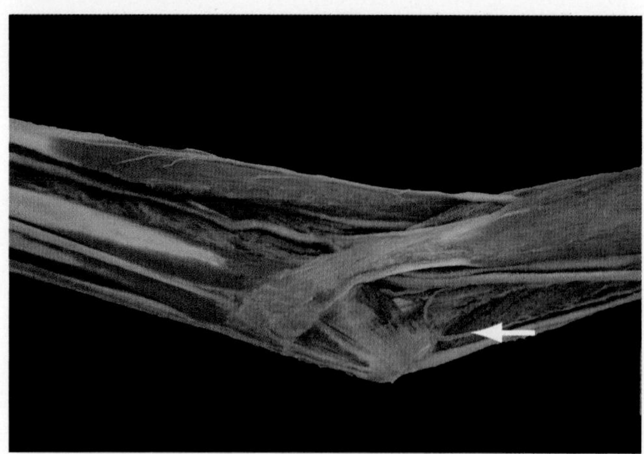

**FIGURE 17-5.** Medial cutaneous nerve of the arm (arrow).

## Medial Cutaneous Nerve of the Forearm Block

### Anatomy

The medial cutaneous nerve of the forearm originates within the medial cord. This nerve supplies branches to the skin of the medial side of the forearm (Figure 17-5).

### Indications

The medial antebrachial cutaneous nerve is blocked by infiltration of local anesthetic into the subcutaneous tissue on the anteromedial and dorsomedial surfaces of the forearm just below the elbow crease. Along with blockade of the lateral antebrachial cutaneous nerve, this block is appropriate for the insertion of an arteriovenous graft on the forearm or other superficial procedures on the volar surface of the forearm.

### Technique

A 1.5-in, 25-gauge needle is used to infiltrate local anesthetic subcutaneously over the entire medial aspect of the arm just below the elbow crease (Figure 17-4B).

## Lateral Cutaneous Nerve of the Forearm Block

### Anatomy

The lateral cutaneous nerve of the forearm is a cutaneous extension of the musculocutaneous nerve, which originates from C5 through C7 and separates from the brachial plexus off the lateral cord. The musculocutaneous nerve runs through the bodies of the coracobrachialis and biceps muscles, emerges between the biceps and brachioradialis muscles, and pierces the deep brachial fascia just above the elbow crease lateral to the biceps tendon (Figure 17-6). As soon as the nerve emerges above the fascia, it becomes the lateral cutaneous nerve of the forearm and descends on the anterolateral surface of the forearm. The nerve supplies branches to the anterolateral and posterior surfaces of the forearm. Its distal branches reach the lateral surface of the wrist.

### Indications

Blockade of the lateral cutaneous and medial cutaneous nerves of the forearm results in anesthesia of the anterior and lateral surfaces of the forearm. This block is suitable for the insertion of arteriovenous grafts or other superficial procedures on the volar aspect of the forearm. It is also useful for supplementing an axillary brachial plexus block in which a separate musculocutaneous nerve block was not performed or failed.

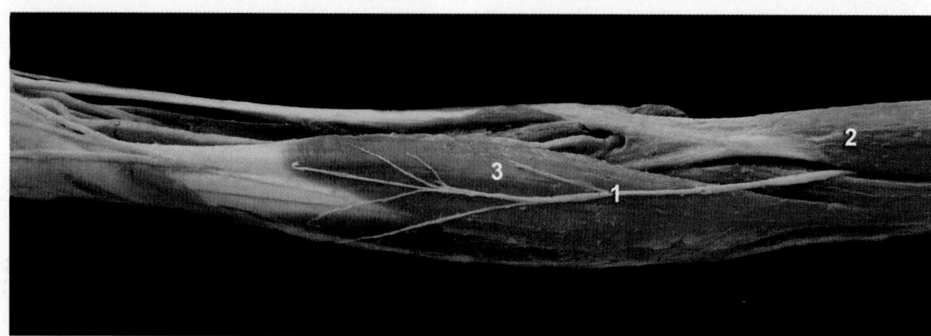


**FIGURE 17-6.** ❶ Lateral cutaneous nerve of the (right) forearm, ❷ Biceps muscle, ❸ Brachioradialis muscle.

### Technique

The nerve can be blocked at the level of the arm (musculocutaneous block; see "Axillary Block" for a description) or when it emerges at the elbow level. To block the lateral cutaneous nerve of the forearm at the *level of the elbow*, a 1.5-in, 25-gauge needle is used to infiltrate local anesthetic subcutaneously over the entire lateral aspect of the arm just below the elbow crease (Figure 17-4C).

## Complications and How to Avoid Them

Complications from cutaneous nerve blocks are few; they are discussed in Table 17-2.

**TABLE 17-2 Complications of Cutaneous Blocks and Preventive Techniques**

| | |
|---|---|
| ***Systemic toxicity of local anesthetic*** | • The risk is small and may be of concern mostly when used in conjunction with other high-dose major conduction blocks. |
| ***Hematoma*** | • Avoid multiple needle insertions.<br>• Avoid inserting the needle through superficial veins. |
| ***Nerve injury*** | • Usually manifested as transient paresthesias or dysesthesias and results from inadvertent intraneural injection.<br>• Injections should not be made when high pressures are felt on injection or when the patient reports pain in the distribution of the nerve. |

# CUTANEOUS NERVE BLOCKS OF THE UPPER EXTREMITY

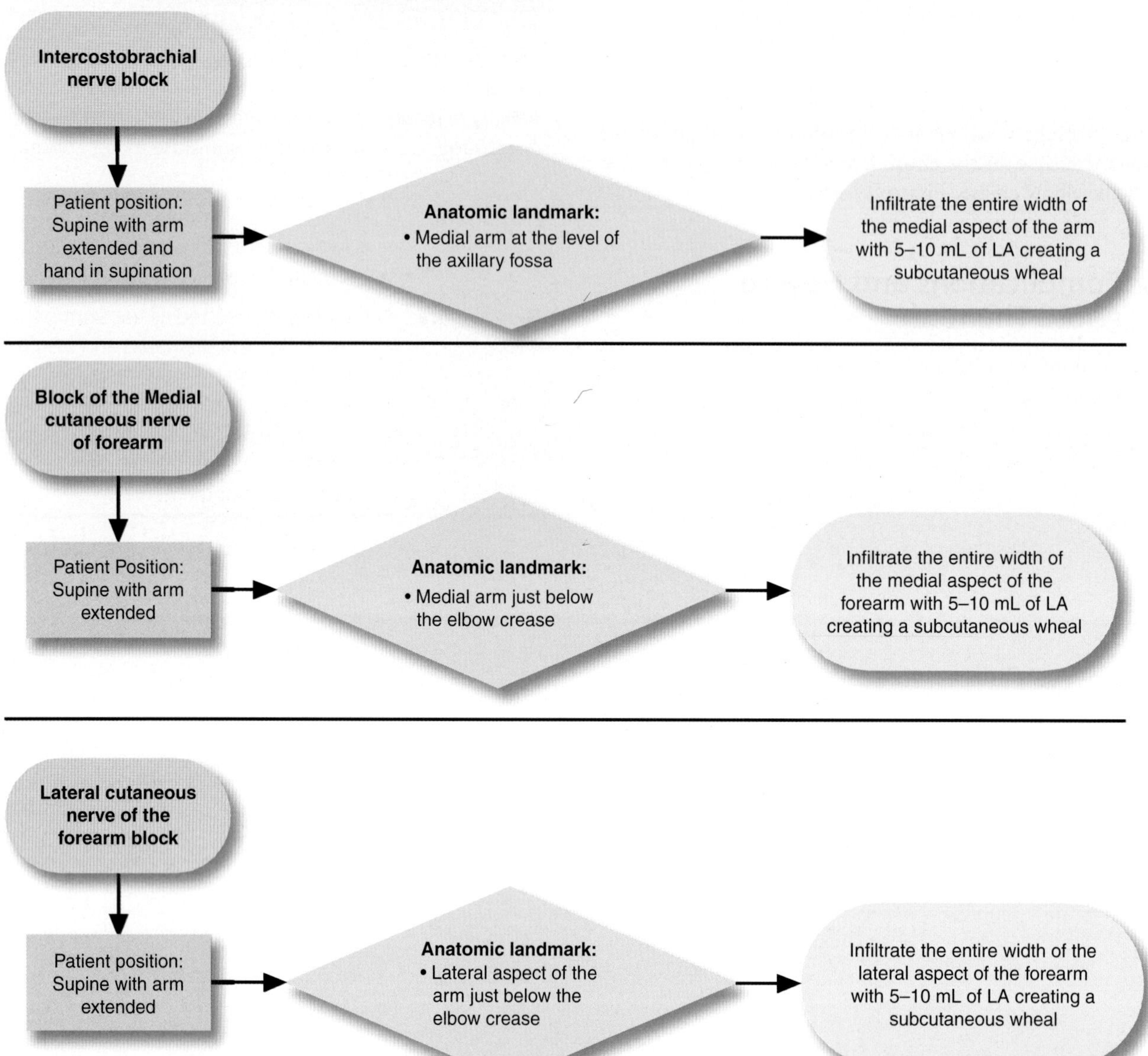

## SUGGESTED READINGS


Agur A, Lee M: Grant's Atlas of Anatomy. Baltimore, Md: Lippincott Williams & Wilkins, 1999.

Coventry DM, Barker KF, Thomson M: Comparison of two neurostimulation techniques for axillary brachial plexus blockade. Br J Anaesth 2001; 86: 80-3.

Cuvillon P, Dion N, Deleuze M, Nouvellon E, Mahamat A, L'Hermite J, Boisson C, Vialles N, Ripart J, de La Coussaye JE: Comparison of 3 intensities of stimulation threshold for brachial plexus blocks at the midhumeral level: a prospective, double-blind, randomized study. Reg Anesth Pain Med 2009; 34: 296-300.

Delaunay L, Chelly JE: Blocks at the wrist provide effective anesthesia for carpal tunnel release. Can J Anaesth 2001; 48: 656-60.

Deleuze A, Gentili ME, Marret E, Lamonerie L, Bonnet F: A comparison of a single-stimulation lateral infraclavicular plexus block with a triple-stimulation axillary block. Reg Anesth Pain Med 2003; 28: 89-94.

Gaertner E, Estebe JP, Zamfir A, Cuby C, Macaire P: Infraclavicular plexus block: multiple injection versus single injection. Reg Anesth Pain Med 2002; 27: 590-4.

Hermanns H, Braun S, Werdehausen R, Werner A, Lipfert P, Stevens MF: Skin temperature after interscalene brachial plexus blockade. Reg Anesth Pain Med 2007; 32: 481-7.

Jandard C, Gentili ME, Girard F, Ecoffey C, Heck M, Laxenaire MC, Bouaziz H: Infraclavicular block with lateral approach and nerve stimulation: extent of anesthesia and adverse effects. Reg Anesth Pain Med 2002; 27: 37-42.

Jankovic D, Wells C: Regional Nerve Blocks. 2nd ed. Wissenchafts-Verlag Berlin, Blackwell Scientific Publications 2001.

Macaire P, Choquet O, Jochum D, Travers V, Capdevila X: Nerve blocks at the wrist for carpal tunnel release revisited: the use of sensory-nerve and motor-nerve stimulation techniques. Reg Anesth Pain Med 2005; 30: 536-40.

March X, Pardina B, Torres-Bahi S, Navarro M, del Mar Garcia M, Villalonga A: A comparison of a triple-injection axillary brachial plexus block with the humeral approach. Reg Anesth Pain Med 2003; 28: 504-8.

Oaklander AL, Siegel SM: Cutaneous innervation: form and function. J Am Acad Dermatol 2005; 53: 1027-37.

Pernkopf E: Atlas of Topographical and Applied Human Anatomy. Vol II: Thorax, Abdomen and Extremities. 2nd ed. Munich, Germany: U&S Saunders, 1980.

Raj P: Textbook of Regional Anesthesia. London, England: Churchill Livingstone 2002.

Salengros JC, Pandin P, Schuind F, Vandesteene A: Intraoperative somatosensory evoked potentials to facilitate peripheral nerve release. Can J Anaesth 2006; 53: 40-5.

Sia S, Lepri A, Ponzecchi P: Axillary brachial plexus block using peripheral nerve stimulator: a comparison between double- and triple-injection techniques. Reg Anesth Pain Med 2001; 26: 499-503.

Viscomi CM, Reese J, Rathmell JP: Medial and lateral antebrachial cutaneous nerve blocks: an easily learned regional anesthetic for forearm arteriovenous fistula surgery. Reg Anesth 1996; 21: 2-5.

# 18 Lumbar Plexus Block

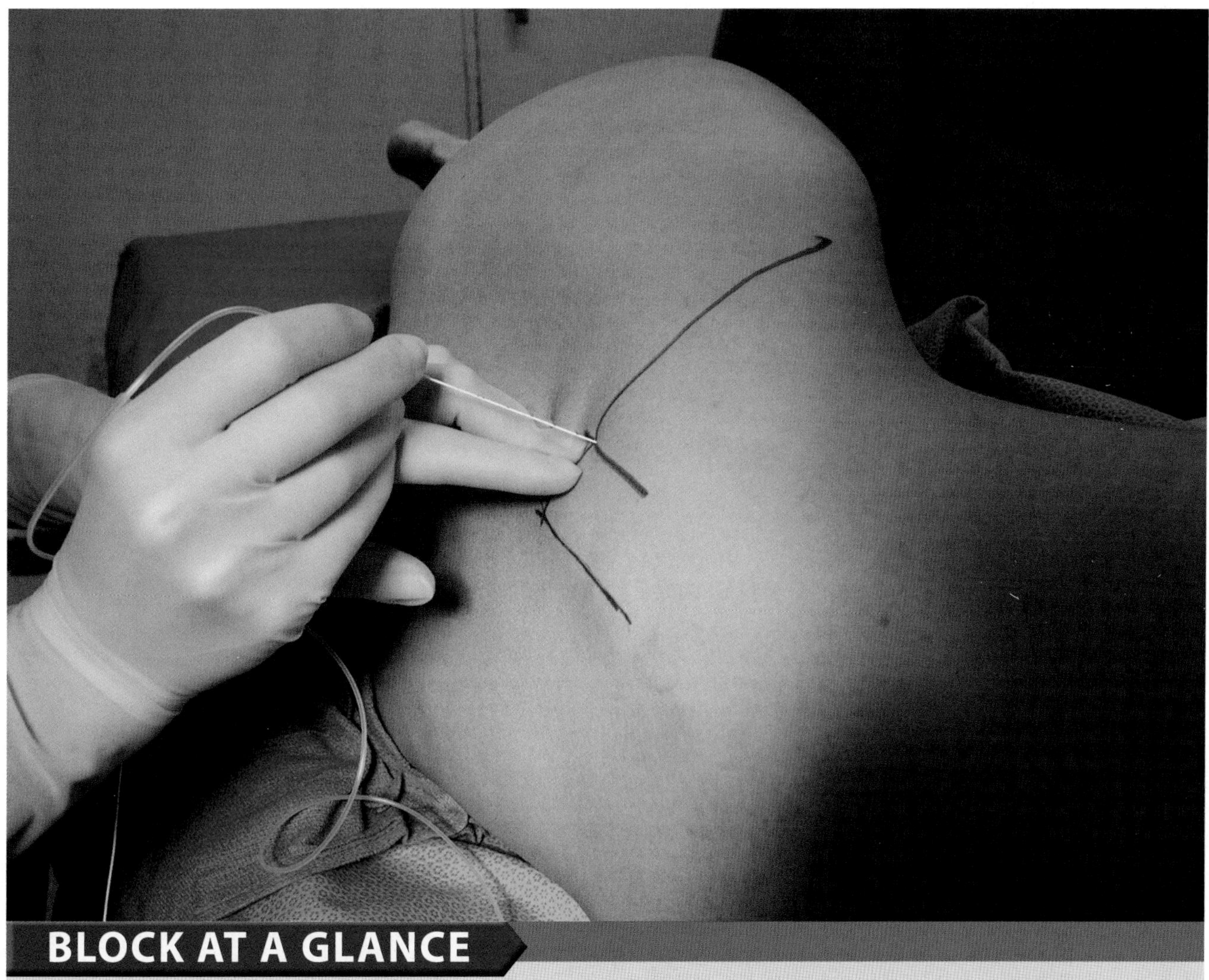

## BLOCK AT A GLANCE

- Indications: surgery on the hip, anterior thigh, and knee
- Landmarks: iliac crest, spinous processes (midline)
- Nerve stimulation: quadriceps muscle at 0.5–1.0 mA
- Local anesthetic: 25–35 mL

**FIGURE 18-1.** To accomplish the lumbar plexus block, a needle is inserted perpendicular to the skin plane, 4 cm lateral to the midline at the level of L3-L5.

## General Considerations

The lumbar plexus block (psoas compartment block) is an advanced nerve block technique. Because the placement of the needle is in the deep muscles, the potential for systemic toxicity is greater than it is with more superficial techniques. The proximity of the lumbar nerve roots to the epidural space also carries a risk of epidural spread of the local anesthetic. For these reasons, care should be taken when selecting the type, volume, and concentration of local anesthetic, particularly in elderly, frail, or obese patients. The lumbar plexus block provides anesthesia or analgesia to the entire distribution of the lumbar plexus, including the anterolateral and medial thigh, the knee, and the saphenous nerve below the knee. When combined with a sciatic nerve block, anesthesia of the entire leg can be achieved. Because of the complexity of the technique, potential for complications, and existence of simpler alternatives (e.g. fascia iliaca or femoral blocks), the benefits of lumbar plexus block should always be weighed against the risks.

## Functional Anatomy

The lumbar plexus is composed of five to six peripheral nerves that have their origins in the spinal roots of L1 to L4, with a contribution from T12 (Figures 18-2 and 18-3). After the roots emerge from the intervertebral foramina, they divide into anterior and posterior branches. The small posterior branches supply innervation to the skin of the lower back and paravertebral muscles. The anterior branches form the lumbar plexus within the substance of the psoas muscle and emerge from the muscle as individual nerves in the pelvis.

The major branches of the lumbar plexus are the iliohypogastric (L1), ilioinguinal (L1), genitofemoral nerve (L1/L2), lateral femoral cutaneous nerve (L2/L3), and the femoral and obturator nerves (L2,3,4). Although not a lumbar nerve root, the T12 spinal nerve contributes to the iliohypogastric nerve in about 50% of cases.

## Distribution of Blockade

The femoral nerve supplies the quadriceps muscle (knee extension), the skin of the anteromedial thigh, and the medial aspect of the leg below the knee and foot (Figure 18-4A and B). The obturator nerve sends motor branches to the adductors of the hip and a variable cutaneous area over the medial thigh or knee joint. The lateral femoral cutaneous, iliohypogastric, ilioinguinal, and genitofemoral nerves are superficial sensory nerves.

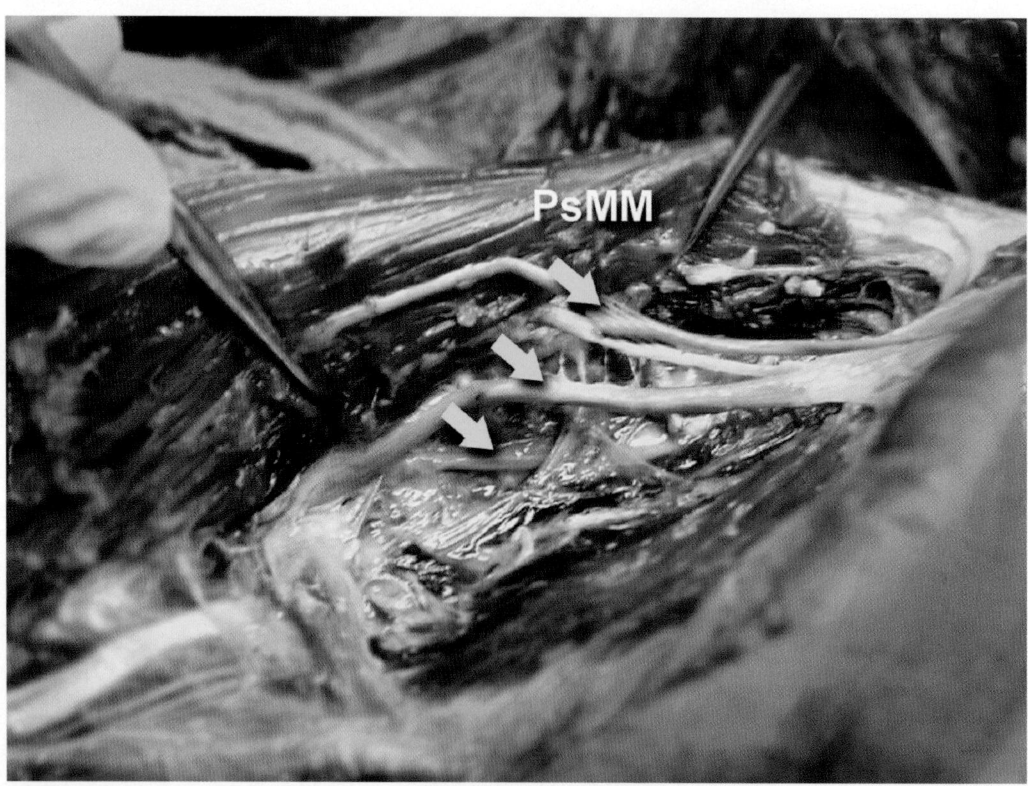


**FIGURE 18-2.** Anatomy of the lumbar plexus. Roots of the lumbar plexus (arrows) are seen within the substance of the psoas major muscle (PsMM); the lumbar plexus is exposed through the abdominal cavity.

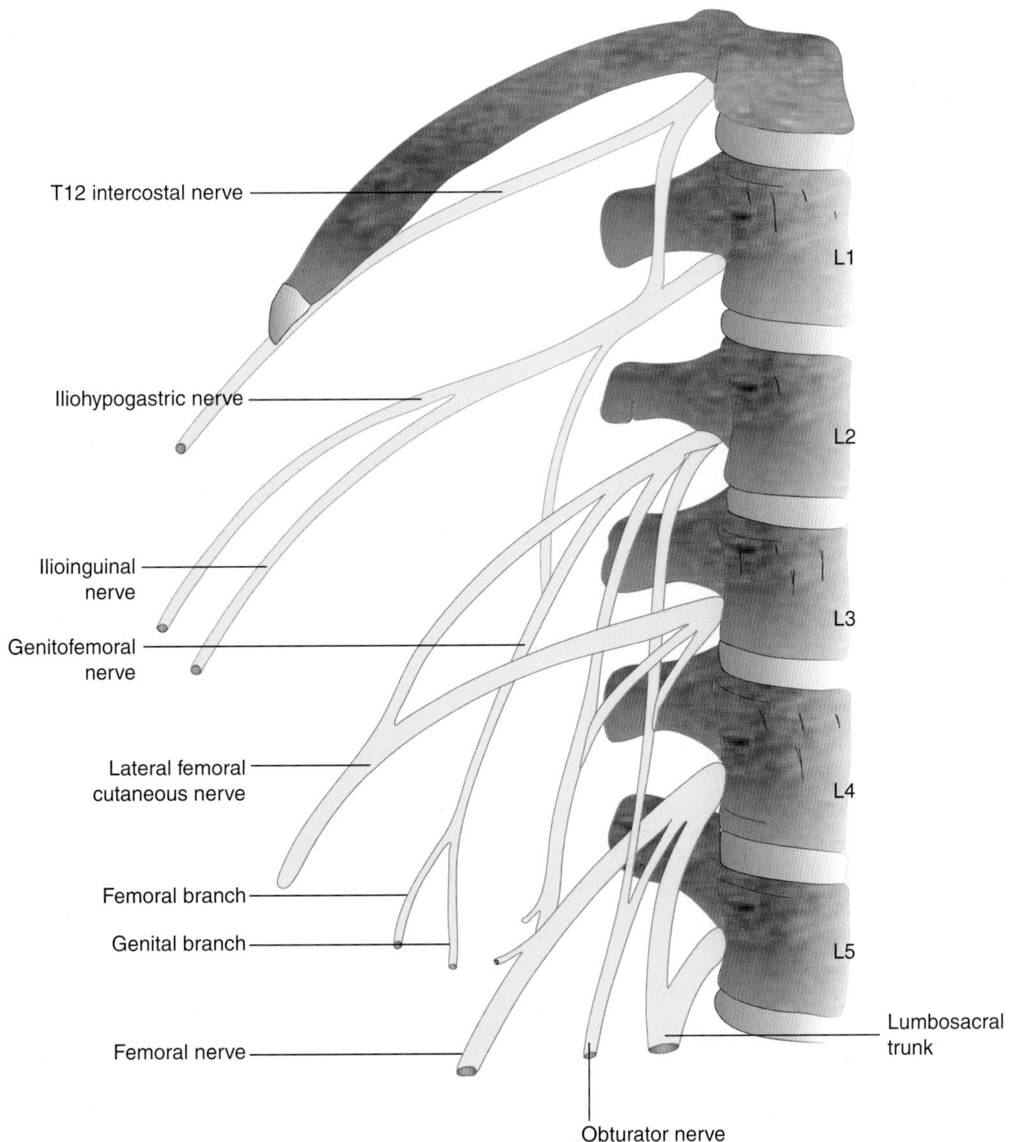


**FIGURE 18-3.** Organization of the Lumbar Plexus into peripheral nerves.

## Single-Injection Lumbar Plexus Block

### Equipment

A standard regional anesthesia tray is prepared with the following equipment:

- Sterile towels and gauze packs
- Two 20-mL syringes with local anesthetic
- A 10-mL syringe plus a 25-gauge needle with local anesthetic for skin infiltration
- A 10-cm, 21-gauge short-bevel insulated stimulating needle
- Peripheral nerve stimulator
- Sterile gloves; marking pen

## Landmarks and Patient Positioning

The patient is in the lateral decubitus position with a slight forward tilt (Figure 18-5). The foot on the side to be blocked should be positioned over the dependent leg so that twitches of the quadriceps muscle and patella can be seen easily. The operator should assume a position from which these responses are visible. Palpation of the anterior thigh can be useful to make sure the motor response is indeed that of the quadriceps muscles.

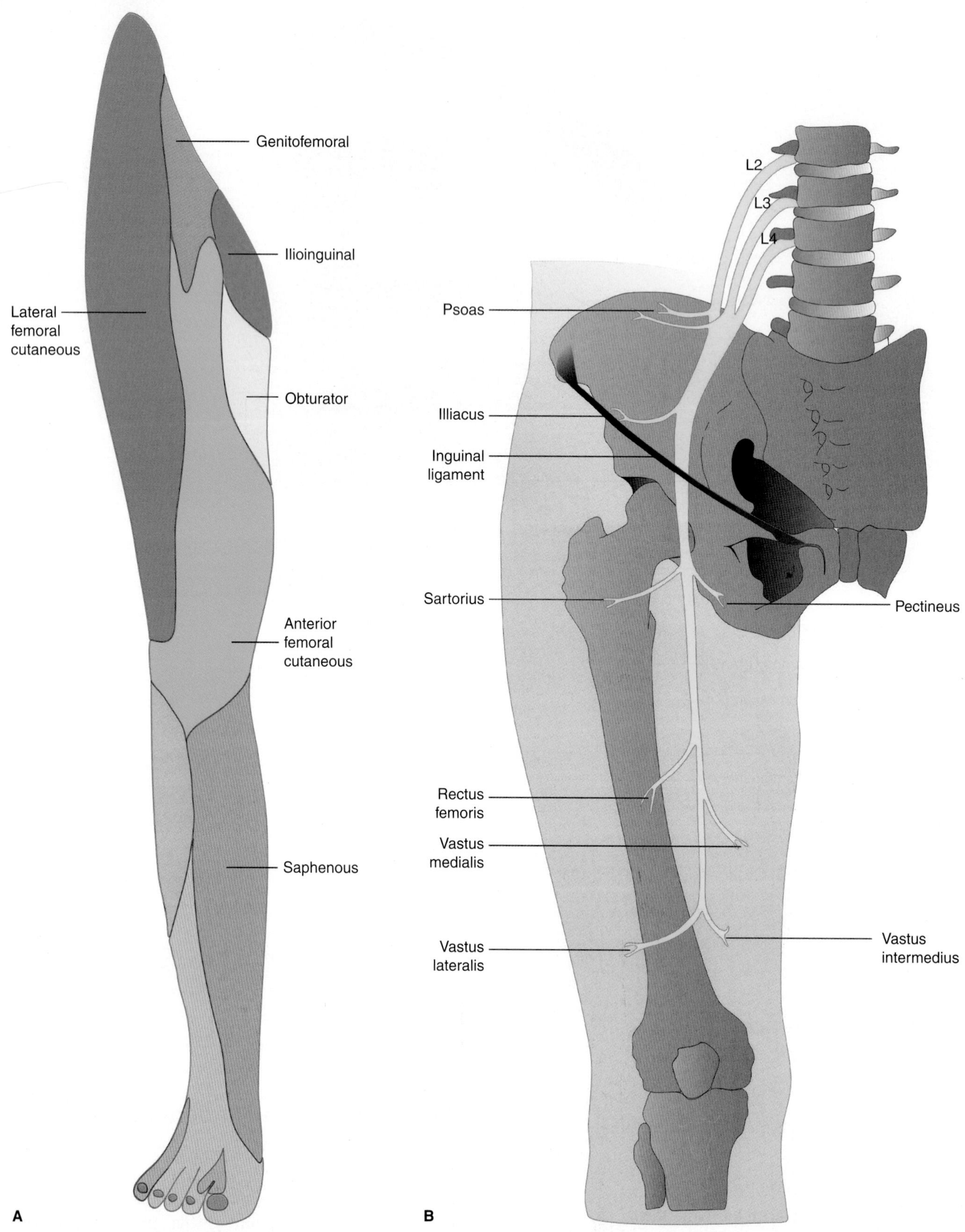


**FIGURE 18-4.** (A) Cutaneous distribution of the lumbar plexus to the lower extremity. (B) Motor innervation of the lumbar plexus to the lower extremity.

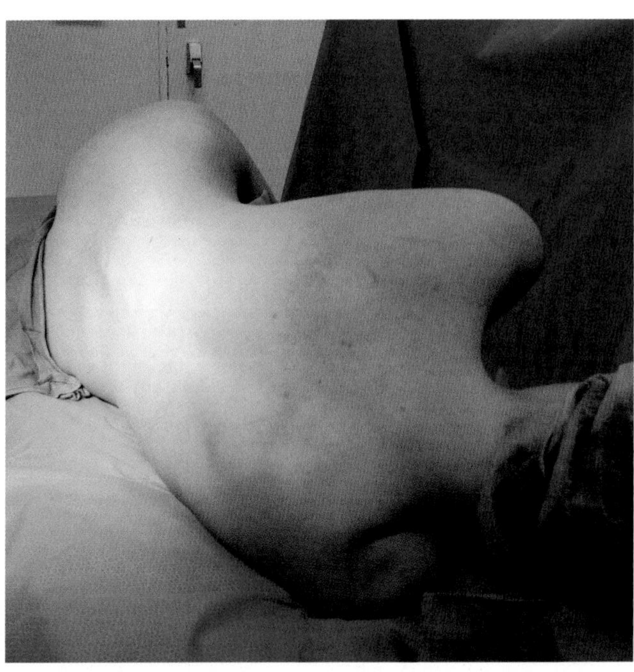

FIGURE 18-5. Patient position for the lumbar plexus block.

**TIP**

- A slight tilt of the pelvis forward allows for a more ergonomic position for the operator.

The anatomical landmarks are as follows (Figure 18-6):

1. Iliac crests (intercristal line)
2. Spinous processes (midline)
3. A point 3–4 cm lateral to the intersection of landmarks 1 and 2 (needle insertion point)

**TIPS**

- Because the gluteal crease tends to sag to a dependent position, it should never be considered as the midline.
- Instead, spinous processes should be relied on to determine the midline more accurately.

## Maneuvers to Facilitate Landmark Identification

The identification of the iliac crest can be facilitated by the following maneuvers:

- Placing the palpating hand over the ridge of the pelvic bone and pressing firmly against it (Figure 18-7).
- To better estimate the location of the iliac crest, the thickness of the adipose tissue over the iliac crest should be considered.

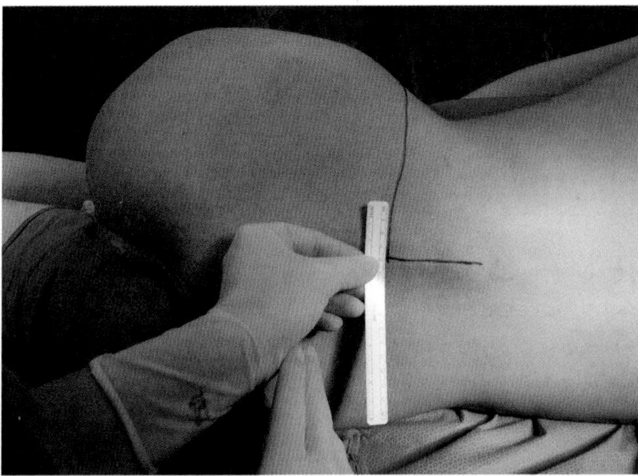

FIGURE 18-6. Landmarks for the lumbar plexus block. The needle insertion site is labeled 3-4 cm lateral to the intersection of the (horizontal) line passing through spinous processes and iliac crest (perpendicular) line.

- Pelvic proportions greatly vary among people; thus a visual "reality check" is always performed. If the estimated iliac crest line appears to be almost at the level of the midtorso or touching the rib cage (too cranial), make an appropriate adjustment to avoid insertion of the needle too cranially.

## Technique

After disinfecting with an antiseptic solution, the skin and paravertebral muscles are anesthetized by infiltrating local anesthetic subcutaneously at site of needle insertion.

The fingers of the palpating hand are firmly pressed against the paravertebral muscles to stabilize the landmark and decrease the skin–nerve distance (Figure 18-8). The palpating hand should not be moved during the entire block procedure so that precise redirections of the angle of needle

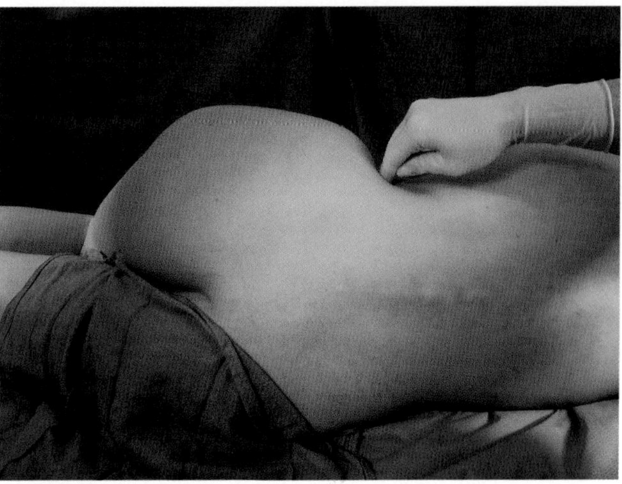

FIGURE 18-7. Technique of palpation of the iliac crest.

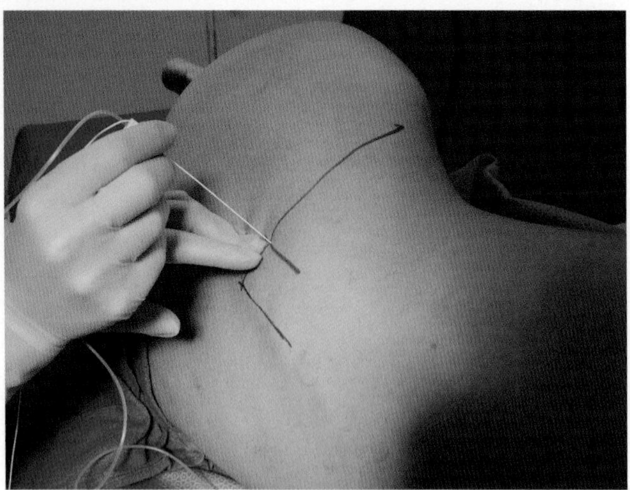

**FIGURE 18-8.** Needle insertion for the lumbar plexus block. The needle is inserted to walkoff the transverse processes and advance the needle 1-2 cm deeper.

insertion can be made, if necessary. The needle is inserted at an angle perpendicular to the skin with the nerve stimulator set initially to deliver a current of 1.5 mA (1.5 mA, 2 Hz, 0.1–0.3 ms). As the needle is advanced, local twitches of the paravertebral muscles are obtained first at a depth of a few centimeters. The needle is advanced further, until twitches of the quadriceps muscle are obtained (usually at a depth of 6–8 cm). After these twitches are observed, the current should be lowered to produce stimulation between 0.5 and 1.0 mA. Motor response should not be present at a current less than 0.5 mA, which could indicate needle placement in the dural sleeve. At this point, 25 to 35 mL of local anesthetic is injected slowly while avoiding resistance to injection and with frequent aspirations to rule out inadvertent intravascular needle placement. A resultant, typical spread of the local anesthetic solution is demonstrated in Figure 18-9.

## GOAL

Visible or palpable twitches of the quadriceps muscle at 0.5 to 1.0 mA.

## TIPS

- A successful lumbar plexus blockade depends on dispersion of the local anesthetic in a fascial plane within the psoas muscle where the roots of the plexus are situated.
- Stimulation at currents <0.5 mA should not be sought when using this technique. Motor stimulation with a low current may indicate placement of the needle inside a dural sleeve. An injection inside this sheath can result in epidural or spinal anesthesia.

**TABLE 18-1 Some Common Responses to Nerve Stimulation and Course of Action for Proper Response**

| RESPONSE OBTAINED | INTERPRETATION | PROBLEM | ACTION |
|---|---|---|---|
| Local twitch of the paravertebral muscles | Direct stimulation of the paravertebral muscles | The needle is placed too superficially | Continue advancement of the needle deeper |
| Needle contacts bone at a 4- to 6-cm depth; no twitches are seen | Needle advancement is stopped by the transverse process | Needle placement probably correct but requires redirection to walk off the transverse process | Withdraw the needle to the skin level and redirect it 15° cranially or caudally |
| Twitches of the hamstring muscles are seen; needle is inserted 6–8 cm | Stimulation of the roots of the sciatic plexus (sciatic nerve) | Needle inserted too caudally | Withdraw the needle and reinsert it 3–5 cm cranially |
| Flexion of the thigh at a depth of >6–8 cm | This subtle and often missed response is caused by direct stimulation of the psoas muscle | Needle insertion is too deep (missed the lumbar plexus roots); further advancement may place the needle intraperitoneally | Stop advancing the needle; withdraw the needle and reinsert it using the protocol outlined in the technique description |
| Needle placement is deep (8–10 cm), but twitches were not elicited and bone is not contacted | Needle missed both the transverse process and roots of the lumbar plexus | Too deep placement of needle | Withdraw the needle and re-evaluate. |

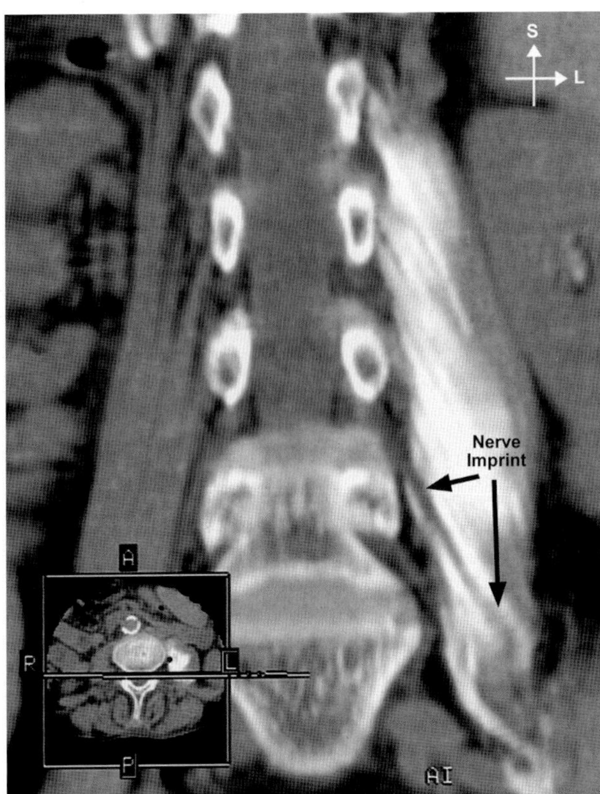


**FIGURE 18-9.** Radiograph demonstrating distribution of the radiopaque solution within the psoas muscle after a lumbar plexus injection.

## Troubleshooting

When insertion of the needle does not result in quadriceps muscle stimulation, the following maneuvers should be followed:

1. Withdraw the needle to the skin level, redirect it 5° to 10° cranially, and repeat the procedure.
2. Withdraw the needle to the skin level, redirect it 5° to 10° caudally, and repeat the procedure.
3. Withdraw the needle to the skin level, redirect it 5° to 10° medially, and repeat the procedure.
4. Withdraw the needle to the skin level, reinsert it 2 cm caudally or cranially, and repeat the procedure.

### TIPS

- Lumbar plexus block carries a higher risk of local anesthetic toxicity than most other nerve block techniques because of its deep location and the close proximity of muscles.
- Consider using a less toxic local anesthetic (e.g., 3% chloroprocaine) or mixtures of two local anesthetics (e.g., mepivacaine or lidocaine with ropivacaine) to decrease the total dose of more toxic, long-acting local anesthetic.

## Block Dynamics and Perioperative Management

A lumbar plexus block can be associated with significant patient discomfort because the needle passes through multiple muscle planes. Adequate sedation and analgesia are necessary to ensure a still and cooperative patient. We often use midazolam 4 to 6 mg after the patient is positioned and alfentanil 500 to 750 μg just before needle insertion. A typical onset time for this block is 20 to 30 minutes, depending on the type, concentration, and volume of local anesthetic and the level at which the needle is placed. The first sign of the onset of blockade is usually a loss of sensation in the saphenous nerve territory (medial skin below the knee).

# Continuous Lumbar Plexus Block

A continuous lumbar plexus blockade is an advanced regional anesthesia technique, and adequate experience with the single-injection technique is a prerequisite to ensure its efficacy and safety. Otherwise, the technique is quite similar to the single-injection procedure, except that a Tuohy-style needle is preferred. The needle opening should be directed caudad and laterally to facilitate threading of the catheter in the direction of the plexus. The technique can be used for postoperative pain management in patients undergoing hip, femur, and knee surgery.

## Equipment

A standard regional anesthesia tray is prepared with the following equipment:

- Sterile towels and gauze packs
- Two 20-mL syringes containing local anesthetic
- Sterile gloves, marking pen, and surface electrode
- A syringe plus 25-gauge needle with local anesthetic for skin infiltration
- Peripheral nerve stimulator
- Catheter kit (including a 8- to 10-cm large-gauge stimulating needle and catheter)

## Landmarks and Patient Positioning

As for the single-injection technique, the patient is positioned in the lateral decubitus position with the side to be blocked up and with a slightly forward pelvic tilt (Figure 18-4). An assistant helps maintain flexion of the spine, as in positioning a patient for an epidural or spinal block in the lateral position.

The landmarks for a continuous lumbar plexus block are the same as for the single-injection technique (Figure 18-6):

1. Iliac crests (intercristal line)
2. Midline (spinous processes)
3. Needle insertion site 4 cm lateral to the intersection of landmarks 1 and 2

## Technique

The skin and subcutaneous tissues are anesthetized with local anesthetic. The needle is attached to the nerve stimulator (1.5 mA, 2 Hz). The palpating hand should be firmly pressed and anchored against the paraspinal muscles to facilitate needle insertion and redirection of the needle when necessary. An 8–10-cm Tuohy-style continuous block needle is inserted at a perpendicular angle and advanced until the quadriceps muscle contractions are obtained at 0.5 to 1.0 mA. A 5–10 mL of local anesthetic or other injectate (e.g., D5W) is injected to "open up" a tissue space and facilitate catheter advancement. The catheter is threaded through the needle for approximately 5 cm beyond the tip of the needle (Figure 18-10). The needle is withdrawn, the catheter secured, and the remaining anesthetic is injected via the catheter. Before administration of the local anesthetic, the needle and/or catheter are checked for inadvertent intravascular and intrathecal placement. This is done by performing an aspiration test and administering a test dose of epinephrine-containing local anesthetic.

### *Continuous Infusion*

Continuous infusion is always initiated after an initial bolus of dilute local anesthetic through the needle or catheter. For this purpose, 0.2% ropivacaine (15 to 20 mL) is used most commonly. The infusion is maintained at 5 mL/h with 5 mL/h patient-controlled regional analgesia bolus dose.

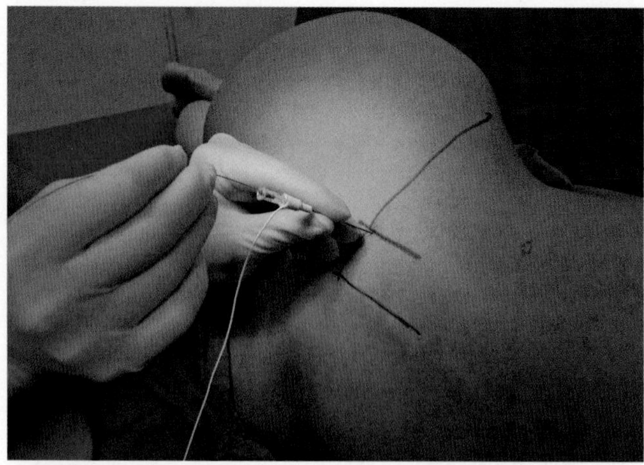

**FIGURE 18-10.** Insertion of the catheter in the lumbar plexus. The catheter is inserted approximately 5 cm beyond the needle tip.

**TIPS**

- Breakthrough pain in patients receiving a continuous infusion is always managed by administering a bolus of local anesthetic. Simply increasing the rate of infusion is rarely adequate.
- For patients on the ward, a shorter-acting local anesthetic (e.g., 1% mepivacaine) is useful to test the functionality of the catheter.

## Complications and How to Avoid Them

The lumbar plexus block is an advanced nerve block technique that carries a potential for serious complications if proper precautions are not strictly followed. Some complications and methods to decrease the risk of them are listed in Table 18-2.

**TABLE 18-2 Complications of Lumbar Plexus Block and How To Avoid Them**

| | |
|---|---|
| ***Infection*** | • A strict aseptic technique is used. |
| ***Hematoma*** | • Reduce the number of needle insertions.<br>• Continuous lumbar plexus blocks are best avoided in patients receiving anticoagulant therapy (i.e., the same considerations as for the use of neuraxial anesthesia in patients on anticoagulant therapy).<br>• The use of antiplatelet therapy is not a contraindication for this block in the absence of spontaneous bleeding. |
| ***Vascular puncture*** | • Vascular puncture is not common with this technique.<br>• Deep needle insertion should be avoided (vena cava, aorta). |
| ***Local anesthetic toxicity*** | • Higher volumes of local anesthetic result in more complete and faster onset blocks; however, high volume/concentration of local anesthetic with this block also carries a higher risk of toxicity.<br>• Large volumes of long-acting anesthetic should be avoided in older and frail patients.<br>• Careful and frequent aspiration should be performed during the injection.<br>• Avoid fast, forceful injection of local anesthetic. Forceful (high-pressure) injections carry a greater risk of systemic toxicity and epidural spread. |
| ***Nerve injury*** | • Local anesthetic should never be injected when the patient complains of pain on injection or when abnormally high resistance (pressure) is noted.<br>• When stimulation is obtained with a current intensity of <0.5 mA, the needle should be pulled back to obtain the same response with a current of 0.5-1 mA before injecting local anesthetic to avoid injection into the dural sleeves and the consequent epidural or spinal spread. |
| ***Hemodynamic consequences*** | • Lumbar plexus blockade results in unilateral sympathectomy.<br>• Spread of the local anesthetic to the epidural space may result in significant hypotension. Avoiding forceful injection helps prevent bilateral and cephalad spread.<br>• Patients receiving a lumbar plexus block should be monitored with the same vigilance as patients receiving epidural anesthesia. |

# LUMBAR PLEXUS BLOCK

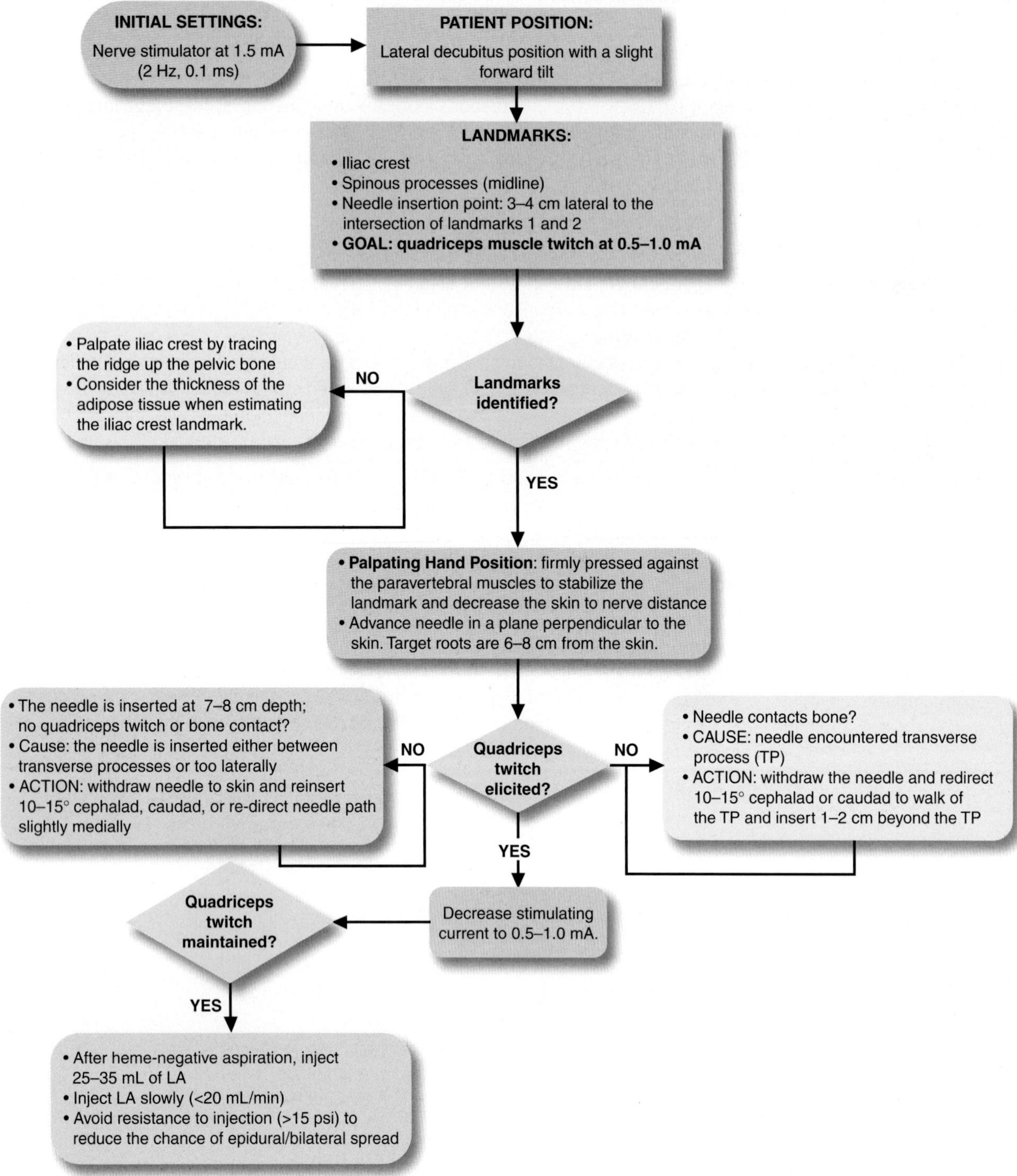

## SUGGESTED READINGS


Altermatt F, Cortinez LI, Munoz H. Plasma levels of levobupivacaine after combined posterior lumbar plexus and sciatic nerve blocks. *Anesth Analg.* 2006;102:1597.

Asakura Y, Kandatsu N, Kato N, Sato Y, Fujiwara Y, Komatsu T. Ultra-sound guided sciatic nerve block combined with lumbar plexus block for infra-inguinal artery bypass graft surgery. *Acta Anaesthesiol Scand.* 2008;52:721-722.

Aveline C, Bonnet F. Delayed retroperitoneal haematoma after failed lumbar plexus block. *Br J Anaesth.* 2004;93:589-591.

Awad IT, Duggan EM. Posterior lumbar plexus block: anatomy, approaches, and techniques. *Reg Anesth Pain Med.* 2005;30:143-149.

Bagry H, de la Cuadra Fontaine JC, Asenjo JF, Bracco D, Carli F. Effect of a continuous peripheral nerve block on the inflammatory response in knee arthroplasty. *Reg Anesth Pain Med.* 2008;33:17-23.

Ben-David B, Joshi R, Chelly JE. Sciatic nerve palsy after total hip arthroplasty in a patient receiving continuous lumbar plexus block. *Anesth Analg.* 2003;97:1180-1182.

Ben-David B, Lee EM. Lumbar plexus or lumbar paravertebral blocks? *Anesthesiology.* 2009;110:1196.

Blumenthal S, Ekatodramis G, Borgeat A. Ropivacaine plasma concentrations are similar during continuous lumbar plexus blockade using two techniques: pharmacokinetics or pharmacodynamics? *Can J Anaesth.* 2004;51:851.

Breslin DS, Martin G, Macleod DB, D'Ercole F, Grant SA. Central nervous system toxicity following the administration of levobupivacaine for lumbar plexus block: a report of two cases. *Reg Anesth Pain Med.* 2003;28:144-147.

Brown DL, Bridenbaugh LD. The upper extremity: somatic block. In: Cousins MJ, Bridenbaugh PO, eds. *Neuronal Blockade in Clinical Anesthesia and Management of Pain.* Philadelphia, PA: Lippincott-Raven; 1988:345-371.

Capdevila X, Biboulet P, Morau D, et al. Continuous three-in-one block for postoperative pain after lower limb orthopedic surgery: where do the catheters go? *Anesth Analg.* 2002;94:1001-1006.

Capdevila X, Coimbra C, Choquet O. Approaches to the lumbar plexus: success, risks, and outcome. *Reg Anesth Pain Med.* 2005;30:150-162.

Capdevila X, Macaire P, Dadure C, et al. Continuous psoas compartment block for postoperative analgesia after total hip arthroplasty: new landmarks, technical guidelines, and clinical evaluation. *Anesth Analg.* 2002;94:1606-1613.

Cappelleri G, Aldegheri G, Ruggieri F, Carnelli F, Fanelli A, Casati A. Effects of using the posterior or anterior approaches to the lumbar plexus on the minimum effective anesthetic concentration (MEAC) of mepivacaine required to block the femoral nerve: a prospective, randomized, up-and-down study. *Reg Anesth Pain Med.* 2008;33:10-16.

Chelly JE. Do we really need an interval between administering fondaparinux and removing a lumbar plexus catheter? *Anesth Analg.* 2009;108:670-671.

Chelly JE, Casati A, Fanelli G. *Continuous Peripheral Nerve Block Techniques: An Illustrated Guide.* London, UK: Mosby International; 2001.

Chelly JE, Szczodry DM, Neumann KJ. International normalized ratio and prothrombin time values before the removal of a lumbar plexus catheter in patients receiving warfarin after total hip replacement. *Br J Anaesth.* 2008;101:250-254.

Cotter JT, Nielsen KC, Guller U, et al. Increased body mass index and ASA physical status IV are risk factors for block failure in ambulatory surgery—an analysis of 9,342 blocks. *Can J Anaesth.* 2004;51:810-816.

Cucchiaro G, Ganesh A. The effects of clonidine on postoperative analgesia after peripheral nerve blockade in children. *Anesth Analg.* 2007;104:532-537.

De Biasi P, Lupescu R, Burgun G, Lascurain P, Gaertner E. Continuous lumbar plexus block: use of radiography to determine catheter tip location. *Reg Anesth Pain Med.* 2003;28:135-139.

de Leeuw MA, Perez RG. Posterior lumbar plexus block in postoperative analgesia for total hip arthroplasty. A comparative study between 0.5% bupivacaine with epinephrine and 0.5% ropivacaine. *Rev Bras Anestesiol* 2010;60:215-216, 124-125.

de Visme V, Picart F, Le Jouan R, Legrand A, Savry C, Morin V. Combined lumbar and sacral plexus block compared with plain bupivacaine spinal anesthesia for hip fractures in the elderly. *Reg Anesth Pain Med.* 2000;25:158-162.

Duarte LT, Beraldo PS, Saraiva RA. Epidural lumbar block or lumbar plexus block combined with general anesthesia: efficacy and hemodynamic effects on total hip arthroplasty. *Rev Bras Anestesiol.* 2009;59:649-664.

Duarte LT, Beraldo PS, Saraiva RA. Effects of epidural analgesia and continuous lumbar plexus block on functional rehabilitation after total hip arthroplasty [in Portuguese]. *Rev Bras Anestesiol.* 2009;59:531-544.

Duarte LT, Paes FC, Fernandes Mdo C, Saraiva RA. Posterior lumbar plexus block in postoperative analgesia for total hip arthroplasty: a comparative study between 0.5% bupivacaine with epinephrine and 0.5% ropivacaine. *Rev Bras Anestesiol.* 2009;59:273-285.

Ekatodramis G, Grimm K, Borgeat A. The effect of lumbar plexus block on blood loss and postoperative pain. *Anesthesiology.* 2001;94:716-717.

Farny J, Drolet P, Girard M. Anatomy of the posterior approach to the lumbar plexus block. *Can J Anaesth.* 1994;41:480-485.

Farny J, Girard M, Drolet P. Posterior approach to the lumbar plexus combined with a sciatic nerve block using lidocaine. *Can J Anaesth.* 1994;41:486-491.

Faust AM, Fournier R, Gamulin Z. Perioperative analgesia with posterior continuous lumbar plexus block for simultaneous ipsilateral total hip and knee arthroplasty. *Reg Anesth Pain Med.* 2006;31:591.

Fowler SJ, Symons J, Sabato S, Myles PS. Epidural analgesia compared with peripheral nerve blockade after major knee surgery: a systematic review and meta-analysis of randomized trials. *Br J Anaesth.* 2008;100:154-164.

Gadsden JC, Lindenmuth DM, Hadžić A, Xu D, Somasundarum L, Flisinski KA. Lumbar plexus block using high-pressure injection leads to contralateral and epidural spread. *Anesthesiology.* 2008;109:683-688.

Goroszeniuk T, di Vadi PP. Repeated psoas compartment blocks for the management of long-standing hip pain. *Reg Anesth Pain Med.* 2001;26:376-378.

Hadžić A, Karaca PE, Hobeika P, et al. Peripheral nerve blocks result in superior recovery profile compared with general anesthesia in outpatient knee arthroscopy. *Anesth Analg.* 2005;100:976-981.

Hanna MH, Peat SJ, D'Costa F. Lumbar plexus block: an anatomical study. *Anaesthesia.* 1993;8:675-678.

Heller AR, Fuchs A, Rossel T, et al. Precision of traditional approaches for lumbar plexus block: impact and management of interindividual anatomic variability. *Anesthesiology.* 2009;111:525-532.

Ho AM, Karmakar MK. Combined paravertebral lumbar plexus and parasacral sciatic nerve block for reduction of hip fracture in a patient with severe aortic stenosis. *Can J Anaesth.* 2002;49:946-950.

Horlocker TT, Hebl JR, Kinney MA, Cabanela ME. Opioid-free analgesia following total knee arthroplasty—a multimodal approach using continuous lumbar plexus (psoas compartment) block, acetaminophen, and ketorolac. *Reg Anesth Pain Med.* 2002;27:105-108.

Hsu DT. Delayed retroperitoneal haematoma after failed lumbar plexus block. *Br J Anaesth.* 2005;94:395.

Huet O, Eyrolle LJ, Mazoit JX, Ozier YM. Cardiac arrest after injection of ropivacaine for posterior lumbar plexus blockade. *Anesthesiology*. 2003;99:1451-1453.

Ilfeld BM, Ball ST, Gearen PF, et al. Ambulatory continuous posterior lumbar plexus nerve blocks after hip arthroplasty: a dual-center, randomized, triple-masked, placebo-controlled trial. *Anesthesiology*. 2008;109:491-501.

Ilfeld BM, Ball ST, Gearen PF, et al. Health-related quality of life after hip arthroplasty with and without an extended-duration continuous posterior lumbar plexus nerve block: a prospective, 1-year follow-up of a randomized, triple-masked, placebo-controlled study. *Anesth Analg*. 2009;109:586-591.

Johr M. The right thing in the right place: lumbar plexus block in children. *Anesthesiology*. 2005;102:865.

Kaloul I, Guay J, Cote C, Fallaha M. The posterior lumbar plexus (psoas compartment) block and the three-in-one femoral nerve block provide similar postoperative analgesia after total knee replacement. *Can J Anaesth*. 2004;51:45-51.

Kaloul I, Guay J, Cote C, Halwagi A, Varin F. Ropivacaine plasma concentrations are similar during continuous lumbar plexus blockade using the anterior three-in-one and the posterior psoas compartment techniques. *Can J Anaesth*. 2004;51:52-56.

Karmakar MK, Ho AM, Li X, Kwok WH, Tsang K, Ngan Kee WD. Ultrasound-guided lumbar plexus block through the acoustic window of the lumbar ultrasound trident. *Br J Anaesth*. 2008;100:533-537.

Kirchmair L, Enna B, Mitterschiffthaler G, et al. Lumbar plexus in children. A sonographic study and its relevance to pediatric regional anesthesia. *Anesthesiology*. 2004;101:445-450.

Kirchmair L, Entner T, Wissel J, Moriggl B, Kapral S, Mitterschiffthaler G. A study of the paravertebral anatomy for ultrasound-guided posterior lumbar plexus block. *Anesth Analg*. 2001;93:477-481.

Kirchmair L, Lirk P, Colvin J, Mitterschiffthaler G, Moriggl B. Lumbar plexus and psoas major muscle: not always as expected. *Reg Anesth Pain Med*. 2008;33:109-114.

Klein SM, Greengrass RA, Grant SA, Higgins LD, Nielsen KC, Steele SM. Ambulatory surgery for multi-ligament knee reconstruction with continuous dual catheter peripheral nerve blockade. *Can J Anaesth*. 2001;48:375-378.

Laguillo Cadenas JL, Martinez Navas A, de la Tabla Gonzalez RO, Ramos Curado P, Echevarria Moreno M. Combined posterior lumbar plexus and sacral block for emergency surgery to treat hip fracture [in Spanish]. *Rev Esp Anestesiol Reanim*. 2009;56:385-388.

Lang S. Posterior lumbar plexus block. *Can J Anaesth*. 1994;41: 1238-1239.

Litz RJ, Vicent O, Wiessner D, Heller AR. Misplacement of a psoas compartment catheter in the subarachnoid space. *Reg Anesth Pain Med*. 2004;29:60-64.

Ludot H, Tharin JY, Belouadah M, Mazoit JX, Malinovsky JM. Successful resuscitation after ropivacaine and lidocaine-induced ventricular arrhythmia following posterior lumbar plexus block in a child. *Anesth Analg*. 2008;106:1572-1574.

Mannion S. Epidural spread depends on the approach used for posterior lumbar plexus block. *Can J Anaesth*. 2004;51:516-517.

Mannion S, Barrett J, Kelly D, Murphy DB, Shorten GD. A description of the spread of injectate after psoas compartment block using magnetic resonance imaging. *Reg Anesth Pain Med*. 2005;30:567-571.

Mannion S, O'Callaghan S, Walsh M, Murphy DB, Shorten GD. In with the new, out with the old? Comparison of two approaches for psoas compartment block. *Anesth Analg*. 2005;101:259-264.

Marhofer P, Nasel C, Sitzwohl C, Kapral S. Magnetic resonance imaging of the distribution of local anesthetic during the three-in-one block. *Anesth Analg*. 2000;90:119-124.

Martin G, Grant SA, Macleod DB, Breslin DS, Brewer RP. Severe phantom leg pain in an amputee after lumbar plexus block. *Reg Anesth Pain Med*. 2003;28:475-478.

Mello SS, Saraiva RA, Marques RS, Gasparini JR, Assis CN, Goncalves MH. Posterior lumbar plexus block in children: a new anatomical landmark. *Reg Anesth Pain Med*. 2007;32:522-527.

Morau D, Lopez S, Biboulet P, Bernard N, Amar J, Capdevila X. Comparison of continuous 3-in-1 and fascia Iliaca compartment blocks for postoperative analgesia: feasibility, catheter migration, distribution of sensory block, and analgesic efficacy. *Reg Anesth Pain Med*. 2003;28:309-314.

Morin AM, Kratz CD, Eberhart LH, et al. Postoperative analgesia and functional recovery after total-knee replacement: comparison of a continuous posterior lumbar plexus (psoas compartment) block, a continuous femoral nerve block, and the combination of a continuous femoral and sciatic nerve block. *Reg Anesth Pain Med*. 2005;30:434-445.

Pandin PC, Vandesteene A, d'Hollander AA. Lumbar plexus posterior approach: a catheter placement description using electrical nerve stimulation. *Anesth Analg*. 2002;95:1428-1431.

Pousman RM, Mansoor Z, Sciard D. Total spinal anesthetic after continuous posterior lumbar plexus block. *Anesthesiology*. 2003;98:1281-1282.

Rose GL, McLarney JT. Retained continuous lumbar plexus block catheter. *J Clin Anesth*. 2009;21:464-465.

Sciard D, Matuszczak M, Gebhard R, Greger J, Al-Samsam T, Chelly JE. Continuous posterior lumbar plexus block for acute postoperative pain control in young children. *Anesthesiology*. 2001;95:1521-1523.

Siddiqui ZI, Cepeda MS, Denman W, Schumann R, Carr DB. Continuous lumbar plexus block provides improved analgesia with fewer side effects compared with systemic opioids after hip arthroplasty: a randomized controlled trial. *Reg Anesth Pain Med*. 2007;32:393-398.

Souron V. A complete block of the knee combines both sacral and lumbar plexus blocks. *Anesth Analg*. 2004;98:1501.

Stevens RD, Van Gessel E, Flory N, Fournier R, Gamulin Z. Lumbar plexus block reduces pain and blood loss associated with total hip arthroplasty. *Anesthesiology*. 2000;93:115-121.

Urmey WF, Grossi P. Use of sequential electrical nerve stimuli (SENS) for location of the sciatic nerve and lumbar plexus. *Reg Anesth Pain Med*. 2006;31:463-469.

Vanterpool S, Steele SM, Nielsen KC, Tucker M, Klein SM. Combined lumbar-plexus and sciatic-nerve blocks: an analysis of plasma ropivacaine concentrations. *Reg Anesth Pain Med*. 2006;31:417-421.

Watson MW, Mitra D, McLintock TC, Grant SA. Continuous versus single-injection lumbar plexus blocks: comparison of the effects on morphine use and early recovery after total knee arthroplasty. *Reg Anesth Pain Med*. 2005;30:541-547.

Weller RS, Gerancher JC, Crews JC, Wade KL. Extensive retroperitoneal hematoma without neurologic deficit in two patients who underwent lumbar plexus block and were later anticoagulated. *Anesthesiology*. 2003;98:581-585.

# 19 Sciatic Block

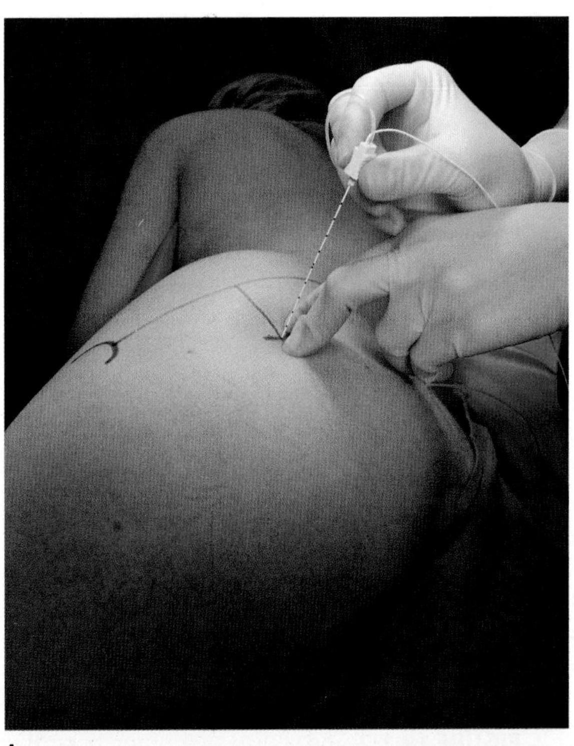

A

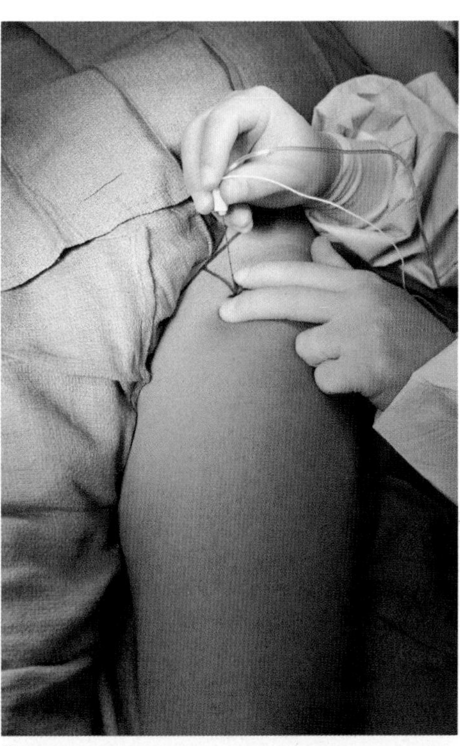

B

## BLOCK AT A GLANCE

TRANSGLUTEAL (POSTERIOR) APPROACH

- Indications: surgery on the knee, tibia, ankle, and foot
- Landmarks: greater trochanter, superior posterior iliac spine, and the midline between the two
- Nerve stimulation: twitch of the hamstring, calf, foot, or toes at 0.2–0.5 mA current
- Local anesthetic: 15–20 mL

ANTERIOR APPROACH

- Indications: surgery on the knee, tibia, fibula, ankle, and foot
- Landmarks: femoral crease, femoral artery
- Nerve stimulation: twitch of the foot or toes at 0.2–0.5 mA
- Local anesthetic: 15–20 mL

**FIGURE 19.1-1.** (A) Needle insertion for the transgluteal (posterior) approach to sciatic nerve block. (B) Needle insertion for anterior sciatic block.

# PART 1: TRANSGLUTEAL APPROACH

## General Considerations

The posterior approach to sciatic nerve block has wide clinical applicability for surgery and pain management of the lower extremity. Consequently, a sciatic block is one of the more commonly used techniques in our practice. In contrast to a common belief, this block is relatively easy to perform and associated with a high success rate. It is particularly well-suited for surgery on the knee, calf, Achilles tendon, ankle, and foot. It provides complete anesthesia of the leg below the knee with the exception of the medial strip of skin, which is innervated by the saphenous nerve. When combined with a femoral nerve or lumbar plexus block, anesthesia of the entire lower extremity can be achieved.

## Functional Anatomy

The sciatic nerve is formed from the L4 through S3 roots. These roots form the sacral plexus on the anterior surface of the lateral sacrum and converge to become the sciatic nerve on the anterior surface of the piriformis muscle. The sciatic nerve is the largest nerve in the body and measures nearly 2 cm in breadth at its origin. The course of the nerve can be estimated by drawing a line on the back of the thigh beginning from the apex of the popliteal fossa to the midpoint of the line joining the ischial tuberosity to the apex of the greater trochanter. The sciatic nerve also gives off numerous articular (hip, knee) and muscular branches.

The sciatic nerve exits the pelvis through the greater sciatic foramen below the piriformis and descends between the greater trochanter of the femur and the ischial tuberosity, superficial to the external rotators of the hip (obturator internus, the gemelli muscles, and quadratus femoris) (Figures 19.1-2 and 19.1-3). On its medial side, the sciatic nerve is accompanied by the posterior cutaneous nerve of the thigh and the inferior gluteal artery. The articular branches of the sciatic nerve arise from the upper part of the nerve and supply the hip joint by perforating the posterior part of its capsule. Occasionally, these branches are derived directly from the sacral plexus. The muscular branches of the sciatic nerve are distributed to the biceps femoris, semitendinosus, and semimembranosus muscles, and to the ischial head of the adductor magnus. The two components of the nerve (tibial and common peroneal) diverge approximately 4 to 10 cm above the popliteal crease to separately continue their paths into the lower leg.

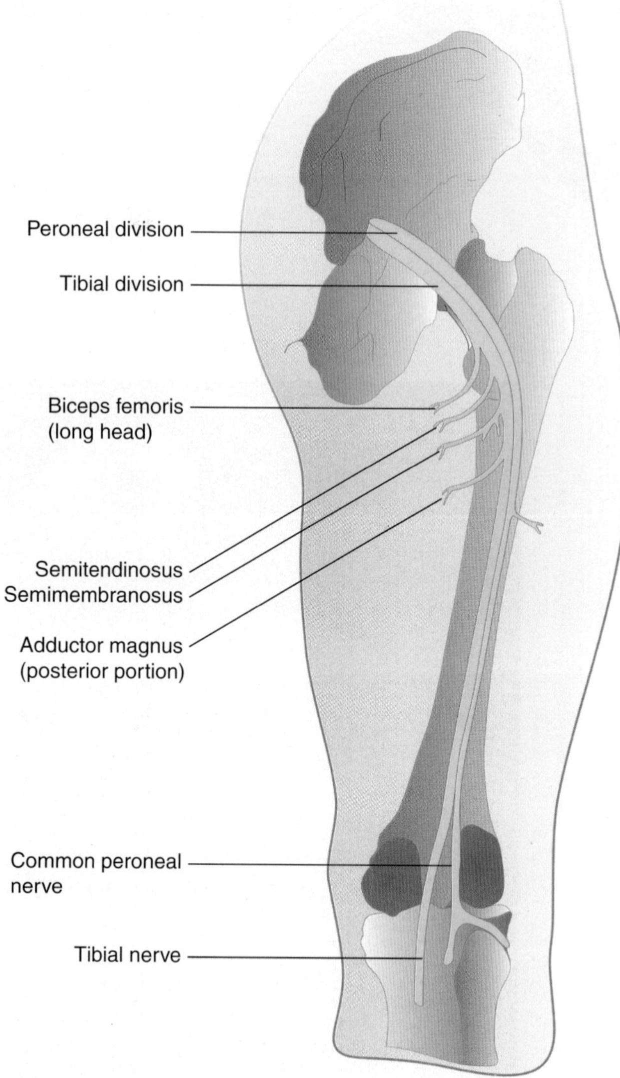


**FIGURE 19.1-2.** The course and motor innervation of the sciatic nerve.

## TIPS

- There are numerous variations in the course of the sciatic nerve through the gluteal region. In about 15% of the population, the piriformis muscle divides the nerve. The common peroneal component passes through or above the muscle, and the tibial component passes below it.
- The components of the sciatic nerve diverge at a variable distance from the knee joint. By and large, most nerves diverge at 4 to 10 cm above the popliteal fossa crease.

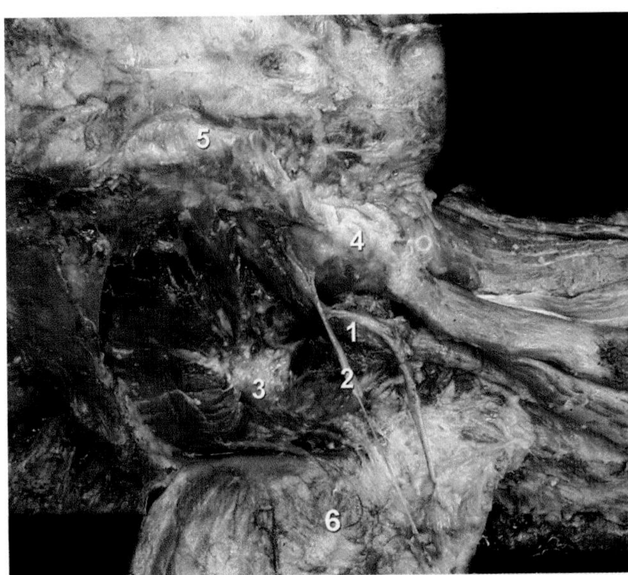


**FIGURE 19.1-3.** Anatomy of the sciatic nerve at the subgluteal location. ❶ sciatic nerve. ❷ nerve branch to the gluteus muscle. ❸ ischial bone. ❹ greater trochanter. ❺ posterior superior iliac spine. ❻ gluteus muscle.

## Distribution of Blockade

A sciatic nerve block results in anesthesia of the skin of the posterior aspect of the thigh, hamstring, and biceps femoris muscles; part of the hip and knee joint; and the entire leg below the knee with the exception of the skin of the medial aspect of the lower leg (Figure 19.1-4). Depending on the level of surgery, the addition of a saphenous or femoral nerve block may be required to provide coverage for this area.

## Single-Injection Sciatic Nerve Block

### Equipment

A standard regional anesthesia tray is prepared with the following equipment:

- Sterile towels and gauze packs
- One 20-mL syringe containing local anesthetic
- A 3- to 5-mL syringe plus 25-gauge needle with local anesthetic for skin infiltration
- A 10-cm, 21-22 gauge short-bevel insulated stimulating needle
- Peripheral nerve stimulator
- Sterile gloves; marking pen

### Landmarks and Patient Positioning

The patient is in the lateral decubitus position tilted slightly forward (Figure 19.1-5). The foot on the side to be blocked should be positioned over the dependent leg so that elicited motor response of the foot or toes can be easily observed.

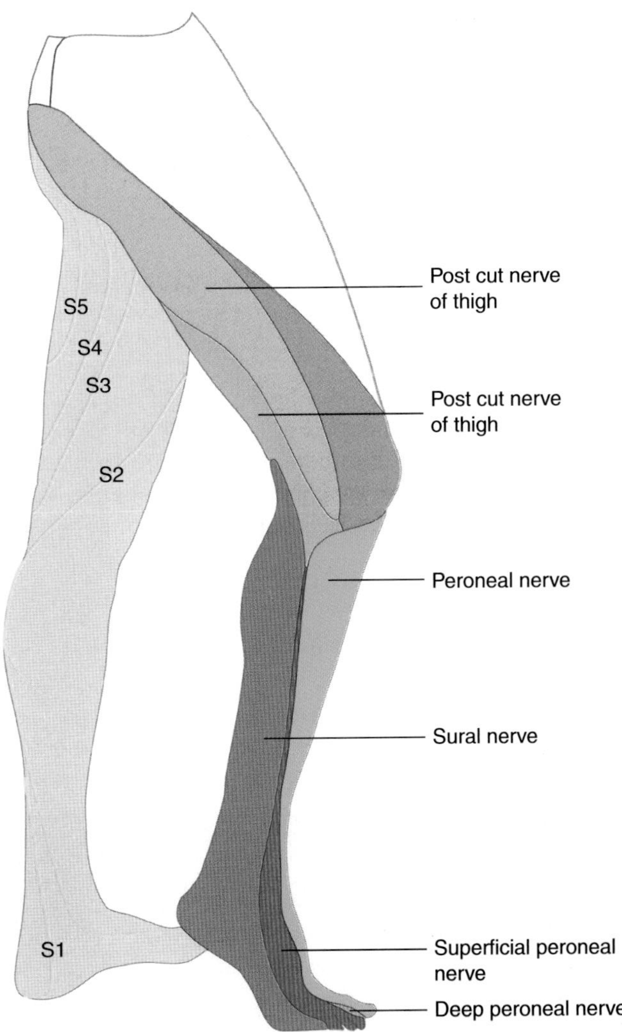


**FIGURE 19.1-4.** Sensory innervation of sciatic nerve and its terminal branches.

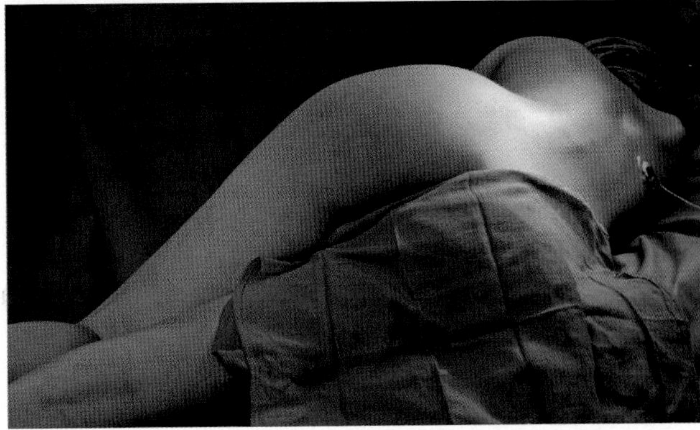

**FIGURE 19.1-5.** The patient is positioned in a lateral oblique position with the dependent leg extended and the leg to be blocked flexed in the knee.

## TIP

- The skin over the gluteal area is easily movable. Therefore, it is important that the patient remains in the same position in which the landmarks are outlined. A small forward or backward tilt of the pelvis can result in a significant shift of the landmarks, leading to difficulty localizing the sciatic nerve.

Landmarks for the posterior approach to a sciatic blockade are easily identified in most patients. A proper palpation technique is important to adhere to because the adipose tissue over the gluteal area can obscure these bony prominences. The landmarks are outlined with a marking pen:

1. Greater trochanter (Figure 19.1-6)
2. Posterior superior iliac spine (PSIS) (Figure 19.1-7)
3. Needle insertion point 4 cm distal to the midpoint between landmarks 1 and 2 (Figure 19.1-8)

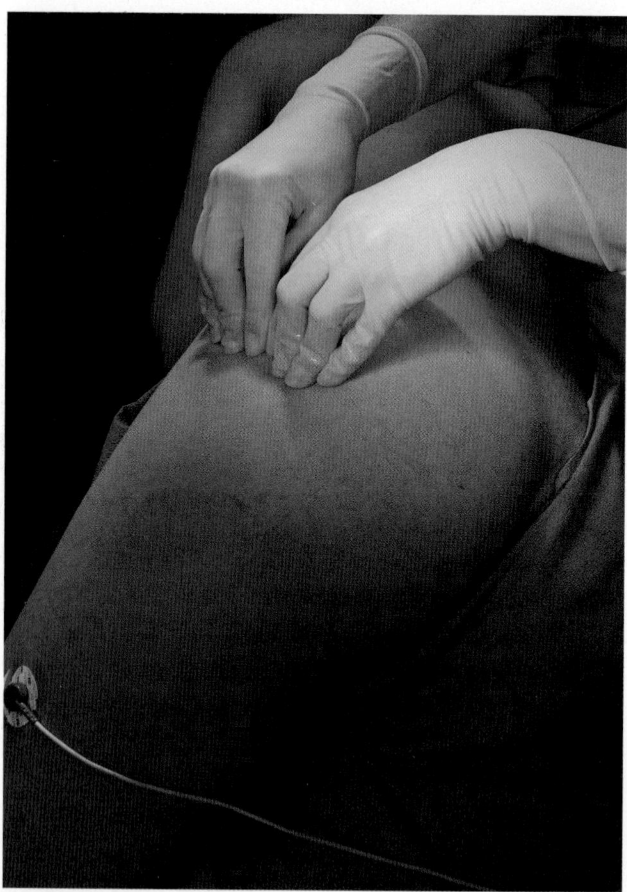

**FIGURE 19.1-6.** Palpation technique for the greater trochanter.

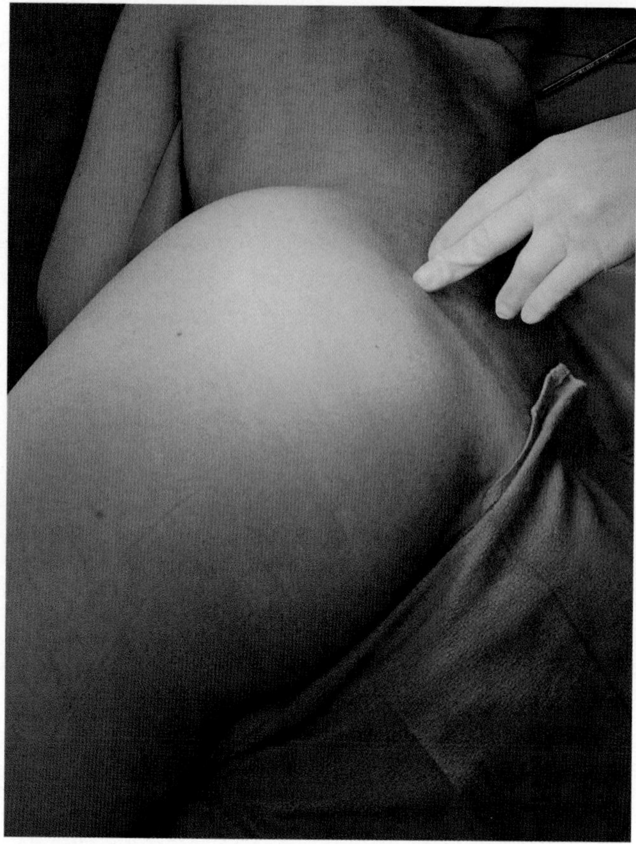

**FIGURE 19.1-7.** Palpation technique for posterior superior iliac spine.

A line between the greater trochanter and the PSIS is drawn and divided in half. Another line passing through the midpoint of this line and perpendicular to it is extended 4 cm caudal and marked as the needle insertion point.

## TIPS

- Palpating the greater trochanter: The osseous prominence of the greater trochanter is best approached from its posterior aspect, Figure 19.1-6.
- Palpating the PSIS: The palpating hand is rolled back from the greater trochanter until the fingers meet the osseous PSIS. This landmark should be labeled on the side facing the great trochanter, Figure 19.1-7.
- Identifying the "inner" aspects of the greater trochanter and the posterior-superior iliac spine results in a shorter line connecting the two and a more accurate approximation of the position of the sciatic nerve.

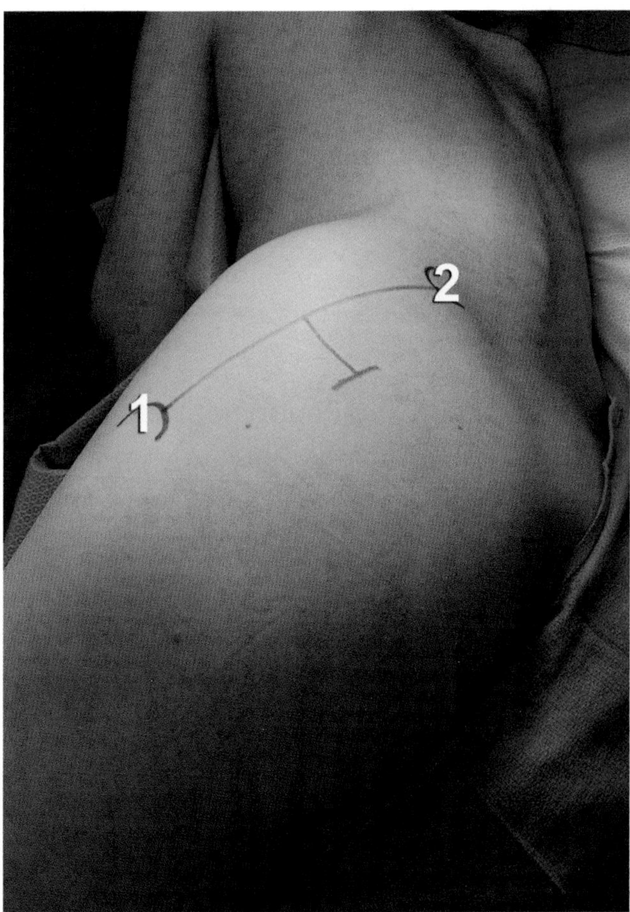


FIGURE 19.1-8. The needle insertion site is marked 5 cm posterior on the line passing through the midpoint between the greater trochanter ❶ and the posterior superior iliac spine ❷.

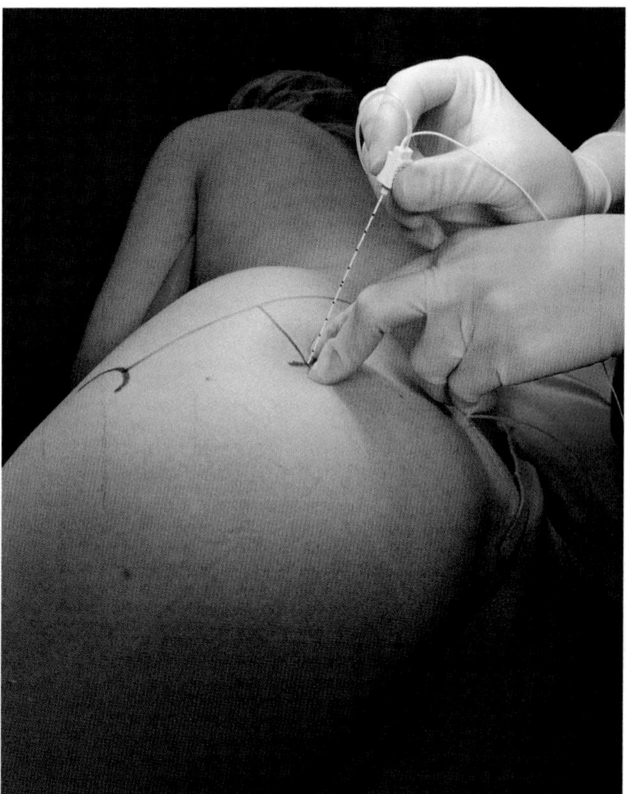

FIGURE 19.1-9. Needle insertion for the transgluteal (posterior) approach to sciatic nerve block.

## Technique

After skin disinfection, local anesthetic is infiltrated subcutaneously at the needle insertion site. The operator should assume an ergonomic position to allow precise needle maneuvering and monitoring of the responses to nerve stimulation.

The fingers of the palpating hand should be firmly pressed on the gluteus area to decrease the skin to nerve distance. Also, the skin between the index and middle fingers should be stretched to allow greater precision during block placement (Figure 19.1-9). The palpating hand should not be moved during the entire procedure. Even small movements of the palpating hand can change the position of the needle insertion site because of the highly movable skin and soft tissues in the gluteal region. The needle is introduced perpendicular to the spherical skin plane. Initially, the nerve stimulator should be set to deliver a current intensity of 1.5 mA to allow for the detection of both twitches of the gluteal muscles as the needle passes through tissue layers and stimulation of the sciatic nerve.

As the needle is advanced, twitches of the gluteal muscles are observed first. These twitches merely indicate the needle position is still too shallow. Once the gluteal twitches disappear, brisk response of the sciatic nerve ensues (hamstring, calf, foot, or toe twitches). After an initial stimulation of the sciatic nerve is obtained, the stimulating current is gradually decreased until twitches are still seen or felt at 0.2 to 0.5 mA. Typically, this occurs at a depth of 5 to 8 cm. At this low current intensity, any observed motor response is from the stimulation of the sciatic nerve, rather than direct muscle stimulation (false twitch). After negative aspiration for blood, 15 to 20 mL of local anesthetic is injected slowly. Any resistance to the injection of local anesthetic should prompt cessation of the injection and withdrawal of the needle by 1 mm before reattempting to inject. Persistent resistance to injection should prompt complete needle withdrawal and flushing to ensure the patency of the needle before reattempting the procedure.

## GOAL

The aim is to obtain visible or palpable twitches of the hamstrings, calf muscles, foot, or toes at 0.2 to 0.5 mA. Twitches of the hamstring are equally acceptable with the transgluteal approach because level of the block is proximal to the departure of the nerve branches to the hamstring muscle.

## Troubleshooting

Table 19.1-1 lists some common responses to nerve stimulation and the course of action to take to obtain the proper response.

## TIP

- Stimulation at a current intensity <0.5 mA may not be possible in some patients. This may occur in elderly patients and in patients with long-standing diabetes mellitus, peripheral neuropathy, sepsis, or severe peripheral vascular disease. In these cases, stimulating currents up to 1.0 mA should be accepted as long as the motor response is distal, specific and clearly seen or felt.
- We do not advise to use epinephrine in sciatic nerve blockade because of the possibility of ischemia of the sciatic nerve that could result due to the combination of stretching or sitting on the anesthetized nerve and the long duration of blockade.

## Block Dynamics and Perioperative Management

This technique may be associated with patient discomfort because the needle passes through the gluteus muscles. Adequate sedation and analgesia are important to ensure the patient is still and tranquil. Typically, we use midazolam 2 to 4 mg after the patient is positioned and alfentanil 500 to 750 μg just before the needle is inserted. A typical onset time for this block is 10 to 25 minutes, depending on the type, concentration, and volume of local anesthetic used. The first signs of onset of the blockade are usually a report by the patient that the foot "feels different" or an inability to wiggle the toes.

**TABLE 19.1-1 Some Common Responses to Nerve Stimulation and Course of Action for Proper Response**

| RESPONSE OBTAINED | INTERPRETATION | PROBLEM | ACTION |
|---|---|---|---|
| Local twitch of the gluteus muscle | Direct stimulation of the gluteus muscle | Needle placement too superficial | Continue advancing the needle |
| Needle contacts bone but local twitch of the gluteus muscle is not elicited | Needle is inserted close to the attachment of the gluteus muscle to the iliac bone | Landmarks are not well estimated/too lateral | Stop the procedure, recheck the patient's position, and reassess the landmarks |
| Needle encounters bone; sciatic twitches not elicited | Needle missed the plane of the sciatic nerve and is stopped by the hip joint or ischial bone | The needle is inserted too laterally (hip joint) or medially (ischial bone) | Withdraw the needle and redirect it slightly medially or laterally (10-15 degrees) |
| Needle placed deep (e.g. 8-10 cm); twitches not elicited; bone is not contacted | Needle has passed through the sciatic notch | Too inferior placement of the needle or insertion adequate but sciatic nerve is missed | Withdraw the needle and redirect it slightly superiorly |
| Hamstring twitch | Stimulation of the main trunk of the sciatic nerve | Acceptable response; these branches are within the sciatic nerve sheath at this level | Accept and inject local anesthetic |
| Twitches of the foot/toes | Stimulation of the sciatic nerve | Best response | Inject local anesthetic |

> **TIP**
>
> - Inadequate skin anesthesia despite an apparently timely onset of the blockade can occur. It can take 30 minutes or more for full sensory-motor anesthesia to develop. However, local infiltration by the surgeon at the site of the incision is often all that is needed to allow the surgery to proceed until the block fully sets up.

## Continuous Sciatic Nerve Block

Adequate experience with the single-injection technique is necessary to ensure efficacy and safety of the continuous block. The procedure is quite similar to the single-injection procedure; however, a slight angulation of the needle caudally is necessary after obtaining the nerve response to facilitate threading of the catheter. This technique can be used for surgery and postoperative pain management in patients undergoing a wide variety of lower leg, foot, and ankle surgeries. In our practice, perhaps the single most important indication for use of this block is for amputation of the lower extremity.

### Equipment

A standard regional anesthesia tray is prepared with the following equipment:

- Sterile towels and gauze packs
- One 20-mL syringe containing local anesthetic
- Sterile gloves, marking pen, and surface electrode
- A 3- to 5-mL syringe plus 25-gauge needle with local anesthetic for skin infiltration
- Peripheral nerve stimulator
- Catheter kit (including an 8- to 10-cm large-gauge stimulating needle and catheter)

Kits come in two varieties based on catheter construction: nonstimulating (conventional) and stimulating catheters. During the placement of a nonstimulating catheter, the needle is advanced first until appropriate twitches are obtained. Then 5 to 10 mL of local anesthetic or other injectate (e.g., D5W) is injected to "open up" a space for the catheter to facilitate its insertion. The catheter is threaded through the needle until approximately 3 to 5 cm is protruding beyond the tip of the needle. The needle is withdrawn, the catheter secured, and the remaining local anesthetic is injected via the catheter. *Stimulating* catheters are insulated and have a filament or core that transmits current to a bare metal tip. After obtaining twitches via the needle, the catheter is advanced with the nerve stimulator guidance while the motor response of the foot, calf, or toes is maintained. With the catheter technique, motor response of ≤1.0 mA is adequate. If the motor response is lost, the catheter can be withdrawn until it reappears, and the catheter is then readvanced while maintaining the response. This method requires that only nonconducting solution be injected through the needle (e.g., dextrose) prior to catheter advancement.

### Landmarks and Patient Positioning

Proper patient positioning at the outset and maintenance of this position during performance of a continuous sciatic nerve blockade is crucial for precise catheter placement.

The patient is placed in the lateral decubitus position similar to the single-injection block. A slightly forward pelvic tilt prevents "sagging" of the soft tissues in the gluteal area and significantly facilitates block placement.

The landmarks for a continuous sciatic block are the same as those in the single-injection technique (Figure 19.1-8):

1. Greater trochanter
2. Posterior superior iliac spine
3. Needle insertion site 4 cm caudal to the midpoint of the line between landmarks 1 and 2

### Technique

The continuous sciatic block technique is similar to the single-injection technique. With the patient in the lateral decubitus position and tilted slightly forward, the landmarks are identified and marked with the pen. After a thorough cleaning of the area with an antiseptic solution, the skin at the needle insertion site is infiltrated with local anesthetic. The palpating hand is positioned and fixed around the site of needle insertion to shorten the skin to nerve distance.

A 10-cm continuous block needle is connected to the nerve stimulator and inserted perpendicularly to the skin (Figure 19.1-10). The initial intensity of the stimulating current should be 1.0 to 1.5 mA.

> **TIP**
>
> - It is useful to inject some local anesthetic intramuscularly to prevent pain during advancement of the needle.
> - When a stimulating catheter is used, motor response at a current intensity ≤1.0 mA is adequate.

As the needle is advanced, twitches of the gluteus muscle are observed first. Deeper needle advancement results in stimulation of the sciatic nerve. The principles of nerve stimulation and needle redirection are identical to those for the single-injection technique. After obtaining the appropriate twitches, the needle is manipulated until the desired response (twitches of the hamstrings muscles or

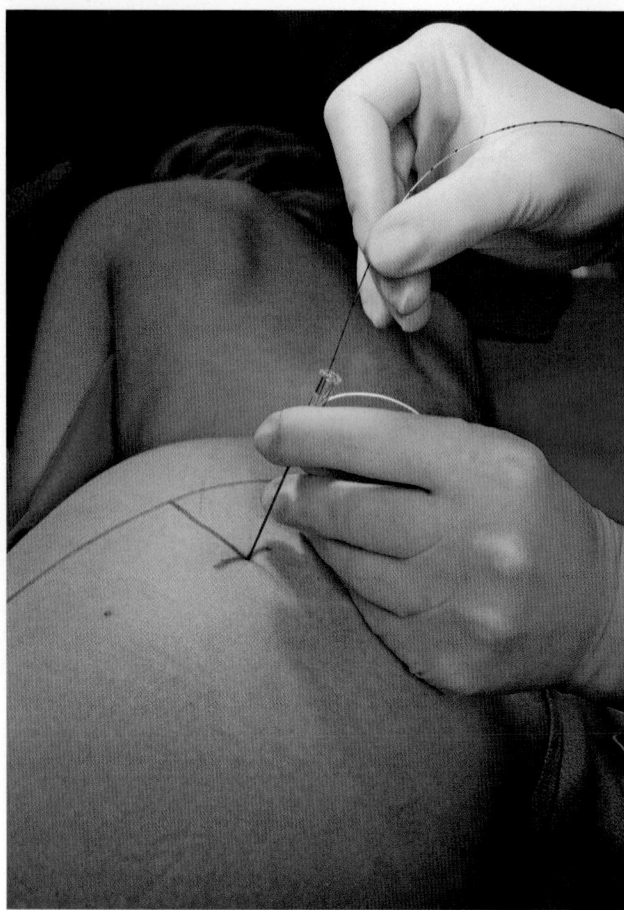

**FIGURE 19.1-10.** Insertion of the catheter for continuous sciatic nerve block.

foot) is seen or felt using a current of 0.5-1.0 mA. The catheter should be advanced 3-5 cm beyond the needle tip. The needle is withdrawn back to the skin level, and the catheter advanced simultaneously to prevent inadvertent removal of the catheter.

The catheter is checked for inadvertent intravascular placement and secured to the buttock using an adhesive skin preparation such as benzoin or Dermabond, followed by application of a clear occlusive dressing. The infusion port should be clearly marked "continuous nerve block."

**TIP**

- When insertion of the catheter proves difficult, lowering the angle of the needle can be helpful.

### *Continuous Infusion*

Continuous infusion is always initiated after administration of an initial bolus of dilute local anesthetic through the needle or catheter. For this purpose, we routinely use 0.2% ropivacaine 15 to 20 mL. Diluted bupivacaine or levobupivacaine are suitable but can result in more pronounced motor blockade. The infusion is maintained at 5 to 10 mL/h when a patient-controlled regional analgesic dose (5 mL every 60 minutes) is planned.

**TIPS**

- Breakthrough pain in patients undergoing a continuous infusion is always managed by administering a bolus of local anesthetic. Simply increasing the rate of infusion is never adequate.
- For patients on the ward, a higher concentration of a shorter acting local anesthetic (e.g., 1% lidocaine) is useful both to treat the pain quickly and to test the position of the catheter.
- When the bolus injection through the catheter fails to result in blockade after 30 minutes, the catheter should be considered dislodged and should be removed.

## Complications and How to Avoid Them

Table 19.1-2 lists some general and specific instructions on possible complications and methods used to avoid them.

| TABLE 19.1-2 | Complications of Sciatic Nerve Block and Preventive Techniques |
|---|---|
| ***Infection*** | • A strict aseptic technique is used. |
| ***Hematoma*** | • Avoid multiple needle insertions, particularly in patients receiving anticoagulant therapy. |
| ***Vascular puncture*** | • Vascular puncture is not common with this technique.<br>• Deep needle insertion should be avoided (pelvic vessels). |
| ***Local anesthetic toxicity*** | • Avoid using large volumes and doses of local anesthetic because of the proximity of the muscle beds and the potential for rapid absorption. |
| ***Nerve injury*** | • A sciatic block has a unique predisposition for mechanical and pressure injury.<br>• Nerve stimulation and slow needle advancement should be employed.<br>• Local anesthetic should never be injected when the patient complains of pain or abnormally high pressure on injection is noted.<br>• When stimulation is obtained with a current intensity of <0.2 mA, the needle should be pulled back to obtain the same response with a current intensity of >0.2 mA before injecting local anesthetic.<br>• Advance the needle slowly when twitches of the gluteus muscle cease to avoid impaling the sciatic nerve on the rapidly advancing needle. |
| ***Other*** | • Instruct the patient and nursing staff on the care of the insensate extremity.<br>• Elevate the heel and rest it on a soft cushion. Evaluate for pressure points on the heel: An insensate patient may not change positions frequently enough to prevent heel ischemia or decubitus formation.<br>• Explain the need for frequent body repositioning to avoid stretching and prolonged ischemia (sitting) on the anesthetized sciatic nerve. |

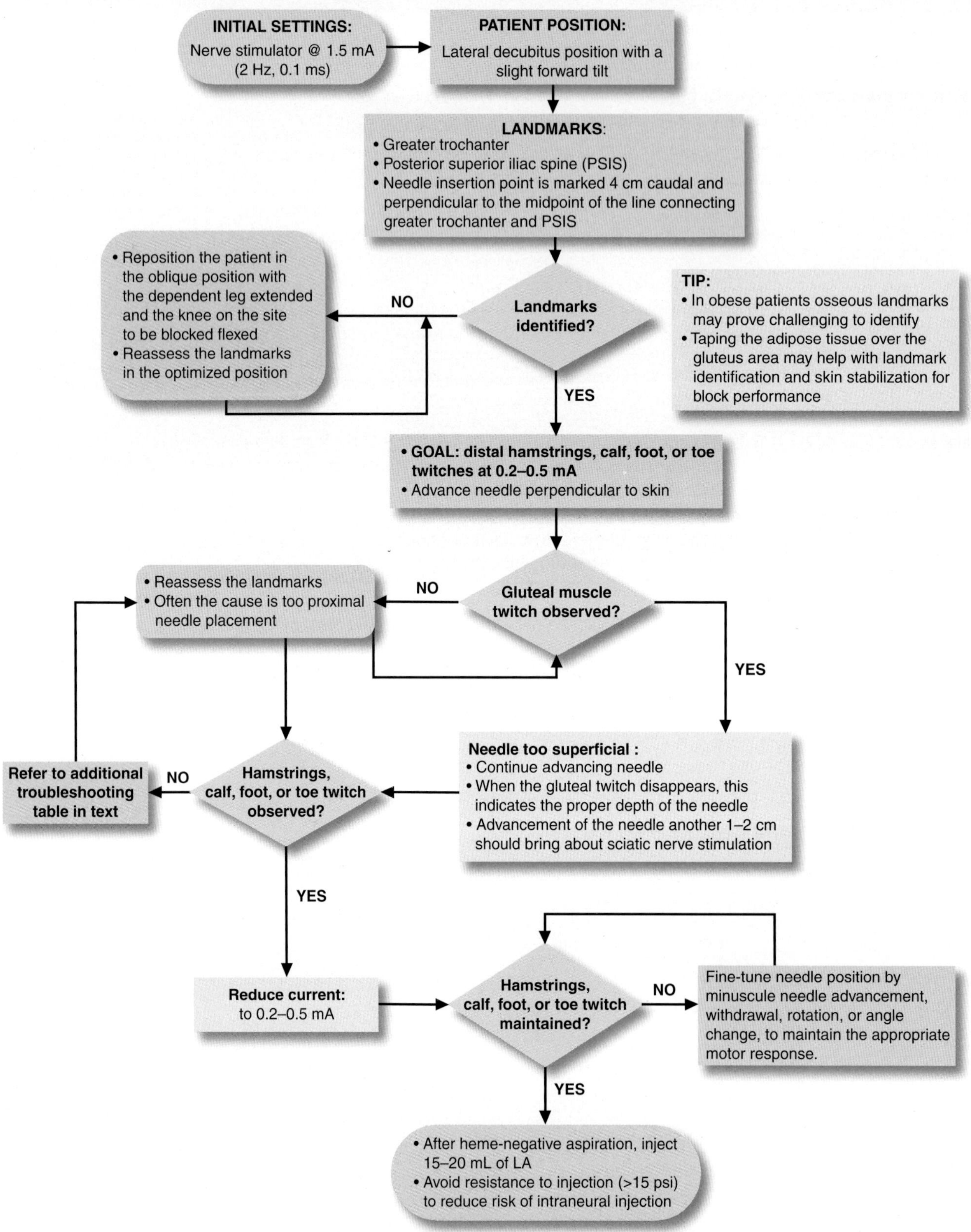
SCIATIC NERVE BLOCK (POSTERIOR APPROACH)
INITIAL SETTINGS:
Nerve stimulator @ 1.5 mA (2 Hz, 0.1 ms)
PATIENT POSITION:
Lateral decubitus position with a slight forward tilt
LANDMARKS:
• Greater trochanter
• Posterior superior iliac spine (PSIS)
• Needle insertion point is marked 4 cm caudal and perpendicular to the midpoint of the line connecting greater trochanter and PSIS
Landmarks identified?
NO
• Reposition the patient in the oblique position with the dependent leg extended and the knee on the site to be blocked flexed
• Reassess the landmarks in the optimized position
TIP:
• In obese patients osseous landmarks may prove challenging to identify
• Taping the adipose tissue over the gluteus area may help with landmark identification and skin stabilization for block performance
YES
• GOAL: distal hamstrings, calf, foot, or toe twitches at 0.2–0.5 mA
• Advance needle perpendicular to skin
Gluteal muscle twitch observed?
NO
• Reassess the landmarks
• Often the cause is too proximal needle placement
YES
Needle too superficial :
• Continue advancing needle
• When the gluteal twitch disappears, this indicates the proper depth of the needle
• Advancement of the needle another 1–2 cm should bring about sciatic nerve stimulation
Hamstrings, calf, foot, or toe twitch observed?
NO
Refer to additional troubleshooting table in text
YES
Reduce current: to 0.2–0.5 mA
Hamstrings, calf, foot, or toe twitch maintained?
NO
Fine-tune needle position by minuscule needle advancement, withdrawal, rotation, or angle change, to maintain the appropriate motor response.
YES
• After heme-negative aspiration, inject 15–20 mL of LA
• Avoid resistance to injection (>15 psi) to reduce risk of intraneural injection

## SUGGESTED READINGS


Altermatt F, Cortinez LI, Munoz H. Plasma levels of levobupivacaine after combined posterior lumbar plexus and sciatic nerve blocks. *Anesth Analg.* 2006;102(5):1597.

Bailey SL, et al. Sciatic nerve block. A comparison of single versus double injection technique. *Reg Anesth.* 1994;19(1):9-13.

Ben-David B, Schmalenberger K, Chelly JE. Analgesia after total knee arthroplasty: is continuous sciatic blockade needed in addition to continuous femoral blockade? *Anesth Analg.* 2004;98(3):747-749.

Bridenbaugh PO, Wedel DJ. The lower extremity: somatic blockade. In: Cousins MJ, Bridenbaugh PO, eds. *Neuronal Blockade in Clinical Anesthesia and Management of Pain.* 3rd ed. Philadelphia, PA: Lippincott-Raven; 1998:375–394.

Brummett CM, et al. Perineural dexmedetomidine added to ropivacaine causes a dose-dependent increase in the duration of thermal antinociception in sciatic nerve block in rat. *Anesthesiology.* 2009;111(5):1111-1119.

Candido KD, Sukhani R, McCarthy RJ. Posterior approach to the sciatic nerve: can "common sense" replace science and logic? *Anesthesiology.* 2003;99(5):1237-1238.

Capdevila X, Ponrouch M, Choquet O. Continuous peripheral nerve blocks in clinical practice. *Curr Opin Anaesthesiol.* 2008;21(5):619-623.

Casati A, et al. A double-blinded, randomized comparison of either 0.5% levobupivacaine or 0.5% ropivacaine for sciatic nerve block. *Anesth Analg.* 2002;94(4):987-990.

Casati A, et al. Levobupivacaine 0.2% or 0.125% for continuous sciatic nerve block: a prospective, randomized, double-blind comparison with 0.2% ropivacaine. *Anesth Analg.* 2004;99(3):919-923.

Casati A, et al. Using stimulating catheters for continuous sciatic nerve block shortens onset time of surgical block and minimizes postoperative consumption of pain medication after halux valgus repair as compared with conventional nonstimulating catheters. *Anesth Analg.* 2005;101(4):1192-1197.

Chan VW, et al. Ultrasound examination and localization of the sciatic nerve: a volunteer study. *Anesthesiology.* 2006; 104(2):309-314.

Crabtree EC, et al. A method to estimate the depth of the sciatic nerve during subgluteal block by using thigh diameter as a guide. *Reg Anesth Pain Med.* 2006;31(4):358-362.

Cuvillon P, et al. Comparison of the parasacral approach and the posterior approach, with single- and double-injection techniques, to block the sciatic nerve. *Anesthesiology.* 2003;98(6):1436-1441.

Dalens B, Tanguy A, Vanneuville G. Sciatic nerve blocks in children: comparison of the posterior, anterior, and lateral approaches in 180 pediatric patients. *Anesth Analg.* 1990;70(2):131-137.

Danelli G, et al. Ultrasound vs nerve stimulation multiple injection technique for posterior popliteal sciatic nerve block. *Anaesthesia.* 2009;64(6):638-642.

di Benedetto P, et al. A new posterior approach to the sciatic nerve block: a prospective, randomized comparison with the classic posterior approach. *Anesth Analg.* 2001;93(4): 1040-1044.

di Benedetto P, et al. Postoperative analgesia with continuous sciatic nerve block after foot surgery: a prospective, randomized comparison between the popliteal and subgluteal approaches. *Anesth Analg.* 2002;94(4):996–1000.

di Benedetto P, et al. Continuous sciatic nerve block: how to choose among different proximal approaches? Gluteal or subgluteal continuous sciatic nerve block. *Anesth Analg.* 2003;97(1):296-297.

di Benedetto P, Casati A, Bertini L. Continuous subgluteus sciatic nerve block after orthopedic foot and ankle surgery: comparison of two infusion techniques. *Reg Anesth Pain Med.* 2002;27(2): 168-172.

Ericksen ML, Swenson JD, Pace NL. The anatomic relationship of the sciatic nerve to the lesser trochanter: implications for anterior sciatic nerve block. *Anesth Analg.* 2002;95(4):1071-1074.

Farny J, Girard M, Drolet P. Posterior approach to the lumbar plexus combined with a sciatic nerve block using lidocaine. *Can J Anaesth.* 1994;41(6):486-491.

Floch H, et al. Computed tomography scanning of the sciatic nerve posterior to the femur: practical implications for the lateral midfemoral block. *Reg Anesth Pain Med.* 2003;28(5):445-449.

Fournier R, et al. Levobupivacaine 0.5% provides longer analgesia after sciatic nerve block using the Labat approach than the same dose of ropivacaine in foot and ankle surgery. *Anesth Analg.* 2010;110(5):1486-1489.

Franco CD. Posterior approach to the sciatic nerve in adults: is euclidean geometry still necessary? *Anesthesiology.* 2003;98(3):723-728.

Franco CD, et al. A subgluteal approach to the sciatic nerve in adults at 10 cm from the midline. *Reg Anesth Pain Med.* 2006;31(3):215-220.

Franco CD, Tyler SG. Modified subgluteal approach to the sciatic nerve. *Anesth Analg.* 2003;97(4):1197.

Fuzier R, et al. Does the sciatic nerve approach influence thigh tourniquet tolerance during below-knee surgery? *Anesth Analg.* 2005;100(5):1511-1514.

Gaertner E, et al. Continuous parasacral sciatic block: a radiographic study. *Anesth Analg.* 2004;98(3):831-834; table of contents.

Hadžić A, et al. The practice of peripheral nerve blocks in the United States: a national survey. *Reg Anesth Pain Med.* 1998;23(3):241-246.

Hagon BS, et al. Parasacral sciatic nerve block: does the elicited motor response predict the success rate? *Anesth Analg.* 2007;105(1):263-266.

Hanks RK, et al. The effect of age on sciatic nerve block duration. *Anesth Analg.* 2006;102(2):588-592.

Helayel PE, et al. Urinary incontinence after bilateral parasacral sciatic-nerve block: report of two cases. *Reg Anesth Pain Med.* 2006;31(4):368-371.

Jochum D, et al. Adding a selective obturator nerve block to the parasacral sciatic nerve block: an evaluation. *Anesth Analg.* 2004;99(5):1544-1549.

Kilpatrick AW, Coventry DM, Todd JG. A comparison of two approaches to sciatic nerve block. *Anaesthesia.* 1992;47(2):155-157.

Klein SM, et al. Ambulatory surgery for multi-ligament knee reconstruction with continuous dual catheter peripheral nerve blockade. *Can J Anaesth.* 2001;48(4):375-378.

Kumar A. Evaluation of a new posterior subgluteus approach to sciatic nerve. *Anesth Analg.* 2002;95(3):780.

Latzke D, et al. Minimal local anaesthetic volumes for sciatic nerve block: evaluation of ED 99 in volunteers. *Br J Anaesth.* 2010;104(2):239-244.

Levesque S, Delbos A. Sciatic nerve block for total-knee replacement: is it really necessary in all patients? *Reg Anesth Pain Med.* 2005;30(4):410-411.

Mansour NY, Bennetts FE. An observational study of combined continuous lumbar plexus and single-shot sciatic nerve blocks for post-knee surgery analgesia. *Reg Anesth.* 1996;21(4):287-291.

Merchan MC, et al. The sciatic nerve block: a new posterior approach to sacral plexus. *Reg Anesth Pain Med.* 2002;27(3):333-334.

Moayeri N, Groen GJ. Differences in quantitative architecture of sciatic nerve may explain differences in potential vulnerability to nerve injury, onset time, and minimum effective anesthetic volume. *Anesthesiology.* 2009;111(5):1128-1134.

Morin AM, et al. Postoperative analgesia and functional recovery after total-knee replacement: comparison of a continuous posterior lumbar plexus (psoas compartment) block, a continuous femoral nerve block, and the combination of a continuous femoral and sciatic nerve block. *Reg Anesth Pain Med.* 2005;30(5):434-445.

Morrow MJ. The lateral approach to the sciatic nerve. *Anesth Analg.* 2000;90(3):770.

Nader A, et al, Sensory testing of distal sural and posterior tibial nerves provides early prediction of surgical anesthesia after single-injection infragluteal-parabiceps sciatic nerve block. *Anesth Analg.* 2010;110(3):951-957.

Navas AM, de la Tabla Gonzalez RO, Gutierrez TV. Combined femoral-sciatic catheters for postoperative pain treatment after total knee replacement. *Anesth Analg.* 2007;105(1):288.

Pham Dang C, et al. The value of adding sciatic block to continuous femoral block for analgesia after total knee replacement. *Reg Anesth Pain Med.* 2005;30(2):128-133.

Ripart J, et al. Parasacral approach to block the sciatic nerve: a 400-case survey. *Reg Anesth Pain Med.*, 2005;30(2):193-197.

Robards C, et al. Sciatic nerve catheter placement: success with using the Raj approach. *Anesth Analg.* 2009;109(3):972-975.

Rodriguez J, et al. Intraneural catheterization of the sciatic nerve in humans: a pilot study. *Reg Anesth Pain Med.* 2008;33(4):285-290.

Sala-Blanch X, et al. Structural injury to the human sciatic nerve after intraneural needle insertion. *Reg Anesth Pain Med.* 2009;34(3):201-205.

Sciard D, Lam N, Hussain M. Continuous sciatic nerve block and total-knee arthroplasty. *Reg Anesth Pain Med.* 2005;30(4):411-412.

Smith BE, Siggins D. Low volume, high concentration block of the sciatic nerve. *Anaesthesia.* 1988;43(1):8-11.

Souron V, Eyrolle L, Rosencher N. The Mansour's sacral plexus block: an effective technique for continuous block. *Reg Anesth Pain Med.* 2000;25(2):208-209.

Sukhani R, et al. Infragluteal-parabiceps sciatic nerve block: an evaluation of a novel approach using a single-injection technique. *Anesth Analg.* 2003;96(3):868-873.

Sukhani R, et al. Nerve stimulator-assisted evoked motor response predicts the latency and success of a single-injection sciatic block. *Anesth Analg.* 2004;99(2):584-588.

Suresh S, et al. Anatomical location of the bifurcation of the sciatic nerve in the posterior thigh in infants and children: a formula derived from MRI imaging for nerve localization. *Reg Anesth Pain Med.* 2007;32(4):351-353.

Sutherland ID. Continuous sciatic nerve infusion: expanded case report describing a new approach. *Reg Anesth Pain Med.* 1998;23(5):496-501.

Taboada M, et al. The effects of three different approaches on the onset time of sciatic nerve blocks with 0.75% ropivacaine. *Anesth Analg.* 2004;98(1):242-247.

Taboada M, et al. Plantar flexion seems more reliable than dorsiflexion with Labat's sciatic nerve block: a prospective, randomized comparison. *Anesth Analg.* 2005;100(1):250-254.

Taboada M, et al. Does the site of injection distal to the greater trochanter make a difference in lateral sciatic nerve blockade? *Anesth Analg.* 2005;101(4):1188-1191.

Taboada M, et al. What is the minimum effective volume of local anesthetic required for sciatic nerve blockade? A prospective, randomized comparison between a popliteal and a subgluteal approach. *Anesth Analg.* 2006;102(2):593-597.

Taboada M, et al. A prospective, randomized comparison between the popliteal and subgluteal approaches for continuous sciatic nerve block with stimulating catheters. *Anesth Analg.* 2006;103(1):244-247.

Taboada M, et al. Two unusual cases of urinary incontinence during continuous sciatic nerve block with stimulating catheters. *Anesth Analg.* 2009;108(3):1042-1043.

Taboada Muniz M, et al. Low volume and high concentration of local anesthetic is more efficacious than high volume and low concentration in Labat's sciatic nerve block: a prospective, randomized comparison. *Anesth Analg.* 2008;107(6):2085-2088.

Tobe M, et al. Long-term effect of sciatic nerve block with slow-release lidocaine in a rat model of postoperative pain. *Anesthesiology.* 2010;112(6):1473-1481.

Tran D, Clemente A, Finlayson RJ. A review of approaches and techniques for lower extremity nerve blocks. *Can J Anaesth.* 2007;54(11):922-934.

Tsai TP, et al. Intensity of the stimulating current may not be a reliable indicator of intraneural needle placement. *Reg Anesth Pain Med.* 2008;33(3):207-210.

Urmey WF, Grossi P. Use of sequential electrical nerve stimuli (SENS) for location of the sciatic nerve and lumbar plexus. *Reg Anesth Pain Med.* 2006;31(5):463-469.

Vanterpool S, et al. Combined lumbar-plexus and sciatic-nerve blocks: an analysis of plasma ropivacaine concentrations. *Reg Anesth Pain Med.* 2006;31(5):417-421.

Voelckel WG, et al. Signs of inflammation after sciatic nerve block in pigs. *Anesth Analg.* 2005;101(6):1844-1846.

Wang CF, et al. An absorbable local anesthetic matrix provides several days of functional sciatic nerve blockade. *Anesth Analg.* 2009;108(3):1027-1033.

Williams BA, et al. Femoral-sciatic nerve blocks for complex outpatient knee surgery are associated with less postoperative pain before same-day discharge: a review of 1,200 consecutive cases from the period 1996–1999. *Anesthesiology.* 2003;98(5):1206-1213.

Yung E, et al. Bicarbonate plus epinephrine shortens the onset and prolongs the duration of sciatic block using chloroprocaine followed by bupivacaine in sprague-dawley rats. *Reg Anesth Pain Med.* 2009;34(3):196-200.

Zaric D, et al. A comparison of epidural analgesia with combined continuous femoral-sciatic nerve blocks after total knee replacement. *Anesth Analg.* 2006;102(4):1240-1246.

# PART 2: ANTERIOR APPROACH

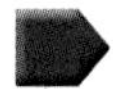

## General Considerations

The anterior approach to sciatic block is an advanced nerve block technique. The block is well-suited for surgery on the leg below the knee, particularly on the ankle and foot. It provides complete anesthesia of the leg below the knee with the exception of the medial strip of skin, which is innervated by the saphenous nerve. When combined with a femoral nerve block, this procedure results in anesthesia of the entire knee and leg. It should be noted that the anterior approach may have less utility compared with the posterior approach. The sciatic nerve is blocked more distally, and a higher level of skill is required to achieve reliable anesthesia. Consequently, we reserve the use of this block for patients who cannot be repositioned into the lateral position needed for the posterior approach. This technique is not ideal for catheter insertion because of the deep location and perpendicular angle of insertion required to reach the sciatic nerve.

## Functional Anatomy

The sciatic nerve is formed from the L4 through S3 roots. The roots of the sacral plexus combine on the anterior surface of the sacrum and are assembled into the sciatic nerve on the anterior surface of the piriformis muscle. The course of the nerve can be estimated by drawing a line on the back of the thigh from the apex of the popliteal fossa to the midpoint of a line joining the ischial tuberosity to the apex of the greater trochanter. The nerve exits the pelvis through the greater sciatic notch and gives off numerous articular (hip, knee) and muscular branches. Once in the upper thigh, it continues its descent behind the lesser trochanter and becomes completely covered by the femur. The only part of the nerve accessible to blockade through an anterior approach is a short segment slightly above and below the lesser trochanter. The muscular branches of the sciatic nerve are distributed to the biceps femoris, semitendinosus, and semimembranosus, and to the ischial head of the adductor magnus.

**TIP**

- Because the level of the blockade with the anterior approach to sciatic block is often below the departure of the muscular branches, twitches of the hamstring muscles *cannot* be accepted as a reliable sign of localization of the main trunk of the sciatic nerve.

## Distribution of Blockade

A sciatic nerve block through the anterior approach results in anesthesia of the hamstring muscles below the blockade and the entire leg below the knee (including the ankle and foot) except for a strip of skin over the medial aspect. The distal two thirds of the hamstring muscles are also anesthetized. Neither the posterior cutaneous nerve of the thigh and articular branches of the hip are anesthetized, nor the skin over the medial aspect of the leg below, because it is innervated by the saphenous nerve, a branch of the femoral nerve. Consequently, the anterior approach to sciatic block should be chosen for selected patients undergoing knee or below-knee surgery who also are unable to be positioned for the posterior approach. A proximal thigh tourniquet should be reconsidered with this technique because of the risk of prolonged ischemia of the sciatic nerve, particularly when epinephrine-containing solutions of local anesthetics are used.

### Equipment

A standard regional anesthesia tray is prepared with the following equipment:

- Sterile towels and gauze packs
- One 20-mL syringe containing local anesthetic
- A 3- to 5-mL syringe plus a 25-gauge needle with local anesthetic for skin infiltration
- A 1.5-mm, 22-gauge short-bevel insulated stimulating needle
- Peripheral nerve stimulator
- Sterile gloves; marking pen

### Landmarks and Patient Positioning

The patient is in the supine position with both legs fully extended.

**TIP**

- Placing a pillow underneath the patient's hips can be useful to optimize access to the groin and landmarks for the block.

The following landmarks should be outlined routinely using a marking pen:

1. Femoral crease (Figure 19.2-1).
2. Femoral artery pulse (Figure 19.2-2).
3. Needle insertion point is marked 4 to 5 cm distally to the femoral crease on a line passing through the pulse of the femoral artery and perpendicularly to the femoral crease (Figures 19.2-3 and 19.2-4).

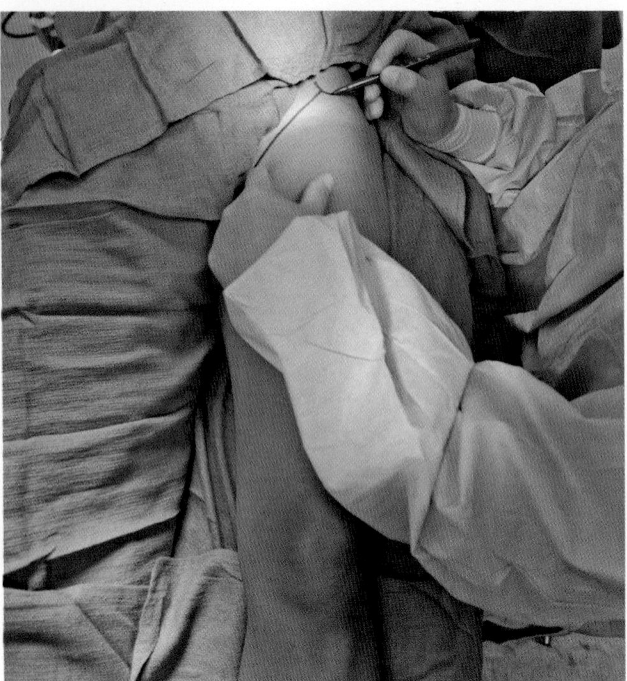

**FIGURE 19.2-1.** Landmarks for anterior sciatic block. Femoral crease is outlined as a line connecting anterior superior iliac spine (semicircle) and the finger palpating the pubic bone.

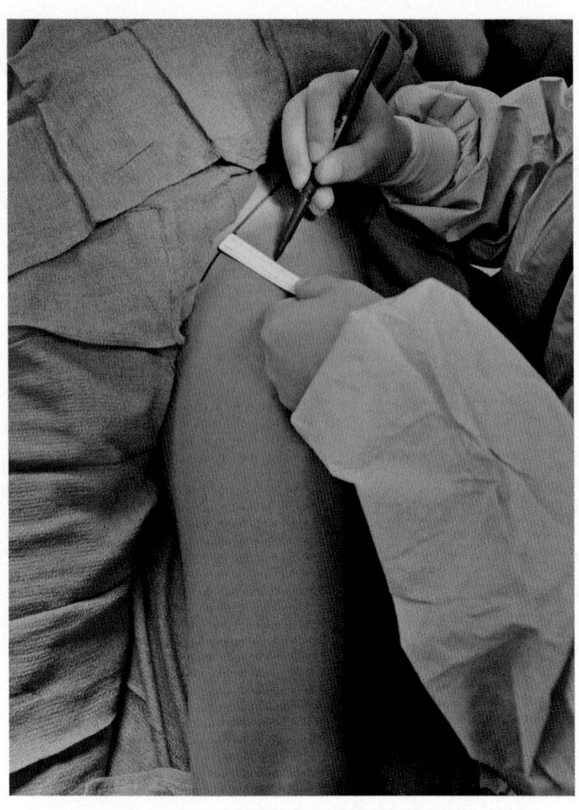

**FIGURE 19.2-3.** A line passing through the pulse of the femoral artery and perpendicular to the femoral crease is drawn.

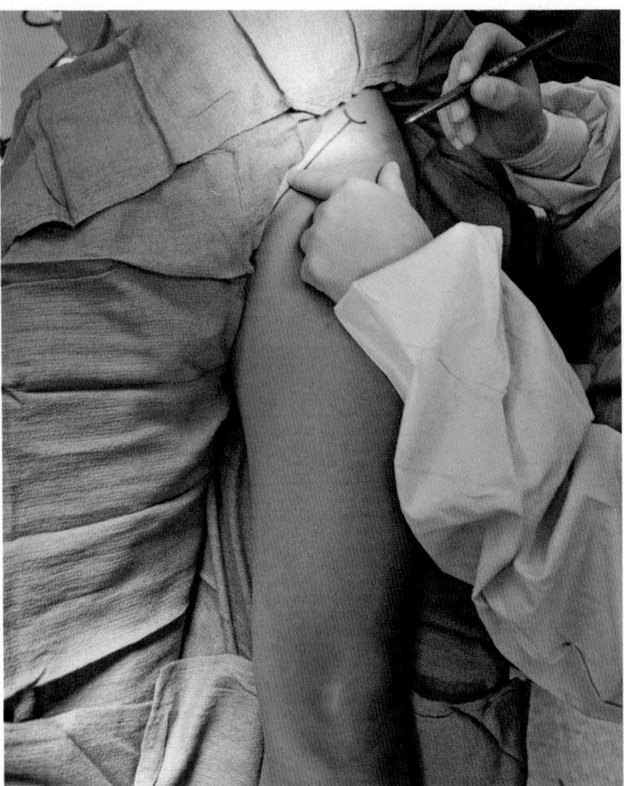

**FIGURE 19.2-2.** Landmarks for the anterior sciatic nerve block. The index finger is on the pulse of the femoral artery.

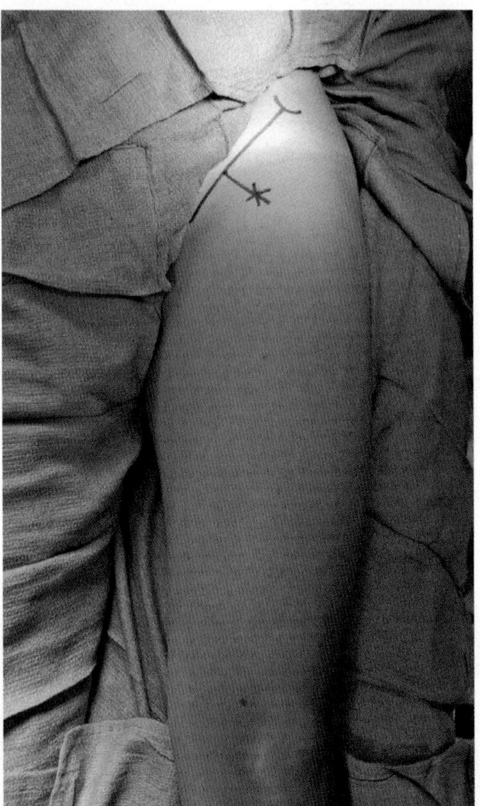

**FIGURE 19.2-4.** Point of needle insertion is labeled 4-5 cm from the femoral crease on the perpendicular line that passes through the femoral pulse

## TIP

- Avoid displacing the soft tissues laterally or medially during palpation of the femoral artery. The skin and subcutaneous tissue in this area are highly movable, and lateral or medial displacement of the tissues can skew the femoral artery landmark.

## Technique

After cleaning the area with an antiseptic solution, local anesthetic is infiltrated subcutaneously at the determined needle insertion site. The operator should stand on the side of the patient to be blocked and have the ipsilateral foot in the line of vision to be able to monitor the patient and the responses to nerve stimulation.

The fingers of the palpating hand should be firmly pressed against the quadriceps muscle to decrease the skin-nerve distance and stabilize the needle path. The needle is introduced at an angle perpendicular to the skin plane (Figure 19.2-5).

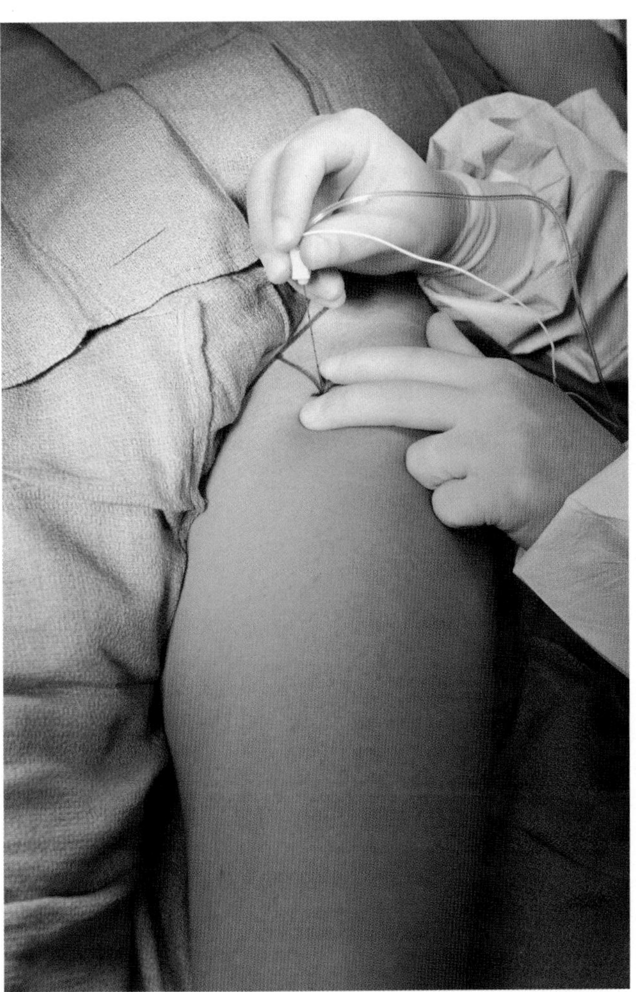

**FIGURE 19.2-5.** Needle insertion for anterior sciatic block.

Initially, the nerve stimulator should be set to deliver a 1.5-mA current, as with all "deep" blocks. The current of higher intensity results in an exaggerated motor response, decreasing the chance of missing this twitch of the foot or toes during nerve localization.. The twitch of the foot or toes typically occurs at a depth of 10 to 12 cm. After obtaining negative results from an aspiration test for blood, 15 to 20 mL of local anesthetic is slowly injected. Any resistance to the injection of local anesthetic should prompt cessation of the injection attempt, followed by slight withdrawal. Persistent resistance to injection should prompt complete needle withdrawal and flushing of the needle before reattempting the block; see "tips" for more explanation of the importance of this strategy.

## TIP

- Because the needle transverses muscle planes, it is occasionally obstructed by muscle fibers. However, when resistance to injection is met, it is never correct to assume the needle is obstructed. The proper action is to withdraw the needle and check its patency by flushing before reinserting it.

## GOAL

Visible or palpable twitches of the calf muscles, foot, or toes at 0.2 to 0.5 mA.

## TIPS

- Local twitches of the quadriceps muscle are elicited often during needle advancement. The needle should be advanced past these twitches.
- Although there is a concern about femoral nerve injury with further needle advancement, this concern is theoretical. At this level, the femoral nerve is divided into smaller terminal branches that are mobile and are unlikely to be penetrated by a slowly advancing, short-beveled needle.
- Resting the heel on the bed surface may prevent the foot from twitching even when the sciatic nerve is stimulated. This can be prevented by placing the ankle on a footrest or by having an assistant continuously palpate the calf or Achilles' tendon.

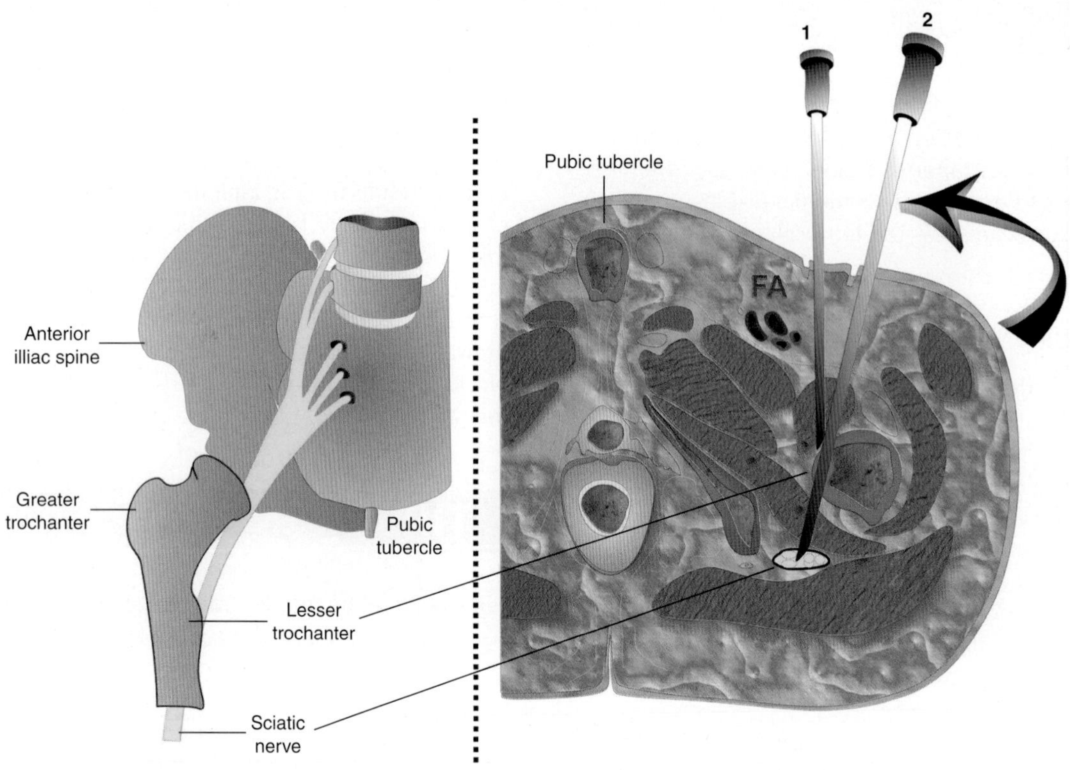


**FIGURE 19.2-6.** Needle pass required to reach the sciatic nerve through the anterior approach. Note that the lesser trochanter of the femur partially obscures the sciatic nerve. ❶ Internal rotation of the leg (arrow) is beneficial in allowing access of the needle to the sciatic nerve ❷.

- Because branches to the hamstring muscle may leave the main trunk of the sciatic nerve before the level of needle insertion, twitches of the hamstring should not be accepted as a reliable sign of sciatic nerve localization Figure 19.1-2.
- Bone contact is frequently encountered during needle advancement, indicating the needle has contacted the femur (usually the lesser trochanter) (Figure 19.2-6). When the needle is stopped by the bone, the following algorithm is used:
  - Withdraw the needle back to the subcutaneous tissue.
  - Rotate the foot inward (internal rotation).
  - Advance the needle to bypass the lesser trochanter. The internal rotation of the leg also rotates the lesser trochanter posteriorly and away from the path of the needle and often allows passage of the needle toward the sciatic nerve.
  - When steps 1-3 fail to facilitate passage of the needle, the needle is withdrawn back to the skin and reinserted 1-2 cm medial to the initial insertion site and at a slightly medial angulation (Figure 19.2-7).

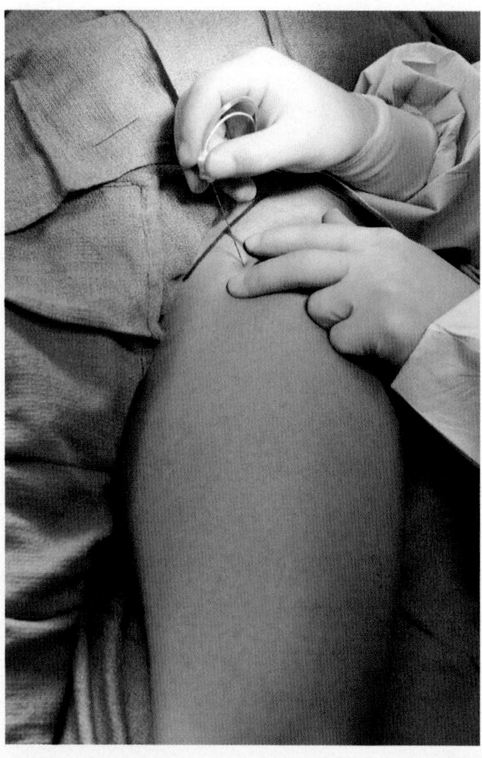

**FIGURE 19.2-7.** When the needle fails to pass by the trochanter minor despite internal leg rotation, the needle is inserted 1–2 cm medial to the initial insertion and advanced in a slight medial to lateral direction to reach the sciatic nerve.

**TABLE 19.2-1 Common Responses to Nerve Stimulation and Course of Action for Proper Response**

| RESPONSE OBTAINED | INTERPRETATION | PROBLEM | ACTION |
|---|---|---|---|
| Twitch of the quadriceps muscle (patella twitch) | Common; stimulation of the branches of the femoral nerve | Needle placement too shallow (superficial) | Continue advancing the needle |
| Local twitch at the femoral crease area | Direct stimulation of the iliopsoas or pectineus muscles | Too cephalad insertion of the needle | Stop the procedure and reassess the landmarks |
| Hamstring twitch | The needle may be stimulating branch(es) of the sciatic nerve to the hamstring muscle; direct stimulation of the hamstring with higher current is also possible | Unreliable | Withdraw needle and redirect it slightly medially or laterally (5–10°) |
| The needle is placed deep (12–15 cm), but twitches were not elicited and bone is not contacted | The needle is likely inserted too medial | | Withdraw needle and redirect it slightly laterally |
| Twitches of the calf, foot, or toes | Stimulation of the sciatic nerve | None | Accept and inject local anesthetic |

## Troubleshooting

Some common responses to nerve stimulation and the course of action to take to obtain the proper response are given in Table 19.2-1.

**TIP**

- **We avoid the use of epinephrine for the anterior approach to a sciatic nerve block because of the perceived risk of nerve ischemia due to the combined effects of the vasoconstrictive action of epinephrine and application of a tourniquet.**

## Block Dynamics and Perioperative Management

Performance of the anterior approach to a sciatic block is associated with patient discomfort because the needle must transverse multiple muscle planes on its way to the sciatic nerve. The administration of midazolam 2 to 4 mg after the patient is positioned and alfentanil 500–1000 mg just before infiltration of local anesthetic is beneficial to allay anxiety and decrease discomfort during the procedure in most patients. A typical onset time for this block is 20 to 30 minutes, depending on the type, concentration, and volume of local anesthetic used. The first sign of blockade onset is usually a report by the patient that the foot "feels different" or an inability to wiggle the toes.

**TIP**

- **When indicated, the femoral block is performed first, resulting in anesthesia of the skin and muscle overlying the needle path for the anterior sciatic block and less patient discomfort.**

## Complications and How to Avoid Them

Table 19.2-2 lists some general and specific instructions on possible complications and methods that can be used to avoid them.

**TABLE 19.2-2 Complications of Anterior Approach to Sciatic Nerve Block and Preventive Techniques**

| | |
|---|---|
| ***Infection*** | • A strict aseptic technique should always be used. |
| ***Hematoma*** | • Avoid multiple needle insertions.<br>• This technique should be avoided in patients receiving anticoagulant therapy. |
| ***Vascular puncture*** | • Vascular puncture is not common with this technique; when it occurs, it is usually because of too medial a placement of the needle (femoral artery and vein). |
| ***Local anesthetic toxicity*** | • Systemic toxicity after sciatic blockade is not common due to the lower volume; however, it is important to avoid injecting large volumes and doses of local anesthetic because of the proximity of the muscle beds and the potential for rapid absorption. |
| ***Nerve injury*** | • A sciatic block appears to be uniquely sensitive to mechanical and pressure injury.<br>• Nerve stimulation and slow needle advancement should be employed.<br>• Local anesthetic should never be injected when a patient complains of pain.<br>• Never forcefully inject local anesthetic when an abnormally high pressure on injection (>15 psi) is noted.<br>• It is never correct to assume that the needle is obstructed with tissue debris when resistance to injection is met; the needle should be taken out and checked for the patency (flush) before reinsertion and another attempt is made to inject.<br>• When stimulation is obtained with current intensity of <0.2 mA, the needle should be pulled back to obtain the same response with a current intensity of 0.2–0.5 mA before injecting local anesthetic. |
| ***Tourniquet*** | • Avoid the use of a tourniquet when possible.<br>• Injection of the local anesthetic within the sciatic nerve sheath, epinephrine, and a tourniquet over the site of injection can all combine to cause ischemia of the sciatic nerve. |
| ***Other*** | • Instruct the patient and nursing staff on care of the insensate extremity.<br>• Explain to the patient that frequent body repositioning is needed to avoid stretching and prolonged ischemia (sitting) of the anesthetized sciatic nerve.<br>• Advise the use of heel padding during prolonged bed rest or sleep. |

# SCIATIC NERVE BLOCK (ANTERIOR APPROACH)

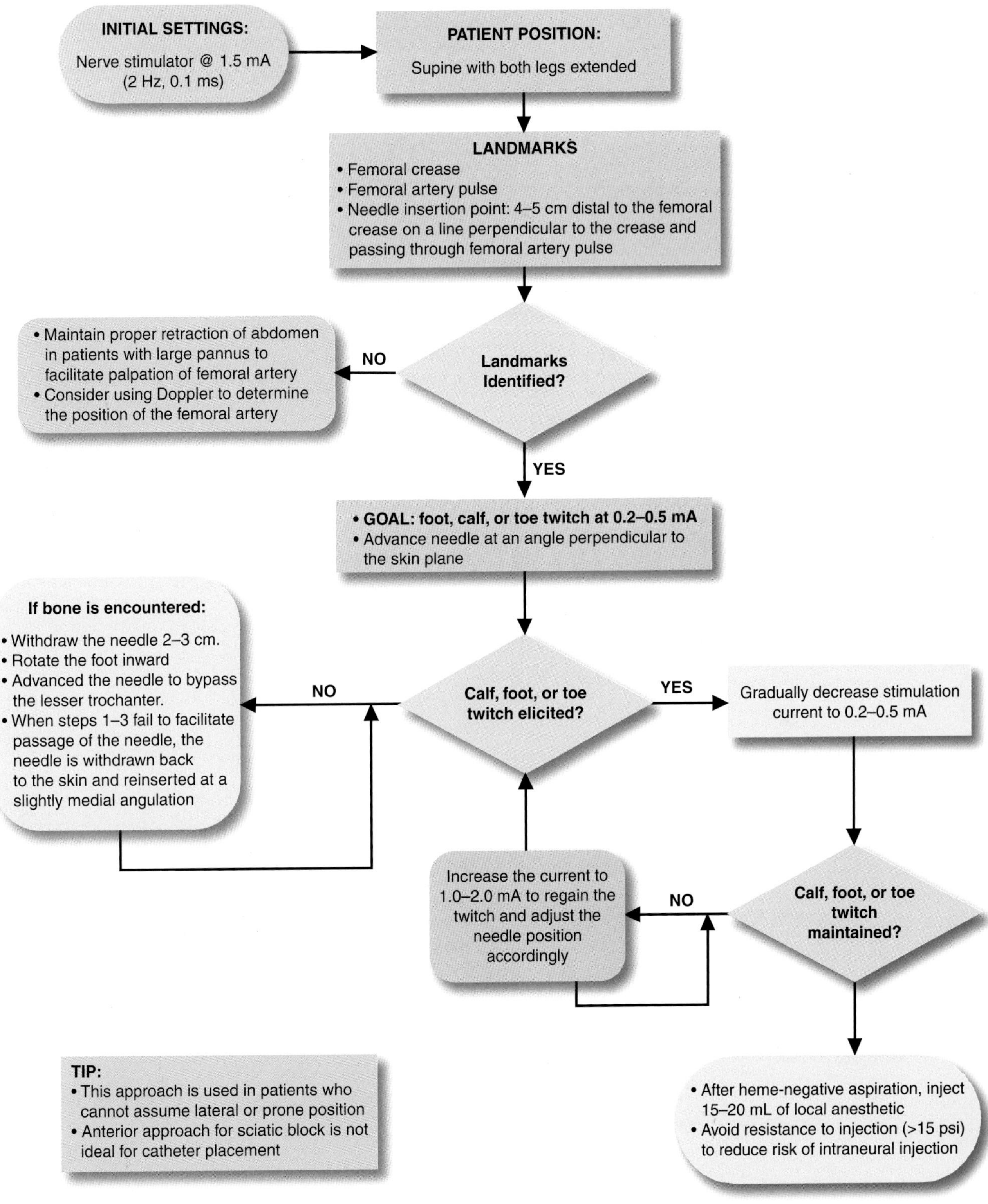

## SUGGESTED READINGS


Barbero C, Fuzier R, Samii K. Anterior approach to the sciatic nerve block: adaptation to the patient's height. *Anesth Analg.* 2004;98(6):1785-1788.

Blumenthal S, Lambert M, Borgeat A. Intraneural injection during anterior approach for sciatic nerve block: what have we learned and where to go from here? *Anesthesiology.* 2005;102(6):1283.

Chelly JE, Delaunay L. A new anterior approach to the sciatic nerve block. *Anesthesiology.* 1999;91(6):1655-1660.

Ericksen ML, Swenson JD, Pace NL. The anatomic relationship of the sciatic nerve to the lesser trochanter: implications for anterior sciatic nerve block. *Anesth Analg.* 2002;95(4):1071-1074.

Magora F, Pessachovitch B, Shoham I. Sciatic nerve block by the anterior approach for operations on the lower extremity. *Br J Anaesth.* 1974;46(2):121-123.

Mansour NY. Anterior approach revisited and another new sciatic nerve block in the supine position. *Reg Anesth.* 1993;18(4):265-266.

McNicol LR. Sciatic nerve block for children. Sciatic nerve block by the anterior approach for postoperative pain relief. *Anaesthesia.* 1985;40(5):410-414.

McNicol LR. Anterior approach to sciatic nerve block in children: loss of resistance or nerve stimulator for identifying the neurovascular compartment. *Anesth Analg.* 1987;66(11):1199-1200.

Moore CS, Sheppard D, Wildsmith JA. Thigh rotation and the anterior approach to the sciatic nerve: a magnetic resonance imaging study. *Reg Anesth Pain Med.* 2004;29(1):32-35.

Pandin P, et al. The anterior combined approach via a single skin injection site allows lower limb anesthesia in supine patients. *Can J Anaesth.* 2003;50(8):801-804.

Plante T Jr, Chaubard M, Delbos A. Unintentional transient sciatic nerve block after knee infiltration with local anesthetics. *Reg Anesth Pain Med.* 2007;32(6):547-548.

Sala-Blanch X, et al. Intraneural injection during anterior approach for sciatic nerve block. *Anesthesiology*. 2004;101(4): 1027-1030.

Shah S, et al. Neurologic complication after anterior sciatic nerve block. *Anesth Analg.* 2005;100(5):1515-1517.

Thota RS, et al. The anterior approach to sciatic nerve block using fluoroscopic guidance and radio-opaque dye. *Anesth Analg.* 2007;104(2):461-462.

Tran D, Clemente A, Finlayson RJ, A review of approaches and techniques for lower extremity nerve blocks. *Can J Anaesth.* 2007;54(11):922-934.

Tran KM, et al. Intraarticular bupivacaine-clonidine-morphine versus femoral-sciatic nerve block in pediatric patients undergoing anterior cruciate ligament reconstruction. *Anesth Analg.* 2005;101(5):1304-1310.

Valade N, et al. Does sciatic parasacral injection spread to the obturator nerve? An anatomic study. *Anesth Analg.* 2008;106(2):664-667.

Van Elstraete AC, et al. New landmarks for the anterior approach to the sciatic nerve block: imaging and clinical study. *Anesth Analg.* 2002;95(1):214-218.

Vloka JD, et al. Anterior approach to the sciatic nerve block: the effects of leg rotation. *Anesth Analg.* 2001;92(2):460-462.

Wiegel M, et al. Anterior sciatic nerve block—new landmarks and clinical experience. *Acta Anaesthesiol Scand.* 2005;49(4):552-557.

# 20 Popliteal Sciatic Block

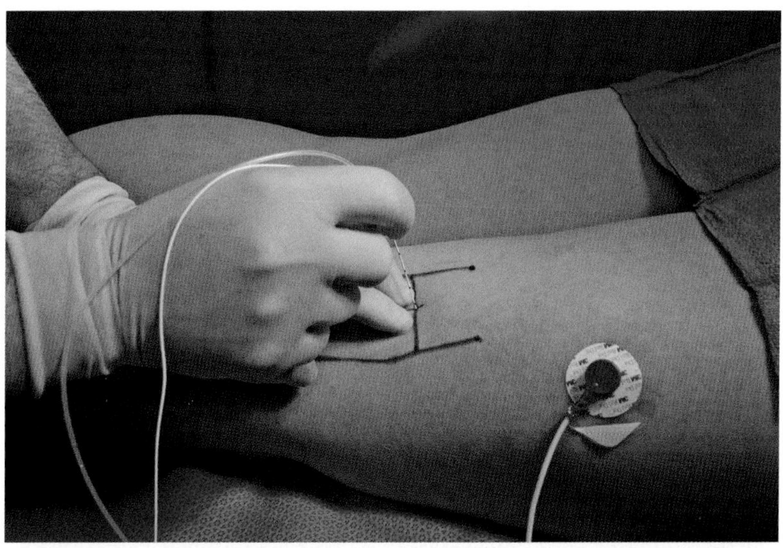

A

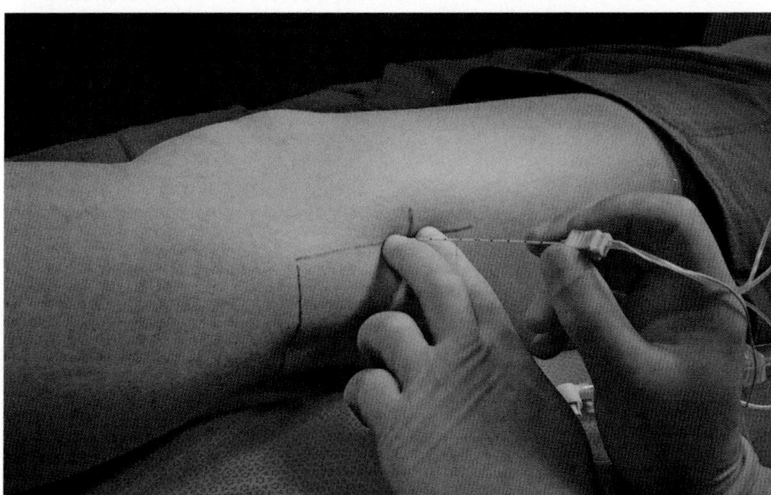

B

## BLOCK AT A GLANCE

- Indications: ankle and foot surgery
- Landmarks for intertendinous approach: popliteal fossa crease, tendons of the semitendinosus and semimembranosus muscles
- Landmarks for lateral approach: popliteal fossa crease, vastus lateralis, and biceps femoris muscles
- Nerve stimulation: twitch of the foot or toes at 0.2–0.5 mA
- Local anesthetic: 30–40 mL

**FIGURE 20.1-1.** (A) Needle insertion for the popliteal intertendinous approach. (B) Needle insertion for lateral approach to popliteal block.

# PART 1: INTERTENDINOUS APPROACH

## General Considerations

The popliteal block is a block of the sciatic nerve at the level of the popliteal fossa. This block is one of the most useful blocks in our practice. Common indications include corrective foot surgery, foot debridement, and Achilles tendon repair. A sound knowledge of the principles of nerve stimulation and the anatomic characteristics of the connective tissue sheaths of the sciatic nerve in the popliteal fossa are essential for its successful implementation.

## Functional Anatomy

The *sciatic nerve* is a nerve bundle consisting of two separate nerve trunks, the tibial and the common peroneal nerves (Figure 20.1-2). A common epineural sheath envelops these two nerves at their outset in pelvis. As the sciatic nerve descends toward the knee, the two components eventually diverge in the popliteal fossa to continue their paths separately as the tibial and the common peroneal nerves. This division of the sciatic nerve usually occurs between 4 and 10 cm proximal to the popliteal fossa crease. From its divergence from the sciatic nerve, the *common peroneal nerve* continues its path downward and laterally, descending along the head and neck of the fibula, Figure 20.1-2. Its major branches in this region are branches to the knee joint and cutaneous branches to the sural nerve. Its terminal branches are the superficial and deep peroneal nerves. The *tibial nerve* is the larger of the two divisions of the sciatic nerve. It continues its path vertically through the popliteal fossa, and its terminal branches are the medial and lateral plantar nerves, Figure 20.1-2. Its collateral branches give rise to the medial cutaneous sural nerve, muscular branches to the muscles of the calf, and articular branches to the ankle joint. It is important to note that the sciatic nerve in the popliteal fossa is lateral and superficial to the popliteal artery and vein, and it is contained in its own tissue (epineural) sheath rather than in a common neurovascular tissue sheath. This anatomic characteristic explains the relatively low risk of systemic toxicity and vascular punctures with a popliteal block (Figure 20.1-3). However, the proximity of the large vessels, popliteal artery, and vein still makes it imperative to carefully rule out an intravascular needle placement by careful aspiration and meticulously slow injection (e.g., ≤20 mL/min).

## Distribution of Blockade

A popliteal block results in anesthesia of the entire distal two thirds of the lower leg, with the exception of the skin on the medial aspect. Cutaneous innervation of the medial leg below the knee is provided by the saphenous nerve, a cutaneous terminal extension of the femoral nerve. When the surgery is on the medial aspect of the leg, the addition of a saphenous nerve block or local anesthetic infiltration at the incision site may be required for complete anesthesia. Popliteal block alone is usually sufficient for tourniquet on the calf because the tourniquet discomfort is the result of pressure and ischemia of the deep muscle beds and not of the skin and subcutaneous tissues.

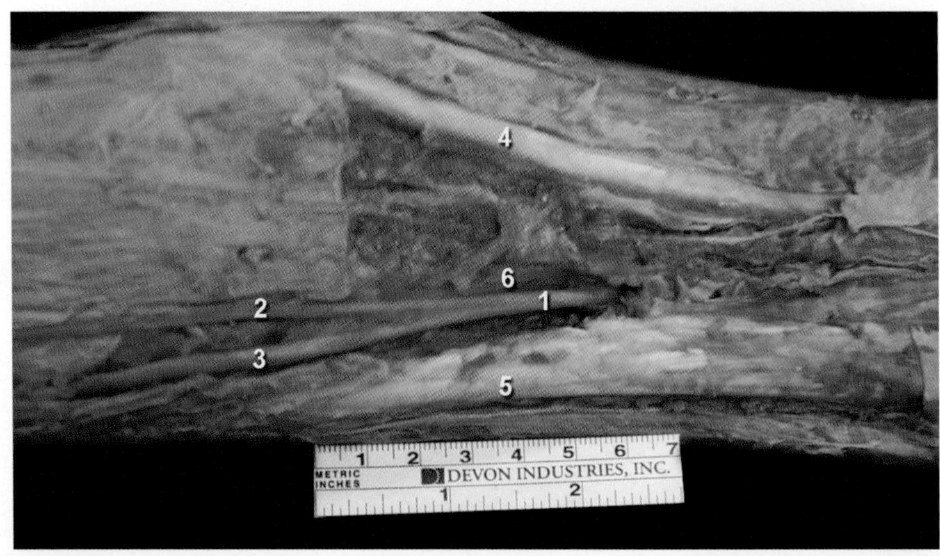


**FIGURE 20.1-2.** Anatomy of the sciatic nerve in the popliteal fossa. The sciatic nerve (1) is shown with its two divisions, tibial (2) and common peroneal (3) nerves. The common sciatic nerve (1) is is seen between semitendinosus ((4), medially) and biceps ((5), laterally) muscles enveloped by the thick epineural sheath (6).

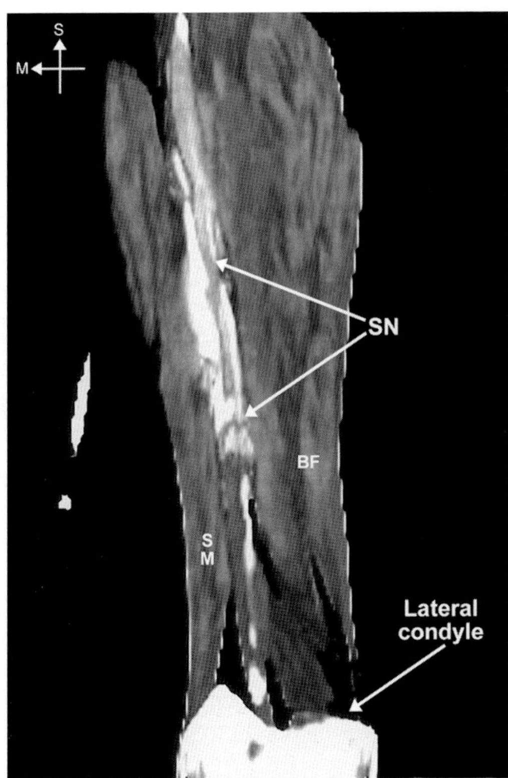


FIGURE 20.1-3. The spread of the contrast solution after injection into the common epineural sheath of the sciatic nerve (SN). The sciatic nerve is positioned between the biceps femoris (BF) and semimembranosus (SM) muscles. An extensive spread within the epineural sheath is seen.

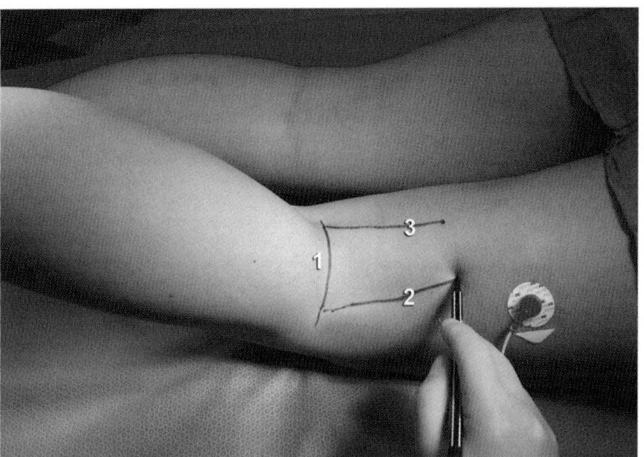


FIGURE 20.1-4. Landmarks for the popliteal block. ❶ popliteal fossa crease. ❷ biceps femoris tendon. ❸ semitendinosus semimembranous muscles.

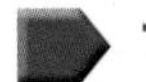

## Technique

### Equipment

A standard regional anesthesia tray is prepared with the following equipment:

- Sterile towels and gauze packs
- Two 20-mL syringes containing local anesthetic
- A 3- to 5-mL syringe plus 25-gauge needle with local anesthetic for skin infiltration
- A 50 cm, 22-gauge short-bevel insulated stimulating needle
- Peripheral nerve stimulator
- Sterile gloves; marking pen

### Landmarks and Patient Positioning

The patient is in the prone position. The foot on the side to be blocked should be positioned so that even the slightest movements of the foot or toes can be easily observed. This is best achieved by allowing the foot to extend beyond the operating room bed.

Landmarks for the intertendinous approach to a popliteal block are easily recognizable even in obese patients (Figure 20.1-4):

1. Popliteal fossa crease
2. Tendon of the biceps femoris muscle (laterally)
3. Tendons of the semitendinosus and semimembranosus muscles (medially)

#### *Maneuvers to Facilitate Landmark Identification*

The anatomic structures are best accentuated by asking the patient to elevate the foot while palpating muscles against resistance. This allows for easier and more reliable identification of the hamstring tendons. All three landmarks should be outlined with a marking pen.

**TIPS**

- Relying on tendons rather than on a subjective interpretation of the popliteal fossa "triangle" results in a more precise and consistent localization of the sciatic nerve.
- In obese patients, it is easier to start tracing the tendons cephalad from their attachment at the knee.

The needle insertion point is marked at 7 cm above the popliteal fossa crease at the midpoint between the two tendons (Figure 20.1-5).

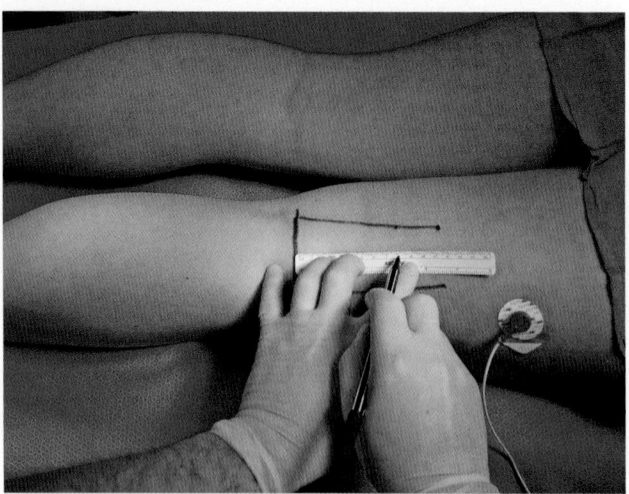

**FIGURE 20.1-5.** The point of needle insertion (circle) is marked at 7 cm above the popliteal crease between tendons of semitendinosus and semimembranosus muscles.

## Technique

After a thorough cleaning of the injection site with an antiseptic solution, local anesthetic is infiltrated subcutaneously. The anesthesiologist stands at the side of the patient with the palpating hand on the biceps femoris muscle. The needle is introduced at the midpoint between the tendons (Figure 20.1-6). This position allows the anesthesiologist to both observe the responses to nerve stimulation and monitor the patient. The nerve stimulator should be initially set to deliver a current of 1.5 mA (2 Hz, 0.1 ms) because this higher current allows the detection of inadvertent needle placement into the hamstring muscles (local twitches). When the needle is inserted in the correct plane, its advancement should not result in any local muscle twitches; the first response to nerve stimulation is typically that of the sciatic nerve (a foot twitch).

## TIPS

- Keeping the fingers of the palpating hand on the biceps muscle is important for the early detection of muscle twitches.
- These local twitches are the result of direct muscle stimulation when the needle is placed too laterally or medially, respectively.
- Local twitches of the semitendinosus muscle indicate that the needle has been inserted too medially. The needle should be withdrawn to skin level and reinserted laterally. Figure 20.1-7
- When local stimulation of the biceps muscle is felt under the fingers, the needle should be redirected medially. Figure 20.1-8

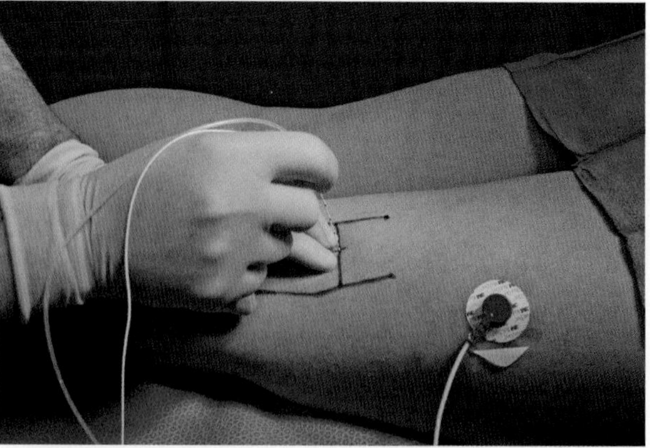

**FIGURE 20.1-6.** Needle insertion for the popliteal intertendinous approach. Needle is inserted at the midpoint between the biceps femoris laterally and semitendinosus muscles medially.

After initial stimulation of the sciatic nerve is obtained, the stimulating current is gradually decreased until twitches are still seen or felt at 0.2 to 0.5 mA. This typically occurs at a depth of 3 to 5 cm. After obtaining negative results from an aspiration test for blood, 30 to 40 mL of local anesthetic is slowly injected.

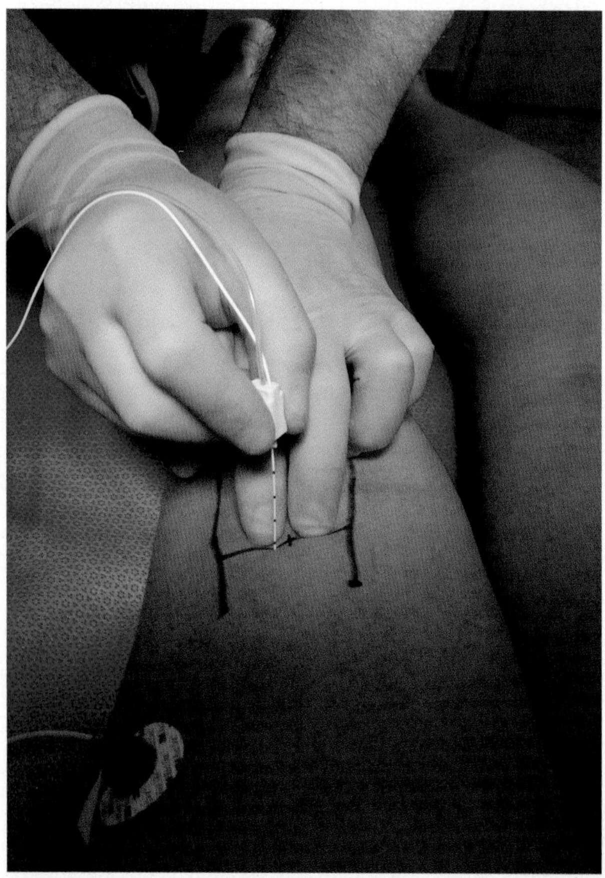

**FIGURE 20.1-7.** The needle is re-oriented laterally when the contractions of the local twitches of the semitendinosus and semimembranous muscles are elicited.

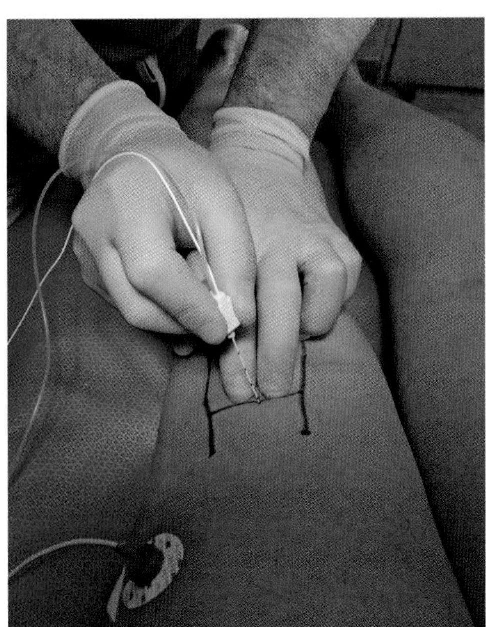

**FIGURE 20.1-8.** The needle is re-oriented medially when local twitches of the biceps femoris muscle are elicited.

## GOAL

The aim is visible or palpable twitches of the foot or toes at 0.2 to 0.5 mA. There are two common types of foot twitches:

- Common peroneal nerve stimulation results in dorsiflexion and eversion of the foot.
- Stimulation of the tibial nerve results in plantar flexion and inversion of the foot.
- Tibial nerve response is the preferred response.

## TIPS

- Stimulation at a current intensity <0.5 mA may not be possible in some patients. This is occasionally (but not frequently) the case in patients with long-standing diabetes mellitus, peripheral neuropathy, sepsis, or severe peripheral vascular disease. In these cases, stimulating currents up to 1.0 mA can be accepted as long as the motor response is specific and clearly seen or felt.
- Occasionally, a very small (e.g., 1 mm) movement of the needle results in a change in the motor response from that of the popliteal nerve (plantar flexion of the foot) to that of the common peroneal nerve (dorsiflexion of the foot). This indicates needle placement at a level before the divergence of the sciatic nerve and should be accepted as the most reliable sign of localization of the common trunk of the sciatic nerve.

## Troubleshooting

When insertion of the needle does not result in stimulation of the sciatic nerve (foot twitches), implement the following maneuvers:

1. Keep the palpating hand in the same position.
2. Withdraw the needle to skin level, redirect it 15° laterally, and reinsert it.
3. When step 2 fails to result in sciatic nerve stimulation, withdraw the needle to skin level, reinsert it 1 cm laterally, and repeat the procedure first with perpendicular needle insertion.
4. When the step 3 fails, reinsert the needle 15° laterally. These maneuvers should facilitate localization of the sciatic nerve when it proves to be challenging.

## TIPS

- When obtaining the motor response is possible only with higher current intensity (≥0.5 mA), stimulation of the tibial nerve (plantar flexion) is more reliable.
- Isolated twitches of the calf muscles should not be accepted because they may result from stimulation of the sciatic nerve branches to calf muscles outside the sciatic nerve sheath.

Table 20.1-1 lists some common responses to nerve stimulation and the course of action to take to obtain the proper response.

## Block Dynamics and Perioperative Management

This technique is associated with minor patient discomfort because the needle passes only through the adipose tissue of the popliteal fossa. Administration of midazolam 1 to 2 mg after the patient is positioned and alfentanil 250 to 500 μg just before block placement suffice as premedication for most patients. A typical onset time for this block is 15 to 30 minutes, depending on the type, concentration, and volume of local anesthetic used. The first signs of the onset of blockade are usually reports by the patient's of inability to move their toes or that the foot "feels different." With this block, sensory anesthesia of the skin is often the last to develop. Inadequate skin anesthesia despite the apparently timely onset of the blockade is common and it may take up to 30 minutes to develop. Thus local infiltration by the surgeon at the site of the incision is often all that is needed to allow the surgery to proceed.

**TABLE 20.1-1 Common Responses to Nerve Stimulation and the Course of Action to Obtain the Proper Response**

| RESPONSE OBTAINED | INTERPRETATION | PROBLEM | ACTION |
|---|---|---|---|
| Local twitch of the biceps femoris muscle | Direct stimulation of the biceps femoris muscle | Too lateral a placement of needle | Withdraw the needle and redirect it slightly medially (5–10°) |
| Local twitch of the semi-tendinosus or semimem-branosus muscle | Direct stimulation of the semitendinosus or semi-membranosus muscle | Too medial a placement of needle | Withdraw the needle and redirect it slightly laterally (5–10°) |
| Twitch of the calf muscles without foot or toe movement | Stimulation of the muscu-lar branches of the sciatic nerve | These branches may have departed the sciatic sheath | Continue advancing the needle until foot or toe twitches are obtained |
| Vascular puncture | Blood in the syringe most commonly indicates place-ment into the popliteal artery or vein | Too medial and or too deep placement of the needle | Withdraw the needle and redirect it laterally |
| Bone contact | Needle has encountered the femur | Too deep a needle inser-tion; the nerve was missed or twitches not noticed | Withdraw the needle slowly and look for a foot twitch; if twitches are not seen, follow the previously described troubleshooting procedure |

## Continuous Popliteal Block

The technique is similar to a single-injection procedure; however, slight angulation of the needle cephalad is necessary to facilitate threading the catheter. Securing and maintaining the catheter is easy and convenient. This technique can be used for surgery and postoperative pain management in patients undergoing a wide variety of lower leg, foot, and ankle surgeries.

### Equipment

A standard regional anesthesia tray is prepared with the following equipment:

- Sterile towels and gauze packs
- Two 20-mL syringes containing local anesthetic
- Sterile gloves, marking pen, and surface electrode
- A 3- to 5-mL syringe plus 25-gauge needle with local anesthetic for skin infiltration
- Peripheral nerve stimulator
- Catheter kit (including an 8- to 10-cm large-gauge stimulating needle and catheter).

Kits come in two varieties based on catheter construction: nonstimulating (conventional) and stimulating catheters. During the placement of a conventional nonstimulating catheter, the stimulating needle is first advanced until appropriate twitches are obtained. Then 5–10 mL of local anesthetic or other injectate (e.g., D5W) is then injected to "open up" a space for the catheter to advance freely without resistance. The catheter is then threaded through the needle until approximately 3 to 5 cm is protruding beyond the tip of the needle. The needle is then withdrawn, the catheter secured, and the remaining local anesthetic injected via the catheter. Stimulating catheters are insulated and have a filament or core that transmits current to a bare metal tip. After obtaining twitches with the needle, the catheter is advanced with the nerve stimulator connected until the sought motor response is obtained. This method requires that no conducting solution (i.e., local anesthetic, saline) be injected through the needle prior to catheter advancement, or difficulty obtaining a motor response will result.

### Landmarks and Patient Positioning

The patient is positioned in the prone position with the feet extending beyond the table to facilitate monitoring of foot or toe responses to nerve stimulation.

The landmarks for a continuous popliteal block are essentially the same as those for the single-injection technique (Figure 20.1-4). These include the following:

1. Popliteal fossa crease
2. Tendon of the biceps femoris muscle (laterally)
3. Tendons of the semitendinosus and semimembranosus muscles (medially)

The needle insertion site is marked 7 cm proximal to the popliteal fossa crease and between the tendons of the biceps femoris and semitendinosus muscles (Figure 20.1-5).

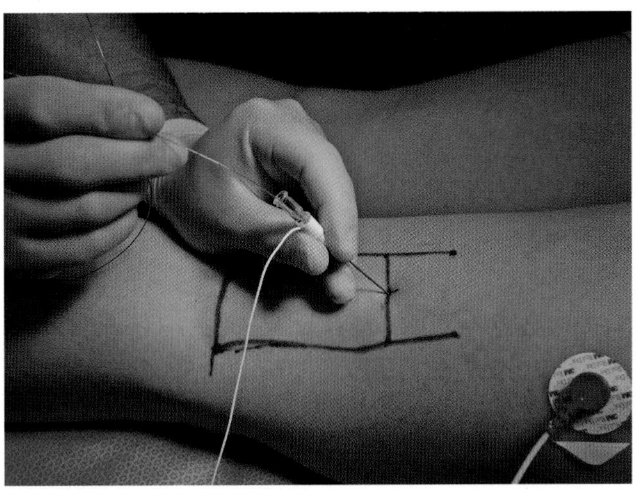

**FIGURE 20.1-9.** Needle direction and insertion of the catheter for continuous popliteal sciatic block. The catheter is inserted 3–5 cm beyond the needle tip.

## Technique

The continuous popliteal block technique is similar to the single-injection technique. With the patient in the prone position, infiltrate the skin with local anesthetic using a 25-gauge needle at an injection site 7 cm above the popliteal fossa crease and between the tendons of biceps femoris and semitendinosus muscles. An 8- to 10-cm needle connected to the nerve stimulator (1.5 mA current) is inserted at the midpoint between the tendons of the biceps femoris and semitendinosus muscles. Advance the block needle slowly in a slightly cranial direction while observing the patient for rhythmic plantar or dorsiflexion of the foot or toes. After appropriate twitches are noted, continue manipulating the needle until the desired response is seen or felt using a current ≤0.5 mA. The catheter should be advanced no more than 5 cm beyond the needle tip (Figure 20.1-9). The needle is then withdrawn back to skin level while advancing the catheter simultaneously to prevent inadvertent removal of the catheter.

The catheter is checked for inadvertent intravascular placement and secured using an adhesive skin preparation, followed by application of a clear dressing. The infusion port should be clearly marked "continuous nerve block."

**TIP**

- When insertion of the catheter proves difficult, lowering the angle of the needle or rotating the needle may facilitate the catheter insertion.

### *Continuous Infusion*

Continuous infusion is initiated after injection of an initial bolus of local anesthetic through the catheter or needle. For this purpose, we routinely use 0.2% ropivacaine 15 to 20 mL. Diluted bupivacaine or levobupivacaine are also suitable but may result in greater degree of motor blockade. The infusion is maintained at 5 to 10 mL/h with a 5-mL patient-controlled bolus hourly.

## Complications and How to Avoid Them

Complications following a popliteal block are uncommon. Table 20.1-2 lists some general and specific instructions on possible complications and how to avoid them.

**TABLE 20.1-2 Complications of Popliteal Sciatic Nerve Block and Preventive Techniques**

| | |
|---|---|
| ***Infection*** | • Use a strict aseptic technique. |
| ***Local anesthetic toxicity*** | • Systemic toxicity after a popliteal block is uncommon.<br>• Use slow injection with frequent aspiration. |
| ***Hematoma*** | • Stop insertion of the needle when the patient complains of pain. This typically indicates that the needle has been inserted through the biceps or semitendinosus muscle. |
| ***Vascular puncture*** | • Avoid medial redirection of the needle because the vascular sheath is positioned medially. |
| ***Nerve injury*** | • Abort attempts to inject when the patient complains of pain:<br>• Abort or when high resistance to injection are met on injection<br>• Do not inject when stimulation is obtained at <0.2 mA (100 ms). |
| ***Other*** | • Instruct the patient on care of the insensate extremity. |

## INTERTENDINOUS POPLITEAL SCIATIC NERVE BLOCK

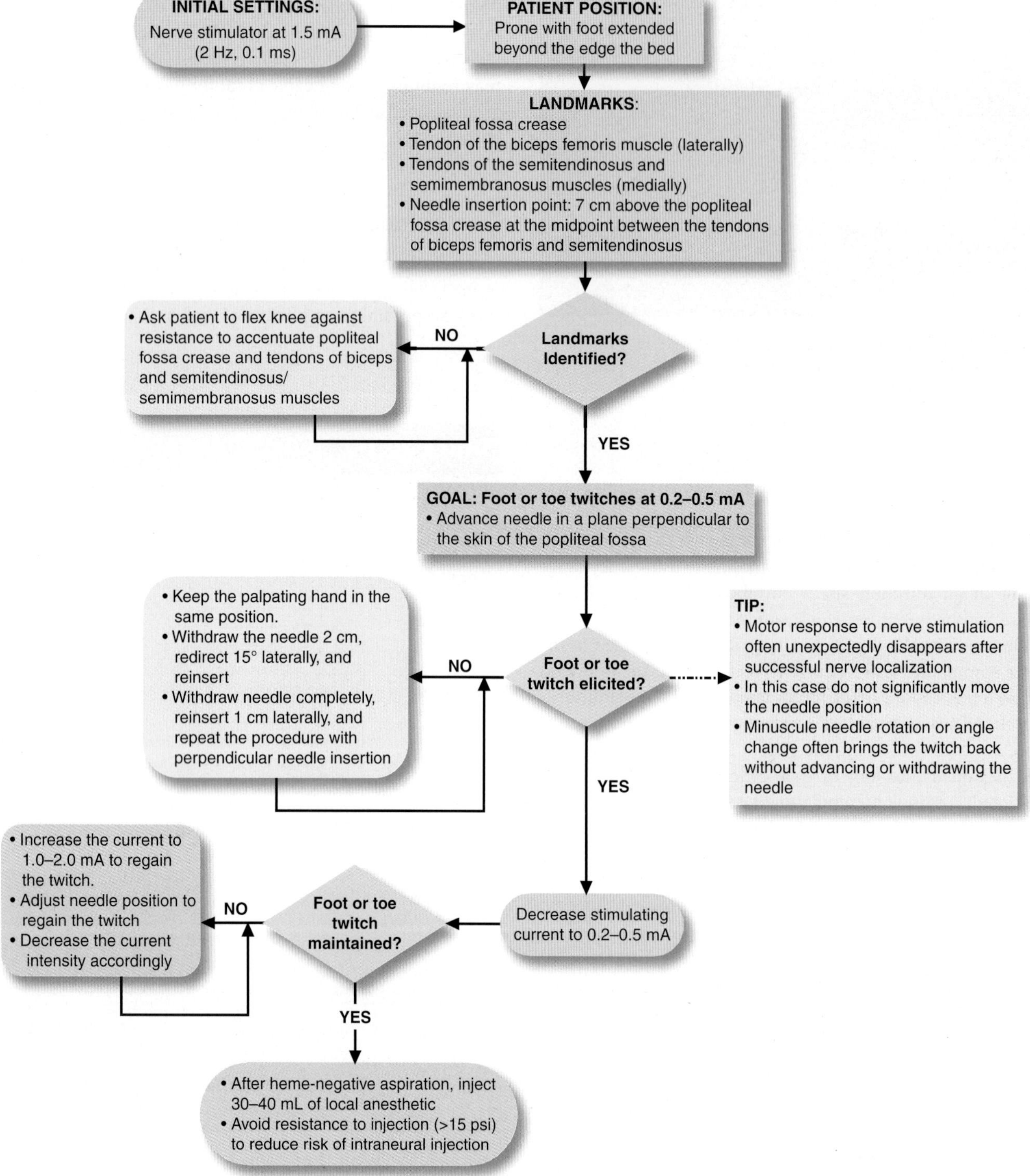

## SUGGESTED READING


Benzon HT, Kim C, Benzon HP, et al. Correlation between evoked motor response of the sciatic nerve and sensory blockade. *Anesthesiology.* 1997;87:547-552.

Borgeat A, Blumenthal S, Karovic D, Delbos A, Vienne P. Clinical evaluation of a modified posterior anatomical approach to performing the popliteal block. *Reg Anesth Pain Med.* 2004;29:290-296.

Borgeat A, Blumenthal S, Lambert M, Theodorou P, Vienne P. The feasibility and complications of the continuous popliteal nerve block: a 1001-case survey. *Anesth Analg.* 2006;103:229-233.

Capdevila X, Dadure C, Bringuier S, et al. Effect of patient-controlled perineural analgesia on rehabilitation and pain after ambulatory orthopedic surgery: a multicenter randomized trial. *Anesthesiology.* 2006;105:566-573.

Cappelleri G, Aldegheri G, Ruggieri F, Mamo D, Fanelli G, Casati A. Minimum effective anesthetic concentration (MEAC) for sciatic nerve block: subgluteus and popliteal approaches. *Can J Anaesth.* 2007;54:283-289.

Compere V, Rey N, Baert O, et al. Major complications after 400 continuous popliteal sciatic nerve blocks for post-operative analgesia. *Acta Anaesthesiol Scand.* 2009;53:339-345.

di Benedetto P, Casati A, Bertini L, Fanelli G, Chelly JE. Postoperative analgesia with continuous sciatic nerve block after foot surgery: a prospective, randomized comparison between the popliteal and subgluteal approaches. *Anesth Analg.* 2002;94:996-1000.

Ekatodramis G, Nadig M, Blumenthal S, Borgeat A. Continuous popliteal sciatic nerve block. How to be sure the catheter works? *Acta Anaesthesiol Scand.* 2004;48:1342-1343.

Eurin M, Beloeil H, Zetlaoui PJ. A medial approach for a continuous sciatic block in the popliteal fossa [in French]. *Can J Anaesth.* 2006;53:1165-1166.

Fernandez-Guisasola J. Popliteal block as an alternative to Labat's approach. *Anesth Analg.* 2002;95:252-253.

Fernandez-Guisasola J, Andueza A, Burgos E, et al. A comparison of 0.5% ropivacaine and 1% mepivacaine for sciatic nerve block in the popliteal fossa. *Acta Anaesthesiol Scand.* 2001;45:967-970.

Fournier R, Weber A, Gamulin Z. Posterior labat vs. lateral popliteal sciatic block: posterior sciatic block has quicker onset and shorter duration of anaesthesia. *Acta Anaesthesiol Scand.* 2005;49:683-686.

Gouverneur JM. Sciatic nerve block in the popliteal fossa with atraumatic needles and nerve stimulation. *Acta Anaesthesiol Belg.* 1985;36:391-399.

Guntz E, Herman P, Debizet E, Delhaye D, Coulic V, Sosnowski M. Sciatic nerve block in the popliteal fossa: description of a new medial approach. *Can J Anaesth.* 2004;51:817-820.

Hadžić A, Vloka JD. A comparison of the posterior versus lateral approaches to the block of the sciatic nerve in the popliteal fossa. *Anesthesiology.* 1998;88:1480-1486.

Hadžić A, Vloka JD, Singson R, Santos AC, Thys DM. A comparison of intertendinous and classical approaches to popliteal nerve block using magnetic resonance imaging simulation. *Anesth Analg.* 2002;94:1321-1324.

Ilfeld BM, Loland VJ, Gerancher JC, et al. The effects of varying local anesthetic concentration and volume on continuous popliteal sciatic nerve blocks: a dual-center, randomized, controlled study. *Anesth Analg.* 2008;107:701-707.

Ilfeld BM, Morey TE, Wang RD, Enneking FK. Continuous popliteal sciatic nerve block for postoperative pain control at home: a randomized, double-blinded, placebo-controlled study. *Anesthesiology.* 2002;97:959-965.

Ilfeld BM, Thannikary LJ, Morey TE, Vander Griend RA, Enneking FK. Popliteal sciatic perineural local anesthetic infusion: a comparison of three dosing regimens for postoperative analgesia. *Anesthesiology.* 2004;101:970-977.

Kilpatrick AW, Coventry DM, Todd JG. A comparison of two approaches to sciatic nerve block. *Anaesthesia.* 1992;47:155-157.

March X, Pineda O, Garcia MM, Carames D, Villalonga A. The posterior approach to the sciatic nerve in the popliteal fossa: a comparison of single- versus double-injection technique. *Anesth Analg.* 2006;103:1571-1573.

Moayeri N, Groen GJ. Differences in quantitative architecture of sciatic nerve may explain differences in potential vulnerability to nerve injury, onset time, and minimum effective anesthetic volume. *Anesthesiology.* 2009;111:1128-1134.

Nader A, Kendall MC, Candido KD, Benzon H, McCarthy RJ. A randomized comparison of a modified intertendinous and classic posterior approach to popliteal sciatic nerve block. *Anesth Analg.* 2009;108:359-363.

Navas AM. Stimulating catheters in continuous popliteal block. *Anesth Analg.* 2006;102:1594; author reply 1594-1595.

Palmisani S, Ronconi P, De Blasi RA, Arcioni R. Lateral or posterior popliteal approach for sciatic nerve block: difference is related to the anatomy. *Anesth Analg.* 2007;105:286.

Paqueron X, Narchi P, Mazoit JX, Singelyn F, Benichou A, Macaire P. A randomized, observer-blinded determination of the median effective volume of local anesthetic required to anesthetize the sciatic nerve in the popliteal fossa for stimulating and nonstimulating perineural catheters. *Reg Anesth Pain Med.* 2009;34:290-295.

Rodriguez J, Taboada M, Carceller J, Lagunilla J, Barcena M, Alvarez J. Stimulating popliteal catheters for postoperative analgesia after hallux valgus repair. *Anesth Analg.* 2006;102:258-262.

Rorie DK, Byer DE, Nelson DO, Sittipong R, Johnson KA. Assessment of block of the sciatic nerve in the popliteal fossa. *Anesth Analg.* 1980;59:371-376.

Singelyn FJ, Aye F, Gouverneur JM. Continuous popliteal sciatic nerve block: an original technique to provide postoperative analgesia after foot surgery. *Anesth Analg.* 1997;84:383-386.

Sunderland S. The sciatic nerve and its tibial and common peroneal divisions: anatomical features. In: Sunderland S, ed. *Nerves and Nerve Injuries.* Edinburgh, UK: E&S Livingstone; 1968.

Suresh S, Simion C, Wyers M, Swanson M, Jennings M, Iyer A. Anatomical location of the bifurcation of the sciatic nerve in the posterior thigh in infants and children: a formula derived from MRI imaging for nerve localization. *Reg Anesth Pain Med.* 2007;32:351-353.

Taboada M, Rodriguez J, Alvarez J, Cortés J, Gude F, Atanassoff PG. Sciatic nerve block via posterior Labat approach is more efficient than lateral popliteal approach using a double-injection technique: a prospective, randomized comparison. *Anesthesiology.* 2004;101:138-142.

Taboada M, Rodriguez J, Bermudez M, et al. A "new" automated bolus technique for continuous popliteal block: a prospective, randomized comparison with a continuous infusion technique. *Anesth Analg.* 2008;107:1433-1437.

Taboada M, Rodriguez J, Bermudez M, et al. Comparison of continuous infusion versus automated bolus for postoperative patient-controlled analgesia with popliteal sciatic nerve catheters. *Anesthesiology.* 2009;110:150-154.

Tran D, Clemente A, Finlayson RJ. A review of approaches and techniques for lower extremity nerve blocks. *Can J Anaesth.* 2007;54:922-934.

Vloka JD, Hadžić A, April E, Thys DM. The division of the sciatic nerve in the popliteal fossa: anatomical implications for popliteal nerve blockade. *Anesth Analg.* 2001;92:215-217.

Vloka JD, Hadžić A, Koorn R, Thys D. Supine approach to the sciatic nerve in the popliteal fossa. *Can J Anaesth.* 1996;43:964-967.

Vloka JD, Hadžić A, Lesser JB, et al. A common epineural sheath for the nerves in the popliteal fossa and its possible implications for sciatic nerve block. *Anesth Analg.* 1997;84:387-390.

Vloka JD, Hadžić A, Mulcare R, Lesser JB, Koorn R, Thys DM. Combined popliteal and posterior cutaneous nerve of the thigh blocks for short saphenous vein stripping in outpatients: an alternative to spinal anesthesia. *J Clin Anesth.* 1997;9:618-622.

White PF, Issioui T, Skrivanek GD, Early JS, Wakefield C. The use of a continuous popliteal sciatic nerve block after surgery involving the foot and ankle: does it improve the quality of recovery? *Anesth Analg.* 2003;97:1303-1309.

Zaric D, Boysen K, Christiansen J, Haastrup U, Kofoed H, Rawal N. Continuous popliteal sciatic nerve block for outpatient foot surgery—a randomized, controlled trial. *Acta Anaesthesiol Scand.* 2004;48:337-341.

# PART 2: LATERAL APPROACH

## General Considerations

The lateral approach to a popliteal blockade is similar to the intertendinous block in many aspects. The main difference is that the technique involves placement of the needle from the lateral aspect of the leg, therefore obviating the need to position the patient in the prone position. Nerve stimulation principles, volume requirements, and block onset time are the same. The block is well suited for surgery on the calf, Achilles tendon, ankle, and foot. It also provides adequate analgesia for a calf tourniquet.

## Functional Anatomy

The *sciatic nerve* consists of two separate nerve trunks, the tibial and common peroneal nerves (Figure 20.2-1). A common epineural sheath envelops these two nerves at their outset in the pelvis. As the sciatic nerve descends toward the knee, the two components eventually diverge in the popliteal fossa, giving rise to the tibial and common peroneal nerves. This division of the sciatic nerve usually occurs 5–7 cm proximal to the popliteal fossa crease.

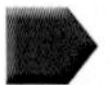

## Distribution of Blockade

The lateral approach to popliteal block also results in anesthesia of the entire distal two thirds of the lower extremity with the exception of the skin on the medial aspect of the leg (Figure 20.2-2). Cutaneous innervation of the medial leg below the knee is provided by the saphenous nerve, the terminal extension of the femoral nerve. Depending on the level of surgery, the addition of a saphenous nerve block may be required for complete surgical anesthesia.

## Single-Injection Popliteal Block (Lateral Approach)

### Equipment

A standard regional anesthesia tray is prepared with the following equipment:

- Sterile towels and gauze packs
- Two 20-mL syringes containing local anesthetic
- A 3- to 5-mL syringe plus 25-gauge needle with local anesthetic for skin infiltration
- A 10-cm, 21-gauge short-bevel insulated stimulating needle
- Peripheral nerve stimulator
- Sterile gloves; marking pen

### Landmarks and Patient Positioning

The patient is in the supine position. The foot on the side to be blocked should be positioned so that the motor response of the foot or toes can be easily observed (Figure 20.2-3). This is best achieved by placing the leg on a footrest with the heel and the foot protruding beyond the footrest. This positioning allows for easy visualization of foot twitches during nerve localization. The foot should form a 90° angle to the horizontal plane of the table.

Landmarks for the lateral approach to a popliteal block include the following (Figure 20.2-4 and 20.2-5):

1. Popliteal fossa crease
2. Vastus lateralis muscle
3. Biceps femoris muscle

The needle insertion site is marked in the groove between the vastus lateralis and biceps femoris muscles 7-8 cm above the popliteal fossa crease. Note that the lateral femoral epicondyle is another landmark that can be used with this technique. It is easily palpated on the lateral aspect of the knee 1 cm cephalad to the popliteal fossa crease (Figures 20.2-6 and 20.2-7).

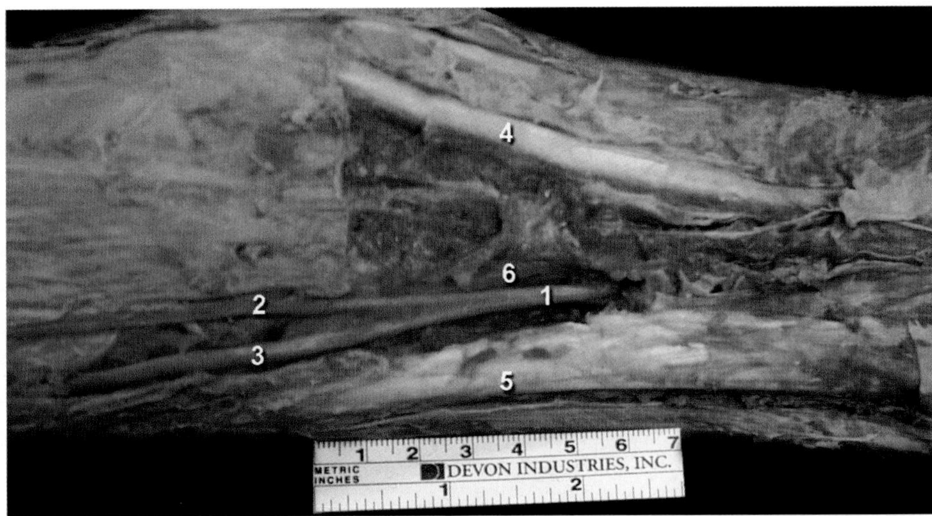


**FIGURE 20.2-1.** Anatomy of the popliteal fossa crease. ❶ tibial nerve. ❷ common peroneal nerve before its division. ❸ epineural sheath of the common sciatic nerve. ❹ tendon of semitendinosus and semimembranous. ❺ bicep femoris tendon.

## TIP

- In patients with an atrophic biceps femoris muscle (e.g., prolonged immobility), the iliotibial aponeurosis can prove to be a more consistent landmark). In this case, the needle insertion site is in the groove between the vastus lateralis and the iliotibial tract.

### *Maneuvers to Facilitate Landmark Identification*

Landmarks can be better appreciated using the following steps:

- Lifting the foot off the table accentuates the biceps femoris and vastus lateralis muscles, and helps the recognition of the groove between the two muscles.
- The groove between the vastus lateralis and biceps femoris can be located by firmly pressing the fingers of the palpating hand against the adipose tissue in the groove approximately 8 cm above the popliteal fossa crease.

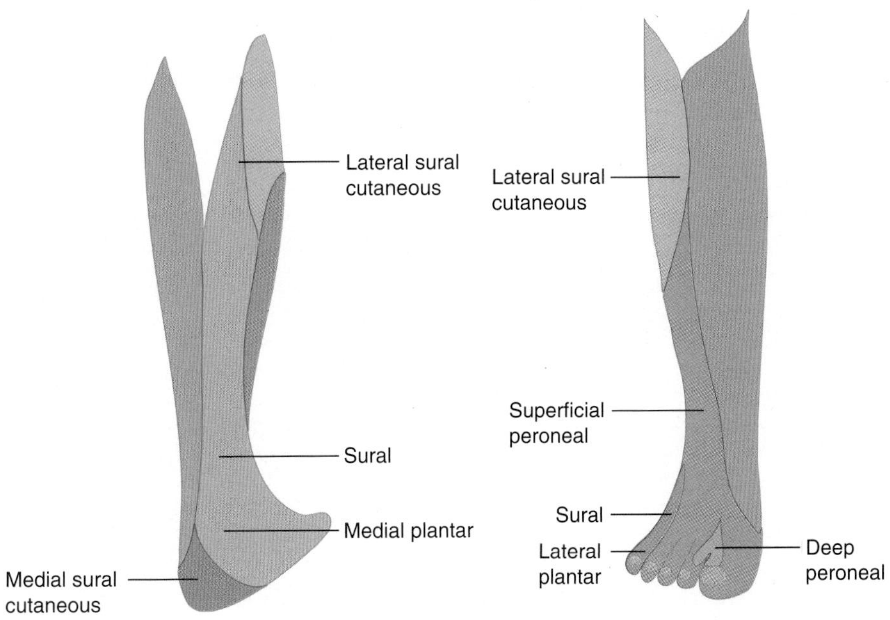


**FIGURE 20.2-2.** Sensory distribution of anesthesia accomplished with popliteal sciatic block. All shaded areas except medial aspect of the leg (blue, saphenous nerve) are anesthetized with the popliteal block.

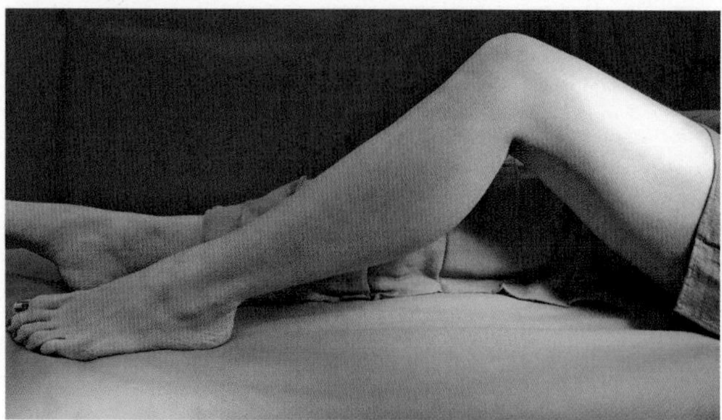

**FIGURE 20.2-3.** Maneuver to accentuate landmarks for popliteal sciatic block. The patient is asked to flex the leg at the knee, which accentuates the popliteal fossa and hamstring muscles.

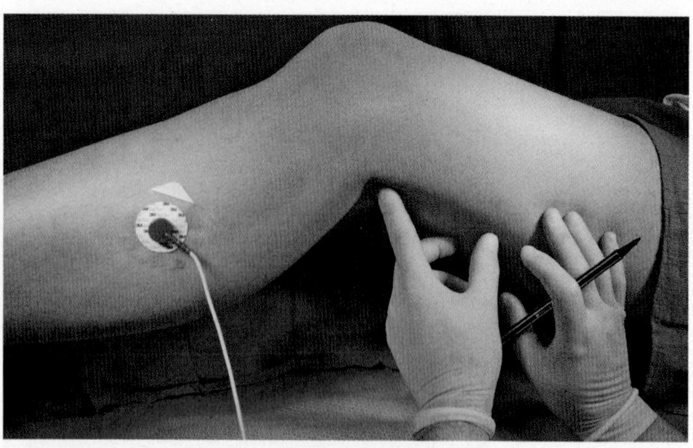

**FIGURE 20.2-4.** Popliteal fossa is marked with the knee flexed.

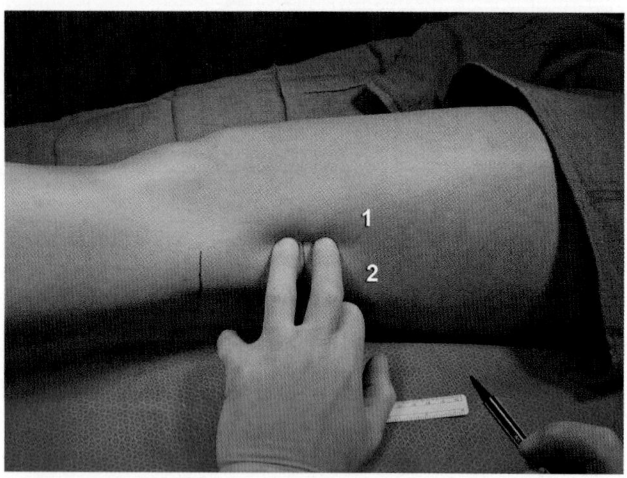


**FIGURE 20.2-5.** The main landmark for popliteal sciatic block is in the groove between the vastus lateralis ❶ and the biceps femoris muscles ❷.

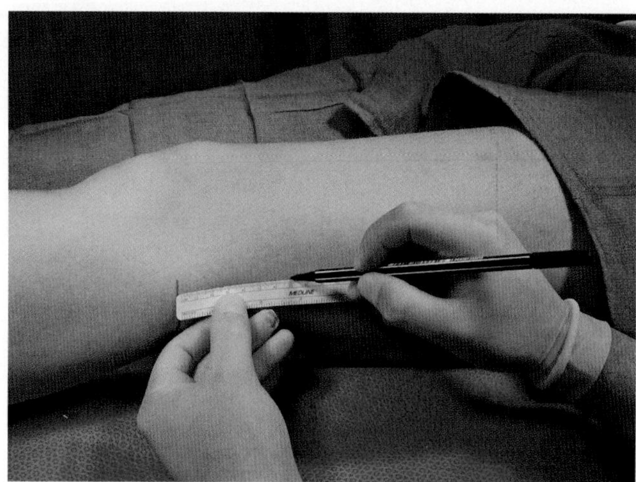

**FIGURE 20.2-6.** Needle insertion site is labeled at 7 cm proximal to the popliteal fossa crease in the groove between the vastus lateralis and bicep femoris muscles.

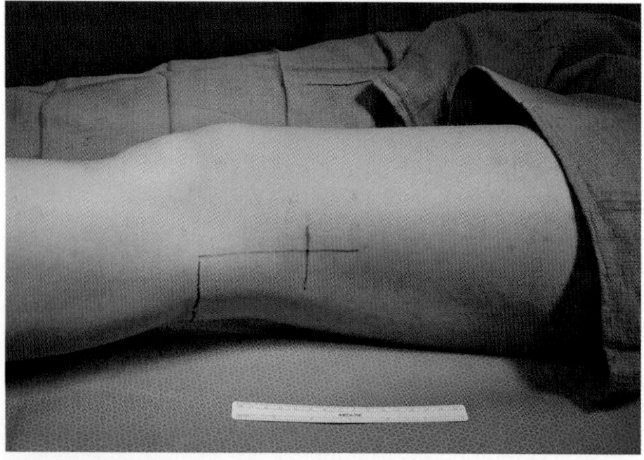

**FIGURE 20.2-7.** A needle insertion point for lateral approach sciatic popliteal block.

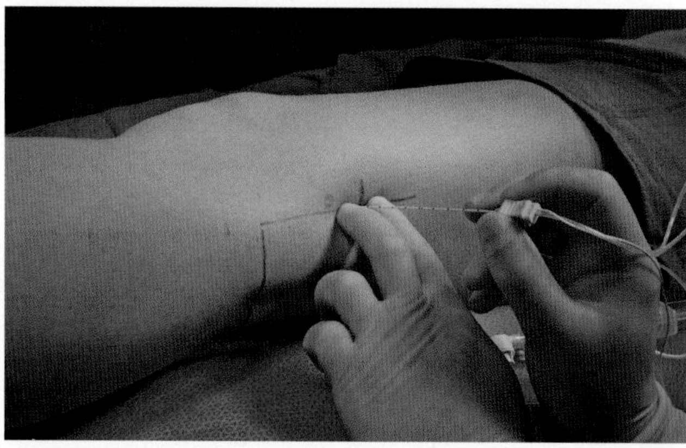

**FIGURE 20.2-8** Needle insertion for lateral approach to popliteal block.

## Technique

The operator should be seated facing the side to be blocked. The height of the patient's bed is adjusted to allow for a more ergonomic position and greater precision during block placement. This position also allows the operator simultaneously to monitor both the patient and the responses to nerve stimulation.

The site of estimated needle insertion is prepared with an antiseptic solution and infiltrated with local anesthetic using a 25-gauge needle. It is useful to infiltrate the skin along a line rather than raise a single skin wheal. This allows needle reinsertion at a different site when necessary without the need to anesthetize the skin again.

A 10-cm, 21-gauge needle is inserted in a horizontal plane perpendicular to the long axis of the leg between the vastus lateralis and biceps femoris muscles (Figure 20.2-8), and it is advanced to contact the femur. Contact with the femur is important because it provides information about the depth of the nerve (typically 1–2 cm beyond the skin to femur distance) and about the angle at which the needle must be redirected posteriorly to stimulate the nerve (Figure 20.2-9). The current intensity is initially set at 1.5 mA. With the fingers of the palpating hand firmly pressed and immobile in the groove, the needle is withdrawn to the skin level, redirected 30° below the horizontal plane, and advanced toward the nerve.

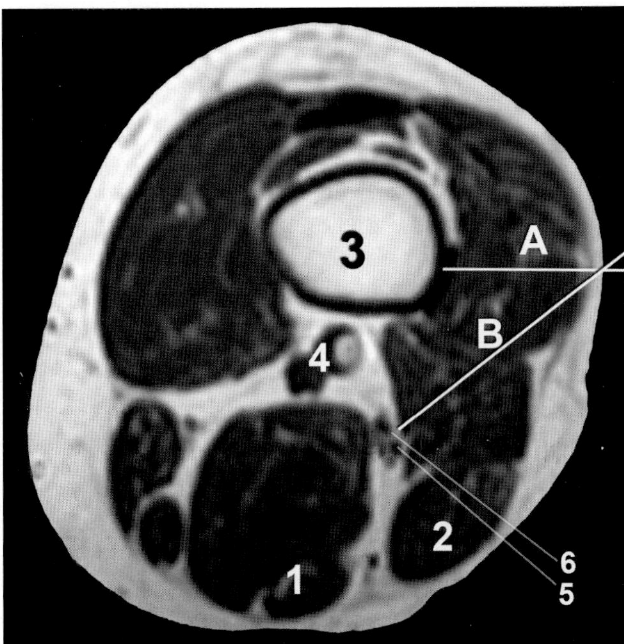


**FIGURE 20.2-9.** Needle insertion strategy for lateral approach to popliteal sciatic block. (A) needle is first inserted to contact femur. (B) After contact with the femur, the needle is withdrawn back to the skin and redirected 30° posteriorly to local the sciatic nerve. Note the needle passage through the biceps femoris muscle before entering the popliteal fossa crease. This explains why local bicep femoris muscle twitch is often obtained during needle advancement.
1 - Semimembranosus-semitendinosus muscles, 2 - Biceps Femoris, 3 - Femur, 4 - Popliteal artery and vein, 5 - Common peroneal nerve, 6 - TIbial nerve

### GOAL

The ultimate goal of nerve stimulation is to obtain visible or palpable twitches of the foot or toes at a current of 0.2–0.5 mA.

### TIPS

- The needle passes through the biceps femoris muscle, often resulting in local twitches of this muscle during needle advancement. Cessation of the local twitches of the biceps muscle should prompt slower needle advancement because this signifies that the needle is in the popliteal fossa and in close proximity to the sciatic nerve.
- When stimulation of the sciatic nerve is not obtained within 2 cm after cessation of the biceps femoris twitches; the needle is probably not in plane with the nerves and should not be advanced further because of the risk of puncturing the popliteal vessels.

After initial stimulation of the sciatic nerve is obtained, the stimulating current is gradually decreased until twitches are still seen or felt at 0.2–0.5 mA. This typically occurs at a depth of 5–7 cm. At this point, the needle should be stabilized and, after aspiration test for blood, 30–40 mL of local anesthetic is injected slowly.

## Troubleshooting

When the sciatic nerve is not localized on the first needle pass, the needle is withdrawn to the skin level and the following algorithm is used:

1. Ensure that the nerve stimulator is functional, properly connected to the patient and to the needle, and set to deliver the current of desired intensity.
2. Ensure that the leg is not externally rotated at the hip joint and that the foot forms a 90° angle to the horizontal plane of the table. A deviation from this angle changes the relationship of the sciatic nerve to the femur and the biceps femoris muscle.
3. Mentally visualize the plane of the initial needle insertion and redirect the needle in a slightly posterior direction (5–10° posterior angulation).
4. If step 3 fails, withdraw the needle and reinsert it with an additional 5–10° posterior redirection.

5. Failure to obtain a foot response to nerve stimulation should prompt reassessment of the landmarks and leg position. In addition, the stimulating current should be increased to 2 mA.

### TIPS

- When motor response can be elicited only with current of ≥0.5 mA, tibial nerve response (Figure 20.2-10) may be associated with a higher success rate of anesthesia of both divisions of the nerve.
- Isolated twitches of the calf muscles should not be accepted as reliable signs because they can be the result of stimulation of the sciatic nerve branches to the calf muscles that may be outside the sciatic nerve sheath.

Table 20.2-1 lists the common responses that can occur during block placement using a nerve stimulator and the proper course of action needed to obtain twitches of the foot.

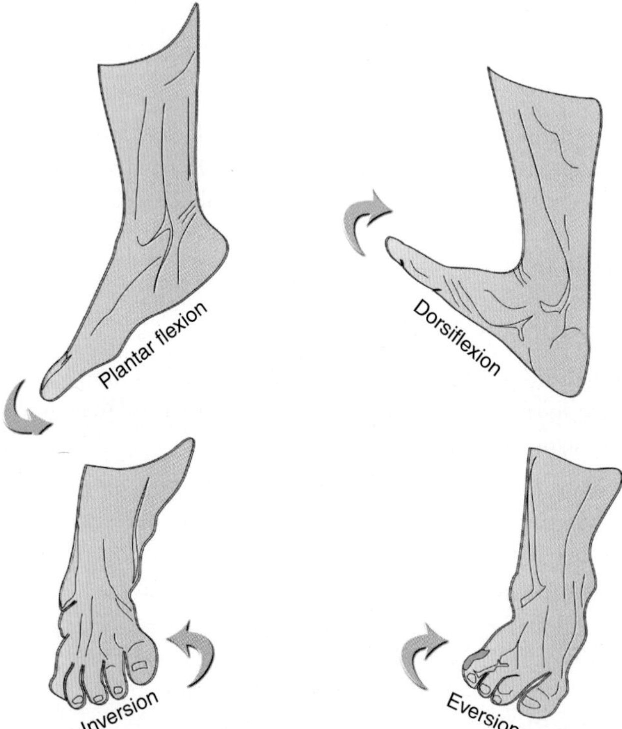


**FIGURE 20.2-10.** Motor responses of the foot obtained with stimulation of the sciatic nerve in the popliteal fossa. Stimulation of the tibial nerve results in plantar flexion and inversion of the foot. Stimulation of the common peroneal nerve results in dorsi flexion and inversion of the foot.

## Block Dynamics and Perioperative Management

This technique may be associated with patient discomfort because the needle transverses the biceps femoris muscle, and adequate sedation and analgesia are necessary. Administration of midazolam (2–4 mg intravenously) and a short-acting narcotic (alfentanil 250–to 750 g) ensures patient comfort and prevents patient movement during needle advancement. Inadequate premedication can make it difficult to interpret the response to nerve stimulation because of patient movement during needle advancement. A typical onset time for this block is 15–30 minutes, depending on the type, concentration, and volume of local anesthetic used. The first signs of onset of the blockade are usually a report by the patient that the foot "feels different" or there is an inability to wiggle their toes. With this block, sensory anesthesia of the skin is often the last to develop. Inadequate skin anesthesia despite an apparently timely onset of the blockade is common, and it can take up to 30 minutes to develop. Local infiltration by the surgeon at the site of the incision is often all that is needed to allow the surgery to proceed.

## Continuous Popliteal Block (Lateral Approach)

The technique is similar to the single-injection except that slight angulation of the needle cephalad is necessary to facilitate threading of the catheter. Securing and maintaining the catheter are easy and convenient with this technique. A lateral popliteal block is suitable for surgery and postoperative pain management in patients undergoing a wide variety of lower leg, foot, and ankle surgeries.

### Equipment

A standard regional anesthesia tray is prepared with the following equipment:

- Sterile towels and gauze packs
- Two 20-mL syringes containing local anesthetic
- Sterile gloves, marking pen, and surface electrode
- A 3- to 5-mL syringe plus 25-gauge needle with local anesthetic for skin infiltration
- Peripheral nerve stimulator
- Catheter kit (including an 8- to 10-cm 18–19 gauge stimulating needle and catheter)

Either nonstimulating (conventional) or stimulating catheters can be used. During the placement of a conventional non-stimulating catheter, the stimulating needle is advanced until appropriate twitches are obtained. Then 5–10 mL of local anesthetic or other injectate (e.g., D5W) is then injected

**TABLE 20.2-1 Some Common Responses to Nerve Stimulation and Course of Action**

| RESPONSE OBTAINED | INTERPRETATION | PROBLEM | ACTION |
|---|---|---|---|
| Local twitch of the biceps femoris muscle | Direct stimulation of the biceps femoris muscle | Too shallow placement of the needle | Advance the needle deeper |
| Local twitch of the vastus lateralis muscle | Direct stimulation of the vastus lateralis muscle | Too anterior a placement of the needle | Withdraw the needle and reinsert it posteriorly |
| Twitch of the calf muscles without foot or toe movement | Stimulation of the motor branches of the sciatic nerve | These small branches are often outside the sciatic sheath | Disregard and continue advancing the needle until foot or toe twitches are obtained |
| Vascular puncture | Blood in the syringe most commonly indicates placement into the popliteal artery or vein | Too deep and too anterior a placement of the needle | Withdraw the needle and redirect it posteriorly |
| Twitches of the foot or toes | Stimulation of the sciatic nerve | None | Accept and inject local anesthetic |

to "open up" a space for the catheter to advance freely without resistance. The catheter is threaded through the needle until approximately 3–5 cm is protruding beyond the tip of the needle. The needle is withdrawn, the catheter secured, and the remaining local anesthetic injected via the catheter. With stimulating catheters, after obtaining desired motor response with stimulation through the needle, the catheter is advanced with the nerve stimulator connected until the anesthesiologist is satisfied with the quality of the motor response. If the response is lost, the catheter can be withdrawn until it reappears and the catheter readvanced. This method requires that no conducting solution be injected through the needle (i.e., local anesthetic, saline) prior to catheter advancement, or difficulty obtaining a motor response will result.

## Landmarks and Patient Positioning

The patient is positioned in the supine position with the feet extending beyond the table to facilitate monitoring of foot or toe responses to nerve stimulation.

The landmarks for a continuous popliteal block with the lateral approach are essentially the same as for the single-injection technique and include the following:

1. Popliteal fossa crease
2. Vastus lateralis
3. Biceps femoris

The needle insertion site is marked at 8 cm proximal to the popliteal fossa crease in the groove between the vastus lateralis and biceps femoris.

## Technique

The continuous popliteal block technique is similar to the single-injection technique. The patient is in the supine position. Using a 25-gauge needle, infiltrate the skin with local anesthetic at the injection site 7–8 cm proximal to the popliteal crease in the groove between the biceps femoris and vastus lateralis muscles. An 8- to 10-cm needle with a Tuohy-style tip for a continuous nerve block is connected to the nerve stimulator (1.5 mA) and inserted to contact the femur (Figure 20.2-11). A slight cephalad orientation to the needle with the opening facing proximally will aid in catheter threading. Once the femur is contacted, the needle is withdrawn to the skin level and redirected in a slightly posterior direction 30°. Then it is advanced slowly while observing the patient for plantar flexion or dorsiflexion of the foot or toes. After obtaining the appropriate twitches, continue manipulating the needle until the desired response is still seen or felt using a current of 0.2–0.5 mA. The catheter should be advanced no more than 5 cm beyond the needle tip. The needle is withdrawn back to the skin level, and the catheter advanced simultaneously to prevent inadvertent removal of the catheter.

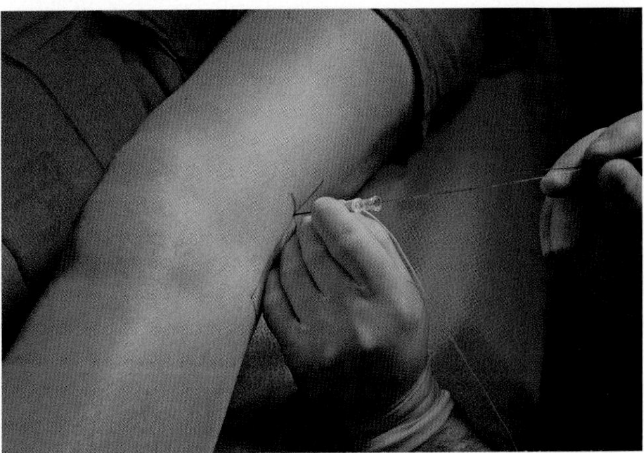

**FIGURE 20.2-11.** Catheter insertion technique for popliteal sciatic block. Technique is similar to that of the single-injection technique. Catheter is inserted 3–5 cm beyond the needle tip.

The catheter is checked for inadvertent intravascular placement and secured to the lateral thigh using an adhesive skin preparation such as benzoin, followed by application of a clear dressing. The infusion port should be clearly marked "continuous nerve block."

**TIPS**

- With a popliteal catheter, a response at 0.5–1.0 mA should be accepted as long as the motor response is specific and clearly seen or felt.
- A very small (e.g., 1 mm) movement of the needle often results in a change in the motor response from that of the tibial nerve (plantar flexion of the foot) to that of the common peroneal nerve (dorsiflexion of the foot). This indicates an intimate needle to nerve relationship at a level before divergence of the sciatic nerve.
- When catheter insertion proves difficult, rotate the needle slightly and try reinserting it again. When these maneuvers do not facilitate insertion of the catheter, angle the needle in a cephalad direction before reattempting to insert the catheter. With this maneuver, care should be taken not to dislodge the needle.

### *Continuous Infusion*

Continuous infusion is initiated after an initial bolus of dilute local anesthetic is administered through the catheter or needle. For this purpose, we routinely use 0.2% ropivacaine 15–20 mL. Diluted bupivacaine or levobupivacaine are suitable but can result in additional motor blockade. The infusion is maintained at 5 mL/h with 5-mL/h patient-controlled regional analgesia.

## Complications and How to Avoid Them

Table 20.2-2 provides specific instructions on some complications and how to avoid them.

**TIPS**

- Breakthrough pain in patients undergoing a continuous infusion is always managed by administering a bolus of local anesthetic. Simply increasing the rate of infusion is not adequate.
- When the bolus injection through the catheter fails to result in blockade after 30 minutes, the catheter should be considered dislodged and should be removed.
- All patients with continuous nerve block infusion should be prescribed an alternative pain management protocol because incomplete analgesia and/or catheter dislodgment can occur.

**TABLE 20.2-2 Complications of Popliteal Block Through the Lateral Approach and Preventive Techniques**

| | |
|---|---|
| ***Infection*** | • Use a strict aseptic technique. |
| ***Hematoma*** | • Avoid multiple needle passes with a continuous block needle; the larger needle diameter and/or Tuohy design can result in a hematoma of the biceps femoris or vastus lateralis muscle.<br>• When the nerve is not localized within a few needle passes, use a smaller gauge, single-injection needle (localization needle) first and then reinsert the continuous block needle using the same angle. |
| ***Vascular puncture*** | • Avoid too deep an insertion of the needle because the popliteal artery and vein are positioned medially and deeper to the sciatic nerve.<br>• When the nerve is not localized within 2 cm after local twitches of the biceps femoris muscle cease, the needle should be withdrawn and reinserted at a different angle rather than advanced deeper. |
| ***Nerve injury*** | • Uncommon.<br>• Advance needle slowly to avoid mechanical nerve injury.<br>• Do not inject when the patient complains of pain or high resistance (pressure >15 psi) is met on injection.<br>• Do not inject when stimulation is obtained at <0.2 mA.<br>• Avoid application of a tourniquet over the injection site to decrease the risk of prolonged ischemia of the nerve. |
| ***Pressure necrosis of the heel*** | • Instruct the patient and nursing staff on care of the insensate extremity.<br>• Use heel padding and frequent repositioning. |

# LATERAL POPLITEAL SCIATIC NERVE BLOCK

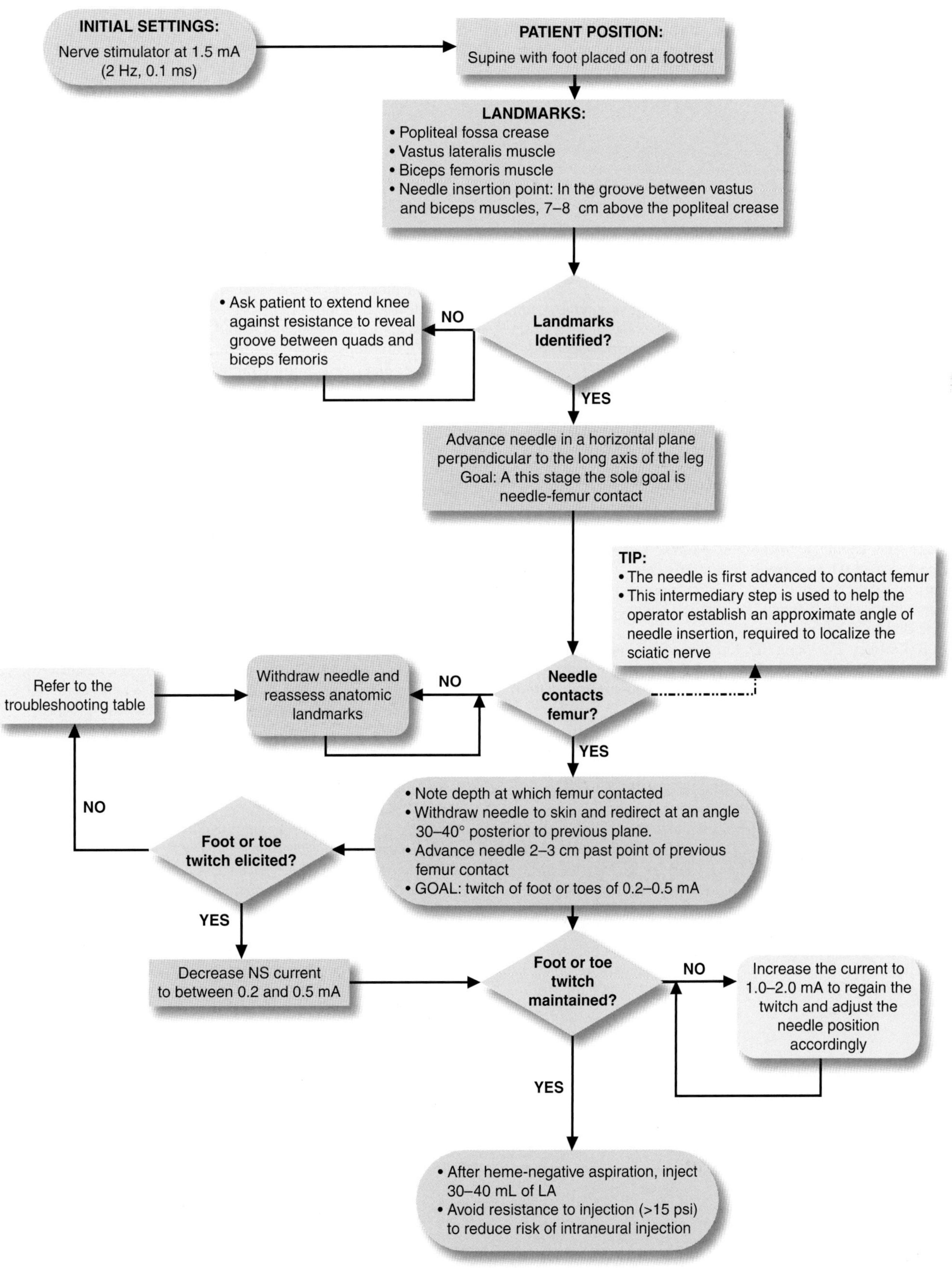

## SUGGESTED READINGS

Arcioni R, Palmisani S, Della Rocca M, et al. Lateral popliteal sciatic nerve block: a single injection targeting the tibial branch of the sciatic nerve is as effective as a double-injection technique. *Acta Anaesthesiol Scand.* 2007;51:115-121.

Benzon HT, Kim C, Benzon HP, et al. Correlation between evoked motor response of the sciatic nerve and sensory blockade. *Anesthesiology.* 1997;87:547-552.

Chelly JE, Casati A, Fanelli G. *Continuous Peripheral Nerve Block Technique: An Illustrated Guide.* London, UK: Mosby International; 2001.

di Benedetto P, Casati A, Bertini L, Fanelli G, Chelly JE. Postoperative analgesia with continuous sciatic nerve block after foot surgery: a prospective, randomized comparison between the popliteal and subgluteal approaches. *Anesth Analg.* 2002;94:996-1000.

Fournier R, Weber A, Gamulin Z. Posterior labat vs. lateral popliteal sciatic block: posterior sciatic block has quicker onset and shorter duration of anaesthesia. *Acta Anaesthesiol Scand.* 2005;49:683-686

Fournier R, Weber A, Gamulin Z. No differences between 20, 30, or 40 mL ropivacaine 0.5% in continuous lateral popliteal sciatic-nerve block. *Reg Anesth Pain Med.* 2006;31:455-459.

Guntz E, Herman P, Debizet E, Delhaye D, Coulic V, Sosnowski M. Sciatic nerve block in the popliteal fossa: description of a new medial approach. *Can J Anaesth.* 2004;51:817-820.

Hadžić A, Vloka JD. A comparison of the posterior versus lateral approaches to the block of the sciatic nerve in the popliteal fossa. *Anesthesiology.* 1998;88:1480-1486.

Hadžić A, Vloka JD, Singson R, Santos AC, Thys DM. A comparison of intertendinous and classical approaches to popliteal nerve block using magnetic resonance imaging simulation. *Anesth Analg.* 2002;94:1321-1324.

Ilfeld BM, Morey TE, Wang RD, Enneking FK. Continuous popliteal sciatic nerve block for postoperative pain control at home: a randomized, double-blinded, placebo-controlled study. *Anesthesiology.* 2002;97:959-965.

Martinez Navas A, Vazquez Gutierrez T, Echevarria Moreno M. Continuous lateral popliteal block with stimulating catheters. *Acta Anaesthesiol Scand.* 2005;49:261-263.

McLeod DH, Wong DH, Claridge RJ, Merrick PM. Lateral popliteal sciatic nerve block compared with subcutaneous infiltration for analgesia following foot surgery. *Can J Anaesth.* 1994;41:673-676.

McLeod DH, Wong DH, Vaghadia H, Claridge RJ, Merrick PM. Lateral popliteal sciatic nerve block compared with ankle block for analgesia following foot surgery. *Can J Anaesth.* 1995;42:765-769.

Minville V, Zegermann T, Hermant N, Eychenne B, Otal .: A modified lateral approach to the sciatic nerve: magnetic resonance imaging simulation and clinical study. *Reg Anesth Pain Med.* 2007;32:157-161.

Nader A, Kendall MC, Candido KD, Benzon H, McCarthy RJ. A randomized comparison of a modified intertendinous and classic posterior approach to popliteal sciatic nerve block. *Anesth Analg.* 2009;108:359-363.

O'Neill T. Lateral popliteal sciatic-nerve block made easy. *Reg Anesth Pain Med.* 2007;32:93-94.

Palmisani S, Ronconi P, De Blasi RA, Arcioni R. Lateral or posterior popliteal approach for sciatic nerve block: difference is related to the anatomy. *Anesth Analg.* 2007;105:286.

Paqueron X, Narchi P, Mazoit JX, Singelyn F, Benichou A, Macaire P. A randomized, observer-blinded determination of the median effective volume of local anesthetic required to anesthetize the sciatic nerve in the popliteal fossa for stimulating and nonstimulating perineural catheters. *Reg Anesth Pain Med.* 2009;34:290-295.

Singelyn FJ, Aye F, Gouverneur JM. Continuous popliteal sciatic nerve block: an original technique to provide postoperative analgesia after foot surgery. *Anesth Analg.* 1997;84:383-386.

Sunderland S. The sciatic nerve and its tibial and common peroneal divisions: anatomical features. In: Sutherland S, ed. *Nerves and Nerve Injuries.* Edinburgh, UK: E&S Livingstone; 1968:1012–1095.

Taboada M, Cortes J, Rodriguez J, Ulloa B, Alvarez J, Atanassoff PG. Lateral approach to the sciatic nerve in the popliteal fossa: a comparison between 1.5% mepivacaine and 0.75% ropivacaine. *Reg Anesth Pain Med.* 2003;28:516-520.

Taboada M, Rodriguez J, Alvarez J, Cortés J, Gude F, Atanassoff PG. Sciatic nerve block via posterior Labat approach is more efficient than lateral popliteal approach using a double-injection technique: a prospective, randomized comparison. *Anesthesiology.* 2004;101:138-142.

Taboada Muniz M, Alvarez J, Cortés J, Rodriguez J, Atanassoff PG. Lateral approach to the sciatic nerve block in the popliteal fossa: correlation between evoked motor response and sensory block. *Reg Anesth Pain Med.* 2003;28:450-445.

Triado VD, Crespo MT, Aguilar JL, Atanassoff PG, Palanca JM, Moro B. A comparison of lateral popliteal versus lateral midfemoral sciatic nerve blockade using ropivacaine 0.5%. *Reg Anesth Pain Med.* 2004;29:23-27.

Vloka JD, Hadžić A, April E, Thys DM. The division of the sciatic nerve in the popliteal fossa: anatomical implications for popliteal nerve blockade. *Anesth Analg.* 2001;92:215-217.

Vloka JD, Hadžić A, Kitain E, et al. Anatomic considerations for sciatic nerve block in the popliteal fossa through the lateral approach. *Reg Anesth.* 1996;21:414-418.

Vloka JD, Hadžić A, Lesser JB, et al. A common epineural sheath for the nerves in the popliteal fossa and its possible implications for sciatic nerve block. *Anesth Analg.* 1997;84:387-390.

Zetlaoui PJ, Bouaziz H. Lateral approach to the sciatic nerve in the popliteal fossa. *Anesth Analg.* 1998;87:79-82.

# 21 Femoral Nerve Block

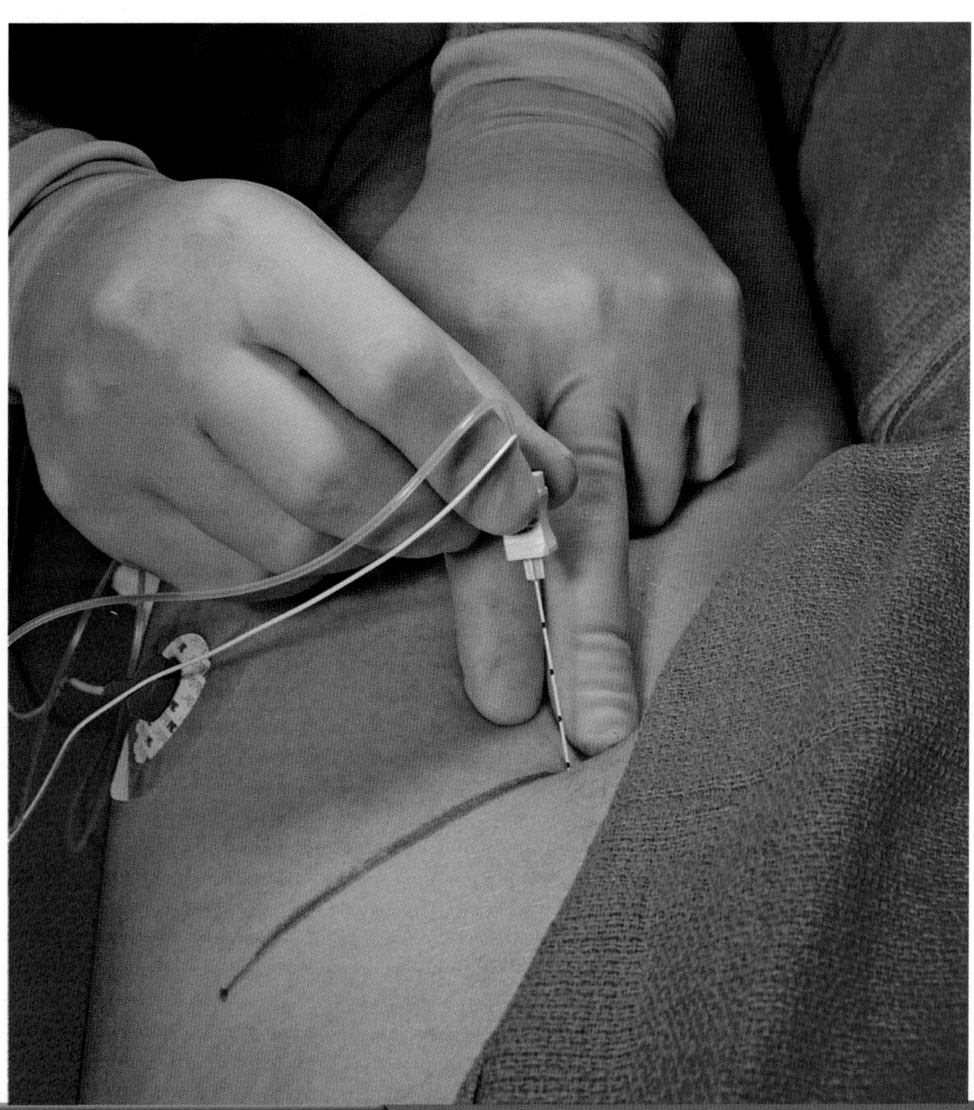

## BLOCK AT A GLANCE

- Indications: surgery of the anterior thigh and knee surgery
- Landmarks: femoral (inguinal) crease, femoral artery pulse
- Nerve stimulation: twitch of the patella (quadriceps) at 0.2–0.5 mA
- Local anesthetic volume: 15–20 mL

**FIGURE 21-1.** Needle insertion for femoral nerve block.

## General Considerations

A femoral nerve block is a quintessential nerve block technique that is easy to master, carries a low risk of complications, and has significant clinical application for surgical anesthesia and postoperative pain management. The femoral block is well-suited for surgery on the anterior thigh and knee, quadriceps tendon repair, and postoperative pain management after femur and knee surgery. When combined with a block of the sciatic nerve, anesthesia of almost the entire lower extremity from the midthigh level can be achieved.

## Functional Anatomy

The femoral nerve is the largest branch of the lumbar plexus, arising from the second, third, and fourth lumbar nerves. The nerve descends through the psoas muscle, emerging from the psoas at the lower part of its lateral border, and it runs downward between the psoas and the iliacus. The femoral nerve eventually passes underneath the inguinal ligament into the thigh, where it assumes a more flattened shape (Figure 21-2). The inguinal ligament is a convergent point of the transversalis fascia (fascial sac lining the deep surface of the anterior abdominal wall) and iliac fascia (fascia covering the posterior abdominal wall). As it passes beneath the inguinal ligament, the nerve is positioned lateral and slightly deeper than the femoral artery between the psoas and iliacus muscles. At the femoral crease, the nerve is on the surface of the iliacus muscle and covered by the fascia iliaca or sandwiched between two layers of fascia iliaca. In contrast, vascular fascia of the femoral artery and vein, a funnel-shaped extension of the transversalis fascia, forms a distinctly different compartment from that of the femoral nerve but often contains the femoral branch of the genitofemoral nerve lateral to the vessels (Figure 21-3). The physical separation of the femoral nerve from the vascular fascia explains the lack of spread of a "blind paravascular" injection of local anesthetic toward the femoral nerve.

### TIP

- It is useful to think of the mnemonic "VAN" (vein, artery, nerve: medial to lateral) when recalling the relationship of the femoral nerve to the vessels in the femoral triangle.

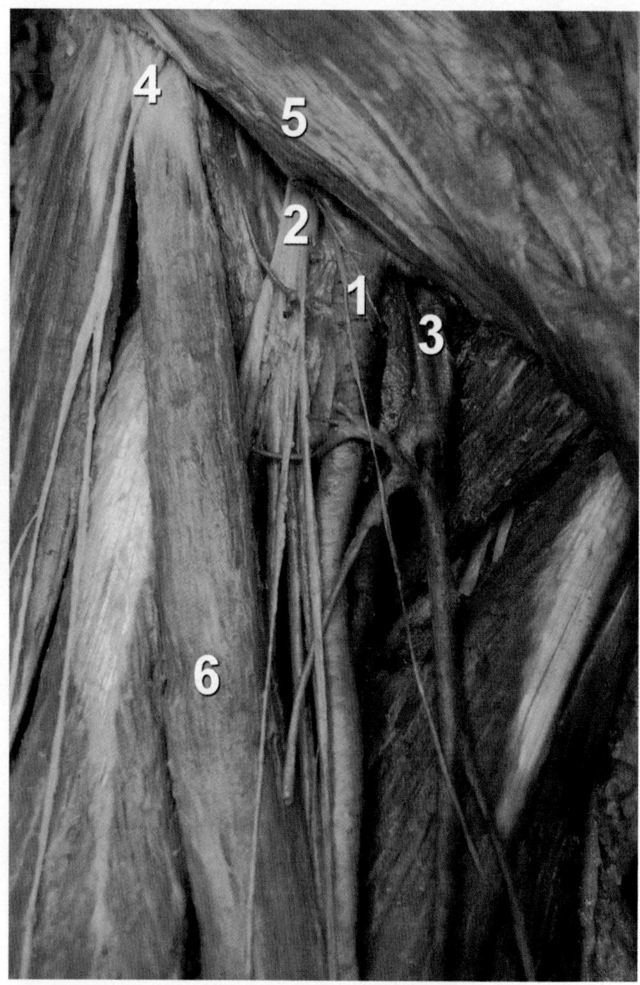


**FIGURE 21-2.** Anatomy of the femoral triangle. ❶ femoral artery. ❷ femoral nerve. ❸ femoral vein. ❹ anterior superior iliac spine. ❺ inguinal ligament. ❻ sartorius.

The branches to the sartorius muscle depart from the anteromedial aspect of the femoral nerve toward the sartorius muscle. Because sartorius muscle twitch may be the result of the stimulation of this specific branch and not the femoral nerve, the sartorius motor response should not be accepted. Although the needle in the proper position (close to the main trunk of the femoral nerve) often results in sartorius muscle twitch, quadriceps twitch results in more consistent blockade, and it routinely should be sought before injecting local anesthetic unless ultrasound is used concomitantly.

The femoral nerve supplies the muscular branches of the iliacus and pectineus and the muscles of the anterior thigh, except for the tensor fascia lata. The nerve also provides cutaneous branches to the front and medial sides of the thigh, the medial leg and foot (saphenous nerve), and the articular branches of the hip and knee joints (Table 21-1).

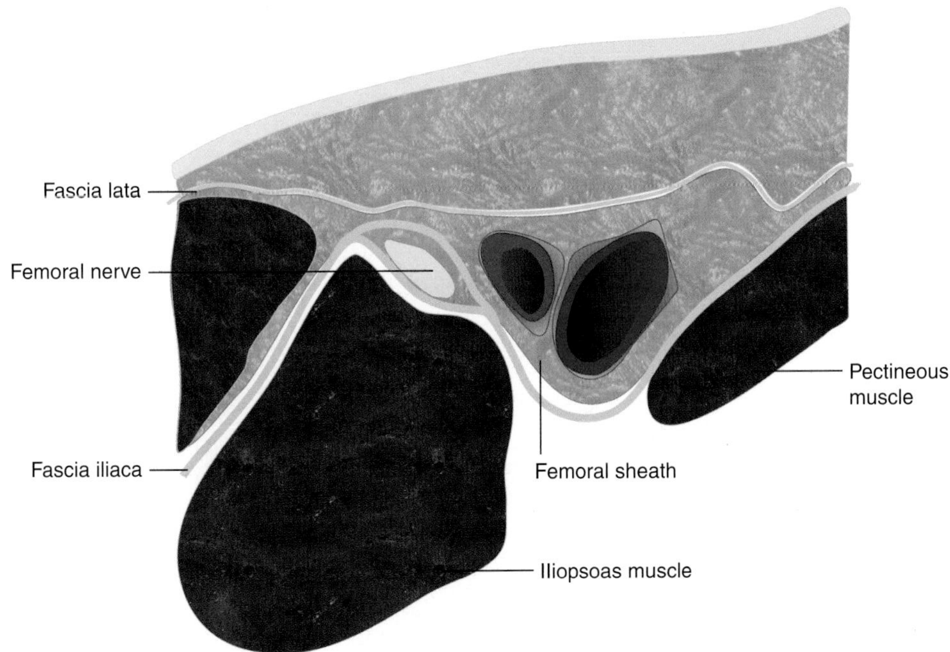


**FIGURE 21-3.** Arrangement of the fascial sheaths at the femoral triangle. Femoral nerve is enveloped by two layers of fascia iliaca, whereas femoral vessels are contained in the vascular (femoral) sheath made up of fascia lata.

## Distribution of Blockade

Femoral nerve block results in anesthesia of the skin and muscles of the anterior thigh and most of the femur and knee joint (Figure 21-4). The block also confers anesthesia of the skin on the medial aspect of the leg below the knee joint (saphenous nerve, a superficial terminal extension of the femoral nerve).

| TABLE 21-1 | Femoral Nerve Branches |
|---|---|
| Anterior division | • Middle cutaneous<br>• Medial cutaneous<br>• Muscular (sartorius) |
| Posterior division | • Saphenous nerve (most medial)<br>• Muscular (individual heads of the quadriceps muscle)<br>• Articular branches (hip and knee) |

## Single-Injection Femoral Nerve Block

### Equipment

A standard regional anesthesia tray is prepared with the following equipment:

- Sterile towels and gauze packs
- One 20-mL syringe containing local anesthetic
- A 3-mL syringe plus 25-gauge needle with local anesthetic for skin infiltration
- A 5-cm, 22-gauge short-bevel insulated stimulating needle
- Peripheral nerve stimulator
- Sterile gloves; marking pen

### Landmarks and Patient Positioning

The patient is in the supine position with both legs extended. In obese patients, a pillow placed underneath the hips can facilitate palpation of the femoral artery and the block performance.

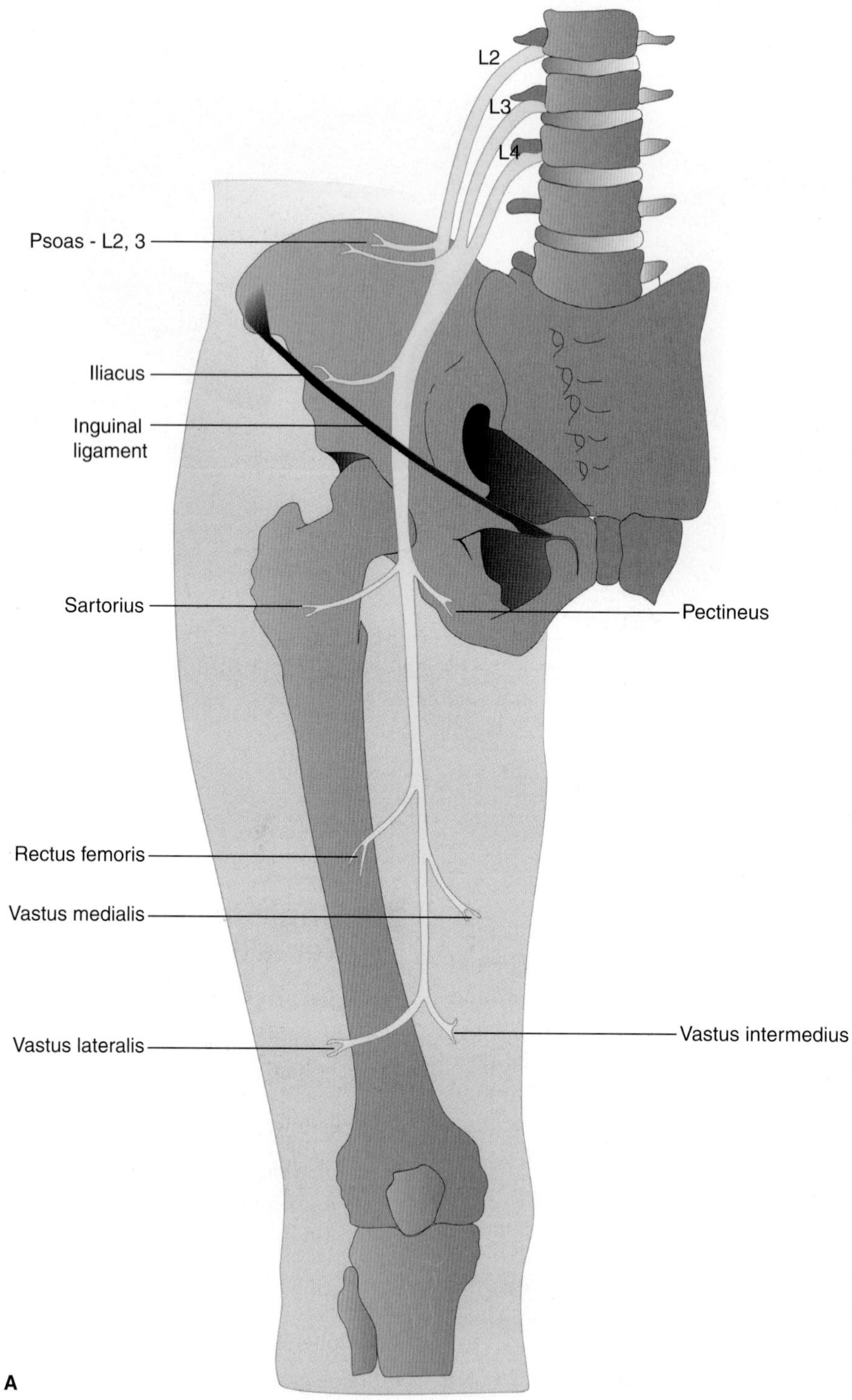


**FIGURE 21-4.** (A) Motor innervation of the femoral nerve. (B) Sensory innervation of the femoral nerve and its cutaneous branches.

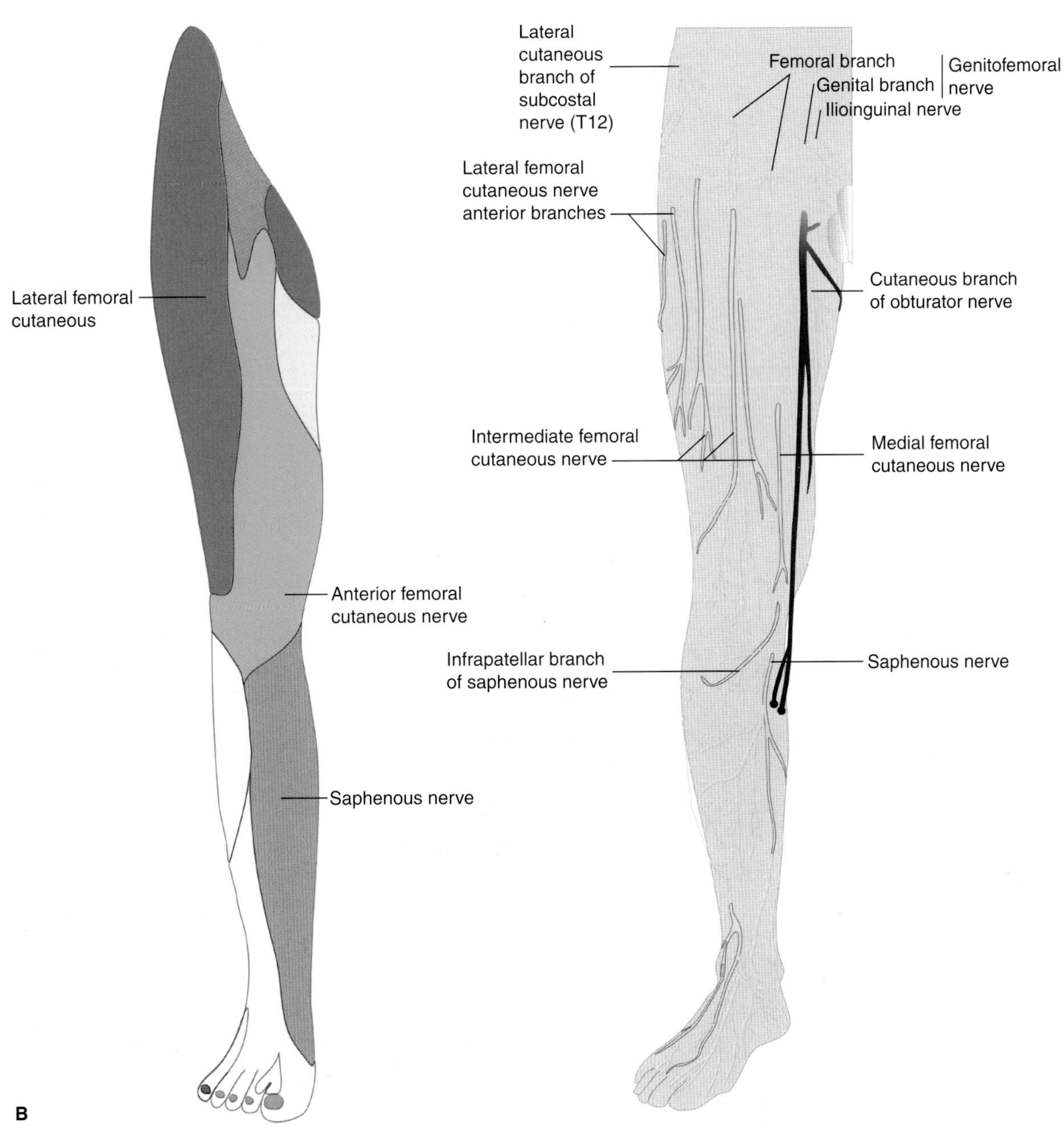


**FIGURE 21-4.** *(Continued)*

Landmarks for the femoral nerve block are easily recognizable in most patients and include the femoral crease (Figure 21-5) and femoral artery pulse (Figure 21-6).

## TIP

- Note that the needle is inserted at the level of the femoral crease, a naturally occurring skin fold positioned a few centimeters *below* the inguinal ligament.

The following maneuvers can be used to facilitate landmark identification:

- The femoral crease can be accentuated in obese patients by having an assistant retract the lower abdomen laterally.
- Retraction of the abdomen should be maintained throughout the procedure to facilitate palpation of the femoral artery and performance of the block.
- Avoid excessive pressure on the crease when palpating for the artery because it can distort the landmarks.

The needle insertion site is labeled immediately lateral to the pulse of the femoral artery (Figure 21-6). All landmarks should be outlined with a marking pen.

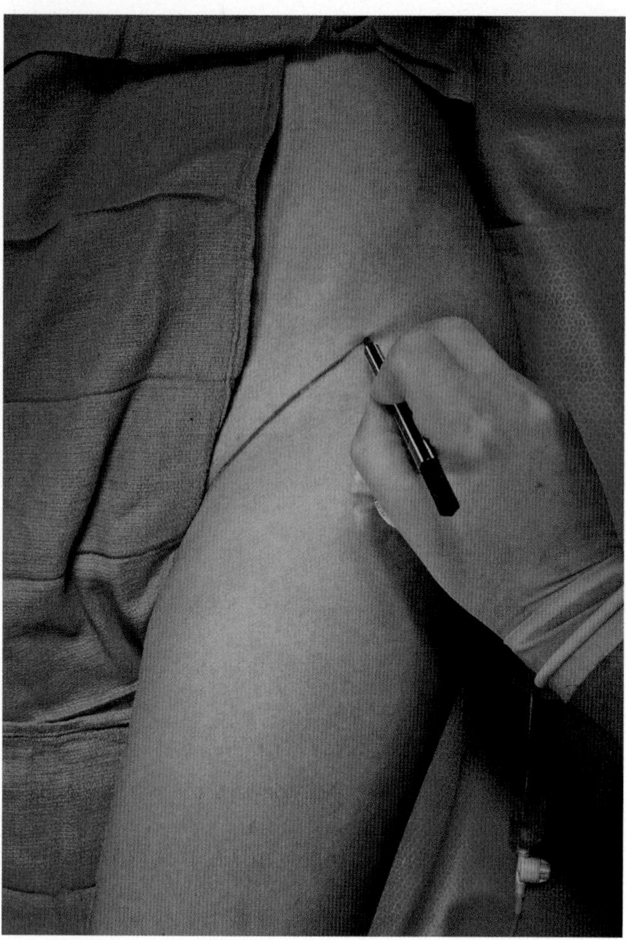

**FIGURE 21-5.** Femoral nerve block is performed at the level of the femoral crease (line).

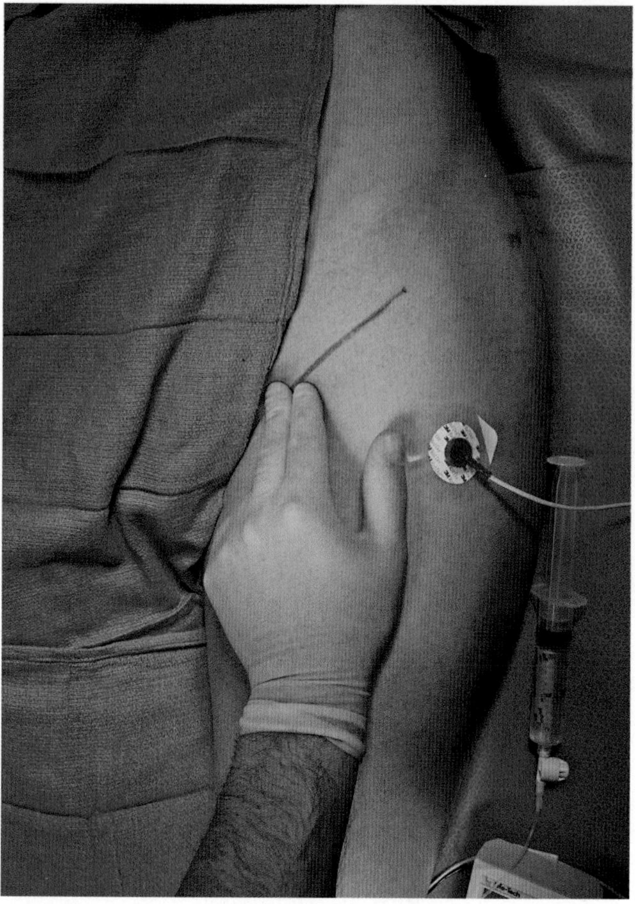

**FIGURE 21-6.** The main landmark for the femoral nerve block is the femoral artery, which is palpated at the level of the femoral crease. Needle insertion point is just lateral to the pulse of the femoral artery.

## Technique

After thorough preparation of the area with an antiseptic solution, local anesthetic is infiltrated subcutaneously at the estimated site of needle insertion. The injection for the skin anesthesia should be shallow and in a line extending laterally to allow for a more lateral needle reinsertion when necessary. The anesthesiologist should stand at the side of the patient with the palpating hand on the femoral artery. The needle is introduced immediately at the lateral border of the artery and advanced in sagittal, slightly cephalad plane (Figure 21-1).

## GOAL

A visible or palpable twitch of the quadriceps muscle (a patella twitch) at 0.2–0.4 mA is the most reliable response.

## TIPS

- A twitch of the sartorius is a common occurence and it is seen as a band-like contraction across the thigh without movement of the patella.
- A sartorius muscle twitch is not a reliable sign because the branches to the sartorius muscle may be outside the femoral sheath (iliacus fascia).
- When a sartorius muscle twitch occurs, simply redirect the needle laterally and advance it several millimeters deeper to obtain patella twitch, assuring that needle tip is in the vicinity of the main trunk of the femoral nerve.

After initial stimulation of the femoral nerve is obtained, the stimulating current is gradually decreased until twitches are still seen or felt at 0.2 to 0.4 mA, which typically occurs at a depth of 2 to 3 cm. After obtaining negative results from an aspiration test for blood, 15 to 20 mL of local anesthetic is injected slowly.

## Troubleshooting

When stimulation of the quadriceps muscle is not obtained on the first needle pass, the palpating hand should not be moved from its position. Instead, visualize the needle plane in which the stimulation was not obtained and:

- Ensure that the nerve stimulator is properly connected and functional.
- Withdraw the needle to skin level, redirect it 10° to 15° laterally, and repeat needle advancement (Figure 21-7).

### TIP

- It is essential to keep the palpating finger in the same position throughout the procedure. This strategy allows for a more organized approach to localize the femoral nerve.

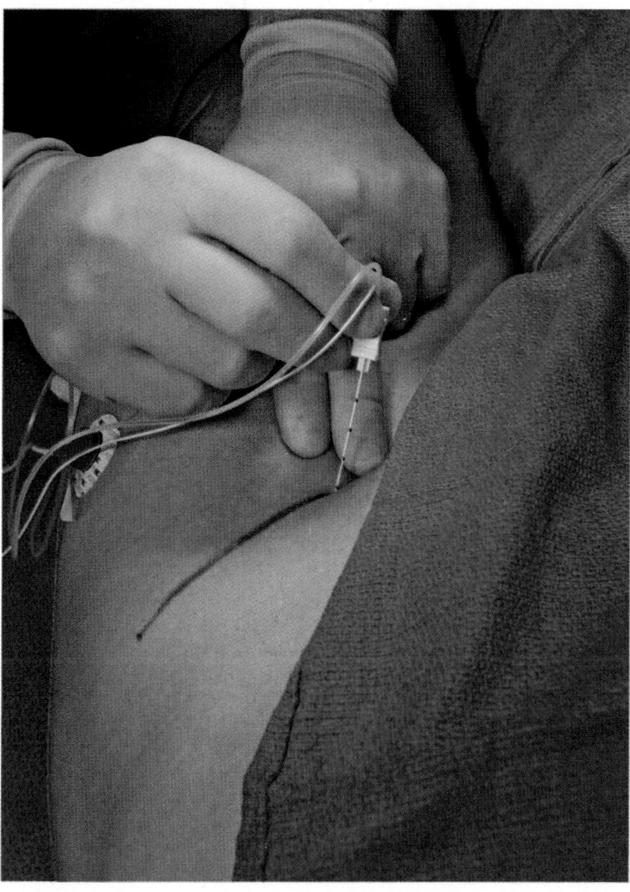

**FIGURE 21-7.** When lateral redirection of the needle does not bring about motor response, the needle is reinserted 1 cm lateral to the original reinsertion point.

When the procedure just described fails to produce a twitch, the needle is withdrawn from the skin and reinserted 1 cm laterally, and the previously described steps are repeated with a progressively more lateral needle insertion.

Table 21-2 shows some common responses to nerve stimulation and the course of action required to obtain the proper response.

## Block Dynamics and Perioperative Management

Femoral nerve blockade is associated with minimal patient discomfort because the needle passes only through the skin and adipose tissue of the femoral inguinal region. However, many patients feel uncomfortable being exposed during palpation of the femoral artery, and appropriate sedation is necessary for the patient's comfort and acceptance. The administration of midazolam 1 to 2 mg after the patient is positioned and alfentanil 250 to 500 μg just before infiltration of the local anesthetic suffices for most patients. A typical onset time for this block is 15 to 20 minutes, depending on the type, concentration, and volume of anesthetic used. The first sign of onset of the blockade is a loss of sensation in the skin over the medial aspect of the leg below the knee (saphenous nerve). Weightbearing on the blocked side is impaired, which should be clearly explained to the patient to prevent falls. Some practitioners advocate the use of large volume of local anesthetic to anesthetize lateral femoral cutaneous and obturator nerves in addition to the femoral nerve. However, such an extensive spread of the local anesthetic has not been substantiated in the literature. Injection of local anesthetic during femoral nerve blockade results primarily in pooling of the injectate around the femoral nerve underneath the fascia iliaca without consistent latera-medial spread (Figure 21-8).

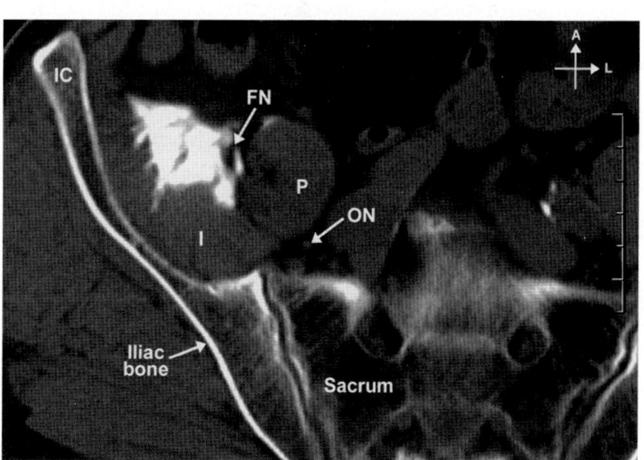


**FIGURE 21-8.** Injection of local anesthetic during femoral nerve blockade results primarily in pooling of the injectate around the femoral nerve underneath the fascia iliaca without consistent latera-medial spread. FN - femoral nerve, IC - Iliac Crest, P - Psoas Muscle, I - Iliacus muscle, ON - Obturator Nerve.

**TABLE 21-2 Common Responses to Nerve Stimulation and Course of Action for Proper Response**

| RESPONSE OBTAINED | INTERPRETATION | PROBLEM | ACTION |
|---|---|---|---|
| No response | Needle is inserted either too medially or too laterally | Femoral artery not properly localized or the palpating hand was moved during the procedure | Re-examine the landmarks and follow the systematic lateral angulation and reinsertion of the needle as described in the technique |
| Bone contact | Needle contacts hip / femur or superior ramus of the pubic bone | Needle is inserted too deeply Femoral nerve is more superficial—typically between 2-3 cm in average size adult patients | Withdraw needle to the skin level and repeat the procedure |
| Local twitch | Direct stimulation of the iliopsoas or pectineus muscle | Needle is inserted too deeply or too cranially | Withdraw the needle, reassess the landmarks, and repeat the procedure |
| Twitch of the sartorius muscle | Stimulation of the nerve branches to the sartorius muscle | Needle tip may be slightly anterior and medial to main trunk of the femoral nerve | Redirect needle laterally and advance it deeper 1–3 mm.<br>Note: Injection after sartorius twitch will result in successful block only if the sartorius branch and femoral nerve are within the same tissue sheath |
| Vascular puncture | Indicates placement into the femoral artery or vein | Needle is inserted too medially | Withdraw needle and reinsert it laterally 1 cm |
| Patella twitch | Stimulation of the main trunk of the femoral nerve | None | Inject local anesthetic |

## Continuous Femoral Nerve Block

The continuous femoral nerve block technique is similar to the single-injection procedure; however, insertion of the needle at a slightly lower angle may be necessary to facilitate threading of the catheter. The most common indications for use of this block are postoperative analgesia after knee arthroplasty, anterior cruciate ligament repair, and femoral fracture repair.

### Equipment

A standard regional anesthesia tray is prepared with the following equipment:

- Sterile towels and gauze packs
- One 20-mL syringes containing local anesthetic
- Sterile gloves, marking pen, and surface electrode
- A 3- to 5-mL syringe plus 25-gauge needle with local anesthetic for skin infiltration
- Peripheral nerve stimulator
- Catheter kit (including a 5- to 8-cm large-gauge stimulating needle and catheter)

Either nonstimulating (conventional) or stimulating catheters can be used. During the placement of a conventional, nonstimulating catheter, the stimulating needle is first advanced until appropriate motor responses are obtained. Five to 10 mL of local anesthetic or nonconducting injectate (e.g., D5W) is injected to "open up" a space for the catheter to advance with less resistance. Then the catheter is threaded through the needle to approximately 3–5 cm beyond the tip of the needle. The needle is withdrawn, the catheter secured, and the remaining local anesthetic is injected via the catheter.

### Landmarks and Patient Positioning

The patient is in the supine position with both legs extended. In obese patients, a pillow placed underneath the hips can facilitate palpation of the femoral artery and the block performance.

The landmarks for a continuous femoral block include:

1. Femoral (inguinal crease)
2. Femoral artery
3. Needle insertion site is marked immediately lateral to the pulse of the femoral artery

## Technique

With the patient in the supine position, the skin is infiltrated with local anesthetic at the injection site using a 25-gauge needle. The palpating hand is used to keep the middle finger on the pulse of the femoral artery while the entire hand slightly pulls the skin caudally to keep it from wrinkling on needle insertion (Figure 21-1). The stimulating needle connected to the nerve stimulator (1.0 mA) is inserted and advanced at a 45° to 60° angle. Care should be taken to avoid insertion of the needle too medially to decrease the risk of a puncture of the femoral artery. The goal is to obtain a quadriceps muscle response (patella twitch) at 0.5 mA. The catheter should be advanced 3 to 5 cm beyond the needle tip (Figure 21-9). The catheter is advanced deeper in obese patients to prevent catheter dislodgement with shifting of the adipose tissue postoperatively. Then the needle is withdrawn back to the skin level, and the catheter is advanced simultaneously to prevent inadvertent removal of the catheter.

The catheter is checked for inadvertent intravascular placement and secured to the thigh using an adhesive skin preparation such as benzoin, followed by application of a clear dressing. The infusion port should be clearly marked "continuous nerve block."

### *Continuous Infusion*

Continuous infusion is always initiated following an initial bolus (15–20 mL) of dilute local anesthetic through the needle or catheter. For this purpose, we routinely use 0.2% ropivacaine. The infusion is maintained at 5 mL/h with a patient-controlled regional analgesic dose of 5 mL/h.

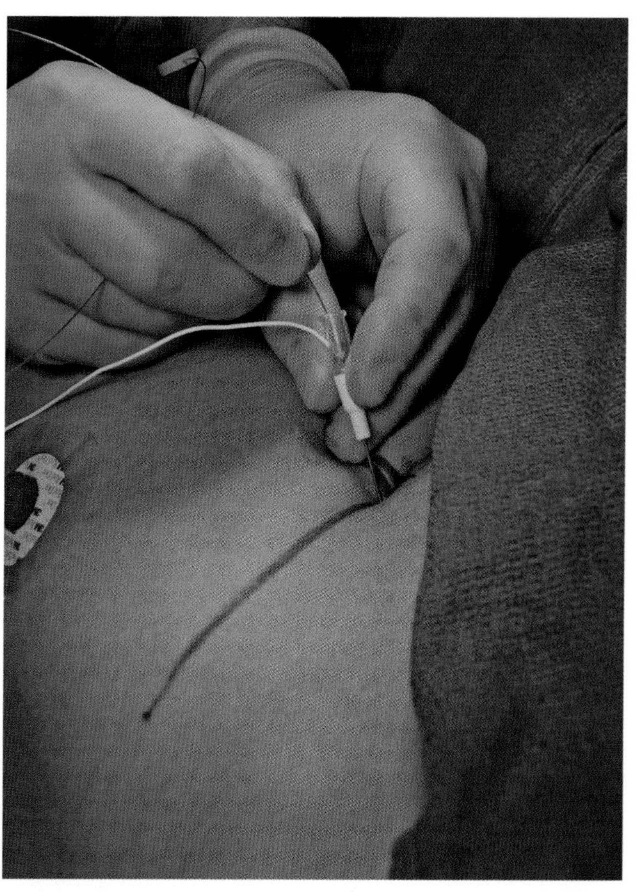

**FIGURE 21-9.** Catheter insertion for continuous femoral nerve block. The catheter is inserted 3–5 cm beyond the needle tip.

## Complications and How to Avoid Them

Table 21-3 provides some general and specific instructions on possible complications and how to avoid them.

**TABLE 21-3 Complications of Femoral Nerve Block and Preventive Techniques**

| | |
|---|---|
| ***Infection*** | • Use a strict aseptic technique.<br>• At the femoral crease, catheters are difficult to keep sterile and should probably be removed after 48–72 h. |
| ***Hematoma*** | • Avoid advancement of the needle when the patient reports pain, which may indicate insertion of the needle through the iliopsoas or pectineus muscle.<br>• When the femoral artery or vein is punctured, the procedure should be stopped and a firm, constant pressure applied over the femoral artery for 2–3 min before proceeding with the blockade.<br>• In a patient with difficult anatomy or severe peripheral vascular disease, use a single-injection smaller gauge needle to localize the femoral nerve before proceeding with a larger gauge needle for the continuous technique. |
| ***Vascular puncture*** | • The needle is first inserted just laterally to the femoral artery, and consequent insertions and redirections should all be made progressively more lateral.<br>• The needle should never be redirected medially! |
| ***Nerve injury*** | • Avoid stimulation at <0.2 mA and advance needle slowly.<br>• Distinct paresthesia is almost never elicited with a femoral nerve block and should not be sought.<br>• Do not inject when the patient complains of pain or when high resistance (injection pressure >15 psi) is present. |
| ***Other*** | • Instruct the patient on the inability to bear weight on the blocked extremity to decrease the risk of falls. |

# NERVE STIMULATOR-GUIDED FEMORAL NERVE BLOCK

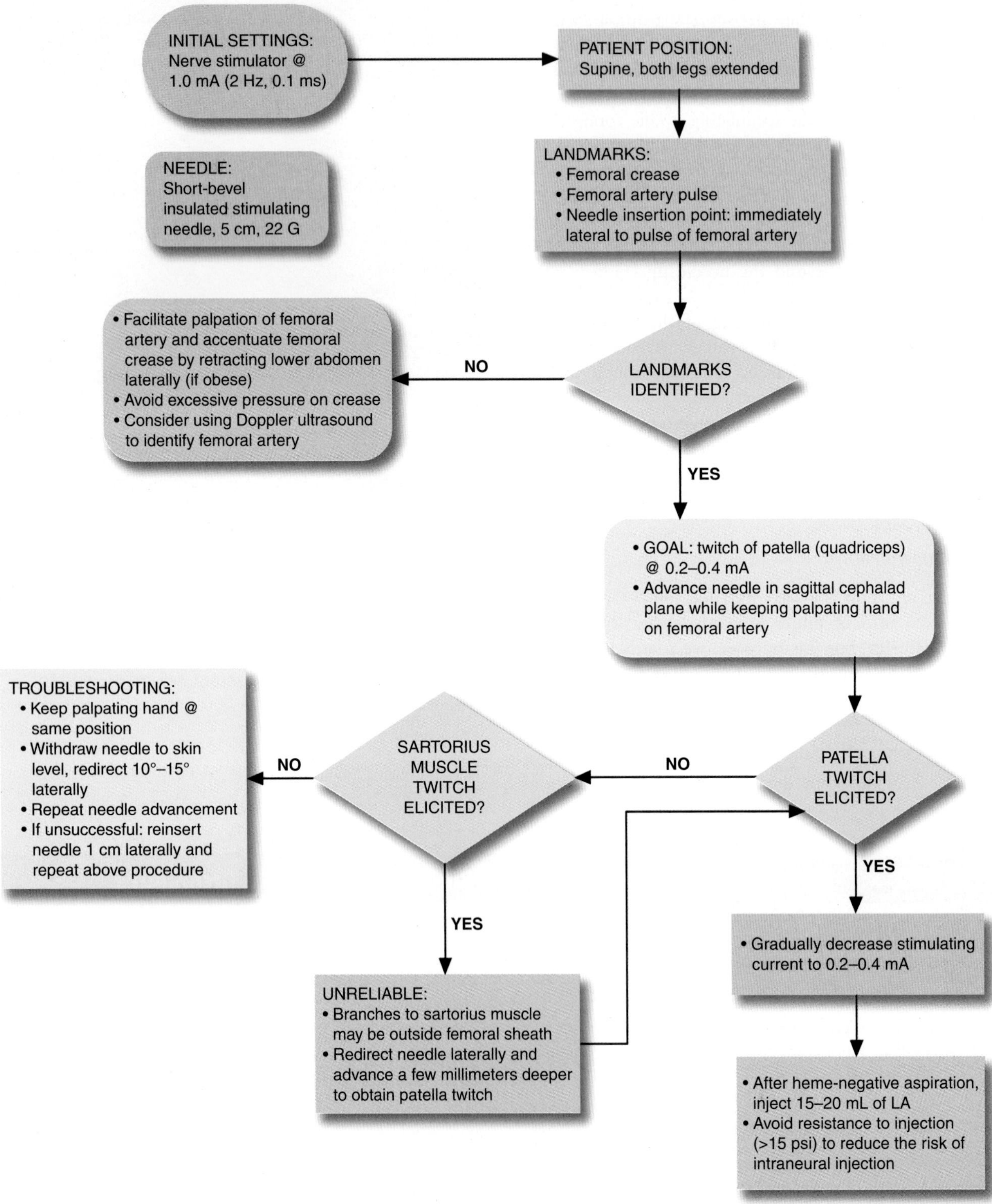

## SUGGESTED READING

### Single-Injection Femoral Nerve Block


Allen HW, Liu SS, Ware PD, Nairn CS, Owens BD. Peripheral nerve blocks improve analgesia after total knee replacement surgery. *Anesth Analg*. 1998;87:93-97.

Beaulieu P, Babin D, Hemmerling T. The pharmacodynamics of ropivacaine and bupivacaine in combined sciatic and femoral nerve blocks for total knee arthroplasty. *Anesth Analg*. 2006;103:768-774.

Biboulet P, Morau D, Aubas P, Bringuier-Branchereau S, Capdevila X. Postoperative analgesia after total-hip arthroplasty: comparison of intravenous patient-controlled analgesia with morphine and single injection of femoral nerve or psoas compartment block. a prospective, randomized, double-blind study. *Reg Anesth Pain Med*. 2004;29:102-109.

de Lima ESR, Correa CH, Henriques MD, de Oliveira CB, Nunes TA, Gomez RS. Single-injection femoral nerve block with 0.25% ropivacaine or 0.25% bupivacaine for postoperative analgesia after total knee replacement or anterior cruciate ligament reconstruction. *J Clin Anesth*. 2008;20:521-527.

Eledjam JJ, Cuvillon P, Capdevila X, et al. Postoperative analgesia by femoral nerve block with ropivacaine 0.2% after major knee surgery: continuous versus patient-controlled techniques. *Reg Anesth Pain Med*. 2002;27:604-611.

Fowler SJ, Symons J, Sabato S, Myles PS. Epidural analgesia compared with peripheral nerve blockade after major knee surgery: a systematic review and meta-analysis of randomized trials. *Br J Anaesth*. 2008;100:154-164.

Hadžić; A, Vloka JD, Kuroda MM, Koorn R, Birnbach DJ. The practice of peripheral nerve blocks in the United States: a national survey [p2e comments]. *Reg Anesth Pain Med*. 1998;23:241-246.

Iskandar H, Benard A, Ruel-Raymond J, Cochard G, Manaud B. Femoral block provides superior analgesia compared with intra-articular ropivacaine after anterior cruciate ligament reconstruction. *Reg Anesth Pain Med*. 2003;28:29-32.

Jansen TK, Miller BE, Arretche N, Pellegrini JE. Will the addition of a sciatic nerve block to a femoral nerve block provide better pain control following anterior cruciate ligament repair surgery? *AANA J*. 2009;77:213-218.

Jochum D, O'Neill T, Jabbour H, Diarra PD, Cuignet-Pourel E, Bouaziz H. Evaluation of femoral nerve blockade following inguinal paravascular block of Winnie: are there still lessons to be learnt? *Anaesthesia*. 2005;60:974-977.

Johnson TW. Will the addition of sciatic nerve block to a femoral nerve block provide better pain control following anterior cruciate ligament repair surgery? *AANA J*. 2009;77:417.

Kardash K, Hickey D, Tessler MJ, Payne S, Zukor D, Velly AM. Obturator versus femoral nerve block for analgesia after total knee arthroplasty. *Anesth Analg*. 2007;105: 853-858.

Lang SA, Yip RW, Chang PC, Gerard MA. The femoral 3-in-1 block revisited. *J Clin Anesth*. 1993;5:292-296.

Macalou D, Trueck S, Meuret P, et al. Postoperative analgesia after total knee replacement: the effect of an obturator nerve block added to the femoral 3-in-1 nerve block. *Anesth Analg*. 2004;99:251-254.

Madej TH, Ellis FR, Halsall PJ. Evaluation of "3 in 1" lumbar plexus block in patients having muscle biopsy. *Br J Anaesth*. 1989;62:515-517.

Marhofer P, Nasel C, Sitzwohl C, Kapral S. Magnetic resonance imaging of the distribution of local anesthetic during the three-in-one block. *Anesth Analg*. 2000;90:119-124.

Martin F, Martinez V, Mazoit JX, et al. Antiinflammatory effect of peripheral nerve blocks after knee surgery: clinical and biologic evaluation. *Anesthesiology*. 2008;109:484-490.

Montes FR, Zarate E, Grueso R, et al. Comparison of spinal anesthesia with combined sciatic-femoral nerve block for outpatient knee arthroscopy. *J Clin Anesth*. 2008;20:415-420.

Mulroy MF, Larkin KL, Batra MS, Hodgson PS, Owens BD. Femoral nerve block with 0.25% or 0.5% bupivacaine improves postoperative analgesia following outpatient arthroscopic anterior cruciate ligament repair. *Reg Anesth Pain Med*. 2001;26:24-29.

Ng HP, Cheong KF, Lim A, Lim J, Puhaindran ME. Intraoperative single-shot "3-in-1" femoral nerve block with ropivacaine 0.25%, ropivacaine 0.5% or bupivacaine 0.25% provides comparable 48-hr analgesia after unilateral total knee replacement. *Can J Anaesth*. 2001;48:1102-1108.

Noiseux N, Prieto I, Bracco D, Basile F, Hemmerling T. Coronary artery bypass grafting in the awake patient combining high thoracic epidural and femoral nerve block: first series of 15 patients. *Br J Anaesth*. 2008;100:184-189.

Parkinson SK, Mueller JB, Little WL, Bailey SL. Extent of blockade with various approaches to the lumbar plexus. *Anesth Analg*. 1989;68:243-248.

Ritter JW. Femoral nerve "sheath" for inguinal paravascular lumbar plexus block is not found in human cadavers. *J Clin Anesth*. 1995;7:470-473.

Rosaeg OP, Krepski B, Cicutti N, Dennehy KC, Lui AC, Johnson DH. Effect of preemptive multimodal analgesia for arthroscopic knee ligament repair. *Reg Anesth Pain Med*. 2001;26:125-130.

Schafhalter-Zoppoth I, Moriggl B. Aspects of femoral nerve block. *Reg Anesth Pain Med*. 2006;31:92-93; author reply 93.

Schiferer A, Gore C, Gorove L, et al. A randomized controlled trial of femoral nerve blockade administered preclinically for pain relief in femoral trauma. *Anesth Analg*. 2007;105:1852-1854; table of contents.

Schulz-Stubner S, Henszel A, Hata JS. A new rule for femoral nerve blocks. *Reg Anesth Pain Med*. 2005;30:473-477.

Seeberger MD, Urwyler A. Paravascular lumbar plexus block: block extension after femoral nerve stimulation and injection of 20 vs. 40 ml mepivacaine 10 mg/ml. *Acta Anaesthesiol Scand*. 1995;39:769-773.

Singelyn FJ, Vanderelst PE, Gouverneur JM. Extended femoral nerve sheath block after total hip arthroplasty: continuous versus patient-controlled techniques. *Anesth Analg*. 2001;92:455-459.

Vloka JD, Hadžić; A, Drobnik L, Ernest A, Reiss W, Thys DM. Anatomical landmarks for femoral nerve block: a comparison of four needle insertion sites. *Anesth Analg*. 1999;89:1467-1470.

Vloka JD, Hadžić; A, Mulcare R, Lesser JB, Kitain E, Thys DM. Femoral and genitofemoral nerve blocks versus spinal anesthesia for outpatients undergoing long saphenous vein stripping surgery. *Anesth Analg*. 1997;84:749-752.

Wang H, Boctor B, Verner J. The effect of single-injection femoral nerve block on rehabilitation and length of hospital stay after total knee replacement. *Reg Anesth Pain Med*. 2002;27:139-144.

Williams BA, Bottegal MT, Kentor ML, Irrgang JJ, Williams JP. Rebound pain scores as a function of femoral nerve block duration after anterior cruciate ligament reconstruction: retrospective analysis of a prospective, randomized clinical trial. *Reg Anesth Pain Med*. 2007;32:186-192.

Williams BA, Kentor ML, Irrgang JJ, Bottegal MT, Williams JP. Nausea, vomiting, sleep, and restfulness upon discharge home after outpatient anterior cruciate ligament reconstruction with regional anesthesia and multimodal analgesia/antiemesis. *Reg Anesth Pain Med.* 2007;32:193-202.

Winnie AP, Ramamurthy S, Durrani Z. The inguinal paravascular technic of lumbar plexus anesthesia: the "3-in-1 block." *Anesth Analg.* 1973;52:989-996.

Wulf H, Lowe J, Gnutzmann KH, Steinfeldt T. Femoral nerve block with ropivacaine or bupivacaine in day case anterior crucial ligament reconstruction. *Acta Anaesthesiol Scand.* 2010;54:414-420.

YaDeau JT, Cahill JB, Zawadsky MW, et al. The effects of femoral nerve blockade in conjunction with epidural analgesia after total knee arthroplasty. *Anesth Analg.* 2005;101:891-895.

Yazigi A, Madi-Gebara S, Haddad F, Hayeck G, Tabet G. Intraoperative myocardial ischemia in peripheral vascular surgery: general anesthesia vs combined sciatic and femoral nerve blocks. *J Clin Anesth.* 2005;17:499-503.

### Continuous Femoral Nerve Block

Allen JG, Denny NM, Oakman N. Postoperative analgesia following total knee arthroplasty: a study comparing spinal anesthesia and combined sciatic femoral 3-in-1 block. *Reg Anesth Pain Med.* 1998;23:142-146.

Barrington MJ, Olive D, Low K, Scott DA, Brittain J, Choong P. Continuous femoral nerve blockade or epidural analgesia after total knee replacement: a prospective randomized controlled trial. *Anesth Analg.* 2005;101:1824-1829.

Barrington MJ, Olive DJ, McCutcheon CA, et al. Stimulating catheters for continuous femoral nerve blockade after total knee arthroplasty: a randomized, controlled, double-blinded trial. *Anesth Analg.* 2008;106:1316-1321.

Birnbaum J, Volk T. Use of a stimulating catheter for femoral nerve block. *Br J Anaesth.* 2006;96:139.

Brodner G, Buerkle H, Van Aken H, et al. Postoperative analgesia after knee surgery: a comparison of three different concentrations of ropivacaine for continuous femoral nerve blockade. *Anesth Analg.* 2007;105:256-262.

Capdevila X, Barthelet Y, Biboulet P, Ryckwaert Y, Rubenovitch J, d'Athis F. Effects of perioperative analgesic technique on the surgical outcome and duration of rehabilitation after major knee surgery. *Anesthesiology.* 1999;91:8-15.

Capdevila X, Biboulet P, Morau D, et al. Continuous three-in-one block for postoperative pain after lower limb orthopedic surgery: where do the catheters go? *Anesth Analg.* 2002;94:1001-1006.

Capdevila X, Pirat P, Bringuier S, et al. Continuous peripheral nerve blocks in hospital wards after orthopedic surgery: a multicenter prospective analysis of the quality of postoperative analgesia and complications in 1,416 patients. *Anesthesiology.* 2005;103:1035-1045.

Cuvillon P, Ripart J, Lalourcey L, et al. The continuous femoral nerve block catheter for postoperative analgesia: bacterial colonization, infectious rate and adverse effects. *Anesth Analg.* 2001;93:1045-1049.

Dauri M, Fabbi E, Mariani P, et al. Continuous femoral nerve block provides superior analgesia compared with continuous intra-articular and wound infusion after anterior cruciate ligament reconstruction. *Reg Anesth Pain Med.* 2009;34:95-99.

Dauri M, Sidiropoulou T, Fabbi E, et al. Efficacy of continuous femoral nerve block with stimulating catheters versus nonstimulating catheters for anterior cruciate ligament reconstruction. *Reg Anesth Pain Med.* 2007;32:282-287.

Eipe N, McCartney CJ, Kummer C. Transient neurological dysfunction after continuous femoral nerve block: should this change our practice? *Anesthesiology.* 2007;107:177-178.

Hadzic A, Houle TT, Capdevila X, Ilfeld BM. Femoral nerve block for analgesia in patients having knee arthroplasty. *Anesthesiology.* 2010;113(5):1014-1015.

Hayek SM, Ritchey RM, Sessler D, et al. Continuous femoral nerve analgesia after unilateral total knee arthroplasty: stimulating versus nonstimulating catheters. *Anesth Analg.* 2006;103:1565-1570.

Hirst GC, Lang SA, Dust WN, Cassidy JD, Yip RW. Femoral nerve block. Single injection versus continuous infusion for total knee arthroplasty. *Reg Anesth.* 1996;21:292-297.

Ilfeld BM, Le LT, Meyer RS, et al. Ambulatory continuous femoral nerve blocks decrease time to discharge readiness after tricompartment total knee arthroplasty: a randomized, triple-masked, placebo-controlled study. *Anesthesiology.* 2008;108:703-713.

Ilfeld BM, Moeller LK, Mariano ER, Loland VJ, Stevens-Lapsley JE, Fleisher AS, Girard PJ, Donohue MC, Ferguson EJ, Ball ST. Continuous peripheral nerve blocks: is local anesthetic dose the only factor, or do concentration and volume influence infusion effects as well? *Anesthesiology.* 2010;112:347-354.

Ilfeld BM, Mariano ER, Williams BA, Woodard JN, Macario A. Hospitalization costs of total knee arthroplasty with a continuous femoral nerve block provided only in the hospital versus on an ambulatory basis: a retrospective, case-control, cost-minimization analysis. *Reg Anesth Pain Med.* 2007;32:46-54.

Ilfeld BM, Meyer RS, Le LT, et al. Health-related quality of life after tricompartment knee arthroplasty with and without an extended-duration continuous femoral nerve block: a prospective, 1-year follow-up of a randomized, triple-masked, placebo-controlled study. *Anesth Analg.* 2009;108:1320-1325.

Ilfeld BM, Moeller LK, Mariano ER, et al. Continuous peripheral nerve blocks: is local anesthetic dose the only factor, or do concentration and volume influence infusion effects as well? *Anesthesiology.* 2010;112:347-354.

Kadic L, Boonstra MC, De Waal Malefijt MC, Lako SJ, Van Egmond J, Driessen JJ. Continuous femoral nerve block after total knee arthroplasty? *Acta Anaesthesiol Scand.* 2009;53:914-920.

Morin AM, Eberhart LH, Behnke HK, et al. Does femoral nerve catheter placement with stimulating catheters improve effective placement? A randomized, controlled, and observer-blinded trial. *Anesth Analg.* 2005;100:1503-1510.

Morin AM, Kratz CD, Eberhart LH, et al. Postoperative analgesia and functional recovery after total-knee replacement: comparison of a continuous posterior lumbar plexus (psoas compartment) block, a continuous femoral nerve block, and the combination of a continuous femoral and sciatic nerve block. *Reg Anesth Pain Med.* 2005;30:434-445.

Paul JE, Arya A, Hurlburt L, Cheng J, Thabane L, Tidy A, Murthy Y. Femoral nerve block improves analgesia outcomes after total knee artheoplasty: meta-analysis of randomized controlled trials. *Anesthesiology.* 2010;113:1144-1162.

Pham Dang C, Difalco C, Guilley J, Venet G, Hauet P, Lejus C. Various possible positions of conventional catheters around the femoral nerve revealed by neurostimulation. *Reg Anesth Pain Med.* 2009;34:285-289.

Pham Dang C, Gautheron E, Guilley J, et al. The value of adding sciatic block to continuous femoral block for analgesia after total knee replacement. *Reg Anesth Pain Med.* 2005;30:128-133.

Pham Dang C, Guilley J, Dernis L, et al. Is there any need for expanding the perineural space before catheter placement in continuous femoral nerve blocks? *Reg Anesth Pain Med.* 2006;31:393-400.

Salinas FV, Liu SS, Mulroy MF. The effect of single-injection femoral nerve block versus continuous femoral nerve block after total knee arthroplasty on hospital length of stay and long-term functional recovery within an established clinical pathway. *Anesth Analg.* 2006;102:1234-1239.

Salinas FV, Neal JM, Sueda LA, Kopacz DJ, Liu SS. Prospective comparison of continuous femoral nerve block with nonstimulating catheter placement versus stimulating catheter-guided perineural placement in volunteers. *Reg Anesth Pain Med.* 2004;29:212-220.

Shum CF, Lo NN, Yeo SJ, Yang KY, Chong HC, Yeo SN. Continuous femoral nerve block in total knee arthroplasty: immediate and two-year outcomes. *J Arthroplasty.* 2009;24:204-209.

Singelyn FJ, Gouverneur JM. Extended "three-in-one" block after total knee arthroplasty: continuous versus patient-controlled techniques. *Anesth Analg.* 2000;91:176-180.

Williams BA, Kentor ML, Vogt MT, et al. Reduction of verbal pain scores after anterior cruciate ligament reconstruction with 2-day continuous femoral nerve block: a randomized clinical trial. *Anesthesiology.* 2006;104:315-327.

# 22 Ankle Block

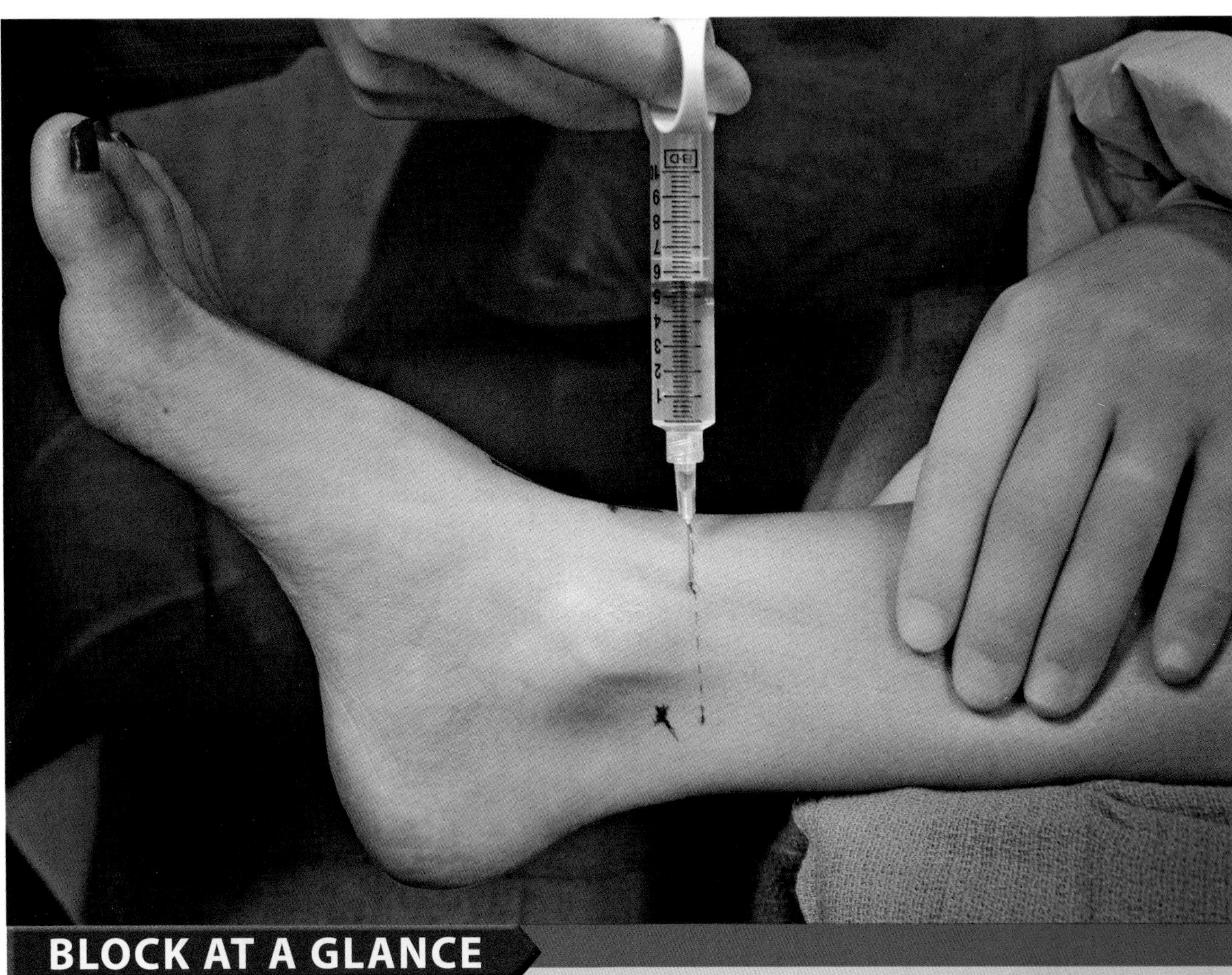

## BLOCK AT A GLANCE

- Indications: surgery of the foot and toes
- Two deep nerves: posterior tibial, deep peroneal
- Three superficial nerves: superficial peroneal, sural, saphenous
- Local anesthetic: 5-6 mL per nerve

**FIGURE 22-1.** Needle insertion for saphenous nerve block of the ankle.

## General Considerations

An ankle block is essentially a block of four terminal branches of the sciatic nerve (deep and superficial peroneal, tibial, and sural) and one cutaneous branch of the femoral nerve (saphenous). Ankle block is simple to perform, essentially devoid of systemic complications, and highly effective for a wide variety of procedures on the foot and toes. For this reason, this technique should be in the arma mentarium of every anesthesiologist. At our institution, an ankle block is most commonly used in podiatric surgery and foot and toe debridement or amputation.

## Functional Anatomy

It is useful to think of the ankle block as a block of two deep nerves (posterior tibial and deep peroneal) and three superficial nerves (saphenous, sural, and superficial peroneal). This concept is important for success of the block because the two deep nerves are anesthetized by injecting local anesthetic under the fascia, whereas the three superficial nerves are anesthetized by a simple subcutaneous injection of local anesthetic.

## Common Peroneal Nerve

The common peroneal nerve separates from the tibial nerve and descends alongside the tendon of the biceps femoris muscle and around the neck of the fibula. Just below the head of the fibula, the common peroneal nerve divides into its terminal branches: the deep peroneal and superficial peroneal nerves. The peroneus longus muscle covers both nerves.

## Deep Peroneal Nerve

The deep peroneal nerve runs downward below the layers of the peroneus longus, extensor digitorum longus, and extensor hallucis longus muscles to the front of the leg (Figure 22-2). At the ankle level, the nerve lies anterior to the tibia and the interosseous membrane and close to the anterior tibial artery. It is usually sandwiched between the tendons of the anterior tibial and extensor digitorum longus muscles. At this point, it divides into two terminal branches for the foot: the medial and the lateral. The medial branch passes over the dorsum of the foot, along the medial side of the dorsalis pedis artery, to the first interosseous space, where it supplies the web space between the first and second toe. The lateral branch of the deep peroneal nerve is directed anterolaterally, penetrates and innervates the extensor digitorum brevis muscle, and terminates as the second, third, and fourth dorsal interosseous nerves. These branches provide innervation to the tarsometatarsal, metatarsophalangeal, and interphalangeal joints of the lesser toes.

## Superficial Peroneal Nerve

The superficial peroneal nerve (also called the musculocutaneous nerve of the leg) provides muscular branches to the peroneus longus and brevis muscles. After piercing the deep fascia covering the muscles, the nerve eventually emerges from the anterolateral compartment of the lower part of the leg and surfaces from beneath the fascia 5 to 10 cm above the lateral malleolus (Figure 22-3). At this point, it divides into terminal cutaneous branches: the medial and the lateral dorsal cutaneous nerves (Figure 22-4A and B). These branches carry sensory innervation to the dorsum of the foot and communicate with the saphenous nerve medially, as well as the deep peroneal nerve in the first web space and the sural nerve on the lateral aspect of the foot.

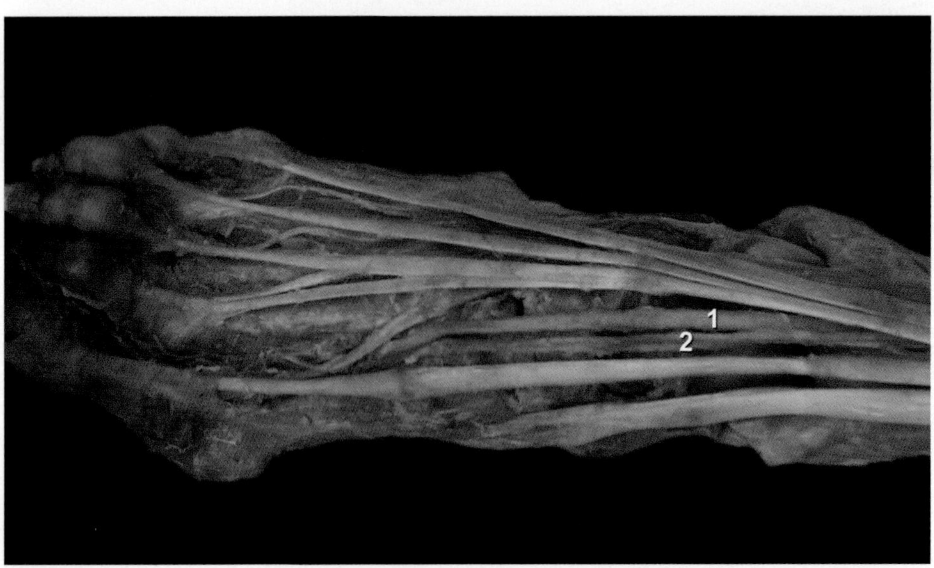


**FIGURE 22-2.** Anatomy of the ankle. ❶ artery dorsal pedis, ❷ deep peroneal nerve.

**FIGURE 22-3.** Anatomy of the ankle. (1) superficial peroneal nerve, (2) sural nerve.

## Tibial Nerve

The tibial nerve separates from the common popliteal nerve proximal to the popliteal fossa crease and joins the tibial artery behind the knee joint. The nerve runs distally in the thick neurovascular fascia and emerges at the inferior third of the leg from beneath the soleus and gastrocnemius muscles on the medial border of the Achilles tendon (Figure 22-5). At the level of the medial malleolus, the tibial nerve is covered by the superficial and deep fasciae of the leg. It is positioned laterally and posteriorly to the posterior tibial artery and midway between the posterior aspect of the medial malleolus and the posterior aspect of the Achilles tendon. Just beneath the malleolus, the nerve divides into lateral and medial plantar nerves. The posterior tibial nerve provides cutaneous, articular, and vascular branches to the ankle joint, medial malleolus, inner aspect of the heel, and Achilles tendon. It also branches to the skin, subcutaneous tissue, muscles, and bones of the sole.

## Sural Nerve

The sural nerve is a sensory nerve formed by a union of the medial sural nerve (a branch of the tibial nerve) and the lateral sural nerve (a branch of the common peroneal nerve).

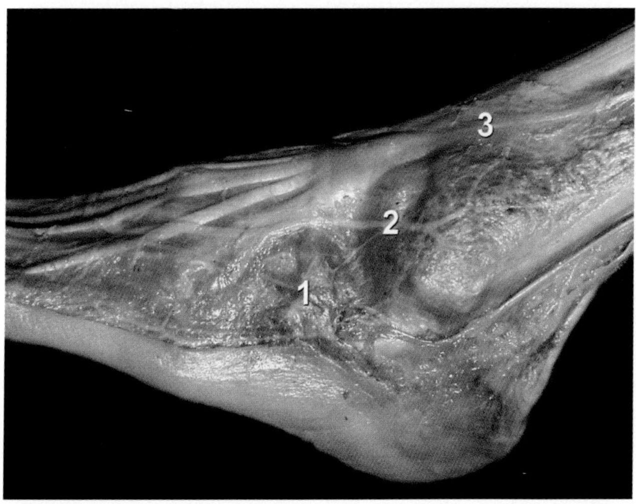


A

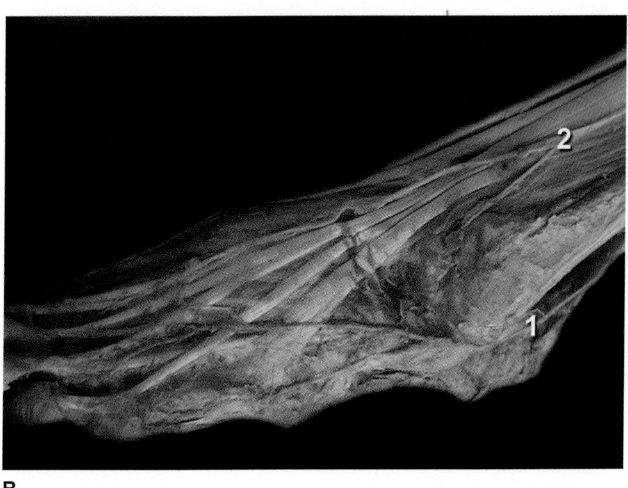


B

**FIGURE 22-4.** (A) Anatomy of the ankle. (1) Sural nerve. (2),(3) Superficial peroneal nerve. (B) Anatomy of the ankle. (1) Sural nerve, (2) Superficial peroneal nerve.

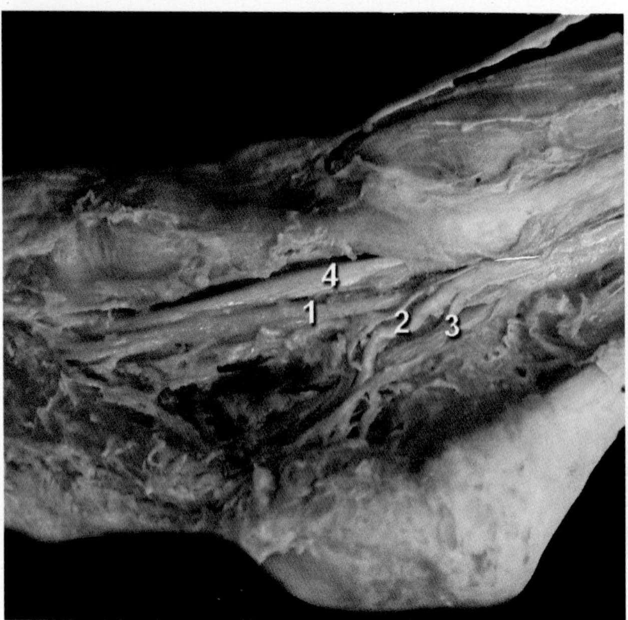


**FIGURE 22-5.** Anatomy of the ankle. ❶ flexor digitorum longus tendon, ❷ posterior tibial artery, ❸ tibial nerve, ❹ flexor hallucis longus.

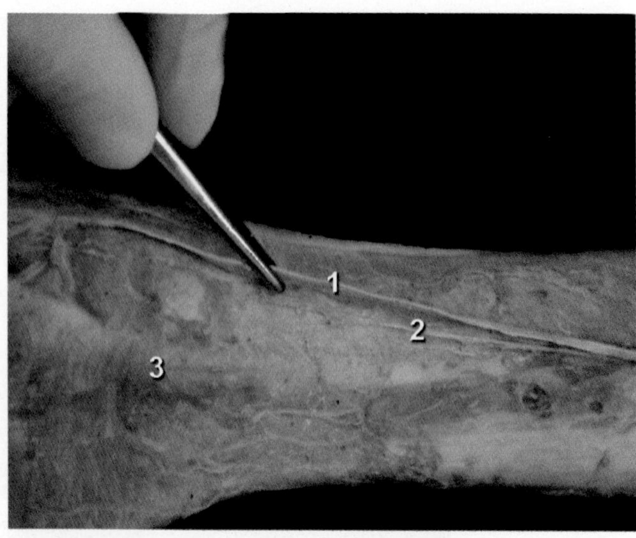


**FIGURE 22-6.** Anatomy of the ankle. ❶, ❷ saphenous nerve, ❸ medial malleolus.

The sural nerve courses between the heads of the gastrocnemius muscle, and after piercing the fascia covering the muscles, it emerges on the lateral aspect of the Achilles tendon 10 to 15 cm above the lateral malleolus (Figure 22-4A and B). After providing lateral calcaneal branches to the heel, the sural nerve descends behind the lateral malleolus, supplying the lateral malleolus, Achilles tendon, and ankle joint. The sural nerve continues on the lateral aspect of the foot, innervating the skin, subcutaneous tissue, fourth interosseous space, and fifth toe.

## Saphenous Nerve

The saphenous nerve is a terminal cutaneous branch (or branches) of the femoral nerve. Its course is in the subcutaneous tissue of the skin on the medial aspect of the ankle and foot (Figure 22-6).

> **TIP**
>
> - All superficial (cutaneous) nerves of the foot should be thought of as a neuronal network rather than as single strings of nerves with a well-defined, consistent anatomic position).

## Distribution of Blockade

An ankle block results in anesthesia of the foot. However, note that an ankle block does not result in anesthesia of the ankle itself. The proximal extension of the blockade is to the level at which the block is performed. The more proximal branches of the tibial and peroneal nerves innervate the deep structures of the ankle joint (see Chapter 01, Essential Regional Anesthesia Anatomy). The two deep nerves (tibial and deep peroneal) provide innervation to the deep structures, bones, and cutaneous coverage of the sole and web between the first and second toes (Figure 22-7).

### Equipment

A standard regional anesthesia tray is prepared with the following equipment:

- Sterile towels and gauze packs
- Three 10-mL syringes containing local anesthetic
- Sterile gloves; marking pen
- 1.5-in, 25-gauge needle

### Landmarks and Patient Positioning

The patient is in the supine position with the foot on a footrest.

> **TIP**
>
> - Position the foot on a footrest to facilitate access to all nerves to be blocked.

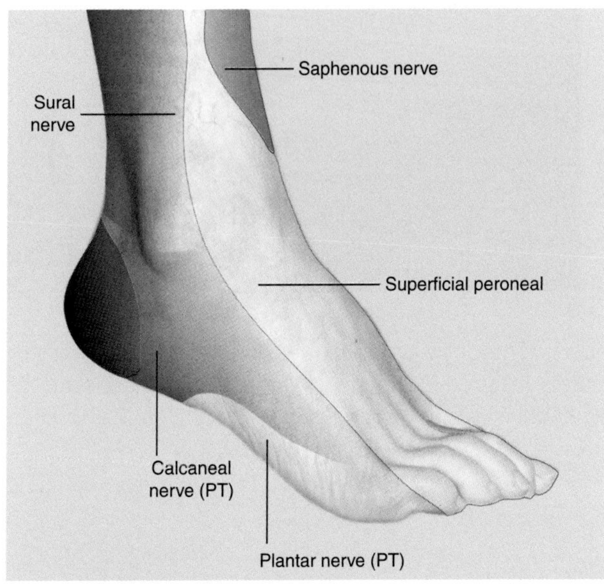


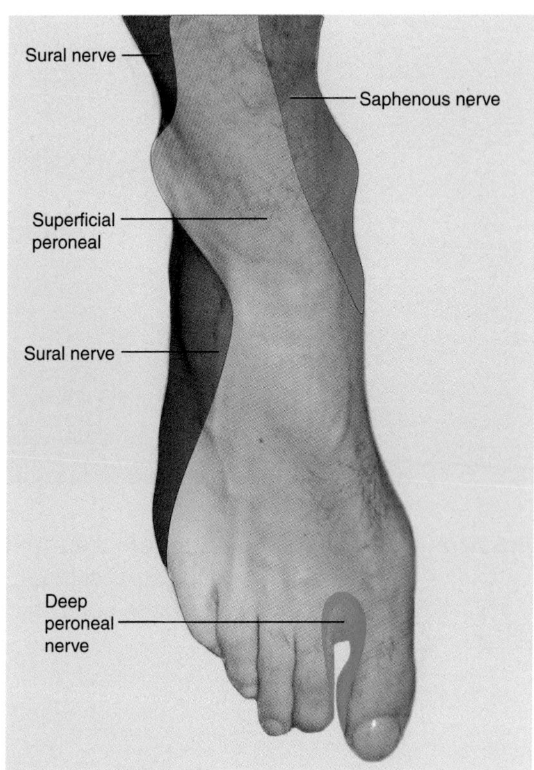


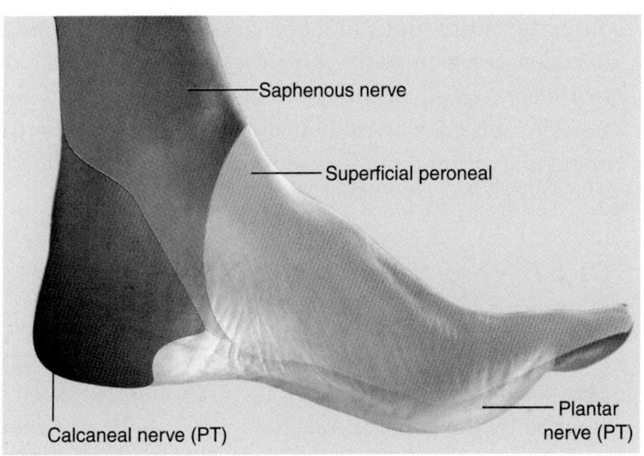


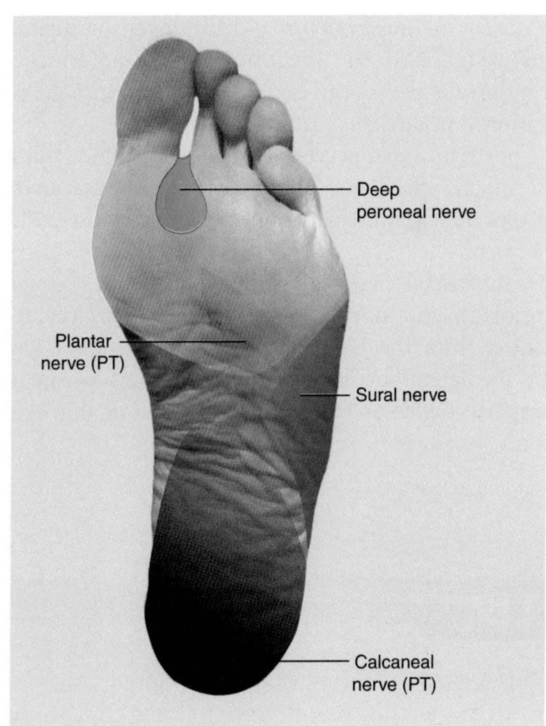


**FIGURE 22-7.** Innervation of the foot.

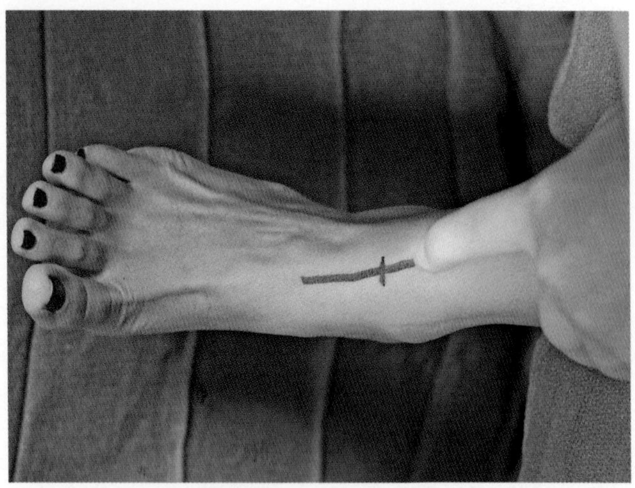
A

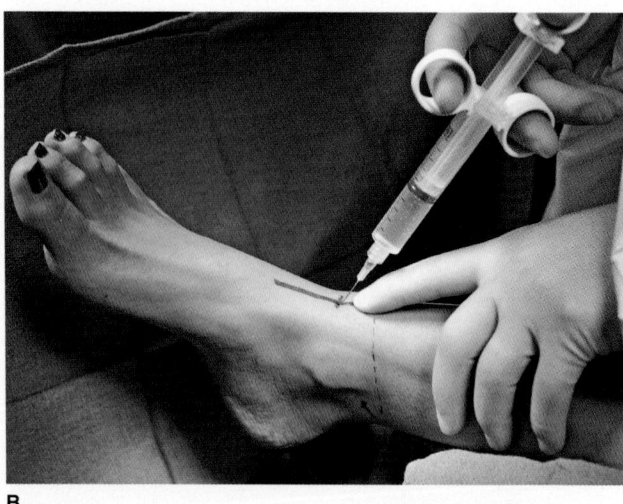
B

**FIGURE 22-8.** (A) Maneuvers to extenuate the extensor tendons. The deep peroneal nerve is located lateral to the hallucis longus tendon (line). (B) Deep peroneal block. The needle is inserted just lateral to the hallucis longus tendon and slowly advanced to contact the bone. Upon bone contact, the needle is withdrawn 2–3 mm, and 5 mL of local anesthetic is injected.

The deep peroneal nerve is located immediately lateral to the tendon of the extensor hallucis longus muscle (between the extensor hallucis longus and the extensor digitorum longus) (Figure 22-8). The pulse of the anterior tibial artery (dorsalis pedis) can be felt at this location; the nerve is positioned immediately lateral to the artery.

The posterior tibial nerve is located just behind and distal to the medial malleolus. The pulse of the posterior tibial artery can be felt at this location; the nerve is just posterior to the artery.

The superficial peroneal, sural, and saphenous nerves are located in the subcutaneous tissue along a circular line stretching from the lateral aspect of the Achilles tendon across the lateral malleolus, anterior aspect of the foot, and medial malleolus to the medial aspect of the Achilles tendon.

## TIP

- The superficial nerves branch out and anastomose extensively; they do not have a single consistently positioned nerve trunk that can be anesthetized by a single precise injection as often taught.

## Techniques

For time-efficient blockade of all five nerves, the operator should walk from one side of the foot to the other during the block procedure instead of bending and leaning over to reach the opposite side. Before beginning the procedure, the entire foot should be cleaned with a disinfectant. It makes sense to begin this procedure with blocks of the two deep nerves because subcutaneous injections for the superficial blocks often deform the anatomy. A controlled or regular syringe can be used.

### *Deep Peroneal Nerve Block*

The finger of the palpating hand is positioned in the groove just lateral to the extensor hallucis longus (Figure 22-8A). The needle is inserted under the skin and advanced until stopped by the bone. At this point, the needle is withdrawn back 1 to 2 mm, and 2 to 3 mL of local anesthetic is injected (Figure 22-8B).

## TIPS

- A deep peroneal block is essentially a "blind" injection of local anesthetic. Instead of relying on a single injection, a "fan" technique is recommended to increase the success rate after the injection.
- The tendon of extensor hallucis longus can be accentuated by asking the patient to dorsiflex the toes.

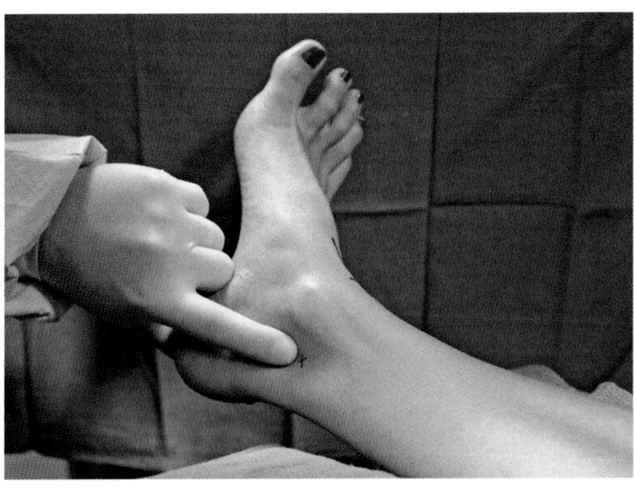
A

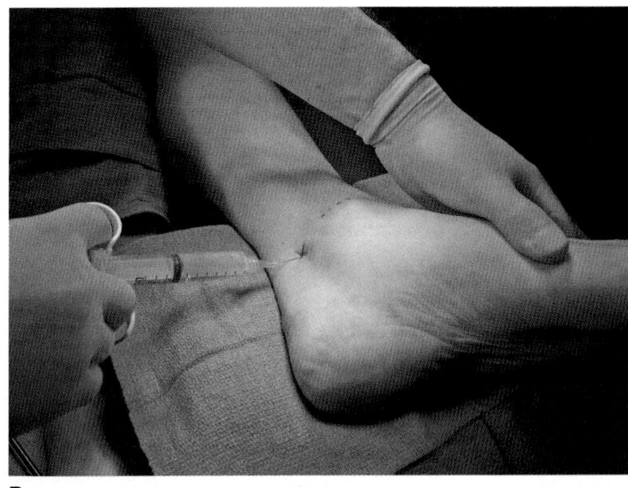
B

**FIGURE 22-9.** (A) Landmark for posterior tibial nerve block is found by palpating the pulse of the tibial artery posterior to the medial malleolus. (B) Posterior tibial nerve block is accomplished by inserting the needle next to the pulse of the tibial artery. The needle is advanced until contact with the bone is established. At this point the needle is withdrawn 2–3 mm, and 5 mL of local anesthetic is injected.

### *Posterior Tibial Nerve Block*

The posterior tibial nerve is anesthetized by injecting local anesthetic just behind the medial malleolus (Figure 22-9A). Similar to that of the deep peroneal nerve, its position is deep to the superficial fascia. The needle is introduced in the groove behind the medial malleolus and advanced until contact with the bone is felt. At this point, the needle is withdrawn back 1 to 2 mm, and 2 to 3 mL of local anesthetic is injected (Figure 22-9B).

**TIP**

- Similar to the procedure used for the deep peroneal nerve, a "fan" technique should be used to increase the success rate. The needle is pulled back to the skin, and two additional boluses of 2 mL of local anesthetic are injected after anterior and posterior needle reinsertions.

### *Blocks of the Superficial Peroneal, Sural, and Saphenous Nerves*

These three nerves are superficial cutaneous extensions of the sciatic and femoral nerves. Because they are positioned superficially to the deep fascia, an injection of local anesthetic in the territory through which they descend to the distal foot is adequate to achieve their blockade. Each nerve is blocked using a simple circumferential injection of local anesthetic subcutaneously (Figures 22-10, 22-11, and 22-12).

To block the *saphenous nerve*, a 1.5 in, 25-gauge needle is inserted at the level of the medial malleolus and a "ring" of local anesthetic is raised from the point of needle entry to the Achilles tendon and anteriorly to the tibial ridge (Figure 22.10). This can be usually accomplished with one or two needle insertions; 5 mL of local anesthetic suffices.

To block the *superficial peroneal* nerve, the needle is inserted at the tibial ridge and extended laterally toward the lateral malleolus (Figure 22-11). It is important to raise a subcutaneous "wheal" during injection, which indicates injection in the proper superficial plane. Five milliliters of local anesthetic is adequate.

To block the *sural nerve*, the needle is inserted at the level of the lateral malleolus and the local anesthetic is infiltrated

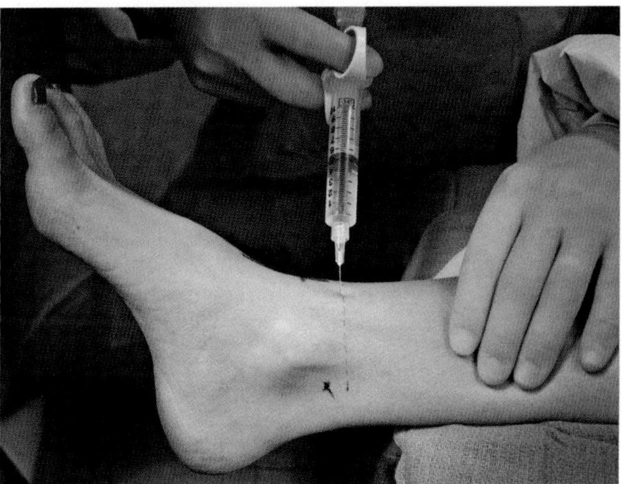

**FIGURE 22-10.** Saphenous nerve block is accomplished by injection of local anesthetic in a circular fashion (line) subcutaneously just above the medial malleolus.

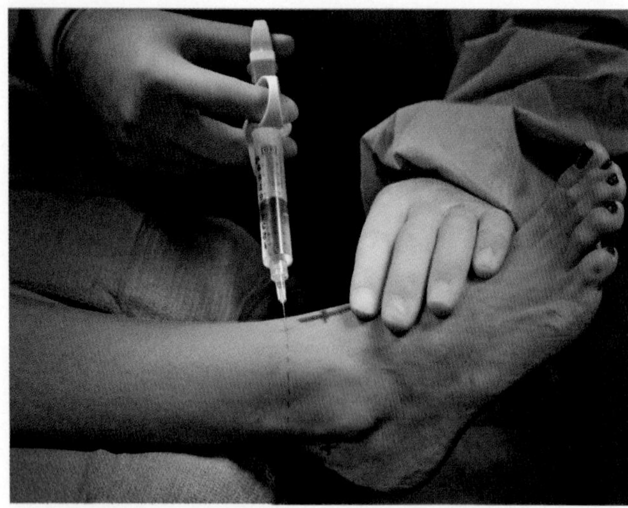

**FIGURE 22-11.** Superficial peroneal nerve block is performed by injecting local anesthetic in a circular fashion at the level of the lateral malleolus and extending from anterior to posterior.

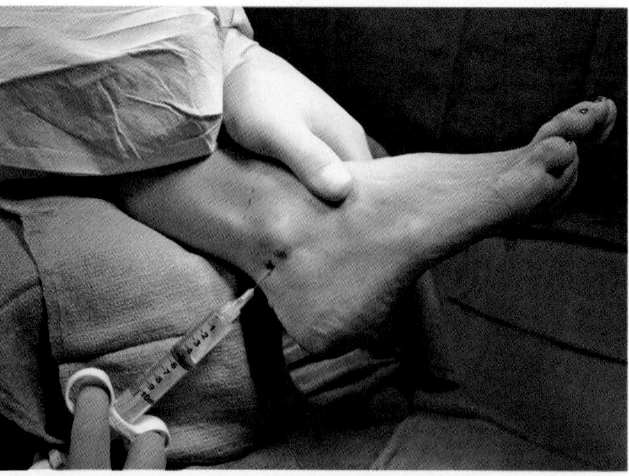

**FIGURE 22-12.** Sural nerve block is accomplished by injecting local anesthetic in a fanwise fashion subcutaneously and below the fascia behind the lateral malleolus.

toward the Achilles tendon (Figure 22-12). Five milliliters of local anesthetic is deposited in a circular fashion to raise a skin "wheal."

**TIP**

- Remember the subcutaneous position of the superficial nerves and think of their blockade as a "field block." A distinct subcutaneous "wheal" should be seen with injection into a proper plane to block the superficial nerves.

## Block Dynamics and Perioperative Management

Ankle block is one of the more uncomfortable block procedures for patients. The reason is that it involves five separate needle insertions, and subcutaneous injections to block the cutaneous nerves result in discomfort due to the pressure distension of the skin and nerve endings. Additionally, the foot is supplied by an abundance of nerve endings and is exquisitely sensitive to needle injections. For these reasons, this block requires significant premedication to make it acceptable to patients. We routinely use a combination of midazolam (2–4 mg intravenously) and a narcotic (500–750 μg alfentanil) to ensure the patient's comfort during the procedure.

A typical onset time for this block is 10 to 25 minutes, depending primarily on the concentration and volume of local anesthetic used. Placement of an Esmarch bandage or a tourniquet at the level of the ankle is well-tolerated and typically does not require additional blockade in sedated patients.

## Complications and How to Avoid Them

Complications following an ankle block are typically limited to residual paresthesias due to inadvertent intraneuronal injection. Systemic toxicity is uncommon because of the distal location of the blockade. Table 22-1 provides more specific instructions on possible complications and corrective measures.

**TABLE 22-1 Complications of Ankle Block and Preventive Techniques**

| | |
|---|---|
| ***Infection*** | • Uncommon with the use of an aseptic technique. |
| ***Hematoma*** | • Avoid multiple needle insertions. (Most superficial blocks can be accomplished with one or two needle insertions.)<br>• Use a small gauge needle and avoid puncturing superficial veins. |
| ***Vascular puncture*** | • Avoid puncturing the greater saphenous vein at the medial malleolus to decrease the risk of local hematoma.<br>• Intermittent aspiration should be performed to avoid intravascular injection. |
| ***Nerve injury*** | • Do not inject when the patient complains of pain or high injection pressure is present.<br>• Do not repeat injections for deep tibial and peroneal nerves. |
| ***Other*** | • Instruct the patient how to care for the insensate extremity.<br>• The use of epinephrine-containing solutions is avoided by many clinicians due to the theoretical risk of foot or digit ischemia. |

## SUGGESTED READING

Delgado-Martinez AD, Marchal JM, Molina M, Palma A. Forefoot surgery with ankle tourniquet: complete or selective ankle block? *Reg Anesth Pain Med.* 2001;26:184-186.

Delgado-Martinez AD, Marchal-Escalona JM. Supramalleolar ankle block anesthesia and ankle tourniquet for foot surgery. *Foot Ankle Int.* 2001;22:836-838.

Hadžić; A, Vloka JD, Kuroda MM, Koorn R, Birnbach DJ. The practice of peripheral nerve blocks in the United States: a national survey. *Reg Anesth Pain Med.* 1998;23:241-246.

Klein SM, Pietrobon R, Nielsen KC, Warner DS, Greengrass RA, Steele SM. Peripheral nerve blockade with long-acting local anesthetics: a survey of the Society for Ambulatory Anesthesia. *Anesth Analg.* 2002;94:71-76.

Mineo R, Sharrock NE. Venous levels of lidocaine and bupivacaine after midtarsal ankle block. *Reg Anesth.* 1992;17:47-49.

Myerson MS, Ruland CM, Allon SM. Regional anesthesia for foot and ankle surgery. *Foot Ankle.* 1992;13:282-288.

Needoff M, Radford P, Costigan P. Local anesthesia for postoperative pain relief after foot surgery: a prospective clinical trial. *Foot Ankle Int.* 1995;16:11-13.

Noorpuri BS, Shahane SA, Getty CJ. Acute compartment syndrome following revisional arthroplasty of the forefoot: the dangers of ankle-block. *Foot Ankle Int.* 2000;21:680-682.

Palmisani S, Arcioni R, Di Benedetto P, De Blasi RA, Mercieri M, Ronconi P. Ropivacaine and levobupivacaine for bilateral selective ankle block in patients undergoing hallux valgus repair. *Acta Anaesthesiol Scand.* 2008;52:841-844.

Reilley TE, Gerhardt MA. Anesthesia for foot and ankle surgery. *Clin Podiatr Med Surg.* 2002;19:125-147, vii.

Reinhart DJ, Stagg KS, Walker KG, et al. Postoperative analgesia after peripheral nerve block for podiatric surgery: clinical efficacy and chemical stability of lidocaine alone versus lidocaine plus ketorolac. *Reg Anesth Pain Med.* 2000;25:506-513.

Rudkin GE, Rudkin AK, Dracopoulos GC. Ankle block success rate: a prospective analysis of 1,000 patients. *Can J Anaesth.* 2005;52:209-210.

Rudkin GE, Rudkin AK, Dracopoulos GC. Bilateral ankle blocks: a prospective audit. *ANZ J Surg.* 2005;75:39-42.

Schabort D, Boon JM, Becker PJ, Meiring JH. Easily identifiable bony landmarks as an aid in targeted regional ankle blockade. *Clin Anat.* 2005;18:518-526.

Schurman DJ. Ankle-block anesthesia for foot surgery. *Anesthesiology.* 1976;44:348-352.

Shah S, Tsai T, Iwata T, Hadžić; A. Outpatient regional anesthesia for foot and ankle surgery. *Int Anesthesiol Clin.* 2005;43: 143-151.

Sharrock NE, Waller JF, Fierro LE. Midtarsal block for surgery of the forefoot. *Br J Anaesth.* 1986;58:37-40.

Tran D, Clemente A, Finlayson RJ. A review of approaches and techniques for lower extremity nerve blocks. *Can J Anaesth.* 2007;54:922-934.

# 23 Thoracic Paravertebral Block

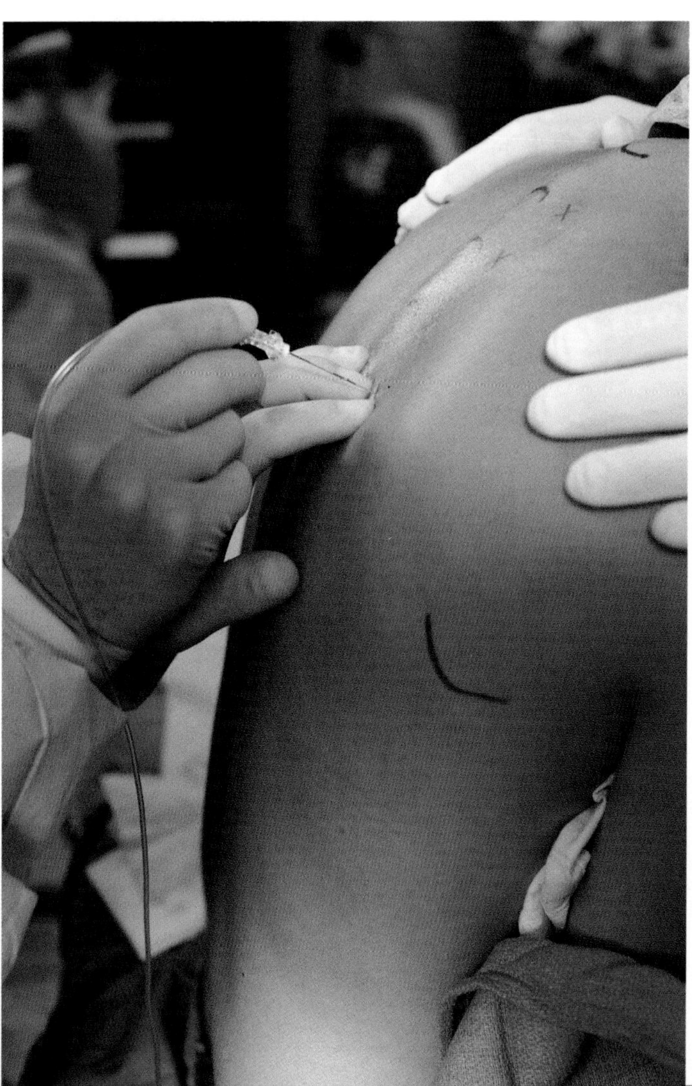

## BLOCK AT A GLANCE

- Indications: breast surgery, analgesia after thoracotomy or in patients with rib fractures
- Landmarks: spinous process at the desired thoracic dermatomal level
- Needle insertion: 2.5 cm lateral to the midline
- Target: needle insertion 1 cm past the transverse process
- Local anesthetic: 5 mL per dermatomal level

**FIGURE 23-1.** Thoracic paravertebral block.

## General Considerations

A thoracic paravertebral block is a technique where a bolus of local anesthetic is injected in the paravertebral space, in the vicinity of the thoracic spinal nerves following their emergence from the intervertebral foramen. The resulting ipsilateral somatic and sympathetic nerve blockade produces anesthesia or analgesia that is conceptually similar to a "unilateral" epidural anesthetic block. Higher or lower levels can be chosen to accomplish a unilateral, bandlike, segmental blockade at the desired levels without significant hemodynamic changes. For a trained regional anesthesia practitioner, this technique is simple to perform and time efficient; however, it is more challenging to teach because it requires stereotactic thinking and needle maneuvering. A certain "mechanical" mind or sense of geometry is necessary to master it. This block is used most commonly to provide anesthesia and analgesia in patients having mastectomy and cosmetic breast surgery, and to provide analgesia after thoracic surgery or in patients with rib fractures. A catheter can also be inserted for continuous infusion of local anesthetic.

## Regional Anesthesia Anatomy

The thoracic paravertebral space is a wedge-shaped area that lies on either side of the vertebral column (Figure 23-2). Its walls are formed by the parietal pleura anterolaterally; the vertebral body, intervertebral disk, and intervertebral foramen medially; and the superior costotransverse ligament posteriorly. After emerging from their respective intervertebral foramina, the thoracic nerve roots divide into dorsal and ventral rami. The dorsal ramus provides innervation to the skin and muscle of the paravertebral region; the ventral ramus continues laterally as the intercostal nerve. The ventral ramus also gives rise to the rami communicantes, which connect the intercostal nerve to the sympathetic chain. The thoracic paravertebral space is continuous with the intercostal space laterally, epidural space medially, and contralateral paravertebral space via the prevertebral fascia. In addition, local anesthetic can also spread longitudinally

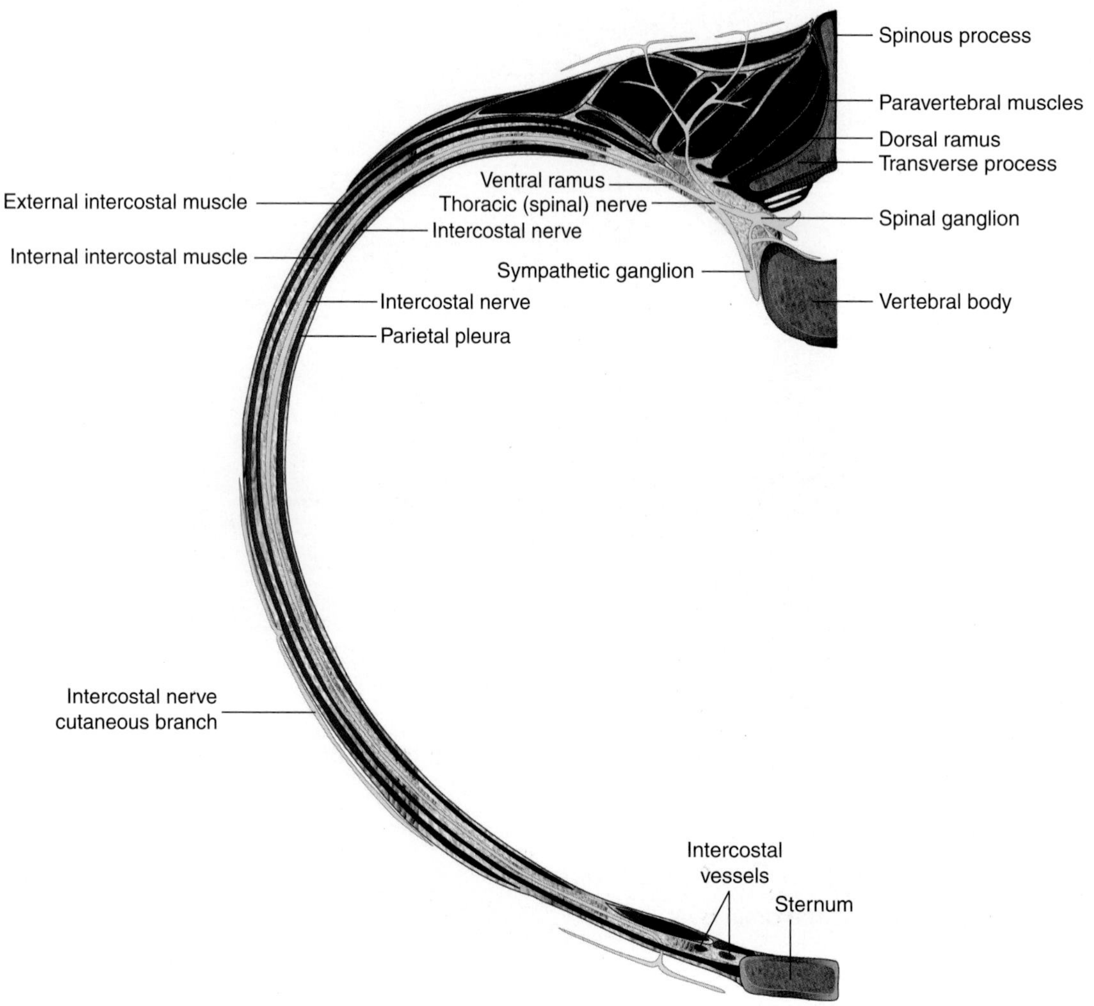


**FIGURE 23-2.** Anatomy of the thoracic spinal nerve (root) and innervation of the chest wall.

either cranially or caudally. The mechanism of action of a paravertebral blockade includes direct action of the local anesthetic on the spinal nerve, lateral extension along with the intercostal nerves and medial extension into the epidural space through the intervertebral foramina.

## Distribution of Anesthesia

Thoracic paravertebral blockade results in ipsilateral anesthesia. The location of the resulting dermatomal distribution of anesthesia or analgesia is a function of the level blocked and the volume of local anesthetic injected (Figure 23-3).

## Single-Injection Thoracic Paravertebral Block

### Equipment

A standard regional anesthesia tray is prepared with the following equipment:

- Sterile towels and gauze packs
- A 20-mL syringe containing local anesthetic
- Sterile gloves and marking pen
- A 10-mL syringe plus 25-gauge needle with local anesthetic for skin infiltration
- An 8-10 cm, 18-gauge Tuohy tip epidural needle for continuous paravertebral block or an 8-10 cm Quincke tip needle for single injection paravertebral block.
- Low-volume extension tubing

**TIP**

- The use of needles with markings to indicate the depth of insertion is suggested for a better monitoring of needle placement.

### Patient Positioning

The patient is positioned in the sitting or lateral decubitus (with the side to be blocked uppermost) position and supported by an attendant (Figure 23-4). The back should assume knee-chest position, similar to the position required for neuraxial anesthesia. The patient's feet rest on a stool to allow greater patient comfort and a greater degree of kyphosis. The positioning increases the distance between the adjacent transverse processes and facilitates advancement of the needle between them.

### Landmarks and Maneuvers to Accentuate Them

The following anatomic landmarks are used to identify spinal levels and estimate the position of the relevant transverse processes (Figure 23-5):

1. Spinous processes (midline)
2. Spinous process of C7 (the most prominent spinous process in the cervical region when the neck is flexed)
3. Lower tips of scapulae (corresponds to T7)

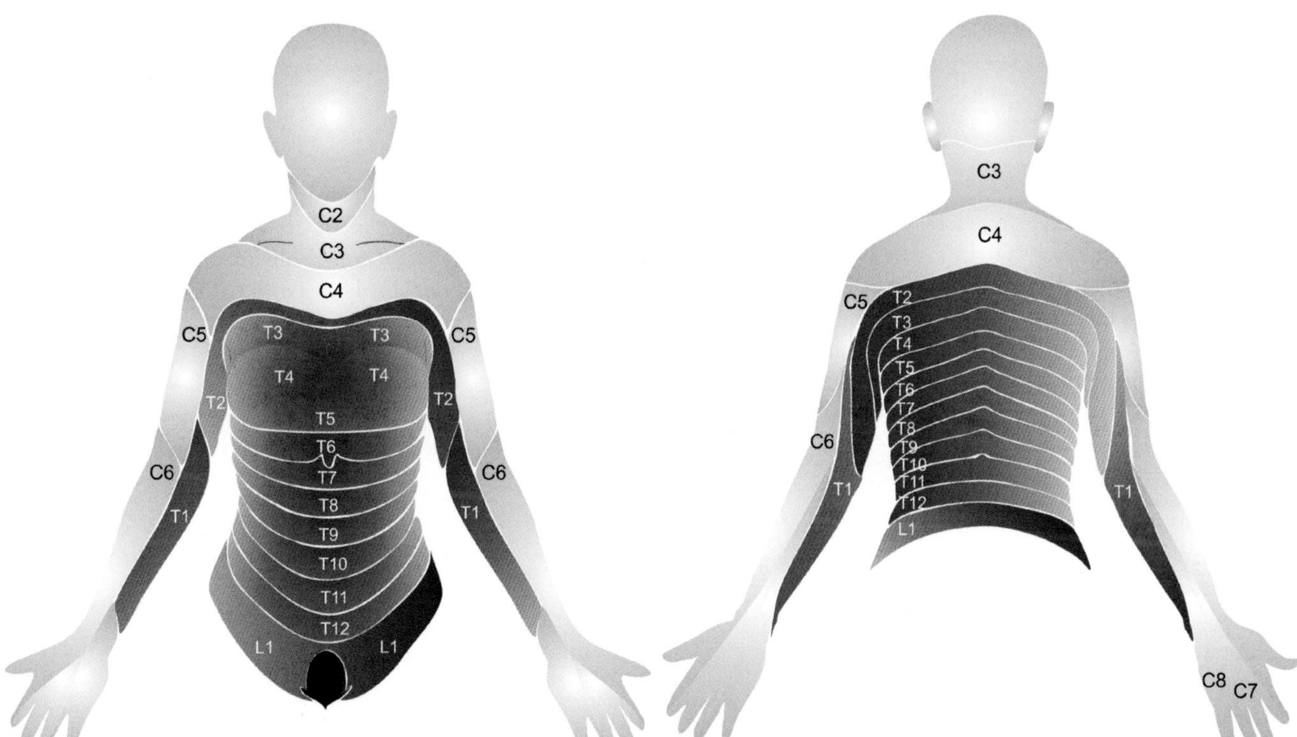


**FIGURE 23-3.** Thoracic dermatomal levels.

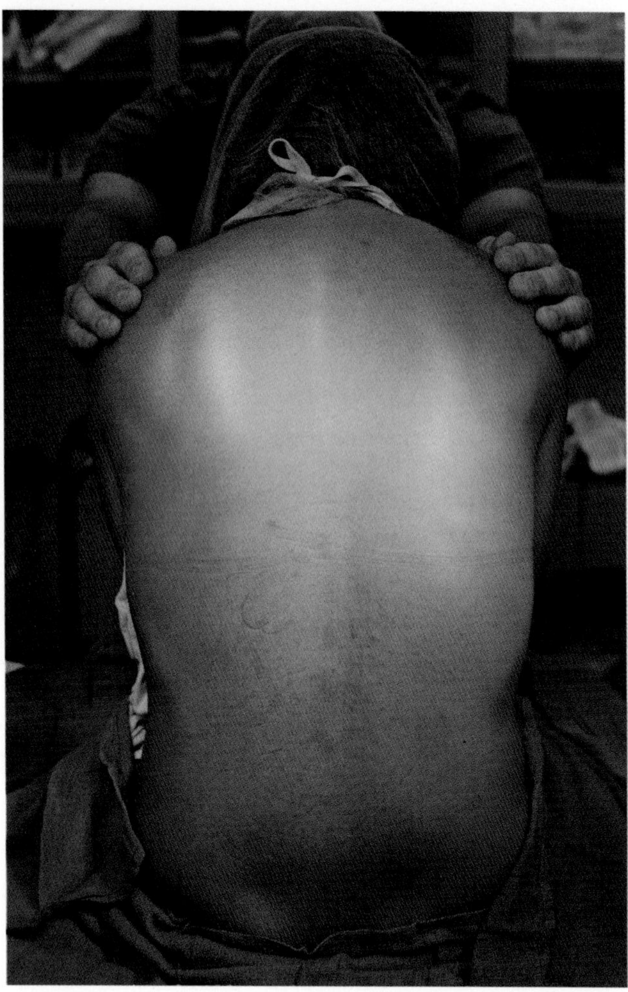

**FIGURE 23-4.** Patient positioning for thoracic paravertebral block. The patient is positioned in a sitting position with feet resting on a stool and assumes a knee-chest position.

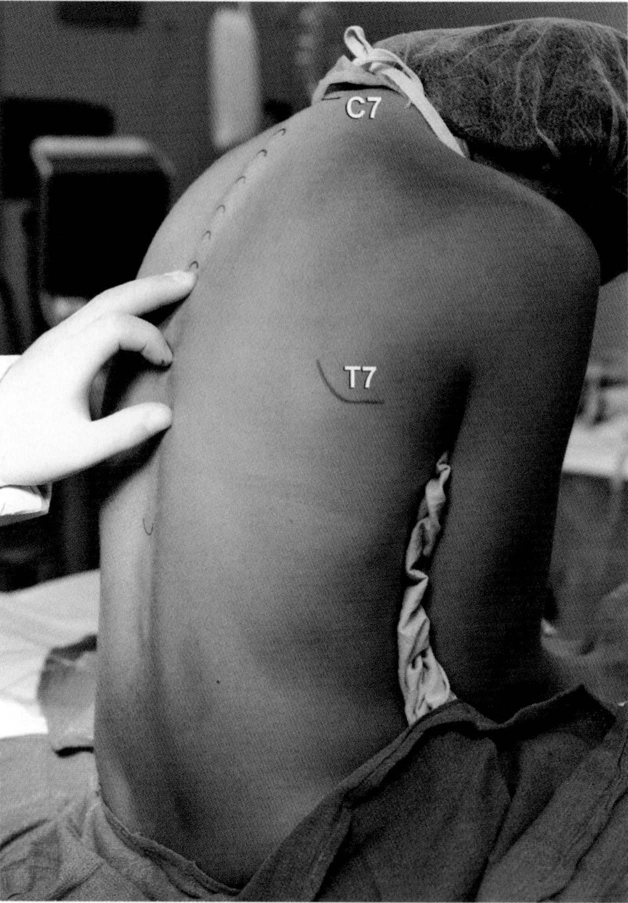


**FIGURE 23-5.** Spinal processes are the main landmarks for the thoracic paravertebral block. Processes are outlined from C7 (the most prominent vertebrate) to T7 (tip of scapulae).

The tips of the spinous processes should be marked on the skin. Then a parasagittal line can be measured and drawn 2.5 cm lateral to the midline (Figure 23-6). For breast surgery, the levels to be blocked are T2 through T6. For thoracotomy, estimates can be made after discussion with the surgeon about the planned approach and length of incision.

## TIP

- Determining the distance between two transverse processes at the level to be blocked is a rough estimation at best. Instead, it is more practical to outline the midline and simply draw an arbitrary line 2.5 cm parallel and lateral to the midline. Once the two first transverse processes are identified on that line, the rest follow a similar cranial-caudal distance between the two processes.

## Technique

After cleaning the skin with an antiseptic solution, 6 to 10 mL of dilute local anesthetic is infiltrated subcutaneously along the line where the injections will be made. The injection should be carried out slowly to avoid pain on injection.

## TIPS

- The addition of a vasoconstrictor helps prevent oozing at the site of injection.
- When more than five or six levels are blocked (e.g., bilateral blocks), the use of alkalinized chloroprocaine or lidocaine for skin infiltration is suggested to decrease the total dose of long-acting local anesthetic.

The subcutaneous tissues and paravertebral muscles are infiltrated with local anesthetic to decrease the discomfort at the site of needle insertion. The fingers of the palpating

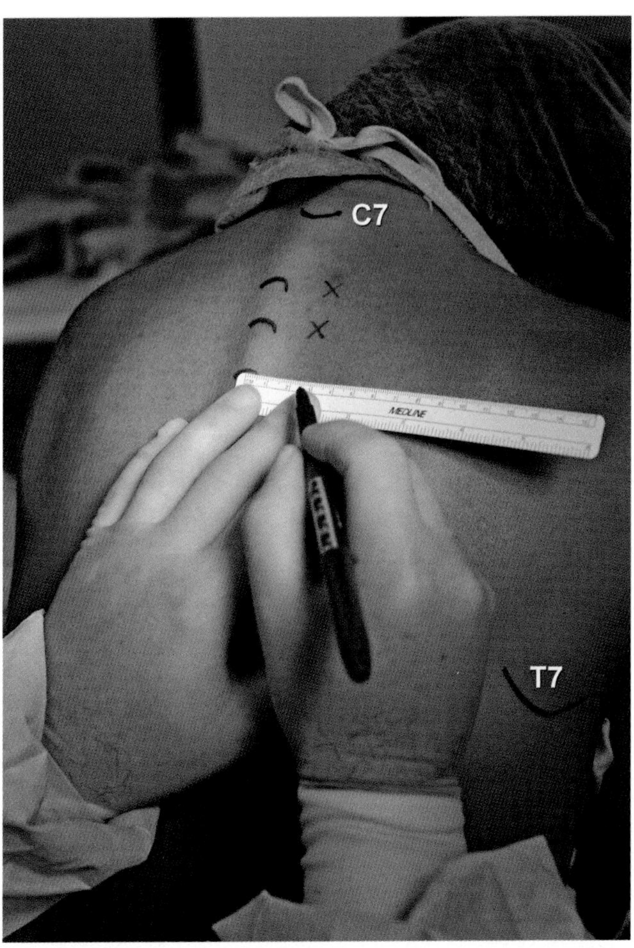


FIGURE 23-6. The needle insertion points for paravertebral block are labeled 2.5 cm lateral to the spinous processes.

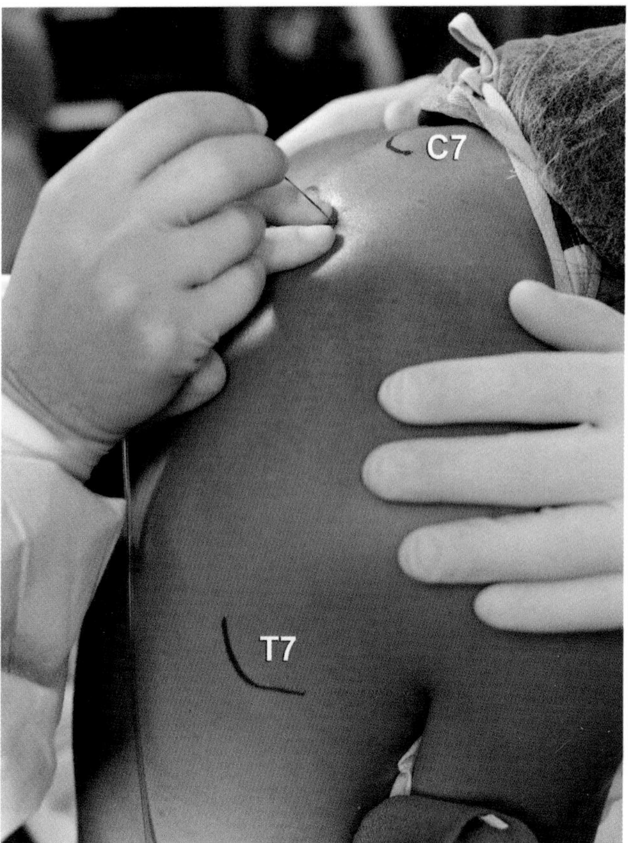


FIGURE 23-7. The technique of thoracic paravertebral block begins with insertion of the needle 2.5 cm lateral to the spinous process with an intention to contact the transverse process.

hand should straddle the paramedian line and fix the skin to avoid medial-lateral skin movement. The needle is attached to a syringe containing local anesthetic via extension tubing and advanced perpendicularly to the skin at the level of the superior aspect of the corresponding spinous process (Figure 23-7). Constant attention to the depth of needle insertion and the slight medial to lateral needle orientation is critical to avoid pneumothorax and direction of the needle toward the neuraxial space, respectively. The utmost care should be taken to avoid directing the needle medially (risk of epidural or spinal injection). The transverse process is typically contacted at a depth of 3 to 6 cm. If it is not, it is possible the needle tip has missed the transverse processes and passed either too laterally or in between the processes. Osseous contact at shallow depth (e.g., 2 cm) is almost always due to a too lateral needle insertion (ribs). In this case, further advancement could result in too deep insertion and possible pleural puncture. Instead, the needle should be withdrawn and redirected superiorly or inferiorly until contact with the bone is made.

After the transverse process is contacted, the needle is withdrawn to the skin level and redirected superiorly or inferiorly to "walk off" the transverse process (Figure 23-8A and B). The ultimate goal is to insert the needle to a depth of 1 cm past the transverse process. A certain loss of resistance to needle advancement often can be felt as the needle passes through the superior costotransverse ligament; however, this is a nonspecific sign and should not be relied on for correct placement.

## TIP

- The block procedure consists of three maneuvers (Figure 23-9):
  - Contact the transverse processes of individual vertebra and note the depth at which the process was contacted (usually 2–4 cm) (Figure 23-9A).
  - Withdraw the needle to the skin level and reinsert it at a 10° caudal or cephalad angulation (Figure 23-9B).
  - Walk off the transverse process, pass the needle 1 cm deeper and inject 5 mL of local anesthetic (Figure 23-9C).

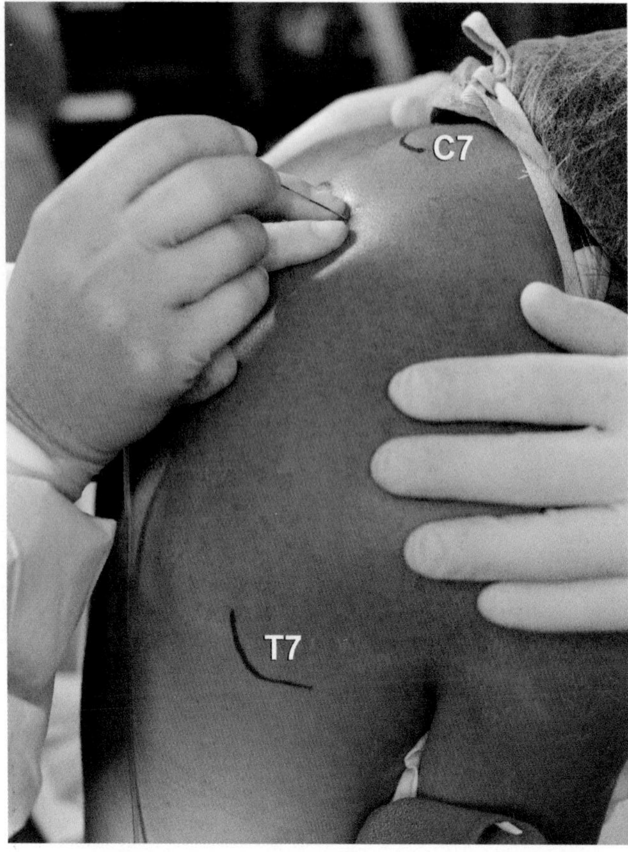


A

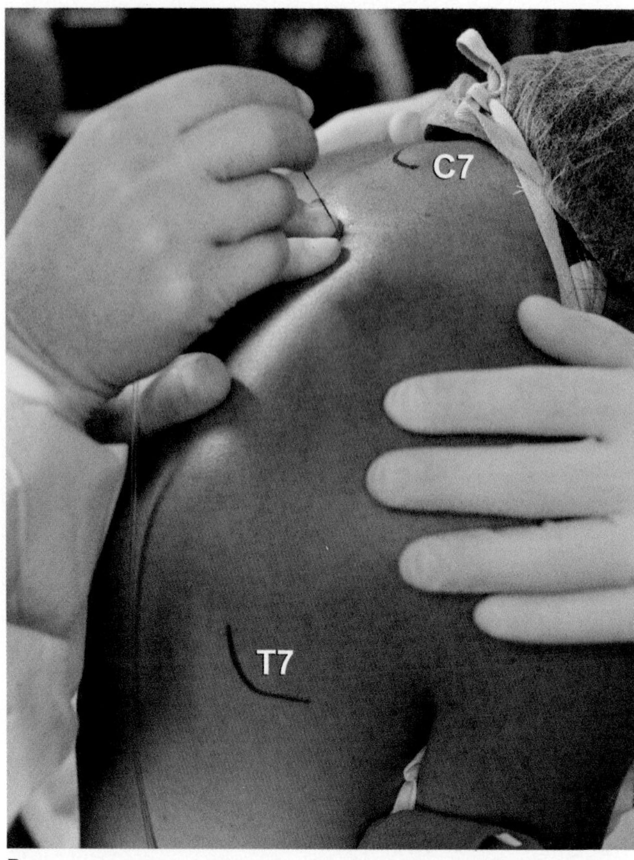


B

**FIGURE 23-8.** (A) Once the transverse process is contacted, the needle is walked-off superiorly or inferiorly and advanced 1–1.5 cm past the transverse process. (B) When walking-off the transverse process superiorly proves difficult, the needle is redirected to walk off inferiorly.

The needle can be redirected to walk off the transverse process superiorly or inferiorly. At levels of T7 and below, however, walking off the inferior aspect of the transverse process is recommended to reduce the risk of intrapleural placement of the needle. Proper handling of the needle is important both for accuracy and safety. Once the transverse process is contacted, the needle should be re-gripped 1 cm away from the skin so that insertion only can be made 1 cm deeper before skin contact with the fingers prevents further advancement.

After aspiration to rule out intravascular or intrathoracic needle tip placement, 5 mL of local anesthetic is injected slowly (Figure 23-10). The process is repeated for the remaining levels to be blocked.

## TIPS

- Loss of resistance technique to identify the paravertebral is subtle. For this reason, we do not rely on the loss of resistance as a marker. Instead, we measure the skin–transverse process distance and simply advance the needle 1 cm past the transverse process.
- Never redirect the needle medially because of the risk of intraforaminal needle passage and consequent spinal cord injury or subarachnoid injection (total spinal).
- Use common sense when advancing the needle. The depth at which the transverse processes are contacted varies with a patient's body habitus and the level at which the block is performed. The deepest levels are at the high thoracic (T1 and T2) and low lumbar levels (L4 and L5), where the transverse process is contacted at a depth of 6 to 8 cm in average-size patients. The shallowest depths are at the midthoracic levels (T5 and T10), where the transverse process is contacted at 3 to 4 cm in an average-size patient.
- Never disconnect the needle from the tubing or the syringe containing local anesthetic while the needle is inserted. Instead, use a stopcock to switch from syringe to syringe during injection. This may prevent the development of a pneumothorax during inspiration in the case of inadvertent puncture of the parietal.

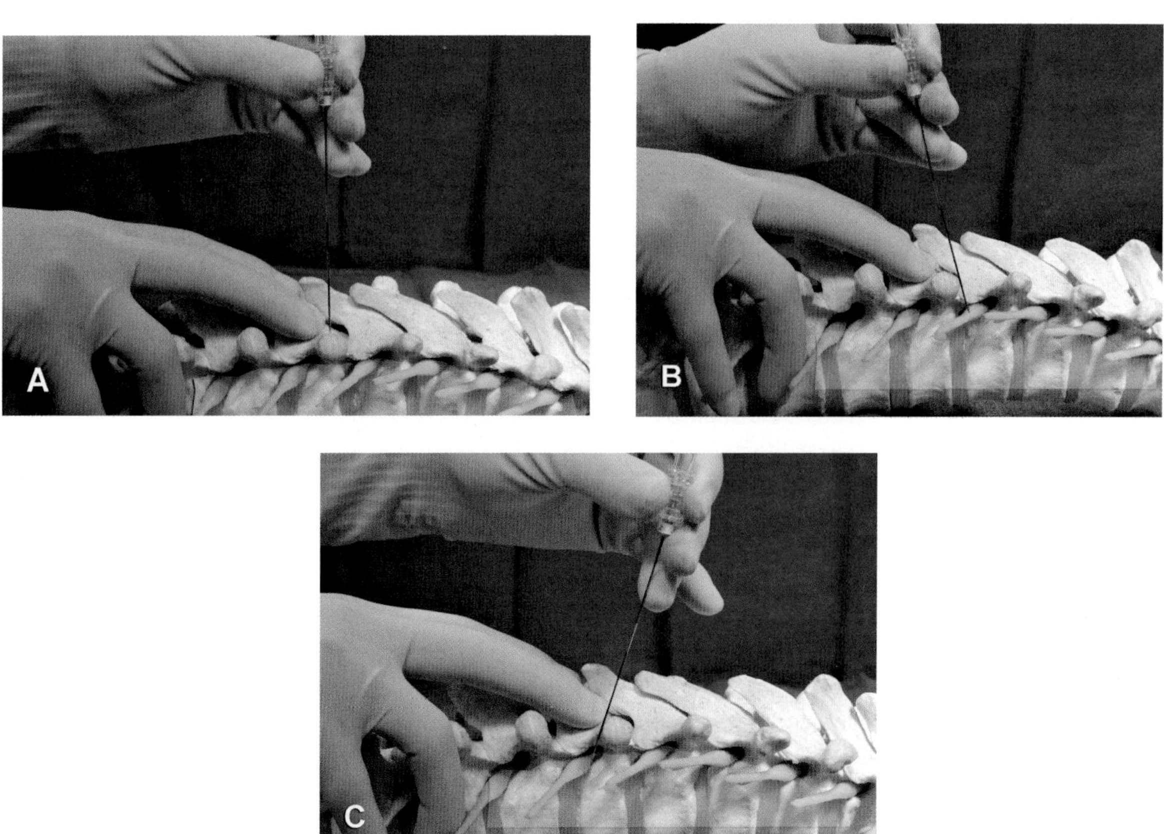


**FIGURE 23-9.** Demonstration of the technique of walking-off the transverse process and needle redirection maneuvers to enter the paravertebral space (lightly shaded area) containing thoracic nerve roots. A. Needle contacts transverse process. B. Needle is "walked off" cephalad to reach paravertebral space. C. Needle is "walked off" to reach paravertebral space.

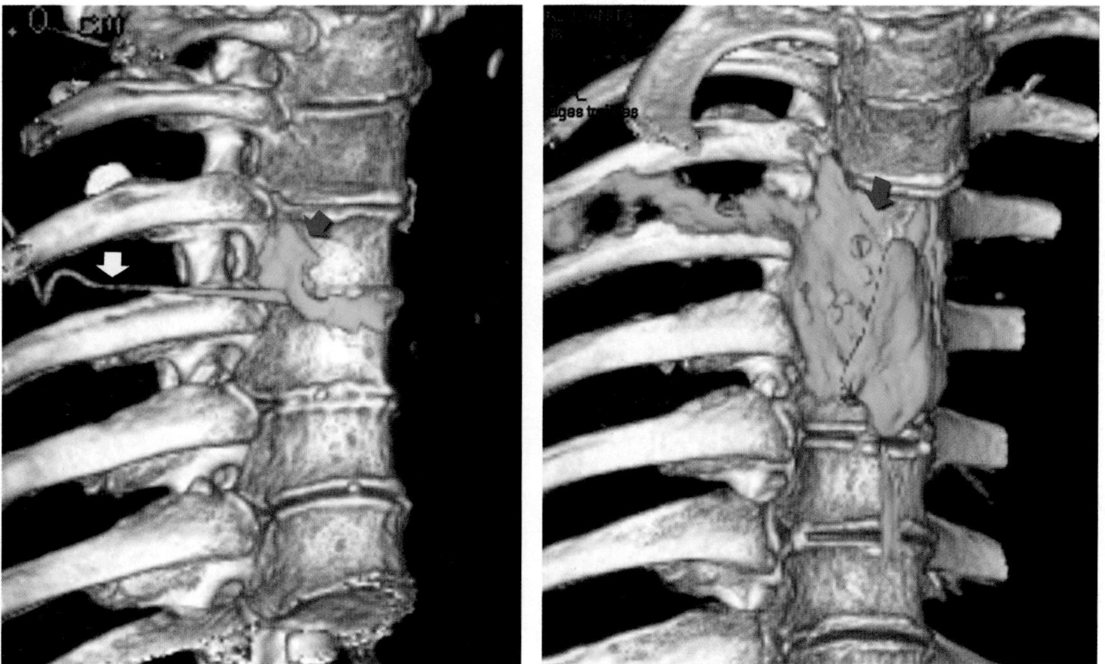

**FIGURE 23-10.** The spread of the contrast-containing local anesthetic in the paravertebral space. White arrow—paravertebral catheter, blue arrows—spread of the contrast. In right image example (5 ml), the contrast spreads somewhat contralaterally and one level above and below the injection.

**TABLE 23-1 Choice of Local Anesthetic for Paravertebral Block**

| ANESTHETIC | ONSET (min) | DURATION OF ANESTHESIA (h) | DURATION OF ANALGESIA (h) |
|---|---|---|---|
| 1.5% mepivacaine (+ $HCO_3$ and epinephrine) | 10–20 | 2–3 | 3–4 |
| 2% lidocaine (+ $HCO_3$ and epinephrine) | 10–15 | 2–3 | 3–4 |
| 0.5% ropivacaine | 15–25 | 3–5 | 8–12 |
| 0.75% ropivacaine | 10–15 | 4–6 | 12–18 |
| 0.5% bupivacaine (+ epinephrine) | 15–25 | 4–6 | 12–18 |
| 0.5% levobupivacaine (+ epinephrine) | 15–25 | 4–6 | 12–18 |

## Choice of Local Anesthetic

It is usually beneficial to achieve longer-acting anesthesia or analgesia in a thoracic paravertebral blockade by using a long-acting local anesthetic. Unless lower lumbar levels (L2 through L5) are part of the planned blockade, paravertebral blocks do not result in extremity motor block and do not impair the patient's ability to ambulate or perform activities of daily living.

Table 23-1 lists some commonly used local anesthetic solutions and their dynamics with this block.

## Block Dynamics and Perioperative Management

Placement of a paravertebral block is associated with moderate patient discomfort, therefore adequate sedation (midazolam 2–4 mg) is necessary for patient comfort. We also routinely administer alfentanil 250 to 750 µg just before beginning the block procedure. However, excessive sedation should be avoided because positioning becomes difficult when patients cannot keep their balance in a sitting position. The efficacy of the block depends on the dispersion of the anesthetic within the space to reach the individual roots at the level of the injection. The first sign of the block is the loss of pinprick sensation at the dermatomal distribution of the root being blocked. The higher the concentration and volume of local anesthetic used, the faster the onset.

# Continuous Thoracic Paravertebral Block

Continuous thoracic paravertebral block is an advanced regional anesthesia technique. Except for the fact that a catheter is advanced through the needle, however, it differs little from the single-injection technique. The continuous thoracic paravertebral block technique is more suitable for analgesia than for surgical anesthesia. The resultant blockade can be thought of as a unilateral continuous thoracic epidural, although bilateral epidural block after injection through the catheter is not uncommon. This technique provides excellent analgesia and is devoid of significant hemodynamic effects in patients following mastectomy, unilateral chest surgery or patients with rib fractures.

## Equipment

A standard regional anesthesia tray is prepared with the following equipment:

- Sterile towels and gauze packs
- A 20-mL syringe containing local anesthetic
- Sterile gloves and marking pen
- A 3- to 5-mL syringe plus 25-gauge needle with local anesthetic for skin infiltration
- Epidural kit with a 10-cm, 18-gauge Tuohy-tip needle and catheter

## Patient Positioning

The patient is positioned in the supine or lateral decubitus position. In our experience, this block is used primarily for patients after various thoracic procedures or for patients undergoing a mastectomy or tumorectomy with axillary lymph node debridement. The ability to recognize spinous processes is crucial.

## Landmarks

The landmarks for a continuous paravertebral block are identical to those for the single-injection technique. The tips of the spinous processes should be marked on the skin. A parasagittal line can then be measured and drawn 2.5 cm lateral to the midline.

**TIP**

- For continuous paravertebral blockade, the catheter is inserted one segmental level below the midpoint of the thoracotomy incision line.

## Technique

The subcutaneous tissues and paravertebral muscles are infiltrated with local anesthetic to decrease the discomfort at the site of needle insertion. The needle is attached to a syringe containing local anesthetic via extension tubing and advanced in a sagittal, slightly cephalad plane to contact the transverse process. Once the transverse process is contacted, the needle is withdrawn back to the skin level and reinserted cephalad at a 10° to 15° angle to walk off 1 cm past the transverse process and enter the paravertebral space. As the paravertebral space is entered, a loss of resistance is sometimes perceived, but it should not be relied on as a marker of correct placement. Once the paravertebral space is entered, the initial bolus of local anesthetic is injected through the needle. The catheter is inserted about 3 to 5 cm beyond the needle tip (Figure 23-11). The catheter is secured using an adhesive skin preparation, followed by application of a clear dressing and clearly labeled "paravertebral nerve block catheter." The catheter should be loss of resistance checked for air, cerebrospinal fluid, and blood before administering a local anesthetic or starting a continuous infusion.

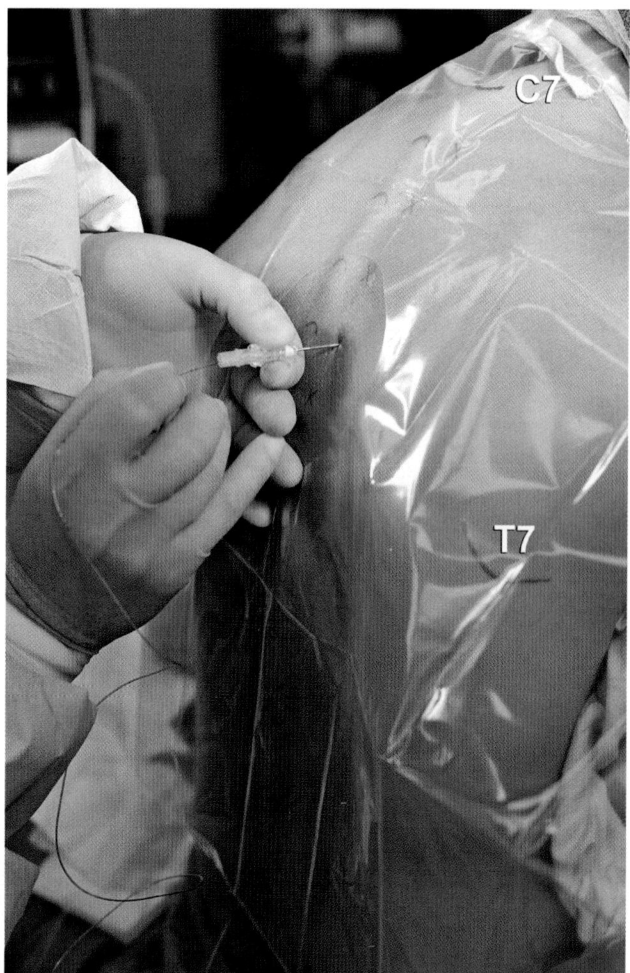


**FIGURE 23-11.** Continuous thoracic paravertebral block. The catheter is inserted 3 cm past the needle tip.

**TIPS**

- Care must be taken to prevent medial orientation of the needle (risk of epidural or subarachnoid placement).
- If it is deemed that the needle is inserted too laterally (inability to advance due to needle-rib contact), the needle should be *reinserted* medially rather than oriented medially (to avoid the risk of the needle entering neuraxial space and spinal cord injury).

## Management of the Continuous Infusion

Continuous infusion is initiated after an initial bolus of dilute local anesthetic is administered through the needle or catheter. The bolus injection consists of a small volume of 0.2% ropivacaine or bupivacaine (e.g., 8 mL). For continuous infusion, 0.2% ropivacaine or 0.25% bupivacaine (levobupivacaine) is also suitable. Local anesthetic is infused at 10 mL/h or 5 mL/h when a patient-controlled regional analgesia dose (5 mL every 60 min) is planned.

**TIPS**

- Breakthrough pain in patients undergoing continuous infusion is always managed by administering a bolus of local anesthetic; increasing the rate of infusion alone is never adequate.
- When the bolus injection through the catheter fails to result in blockade after 30 minutes, the catheter should be considered dislodged and should be removed.

## Complications and How to Avoid Them

Table 23-2 lists the complications and preventive techniques of thoracic paravertebral block.

**TABLE 23-2 Complications of Thoracic Paravertebral Block and Preventive Techniques**

| Complication | Preventive Techniques |
|---|---|
| ***Infection*** | • A strict aseptic technique should be used. |
| ***Hematoma*** | • Avoid multiple needle insertions in patients undergoing anticoagulation therapy. |
| ***Local anesthetic toxicity*** | • Rare.<br>• Large volumes of long-acting anesthetic should be avoided in older and frail patients.<br>• Consider using chloroprocaine for skin infiltration to decrease the total dose of the more toxic, long-acting local anesthetic.<br>• Never inject local anesthetic forcefully; this can lead to a more rapid absorption of local anesthetic. |
| ***Nerve injury*** | • Local anesthetic should never be injected when a patient complains of severe pain or exhibits a withdrawal reaction on injection. |
| ***Total spinal anesthesia*** | • Avoid medial angulation of the needle, which can result in an inadvertent epidural or subarachnoid needle placement.<br>• Aspirate before injection (to detect blood and cerebrospinal fluid).<br>• Do not inject local anesthetic forcefully; this can lead to a greater risk of an epidural spread. |
| ***Paravertebral muscle pain*** | • Paravertebral muscle pain, resembling a muscle spasm, is occasionally seen, particularly in young muscular men and when a larger gauge Tuohy-tip needle is used.<br>• Injection of local anesthetic into the paravertebral muscle before needle insertion and the use of a smaller gauge (e.g., 22 gauge) needle is suggested to avoid this side effect. |

# THORACIC PARAVERTEBRAL BLOCK

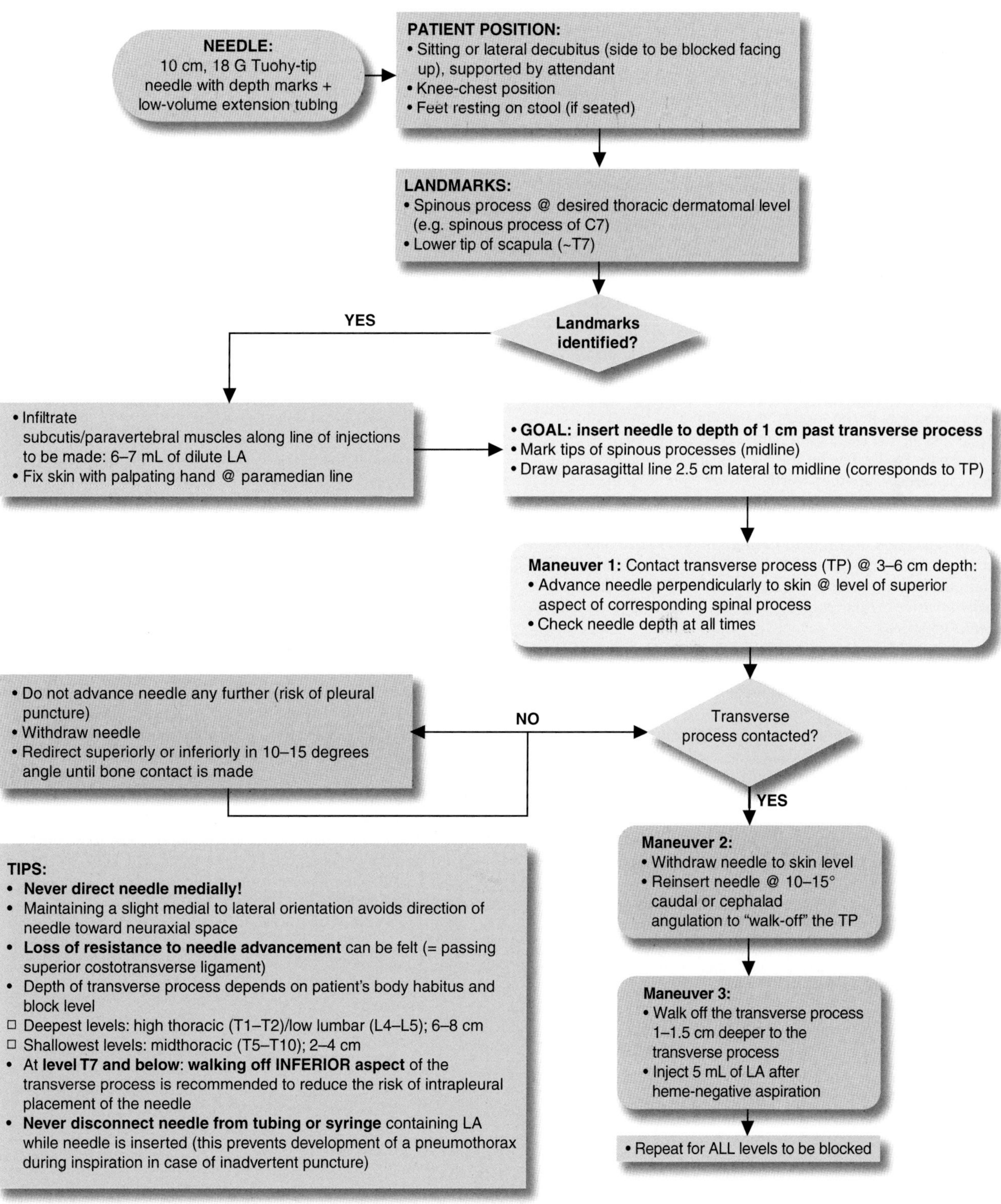

## SUGGESTED READING


Boezaart AP, Raw RM. Continuous thoracic paravertebral block for major breast surgery. *Reg Anesth Pain Med.* 2006;31:470-476.

Buckenmaier CC III, Steele SM, Nielsen KC, Martin AH, Klein SM. Bilateral continuous paravertebral catheters for reduction mammoplasty. *Acta Anaesthesiol Scand.* 2002;46:1042-1045.

Canto M, Sanchez MJ, Casas MA, Bataller ML. Bilateral paravertebral blockade for conventional cardiac surgery. *Anaesthesia.* 2003;58:365-370.

Catala E, Casas JI, Unzueta MC, Diaz X, Aliaga L, Landeira JM. Continuous infusion is superior to bolus doses with thoracic paravertebral blocks after thoracotomies. *J Cardiothorac Vasc Anesth.* 1996;10:586-588.

Cheung SL, Booker PD, Franks R, Pozzi M. Serum concentrations of bupivacaine during prolonged continuous paravertebral infusion in young infants. *Br J Anaesth.* 1997;79:9-13.

Conacher ID, Kokri M. Postoperative paravertebral blocks for thoracic surgery: a radiological appraisal. *Br J Anaesth.* 1987;59:155.

Coveney E, Weltz CR, Greengrass R, et al. Use of paravertebral block anesthesia in the surgical management of breast cancer: experience in 156 cases. *Ann Surg.* 1998;227:496-501.

Daly DJ, Myles PS. Update on the role of paravertebral blocks for thoracic surgery: are they worth it? *Curr Opin Anaesthesiol.* 2009;22:38-43.

Eng J, Sabanathan S. Continuous paravertebral block for postthoracotomy analgesia in children. *J Pediatr Surg.* 1992;27:556-557.

Ganapathy S, Murkin JM, Boyd DW, Dobkowski W, Morgan J. Continuous percutaneous paravertebral block for minimally invasive cardiac surgery. *J Cardiothorac Vasc Anesth.* 1999;13:594-596.

Greengrass RA, Klein SM, D'Ercole FJ, Gleason DG, Shimer CL, Steele SM. Lumbar plexus and sciatic nerve block for knee arthroplasty: comparison of ropivacaine and bupivacaine. *Can J Anaesth.* 1998;45:1094-1096.

Hadžić A, Vloka JD, Kuroda MM, Koorn R, Birnbach DJ. The practice of peripheral nerve blocks in the United States: a national survey. *Reg Anesth Pain Med.* 1998;23:241-246.

Hultman JL, Schuleman S, Sharp T, Gilbert TJ. Continuous thoracic paravertebral block. *J Cardiothorac Anesth.* 1989;3:54.

Johnson LR, Rocco AG, Ferrante FM. Continuous subpleural-paravertebral block in acute thoracic herpes zoster. *Anesth Analg.* 1988;67:1105-1108.

Karmakar MK. Thoracic paravertebral block. *Anesthesiology.* 2001;95:771-780.

Karmakar MK, Booker PD, Franks R. Bilateral continuous paravertebral block used for postoperative analgesia in an infant having bilateral thoracotomy. *Paediatr Anaesth.* 1997;7:469-471.

Klein SM, Bergh A, Steele SM, Georgiade GS, Greengrass RA. Thoracic paravertebral block for breast surgery. *Anesth Analg.* 2000;90:1402-1405.

Kopacz DJ, Thompson GE. Neural blockade of the thorax and abdomen. In: Cousins MJ, Bridenbaugh PO, eds. *Neuronal Blockade in Clinical Anesthesia and Management of Pain.* Philadelphia, PA: Lippincott-Raven; 1988:451-485.

Norum HM, Breivik H. Thoracic paravertebral blockade and thoracic epidural analgesia: two extremes of a continuum. *Anesth Analg.* 2011;112:990; 990-1.

Pintaric TS, Potocnik I, Hadzic A, Stupnik T, Pintaric M, Jankovic VN. Comparison of continuous thoracic epidural with paravertebral block on perioperative analgesia and hemodynamic stability in patients having open lung surgery.*Reg Anesth Pain Med.* 2011;36:256-60.

Pusch F, Wildling E, Klimscha W, Weinstable C. Sonographic measurement of needle insertion depth in paravertebral blocks in women. *Br J Anaesth.* 2002;85:841-843.

Renes SH, Van Geffen GJ, Snoeren MM, Gielen MJ, Groen GJ. "Ipsilateral brachial plexus block and hemidiaphragmatic paresis as adverse effect of a high thoracic paravertebral block. *Reg Anesth Pain Med.* 2011;36:198-201.

Richardson J, Lönnqvist PA, Naja Z. Bilateral thoracic paravertebral block: potential and practice. *Br J Anaesth.* 2011;106:164-71.

Richardson J, Sabanathan S, Jones J, Shah RD, Cheema S, Mearns AJ. A prospective, randomized comparison of preoperative and continuous balanced epidural or paravertebral bupivacaine on post-thoracotomy pain, pulmonary function and stress responses. *Br J Anaesth.* 1999;83:387-392.

Richardson J, Sabanathan S. Thoracic paravertebral analgesia. *Acta Anaesthesiol Scand.* 1995;39:1005-1015.

Schnabel A, Reichl SU, Kranke P, Pogatzki-Zahn EM, Zahn PK.Efficacy and safety of paravertebral blocks in breast surgery: a meta-analysis of randomized controlled trials. Br J Anaesth. 2010;105:842-52.

Terheggen MA, Wille F, Borel Rinkes IH, Ionescu TI, Knape JT. Paravertebral blockade for minor breast surgery. *Anesth Analg.* 2002;94:355-359.

Terheggen MA, Wille F, Borel Rinkes IH, Ionescu TI, Knape JT. Paravertebral blockade for minor breast surgery. *Anesth Analg.* 2002;94:355-359.

Vila H Jr, Liu J, Kavasmaneck D. Paravertebral block: new benefits from an old procedure. *Curr Opin Anaesthesiol.* 2007;20:316-318.

Wheeler LJ. Peripheral nerve stimulation end-point for thoracic paravertebral block. *Br J Anaesth.* 2001;86:598.

# 24 Intercostal Block

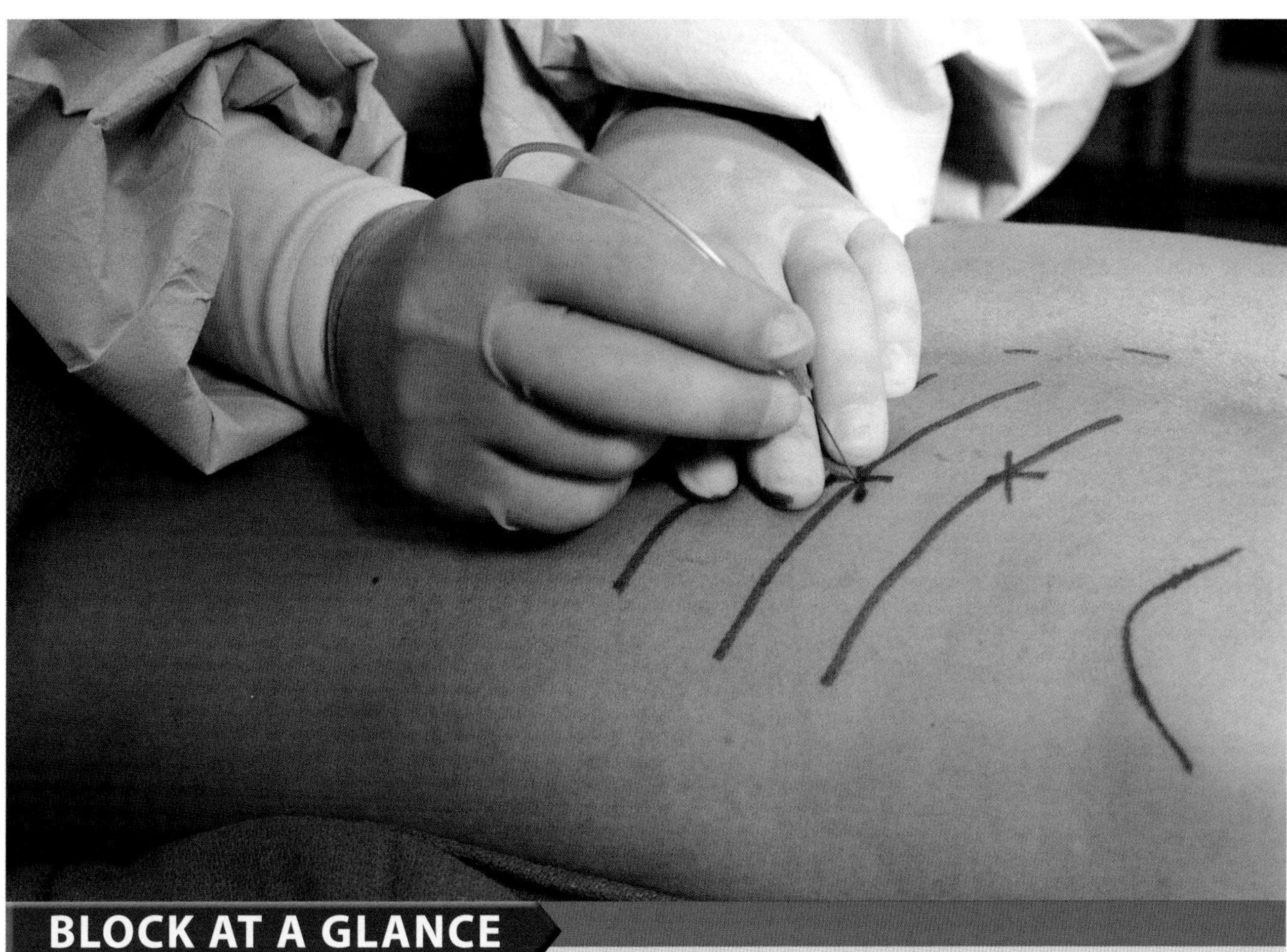

## BLOCK AT A GLANCE

- Indications: thoracic or upper abdominal surgery, rib fractures, breast surgery
- Landmarks: angle of the rib (6–8 cm lateral to the spinous process)
- Needle insertion: Under the rib with approximately 20-30° cephalad angulation
- Target: needle insertion 0.5 cm past the inferior border of the rib
- Local anesthetic: 3–5 mL per intercostal level
- Complexity level: advanced

**FIGURE 24-1.** Intercostal nerve block: Patient position and needle insertion.

## General Considerations

Intercostal block produces discrete bandlike segmental anesthesia in the chosen levels. Intercostal block is an excellent analgesic option for a variety of acute and chronic pain conditions. The beneficial effect of intercostal blockade on respiratory function following thoracic or upper abdominal surgery, or following chest wall trauma, is well documented. Although similar in many ways to the paravertebral block, intercostal blocks are generally simpler to perform because the osseous landmarks are more readily palpable. However, the risks of pneumothorax and local anesthetic systemic toxicity are present, and care must be taken to prevent these potentially serious complications. Intercostal blocks can be more challenging to perform above the level of T7 because the scapula prevents access to the ribs. Although an intercostal block is an excellent choice for analgesic purposes, it is often inadequate as a complete surgical anesthesia. For this application, supplementation with another anesthesia technique usually is required.

## Regional Anesthesia Anatomy

After emerging from their respective intervertebral foramina, the thoracic nerve roots divide into dorsal and ventral rami (Figure 24-2). The dorsal ramus provides innervation to the skin and muscle of the paravertebral region; the ventral ramus continues laterally as the intercostal nerve. This nerve then pierces the posterior intercostal membrane approximately 3 cm lateral to the intervertebral foramen and enters the subcostal groove of the rib, where it travels inferiorly to the intercostal artery and vein. Initially, the nerve lies between the parietal pleura and the inner most intercostal muscle. Immediately proximal to the angle of the rib, it passes into the space between the innermost and internal intercostal muscles, where it remains for much of the remainder of its course. At the midaxillary line, the intercostal nerve gives rise to the lateral cutaneous branch, which pierces the internal and external intercostal muscles and supplies the muscles and skin of the lateral trunk. The continuation of the intercostal nerve terminates as the anterior cutaneous branch, which supplies

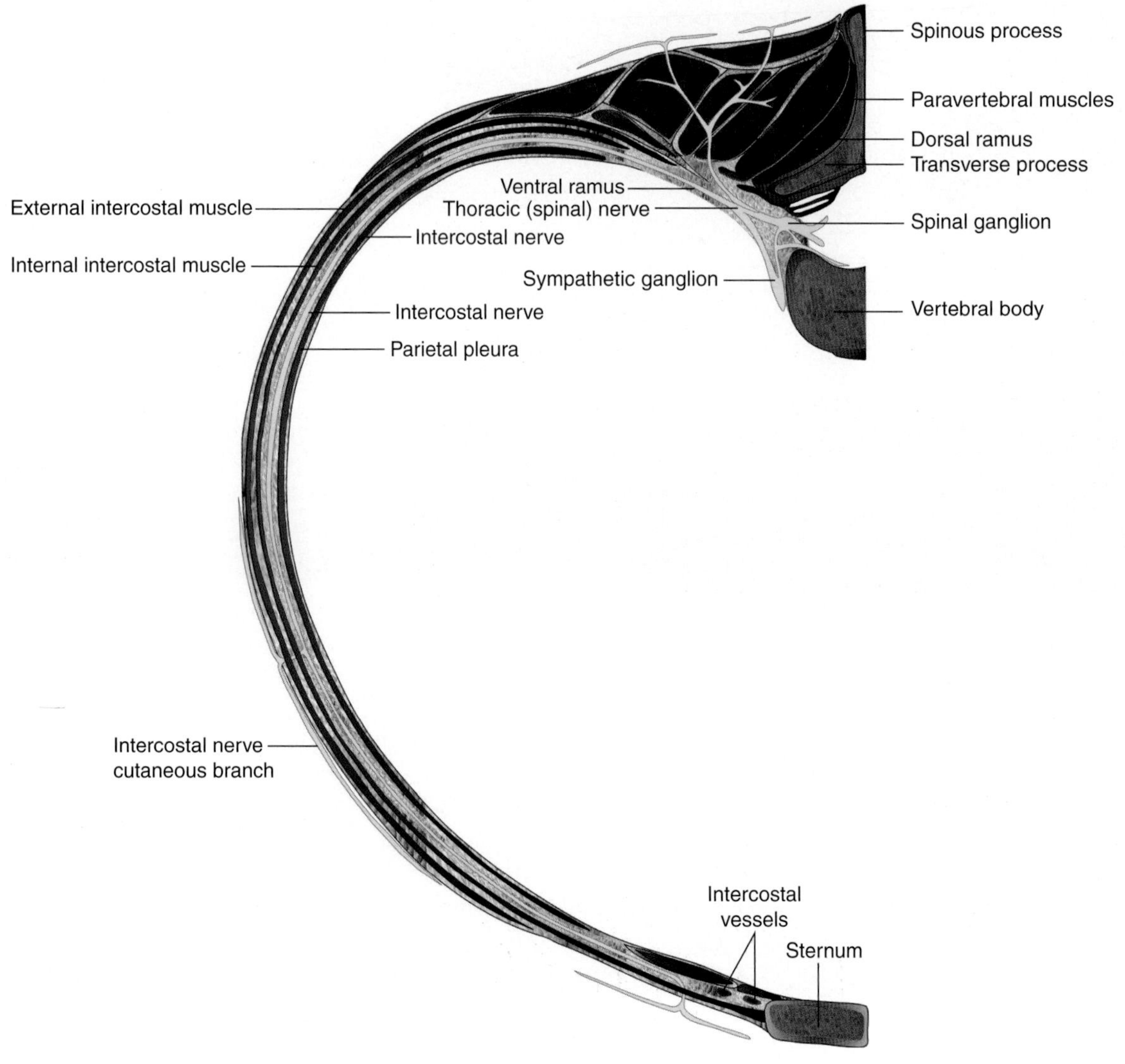


**FIGURE 24-2.** Anatomy of the thoracic spinal and intercostal nerves.

the skin and muscles of the anterior trunk, including the skin overlying the sternum and rectus abdominis.

## Distribution of Anesthesia

Intercostal blockade results in the spread of local anesthetic along the intercostals sulcus underneath the parietal pleura, leading to ipsilateral anesthesia of the blocked intercostals levels (Figure 24-3). A larger volume of local anesthetic or more medial injection may result in backtracking of local anesthetic into the paravertebral space. The extent of the resulting dermatomal distribution of anesthesia or analgesia is simply a function of the level of blockade. In contrast to paravertebral blockade, longitudinal (cephalad-caudad) spread between adjacent levels is much less common, although possible with large volumes of injectate and/or injection sites close to the midline of the back. In such instances, the local anesthetic can spread between the levels via the overflow into the paravertebral space.

### Equipment

A standard regional anesthesia tray is prepared with the following equipment:

- Sterile towels and gauze packs
- 20-mL syringes containing local anesthetic

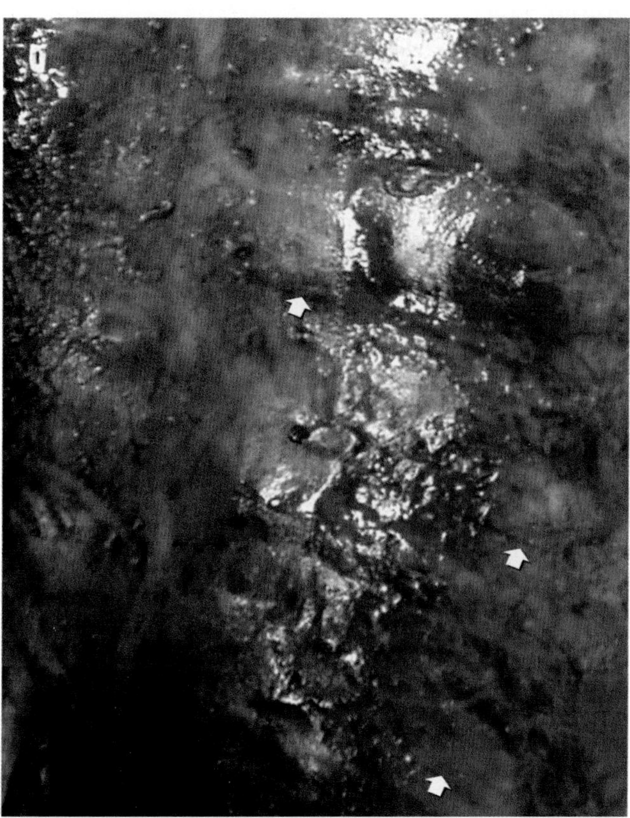

**FIGURE 24-3.** Injection of the local anesthetic (red dye) in intercostal space results in a medial-lateral spread of the local anesthetic in the intercostal space where the intercostal nerves (arrow) are contained.

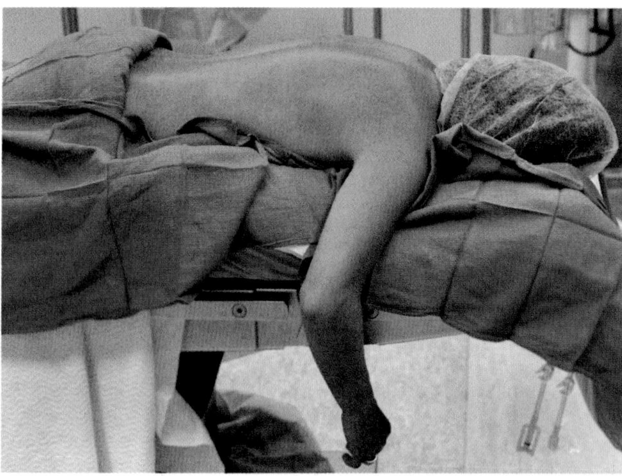

**FIGURE 24-4.** The patient position for intercostal block. A pillow is used as an abdominal/pelvic support. The arms are hanging off the table.

- Sterile gloves and marking pen
- A 10-mL syringe plus 25-gauge needle with local anesthetic for skin infiltration
- A 1.5-in, 22-gauge needle attached to extension tubing

### Patient Positioning

An intercostal block can be performed with the patient in the sitting, lateral decubitus, or prone positions. With the patient in sitting or lateral position, it is helpful to have the patient's spine arched with the arms extended forward. Patients who are prone are best positioned for the block by placing a pillow under the abdomen and with the arms hanging down from the sides of the bed (Figure 24-4). This rotates the scapulae laterally and permits access to the angles of the rib above the level of T7 (Figure 24-5).

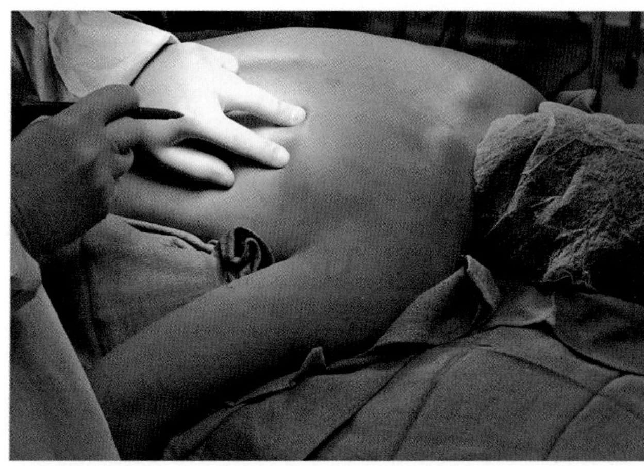

**FIGURE 24-5.** Technique of palpating the intercostal space. The fingers of the palpating hand are firmly pressed in the intercostal space 5–7 cm lateral to the midline.

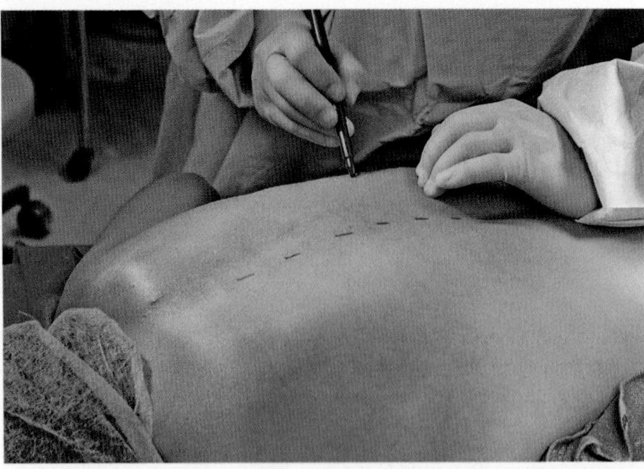

**FIGURE 24-6.** Landmarks for intercostal space are identified first by determining the midline and the spinous processes (skin marks). Intercostal space is then determined by palpation at each level to be blocked, and the insertion point for needle is marked 5–7 cm lateral to the midline.

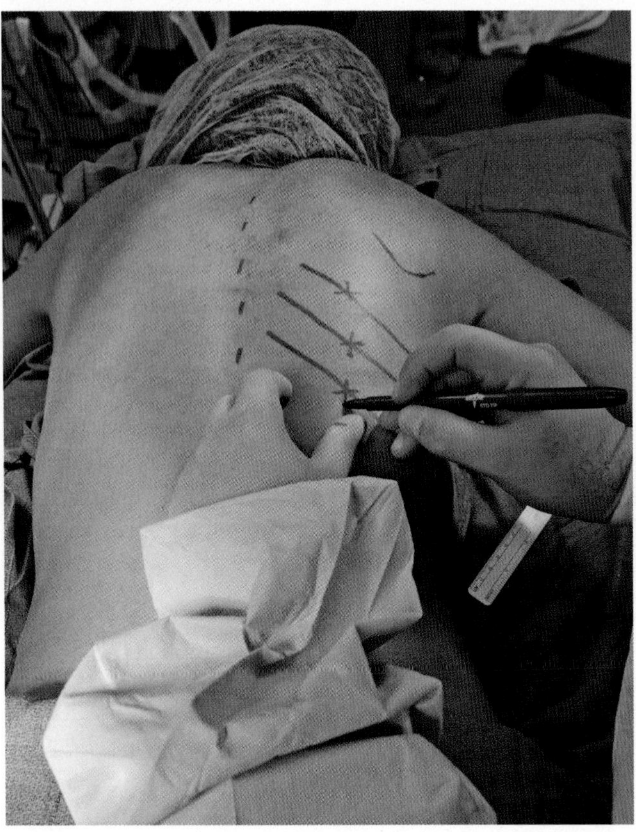

**FIGURE 24-8.** The needle insertion site for intercostal space is labeled 5–7 cm lateral to the midline.

## Landmarks and Maneuvers to Accentuate Them

The following anatomic landmarks are used to estimate the position of the relevant ribs.

1. Twelfth rib (last rib palpable inferiorly) (Figure 24-6)
2. The 7th rib (lowest rib covered by the angle of the scapula) (Figure 24-7)

Once identified by palpation, the inferior border of the corresponding ribs can be marked on the skin (Figure 24-8). An "x" at the angle of the rib identifies the site of needle insertion, usually about 6–8 cm from the midline. For thoracotomy or upper abdominal incisions, an estimate of the levels required for effective analgesia can be made after discussion with the surgeon as to the planned approach and length of incision. Analgesic blocks for rib fractures are planned based on the area of the injury. Typically, in addition to the estimated dermatomal levels, one additional level above and one below the estimated levels are also blocked.

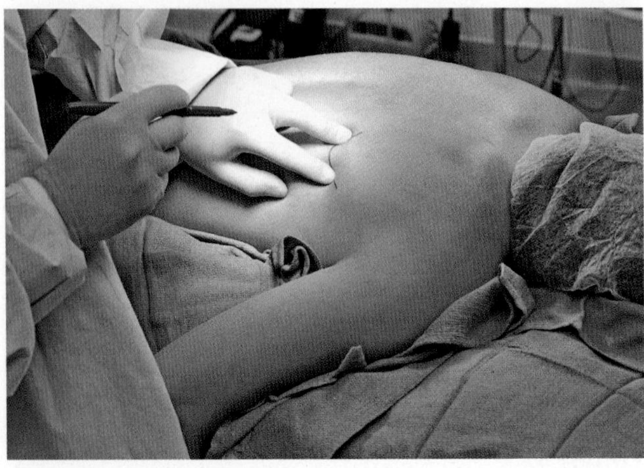

**FIGURE 24-7.** Estimating T7 level at the tip of the scapula.

**TIP**

- Determining the level of the blockade by counting ribs is merely an estimated, rather than a precise, technique.

## Technique

After cleaning the skin with an antiseptic solution, 1–2 mL of dilute local anesthetic is infiltrated subcutaneously at each planned injection site.

The fingers of the palpating hand should straddle the insertion site at the inferior border of the rib and fix the

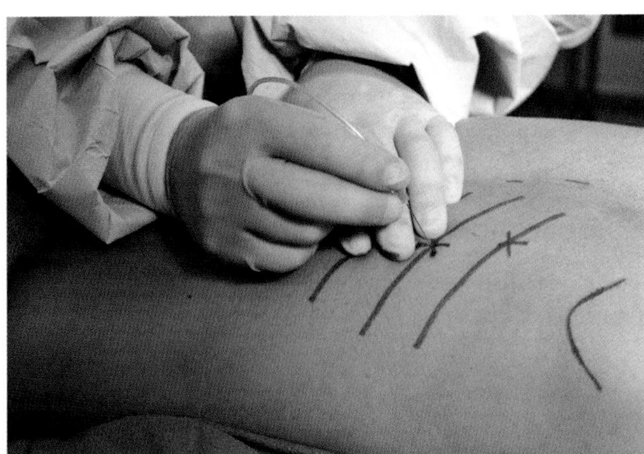

**FIGURE 24-9.** Intercostal nerve block: Patient position and needle insertion.

skin to avoid unwanted skin movement. A 1.5-in, 22-gauge needle is attached to a syringe containing local anesthetic via extension tubing and advanced at an angle of approximately 20° cephalad to the skin (Figure 24-9). Contact with the rib should be made at within 1 cm in most patients. While maintaining the same angle of insertion, the needle is walked off the inferior border of the rib as the skin is allowed to return to its initial position. Then the needle is advanced 3 mm below the inferior margin of the rib, with the goal of placing the tip in the space containing the neurovascular bundle (i.e., between the internal and innermost intercostal muscles). The end point for advancement should be the predetermined distance (3 mm).

Following negative aspiration for blood or air, 3–5 mL of local anesthetic of insertion and the needle withdrawn. The process is repeated for the remaining levels of blockade.

## TIPS

- A perpendicular or caudad angulation of the needle can cause the block failure; maintenance of the 20° cephalad angle increases the chances that the needle tip will be placed in close proximity to the intercostal nerve.
- Use common sense when advancing the needle. The depth at which the ribs are contacted varies with a patient's body habitus, and an absence of bony contact at 1 cm should prompt a reevaluation of landmarks rather than continued advancement.
- Never disconnect the needle from the tubing or the syringe containing local anesthetic while the needle is inserted. Instead, use a stopcock to switch the syringes. In the case of inadvertent puncture of the parietal pleura, this strategy prevents the development of a pneumothorax during inspiration, unless the visceral pleura are punctured also.
- In patients with a multiple-level blockade, consider using alkalinized 3-chloroprocaine for skin infiltration to decrease the total dose of the more toxic, long-acting local anesthetic

## Choice of Local Anesthetic

It is usually beneficial to achieve longer-acting anesthesia or analgesia for intercostal blockade by using a long-acting local anesthetic. Systemic absorption of local anesthetic is high following an intercostal block, and careful consideration of the dose should precede the block performance to decrease the risk of systemic toxicity.

Table 24-1 lists some commonly used local anesthetic solutions and their dynamics with this block..

**TABLE 24-1 Choice of Local Anesthetic for Intercostal Block**

| LOCAL ANESTHETIC | ONSET (min) | DURATION OF ANESTHESIA (h) | DURATION OF ANALGESIA (h) |
|---|---|---|---|
| 1.5% mepivacaine (+ $HCO_3$ and epinephrine) | 10–20 | 2–3 | 3–4 |
| 2% lidocaine (+ $HCO_3$ and epinephrine) | 10–15 | 2–3 | 3–4 |
| 0.5% ropivacaine | 15–25 | 3–5 | 8–12 |
| 0.75% ropivacaine | 10–15 | 4–6 | 12–18 |
| 0.5% bupivacaine (+ epinephrine) | 15–25 | 4–6 | 12–18 |
| 0.5% levobupivacaine (+ epinephrine) | 15–25 | 4–6 | 12–18 |

## Block Dynamics and Perioperative Management

The performance of intercostal blocks is associated with relatively minor patient discomfort, although needle contact with the periosteum can be uncomfortable. A small dose of midazolam (2 mg) and alfentanil (250–500 μg) just before beginning the block procedure is usually adequate to decrease the discomfort. Excessive sedation should be avoided because positioning becomes difficult when patients cannot keep their balance in a sitting position. The first sign of successful blockade is the loss of pinprick sensation at the dermatomal distribution of the nerve being blocked. The higher the concentration and volume of local anesthetic used, the faster the onset.

## Complications and How to Avoid Them

Table 24-2 lists the complications of intercostal block and preventive techniques.

**TABLE 24-2 Complications of Intercostal Block and Preventive Techniques**

| | |
|---|---|
| ***Infection*** | • An aseptic technique should be used. |
| ***Pneumothorax*** | • Avoid intercostal blockade where a pneumothorax would be catastrophic. Limit advancement of needle under the rib.<br>• Maintain precise control of the needle at all times.<br>• The palpating hand should rest firmly on skin to prevent inadvertent movement. |
| ***Peritoneal/visceral injury*** | • Rare. Avoid excessive needle advancement. |
| ***Local anesthetic toxicity*** | • An important concern because systemic absorption can be rapid. Large volumes of long-acting anesthetic should be reconsidered in older and frail patients.<br>• Consider using chloroprocaine for skin infiltration to decrease the total dose of the more toxic, long-acting local anesthetic. |
| ***Spinal anesthesia*** | • Because the dural sleeves can extend up to 8 cm from the midline, there is a small risk of subarachwnoid spread if the needle tip contacts the dural sleeve.<br>• Maintain a high index of suspicion of neuraxial spread. If bilateral block occurs treat hemodynamic/respiratory symptoms accordingly (may mimic tension pneumothorax). |

# INTERCOSTAL NERVE BLOCK

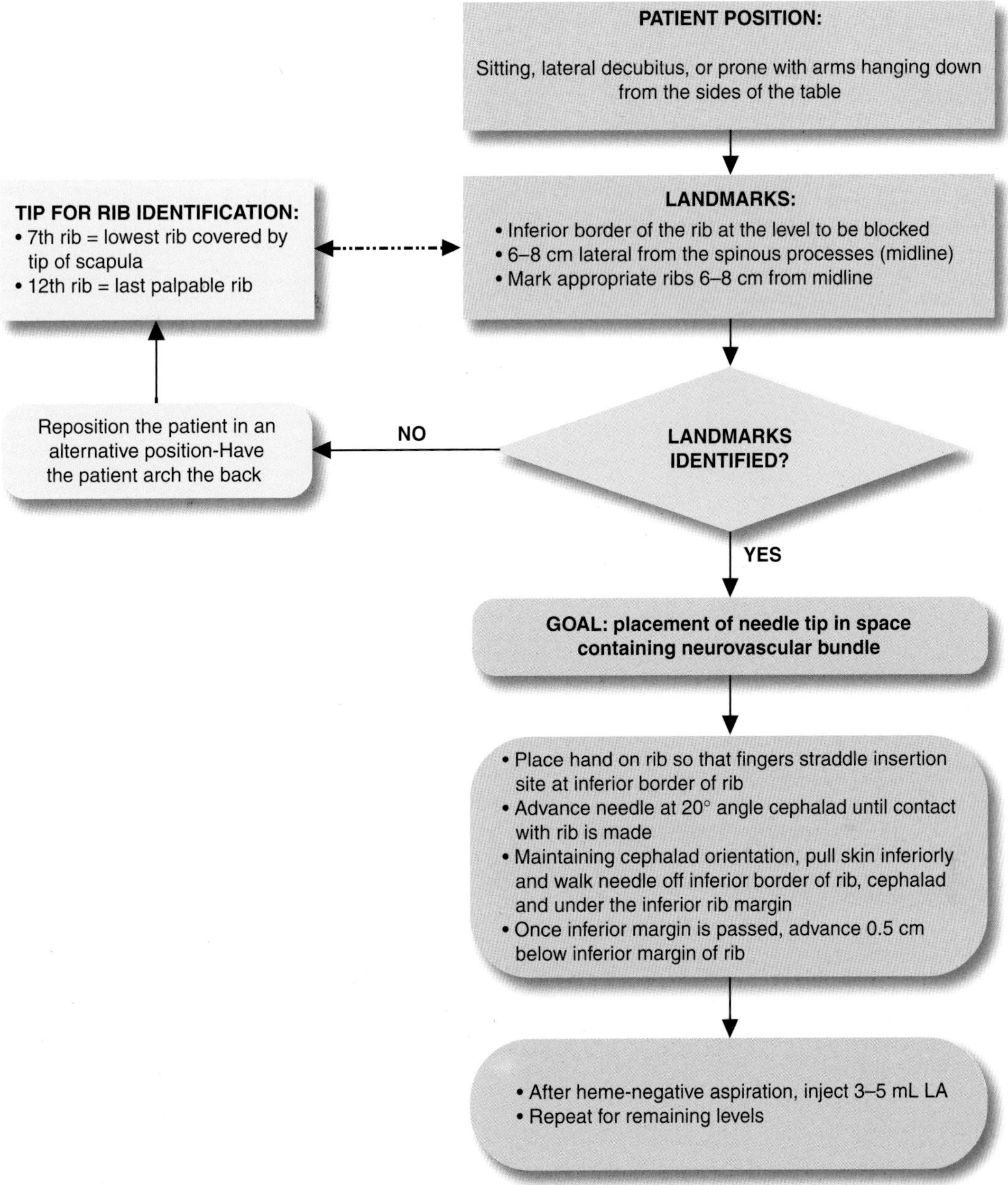

## SUGGESTED READING

Finnerty O, Carney J, McDonnell JG. Trunk blocks for abdominal surgery. *Anaesthesia.* 2010;65(Suppl 1):76-83.

Joshi GP, Bonnet F, Shah R, et al. A systematic review of randomized trials evaluating regional techniques for postthoracotomy analgesia. *Anesth Analg.* 2008;107:1026-1040.

Karmakar MK, Critchley LAH, Ho AMH, et al. Continuous thoracic paravertebral infusion of bupivacaine for pain management in patients with multiple fractured ribs. *Chest.* 2003;123:424-431.

Karmakar MK, Ho AMH. Acute pain management of patients with multiple fractured ribs. *J Trauma.* 2003;54:612-615.

Kopacz DJ, Thompson GE. Intercostal blocks for thoracic and abdominal surgery. *Tech Reg Anesth Pain Manage.* 1998;2:25-29.

Nunn JF, Slavin G. Posterior intercostal nerve block for pain relief after cholecystectomy. Anatomical basis and efficacy. *Br J Anaesth.* 1980;52:253-260.

Osinowo OA, Zahrani M, Softah A. Effect of intercostal nerve block with 0.5% bupivacaine on peak expiratory flow rate and arterial oxygen saturation in rib fractures. *J Trauma.* 2004;56:345-347.

Stromskag KE, Kleiven S. Continuous intercostals and interpleural nerve blockades. *Tech Reg Anesth Pain Manage.* 1998;2:79-89.

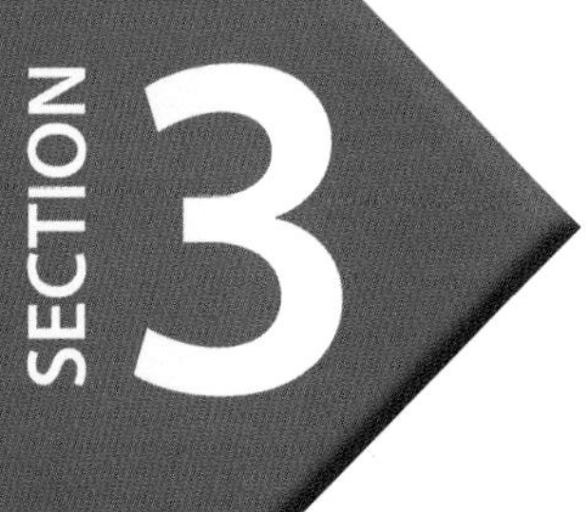


# Intravenous Regional Anesthesia

# 25 Bier Block

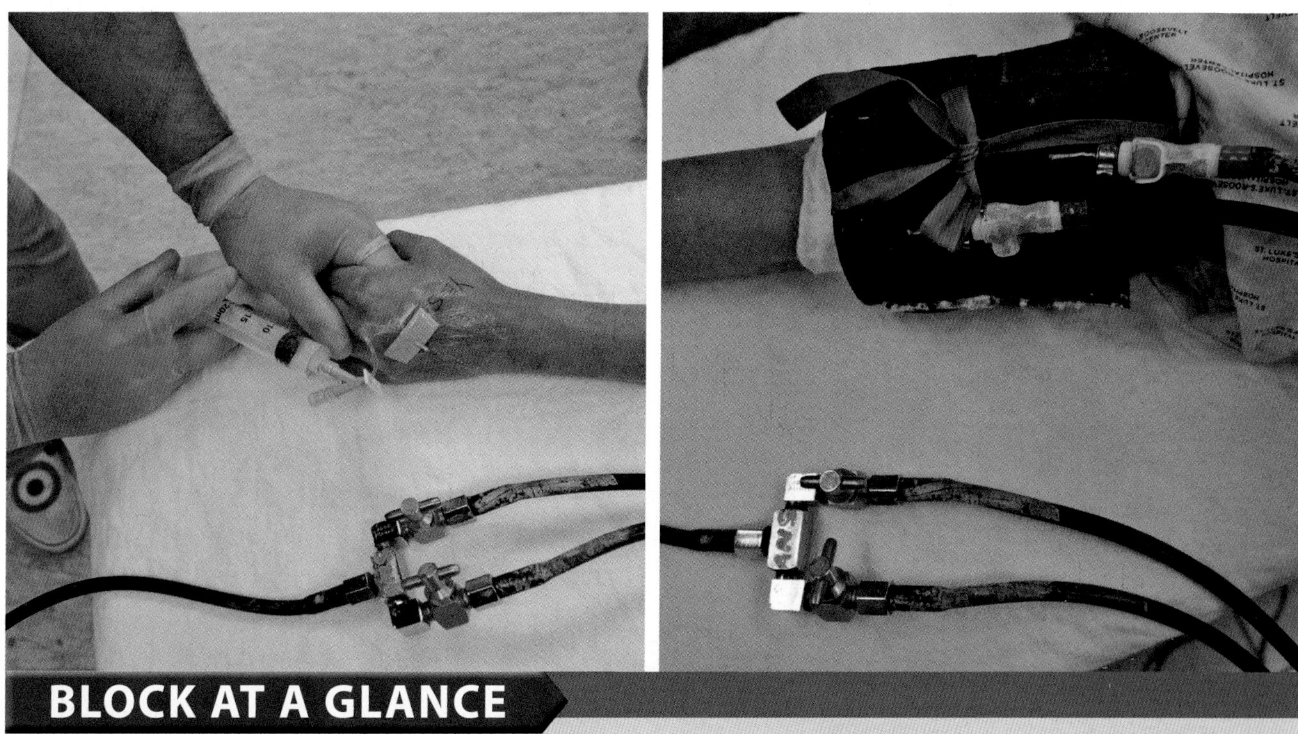

## BLOCK AT A GLANCE

- Indications: short operative procedures for the extremities; pain therapy (e.g., treatment of recurrent complex pain syndrome); treatment of hyperhidrosis
  - Local anesthetic: 12–15 mL of 2% lidocaine for upper extremities (or 30–40 mL of 0.5% lidocaine)
  - Relative contraindications: crush injuries; inability to access peripheral veins; infections (skin, cellulitis); compound fractures; convincing history of allergy to local anesthetics (LAs); severe peripheral vascular disease; atrioventricular shunts; severe hepatic insufficiency; disrupted integrity of venous system; sickle cell disease
  - Complexity level: Basic

**FIGURE 25-1.** Intravenous regional anesthesia: Injection of local anesthetic and placement of the tourniquet.

## General Considerations

Intravenous regional anesthesia (IVRA) was first described in 1908 by the German surgeon A.G. Bier, hence the procedure name Bier block. Originally, anesthesia was obtained by the intravenous injection of procaine in a previously exsanguinated vascular space, isolated from the rest of the circulation by two Esmarch bandages used as tourniquets. After initial enthusiasm, the technique fell into obscurity for >50 years. In 1963, Holmes reintroduced the Bier block with the novel use of lidocaine, describing a series of 30 patients in *The Lancet*. Today, intravenous regional anesthesia of the upper limb remains popular because it is reliable, cost effective, safe, and simple to administer. It is a widely accepted technique well suited for brief minor surgeries such as wrist or hand ganglionectomy, carpal tunnel release, Dupuytren contractures, reduction of fractures, and others. Since the duration of anesthesia depends on the length of time the tourniquet is inflated, there is no need to use long-acting or more toxic agents. Its application for longer surgical procedures is precluded by the discomfort caused by the tourniquet, typically beginning within 30 to 45 minutes. Other disadvantages include incomplete muscle relaxation (where important) and lack of postoperative pain relief. With the implementation of a safety protocol and with meticulous attention to detail, concerns about local anesthetic (LA) toxicity should merely be a theoretical issue.

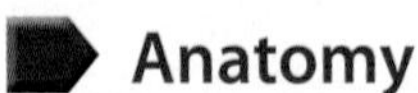

## Anatomy

The only relevant anatomy is the location and distribution of peripheral veins in the extremity to be blocked. By preference, a vein as distal as possible is chosen. The antecubital fossa is an alternative only when more distal peripheral access is lacking.

## Distribution of Anesthesia

The entire extremity below the level of the tourniquet is anesthetized. Numerous radiographic, radioisotope, and neurophysiologic studies looked into the site of action of IVRA. However, the exact mechanism still remains the subject of debate and controversy. The likely mechanism is that the local anesthetic, via the vascular bed, reaches both peripheral nerves and nerve trunks (*vasae nervorum*), and nerve endings (valveless venules). Diffusion of local anesthetic into the surrounding tissues also plays a role. Ischemia and compression of the peripheral nerves at the level of the inflated cuff is probably another contributory component of the mechanism of IVRA. Again, anesthesia achieved by intravenous regional anesthesia is limited only by the inevitable pain due to tourniquet application; and, therefore, it is used typically for procedures lasting 30 to 45 minutes.

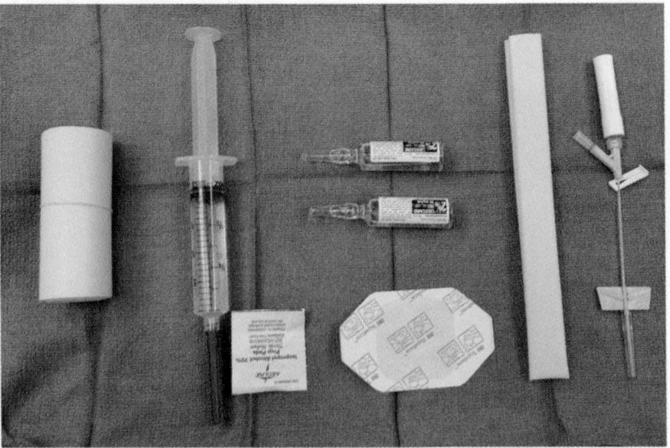

**FIGURE 25-2.** Equipment for intravenous (IV) regional anesthesia consists of IV catheter, Esmarch, and local anesthetic.

## Equipment

Equipment includes the following items (Figure 25-2):

- Local anesthetic agent: lidocaine HCl (0.25–2%)
- Rubber tourniquet
- IV catheters (18- or 20-gauge)
- 500-mL or 1-L bag of IV solution (crystalloid)
- Infusion set
- Pneumatic tourniquet, ideally with a double cuff
- One Esmarch bandage (about 150 cm in length, 10 cm in width)
- Syringes

## Positioning and Preparation

The patient lies in the supine position with the vein selected for block placement readily accessible. Baseline vital signs are assessed; blood pressure, oxygen saturation, and ECG monitoring are applied. Intravenous access in the nonoperated extremity is obtained. Small doses of benzodiazepine for anxiolysis or small aliquots of opioids in case of discomfort, or both, may be administered. Adequate premedication will improve tourniquet tolerance and benzodiazepines can prevent the potential central nervous system signs of mild local anesthetic toxicity should the level of local anesthetic raise. An intact tourniquet system is essential for success and safety. Therefore, pneumatic cuffs always must be checked for air leaks before starting any IVRA procedure.

## Technique

The technique consists of the following steps:

1. An IV cannula is inserted in the extremity opposite to the block side.
2. A double pneumatic tourniquet is placed on a padding layer of soft cloth (stockinette) with the proximal cuff high on the upper arm.
3. An IV cannula is inserted and carefully secured into a peripheral vein of the operative limb, as far distally as feasible. The cannula is flushed with saline before capping (Figure 25-3).
4. The entire arm is elevated for 1 to 2 minutes to allow for passive exsanguination (Figure 25-4). After exsanguination, while still keeping the arm high, a rubber Esmarch bandage is wrapped around the arm, spirally from the hand to the distal cuff of the double tourniquet, to exsanguinate the extremity completely (Figure 25-5).
5. While the axillary artery is digitally occluded, the proximal cuff is inflated to 50 to 100 mm Hg above systolic arterial blood pressure (Figure 25-6).
6. Sequence for initial tourniquet management:
   a. Exsanguinate by elevation and Tourniquet wrapping
   b. Inflate *distal* cuff
   c. Inflate *proximal* cuff
   d. Deflate *distal* cuff
7. Inject local anesthetic.
8. After reaching the correct pressure, the Esmarch bandage is removed and 12 to 15 mL of preservative-free 2% lidocaine HCl (or 30–50 mL of 0.5% lidocaine HCl) is slowly injected via the indwelling extra catheter (20 mL/min) (Figure 25-7). The volume depends on the size of the arm being anesthetized and the concentration of the anesthetic solution. Commonly recommended maximal dose is 3 mg/kg.

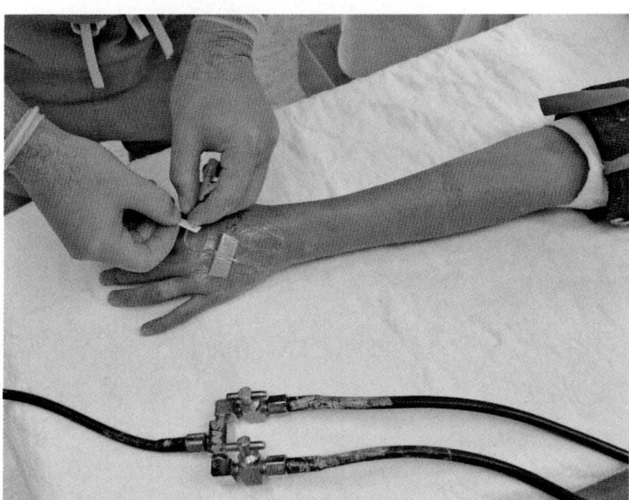

**FIGURE 25-3.** A small gauge intravenous catheter is inserted in the peripheral vein and secured.

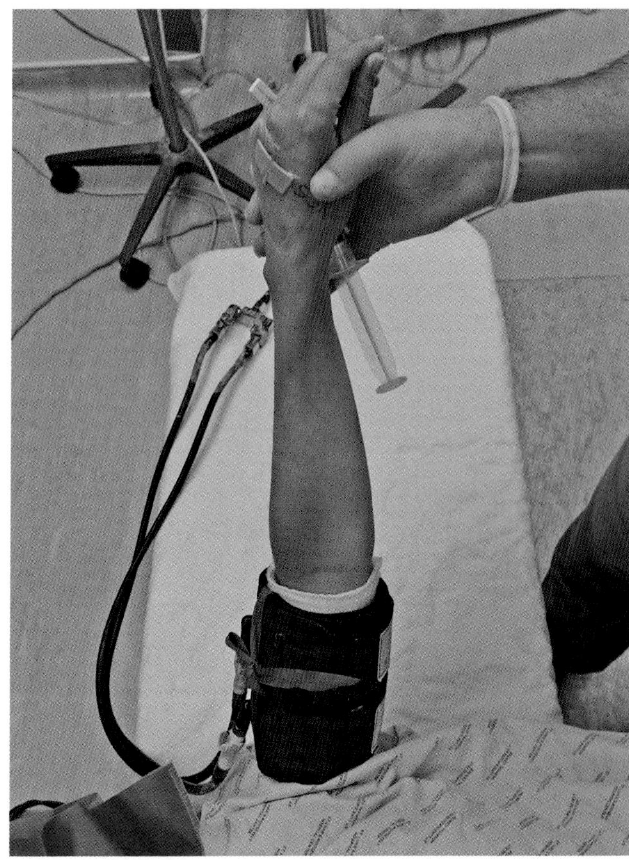

**FIGURE 25-4.** A double well-padded tourniquet is placed on the upper arm. The arm is elevated to allow for passive exsanguinations.

9. After the injection, the arm is lowered to the level of the table. The IV cannula from the anesthetized hand is removed, and in a sterile manner, pressure is quickly applied over the puncture site.

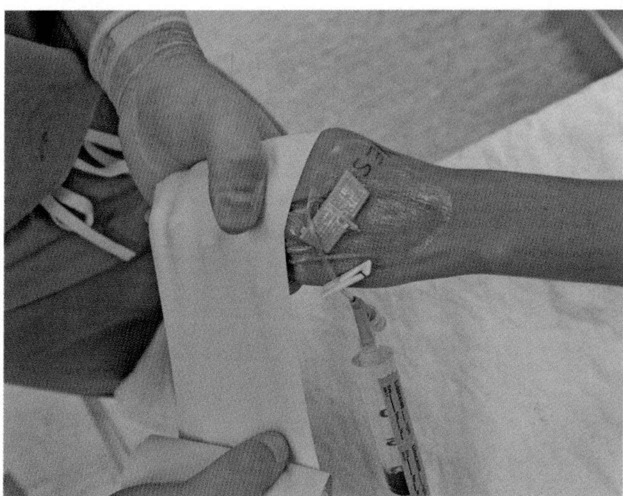

**FIGURE 25-5.** With the arm elevated, an Esmarch bandage is systematically applied from the fingertips to the double tourniquet to help empty the venous bed.

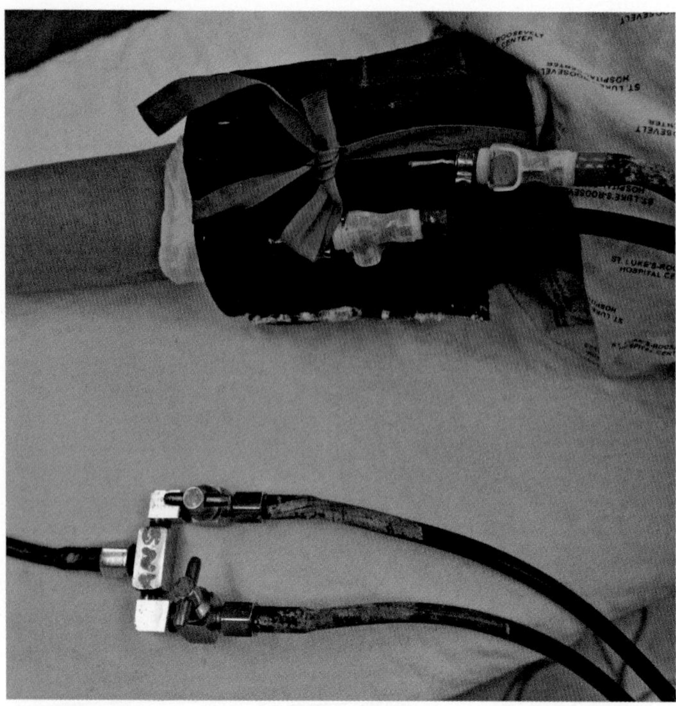

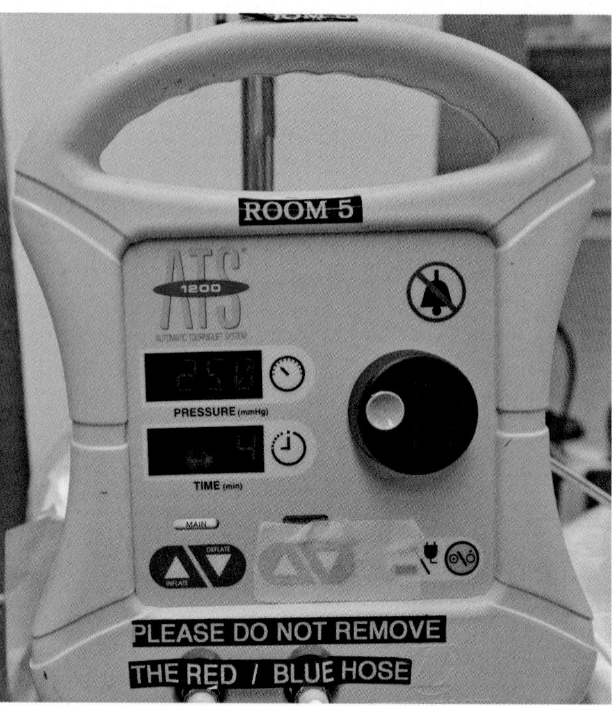


**FIGURE 25-6.** With the Esmarch in place, the double tourniquet is inflated in the following sequence: The distal cuff (red) is inflated first, followed by inflation of the proximal cuff (blue). Once the proximal cuff is inflated and checked for functionality, the distal cuff is deflated. The cuff pressure is determined by the patient's systolic blood pressure; the cuff pressure should be about 100 mmHg above the arterial systolic blood pressure.

10. The onset of anesthesia is almost immediate after injection. When the tourniquet pain is reported by the patient, the distal cuff should be inflated and the proximal cuff deflated about 25 to 30 minutes after the beginning of anesthesia (Figure 25-8).

## TIPS

- Sequence for managing tourniquet pain:
  - Inflate *distal* cuff.
  - Assure that *distal* cuff is inflated.
  - Deflate *proximal* cuff.

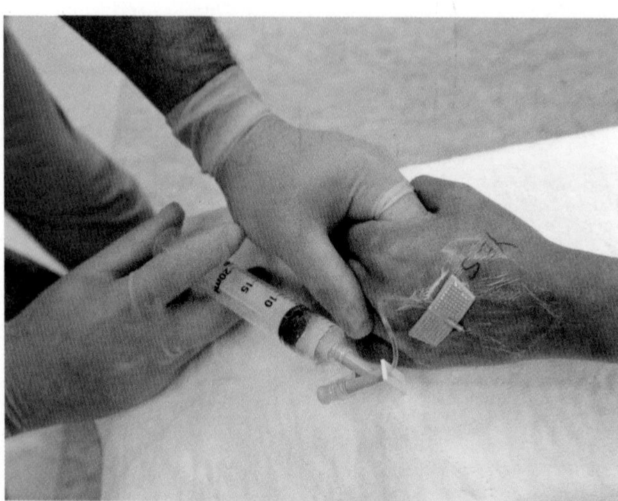

**FIGURE 25-7.** With the extremity exsanguinated and the proximal cuff inflated, local anesthetic is injected to anesthetize the extremity.

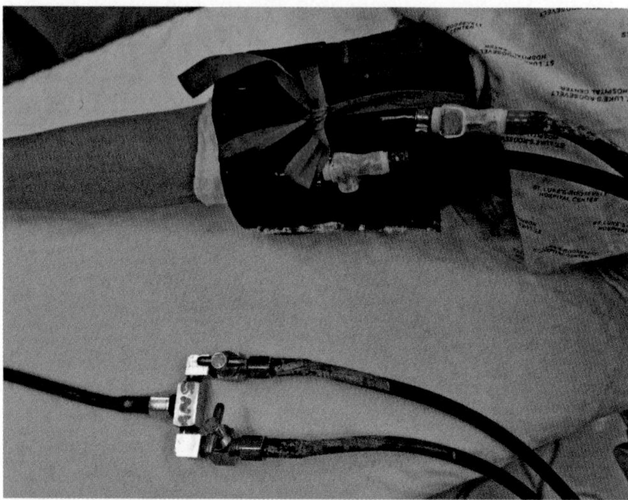

**FIGURE 25-8.** Management of the tourniquet pain. When the patient complains of tourniquet pain, the distal cuff (red) is inflated. Once the distal tourniquet is assured to be inflated and functional, the proximal tourniquet (blue) is deflated. All connectors must be clearly labeled (color coded in our practice) to avoid error in the sequence of inflation/deflation.

## Choice of a Local Anesthetic

Almost all local anesthetic agents have been reported to have been used for IVRA. At present, lidocaine remains the most commonly used local anesthetic of choice in North America. When used in the recommended dose of not more than 3 mg/kg, it appears to be remarkably safe in IV regional blockade. Most researchers report the use of a large volume of a dilute solution of local anesthetic. We often use a smaller volume of a concentrated agent to simplify by avoiding the need for dilution and multiple syringes. By using smaller volumes, we find the procedure tends to be more straightforward and less time consuming; the medication is simpler to prepare and easier to inject.

In some European institutions, prilocaine remains a preferred agent in IVRA. It may be the least toxic of the drugs used currently, and it is better tolerated than lidocaine in terms of systemic and central nervous system side effects. However, because it has been associated with the formation of methemoglobin, prilocaine is not used in North America.

Much research has been done on suitable adjuncts and additives to reduce anesthetic dose and to obtain improved tourniquet tolerance, better muscle relaxation, and prolonged postoperative pain control. Research evidence suggests that some adjuvants may offer some benefits. (e.g., ketorolac, clonidine, meperidine, and muscle relaxants). However, in our opinion, the marginal benefits may not justify the routine use of any additive because they do not outweigh the risk of increased complexity, potential for side effects, and drug error that may occur during addition of adjuvants to local anesthetics.

## Block Dynamics and Perioperative Management

With a Bier block, anesthesia of the extremity typically develops within 5 minutes. Progressive numbness and complete insensitivity are followed by patchy decolorization of the skin and motor paralysis. Some patients report a tingly or cold sensation in the limb. However, with adequate premedication, this sign is often missed. After 30 to 45 minutes, the majority of patients report discomfort at the site of the inflated tourniquet. When this occurs, the distal cuff of the tourniquet should be inflated and the proximal cuff deflated. This maneuver provides immediate and significant relief, and the patient gains an additional 15 to 30 minutes of relative comfort. As soon as the patient gives notice of tourniquet pain, the surgeon should be consulted for information on the expected time necessary to complete the operation. The proximal tourniquet however, should never be released before inflation of the distal cuff. Proper labeling of the proximal and distal cuffs and their respective valves is of the utmost importance. Deflation of the wrong cuff will result in the rapid loss of anesthesia and the risk of systemic local anesthetic toxicity.

With respect to deflating the tourniquet at the end of a short surgical procedure (i.e., <45 minutes), it remains important to proceed cautiously. Several protocols for deflation are published. We adhere to a two-stage deflation: The tourniquet is deflated for 10 seconds and reinflated for 1 minute before the final release. This sequence results in a more gradual washout of the local anesthetic agent, and, as such, it reduces the chances of systemic toxicity.

## Possible Complications

Untoward sequelae are few. Most of the reports of complications are related to equipment failure or other factors not directly attributable to the method itself (e.g., neglecting protocol guidelines). Table 25-1 lists complications and ways to prevent them.

| TABLE 25-1 | Complications and How to Avoid Them |
|---|---|
| ***Systemic toxicity of local anesthetic*** | • The risk mainly comes from an inadequate tourniquet application or equipment failure at the beginning of the procedure.<br>• Every precaution should be undertaken to ensure that the tourniquet is reliable and the pressure is maintained, that is, before the start of the procedure.<br>• Gradually, release the tourniquet in two steps to prevent a massive "washout" of local anesthetic.<br>• When the surgical procedure is completed within 20 min after injection of local anesthetic, gradually release the tourniquet in several steps, with 2-min intervals between deflations.<br>• Do not use long-acting, more toxic LAs (e.g., bupivacaine).<br>• Have intralipid readily available. |
| ***Hematoma*** | • Use a small-gauge IV catheter (22 gauge).<br>• When the superficial veins are punctured during an unsuccessful attempt at placement of the IV catheter, apply firm pressure on the puncture site for 2–3 min. to prevent venous bleeding and possible hematoma during application of the Esmarch. |
| ***Engorgement of the extremity*** | • Ensure that the tourniquet is fully functional and the arterial pulse is absent.<br>• Elevate the limb for a few minutes before winding the Esmarch bandage around it.<br>• Apply digital pressure on the axillary artery before inflating the tourniquet.<br>• Use small volumes of local anesthetic; consider lower placement of tourniquet.<br>• This scenario may be more common in patients with arteriosclerosis; the calcifications in the arterial walls prevent effective functioning of the tourniquet; consequently, the arterial blood continues to enter the distal extremity while the venous blood is unable to escape, resulting in engorgement of the extremity and occasionally ecchymotic hemorrhage in the subcutaneous tissue. This should be considered when discussing selection of anesthesia technique.<br>• In case of engorgement, consider re-exsanguination. Twenty minutes after onset of anesthesia it is possible to rewrap the extremity with an Esmarch bandage, after which the tourniquet can be deflated and reinflated at once. |
| ***Ecchymosis and subcutaneous hemorrhage*** | • The previously described principles apply.<br>• Assure that adequate padding is used over the arm where the application of the tourniquet is planned. |

# INTRAVENOUS REGIONAL ANESTHESIA (UPPER LIMB)

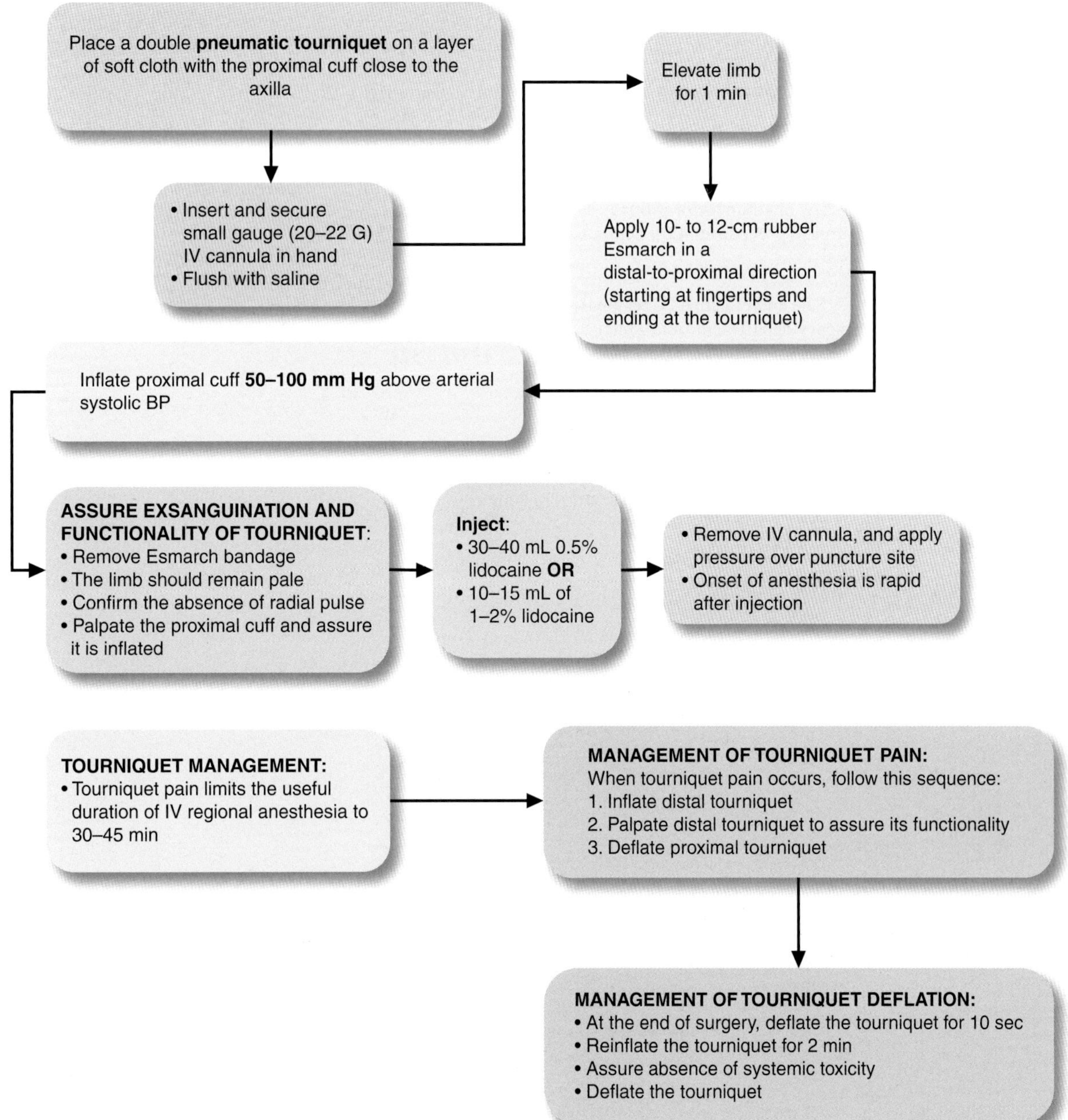

## SUGGESTED READING


Bannister M. Bier's block. *Anaesthesia.* 1997;52:713.

Blyth MJ, Kinninmonth AW, Asante DK. Bier's block: a change of injection site. *J Trauma.* 1995;39:726.

Brown EM, McGriff JT, Malinowski RW. Intravenous regional anaesthesia (Bier block): review of 20 years' experience. *Can J Anaesth.* 1989;36:307.

Casale R, Glynn C, Buonocore M. The role of ischaemia in the analgesia which follows Bier's block technique. *Pain.* 1992;50:169.

Choyce A, Peng P. A systematic review of adjuncts for intravenous regional anesthesia for surgical procedures. *Can J Anesth.* 2002;49:32-45.

de May JC. Bier's block. *Anaesthesia.* 1997;52:713.

Farrell RG, Swanson SL, Walter JR. Safe and effective IV regional anesthesia for use in the emergency department. *Ann Emerg Med.* 1985;14:288.

Hadžić A, Vloka JD, Kuroda MM, Koorn R, Birnbach DJ. The practice of peripheral nerve blocks in the United States: a national survey. *Reg Anesth Pain Med.* 1998;23:241-246.

Hilgenhurst G. The Bier block after 80 years: a historical review. *Reg Anesth.* 1990;15:2.

Holmes CM. Intravenous regional neural blockade. In Cousins MJ, Bridenbaugh PO, eds. *Neuronal Blockade in Clinical Anesthesia and Management of Pain.* Philadelphia, PA: Lippincott-Raven; 1988:395-409.

Hunt SJ, Cartwright PD. Bier's block—under pressure? *Anaesthesia.* 1997;52:188.

Moore DC. Bupivacaine toxicity and Bier block: the drug, the technique, or the anesthetist. *Anesthesiology.* 1984;61:782.

Tramer MR, Glynn CJ. Magnesium Bier's block for treatment of chronic limb pain: a randomised, double-blind, cross-over study. *Pain.* 2002;99:235.

Van Zundert A, Helmstadter A, Goerig M. Centennial of intravenous regional anesthesia. Bier's block (1908–2008). *Reg Anesth Pain Med.* 2008;33:483-489.

Wilson JK, Lyon GD. Bier block tourniquet pressure. *Anesth Analg.* 1989;68:823.

# Foundations Of Ultrasound-Guided Nerve Blocks

# 26 Ultrasound Physics

*Daquan Xu*

## Introduction

Ultrasound application allows for noninvasive visualization of tissue structures. Real-time ultrasound images are integrated images resulting from reflection of organ surfaces and scattering within heterogeneous tissues. Ultrasound scanning is an interactive procedure involving the operator, patient, and ultrasound instruments. Although the physics behind ultrasound generation, propagation, detection, and transformation into practical information is rather complex, its clinical application is much simpler. Understanding the essential ultrasound physics presented in this chapter should be useful for comprehending the principles behind ultrasound-guided peripheral nerve blockade.

## History of Ultrasound

In 1880, French physicists Pierre Curie, and his elder brother Jacques Curie, discovered the piezoelectric effect in certain crystals. Paul Langevin, a student of Pierre Curie, developed piezoelectric materials, which can generate and receive mechanical vibrations with high frequency (therefore *ultrasound*). During WWI, ultrasound was introduced in the navy as a means to detect enemy submarines. In the medical field, however, ultrasound was initially used for therapeutic rather than diagnostic purposes. In the late 1920s, Paul Langevin discovered that high power ultrasound could generate heat in bone and disrupt animal tissues. As a result, ultrasound was used to treat patients with Ménière disease, Parkinson disease, and rheumatic arthritis throughout the early 1950s. Diagnostic applications of ultrasound began through the collaboration of physicians and SONAR engineers. In 1942, Karl Dussik, a neuropsychiatrist and his brother, Friederich Dussik, a physicist, described ultrasound as a diagnostic tool to visualize neoplastic tissues in the brain and the cerebral ventricles. However, limitations of ultrasound instrumentation at the time prevented further development of clinical applications until the early 1970s.

With regard to regional anesthesia, as early as 1978, P. La Grange and his colleagues were the first anesthesiologists to publish a case-series report of ultrasound application for peripheral nerve blockade. They simply used a Doppler transducer to locate the subclavian artery and performed supraclavicular brachial plexus block in 61 patients (Figure 26-1). Reportedly, Doppler guidance led to a high block success rate (98%) and absence of complications such as pneumothorax, phrenic nerve palsy, hematoma, convulsion, recurrent laryngeal nerve block, and spinal anesthesia.

In 1989, P. Ting and V. Sivagnanaratnam reported the use of B-mode ultrasonography to demonstrate the anatomy of the axilla and to observe the spread of local anesthetics during axillary brachial plexus block. In 1994, Stephan Kapral and colleagues systematically explored brachial plexus with B-mode ultrasound. Since that time, multiple teams worldwide have worked tirelessly on defining and improving the application of ultrasound imaging in regional anesthesia. Ultrasound-guided nerve blockade is currently used routinely in the practice of regional anesthesia in many centers worldwide.

Here is a summary of ultrasound quick facts:

- 1880: Pierre and Jacques Curie discovered the piezoelectric effect in crystals.
- 1915: Ultrasound was used by the navy for detecting submarines.

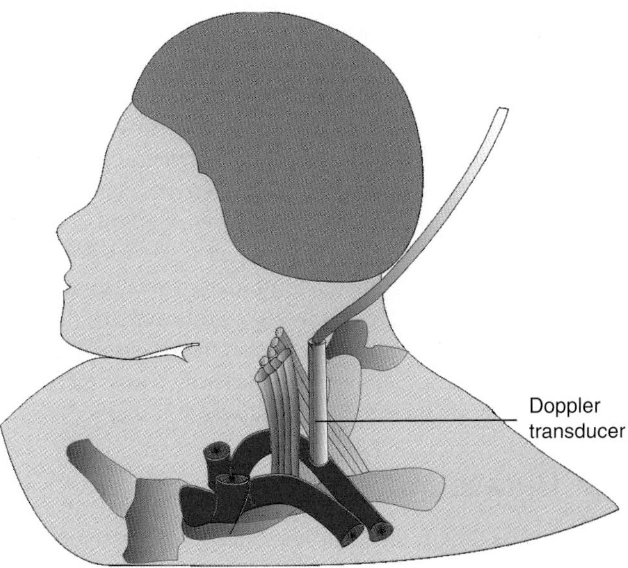


**FIGURE 26-1.** Early application of Doppler ultrasound by LaGrange to perform supraclavicular brachial block.

- 1920s: Paul Langevin discovers that high-power ultrasound can generate heat in osseous tissues and disrupt animal tissues.
- 1942: Karl and Dussik described ultrasound use as a diagnostic tool.
- 1950s: Ultrasound was used to treat patients with Ménière disease, Parkinson disease, and rheumatic arthritis.
- 1978: P. La Grange published the first case-series of ultrasound application for placement of needles for nerve blocks.
- 1989: P. Ting and V. Sivagnanaratnam used ultrasonography to demonstrate the anatomy of the axilla and to observe the spread of local anesthetics during axillary block.
- 1994: Steven Kapral and colleagues explored brachial plexus blockade using B-mode ultrasound.

## Definition of Ultrasound

Sound travels as a mechanical longitudinal wave in which back-and-forth particle motion is parallel to the direction of wave travel. Ultrasound is high-frequency sound and refers to mechanical vibrations above 20 kHz. Human ears can hear sounds with frequencies between 20 Hz and 20 kHz. Elephants can generate and detect the sound with frequencies <20 Hz for long-distance communication; bats and dolphins produce sounds in the range of 20 to 100 kHz for precise navigation (Figure 26-2A and B). Ultrasound frequencies commonly used for medical diagnosis are between 2 MHz and 15 MHz. However, sounds with frequencies above 100 kHz do not occur naturally; only human-developed devices can both generate and detect these frequencies, or ultrasounds.

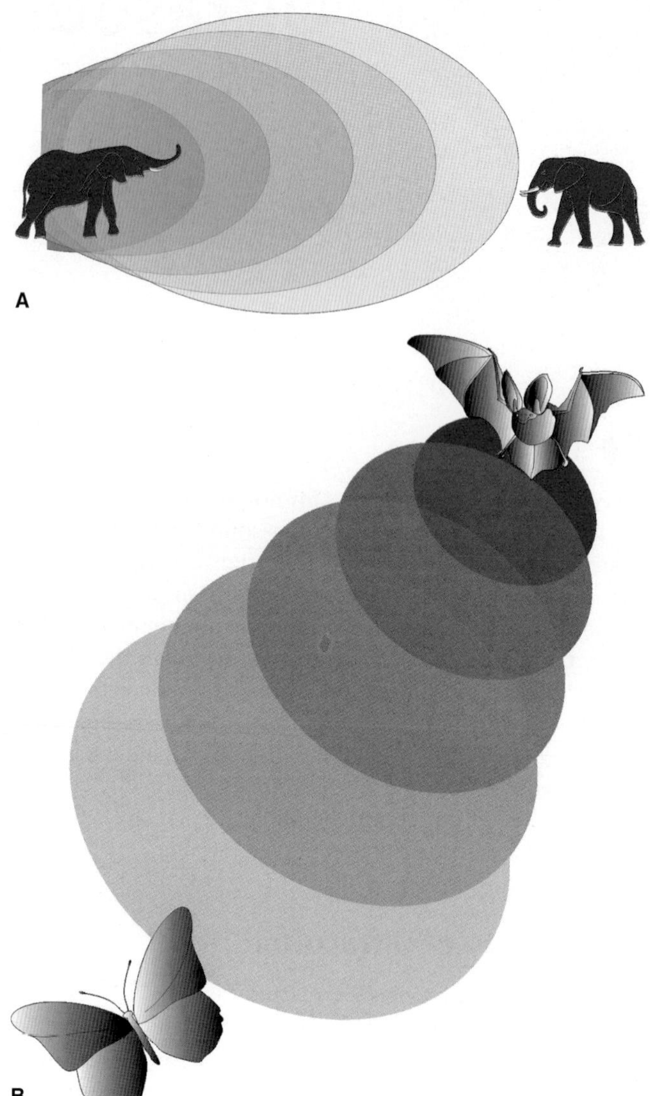


**FIGURE 26-2.** (A) Elephants can generate and detect the sound of frequencies <20 Hz for long-distance communication. (B) Bats and dolphins produce sounds in the range of 20–100 kHz for navigation and spatial orientation.

## Piezoelectric Effect

The piezoelectric effect is a phenomenon exhibited by the generation of an electric charge in response to a mechanical force (squeeze or stretch) applied on certain materials. Conversely, mechanical deformation can be produced when an electric field is applied to such material, also known the piezoelectric effect (Figure 26-3). Both natural and human-made materials, including quartz crystals and ceramic materials, can demonstrate piezoelectric properties. Recently, lead zirconate titanate has been used as piezoelectric material for medical imaging. Lead-free piezoelectric materials are also under development. Individual piezoelectric materials produce a small amount of energy. However, by stacking piezoelectric elements into layers in a transducer, the transducer can convert electric energy into mechanical oscillations more efficiently. These mechanical oscillations are then converted into electric energy.

## Ultrasound Terminology

*Period* is the time it takes for one cycle to occur; the period unit of measure is the microsecond (μs).

*Wavelength* is the length of space over which one cycle occurs; it is equal to the travel distance from the beginning to the end of one cycle.

*Acoustic velocity* is the speed at which a sound wave travels through a medium. It is equal to the frequency times the wavelength. Speed is determined by the density ($\rho$) and stiffness ($\kappa$) of the medium ($c = (\kappa/\rho)^{1/2}$). *Density* is the concentration of medium. *Stiffness* is the resistance of a material to compression. Propagation speed increases if the stiffness is increased or the density is decreased. The average propagation speed in soft tissues is 1540 m/s (ranges from 1400 m/s to 1640 m/s). However, ultrasound cannot penetrate lung or bone tissues.

*Acoustic impedance*($z$) is the degree of difficulty demonstrated by a sound wave being transmitted through a medium; it is equal to density $\rho$ multiplied by acoustic velocity $c$ ($z = \rho c$). It increases if the propagation speed or the density of the medium is increased.

*Attenuation coefficient* is the parameter used to estimate the decrement of ultrasound amplitude in a certain medium

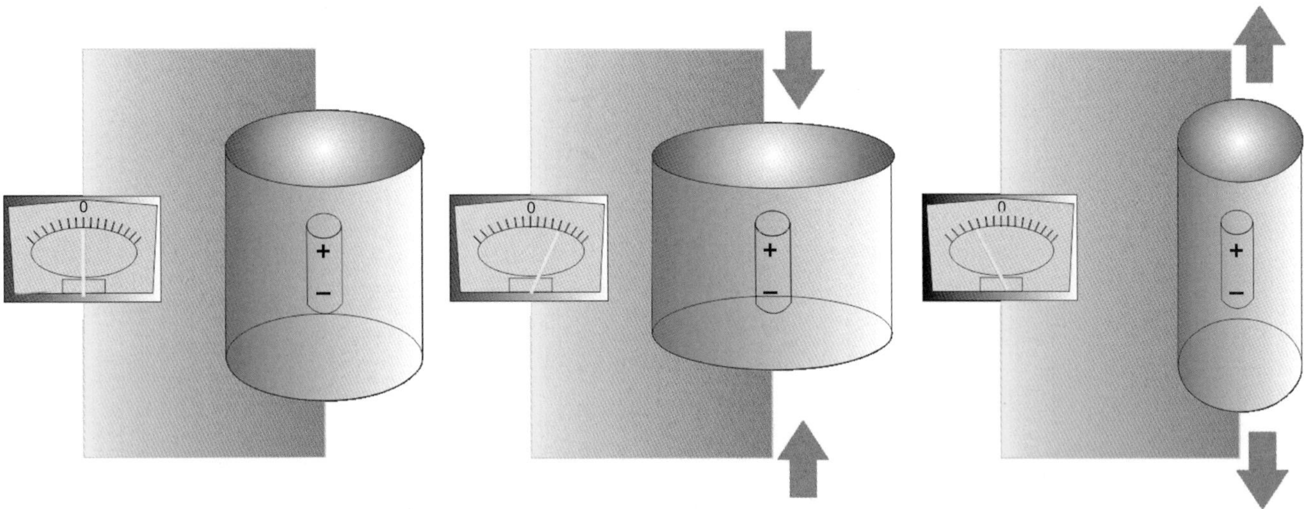


**FIGURE 26-3.** The piezoelectric effect. Mechanical deformation and consequent oscillation caused by an electrical field applied to certain material can produce a sound of high frequency.

as a function of ultrasound frequency. The attenuation coefficient increases with increasing frequency; therefore, a practical consequence of attenuation is that the penetration decreases as frequency increases (Figure 26-4).

Ultrasound waves have a *self-focusing* effect, which refers to the natural narrowing of the ultrasound beam at a certain travel distance in the ultrasonic field. It is a transition level between *near field* and *far field*. The beam width at the transition level is equal to half the diameter of the transducer. At the distance of two times the near-field length, the beam width reaches the transducer diameter. The self-focusing effect amplifies ultrasound signals by increasing acoustic pressure.

In ultrasound imaging, there are two aspects of spatial resolution: axial and lateral. *Axial resolution* is the minimum separation of above-below planes along the beam axis. It is determined by spatial pulse length, which is equal to the product of wavelength and the number of cycles within a pulse. It can be presented in the following formula:

*Axial resolution* = *wavelength* (λ) × *number of cycle per pulse* (*n*) ÷ 2

The number of cycles within a pulse is determined by the damping characteristics of the transducer. The number of cycles within a pulse is usually set between 2 and 4 by the manufacturer of the ultrasound machines. As an example, if a 2-MHz ultrasound transducer is theoretically used to do the scanning, the axial resolution would be between 0.8 and 1.6 mm, making it impossible to visualize a 21-G needle. For a constant acoustic velocity, higher frequency ultrasound can detect smaller objects and provide a better resolution image.

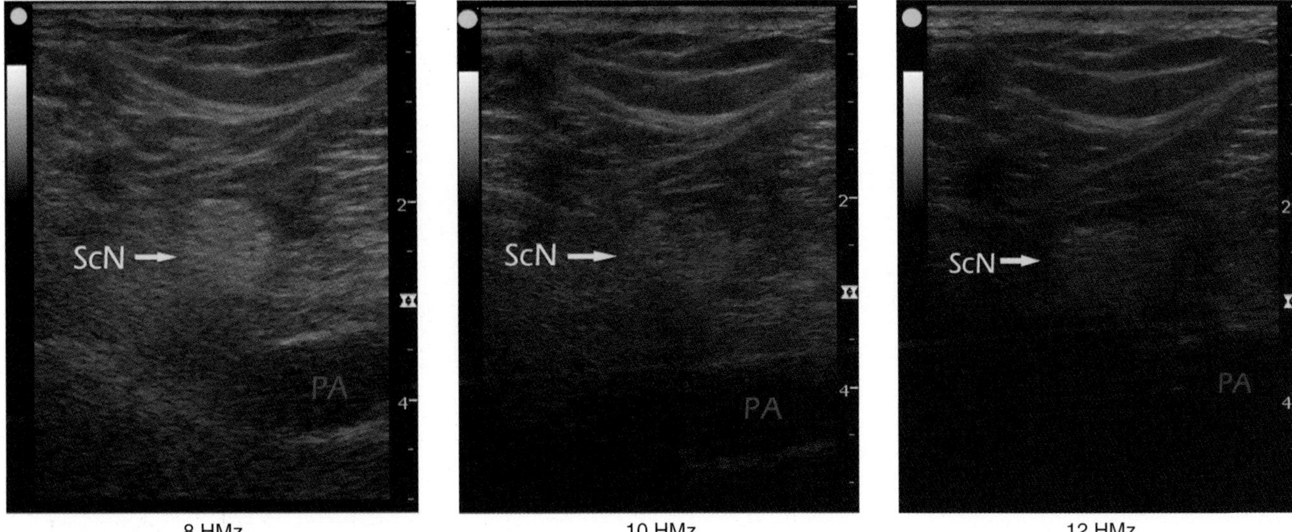


**FIGURE 26-4.** The ultrasound amplitude decreases in certain media as a function of ultrasound frequency, a phenomenon known as attenuation coefficient. ScN-Sciatic nerve, PA - Popliteal artery.

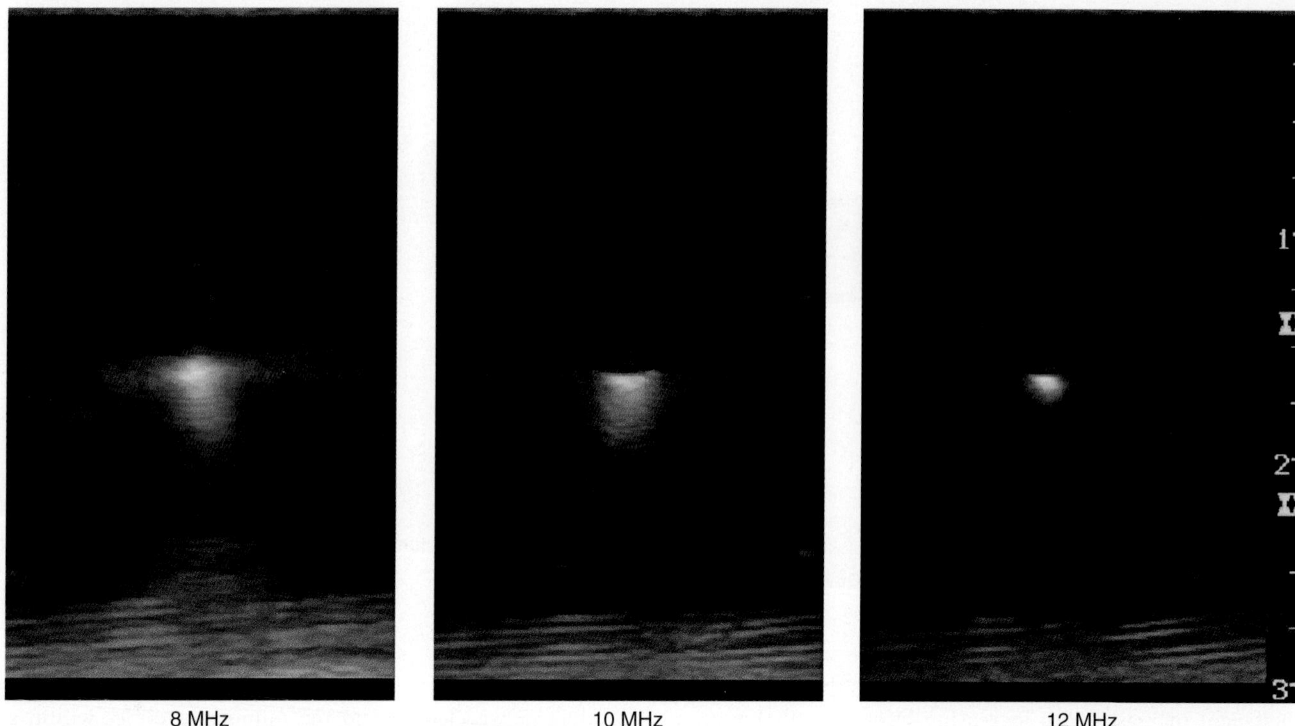


**FIGURE 26-5.** Ultrasound frequency affects the resolution of the imaged object. Resolution can be improved by increasing frequency and reducing the beam width by focusing.

Figure 26-5 shows the images at different resolutions when a 0.5-mm-diameter object is visualized with three different frequency settings. *Lateral resolution* is another parameter of sharpness to describe the minimum side-by-side distance between two objects. It is determined by both ultrasound frequency and beam width. Lateral resolution can be improved by focusing to reduce the beam width.

*Temporal resolution* is also important to observe moving objects, such as blood vessels and the heart. Similar to a movie or cartoon video, the human eye requires that the image be updated at a rate of approximately 25 times a second or higher for an ultrasound image to appear continuous. However, imaging resolution is compromised by increasing the frame rate. Optimizing the ratio of resolution to frame rate is essential to provide the best possible image.

## Interactions of Ultrasound Waves with Tissue

As the ultrasound wave travels through tissue, it is subject to a number of interactions. The most important features are as follows:

- Reflection
- Scatter
- Absorption

When an ultrasound wave encounters boundaries between different media, part of the ultrasound is reflected and other part is transmitted. The reflected and transmitted directions are given by the reflection angle $\theta_r$ and transmission angle $\theta_t$, respectively (Figure 26-6).

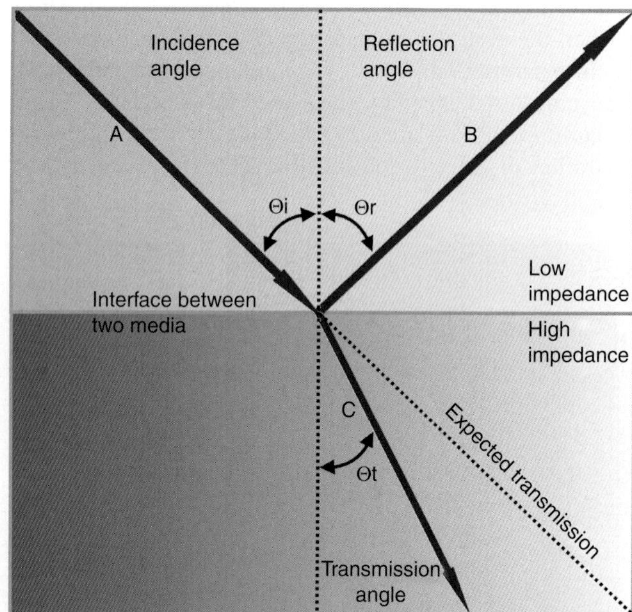


**FIGURE 26-6.** The interaction of ultrasound waves through the media in which they travel is complex. When ultrasound encounters boundaries between different media, part of the ultrasound is reflected and part transmitted. The reflected and transmitted directions depend on the respective angles of reflection and transmission.

*Reflection* of a sound wave is very similar to optical reflection. Some of its energy is sent back into the originating medium. In a true reflection, reflection angle $\theta_r$ must equal incidence angle $\theta_i$. The strength of the reflection from an interface is variable and depends on the difference of impedances between two affinitive media and the incident angle at boundary. If the media impedances are equal, there is no reflection (no echo). If there is a significant difference between media impedances, there will be far greater or nearly complete reflection. For example, an interface between soft tissues and either lung or bone involves a considerable change in acoustic impedance and creates strong echoes. This reflection intensity is also highly angle dependent, meaning that the ultrasound transducer must be placed perpendicularly to the target nerve to visualize it clearly.

A change in sound direction when crossing the boundary between two media is called *refraction*. If the propagation speed through the second medium is slower than it is through the first medium, the refraction angle is smaller than the incident angle. Refraction can cause artifacts such as those that occur beneath large vessels.

During ultrasound scanning, a coupling medium must be used between the transducer and the skin to displace air from the transducer–skin interface. A variety of gels and oils are applied for this purpose. They also act as lubricants, providing a smooth surface scanning.

Most scanned interfaces are somewhat irregular and curved. If boundary dimensions are significantly less than the wavelength or not smooth, the reflected waves will be diffused. *Scattering* is the redirection of sound in any direction by rough surfaces or by heterogeneous media (Figure 26-7). Normally, scattering intensity is much less than mirrorlike reflection intensities and is relatively independent of the direction of the incident sound wave. Therefore, the visualization of the target nerve is not significantly influenced by other nearby scattering.

*Absorption* is defined as the direct conversion of sound energy into heat. In other words, ultrasound scanning generates heat in the tissue. Higher frequencies are absorbed at a greater rate than lower frequencies. However, higher scanning frequency gives better axial resolution. If the ultrasound penetration is not sufficient to visualize the structures of interest, a lower frequency is selected to increase the penetration. The use of longer wavelengths (lower frequency) results in lower resolution because the resolution of ultrasound imaging is proportional to the wavelength of the imaging wave. Frequencies between 6 and 12 MHz typically yield better resolution for imaging of the peripheral nerves because they are located more superficially. Lower imaging frequencies, between 2 and 5 MHz, are usually needed for imaging of neuraxial structures. For most clinical applications, frequencies less than 2 MHz or higher than 15 MHz are rarely used because of insufficient resolution or insufficient penetration, respectfully.

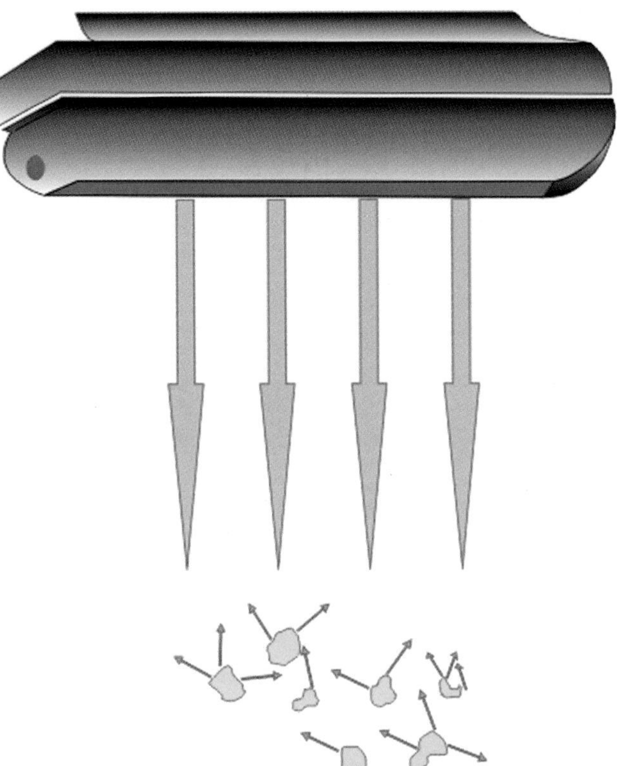

**FIGURE 26-7.** Scattering is the redirection of ultrasound in any direction caused by rough surfaces or by heterogeneous media.

## Ultrasound Image Modes

### A-Mode

The A-mode is the oldest ultrasound modality, dating back to 1930. The transducer sends a single pulse of ultrasound into the medium and waits for the returned signal. Consequently, a simple one-dimensional ultrasound image is generated as a series of vertical peaks corresponding to the depth of the structures at which the ultrasound beam encounters different tissues. The distance between the echoed spikes (Figure 26-8) can be calculated by dividing the speed of the ultrasound in the tissue (1540 m/sec) by half the elapsed time. This mode provides little information on the spatial relationships of the imaged structures, however. Therefore, A-mode ultrasound is not used in regional anesthesia.

### B-Mode

The B-mode supplies a two-dimensional image of the area by simultaneously scanning from a linear array of 100–300 piezoelectric elements rather than a single one, as is the case in A-mode. The amplitude of the echo from a series of A-scans is converted into dots of different brightness in B-mode imaging. The horizontal and vertical directions represent real distances in tissue, whereas the intensity of the grayscale indicates echo strength (Figure 26-9). B mode can provide a cross

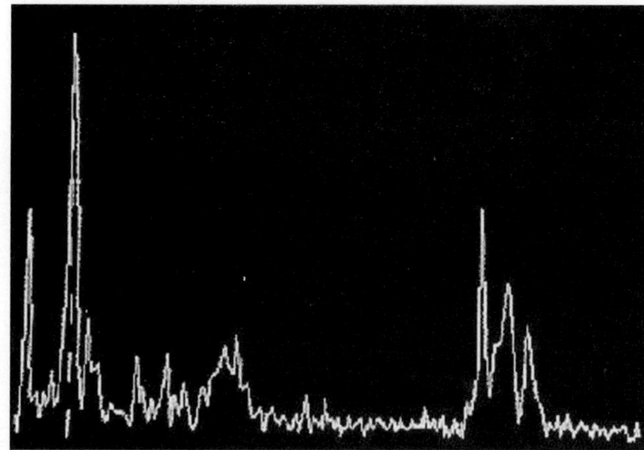

**FIGURE 26-8.** The A-mode of ultrasound consists of a one-dimensional ultrasound image displayed as a series of vertical peaks corresponding to the depth of structures at which the ultrasound encounters different tissues.

sectional image through the area of interest and is the primary mode currently used in regional anesthesia.

## Doppler Mode

The *Doppler effect* is based on the work of Austrian physicist Johann Christian Doppler. The term describes a change in the frequency or wavelength of a sound wave resulting from relative motion between the sound source and the sound receiver. In other words, at a stationary position, the sound frequency is constant. If the sound source moves toward the sound receiver, a higher pitched sound occurs. If the sound source moves away from the receiver, the received sound has a lower pitch (Figure 26-10).

Color Doppler produces a color-coded map of Doppler shifts superimposed onto a B-mode ultrasound image. Blood flow direction depends on whether the motion is toward or away from the transducer. Selected by convention, red and blue colors provide information about the direction and velocity of the blood flow. According to the color map (color bar) in the upper left-hand corner of the figure (Figure 26-11), the red color on the top of the bar denotes the flow coming toward the ultrasound probe, and the blue color on the bottom of the bar indicates the flow away from the probe. In ultrasound-guided peripheral nerve blocks, color Doppler mode is used to detect the presence and nature of the blood vessels (artery vs. vein) in the area of interest. When the direction of the ultrasound beam changes, the color of the arterial flow switches from blue to red, or vice versa, depending on the convention used. Power Doppler is up to five times more sensitive in detecting blood flow than color Doppler and it is less dependent on the scanning angle. Thus power Doppler can be used to identify the smaller blood vessels more reliably. The drawback is that

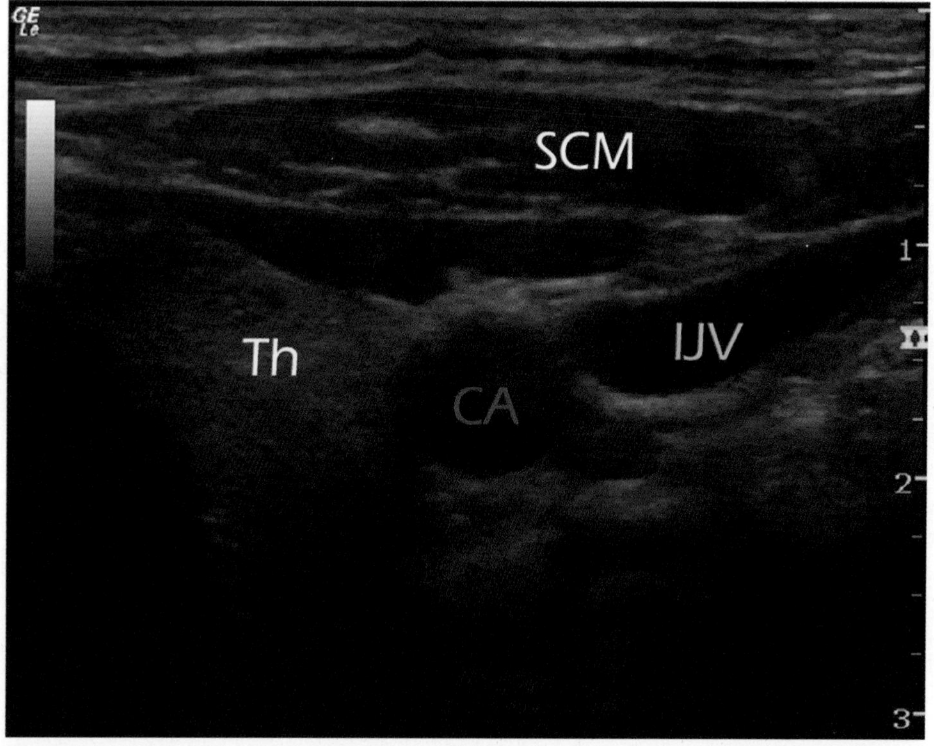


B-Mode

**FIGURE 26-9.** An example of B-mode imaging. The horizontal and vertical directions represent distances and tissues, whereas the intensity of the grayscale indicates echo strength. Scm-sternocleidomastoid muscle, IJV-Internal jugular vein, CA-carotid artery, Th-Thyroid gland.

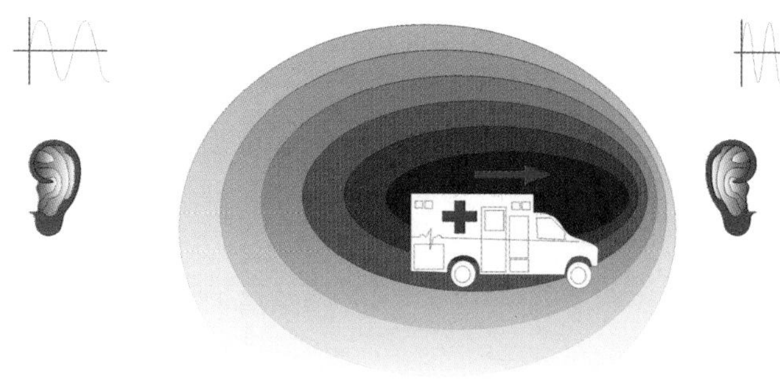

**FIGURE 26-10.** The Doppler effect. When a sound source moves away from the receiver, the received sound has a lower pitch and vice versa.

power Doppler does not provide any information on the direction and speed of blood flow (Figure 26-12).

## M-Mode

A single beam in an ultrasound scan can be used to produce a picture with a motion signal, where movement of a structure such as a heart valve can be depicted in a wave-like manner. M-mode is used extensively in cardiac and fetal cardiac imaging; however, its present use in regional anesthesia is negligible (Figure 26-13).

## Ultrasound Instruments

Ultrasound machines convert the echoes received by the transducer into visible dots, which form the anatomic image on ultrasound screen. The brightness of each dot corresponds to the echo strength, producing what is known as a grayscale image.

Two types of scan transducers are used in regional anesthesia: linear and curved. A linear transducer can produce parallel scan lines and rectangular display, called a linear scan, whereas a curved transducer yields a curvilinear scan and arc-shaped image (Figure 26-14A and B). In clinical scanning, even a very thin layer of air between the transducer and skin may reflect virtually all the ultrasound, hindering any penetration into the tissue. Therefore, a coupling medium, usually an aqueous gel, is applied between surfaces of the transducer and skin to eliminate the air layer. The ultrasound machines currently used in regional anesthesia provide a two-dimensional image, or "slice." Machines capable of producing three-dimensional images have recently been developed. Theoretically, three-dimensional (3D) imaging should help in understanding the relationship of anatomic structures and spread of local anesthetics. (Figure 26-14C and D). At present, however, 3D-real time imaging systems still lack the resolution and simplicity of 2D images, so their practical use in regional anesthesia is limited.

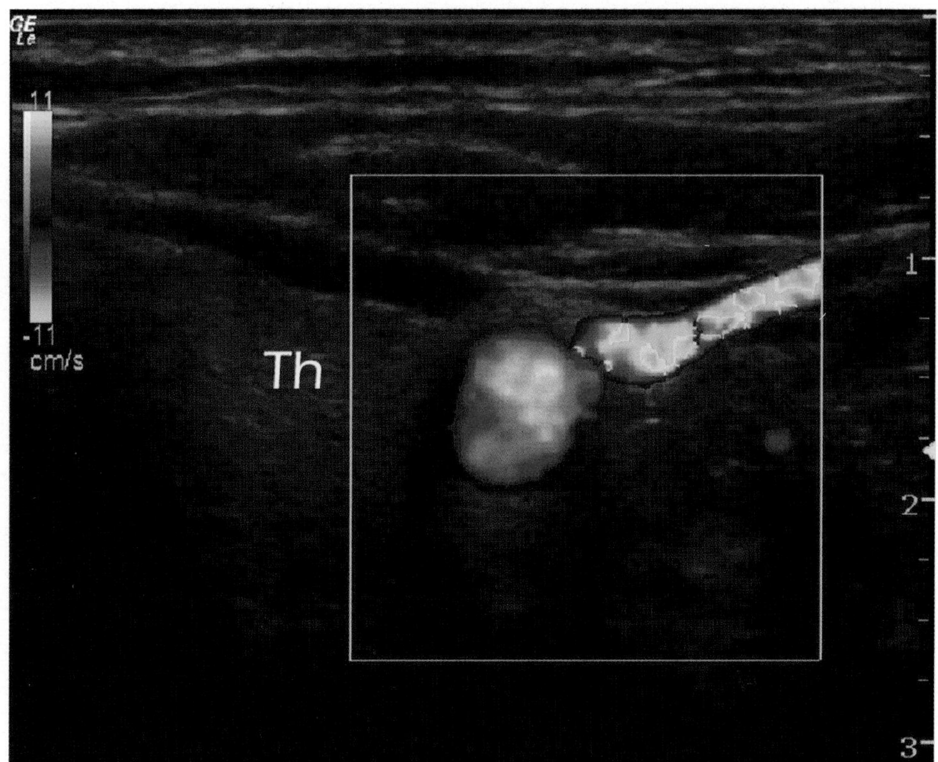


**FIGURE 26-11.** Color Doppler produces a color-coded map of Doppler shapes superimposed onto a B-mode ultrasound image. Selected by convention, red and blue colors provide information about the direction and velocity of the blood flow.

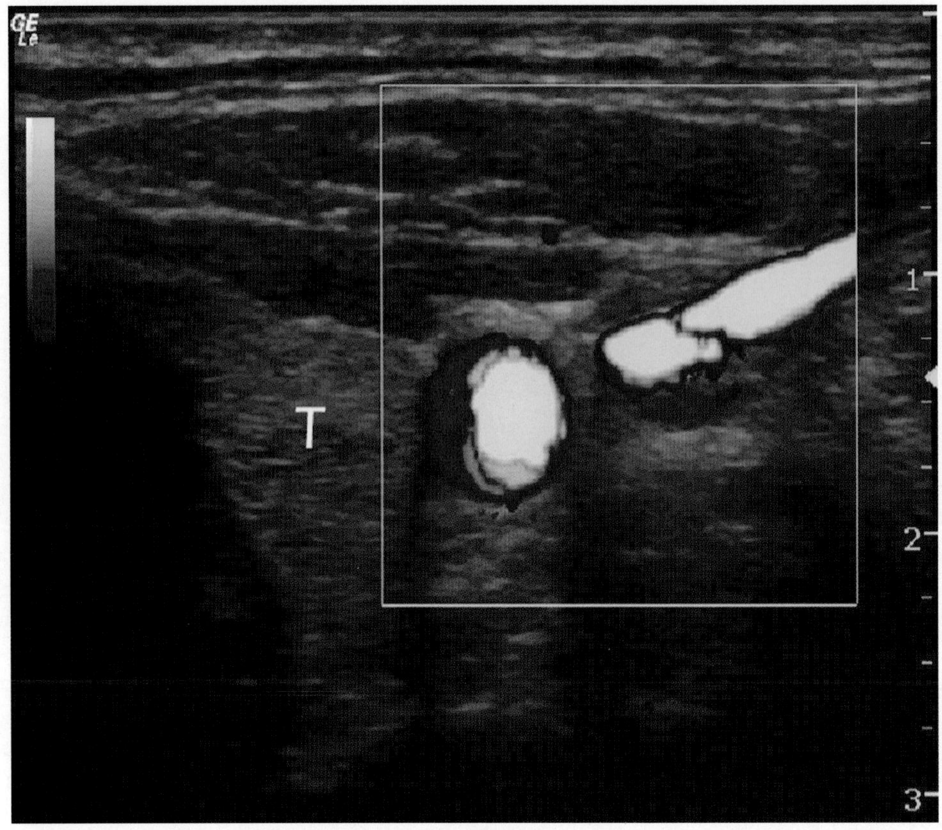


**FIGURE 26-12.** Although the power Doppler may be useful in identifying smaller blood vessels, the drawback is that it does not provided information on the direction and speed of blood flow.

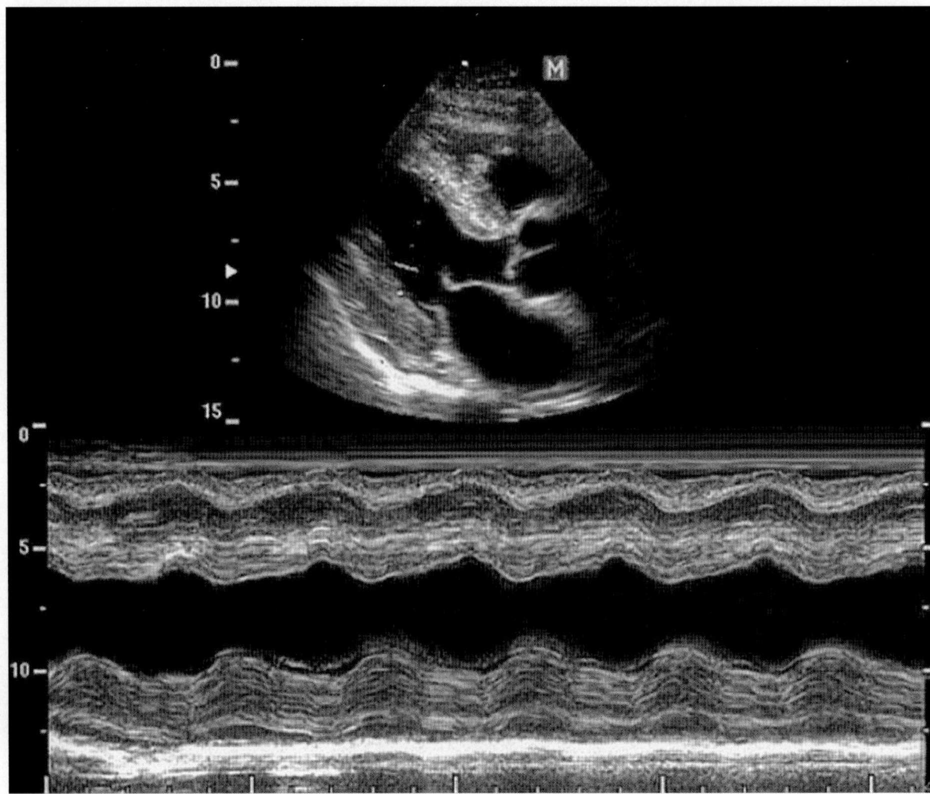


**FIGURE 26-13.** M-mode consists of a single beam used to produce an image with a motion signal. Movement of a structure can be depicted in a wavelike matter.

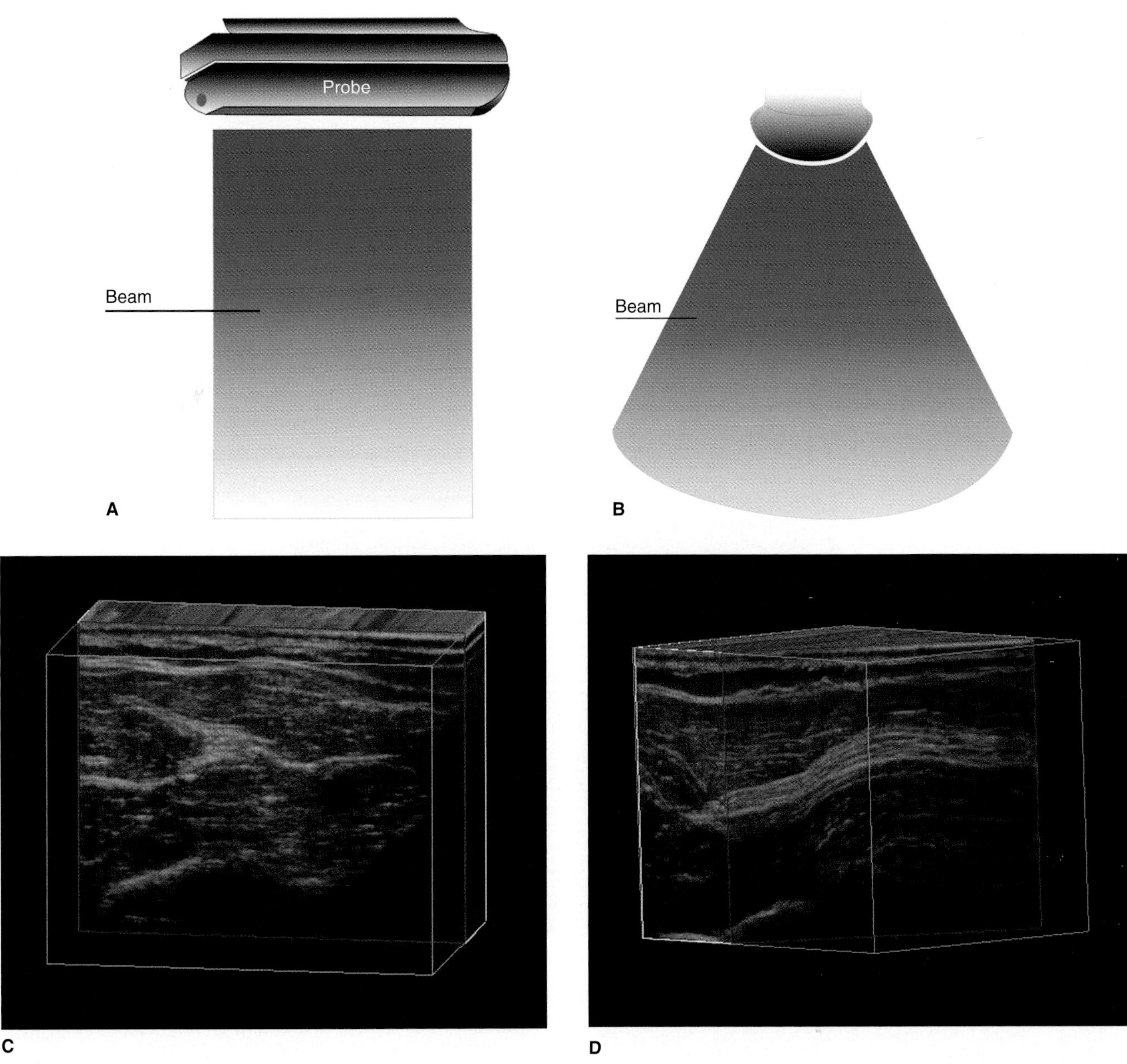


**FIGURE 26-14.** Three-dimensional imaging. (A) A linear transducer produces parallel scan lines and rectangular display; linear scan. (B) A curve "phase array" transducer results in a curvilinear scan and an arch-shaped image. (C) An example of cross-sectional three-dimensional (3D) imaging. (D) An example of longitudinal 3D imaging. Three-dimensional imaging theoretically should provide more spatial orientation of the image structures; however, its current drawback is lower resolution and greater complexity compared with 2D images, which limit its application in the current practice of regional anesthesia.

## Time-Gain Compensation

The echoes exhibit a steady decline in amplitude with increasing depth. This occurs for two reasons: First, each successive reflection removes a certain amount of energy from the pulse, decreasing the generation of later echoes. Second, tissue absorbs ultrasound, so there is a steady loss of energy as the ultrasound pulse travels through the tissues. This can be corrected by manipulating time-gain compensation (TGC) and compression functions.

*Amplification* is the conversion of the small voltages received from the transducer into larger ones that are suitable for further processing and storage. *Gain* is the ratio of output to input electric power. TGC is time-dependent exponential amplification. TGC function can be used to increase the amplitude of incoming signals from various tissue depths. The layout of the TGC controls varies from one machine to another. A popular design is a set of slider knobs; each knob in the slider set controls the gain for a specific depth, which allows for a well-balanced gain scale on the image (Figure 26-15A–C). *Compression* is the process of decreasing the differences between the smallest and largest echo-voltage amplitudes; the optimal compression is between 2 and 4 for maximal scale equal to 6.

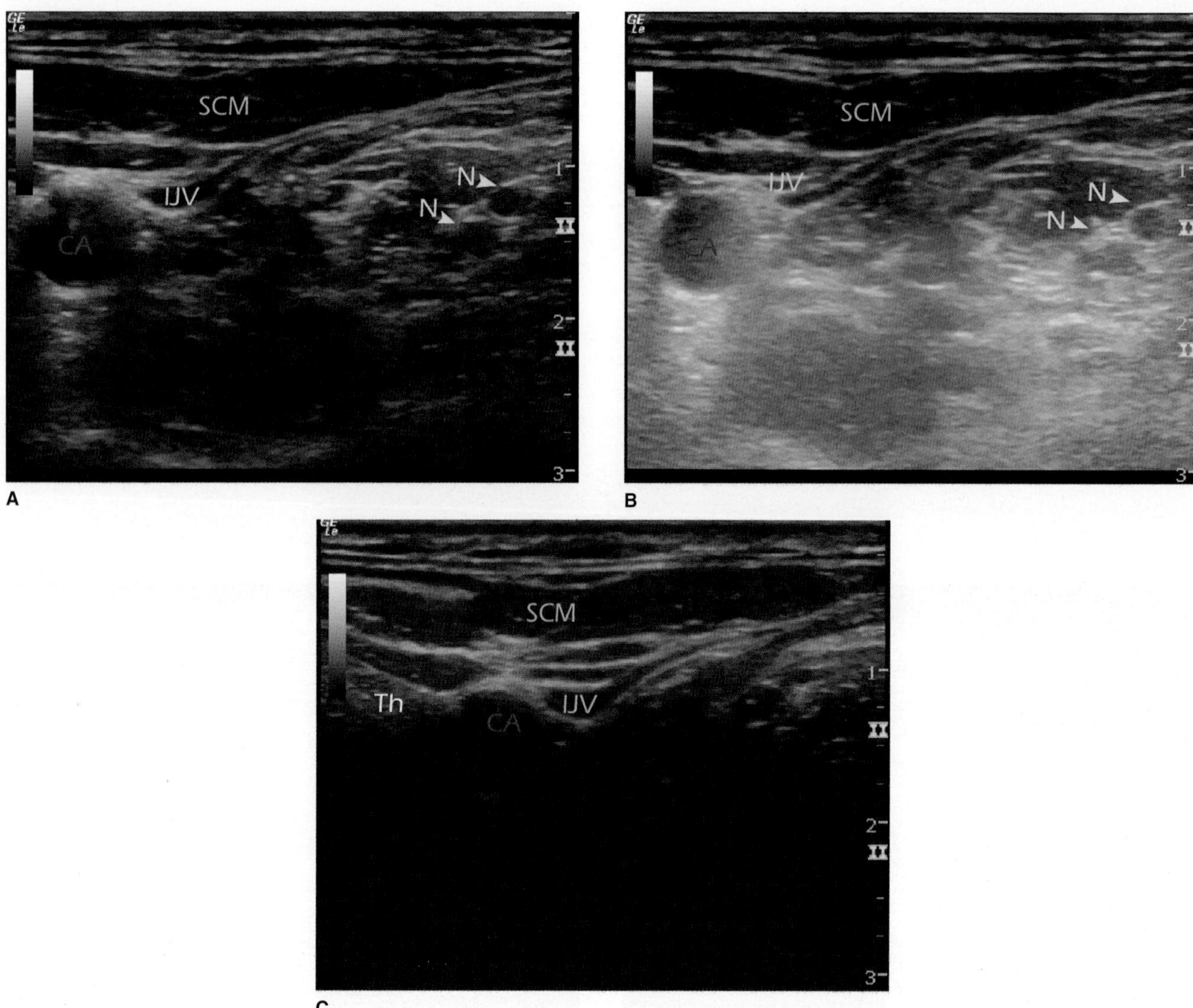


**FIGURE 26-15.** (A–C) The effect of the time-gain compensation settings. Time-gain compensation is a function that allows time (depth) dependent amplification of signals returning from different depths. SCM-sternocleidomastoid muscle, IJV-Internal jugular vein, N-nerve, CA-carotid artery, Th-thyroid gland.

## Focusing

As previously discussed, it is common to use an electronic means to narrow the width of the beam at some depth and achieve a focusing effect similar to that obtained using a convex lens (Figure 26-16). This strategy improves the resolution in the plane because the beam width is converged. However, the reduction in beam width at the selected depth is achieved at the expense of degradation in beam width at other depths, resulting in poorer images below the focal region.

## Bioeffect and Safety

The mechanisms of action by which ultrasound application could produce a biologic effect can be characterized into two aspects: heating and mechanical. The generation of heat increases as ultrasound intensity or frequency is increased. For similar exposure conditions, the expected temperature increase in bone is significantly greater than in soft tissues. Reports in animal models (mice and rats) suggest that application of ultrasound may result in a number of undesired effects, such as fetal weight reduction, postpartum mortality, fetal abnormalities, tissue lesions, hind limb paralysis, blood flow stasis, and tumor regression. Other reported undesired effects in mice are abnormalities in B-cell development and ovulatory response, and teratogenicity. In general, adult tissues are more tolerant of rising temperature than fetal and neonatal tissues. A modern ultrasound machine displays two standard indices: thermal and mechanical. The thermal index (TI) is defined as the transducer acoustic output power divided by the estimated power required to raise tissue

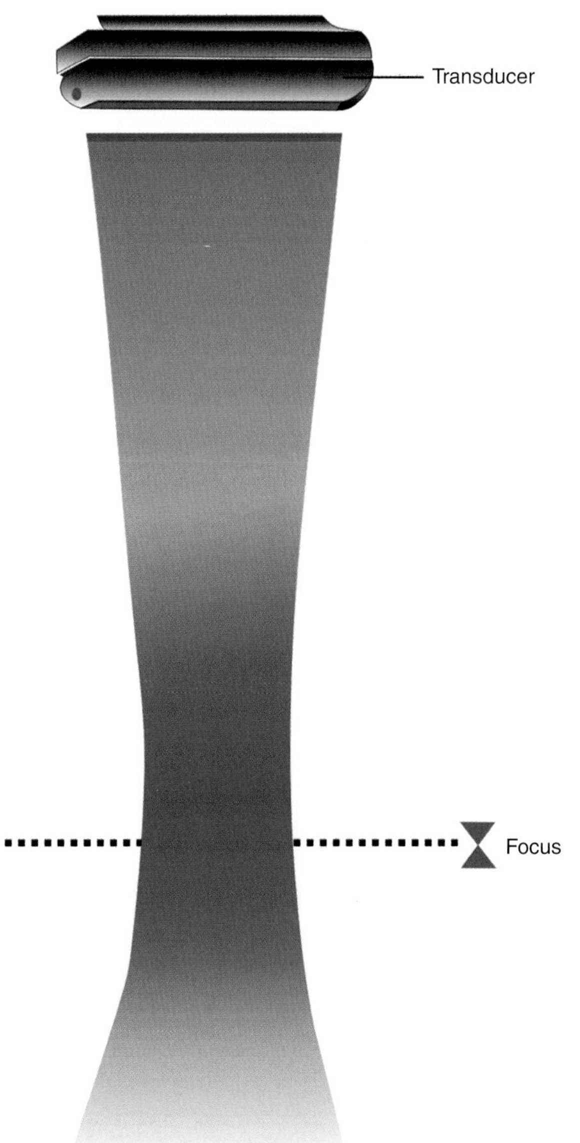


**FIGURE 26-16.** A demonstration of focusing effect. An electronic means can be used to narrow the width of the beam at specific depth resulting in the focusing effect and a greater resolution at a chosen depth.

temperature by 1°C. Mechanical index (MI) is equal to the peak rarefactional pressure divided by the square root of the center frequency of the pulse bandwidth. TI and MI indicate the relative likelihood of thermal and mechanical hazard in vivo, respectively. Either TI or MI >1.0 is hazardous.

Biologic effect due to ultrasound also depends on tissue exposure time. Fortunately, ultrasound-guided nerve block requires the use of only low TI and MI values on the patient for a short period of time. Based on in vitro and in vivo experimental study results to date, there is no evidence that the use of diagnostic ultrasound in routine clinical practice is associated with any biologic risks.

## SUGGESTED READING

Edelman SK. *Understanding Ultrasound Physics.* 3d ed. Woodlands, TX: ESP; 2004.

Hedrick WR, Hykes DL, Starchman DE. *Ultrasound Physics and Instrumentation.* 4th ed. Chicago, IL: Mosby Yearbook; 2004.

Kapral S, Krafft P, Eibenberger K, Fitzgerald R, Gosch M, Weinstabl C. Ultrasound-guided supraclavicular approach for regional anesthesia of the brachial plexus. *Anesth Analg* 1994; 78:507-513.

La Grange PDP, Foster PA, Pretorius LK. Application of the Doppler ultrasound bloodflow detector in supraclavicular brachial plexus block. *Br J Anesth.* 1978;50:965-967.

Marhofer P, Greher M, Kapral S. Ultrasound guidance in regional anaesthesia. *Br J Anesth.* 2005;94:7-17.

O'Neill JM. *Musculoskeletal Ultrasound: Anatomy and Technique.* New York, NY: Springer; 2008.

Ting PL, Sivagnanaratnam V. Ultrasonographic study of the spread of local anaesthetic during axillary brachial plexus block. *Br J Anesth.* 1978;63:326-329.

Zagzebski JA. *Essentials of Ultrasound Physics.* St. Louis, MO: Mosby; 1996.

# 27 Optimizing an Ultrasound Image

*Daquan Xu*

Optimizing an image produced by ultrasound is an essential skill for performance of an ultrasound-guided nerve block. Anatomically, peripheral nerves are often located in the vicinity of an artery or between muscle layers. The echo texture of normal peripheral nerves can have a hyperechoic, hypoechoic, or honeycomb pattern (Figure 27-1). Several scanning steps and techniques can be used to facilitate adequate nerve imaging, including the selection of sonographic modes, adjustment of function keys, needle visualization, and interpretation of image artifacts.

All in all, sonographic imaging modes used for ultrasound-guided regional anesthesia and medical diagnostics are conventional imaging, compound imaging, and tissue harmonic imaging (THI). The *conventional* imaging is generated by a single-element angle beam. The *compound* imaging is implemented by acquiring several (usually three to nine) overlapping frames from different frequencies or from different angles. The *tissue harmonic imaging* acquires the information from harmonic frequencies generated by ultrasound beam transmission through tissue, which improves tissue contrast by suppression of scattering signals. Compound imaging with The *tissue harmonic imaging* can provide images with better resolution, penetration, and interfaces and margin enhancement, compared with those obtained using conventional sonography. In Figure 27-2, compound imaging and conventional imaging was used to view the interscalene brachial plexus. There is a clear margin definition of two hypoechoic oval-shaped nerve structures in compound imaging. As an example, the contrast resolution between the anterior scalene muscle and the surrounding adipose tissue is enhanced in comparison with those made with conventional imaging techniques.

Five function keys on an ultrasound machine are of crucial importance to achieve an optimal image during the performance of peripheral nerve imaging (Figure 27-3A).

1. *Depth*: The depth of the nerve is the first consideration when ultrasound-guided nerve block is performed. The depth at which peripheral nerves are positioned and therefore imaged greatly varies and also depends on a patient's habitus. An optimal depth setting is important for proper focusing properties during imaging. Table 27-1 describes the recommended initial depth settings for common peripheral nerves. The target nerve should be at the center of the ultrasound image to obtain the best resolution of the nerve and reveal other anatomic structures in the vicinity of the nerve. For example, ultrasound imaging during supraclavicular or infraclavicular brachial plexus blockade requires that first rib and pleura are viewed simultaneously to decrease the risk of lung puncture with the needle.

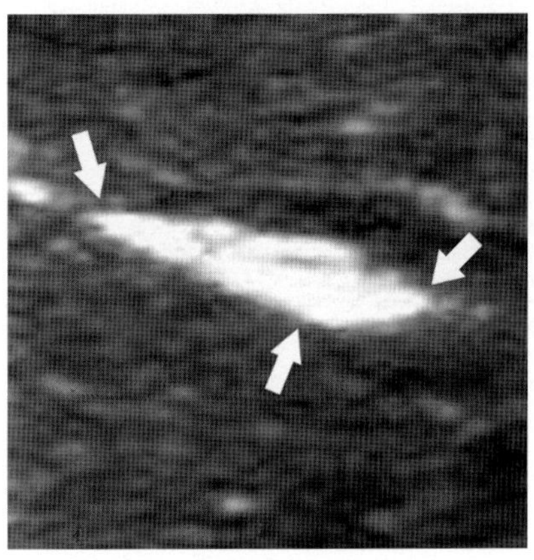

Hyperechoic
(Musculocutaneous nerve)

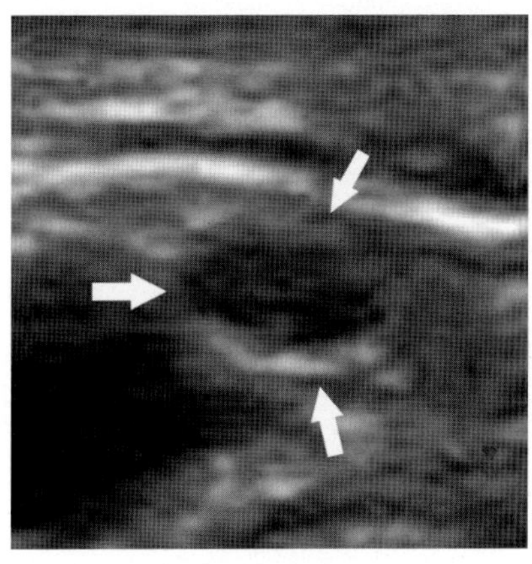

Hypoechoic
(Ulnar nerve)

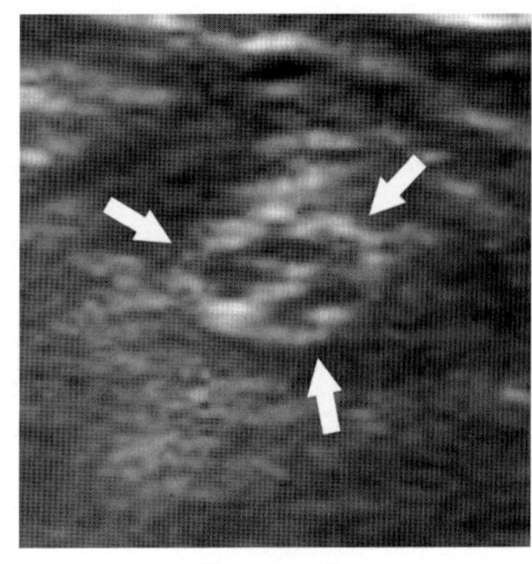

Honeycomb
(median nerve)

**FIGURE 27-1.** Architecture of peripheral nerves.

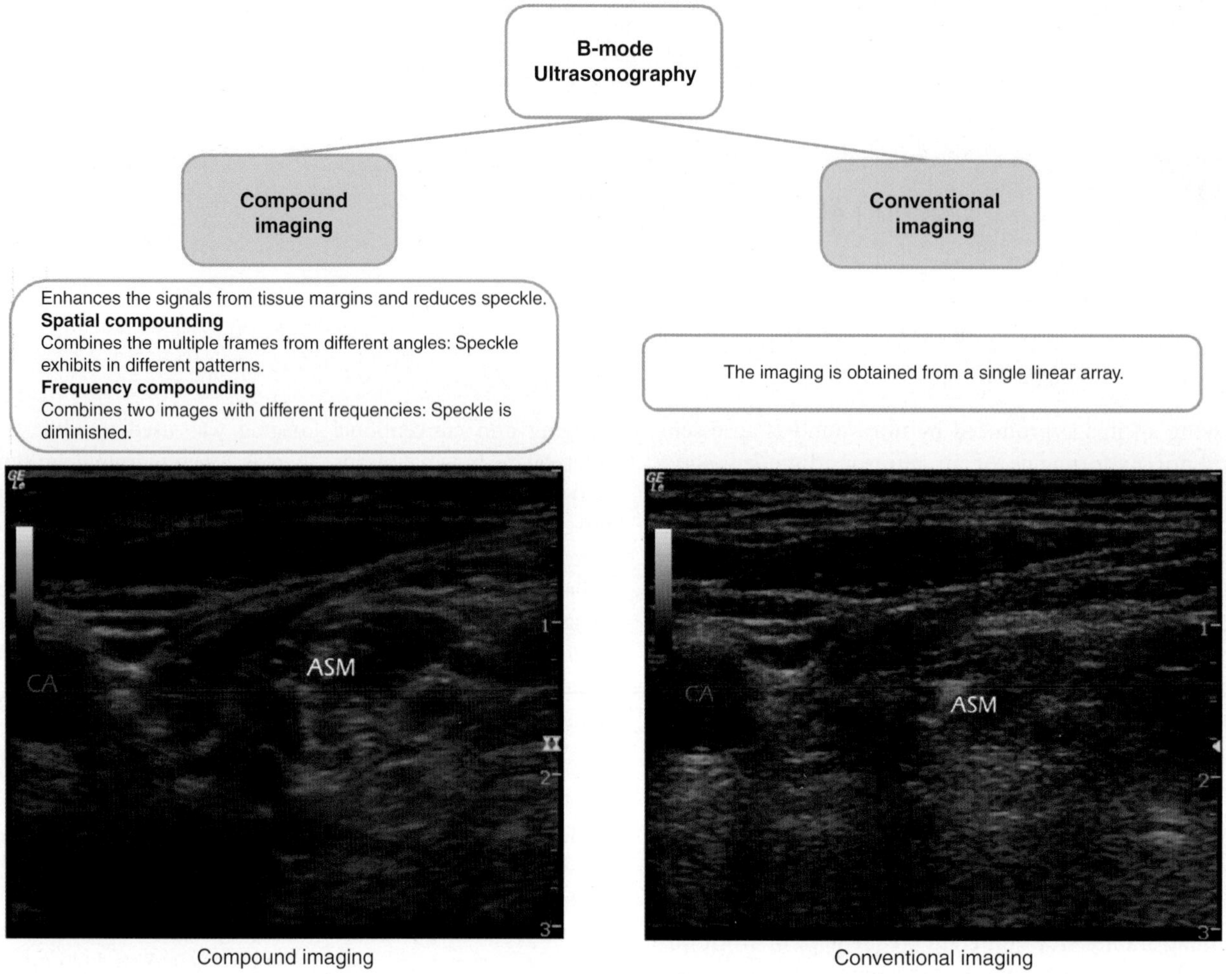

B-mode Ultrasonography

Compound imaging

Conventional imaging

Enhances the signals from tissue margins and reduces speckle.
**Spatial compounding**
Combines the multiple frames from different angles: Speckle exhibits in different patterns.
**Frequency compounding**
Combines two images with different frequencies: Speckle is diminished.

The imaging is obtained from a single linear array.

CA ASM

Compound imaging

CA ASM

Conventional imaging

**FIGURE 27-2.** Examples of image quality typically obtained with conventional versus compound imaging.

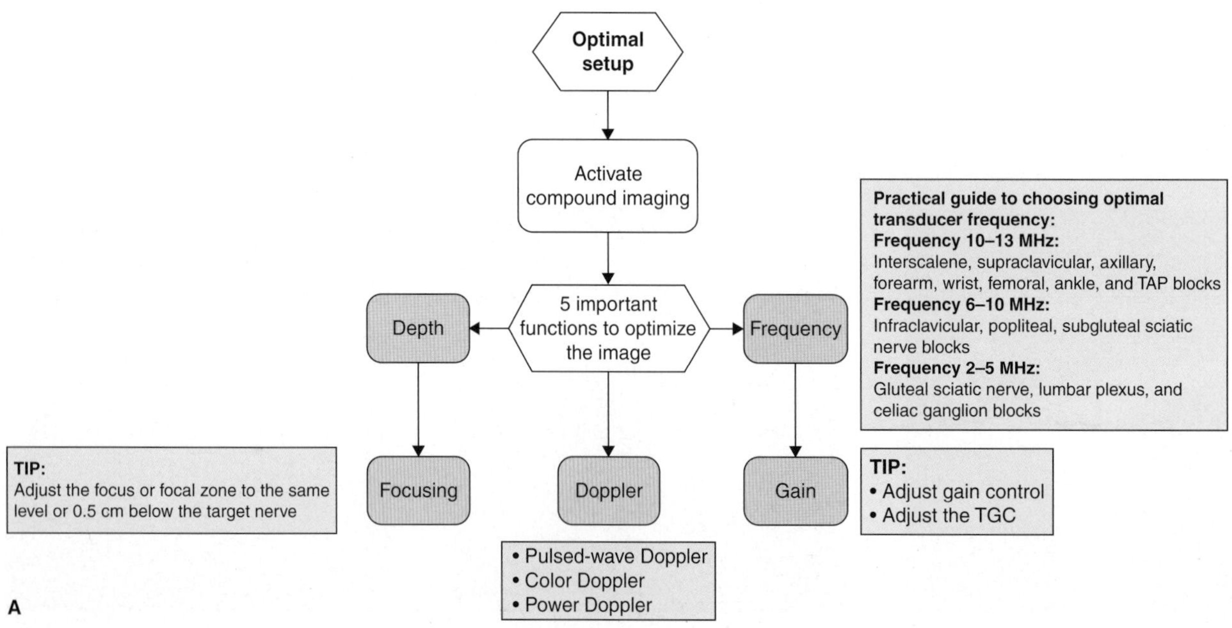


**FIGURE 27-3.** Optimizing an ultrasound image using five key functional adjustments (A) and specific tips on adjusting the focus (B) and gain (C). Some ultrasound models are specifically optimized for regional anesthesia application and may not incorporate user-adjustable focus and/or time gain compensation (TGC).

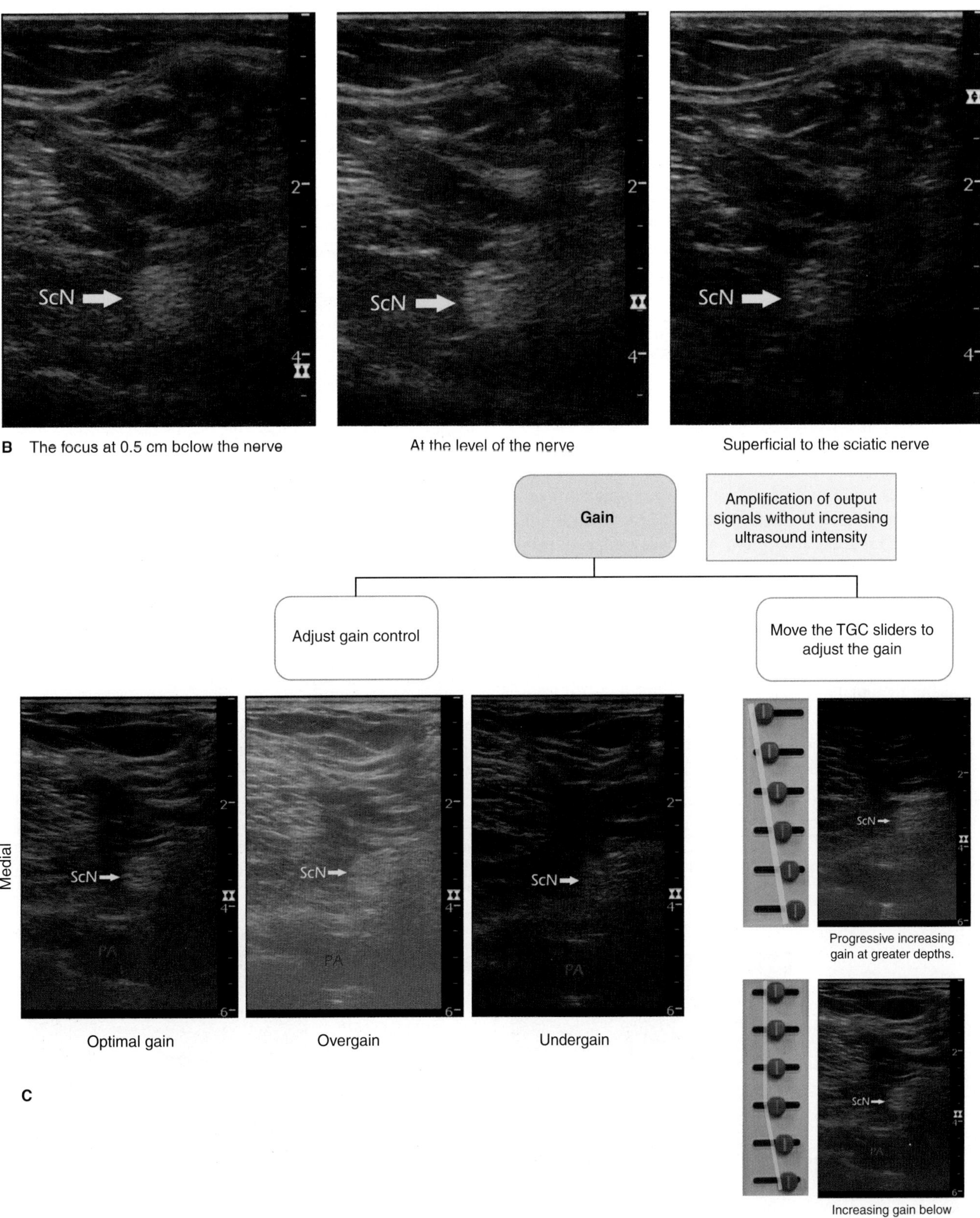


**FIGURE 27-3.** *(Continued)*

**TABLE 27-1 Suggested Optimal Imaging Depth for Common Peripheral Nerve Blocks**

| FIELD DEPTH | PERIPHERAL BLOCKADES |
|---|---|
| <2.0 cm | Wrist, ankle block |
| 2.0–3.0 cm | Interscalene, axillary brachial plexus block |
| 3.0–4.0 cm | Femoral, supraclavicular, transversus abdominis plane block |
| 4.0–7.0 cm | Infraclavicular, popliteal, subgluteal sciatic nerve blocks |
| 7.0–10.0 cm | Pudendal, gluteal sciatic nerve, lumbar plexus block |
| >10.0 cm | Anterior approach to sciatic nerve |

2. *Frequency*: The ultrasound transducer with the optimal frequency range should be selected to best visualize the target nerves. Ultrasound energy is absorbed gradually by the transmitted tissue; the higher the frequency of ultrasound, the more rapid the absorption, and the less distance propagation. Therefore, a low-frequency transducer is used to scan structures at a deeper location. Unfortunately, this is at the expense of reduced image resolution.
3. *Focusing*: Lateral resolution can be improved by choosing the higher frequency as well as by focusing the ultrasound beam. In actual practice, the focus is adjusted at the level of the target nerve; the best image quality for a given nerve is obtained by choosing an appropriate frequency transducer and the focal zone (Figure 27-3B).
4. *Gain*: Screen brightness can be adjusted manually by two function buttons: gain and time-gain compensation (TGC). Excessive or inadequate gain can cause both a blurring of tissue boundaries and a loss of information. Optimal gain for scanning peripheral nerves is typically the gain at which the best contrast is obtained between the muscles and the adjacent connective tissue. This is because muscles are well-vascularized tissue invested with connective tissue fibers, whereas, the echo texture of connective tissue is similar to that of nerves. In addition, increasing gain below the focus works well with the TGC control to visualize both the target nerve and the structures below it. Figure 27-3C shows the same section with both correct and incorrect gain and TGC settings.
5. *Doppler*: In regional anesthesia, Doppler ultrasound is used to detect vascular structures or the location of the spread of the local anesthetic injection. Doppler velocity is best set between 10 and 20 cm/s to reduce aliasing of color Doppler imaging and artifacts of color. Of note, power Doppler is more sensitive for detecting blood flow than color Doppler.

Two needle insertion techniques with relevance to the needle–transducer relationship are commonly used in ultrasound-guided nerve block: the in-plane and out-of-plane techniques (Figure 27-4). *In-plane* technique means the needle is placed in the plane of ultrasound beam; as a result, the needle shaft and the tip can be observed in the longitudinal view real time as the needle is advanced toward the target nerve. When the needle is not visualized on the image, the needle advancement should be stopped. Tilting or rotating the transducer can bring the ultrasound beam into alignment with the needle and help with its visualization. Additionally, a subtle, fast needle shake and or injection of small amount of injectate may help depict the needle location. The *out-of-plane* technique involves needle insertion perpendicularly to the transducer. The needle shaft is imaged in a cross-section plane and can be identified as a bright dot in the image. Visualization of the tip of the needle, however, is difficult and unreliable. The method used to visualize the tip of the needle is as follows: Once a bright dot (shaft) is seen in the image, the needle can be shaken slightly and/or the transducer can be tilted toward the direction of needle

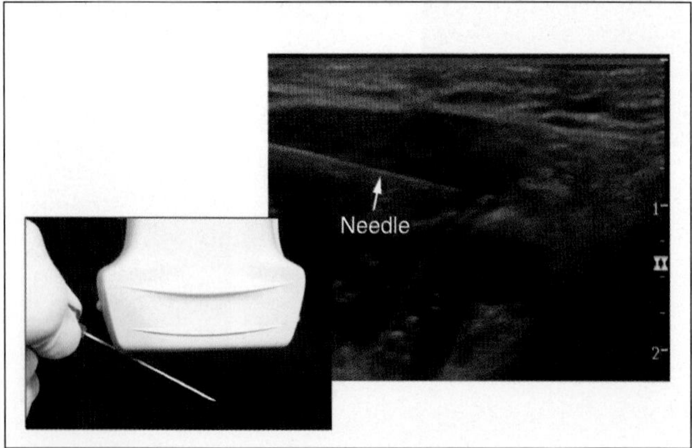


In-plane (long axis) approach

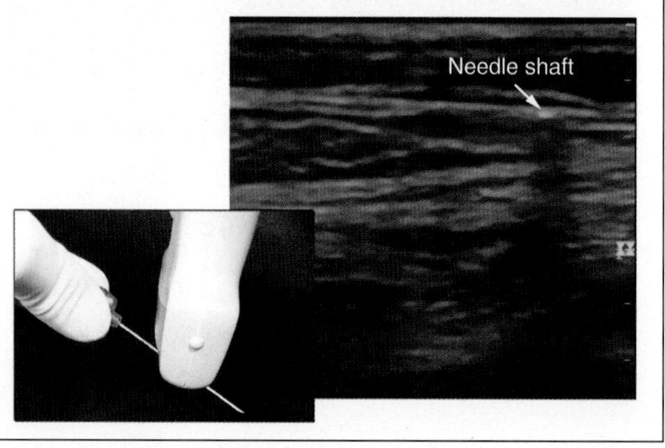


Out-of-plane (short axis) approach

**FIGURE 27-4.** In-plane and out-of-plane needle insertion and corresponding ultrasound image.

insertion simultaneously until the dot disappears. Shaking the needle helps differentiate the echo as emanating from the needle or from the surrounding tissue. The last capture of the hyperechoic dot is its tip. A small amount of injectate can be used to confirm the location of needle tip. Whenever injectate is used to visualize the needle tip, attention must be paid to avoid resistance (pressure) to injection because when the needle–nerve interface is not well seen, there is a risk for an intraneural injection.

By definition, ultrasound artifact is any image aberration that does not represent the correct anatomic arrangement. The five artifacts often seen in regional anesthesia practice (Figure 27-5) are as follows.

1. *Shadowing* is a significant reduction of ultrasound energy lying below solid objects (e.g., osseous structures, gallstone). This is manifested by attenuation of the echo signals as seen in an abnormal decrease of the brightness, which appear as a shadow on the image.
2. *Enhancement* manifests as overly intense echogenicity behind an object (such as vessel, cyst) that is less attenuating than the surrounding soft tissues. The echo signals are enhanced in brightness disproportional to the echo strength. Scanning from different angles or from different planes may help to decrease shadowing/enhancement artifacts and to visualize the target nerve.
3. *Reverberation* is a set of equally spaced bright linear echoes behind the reflectors in the near field of the image. It may be attenuated or eliminated when scanning direction is changed or ultrasound frequency is decreased.
4. *Mirror image* artifact results from an object located on one side of a highly reflective interface, appearing on the other side as well. Both virtual and artifactual images have an equal distance to the reflector from opposite directions. Changing scanning direction may decrease the artifact.
5. *Velocity error* is the displacement of the interface, which is caused by the difference of actual velocity of ultrasound in human soft tissue, compared with the calibrated speed, which is assumed to be 1540 m/sec in the ultrasound system.

The inherent artifact in the process of scanning cannot be completely eliminated in all cases by manipulating ultrasound devices or changing the settings. However, recognizing and understanding ultrasound artifacts help the operator avoid misinterpretation of images.

Here is an acronym, SCANNING, for preparing to scan:

S: **S**upplies

C: **C**omfortable positioning

A: **A**mbiance

N: **N**ame and procedure

N: **N**ominate transducer

I: **I**nfection control

N: **N**ote lateral/medial side on screen

G: **G**ain depth

1. **Gather supplies:** All equipment necessary for ultrasound scanning should be prepared. Equipment may differ slightly depending on the area to be scanned; however some necessary equipment includes:
   a. Ultrasound machine
   b. Transducer covers
   c. Nerve block kit, nerve stimulator
   d. Sterile work trolley
   e. Local anesthetic drawn up and labeled
   f. Whenever possible, connect the ultrasound machine to the power outlet to prevent the machine from powering down during a procedure
2. **Comfortable patient position:** Patient should be positioned in such a way that the patient, the anesthesiologist, the ultrasound machine, and the sterile block tray are all arranged in an ergonomic position that allows for a time-efficient performance of the procedure.
   a. The ultrasound machine should be set up on the opposite side of the patient with the screen at the operator's eye level.
   b. Block tray should be positioned close enough to the operator so it eliminates the need to reach for needle, gel, and other supplies but should not interfere with the scanning procedure.
3. **Ambiance—set room settings:** Adjust the lights in the room in order to view the ultrasound machine and procedural site adequately.
   a. Dim lighting optimizes visualization of the image on the screen; more lighting is typically needed for the procedural site.
   b. Adjust the room light settings to allow for proper lighting to both areas, as well for safe monitoring of the patient.
4. **Name of patient, procedure, and site of procedure:** Before performing a scan take a "time-out" to ensure patient information is correct, the operation being done is confirmed, and the side in which the procedure is being done is validated. Checking that patient informati on is entered into the ultrasound machine and matches the information on the patient's wristband not only confirms identity but also allows for images to be saved during the scanning process for documentation.
5. **Select transducer:** Select the transducer that best fits the scheduled procedure to be done.
   a. A linear transducer is best scanning superficial anatomic structures; a curved (phased array) transducer displays a sector image and is typically better for deeper positioned structures.
6. **Disinfection:** Disinfect the patient's skin using a disinfectant solution to reduce the risk of contamination and infection.

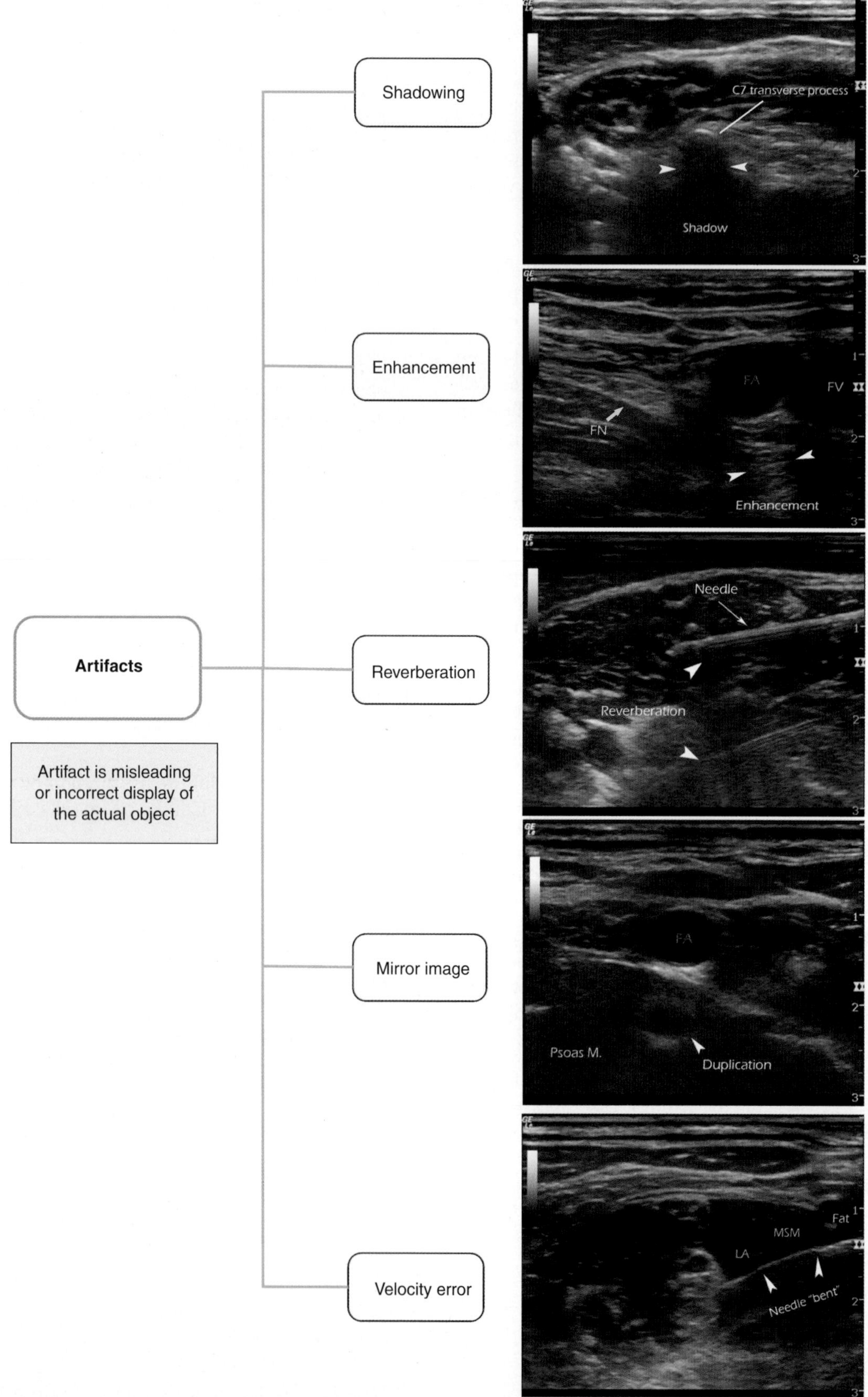


**FIGURE 27-5.** Common artifacts during ultrasound imaging. LA - local anesthetic, MSM - middle scalene muscle.

7. **Orient transducer and apply gel:** The operator should orient the transducer to match the medial-lateral orientation of the patient. This is conventionally not done by radiologists/sonographers, but it is very useful for intervention-oriented regional anesthesia procedures.
   a. Touch one edge of the transducer to orient the side of the transducer so the medial-lateral orientation on the patient corresponds to that on the screen.
   b. A sufficient amount of gel is applied to either the transducer or the patient's skin to allow for transmission of the ultrasound. A copious amount of disinfectant solution can be used instead of gel in many instances.
   c. Insufficient quality of gel will decrease reflection-absorption rates and may result in unclear/blurry images on the ultrasound image being displayed.
8. **Place transducer on the patient's skin and adjust ultrasound machine settings:**
   a. The gain should be adjusted with the general gain setting and/or by using TGC.
   b. The depth is adjusted to optimize imaging of structures of interest.
   c. Where available, focus point is adjusted at the desired level.
   d. Scanning mode can be switched to aid in the recognition of the structures as necessary (e.g., color Doppler can help depict blood vessels, M-mode can distinguish between arteries and veins).

## SUGGESTED READING

Chudleigh T, Thilaganathan B. *Obstetric Ultrasound: How, Why and When.* 3rd ed. Edinburgh, UK: Elsevier Churchill Livingstone; 2004.

Grau T. Ultrasonography in the current practice of regional anaesthesia. *Best Pract Res Clin Anaesthesiol.* 2005;19:175-200.

Gray AT. Ultrasound-guided regional anesthesia: current state of the art. *Anesthesiology.* 2006;104(2):368-373.

Sites BD, Brull R, Chan VW, et al. Artifacts and pitfall errors associated with ultrasound-guided regional anesthesia. Part I: understanding the basic principles of ultrasound physics and machine operations. *Reg Anesth Pain Med.* 2007;32(5):412-418.

Sites BD, Brull R, Chan VW, et al. Artifacts and pitfall errors associated with ultrasound-guided regional anesthesia. Part II: a pictorial approach to understanding and avoidance. *Reg Anesth Pain Med.* 2007;32(5):419-433.

SECTION 5

# Ultrasound-Guided Nerve Blocks

# 28 Ultrasound-Guided Cervical Plexus Block

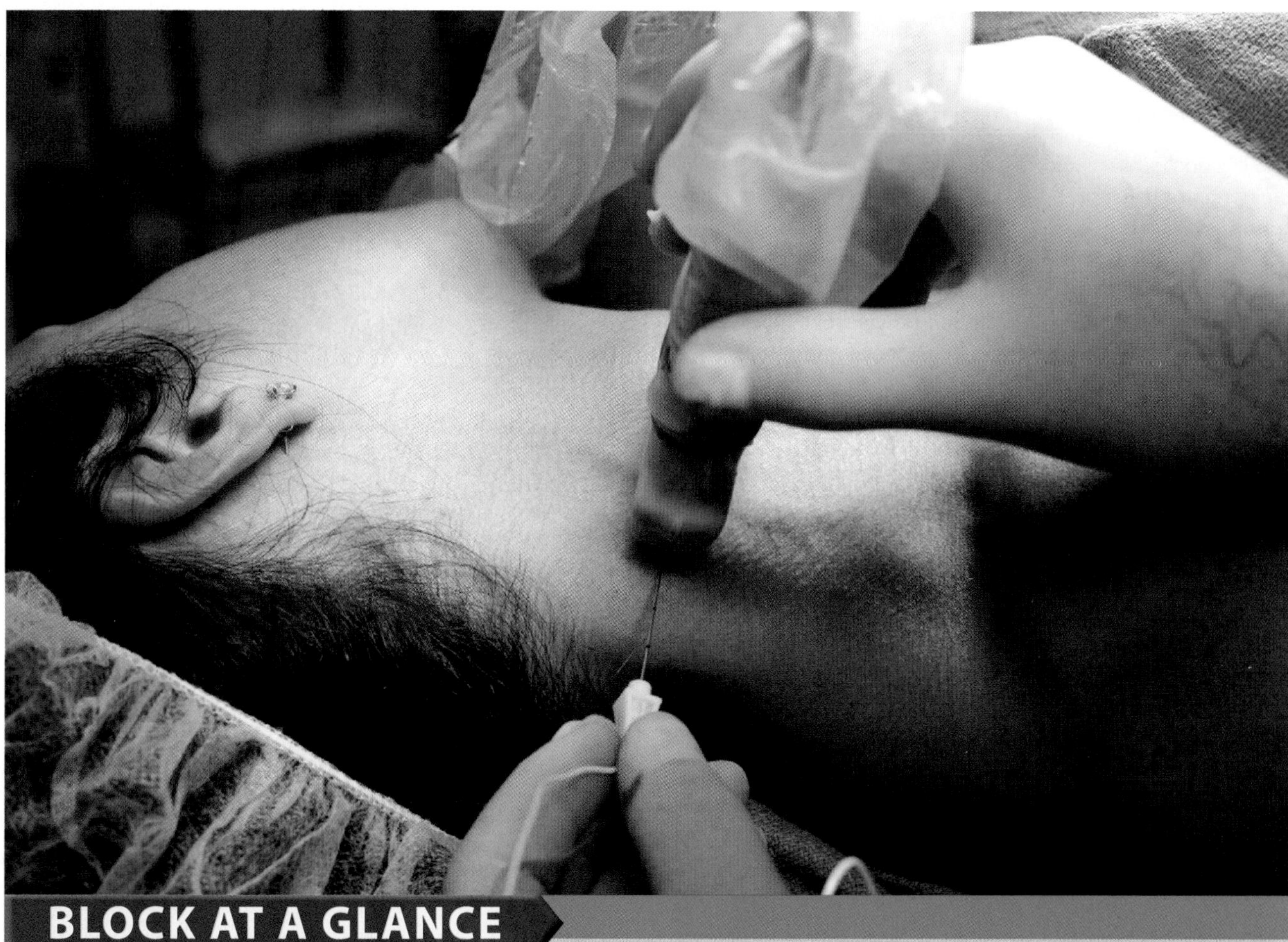

## BLOCK AT A GLANCE

- Indications: carotid endarterectomy, superficial neck surgery
- Transducer position: transverse over the midpoint of the sternocleidomastoid muscle (posterior border)
- Goal: local anesthetic spread around the superficial cervical plexus *or* deep to the sternocleidomastoid muscle
- Local anesthetic: 10–15 mL

**FIGURE 28-1.** Needle and transducer position to block the superficial cervical plexus using a transverse view.

## General Considerations

The goal of the ultrasound-guided technique of superficial cervical plexus block is to deposit local anesthetic in the vicinity of the sensory branches of the nerve roots C2, C3, and C4. Advantages over the landmark-based technique include the ability to ensure the spread of local anesthetic in the correct plane and therefore increase the success rate and avoid too deep needle insertion and/or inadvertent puncture of neighboring structures. Both in-plane and out-of-plane approaches can be used. The experience with ultrasound-guided deep cervical plexus is still in its infancy and not described here.

## Ultrasound Anatomy

The sternocleidomastoid muscle (SCM) forms a "roof" over the nerves of the superficial cervical plexus (C2-4). The roots combine to form the four terminal branches (lesser occipital, greater auricular, transverse cervical, and supraclavicular nerves) and emerge from behind the posterior border of the SCM (Figure 28-2). The plexus can be visualized as a small collection of hypoechoic nodules (honeycomb appearance or hypo-echoic [dark] oval structures) immediately deep or lateral to the posterior border of the SCM (Figure 28-3), but this is not always apparent. Occasionally, the greater auricular nerve is visualized (Figure 28-4) on the superficial surface of the SCM muscle as a small, round hypoechoic structure. The SCM is separated from the brachial plexus and the scalene muscles by the prevertebral fascia, which can be seen as a hyperechoic linear structure. The superficial cervical plexus lies posterior to the SCM muscle, and immediately underneath the prevertebral fascia overlying the interscalene groove. (Figure 28-3).

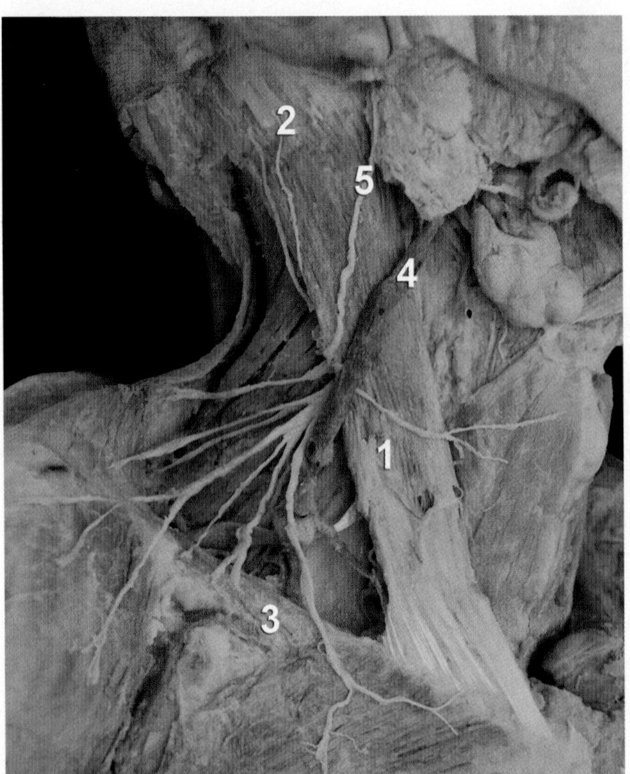


**FIGURE 28-2.** Anatomy of the superficial cervical plexus. ❶ sternocleidomastoid muscle. ❷ mastoid process. ❸ clavicle. ❹ external jugular vein. Superficial cervical plexus is seen emerging behind the posterior border of the sternocleidomastoid muscle at the intersection of the muscle with the external jugular vein. ❺ Greater auricular nerve.

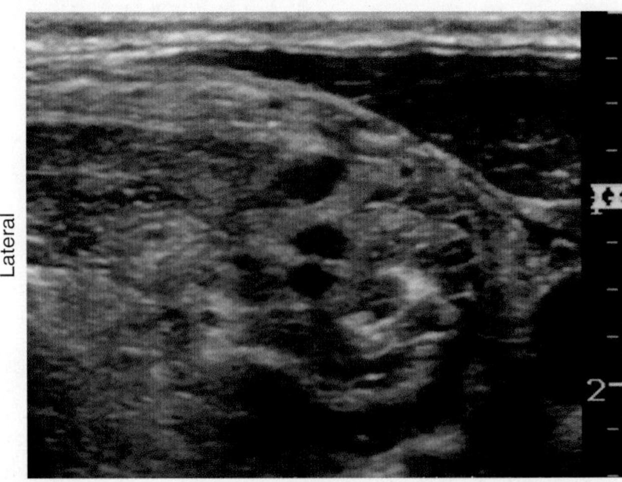


**FIGURE 28-3.** Superficial cervical plexus-transverse view.

## Distribution of Blockade

The superficial cervical plexus block results in anesthesia of the skin of the anterolateral neck and the anteauricular and retroauricular areas, as well as the skin overlying and immediately inferior to the clavicle on the chest wall (Figure 28-5).

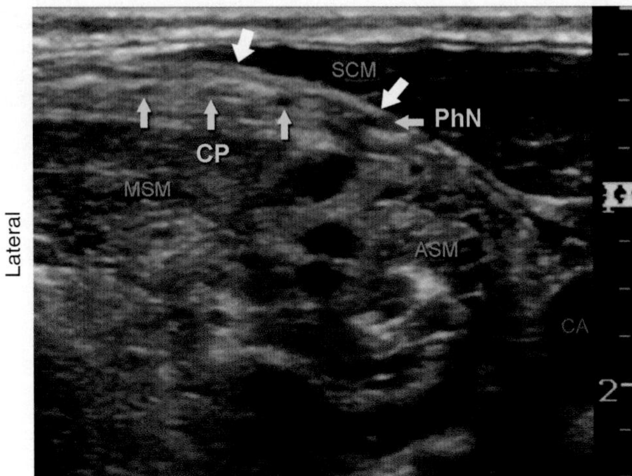


**FIGURE 28-4.** Branches of the superficial cervical plexus (CP) emerging behind the prevertebral fascia that covers the middle (MSM) and anterior (ASM) scalene muscles, and posterior to the sternocleidomastoid muscle (SCM). White arrows, Prevertebral Fascia; CA, carotid artery; PhN, phrenic nerve.

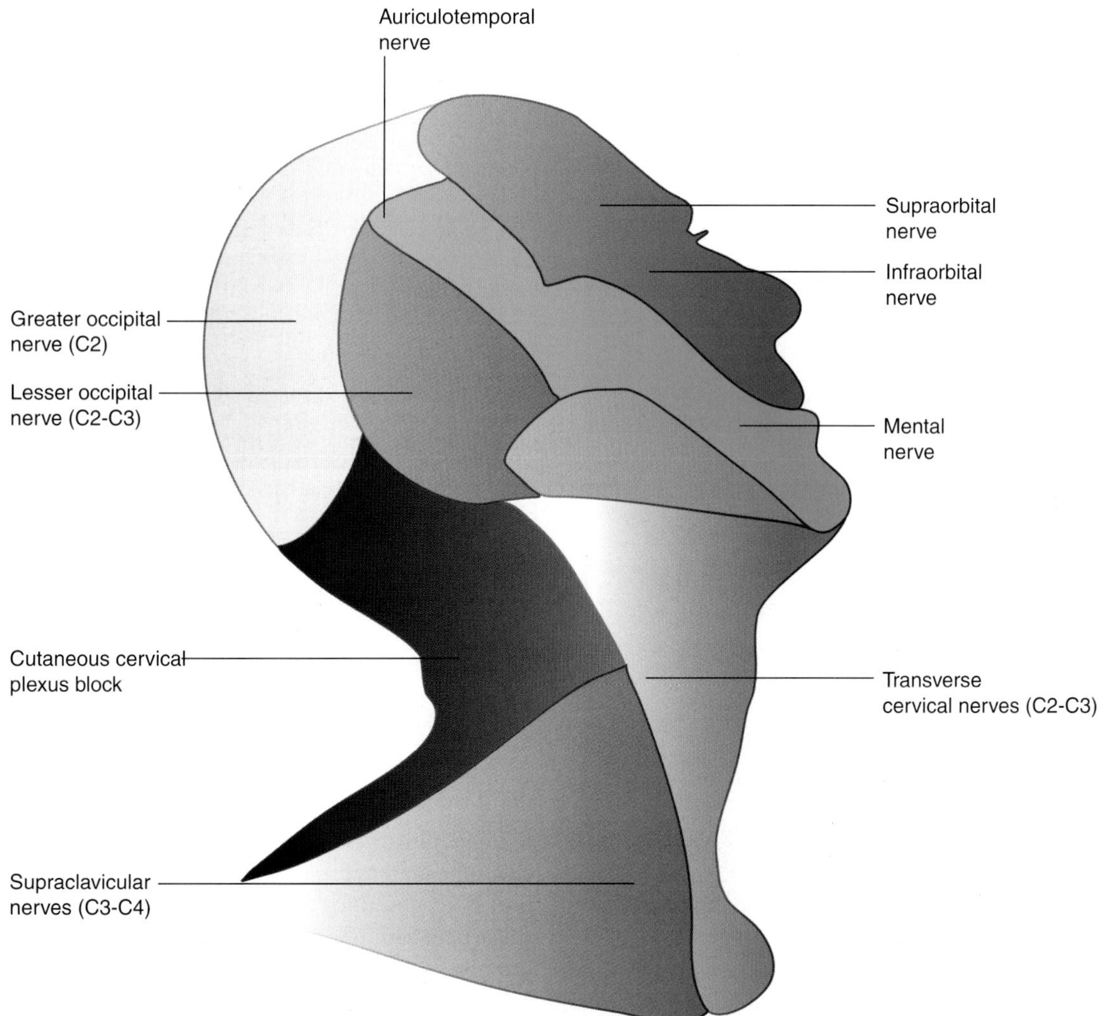


**FIGURE 28-5.** Sensory distribution of the cervical plexus and innervation of the lateral aspect of the face.

## Equipment

Equipment needed includes the following:

- Ultrasound machine with linear transducer (8–18 MHz), sterile sleeve, and gel
- Standard nerve block tray (described in the equipment section)
- Two 10-mL syringes containing local anesthetic
- A 2.5-in, 23- to 25-gauge needle attached to low-volume extension tubing
- Sterile gloves

## Landmarks and Patient Positioning

Any patient position that allows for comfortable placement of the ultrasound transducer and needle advancement is appropriate. This block is typically performed in the supine or semi-sitting position, with the head turned slightly away from the side to be blocked to facilitate operator access (Figure 28-6A and B). The patient's neck and upper chest should be exposed so that the relative length and position of the SCM can be assessed.

## GOAL

The goal is to place the needle tip immediately adjacent to the superficial cervical plexus. If it is not easily visualized, the local anesthetic can be deposited in the plane immediately deep to the SCM and underneath the prevertebral fasica. A volume of 10 to 15 mL of local anesthetic usually suffices.

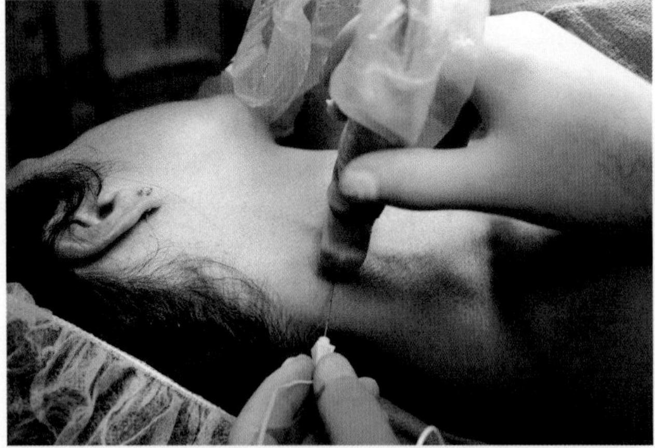


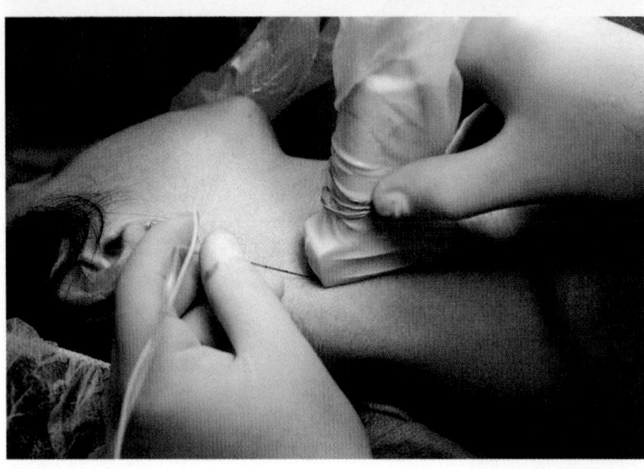


**FIGURE 28-6.** Superficial cervical plexus block. A) Transverse approach with an in-plane needle advancement. B) Longitudinal approach.

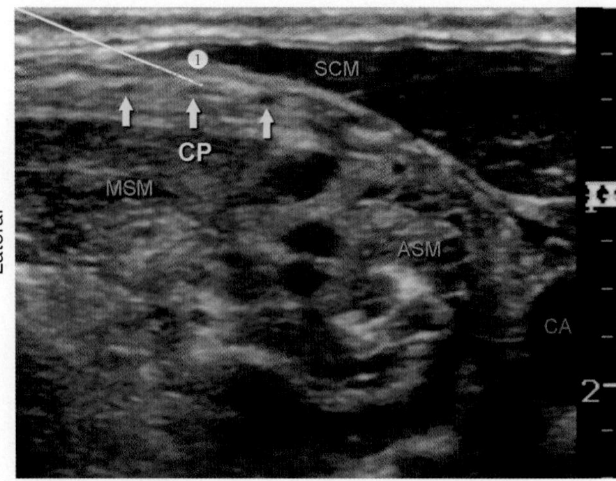


**FIGURE 28-7.** Needle path (1) and position to block the superficial cervical plexus (CP), transverse view. The needle is seen positioned underneath the lateral border of the sternocleidomastoid muscle (SCM) and underneath the prevertebral fascia with the transducer in a transverse position (Figure 28-1). ASM, anterior scalene muscle; CA, carotid artery; MSM, middle scalene muscle.

## Technique

With the patient in the proper position, the skin is disinfected and the transducer is placed on the lateral neck, overlying the SCM at the level of its midpoint (approximately the level of the cricoid cartilage). Once the SCM is identified, the transducer is moved posteriorly until the tapering posterior edge is positioned in the middle of the screen. At this point, an attempt should be made to identify the brachial plexus and/or the interscalene groove between the anterior and middle scalene muscles. The plexus is visible as a small collection of hypoechoic nodules (honeycomb appearance) immediately underneath the prevertebral fascia that overlies the interscalene groove (Figures 28-3 and 28-4).

Once identified, the needle is passed through the skin, platysma and prevertebral fascia, and the tip placed adjacent to the plexus (Figure 28-7). Because of the relatively shallow position of the target, both in-plane (from medial or lateral sides) and out-of-plane approaches can be used. Following negative aspiration, 1 to 2 mL of local anesthetic is injected to confirm the proper injection site. Then the remainder of the local anesthetic (10–15 mL) is administered to envelop the plexus (Figure 28-8).

If the plexus is not visualized, an alternative substernocleidomastoid approach can be used. In this case, the needle is passed behind the SCM and the tip is directed to lie in the space between the SCM and the prevertebral fascia, close to the posterior border of the SCM (Figures 28-6B, 28-9, and 28-10). Local anesthetic (10–15 mL) is administered and

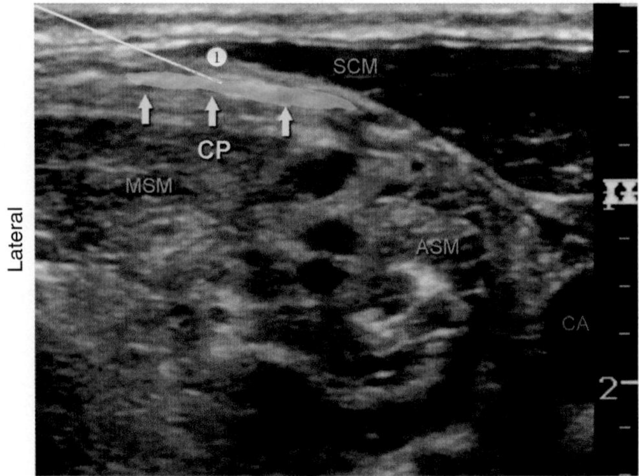


**FIGURE 28-8.** Desired distribution of the local anesthetic (area shaded in blue) to block the superficial cervical plexus. ASM, anterior scalene muscle; CA, carotid artery; CP, cervical plexus; MSM, middle scalene muscle; SCM, sternocleidomastoid muscle.

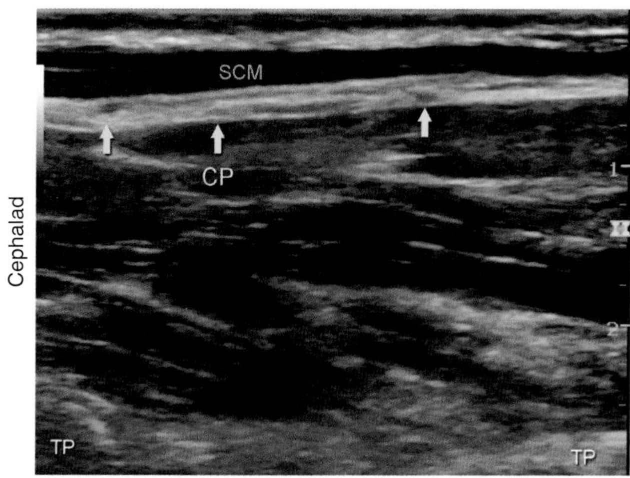


Superficial cervical plexus-longitudinal view

**FIGURE 28-9.** Longitudinal view of the superficial cervical plexus (CP) underneath the lateral border of the sternocleidomastoid muscle (SCM).

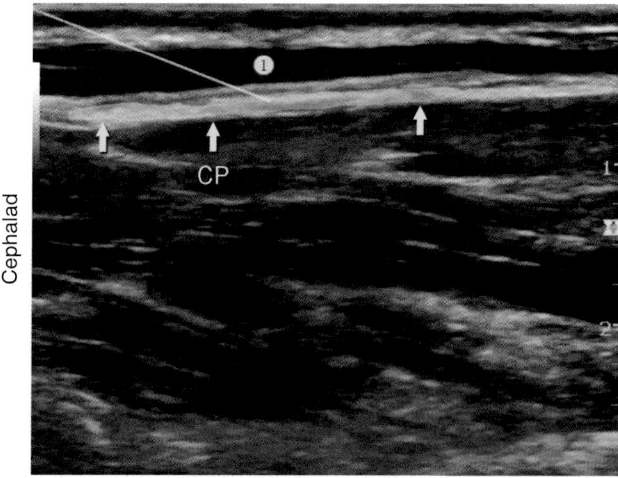


Superficial cervical plexus-longitudinal view

**FIGURE 28-11.** Desired spread of the local anesthetic under the cervical fascia to block the cervical plexus (CP).

should be visualized layering out between the SCM and the underlying prevertebral fascia (Figure 28-11). If injection of the local anesthetic does not appear to result in an appropriate spread, additional needle repositioning and injections may be necessary. Because the superficial cervical plexus is made up of purely sensory nerves, high concentrations of local anesthetic are usually not required; 0.25%-0.5% ropivacaine, bupivacaine 0.25%, or lidocaine 1% are examples of good choices.

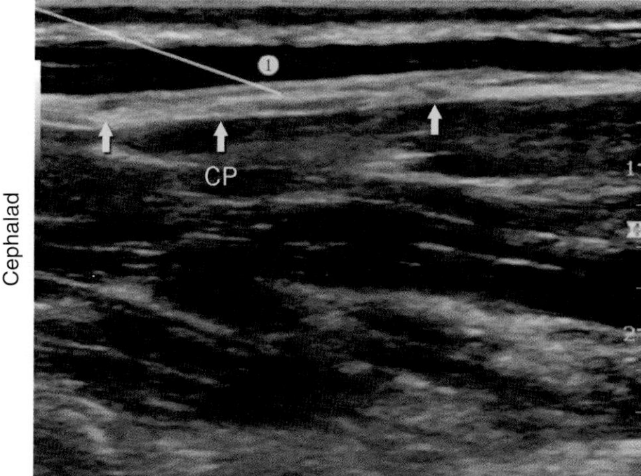


Superficial cervical plexus-longitudinal view

**FIGURE 28-10.** Needle position to block the cervical plexus (CP), longitudinal view.

## TIPS

- Visualization of the plexus is *not* necessary to perform this block because it may not be always readily apparent. Administration of 10 to 15 mL of local anesthetic deep to the SCM provides a reliable block without confirming the position of the plexus.
- The superficial cervical plexus overlies the brachial plexus (i.e., immediately superficial to the interscalene groove and underneath the prevertebral fascia). This can serve as a sonographic landmark by identifying the scalene muscles, the trunks of the brachial plexus, and/or the groove itself and the prevertebral fascia.

# ULTRASOUND-GUIDED SUPERFICIAL CERVICAL PLEXUS BLOCK

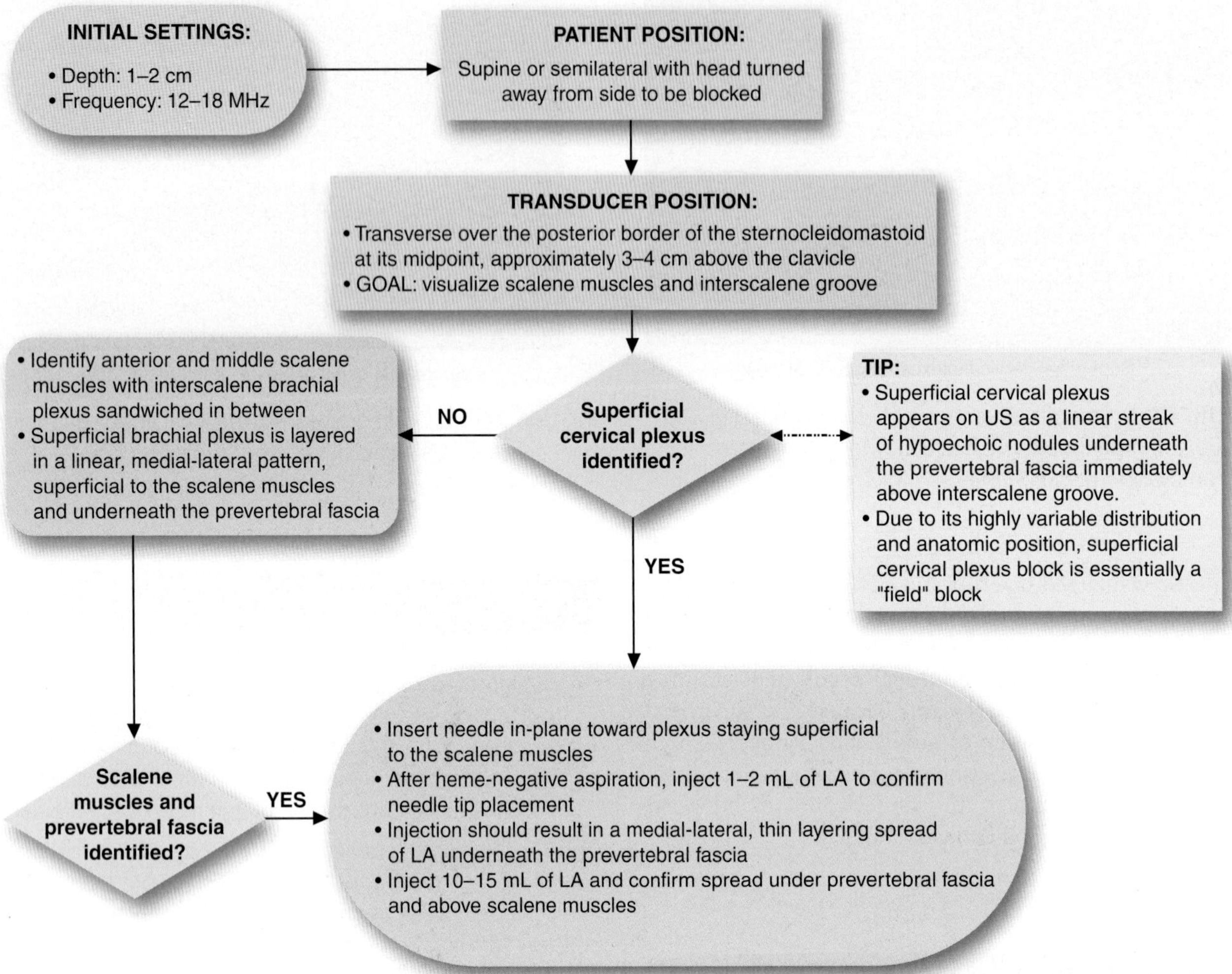

## SUGGESTED READING

Aunac S, Carlier M, Singelyn F, De Kock M. The analgesic efficacy of bilateral combined superficial and deep cervical plexus block administered before thyroid surgery under general anesthesia. *Anesth Analg.* 2002;95:746-750.

Demondion X, Herbinet P, Boutry N, et al. Sonographic mapping of the normal brachial plexus. *Am J Neuroradiol.* 2003;24: 1303-1309.

Eti Z, Irmak P, Gulluoglu BM, Manukyan MN, Gogus FY. Does bilateral superficial cervical plexus block decrease analgesic requirement after thyroid surgery? *Anesth Analg.* 2006;102:1174-1176.

Guay J. Regional anesthesia for carotid surgery. *Curr Opin Anaesthesiol.* 2008;21:638-644.

Narouze S. Sonoanatomy of the cervical spinal nerve roots: implications for brachial plexus block. *Reg Anesth Pain Med.* 2009;34:616.

Roessel T, Wiessner D, Heller AR, et al. High-resolution ultrasound-guided high interscalene plexus block for carotid endarterectomy. *Reg Anesth Pain Med.* 2007;32:247-253.

Sandeman DJ, Griffiths MJ, Lennox AF. Ultrasound guided deep cervical plexus block. *Anaesth Intensive Care.* 2006;34:240-244.

Soeding P, Eizenberg N. Review article: anatomical considerations for ultrasound guidance for regional anesthesia of the neck and upper limb. *Can J Anaesth.* 2009;56:518-533.

Usui Y, Kobayashi T, Kakinuma H, Watanabe K, Kitajima T, Matsuno K. An anatomical basis for blocking of the deep cervical plexus and cervical sympathetic tract using an ultrasound-guided technique. *Anesth Analg.* 2010;110:964-968.

# 29 Ultrasound-Guided Interscalene Brachial Plexus Block

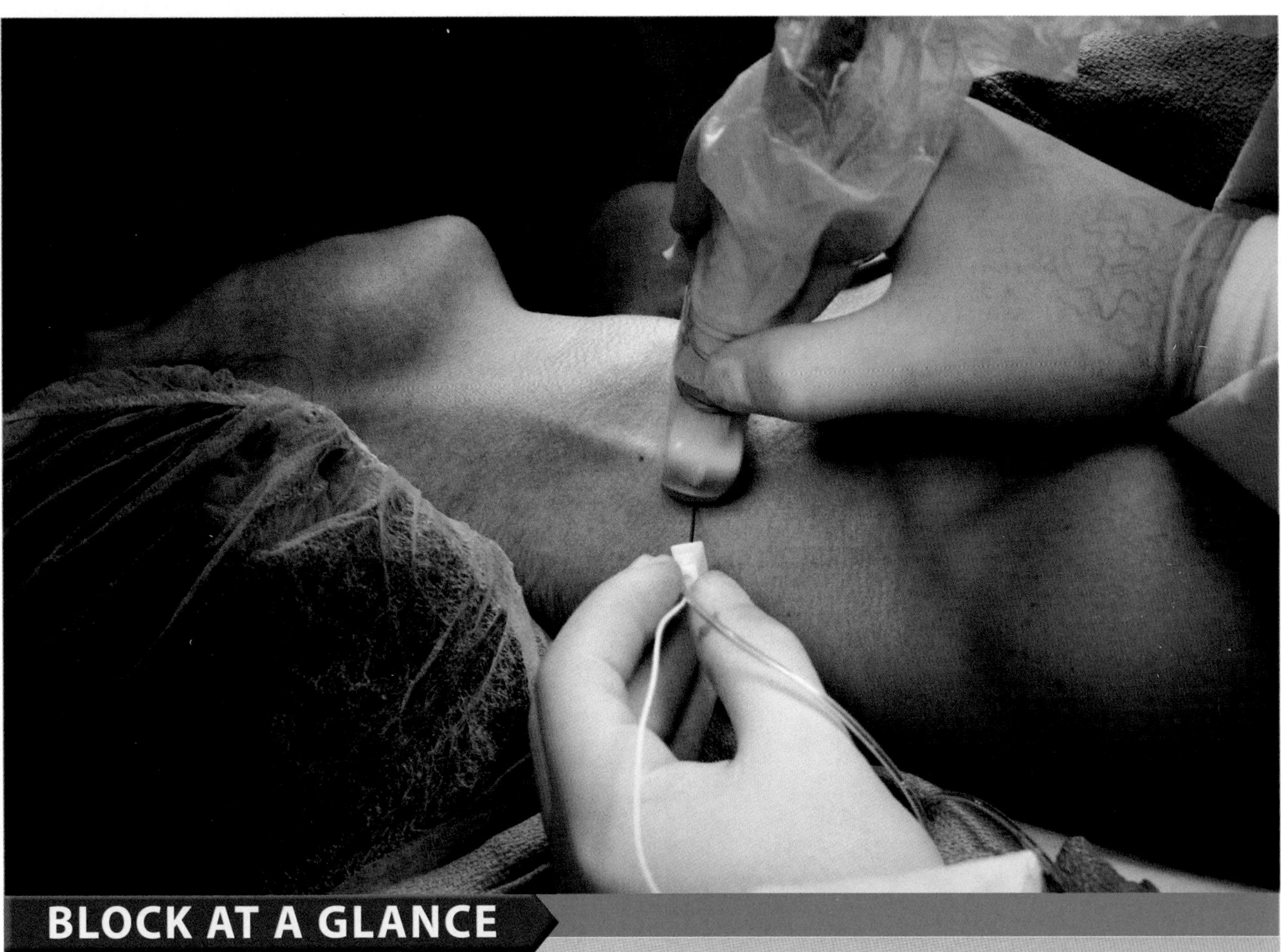

## BLOCK AT A GLANCE

- Indications: shoulder and upper arm surgery
- Transducer position: transverse on neck, 3–4 cm superior to clavicle, over external jugular vein
- Goal: local anesthetic spread around superior and middle trunks of brachial plexus, between anterior and middle scalene muscles
- Local anesthetic: 15–25 mL

**FIGURE 29-1.** Ultrasound-guided interscalene brachial plexus block; transducer and needle position to obtain the desired ultrasound image for an in-plane approach.

## General Considerations

The ultrasound-guided technique of interscalene brachial plexus block differs from nerve stimulator or landmark-based techniques in several important aspects. Most importantly, distribution of the local anesthetic is visualized to assure adequate spread around the brachial plexus. Ultrasound guidance allows multiple injections around the brachial plexus, therefore eliminating the reliance on a single large injection of local anesthetic for block success as is the case with non–ultrasound-guided techniques. Ability to inject multiple aliquots of local anesthetic also may allow for the reduction in the volume of local anesthetic required to accomplish the block. Repetition of the block in case of inadequate anesthesia is also possible, a management option that is unpredictable without ultrasound guidance. Finally, the risk of major vessel and nerve puncture during nerve block performance is reduced.

## Ultrasound Anatomy

The brachial plexus at the interscalene level is seen lateral to the carotid artery, between the anterior and middle scalene muscles (Figures 29-2, 29-3, and 29-4). Prevertebral fascia, superficial cervical plexus and sternocleidomastoid muscle are seen superficial to the plexus. The transducer is moved in the superior-inferior direction until two or more of the brachial plexus trunks are seen in the space between the scalene muscles. Depending on the depth of field selected and the level at which the scanning is performed, first rib and/or apex of the lung may be seen. The brachial plexus is typically visualized at a depth of 1 to 3 cm.

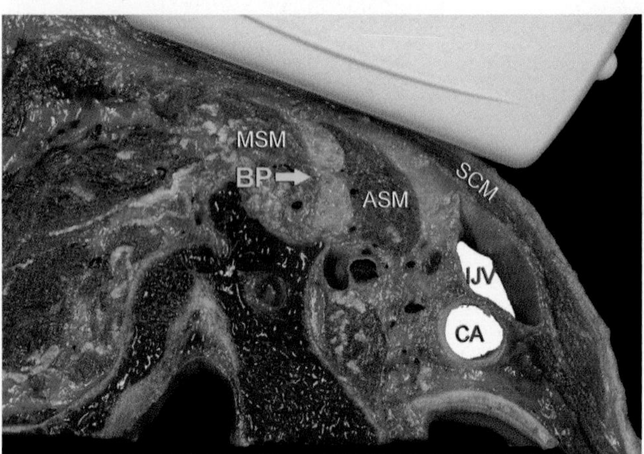


**FIGURE 29-2.** Relevant anatomy for interscalene brachial block and transducer position to obtain the desired views. Brachial plexus (BP) is seen sandwiched between middle scalene muscle (MSM) laterally and anterior scalene muscle (ASM) medially. Ultrasound image often includes a partial view of the lateral border of the sternocleidomastoid muscle (SCM) as well as the internal jugular vein (IJV) and carotid artery (CA). The transverse process of one of the cervical vertebrae is also often seen.

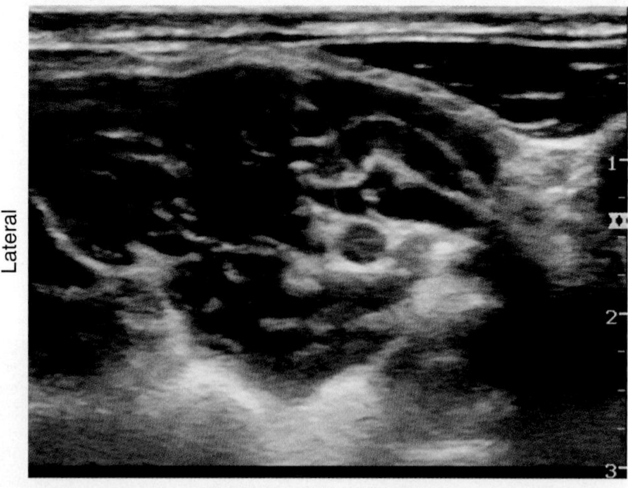


**FIGURE 29-3.** Interscalene brachial plexus is seen between middle scalene muscle and anterior scalene muscle. Carotid artery is seen medial at 1 cm depth in this image.

## Distribution of Blockade

The interscalene approach to brachial plexus blockade results in anesthesia of the shoulder and upper arm. Inferior trunk for more distal anesthesia can also be blocked by additional, selective injection, deeper in the plexus. This is accomplished either by controlled needle redirection inferiorly or by additional scanning to visualize the inferior trunk and another needle insertion and targeted injection. For a more comprehensive review of the brachial plexus distribution, see Chapter 1 on Essential Regional Anesthesia Anatomy.

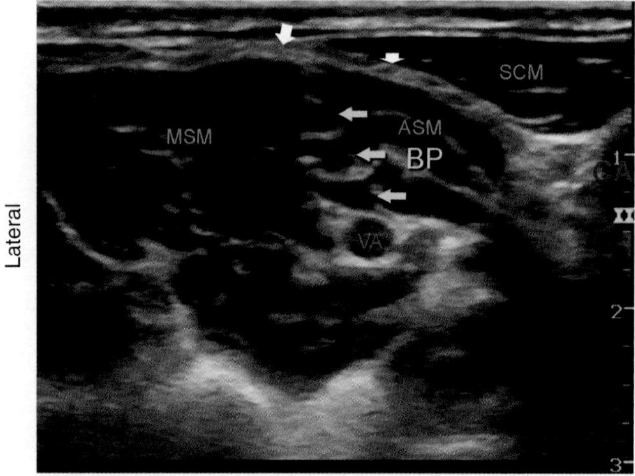


**FIGURE 29-4.** Typical image of the brachial plexus (BP). The BP is seen positioned between the anterior scalene muscle (ASM) and the middle scalene muscle (MSM). The superficial cervical plexus (white arrowhead) can be seen posterior to the SCM and underneath the prevertebral fascia. In this particular image, the vertebral artery (VA), carotid artery (CA), as well as the transverse process of C6 are also seen.

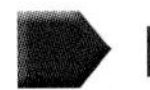

## Equipment

Equipment needed includes the following:

- Ultrasound machine with linear transducer (8–14 MHz), sterile sleeve, and gel
- Standard nerve block tray (described in the equipment section)
- One 20-mL syringe containing local anesthetic
- 5-cm, 22-gauge short-bevel insulated stimulating needle
- Peripheral nerve stimulator
- Sterile gloves

## Landmarks and Patient Positioning

Any position that allows comfortable placement of the ultrasound transducer and needle advancement is appropriate. The block is typically performed with the patient in supine, semisitting, or semilateral decubitus position, with the patient's head facing away from the side to be blocked. The latter position may prove ergonomically more convenient, especially during an in-plane approach from the lateral side, in which the needle is entering the skin at the posterolateral aspect of the neck. A slight elevation of the head of the bed is often more comfortable for the patient, and it allows for better drainage and less prominence of the neck veins.

Adherence to strict anatomic landmarks is of lesser importance for the ultrasound-guided interscalene block than it is the case for the surface anatomy-based techniques. Regardless, knowledge of the underlying anatomy and the position of the brachial plexus is important to facilitate recognition of the ultrasound anatomy. Scanning usually begins just below the level of the cricoid cartilage and medial to the sternocleidomastoid muscle with a goal to identify the carotid artery.

**GOAL**

The goal is to place the needle in the tissue space between the anterior and middle scalene muscles and inject local anesthetic until the spread around the brachial plexus is documented by ultrasound.The volume of the local anesthetic and number of needle insertions are determined during the procedure and depend on the adequacy of the observed spread of the local anesthetic.

## Technique

With the patient in the proper position, the skin is disinfected and the transducer is positioned in the transverse plane to identify the carotid artery (Figure 29-5). Once the artery is identified, the transducer is moved slightly laterally across the neck (see algorithm at end of chapter). The goal is to identify the scalene muscles and the brachial plexus that is sandwiched between the anterior and middle scalene muscles.

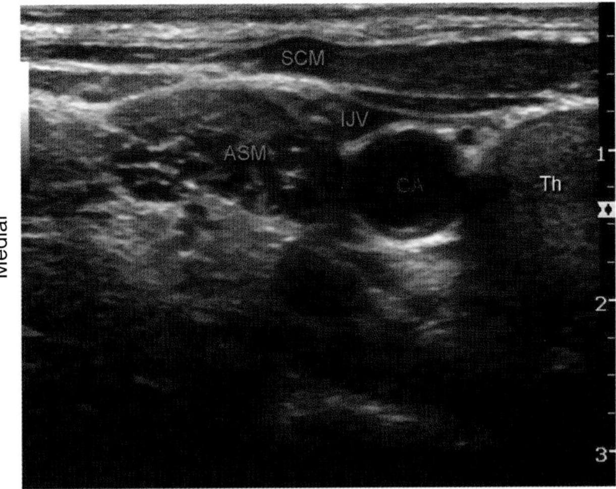


**FIGURE 29-5.** Ultrasound image just below the level of the cricoid cartilage and medial to the sternocleidomastoid muscle. ASM, anterior scalene muscle; SCM, sternocleidomastoid muscle; IJV, internal jugular vein; CA, carotid artery; Th, thyroid gland.

**TIP**

- When the visualization of the brachial plexus between the scalene muscles proves difficult, the transducer is lowered to the supraclavicular fossa. At this position, the brachial plexus is identified lateral and superficial to the subclavian artery, (Figure 29-6). From here, the brachial plexus is traced cranially to the desired level.

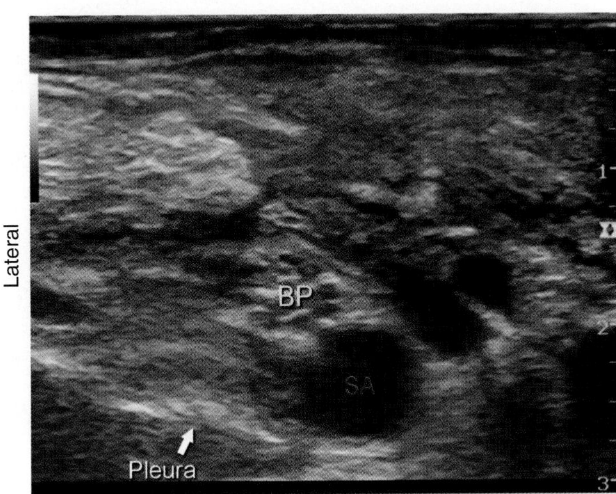


**FIGURE 29-6.** View of the brachial plexus (BP) at the supraclavicular fossa. When identification of the brachial plexus at the interscalene level proves difficult, the transducer is positioned at the supraclavicular fossa to identify the BP superficial and lateral to the subclavian artery (SA). The transducer is then slowly moved cephalad while continuously visualizing the brachial plexus until the desired level is reached.

The needle is then inserted in-plane toward the brachial plexus, typically in a lateral-to-medial direction (Figure 29-7), although medial-to-lateral needle orientation also can be chosen if more convenient. As the needle passes through the prevertebral fascia, a certain "give" is often appreciated. When nerve stimulation is used (0.5 mA, 0.1 msec), the entrance of the needle in the interscalene groove is often associated with a motor response of the shoulder, arm, or forearm as another confirmation of the proper needle placement. After a careful aspiration to rule out an intravascular needle placement, 1 to 2 mL of local anesthetic is injected to document the proper needle placement (Figure 29-8A). Injection of several milliliters of local anesthetic often displaces the brachial plexus away from the needle.

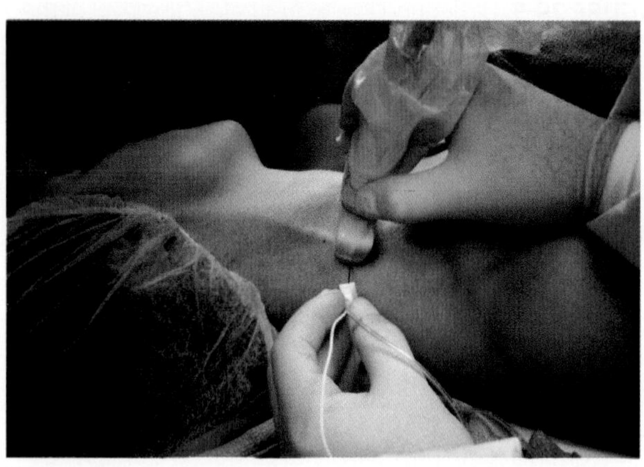

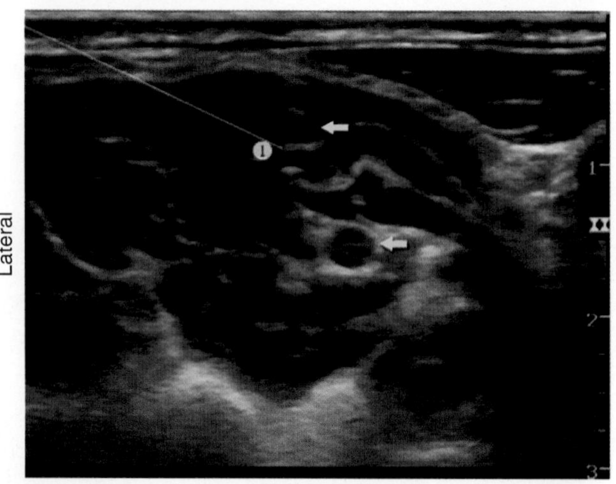


**FIGURE 29-7.** (A) Transducer placement and needle insertion. (B) Position of the needle (1) for the interscalene brachial plexus block using an in-plane approach. The needle tip is seen in contact with the superior trunk of the brachial plexus (yellow arrows); this always results in high injection pressure (>15 psi)—indicating that the needle should be withdrawn slightly away from the trunk.

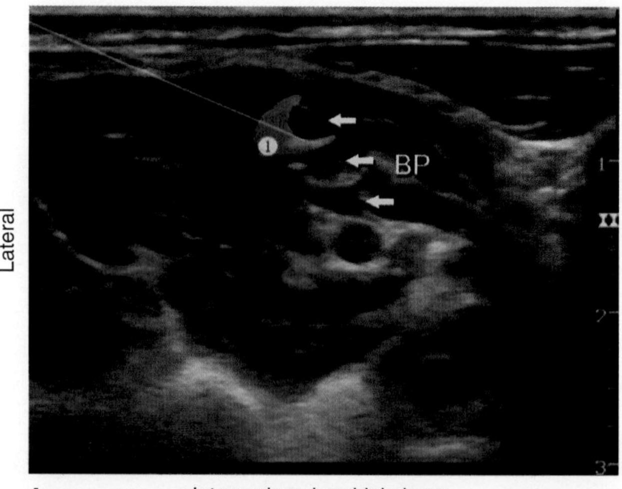


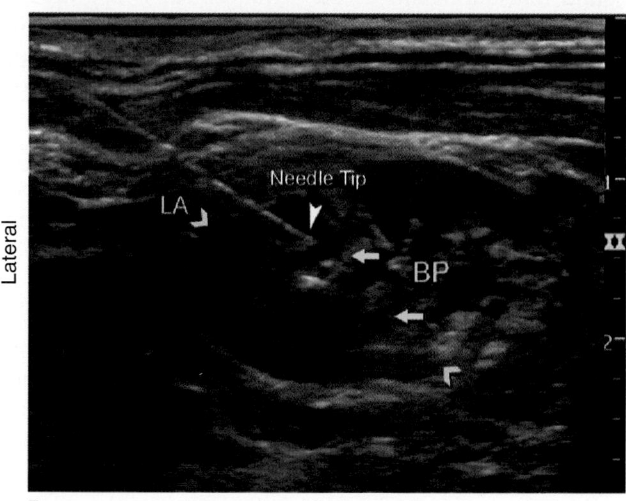


**FIGURE 29-8.** (A) A small amount of local anesthetic (blue shaded area) is injected through the needle to confirm the proper needle placement. A properly placed needle tip will result in distribution of the local anesthetic between and/or alongside roots of the brachial plexus (BP). (B) An actual needle (white arrowhead) placement in the interscalene groove with the dispersion of the local anesthetic (LA; blue shaded area or arrows) surrounding the BP.

An additional advancement of the needle 1 to 2 mm toward the brachial plexus may be beneficial to assure a proper spread of the local anesthetic (Figure 29-8B). Whenever the needle is further advanced, or multiple injections used, assure that high resistance to injection is absent to decrease the risk of an intrafascicular injection. When injection of the local anesthetic does not appear to result in a spread around the brachial plexus, additional needle repositions and injections may be necessary.

## TIPS

- The presence of the motor response to nerve stimulation is useful but not necessary to elicit if the plexus, needle, and local anesthetic spread are well-visualized.
- The neck is a very vascular area, and care must be exercised to avoid needle placement or injection into the vascular structures. Of particular importance is to avoid the vertebral artery, and branches of the thyrocervical trunk: inferior thyroid artery, suprascapular artery, and transverse cervical artery.
- Never inject against high resistance (>15 psi) because this may indicate a needle-nerve contact or an intrafascicular injection.
- Pro and con of multiple injections:
  - Pro: May increase the speed of onset and success rate of the interscalene block.
  - Pro: May allow for a reduction in the total volume and dose of local anesthetic required to accomplish block.
  - Con: May carry a higher risk of nerve injury because part of the plexus may be anesthetized by the time consecutive injections are made.
  - NOTE: Avoidance of high resistance to injection and needle–nerve contact is essential to avoid intrafascicular injection because reliance on nerve stimulation with multiple injections is diminished.

In an adult patient, 15 to 25 mL of local anesthetic is usually adequate for successful and rapid onset of blockade. Smaller volumes of local anesthetics can also be effective, however, their success rate in everyday clinical practice may be inferior to those reported in meticulously conducted clinical trials. The block dynamics and perioperative management are similar to those described in Chapter 12.

## Continuous Ultrasound-Guided Interscalene Block

The goal of the continuous interscalene block is similar to the non–ultrasound-based techniques: to place the catheter in the vicinity of the trunks of the brachial plexus between the scalene muscles. The procedure consists of three phases: needle placement, catheter advancement, and securing of the catheter. For the first two phases of the procedure, ultrasound can be used to assure accuracy. The needle is typically inserted in-plane from the lateral-to-medial direction and underneath the prevertebral fascia to enter the interscalene space (Figure 29-9), although other needle directions could be used.

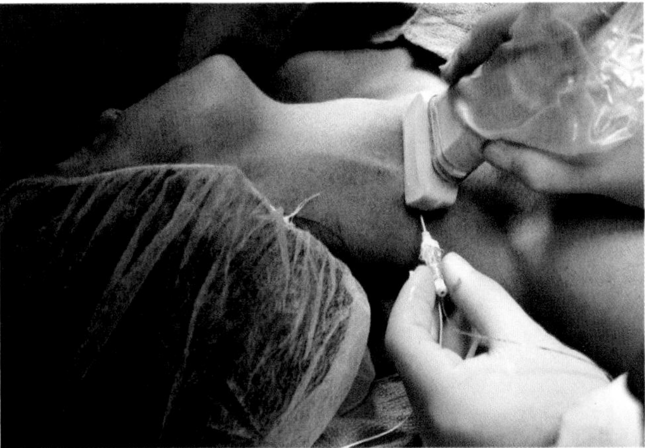

**FIGURE 29-9.** Continuous brachial plexus block. Needle is inserted in the interscalene space using an in-plane approach. Please note that for better demonstration, sterile drapes are not used in the model in this figure.

## TIP

- Both stimulating and nonstimulating catheters can be used, although for simplicity we prefer nonstimulating catheters for ultrasound-guided continuous interscalene block.

Proper placement of the needle can also be confirmed by obtaining a motor response of the deltoid muscle, arm, or forearm (0.5 mA, 0.1 msec) at which point 4 to 5 mL of local anesthetic can be injected. This small dose of local anesthetic serves to assure adequate distribution of the local anesthetic as well as to make the advancement of the catheter more comfortable to the patient. This first phase of the procedure does not significantly differ from the single-injection technique. The second phase of the procedure involves maintaining the needle in the proper position and inserting the catheter 2 to 3 cm into the interscalene space in the vicinity of the brachial plexus (Figure 29-10). Insertion of the catheter can be accomplished by a single operator or with a helper. Proper location of the catheter can be determined either by visualizing the course of the catheter or by an injection of the local anesthetic through the catheter. When this proves difficult, alternatively, a small amount of air (1 mL) can be injected to confirm the catheter tip location.

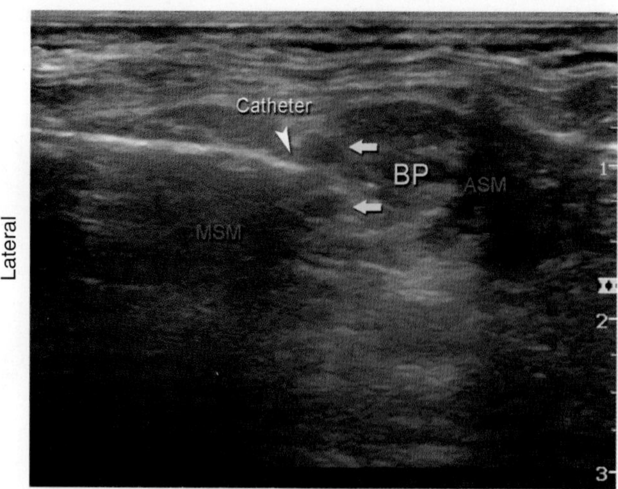


**FIGURE 29-10.** An ultrasound image demonstrating needle and catheter (white arrow) inserted in the interscalene space between the anterior (ASM) and middle (MSM) scalene muscles. BP, brachial plexus.

There is no agreement on what constitutes the ideal catheter securing system. The catheter is secured by either taping to the skin or tunneling. Some clinicians prefer one over the other. However, the decision about which method to use could be based on the patient's age, duration of the catheter therapy, and anatomy. Tunneling could be preferred in older patients with obesity or mobile skin over the neck and when longer duration of catheter infusion is expected. Two main disadvantages of tunneling are the risk of catheter dislodgment during the tunneling and the potential for scar formation. Fortunately, a number of catheter-securing devices are available to help stabilize the catheter.

# ULTRASOUND-GUIDED INTERSCALENE BLOCK

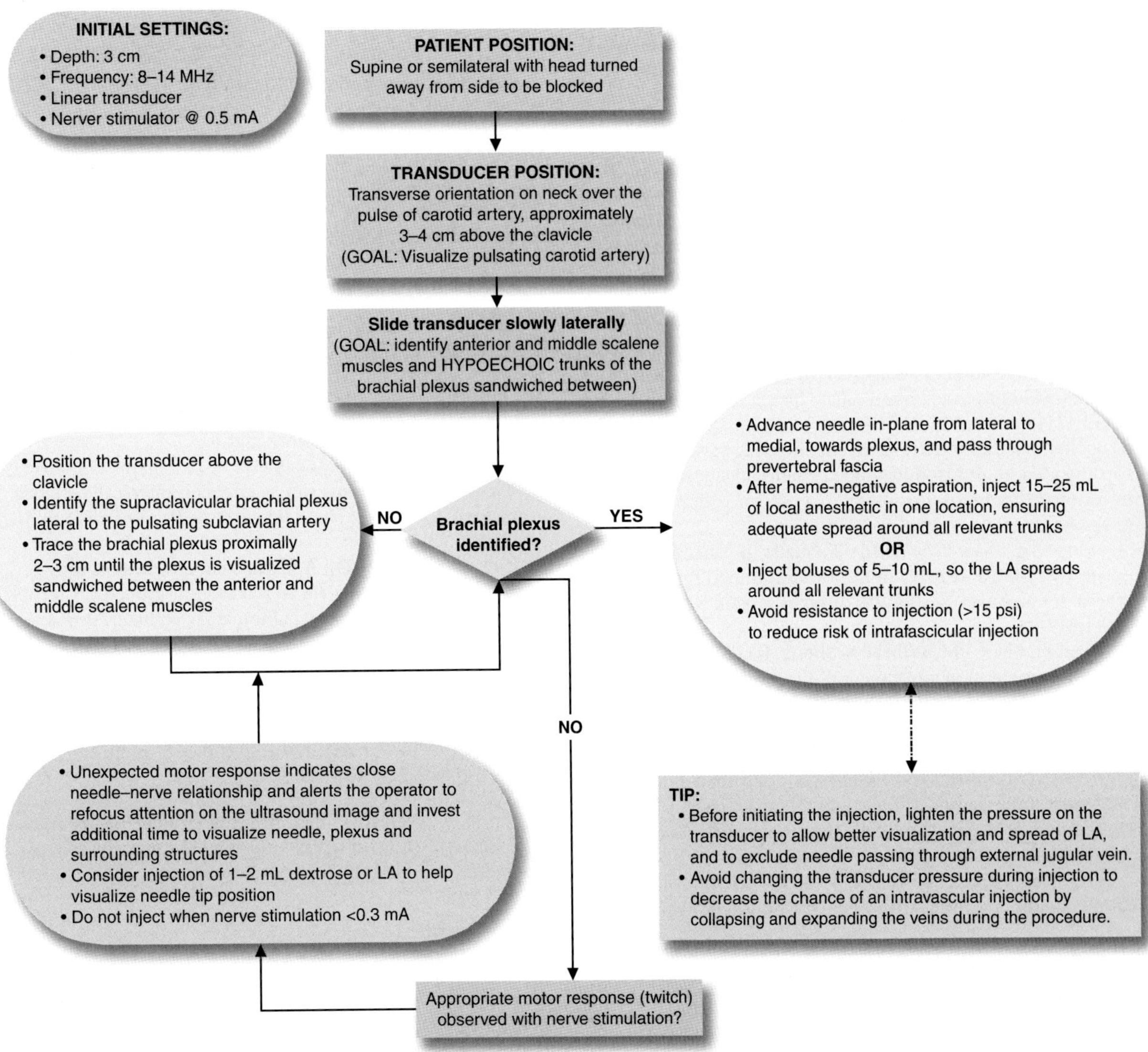

## SUGGESTED READING

### Single Injection UG-IS block


Fredrickson MJ, Ball CM, Dalgleish AJ. Posterior versus anterolateral approach interscalene catheter placement: a prospective randomized trial. *Reg Anesth Pain Med.* 2011;36:125-33.

Fredrickson MJ, Ball CM, Dalgleish AJ, Stewart AW, Short TG. A prospective randomized comparison of ultrasound and neurostimulation as needle end points for interscalene catheter placement. *Anesth Analg.* 2009;108:1695-700.

Fredrickson MJ, Kilfoyle DH. Neurological complication analysis of 1000 ultrasound guided peripheral nerve blocks for elective orthopaedic surgery: a prospective study. *Anaesthesia.* 2009; 64:836-44.

Gadsden J, Hadzic A, Gandhi K, Shariat A, Xu D, Maliakal T, Patel V. The effect of mixing 1.5% mepivacaine and 0.5% bupivacaine on duration of analgesia and latency of block onset in ultrasound-guided interscalene block. *Anesth Analg.* 2011;112:471-6.

Koff MD, Cohen JA, McIntyre JJ, Carr CF, Sites BD. Severe brachial plexopathy after an ultrasound-guided single-injection nerve block for total shoulder arthroplasty in a patient with multiple sclerosis. *Anesthesiology.* 2008;108:325-8.

Liu SS, Gordon MA, Shaw PM, Wilfred S, Shetty T, Yadeau JT. A prospective clinical registry of ultrasound-guided regional anesthesia for ambulatory shoulder surgery. *Anesth Analg.* 2010;111:617-23.

Liu SS, YaDeau JT, Shaw PM, Wilfred S, Shetty T, Gordon M. Incidence of unintentional intraneural injection and postoperative neurological complications with ultrasound-guided interscalene and supraclavicular nerve blocks. *Anaesthesia.* 2011;66:168-74.

Marhofer P, Harrop-Griffiths W, Willschke H, Kirchmair L. Fifteen years of ultrasound guidance in regional anaesthesia: Part 2-recent developments in block techniques. *Br J Anaesth.* 2010;104:673-83.

McNaught A, Shastri U, Carmichael N, Awad IT, Columb M, Cheung J, Holtby RM, McCartney CJ. Ultrasound reduces the minimum effective local anaesthetic volume compared with peripheral nerve stimulation for interscalene block. *Br J Anaesth.* 2011;106:124-30.

Orebaugh SL, McFadden K, Skorupan H, Bigeleisen PE. Subepineurial injection in ultrasound-guided interscalene needle tip placement. *Reg Anesth Pain Med.* 2010;35:450-4.

Renes SH, van Geffen GJ, Rettig HC, Gielen MJ, Scheffer GJ.Minimum effective volume of local anesthetic for shoulder analgesia by ultrasound-guided block at root C7 with assessment of pulmonary function. *Reg Anesth Pain Med.* 2010;35:529-34.

Spence BC, Beach ML, Gallagher JD, Sites BD. Ultrasound-guided interscalene blocks: understanding where to inject the local anaesthetic. *Anaesthesia.* 2011;66:509-14.


### Continuous US-IS Block


Antonakakis JG, Sites BD, Shiffrin J. Ultrasound-guided posterior approach for the placement of a continuous interscalene catheter. *Reg Anesth Pain Med.* 2009;34:64-8.

Fredrickson MJ, Ball CM, Dalgleish AJ. Analgesic effectiveness of a continuous versus single-injection interscalene block for minor arthroscopic shoulder surgery. *Reg Anesth Pain Med.* 2010;35:28-33.

Fredrickson MJ, Price DJ. Analgesic effectiveness of ropivacaine 0.2% vs 0.4% via an ultrasound-guided C5-6 root/ superior trunk perineural ambulatory catheter. *Br J Anaesth.* 2009;103:434-9.

Mariano ER, Afra R, Loland VJ, Sandhu NS, Bellars RH, Bishop ML, Cheng GS, Choy LP, Maldonado RC, Ilfeld BM. Continuous interscalene brachial plexus block via an ultrasound-guided posterior approach: a randomized, triple-masked, placebo-controlled study. *Anesth Analg.* 2009;108:1688-94.

Mariano ER, Loland VJ, Ilfeld BM. Interscalene perineural catheter placement using an ultrasound-guided posterior approach. *Reg Anesth Pain Med.* 2009;34:60-3.

# Ultrasound-Guided Supraclavicular Brachial Plexus Block

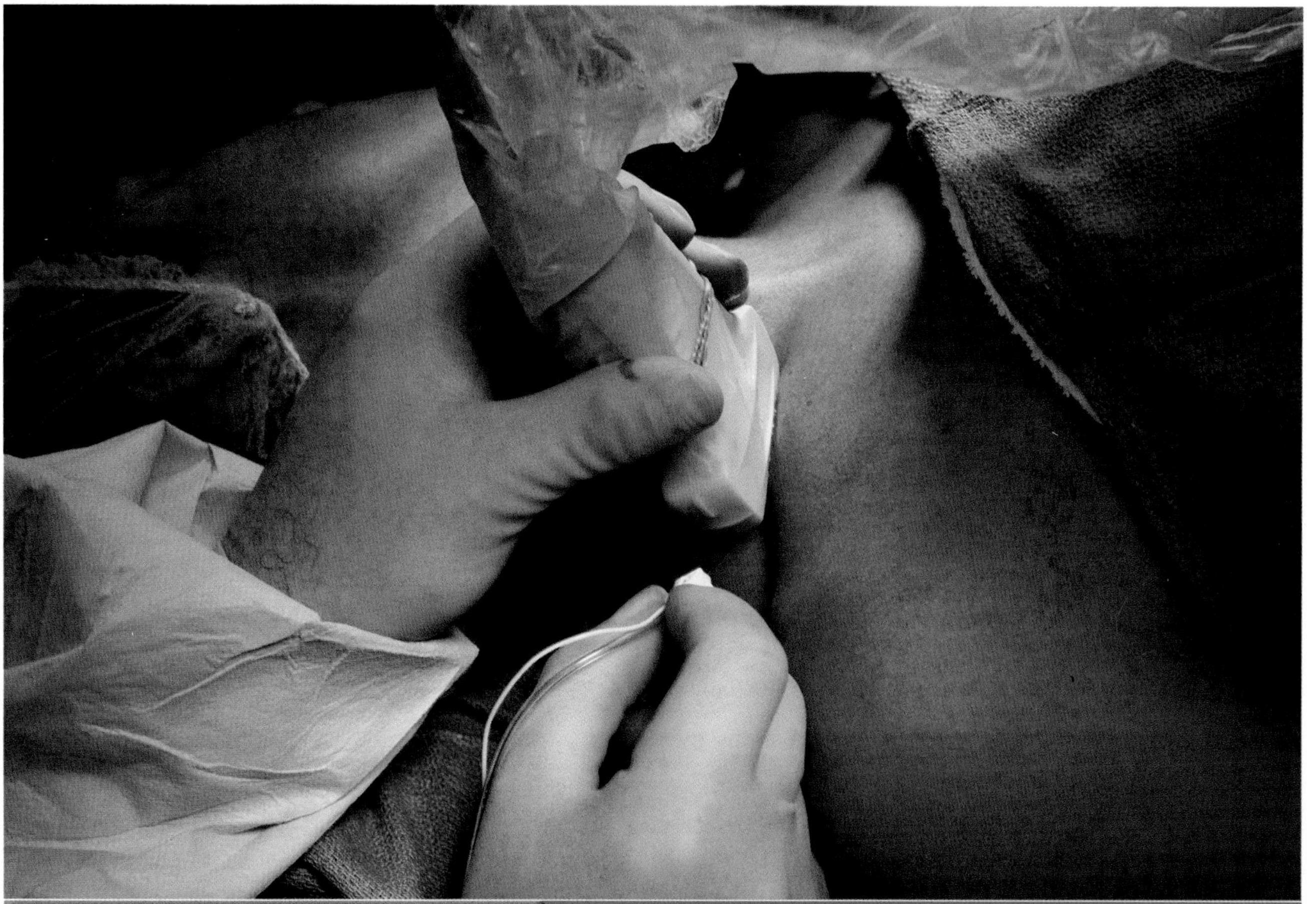

## BLOCK AT A GLANCE

- Indications: arm, elbow, forearm, and hand surgery
- Transducer position: transverse on neck, just superior to the clavicle at midpoint
- Goal: local anesthetic spread around brachial plexus, lateral and superficial to subclavian artery
- Local anesthetic: 20–25 mL

**FIGURE 30-1.** Supraclavicular brachial plexus; transducer position and needle insertion.

## General Considerations

The proximity of the brachial plexus at this location to the chest cavity and pleura, has been of concern to many practitioners (Figure 30-2). However, ultrasound guidance has resulted in a resurgence of interest in the supraclavicular approach to the brachial plexus. The ability to image the plexus, rib, pleura, and subclavian artery with ultrasound guidance has increased safety due to better monitoring of anatomy and needle placement. Because the trunks and divisions of the brachial plexus are relatively close as they travel over the first rib, the onset and quality of anesthesia is fast and complete. For these reasons, the supraclavicular block has become a popular technique for surgery below the shoulder.

## Ultrasound Anatomy

The subclavian artery crosses over the first rib between the insertions of the anterior and middle scalene muscles, at approximately the midpoint of the clavicle. The pulsating subclavian artery is readily apparent, whereas the parietal pleura and the first rib can be seen as a linear hyperechoic structure immediately lateral and deep to it, respectively (Figure 30-3). The rib, as an osseous structure, casts an acoustic shadow, so that the image field deep to the rib appears anechoic, or dark. A reverberation artifact (refer to Chapter 26) often occurs, mimicking a second subclavian artery beneath the rib. The brachial plexus can be seen as a bundle of hypoechoic round nodules (e.g., "grapes") just lateral and superficial to the artery (Figures 30-3, 30-4, 30-5A and B). It is often possible to see the fascial sheath enveloping the brachial plexus. Depending at the level at which the plexus is scanned and the transducer orientation, brachial plexus can have an oval or flattened appearance (Figure 30-5A and B). Two different sonographic appearances of the brachial plexus (one oval and one flattened) are easily seen by changing the angle of the transducer orientation during imaging. Lateral and medial to the first rib is the hyperechoic pleura, with lung tissue deep to it. This structure can be confirmed by observation of a "sliding" motion of the viscera pleura with the patient's respiration. The brachial plexus is typically visualized at a 1- to 2-cm depth at this location, an important anatomical characteristic of the plexus that must be kept in mind throughout the procedure.

## Distribution of Blockade

The supraclavicular approach to the brachial plexus blockade results in anesthesia of the upper limb below the shoulder because all trunks and divisions can be anesthetized. The medial skin of the upper arm (intercostobrachial nerve, T2), however, is never anesthetized by any technique of the brachial plexus block and when needed can be blocked by an additional subcutaneous injection just distal to the axilla. For a more comprehensive review of the brachial plexus anatomy and distribution, see Chapter 1, Essential Regional Anesthesia Anatomy.

## Equipment

Equipment needed includes the following:

- Ultrasound machine with linear transducer (8–14 MHz), sterile sleeve, and gel (or other coupling medium; e.g. saline)
- Standard nerve block tray (described in Chapter 3)

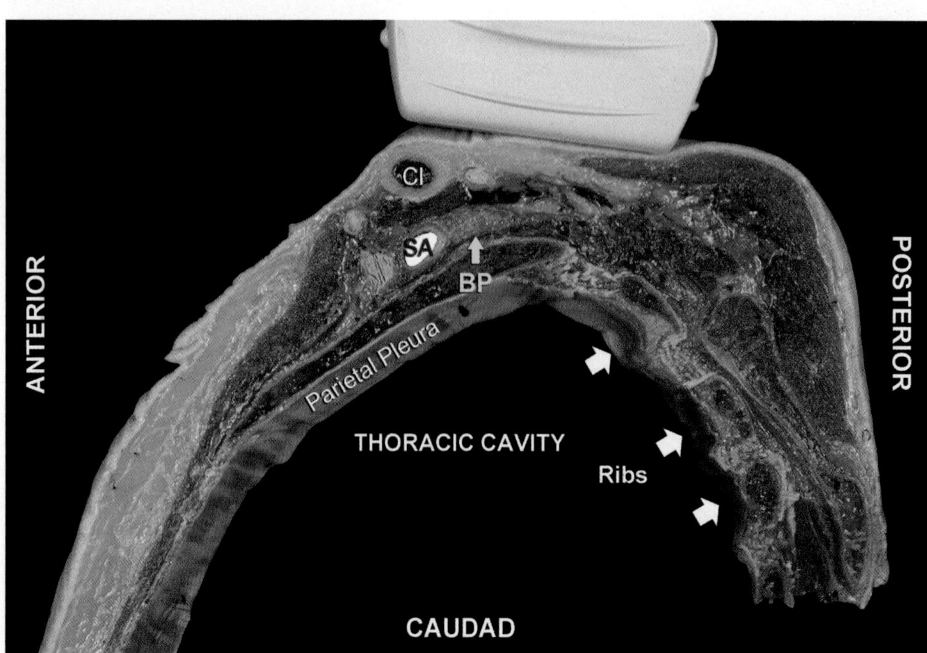


**FIGURE 30-2.** Anatomy of the supraclavicular brachial plexus with proper transducer placement slightly obliquely above the clavicle (Cl). SA, subclavian artery; arrow, brachial plexus (BP).

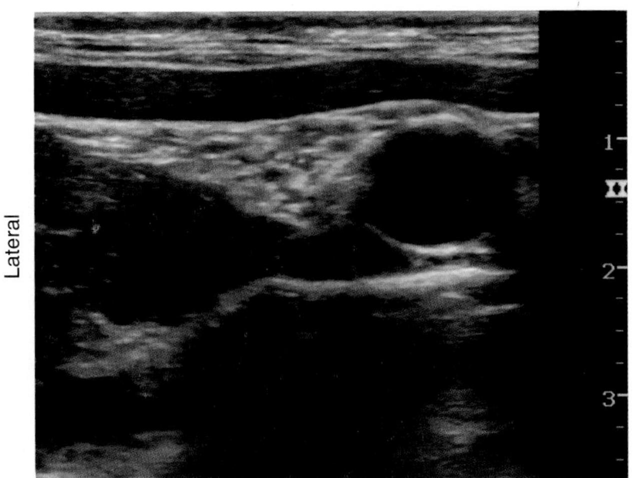


**FIGURE 30-3.** Unlabeled ultrasound image of the supraclavicular brachial plexus.

- 20 to 25 mL local anesthetic
- 5-cm, 22-gauge short-bevel insulated stimulating needle
- Peripheral nerve stimulator
- Sterile gloves

## Landmarks and Patient Positioning

Any position that allows comfortable placement of the ultrasound transducer and needle advancement is appropriate. This block can be performed with the patient in the supine, semi-sitting (our favorite), or slight oblique position, with the patient's head turned away from the side to be blocked. When possible, asking the patient to reach for the ipsilateral knee will depress the clavicle slightly and allow better access to the structures of the anterolateral neck. Also, a slight elevation of the head of the bed is often more comfortable for the patient and allows for better drainage and less prominence of the neck veins (Figure 30-1).

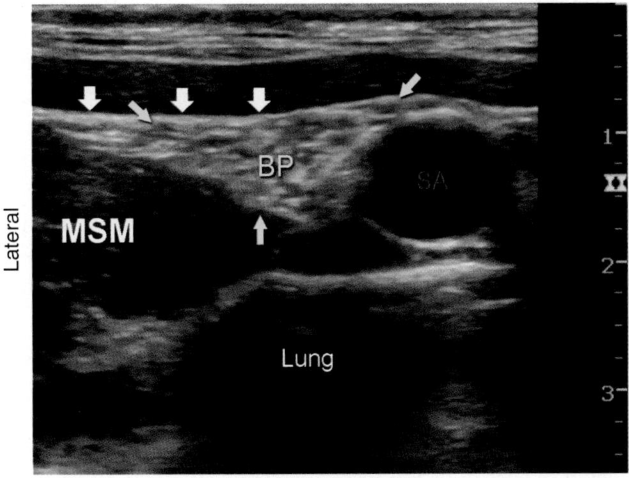


**FIGURE 30-4.** Supraclavicular brachial plexus (BP) is seen slightly superficial and lateral to the subclavian artery (SA). Brachial plexus is enveloped by a tissue sheath (white arrows). Note the intimate location of the pleura and lung to the brachial plexus and subclavian artery. Middle scalene muscle (MSM). White arrows: Prevertebral fascia.

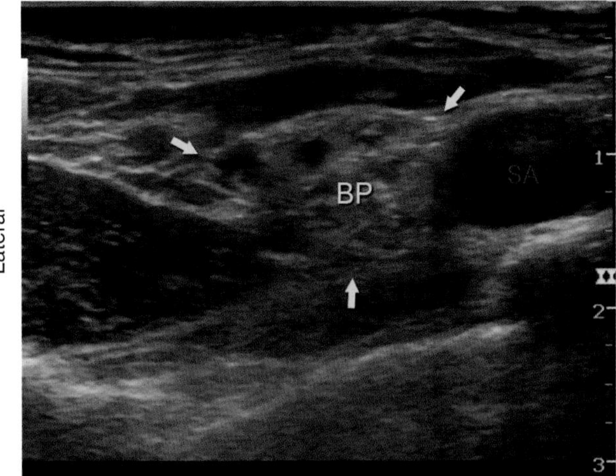


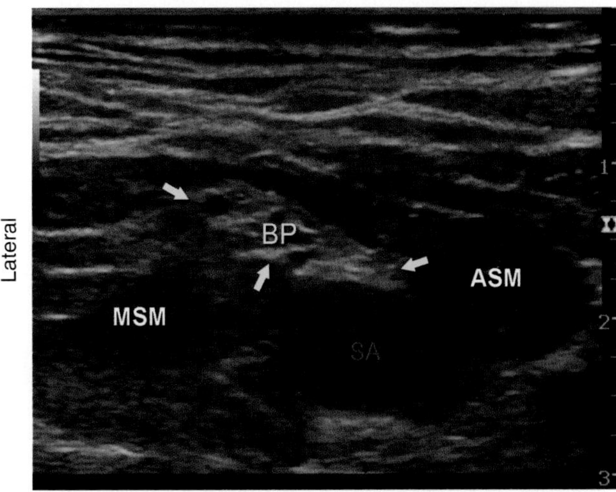


**FIGURE 30-5.** (A) Ultrasound image of the brachial plexus (BP) assuming an oval shape and circled by the tissue sheath (yellow arrows). (B) Ultrasound image of the BP at the supraclavicular fossa with the downward orientation of the transducer. The brachial plexus assumes a flatter configuration as it descends underneath the clavicle into the infraclavicular fossa. SA, subclavian artery. ASM, anterior scalene muscle.

Adherence to strict anatomic landmarks is of lesser importance for the ultrasound-guided supraclavicular block than for the surface anatomy techniques. However, knowledge of the underlying anatomy and the position of the brachial plexus in relation to the subclavian artery, first rib, and pleura are important for the success and safety of the technique. Scanning is usually started just above the clavicle at approximately its midpoint.

## GOAL

The goal is to place the needle in the brachial plexus sheath in the vicinity of the subclavian artery and inject local anesthetic until the spread within the brachial plexus is documented by observing the centrifugal displacement of the trunks and divisions on the ultrasound.

## Technique

With the patient in the proper position (we prefer semi-sitting position), the skin is disinfected and the transducer is positioned in the transverse plane immediately superior to the clavicle at approximately its midpoint. The transducer is tilted caudally to obtain a cross-sectional view of the subclavian artery (Figures 30-6). The brachial plexus is seen as a collection of hypoechoic oval structures lateral and superficial to the artery.

## TIP

- To achieve the best possible view, the transducer often must be tilted slightly inferiorly, rather than perpendicular to the skin. The goal is to see the artery as a pulsating circular structure (transverse view), rather than an oval or linear structure.

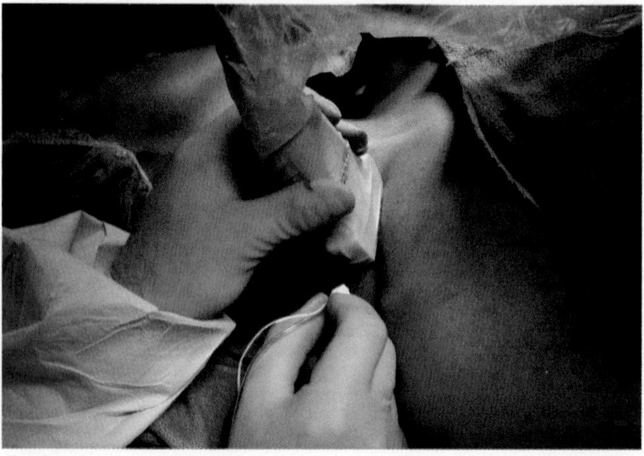

**FIGURE 30-6.** Supraclavicular brachial plexus; transducer position and needle insertion.

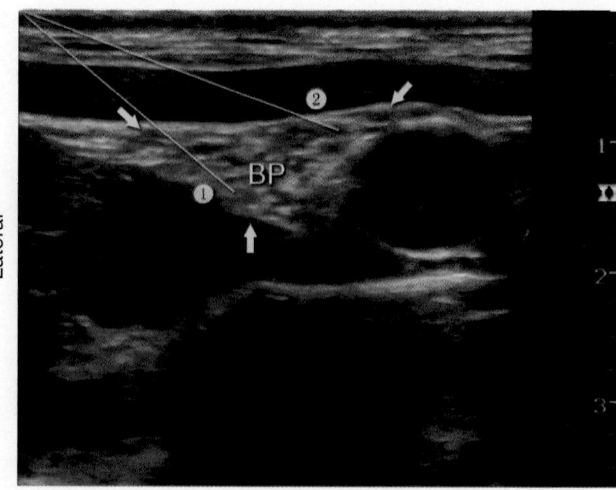


**FIGURE 30-7.** Supraclavicular brachial plexus. Needle path and two separate injections required for block of the supraclavicular brachial plexus. Shown are two needle positions (1 and 2) used to inject local anesthetic within the tissue sheath (arrows) containing the brachial plexus (BP).

Using a 25- to 27-gauge needle, 1 to 2 mL of local anesthetic is injected into the skin 1 cm lateral to the transducer to decrease the discomfort during needle insertion. Local infiltration may not be necessary in well premedicated patients. The needle should never be inserted deeper than 1 cm to avoid inadvertent puncture of and injection into the brachial plexus. Always observe the distribution of the local anesthetic during administration by injecting small amounts of the local anesthetic as the needle advances through tissue layers (hydro-localization). The block needle is then inserted in-plane toward the brachial plexus, in a lateral-to-medial direction (Figures 30-6 and 30-7). When nerve stimulation is used (0.5 mA, 0.1 msec), the entrance of the needle into the brachial plexus sheath is often associated with a palpable "pop" as the needle passes through the paravertebral fascia/brachial plexus sheath. In addition, a motor response of the arm, forearm, or hand as another confirmation of the proper needle placement. Note, however, that motor response may be absent despite the adequate needle placement. Tilting the needle slightly within the plexus and/or increasing the current intensity (e.g., 1.0–1.5 mA) will bring about the motor response, if required. After a careful aspiration, 1 to 2 mL of local anesthetic is injected to document the proper needle placement. When the injection displaces the brachial plexus away from the needle, an additional advancement of the needle 1 to 2 mm deeper may be required to accomplish adequate spread of the local anesthetic (Figures 30-8, 30-9, and 30-10). When injection of the local anesthetic does not appear to result in a spread in and around the brachial plexus, additional needle repositioning and injections may be necessary. The required volume of local anesthetic should not be premeditated but rather determined based on the adequacy of the spread. In our practice, 20 to 25 mL is the most common total volume used.

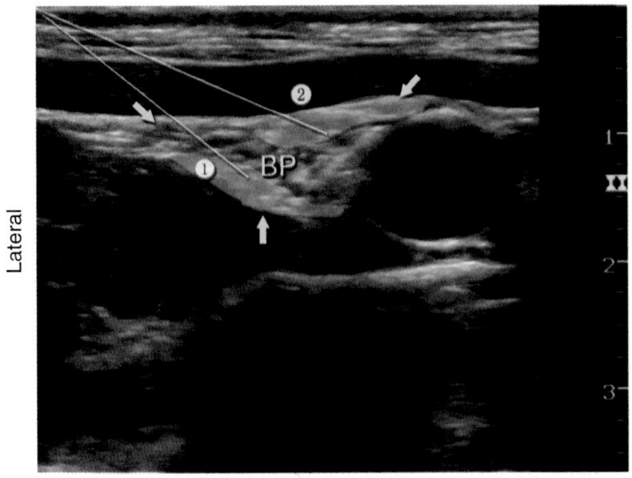

Supraclavicular block

**FIGURE 30-8.** Desired spread of the local anesthetic (areas shaded in blue) through two different needle positions (1 and 2), to accomplish brachial plexus (BP) block. Local anesthetic should freely spread within the tissue sheath resulting in separation of the BP cords.

## TIPS

- The presence of the motor response to nerve stimulation is useful but not necessary to elicit if the plexus, needle, and local anesthetic spread are well visualized.
- The neck is a very vascular area and care must be exercised to avoid needle placement or injection into the vascular structures. Of particular importance is to note the intimately located internal jugular vein, inferior carotid artery, subclavian artery and the dorsal scapular artery which often crosses the supraclavicular brachial plexus at this level. The use of color Doppler before needle placement and injection is suggested.
- Never inject against high resistance (>15 psi) to injection because this may signal an intrafascicular injection.
- Multiple injections:
    - May increase the speed of onset and success rate.
    - May allow for a reduction in the required volume of local anesthetic.
    - May carry a higher risk of nerve injury because part of the plexus may be anesthetized by the previous injections.

In an adult patient, 20 to 25 mL of local anesthetic is usually adequate for successful and rapid onset of blockade; however, when necessary, higher volumes may be used.

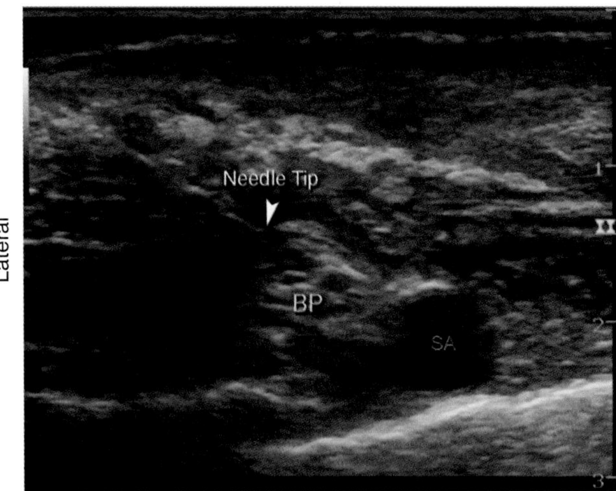


Supraclavicular block, needle placement

**FIGURE 30-9.** Supraclavicular brachial plexus (BP) with an actual needle passing the tissue sheath surrounding brachial plexus. Needle is seen within the BP, although its tip is not visualized. Injection at this location often results in deterioration of the ultrasound image; reliance on additional monitoring (injection pressure, nerve stimulation) to avoid intrafascicular injection is essential.

Some clinicians recommend injecting a single bolus at the point where the subclavian artery meets the first rib. This is thought to "float" the plexus superficially and result in more reliable blockade of the inferior divisions of the plexus. However, we do not find this useful or safe (risk of pleura puncture); instead it is always beneficial to inject two to three smaller aliquots at different locations within the plexus

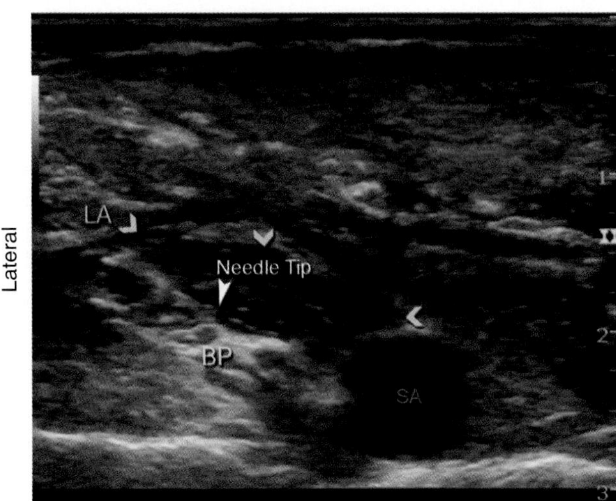


Supraclavicular block, injecting LA

**FIGURE 30-10.** Proper dispersion of the local anesthetic (LA; blue arrows after its injection within the tissue sheath containing the brachial plexus (BP).

sheath to assure spread of the local anesthetic solution in all planes containing brachial plexus. In our program, we simply administer two aliquots of local anesthetics at two separate locations within the plexus sheath as seen in Figure 30-8. The block dynamics and perioperative management are similar to those described in Chapter 13.

## Continuous Ultrasound-Guided Supraclavicular Block

The ultrasound-guided continuous supraclavicular block is in many ways similar to the technique for interscalene catheter placement. The goal is to place the catheter in the vicinity of the trunks/divisions of the brachial plexus adjacent to the subclavian artery. The procedure consists of three phases: needle placement, catheter advancement, and securing of the catheter. For the first two phases of the procedure, ultrasound can be used to assure accuracy in most patients. The needle is typically inserted in-plane from the lateral-to-medial direction so that the tip is just lateral to the brachial plexus sheath. The needle is then advanced to indent and transverse the sheath, followed by placement of the catheter.

### TIP

- When the needle approaches the brachial plexus, extra force is required to penetrate the prevertebral fascia and enter the brachial plexus "sheath". The entrance of the needle into the sheath is always associated with a distinct "pop" sensation as the needle breaches the fascial layer.

Proper placement of the needle can also be confirmed by obtaining a motor response of the arm, forearm, or hand, at which point 4–5 mL of local anesthetic is injected. This small dose of local anesthetic serves to assure adequate distribution of the local anesthetic as well as to make the advancement of the catheter more comfortable to the patient. This first

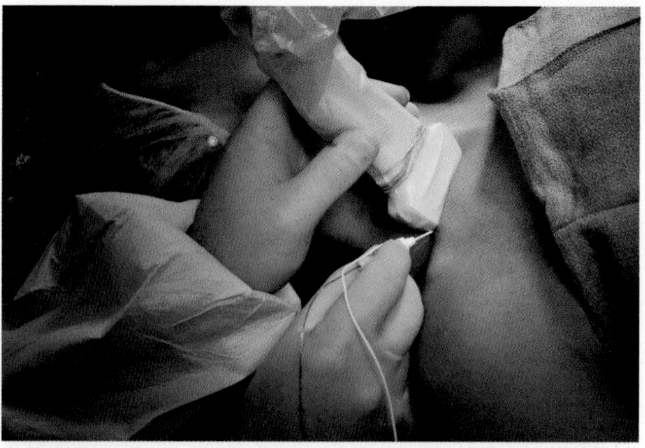

**FIGURE 30-11.** A needle insertion for the continuous supraclavicular brachial plexus block. The catheter is inserted 3–5 cm beyond the needle tip and injected with 3–5 mL of local anesthetic to document the proper dispersion of the local anesthetic within the brachial plexus sheath.

phase of the procedure does not significantly differ from the single-injection technique. The second phase of the procedure involves maintaining the needle in the proper position and inserting the catheter 2 to 3 cm into the sheath of the brachial plexus (Figure 30-11 shows the preloaded needle with the catheter). Care must be taken not to advance the catheter too far, which may result in the catheter exiting the brachial plexus and the consequent failure to provide analgesia. Insertion of the catheter can be accomplished by either a single operator or a with a helper.

The catheter is secured by either taping to the skin or tunneling. Some clinicians prefer one over the other. The decision about which method to use could be based on the patient's age, duration of the catheter therapy, and anatomy. Tunneling could be preferred in older patients with obesity or mobile skin over the neck and longer planned duration of the catheter infusion. Two main disadvantages of the tunneling are the risk of catheter dislodgment during the tunneling and the potential for scar formation. A number of devices are commercially available to help secure the catheter. The starting infusion regimen is typically 5 mL/hour of 0.2% ropivacaine with 5-mL patient-controlled boluses hourly.

## ULTRASOUND-GUIDED SUPRACLAVICULAR BLOCK

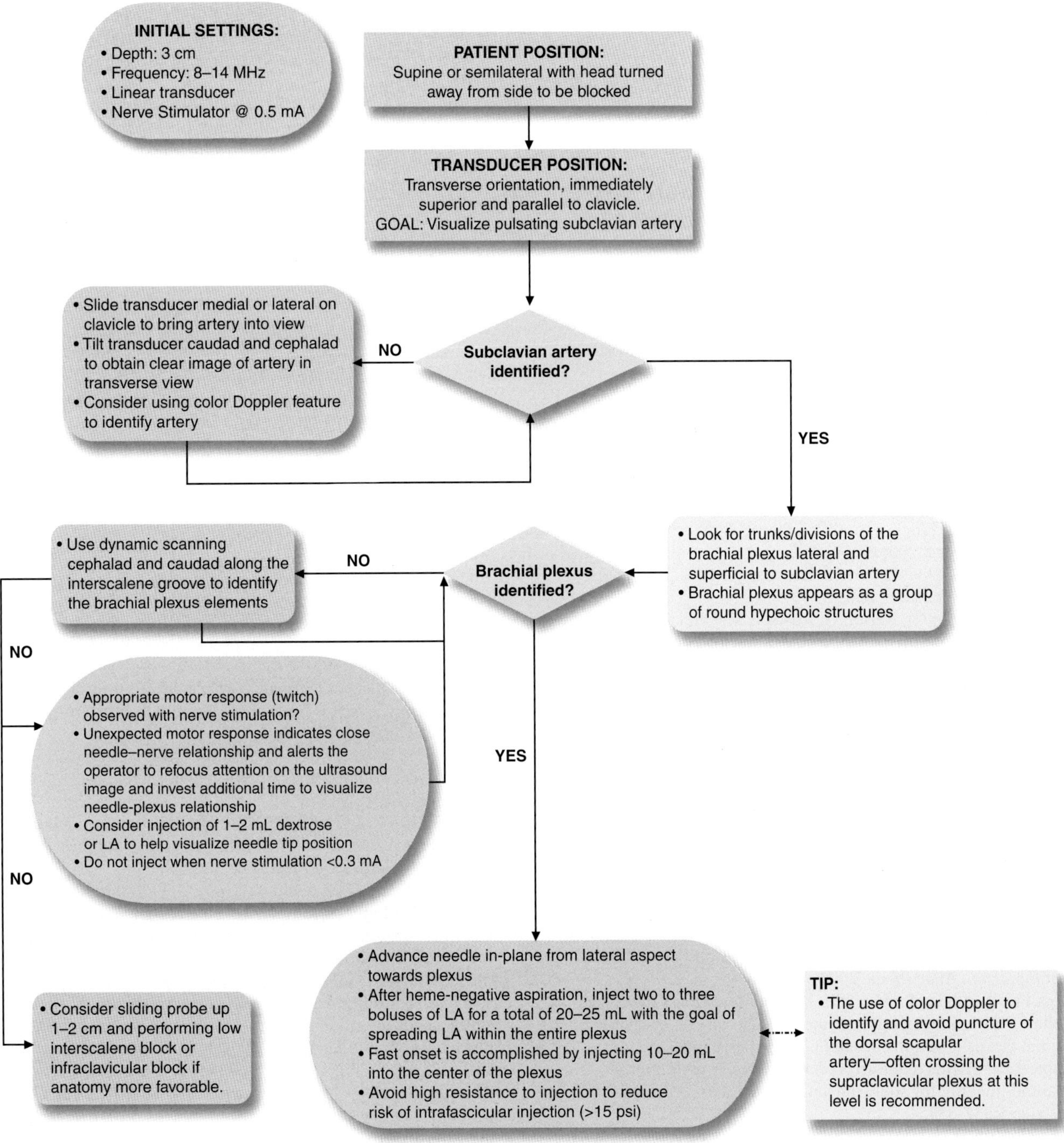

## SUGGESTED READING


Aguirre J, Ekatodramis G, Ruland P, Borgeat A: Ultrasound-guided supraclavicular block: is it really safer? *Reg Anesth Pain Med.* 2009;34:622.

Arcand G, Williams SR, Chouinard P, et al. Ultrasound-guided infraclavicular versus supraclavicular block. *Anesth Analg.* 2005;101:886-890.

Beach ML, Sites BD, Gallagher JD. Use of a nerve stimulator does not improve the efficacy of ultrasound-guided supraclavicular nerve blocks. *J Clin Anesth.* 2006;18:580-584.

Bigeleisen PE, Moayeri N, Groen GJ. Extraneural versus intraneural stimulation thresholds during ultrasound-guided supraclavicular block. *Anesthesiology.* 2009;110:1235-1243.

Chan VW, Perlas A, Rawson R, Odukoya O. Ultrasound-guided supraclavicular brachial plexus block. *Anesth Analg.* 2003;97:1514-1517.

Chin KJ, Niazi A, Chan V. Anomalous brachial plexus anatomy in the supraclavicular region detected by ultrasound. *Anesth Analg.* 2008;107:729-731.

Chin KJ, Singh M, Velayutham V, Chee V. Infraclavicular brachial plexus block for regional anaesthesia of the lower arm. *Cochrane Database Syst Rev.* 2010;2:CD005487.

Chin J, Tsui BC. No change in impedance upon intravascular injection of D5W. *Can J Anaesth.* 2010;57:559-564.

Collins AB, Gray AT, Kessler J. Ultrasound-guided supraclavicular brachial plexus block: a modified Plumb-Bob technique. *Reg Anesth Pain Med.* 2006;31:591-592.

Cornish P. Supraclavicular block—new perspectives. *Reg Anesth Pain Med.* 2009;34:607-608.

Cornish PB, Leaper CJ, Nelson G, Anstis F, McQuillan C, Stienstra R. Avoidance of phrenic nerve paresis during continuous supraclavicular regional anaesthesia. *Anaesthesia.* 2007;62:354-358.

Duggan E, Brull R, Lai J, Abbas S. Ultrasound-guided brachial plexus block in a patient with multiple glomangiomatosis. *Reg Anesth Pain Med.* 2008;33:70-73.

Duggan E, El Beheiry H, Perlas A, et al. Minimum effective volume of local anesthetic for ultrasound-guided supraclavicular brachial plexus block. *Reg Anesth Pain Med.* 2009;34:215-218.

Fredrickson MJ, Kilfoyle DH. Neurological complication analysis of 1000 ultrasound guided peripheral nerve blocks for elective orthopaedic surgery: a prospective study. *Anaesthesia.* 2009;64:836-844.

Fredrickson MJ, Patel A, Young S, Chinchanwala S. Speed of onset of 'corner pocket supraclavicular' and infraclavicular ultrasound guided brachial plexus block: a randomised observer-blinded comparison. *Anaesthesia.* 2009;64:738-744.

Gupta PK, Pace NL, Hopkins PM. Effect of body mass index on the ED50 volume of bupivacaine 0.5% for supraclavicular brachial plexus block. *Br J Anaesth.* 2010;104:490-495.

Hebbard PD. Artifactual mirrored subclavian artery on ultrasound imaging for supraclavicular block. *Can J Anaesth.* 2009;56:537-538.

Jeon DG, Kim WI. Cases series: ultrasound-guided supraclavicular block in 105 patients. *Korean J Anesthesiol.* 2010;58:267-271.

Kapral S, Krafft P, Eibenberger K, Fitzgerald R, Gosch M, Weinstabl C. Ultrasound-guided supraclavicular approach for regional anesthesia of the brachial plexus. *Anesth Analg.* 1994;78:507-513.

Klaastad O, Sauter AR, Dodgson MS. Brachial plexus block with or without ultrasound guidance. *Curr Opin Anaesthesiol.* 2009;22:655-660.

la Grange P, Foster PA, Pretorius LK. Application of the Doppler ultrasound bloodflow detector in supraclavicular brachial plexus block. *Br J Anaesth.* 1978;50:965-967.

Lasserre A, Tran-Van D, Gaertner E, Labadie P, Fontaine B: Ultrasound guided locoregional anaesthesia: realization and diagnosis of complications [in French]. *Ann Fr Anesth Reanim.* 2009;28:584-587.

Macfarlane AJ, Perlas A, Chan V, Brull R. Eight ball, corner pocket ultrasound-guided supraclavicular block: avoiding a scratch. *Reg Anesth Pain Med.* 2008;33:502-503.

Manickam BP, Oosthuysen SA, Parikh MK. Supraclavicular brachial plexus block-variant relation of brachial plexus to subclavian artery on the first rib. *Reg Anesth Pain Med.* 2009;34:383-384.

Marhofer P, Schrogendorfer K, Koinig H, Kapral S, Weinstabl C, Mayer N. Ultrasonographic guidance improves sensory block and onset time of three-in-one blocks. *Anesth Analg.* 1997;85:854-857.

Morfey D, Brull R. Ultrasound-guided supraclavicular block: What is intraneural? *Anesthesiology.* 2010;112:250-251.

Morfey DH, Brull R. Finding the corner pocket: landmarks in ultrasound-guided supraclavicular block. *Anaesthesia.* 2009;64:1381.

Neal JM, Moore JM, Kopacz DJ, Liu SS, Kramer DJ, Plorde JJ. Quantitative analysis of respiratory, motor, and sensory function after supraclavicular block. *Anesth Analg.* 1998;86:1239-1244.

Perlas A, Chan VW, Simons M. Brachial plexus examination and localization using ultrasound and electrical stimulation: a volunteer study. *Anesthesiology.* 2003;99:429-435.

Perlas A, Lobo G, Lo N, Brull R, Chan VW, Karkhanis R. Ultrasound-guided supraclavicular block: outcome of 510 consecutive cases. *Reg Anesth Pain Med.* 2009;34:171-176.

Plunkett AR, Brown DS, Rogers JM, Buckenmaier CC 3rd. Supraclavicular continuous peripheral nerve block in a wounded soldier: when ultrasound is the only option. *Br J Anaesth.* 2006;97:715-717.

Renes SH, Spoormans HH, Gielen MJ, Rettig HC, van Geffen GJ. Hemidiaphragmatic paresis can be avoided in ultrasound-guided supraclavicular brachial plexus block. *Reg Anesth Pain Med.* 2009; 34:595-599.

Samet R, Villamater E. Eight ball, corner pocket for ultrasound-guided supraclavicular block: high risk for a scratch. *Reg Anesth Pain Med.* 2008;33:87.

Shorthouse JR, Danbury CM. Ultrasound-guided supraclavicular brachial plexus block in Klippel-Feil syndrome. *Anaesthesia.* 2009;64:693-694.

Soares LG, Brull R, Lai J, Chan VW. Eight ball, corner pocket: the optimal needle position for ultrasound-guided supraclavicular block. *Reg Anesth Pain Med.* 2007;32:94-95.

Tran de QH, Munoz L, Zaouter C, Russo G, Finlayson RJ. A prospective, randomized comparison between single- and double-injection, ultrasound-guided supraclavicular brachial plexus block. *Reg Anesth Pain Med.* 2009;34:420-424.

Tran de QH, Russo G, Munoz L, Zaouter C, Finlayson RJ. A prospective, randomized comparison between ultrasound-guided supraclavicular, infraclavicular, and axillary brachial plexus blocks. *Reg Anesth Pain Med.* 2009;34:366-371.

Tsui BC, Doyle K, Chu K, Pillay J, Dillane D. Case series: ultrasound-guided supraclavicular block using a curvilinear probe in 104 day-case hand surgery patients. *Can J Anaesth.* 2009;56:46-51.

Tsui BC, Twomey C, Finucane BT. Visualization of the brachial plexus in the supraclavicular region using a curved ultrasound probe with a sterile transparent dressing. *Reg Anesth Pain Med.* 2006;31:182-184.

VadeBoncouer TR, Weinberg GL, Oswald S, Angelov F. Early detection of intravascular injection during ultrasound-guided supraclavicular brachial plexus block. *Reg Anesth Pain Med.* 2008;33:278-279.

Williams SR, Chouinard P, Arcand G, et al. Ultrasound guidance speeds execution and improves the quality of supraclavicular block. *Anesth Analg.* 2003;97:1518-1523.

# Ultrasound-Guided Infraclavicular Brachial Plexus Block

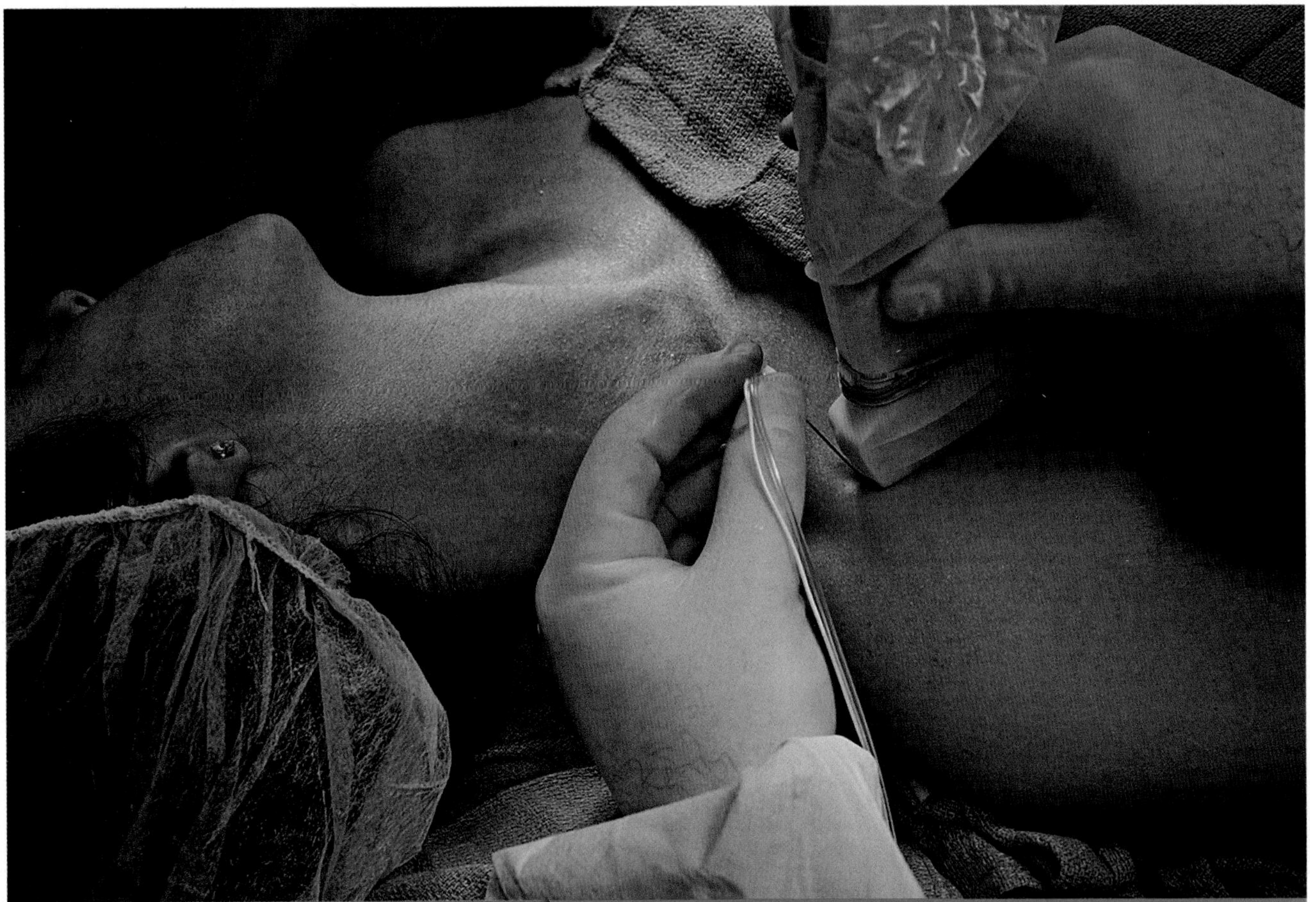

## BLOCK AT A GLANCE

- Indications: arm, elbow, forearm, and hand surgery
- Transducer position: approximately parasagittal, just medial to coracoid process, inferior to clavicle
- Goal: local anesthetic spread around axillary artery
- Local anesthetic volume: 20–30 mL

**FIGURE 31-1.** In-plane needle insertion technique during infraclavicular brachial plexus block.

## General Considerations

The ultrasound-guided infraclavicular brachial plexus block is in some ways both simple and challenging. It is simple in the sense that geometric measuring of distances and angles on the surface of the patient, as is the case with the nerve stimulator–based technique, is not required. Identification of the arterial pulse on the sonographic image is an easy primary goal in establishing the landmark. However, the plexus at this level is situated deeper, and the angle of approach is more acute, making simultaneous visualization of the needle and the relevant anatomy more challenging. Fortunately, although it is not always possible to reliably identify the three cords of the plexus at this position, adequate block can be achieved by simply depositing the local anesthetic in a "U" shape around the artery. Infraclavicular block is well-suited for catheter technique because the musculature of the chest wall helps stabilize the catheter and prevents its dislodgment compared with the more superficial location with the interscalene or supraclavicular approaches.

## Ultrasound Anatomy

The axillary artery can be identified deep to the pectoralis major and minor muscles. An effort needs to be made to obtain clear views of both pectoralis muscles and their respective fasciae. This is important because the area of interest lies underneath the fascia of the pectoralis minor muscle. Surrounding the artery are the three cords of the brachial plexus: the lateral, posterior, and medial cords. These are named for their usual position relative to the axillary artery, although there is a great deal of anatomic variation. With the left side of the screen corresponding to the cephalad aspect, the cords can often be seen as round hyperechoic structures at approximately 9 o'clock (lateral cord), 7 o'clock (posterior cord), and 5 o'clock (medial cord) (Figures 31-2, 31-3, and 31-4). The axillary vein is seen as a compressible hypoechoic structure that lies inferior, or slightly superficial, to the axillary artery. Multiple other, smaller vessels (e.g., the cephalic vein) are often present as well. The transducer is moved in the superior-inferior direction until the artery is identified in cross-section. Depending on the depth of field selected and the level at which the scanning is performed, the chest wall and lung may be seen in the inferior aspect of the image. The axillary artery and/or brachial plexus are typically identified at a depth of 3 to 5 cm in average size patients.

## Distribution of Blockade

The infraclavicular approach to brachial plexus blockade results in anesthesia of the upper limb below the shoulder. The medial skin of the upper arm (intercostobrachial nerve, T2), if required, can be blocked by an additional subcutaneous injection on the medial aspect of the arm just distal to the axilla. A simpler approach is for surgeons to infiltrate the skin with the local anesthetic directly over the incision line, if necessary. For a more comprehensive review of the brachial plexus distribution, see Chapter 1, Essential Regional Anesthesia Anatomy.

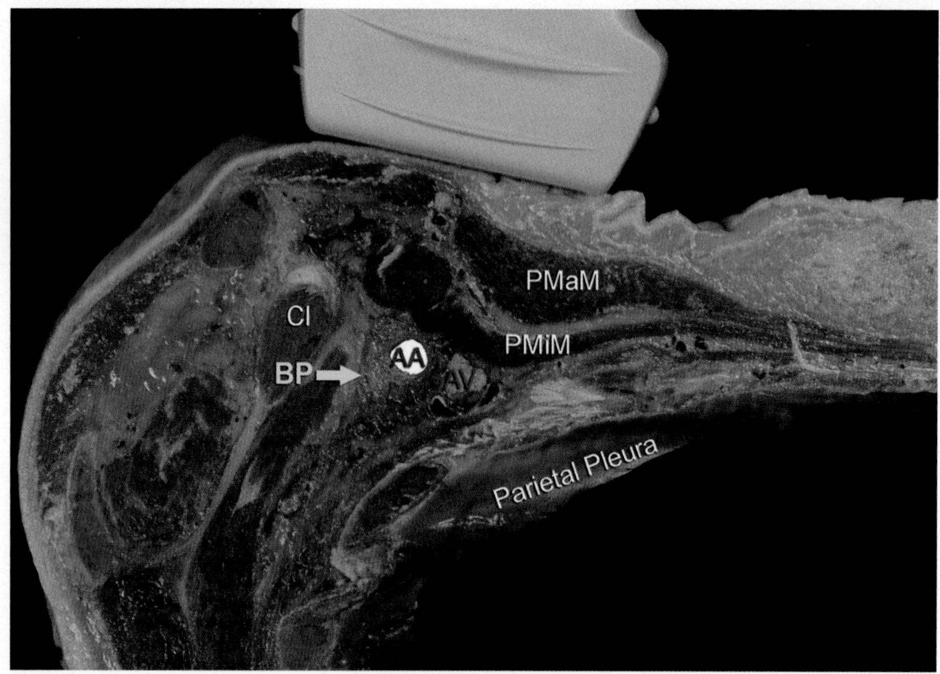


**FIGURE 31-2.** Anatomy of the infraclavicular brachial plexus and the position of the transducer. Brachial plexus (BP) is seen surrounding the axillary artery (AA) underneath the clavicle (CI) and pectoralis minor muscle (PMiM). Note that the injection of local anesthetic should take place below the fascia of the PMiM to spread around the AA. PMaM, pectoralis major muscle.

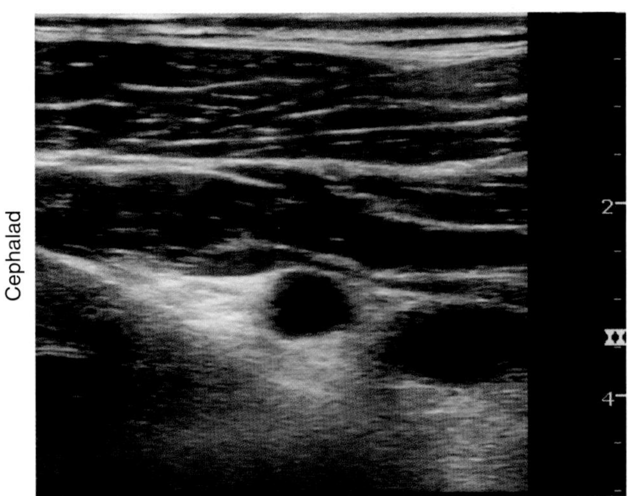


**FIGURE 31-3.** Unlabeled ultrasound image of the infraclavicular fossa demonstrating pectoralis muscles, their respective sheets, axillary (subclavian) vessels, and the chest wall.

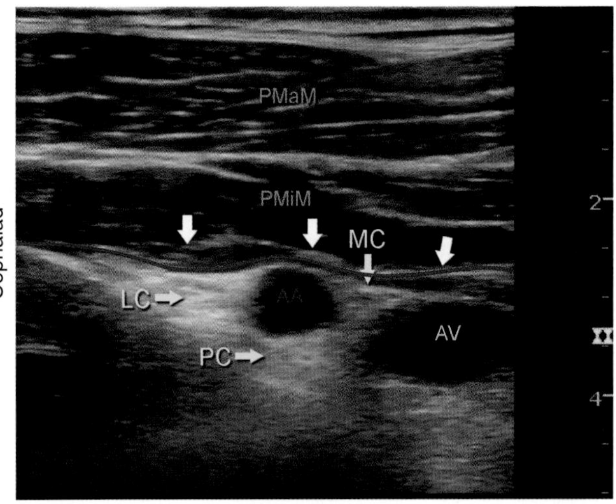


**FIGURE 31-4.** Labeled ultrasound image of the brachial plexus (BP) in the infraclavicular fossa. LC, lateral cord; PC, posterior cord; MC, medial cord. Note that the brachial plexus and the axillary artery (AA) are located below the fascia (red line) of the pectoralis minor muscle (PMiM). PMaM, pectoralis major muscle.

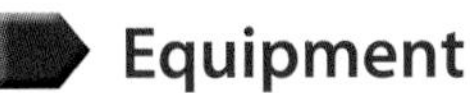

## Equipment

Equipment needed for this block includes the following:

- Ultrasound machine with linear transducer (8–14 MHz), sterile sleeve, and gel
- Standard nerve block tray
- 20 to 30 mL of local anesthetic drawn up in syringes
- 8- to 10-cm long, 21-22 gauge short-bevel insulated stimulating needle
- Peripheral nerve stimulator
- Sterile gloves

## Landmarks and Patient Positioning

Any position that allows comfortable placement of the ultrasound transducer and needle advancement is appropriate. The block is typically performed with the patient in supine position with the head turned away from the side to be blocked (Figure 31-5). The arm is abducted to 90° and the elbow flexed. This maneuver reduces the depth from the skin to the plexus and substantially facilitates visualization of the pectoralis muscles as well as the cords of the brachial plexus.

The coracoid process is an important landmark and can be easily identified by palpating the bony prominence just medial to the shoulder while the arm is elevated and lowered. As the arm is lowered, the coracoid process meets the fingers of the palpating hand. Scanning is usually begun just medial to the coracoid process and inferior to the clavicle. As scanning experience increases, it eventually becomes unnecessary to identify the coracoids process before scanning.

## GOAL

**The goal of the technique is to inject local anesthetic until the spread around the artery is documented by ultrasound. It is not necessary to identify and target individual cords. Instead, injection of the local anesthetic to surround the artery in a U-shape pattern (cephalad, caudad, and posterior) suffices for block of all three cords.**

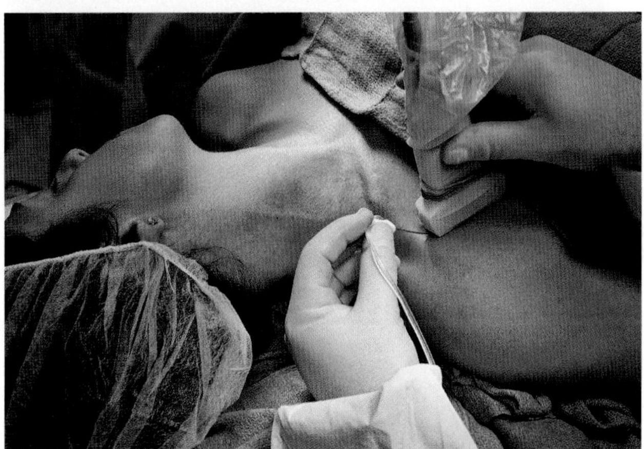

**FIGURE 31-5.** Patient position in needle insertion for infraclavicular brachial plexus block. The transducer is positioned parasagittally just medial to the coracoid process and inferior to the clavicle.

## Technique

With the patient in the proper position, the skin is disinfected and the transducer is positioned in the parasagittal plane to identify the axillary artery (Figures 31-3 and 31-4, and 31-5). This may require adjustment of the depth, depending on the thickness of the patient's chest wall musculature. The axillary artery (or the transition of the subclavian to axillary artery) is typically seen between 3 and 5 cm. Once the artery is identified, an attempt is made to identify the hyperechoic cords of the brachial plexus and their corresponding positions relative to the artery, although these may not always be identifiable. Fortunately, exhaustive efforts to visualize the cords are not necessary for successful blockade.

### TIP

- Reverberation artifact posterior to the artery is often misinterpreted as the posterior cord. Figure 31-7 demonstrate such a dilemma where the structured labeled as posterior cord (PC) can easily represent a mere reverberation artifact.

The needle is inserted in-plane from the cephalad aspect, with the insertion point just inferior to the clavicle (Figure 31-5). The needle is aimed toward the posterior aspect of the axillary artery and passes through the pectoralis major and minor muscles. If nerve stimulation is used concurrently (0.5-0.8 mA, 0.1 msec), the first motor response is often from the lateral cord (either elbow flexion or finger flexion). As the needle is further advanced beneath the artery, a posterior cord motor response may appear (finger and wrist extension). After careful aspiration, 1 to 2 mL of local anesthetic is injected to confirm the proper needle placement and spread. The injectate should spread cephalad and caudad to cover the lateral and medial cords, respectively (Figure 31-6). When injection of the local anesthetic with a single injection does not appear to result in adequate spread, additional needle repositions and injections around the axillary artery may be necessary (Figure 31-7).

### TIPS

- A caudad to cephalad needle insertion is also possible but may carry a higher risk of peumothorax and venous puncture.
- To decrease the risk of complications:
  - Aspirate every 5 mL to decrease a risk of an intravascular injection.
  - Do not inject if the resistance to injection is high.
  - Do not change the transducer pressure throughout the injection (this can "open and close" veins in the area and possibly increase the risk of an intravascular injection).

Infraclavicular block

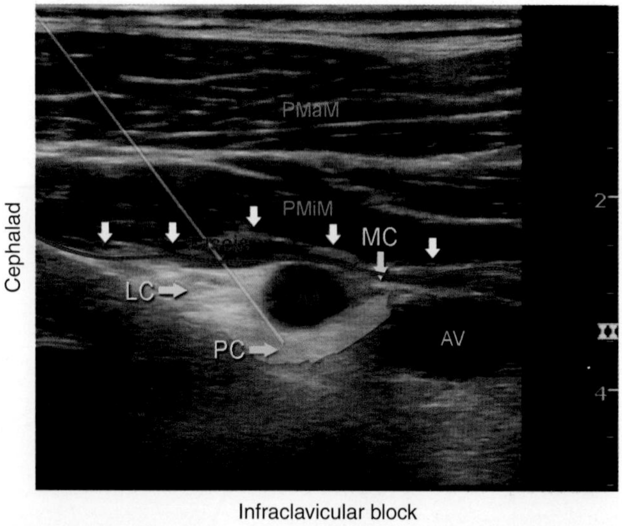

**FIGURE 31-6.** Ultrasound image demonstrating an ideal needle path for the infraclavicular brachial plexus block. Blue-shaded area mimics an ideal spread of the local anesthetic around axillary artery (AA) and reaching all three cords of the brachial plexus (LC, PC, MC) below the fascia (red line) of the pectoralis minor muscle. PMaM, pectoralis major muscle; PMiM, pectoralis minor muscle.

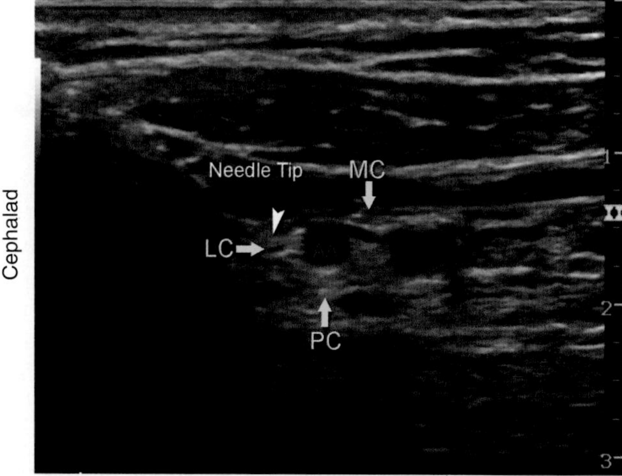


**FIGURE 31-7.** An ultrasound image demonstrating an actual needle placement above (cephalad) the axillary artery (AA) and an injection of local anesthetic (2 mL; blue shadow) to document the proper needle tip placement. LC, lateral cord; MC, medial cord; PC, posterior cord.

In an adult patient, 20 to 30 mL of local anesthetic is usually adequate for successful blockade. Although a single injection of such large volumes of local anesthetic often suffices, it may be beneficial to inject two to three smaller aliquots at different locations to assure spread of the local anesthetic solution in all planes containing brachial plexus. The block dynamics and perioperative management are similar to those described in Chapter 14.

## Continuous Ultrasound-Guided Infraclavicular Block

The goal of the continuous infraclavicular block is similar to the non–ultrasound-based techniques: to place the catheter in the vicinity of the cords of the brachial plexus beneath the pectoral muscles. The procedure consists of three phases: needle placement, catheter advancement, and securing of the catheter. For the first two phases of the procedure, ultrasound can be used to assure accuracy in most patients. The needle is typically inserted in-plane from the cephalad-to-caudad direction, similar to the single-injection technique (Figure 31-8).

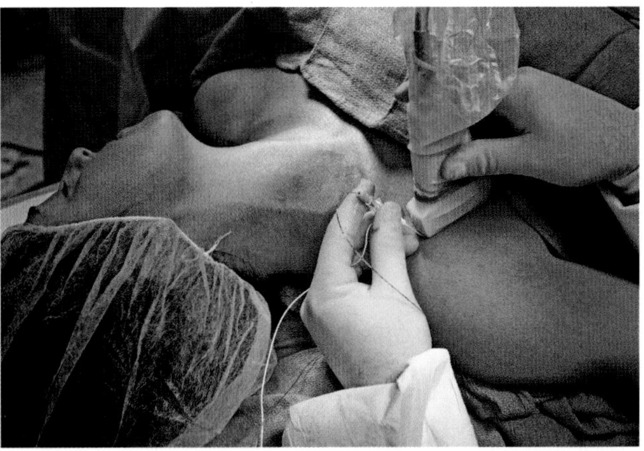

**FIGURE 31-8.** Patient position, imaging and needle placement for continuous infraclavicular brachial plexus block are similar to those in a single-injection technique. Once the proper needle tip is determined by injection of a small volume of local anesthetic, the catheter is inserted 2–4 cm beyond the needle tip.

As with the single injection technique, the needle tip should be placed posterior to the axillary artery prior to injection and catheter advancement. Proper placement of the needle can also be confirmed by obtaining a motor response of the posterior cord (finger or wrist flexion) at which point 1 to 2 mL of local anesthetic is injected. This small dose of local anesthetic serves to document the proper placement of the needle tip as evidenced by adequate distribution of the local anesthetic. The injection also may make the advancement of the catheter more comfortable to the patient. This first phase of the procedure does not significantly differ from the single-injection technique. The second phase of the procedure involves maintaining the needle in the proper position and advancing the catheter 2 to 4 cm beyond the needle tip, in the vicinity of the posterior cord. Insertion of the catheter can be accomplished by either single operator or a with a helper (Figure 31-8). A typical starting infusion regimen is 5 mL/hour with 8-mL patient-controlled boluses every hour. The larger bolus volume is necessary for the adequate spread of the injectate around the artery to reach all cords of the brachial plexus. The catheter is secured by either taping to the skin or tunneling. Some clinicians prefer one over the other. However, the decision on which method to use could be based on the patient's age, duration of the catheter therapy, and anatomy. Tunneling could be preferred in older patients with obesity or mobile skin over the neck and longer planned duration of the catheter infusion. One advantage to catheter placement with the infraclavicular approach is that the pectoralis muscles tend to stabilize the catheter and prevent dislodgment.

# ULTRASOUND-GUIDED INFRACLAVICULAR BLOCK

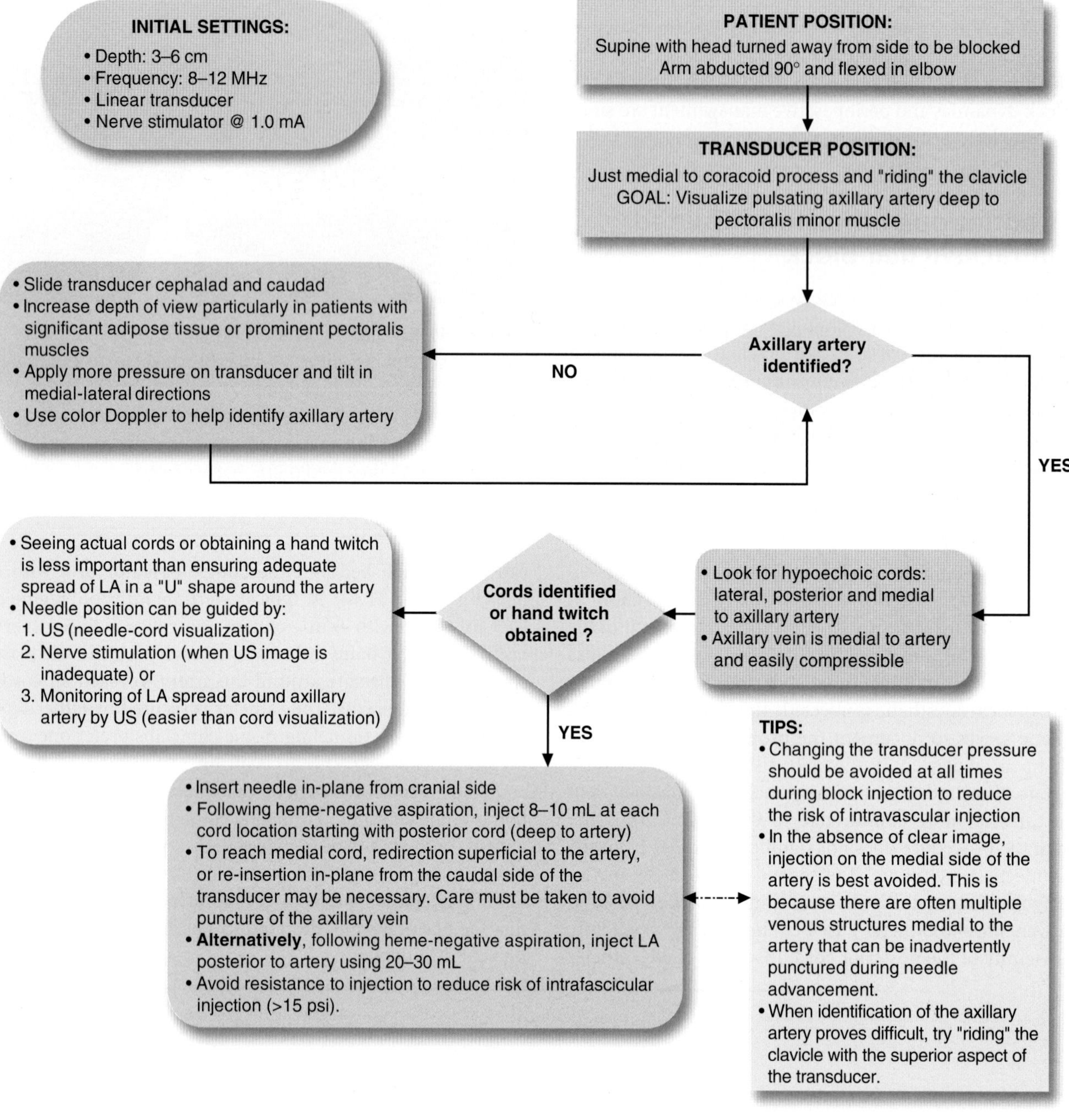

## SUGGESTED READING


Aguirre J, Baulig B, Borgeat A. Does ultrasound-guided infraclavicular block meet users' expectations? *Can J Anaesth.* 2010;57:176-177.

Akyildiz E, Gurkan Y, Caglayan C, Solak M, Toker K. Single vs. double stimulation during a lateral sagittal infraclavicular block. *Acta Anaesthesiol Scand.* 2009;53:1262-1267.

Arcand G, Williams SR, Chouinard P, et al. Ultrasound-guided infraclavicular versus supraclavicular block. *Anesth Analg.* 2005;101:886-890.

Bigeleisen P, Wilson M. A comparison of two techniques for ultrasound guided infraclavicular block. *Br J Anaesth.* 2006;96:502-507.

Bigeleisen PE. Ultrasound-guided infraclavicular block in an anticoagulated and anesthetized patient. *Anesth Analg.* 2007;104:1285-1287.

Bloc S, Garnier T, Komly B, et al. Spread of injectate associated with radial or median nerve-type motor response during infraclavicular brachial-plexus block: an ultrasound evaluation. *Reg Anesth Pain Med.* 2007;32:130-135.

Bowens C Jr, Gupta RK, O'Byrne WT, Schildcrout JS, Shi Y, Hawkins JJ, Michaels DR, Berry JM. *Selective local anesthetic placement using ultrasound guidance and neurostimulation for infraclavicular brachial plexus block.* Anesth Analg. 2010;110:1480-5.

Bowens C Jr, Gupta RK, O'Byrne WT, et al. Selective local anesthetic placement using ultrasound guidance and neurostimulation for infraclavicular brachial plexus block. *Anesth Analg.* 2010;110:1480-1485.

Brull R, Lupu M, Perlas A, Chan VW, McCartney CJ. Compared with dual nerve stimulation, ultrasound guidance shortens the time for infraclavicular block performance. *Can J Anaesth.* 2009;56:812-818.

Brull R, McCartney CJ, Chan VW. A novel approach to infraclavicular brachial plexus block: the ultrasound experience. *Anesth Analg.* 2004;99:950.

Chin KJ, Singh M, Velayutham V, Chee V. Infraclavicular brachial plexus block for regional anaesthesia of the lower arm. *Cochrane Database Syst Rev* 2010;2:CD005487.

Chin KJ, Singh M, Velayutham V, Chee V. *Infraclavicular brachial plexus block for regional anaesthesia of the lower arm. Anesth Analg.* 2010;111:1072.

Desgagnes MC, Levesque S, Dion N, et al. A comparison of a single or triple injection technique for ultrasound-guided infraclavicular block: a prospective randomized controlled study. *Anesth Analg.* 2009;109:668-672.

De Tran QH, Bertini P, Zaouter C, Munoz L, Finlayson RJ. A prospective, randomized comparison between single- and double-injection ultrasound-guided infraclavicular brachial plexus block. *Reg Anesth Pain Med.* 2010;35:16-21.

Dhir S, Ganapathy S. Use of ultrasound guidance and contrast enhancement: a study of continuous infraclavicular brachial plexus approach. *Acta Anaesthesiol Scand.* 2008;52:338-342.

Dhir S, Ganapathy S. Comparative evaluation of ultrasound-guided continuous infraclavicular brachial plexus block with stimulating catheter and traditional technique: a prospective-randomized trial. *Acta Anaesthesiol Scand.* 2008;52:1158-1166.

Dhir S, Singh S, Parkin J, Hannouche F, Richards RS. Multiple finger joint replacement and continuous physiotherapy using ultrasound guided, bilateral infraclavicular catheters for continuous bilateral upper extremity analgesia. *Can J Anaesth.* 2008;55:880-881.

Dingemans E, Williams SR, Arcand G, et al. Neurostimulation in ultrasound-guided infraclavicular block: a prospective randomized trial. *Anesth Analg.* 2007;104:1275-1280.

Dolan J. Ultrasound-guided infraclavicular nerve block and the cephalic vein. *Reg Anesth Pain Med.* 2009;34:528-529.

Dolan J. Fascial planes inhibiting the spread of local anesthetic during ultrasound-guided infraclavicular brachial plexus block are not limited to the posterior aspect of the axillary artery. *Reg Anesth Pain Med.* 2009;34:612-613.

Fredrickson MJ, Wolstencroft P, Kejriwal R, Yoon A, Boland MR, Chinchanwala S. *Single versus triple injection ultrasound-guided infraclavicular block: confirmation of the effectiveness of the single injection technique.* Anesth Analg. 2010;111:1325-7.

Fredrickson MJ, Patel A, Young S, Chinchanwala S. Speed of onset of 'corner pocket supraclavicular' and infraclavicular ultrasound guided brachial plexus block: a randomised observer-blinded comparison. *Anaesthesia.* 2009;64:738-744.

Gurkan Y, Acar S, Solak M, Toker K. Comparison of nerve stimulation vs. ultrasound-guided lateral sagittal infraclavicular block. *Acta Anaesthesiol Scand.* 2008;52:851-855.

Gurkan Y, Ozdamar D, Hosten T, Solak M, Toker K. Ultrasound guided lateral sagital infraclavicular block for pectoral flap release. *Agri.* 2009;21:39-42.

Gurkan Y, Tekin M, Acar S, Solak M, Toker K. Is nerve stimulation needed during an ultrasound-guided lateral sagittal infraclavicular block? *Acta Anaesthesiol Scand.* 2010;54:403-407.

Jiang XB, Zhu SZ, Jiang Y, Chen QH, Xu XZ. Optimal dose of local anesthetic mixture in ultrasound-guided infraclavicular brachial plexus block via coracoid approach: analysis of 160 cases [in Chinese]. *Zhonghua Yi Xue Za Zhi.* 2009;89:449-452.

Koscielniak-Nielsen ZJ, Frederiksen BS, Rasmussen H, Hesselbjerg L. A comparison of ultrasound-guided supraclavicular and infraclavicular blocks for upper extremity surgery. *Acta Anaesthesiol Scand.* 2009;53:620-626.

Koscielniak-Nielsen ZJ, Rasmussen H, Hesselbjerg L. Pneumothorax after an ultrasound-guided lateral sagittal infraclavicular block. *Acta Anaesthesiol Scand.* 2008;52:1176-1177.

Levesque S, Dion N, Desgagne MC. Endpoint for successful, ultrasound-guided infraclavicular brachial plexus block. *Can J Anaesth.* 2008;55:308.

Marhofer P, Harrop-Griffiths W, Willschke H, Kirchmair L. Fifteen years of ultrasound guidance in regional anaesthesia: Part 2-recent developments in block techniques. *Br J Anaesth.* 2010;104:673-683.

Mariano ER, Loland VJ, Bellars RH, et al. Ultrasound guidance versus electrical stimulation for infraclavicular brachial plexus perineural catheter insertion. *J Ultrasound Med.* 2009;28:1211-1218.

Martinez Navas A, DE LA Tabla Gonzalez RO. Ultrasound-guided technique allowed early detection of intravascular injection during an infraclavicular brachial plexus block. *Acta Anaesthesiol Scand.* 2009;53:968-970.

Moayeri N, Renes S, van Geffen GJ, Groen GJ. Vertical infraclavicular brachial plexus block: needle redirection after elicitation of elbow flexion. *Reg Anesth Pain Med.* 2009;34:236-241.

Morimoto M, Popovic J, Kim JT, Kiamzon H, Rosenberg AD. Case series: Septa can influence local anesthetic spread during infraclavicular brachial plexus blocks. *Can J Anaesth.* 2007;54:1006-1010.

Nadig M, Ekatodramis G, Borgeat A. Ultrasound-guided infraclavicular brachial plexus block. *Br J Anaesth.* 2003;90:107-108.

Ootaki C, Hayashi H, Amano M. Ultrasound-guided infraclavicular brachial plexus block: an alternative technique to anatomical landmark-guided approaches. *Reg Anesth Pain Med.* 2000;25:600-604.

Perlas A, Chan VW, Simons M. Brachial plexus examination and localization using ultrasound and electrical stimulation: a volunteer study. *Anesthesiology.* 2003;99:429-435.

Ponde VC, Diwan S. Does ultrasound guidance improve the success rate of infraclavicular brachial plexus block when compared with nerve stimulation in children with radial club hands? *Anesth Analg.* 2009;108:1967-1970.

Porter JM, McCartney CJ, Chan VW. Needle placement and injection posterior to the axillary artery may predict successful infraclavicular brachial plexus block: a report of three cases. *Can J Anaesth.* 2005;52:69-73.

Punj J, Joshi A, Darlong V, Pandey R. Ultrasound characteristics of spread during infraclavicular plexus block. *Reg Anesth Pain Med.* 2009;34:73.

Renes S, Clark L, Gielen M, Spoormans H, Giele J, Wadhwa A. A simplified approach to vertical infraclavicular brachial plexus blockade using hand-held Doppler. *Anesth Analg.* 2008;106:1012-1014.

Ruiz A, Sala X, Bargallo X, Hurtado P, Arguis MJ, Carrera A. The influence of arm abduction on the anatomic relations of infraclavicular brachial plexus: an ultrasound study. *Anesth Analg.* 2009;108:364-366.

Sahin L, Gul R, Mizrak A, Deniz H, Sahin M, Koruk S, Cesur M, Goksu S. Ultrasound-guided infraclavicular brachial plexus block enhances postoperative blood flow in arteriovenous fistulas. J Vasc Surg. 2011; Feb 28.

Sandhu NS, Capan LM. Ultrasound-guided infraclavicular brachial plexus block. *Br J Anaesth.* 2002;89:254-259.

Sandhu NS, Maharlouei B, Patel B, Erkulwater E, Medabalmi P. Simultaneous bilateral infraclavicular brachial plexus blocks with low-dose lidocaine using ultrasound guidance. *Anesthesiology.* 2006;104:199-201.

Sandhu NS, Sidhu DS, Capan LM. The cost comparison of infraclavicular brachial plexus block by nerve stimulator and ultrasound guidance. *Anesth Analg.* 2004;98:267-268.

Sauter AR, Dodgson MS, Stubhaug A, Halstensen AM, Klaastad O. Electrical nerve stimulation or ultrasound guidance for lateral sagittal infraclavicular blocks: a randomized, controlled, observer-blinded, comparative study. *Anesth Analg.* 2008;106:1910-1915.

Sauter AR, Smith HJ, Stubhaug A, Dodgson MS, Klaastad O. Use of magnetic resonance imaging to define the anatomical location closest to all three cords of the infraclavicular brachial plexus. *Anesth Analg.* 2006;103:1574-1576.

Slater ME, Williams SR, Harris P, et al. Preliminary evaluation of infraclavicular catheters inserted using ultrasound guidance: through-the-catheter anesthesia is not inferior to through-the-needle blocks. *Reg Anesth Pain Med.* 2007;32:296-302.

Taboada M, Rodriguez J, Amor M, et al. Is ultrasound guidance superior to conventional nerve stimulation for coracoid infraclavicular brachial plexus block? *Reg Anesth Pain Med.* 2009;34:357-360.

Tedore TR, YaDeau JT, Maalouf DB, et al. Comparison of the transarterial axillary block and the ultrasound-guided infraclavicular block for upper extremity surgery: a prospective randomized trial. *Reg Anesth Pain Med.* 2009;34:361-365.

Tran de QH, Dugani S, Dyachenko A, Correa JA, Finlayson RJ. *Minimum effective volume of lidocaine for ultrasound-guided infraclavicular block.* Reg Anesth Pain Med. 2011;36:190-4.

Tran de QH, Clemente A, Tran DQ, Finlayson RJ. A comparison between ultrasound-guided infraclavicular block using the "double bubble" sign and neurostimulation-guided axillary block. *Anesth Analg.* 2008;107:1075-1078.

Tran de QH, Russo G, Munoz L, Zaouter C, Finlayson RJ. A prospective, randomized comparison between ultrasound-guided supraclavicular, infraclavicular, and axillary brachial plexus blocks. *Reg Anesth Pain Med.* 2009;34:366-371.

# 32 Ultrasound-Guided Axillary Brachial Plexus Block

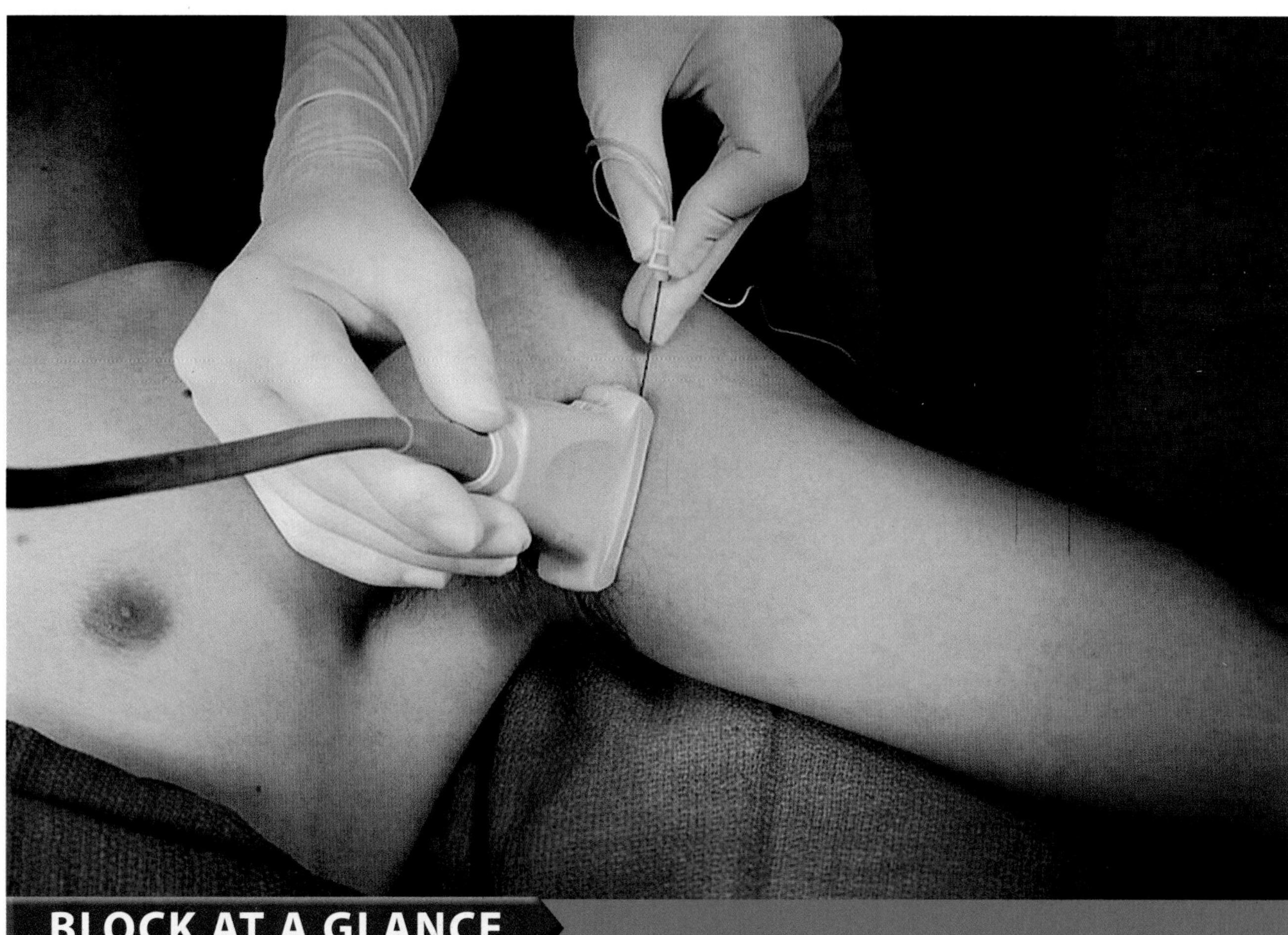

## BLOCK AT A GLANCE

- Indications: forearm and hand surgery
- Transducer position: short axis to arm, just distal to pectoralis major insertion
- Goal: local anesthetic spread around axillary artery
- Local anesthetic: 20-25 mL

**FIGURE 32-1.** Transducer position and needle insertion in ultrasound-guided axillary brachial plexus block.

## General Considerations

The axillary brachial plexus block offers several advantages over the other approaches to the brachial plexus. The technique is relatively simple to perform, and may be associated with a relatively lower risk of complications as compared with interscalene (e.g., spinal cord or vertebral artery puncture) or supraclavicular brachial plexus block (e.g., pneumothorax). In clinical scenarios in which access to the upper parts of the brachial plexus is difficult or impossible (e.g, local infection, burns, indwelling venous catheters), the ability to anesthetize the plexus at a more distal level may be important. The axillary brachial plexus block is also relatively simple to perform with ultrasound because of its superficial location. Although individual nerves can usually be identified in the vicinity of the axillary artery, this is not necessary because the deposition of local anesthetic around the axillary artery is sufficient for an effective block.

## Ultrasound Anatomy

The structures of interest are superficial (1–3 cm), and the pulsating axillary artery can be identified usually within a centimeter of the skin surface on the anteromedial aspect of the proximal arm, Figure 32-2. The artery can be associated with one or more axillary veins, often located medially to the artery. Importantly, an undue pressure with the transducer during imaging may obliterate the veins, rendering veins invisible and prone to puncture with the needle if care is not taken to avoid it. Surrounding the axillary artery are three of the four principal branches of the brachial plexus: the median (superficial and lateral to the artery), the ulnar (superficial and medial to the artery), and the radial (posterior and lateral or medial to the artery) nerves (Figure 32-2). These are seen as round hyperechoic structures, and although the previously mentioned locations relative to the artery are frequently encountered, there is considerable anatomic variation from individual to individual,. Three muscles surround the neurovascular bundle: the biceps brachii (lateral and superficial), the wedge-shaped coracobrachialis (lateral and deep), and the triceps brachii (medial and posterior). The fourth principal nerve of the brachial plexus, the musculocutaneous nerve, is found in the fascial layers between biceps and coracobrachialis muscles, though its location is variable and can be seen within either muscle. It is usually seen as a hypoechoic flattened oval with a bright hyperechoic rim. Moving the transducer proximally and distally along the long axis of the arm, the musculocutaneous nerve will appear to move toward or away from the neurovascular bundle in the fascial plane between the two muscles. Refer to Chapter 1, Essential Regional Anesthesia Anatomy for additional information on the anatomy of the axillary brachial plexus and its branches.

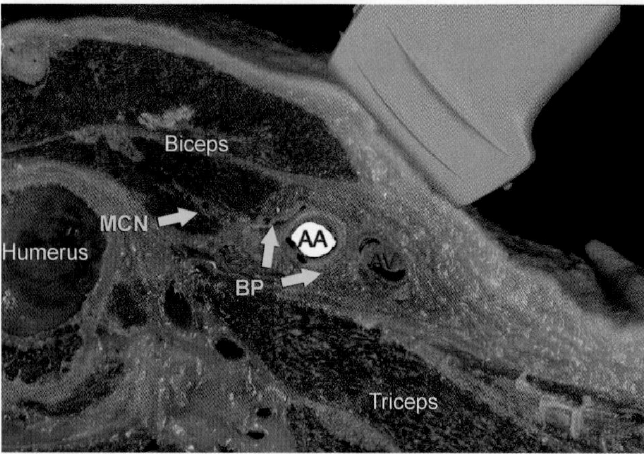


**FIGURE 32-2.** Cross-sectional anatomy of the axillary fossa and the transducer position to image the brachial plexus. The brachial plexus (BP) is seen scattered around the axillary artery and enclosed in the adipose tissue compartment containing BP, axillary artery (AA), and axillary vein (AV). MCN, musculocutaneous nerve.

## Distribution of Blockade

The axillary approach to brachial plexus blockade (including musculocutaneous nerve) results in anesthesia of the upper limb from the midarm down to and including the hand. The axillary nerve itself is not blocked because it departs from the posterior cord high up in the axilla. As a result, the skin over the deltoid muscle is not anesthetized. With nerve stimulator and landmark-based techniques, the blockade of the musculocutaneous is often unreliable, leading to a lack of blockade on the lateral side of the forearm and wrist. This problem is remedied easily with the ultrasound-guided approach because the musculocutaneous nerve is readily apparent and reliably anesthetized. When required, the medial skin of the upper arm (intercostobrachial nerve, T2) can be blocked by an additional subcutaneous injection just distal to the axilla, if required. For a more comprehensive review of the brachial plexus distribution, see Chapter 1.

## Equipment

Equipment needed includes the following:

- Ultrasound machine with linear transducer (8–14 MHz), sterile sleeve, and gel
- Standard nerve block tray (described in the equipment section)
- Syringes with local anesthetic (20–25 mL)
- 4-cm, 22-gauge short-bevel insulated stimulating needle
- Peripheral nerve stimulator
- Sterile gloves

## Landmarks and Patient Positioning

The axillary brachial plexus block requires access to the axilla. Therefore abduction of the arm 90° is an appropriate

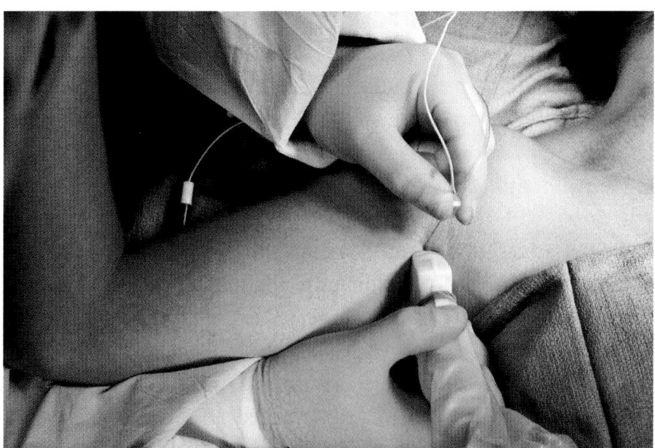

**FIGURE 32-3.** Patient position and insertion of the needle for ultrasound-guided (in plane) axillary brachial plexus block. All needle redirections except occasionally for the musculocutaneous nerve are done through the same needle insertion site. Seldom, another insertion of the needle is made to block the musculocutaneous nerve.

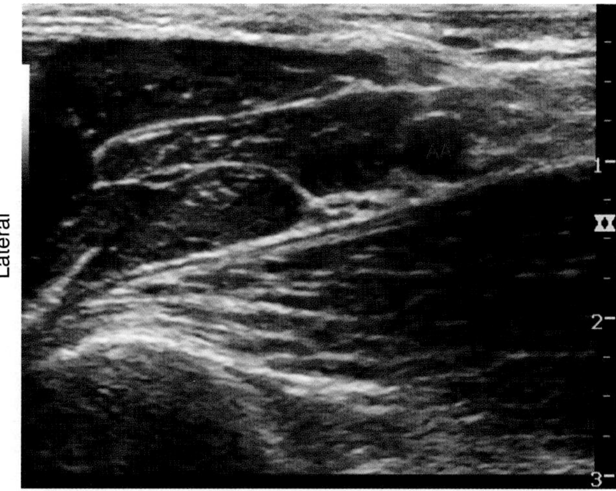


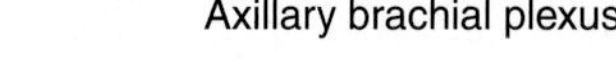

A Axillary brachial plexus

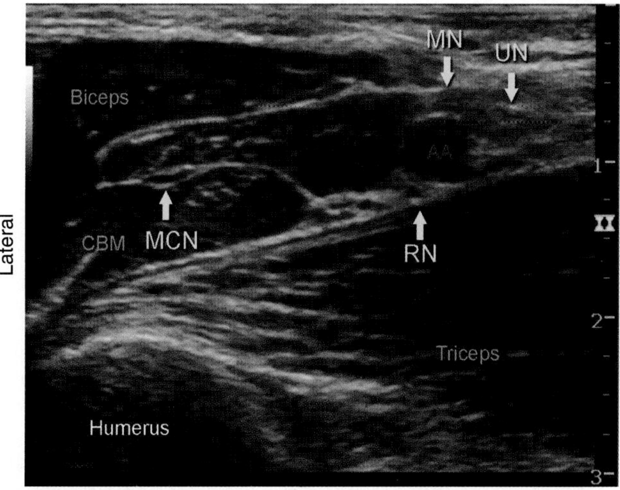


B Axillary brachial plexus with anatomical structures labeled

**FIGURE 32-4.** (A,B) Median (MN), ulnar (UN), and radial (RN) nerves are seen scattered around the axillary artery with the tissue sheath (white-appearing tissue fasciae around the artery) containing nerves and axillary vessels. The musculocutaneous nerve (MCN) is seen between the biceps and coracobrachialis (CBM) away from the rest of the brachial plexus. AA, axillary artery.

position that allows for transducer placement and needle advancement, as well as patient comfort (Figure 32-3). Care should be taken not to overabduct the arm because that may cause discomfort as well as produce tension on the brachial plexus, theoretically making it more vulnerable to needle or injection injury during the block procedure.

The pectoralis major muscle is palpated as it inserts onto the humerus, and the transducer is placed on the skin immediately distal to that point perpendicular to the axis of the arm. The starting point should result in part of the transducer overlying both the biceps and the triceps muscles (i.e., on the medial aspect of the arm). Sliding the transducer across the axilla will bring the axillary artery and brachial plexus into view, if not readily apparent.

## GOAL

The goal is to deposit local anesthetic around the axillary artery. Sometimes, a single injection is sufficient to spread in a "doughnut" shape around the artery; more commonly, two or three injections are required. In addition, an aliquot of local anesthetic should be injected adjacent to the musculocutaneous nerve.

## Technique

With the patient in the proper position, the skin is disinfected and the transducer is positioned in the short axis orientation to identify the axillary artery (Figure 32-4A about 1 to 3 cm from the skin surface. Once the artery is identified, an attempt is made to identify the hyperechoic median, ulnar, and radial nerves (Figure 32-4B). However, these may not be always well seen on an ultrasound image. Frequently present, a reverberation artifact deep to the artery is often misinterpreted for the radial nerve. Prescanning should also reveal the position of the musculocutaneous nerve, in the plane between the coracobrachialis and biceps muscles (a slight proximal-distal movement of the transducer is often required to bring this nerve into view) (Figure 32-5).

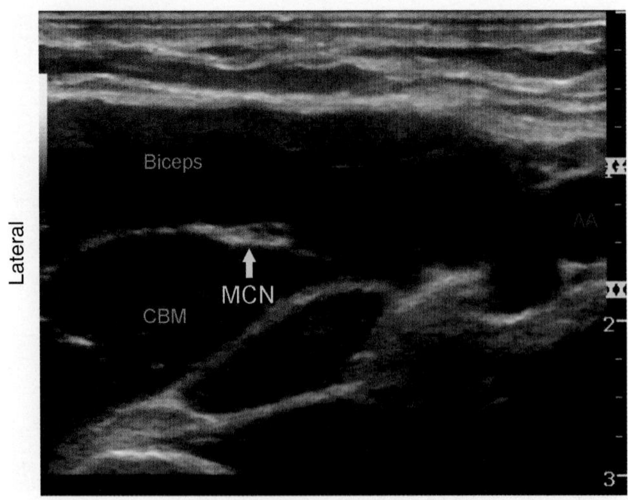


**FIGURE 32-5.** Musculocutaneous nerve (MCN) is seen approximately 3 cm from the axillary neurovascular bundle (around AA). MCN in this image is positioned between the biceps and coracobrachialis muscles (CBM). MCN must be blocked with a separate injection of local anesthetic for a complete axillary brachial plexus block.

The needle is inserted in-plane from the cephalad aspect (Figures 32-1 and 32-3) and directed toward the posterior aspect of the axillary artery (Figure 32-6).

As nerves and vessels are positioned together in the neurovascular bundle by adjacent musculature, advancement of the needle through the axilla may require careful hydrodissection with a small amount of local anesthetic or other injectate. This technique involves the injection of 0.5 to 2 mL, which "peels apart" the plane in which the needle tip is continuously inserted. The needle is then advanced a few millimeters and more injectate is administered.

Local anesthetic should be deposited posterior to the artery first, to avoid displacing the structures of interest deeper and obscuring the nerves, which is often the case if the median or ulnar nerves are injected first. Once 5 to 10 mL is administered, the needle is withdrawn almost to the level of the skin, redirected toward the median and ulnar nerves, and a further 10 to 15 mL is injected in these areas to complete the circle around the artery. The described sequence of injection is demonstrated in Figure 32-7.

Finally, the needle is once again withdrawn to the biceps and redirected toward the musculocutaneous nerve. Once adjacent to the nerve (stimulation will result in elbow flexion), 5 to 7 mL of local anesthetic is deposited.

In an adult patient, 20 to 25 mL of local anesthetic is usually adequate for successful blockade. Complete spread around the artery is necessary for success but infrequently seen with a single injection. Two to three redirections and injections are usually necessary for reliable blockade, as well as a separate injection to block the musculocutaneous nerve. The block dynamics and perioperative management are similar to those described in Chapter 15.

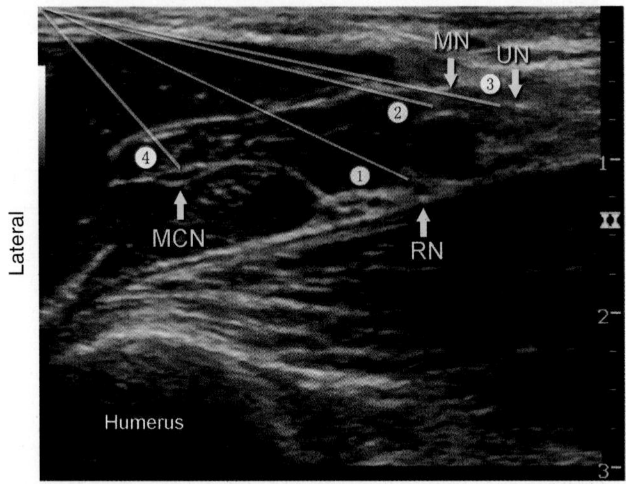


**FIGURE 32-6.** Needle insertions for axillary brachial plexus block. Axillary brachial block can be accomplished by two to four separate injections (1–4) to accomplish a block of the entire brachial plexus. MCN, musculocutaneous nerve; RN, radial nerve; MN, median nerve; UN, ulnar nerve.

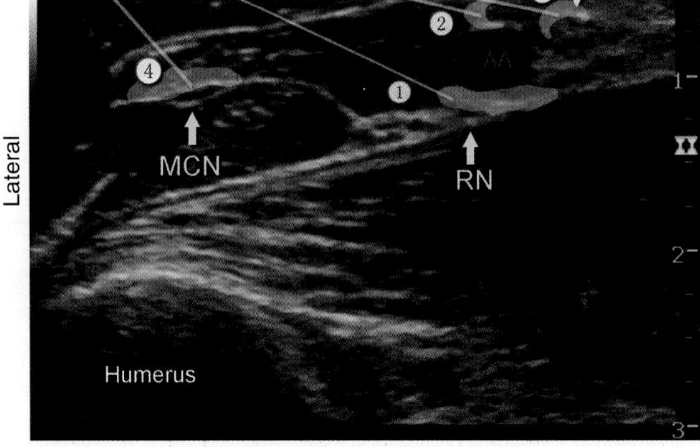


**FIGURE 32-7.** An image demonstrating the ideal distribution patterns of local anesthetic spread after three separate injections (1–3) to surround the axillary artery with local anesthetic and block the radial nerve (RN), median nerve (MN), and ulnar nerve (UN). Musculocutaneous nerve (MCN) is blocked with a separate injection (4) because it is often outside the axillary neurovascular tissue sheath. AA, axillary artery.

TIPS

- Frequent aspiration and slow administration of local anesthetic are critical to decrease the risk of an intravascular injection.
  - Cases of systemic toxicity have been reported after apparently straightforward ultrasound-guided axillary brachial plexus blocks.
  - Keep the pressure applied on the transducer steady to avoid opening and closing of the multitude of veins in the axilla and reduce the risk of an intravascular injection.

## Continuous Ultrasound-Guided Axillary Block

The continuous axillary catheter is a useful technique for analgesia and a sympathetic block, such as following finger reimplantation surgery. The goal of the continuous axillary block is similar to the non–ultrasound-based techniques: to place the catheter in the vicinity of the branches of the brachial plexus (i.e., within the "sheath" of the brachial plexus). The procedure consists of three phases—(1) needle placement, (2) catheter advancement, and (3) securing of the catheter. For the first two phases of the procedure, ultrasound can be used to assure accuracy in most patients. The needle is typically inserted in plane from the cephalad-to-caudad direction, just as in the single-injection technique (Figure 32-8).

After an initial injection of the local anesthetic to confirm the proper position of the needle-tip, the catheter is inserted 2 to 3 cm beyond the needle tip. Injection is then repeated through the catheter to document adequate spread of the local anesthetic. Alternatively, the axillary artery can be visualized in the longitudinal view and the catheter is inserted in the longitudinal plane alongside the axillary artery 4 to 5 cm. The longitudinal approach requires a significantly greater degree of ultrasonographic skill, yet no data exist at this time suggesting that one approach is more efficient or better than the other one.

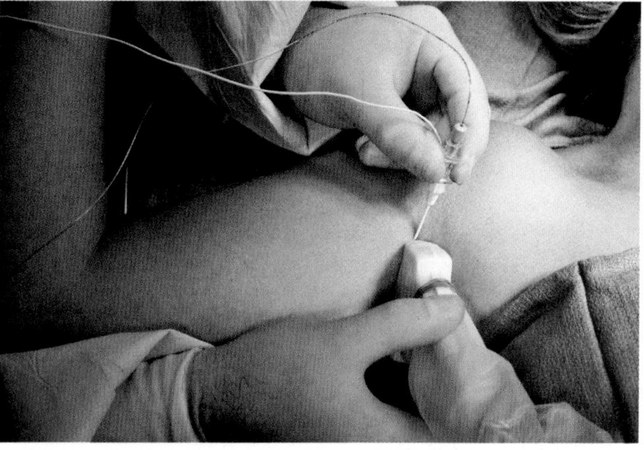

**FIGURE 32-8.** Continuous axillary brachial plexus block is performed using a similar technique as in the single-injection method. After injection of a small volume of local anesthetic through the needle to document its proper placement, the catheter is advanced 2-3 cm beyond the needle tip.

TIP

- Tunneling of the catheter or taping on the shaved skin using transparent occlusive dressing are commonly used methods of securing the catheter.

# ULTRASOUND-GUIDED AXILLARY NERVE BLOCK

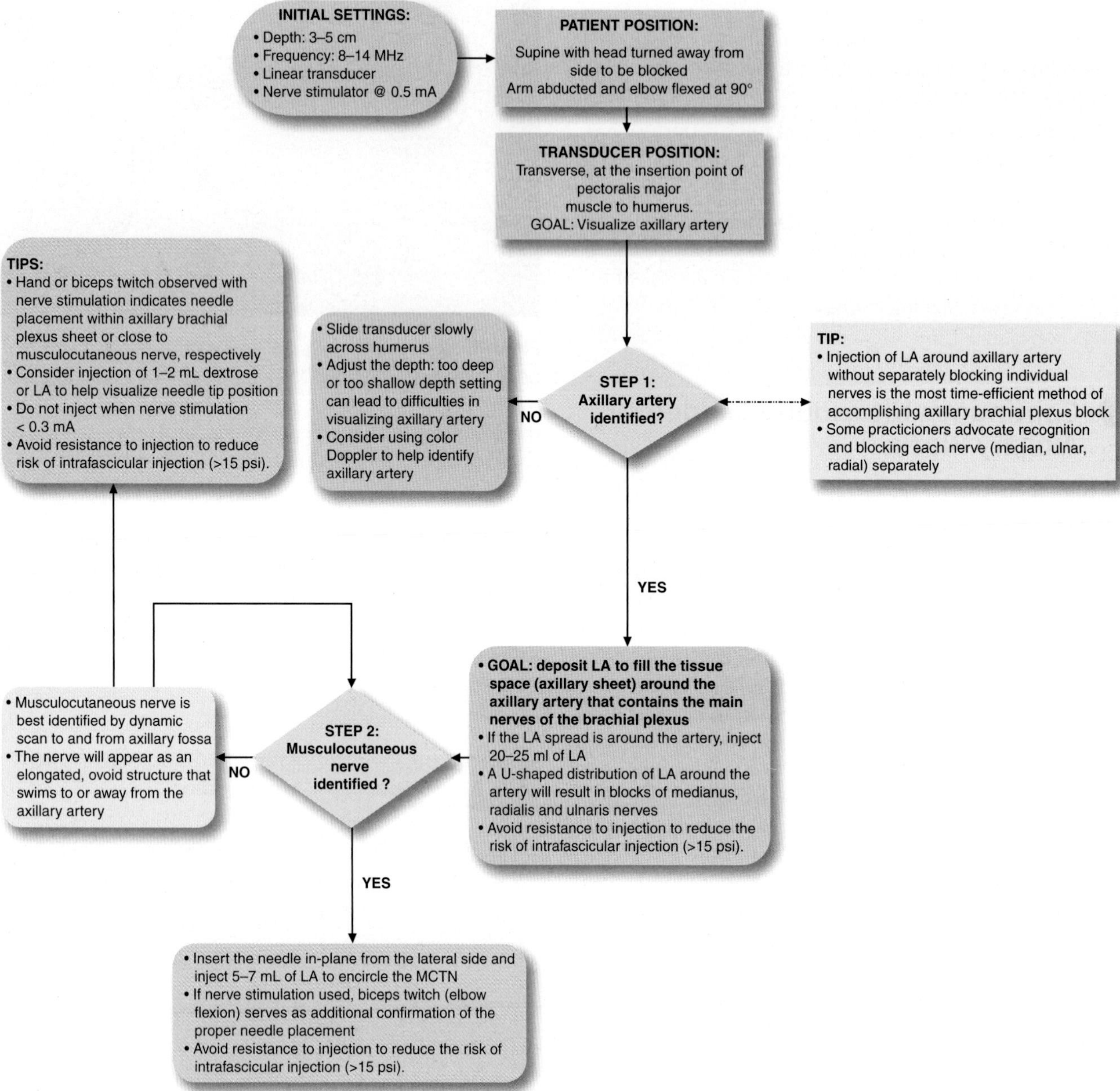

## SUGGESTED READING

Aguirre J, Blumenthal S, Borgeat A. Ultrasound guidance and success rates of axillary brachial plexus block—I. *Can J Anaesth.* 2007;54:583.

Baumgarten RK, Thompson GE. Is ultrasound necessary for routine axillary block? *Reg Anesth Pain Med.* 2006;31:88-9.

Bigeleisen PE. Nerve puncture and apparent intraneural injection during ultrasound-guided axillary block does not invariably result in neurologic injury. *Anesthesiology.* 2006;105:779-783.

Bruhn J, Fitriyadi D, van Geffen GJ. A slide to the radial nerve during ultrasound-guided axillary block. *Reg Anesth Pain Med.* 2009;34:623; author reply 623-624.

Campoy L, Bezuidenhout AJ, Gleed RD, et al. Ultrasound-guided approach for axillary brachial plexus, femoral nerve, and sciatic nerve blocks in dogs. *Vet Anaesth Analg.* 2010;37:144-153.

Casati A, Danelli G, Baciarello M, et al. A prospective, randomized comparison between ultrasound and nerve stimulation guidance for multiple injection axillary brachial plexus block. *Anesthesiology.* 2007;106:992-996.

Chan VW, Perlas A, McCartney CJ, Brull R, Xu D, Abbas S. Ultrasound guidance improves success rate of axillary brachial plexus block. *Can J Anaesth.* 2007;54:176-182.

Christophe JL, Berthier F, Boillot A, et al. Assessment of topographic brachial plexus nerves variations at the axilla using ultrasonography. *Br J Anaesth.* 2009;103:606-612.

Clendenen SR, Riutort K, Ladlie BL, Robards C, Franco CD, Greengrass RA. Real-time three-dimensional ultrasound-assisted axillary plexus block defines soft tissue planes. *Anesth Analg.* 2009;108:1347-1350.

Dibiane C, Deruddre S, Zetlaoui PJ. A musculocutaneous nerve variation described during ultrasound-guided axillary nerve block. *Reg Anesth Pain Med.* 2009;34:617-618.

Dolan J, McKinlay S. Early detection of intravascular injection during ultrasound-guided axillary brachial plexus block. *Reg Anesth Pain Med.* 2009;34:182.

Dufour E, Laloe PA, Culty T, Fischler M. Ultrasound and neurostimulation-guided axillary brachial plexus block for resection of a hemodialysis fistula aneurysm. *Anesth Analg.* 2009;108:1981-1983.

Errando CL, Pallardo MA, Herranz A, Peiro CM, de Andres JA. Bilateral axillary brachial plexus block guided by multiple nerve stimulation and ultrasound in a multiple trauma patient [in Spanish]. *Rev Esp Anestesiol Reanim.* 2006;53:383-386.

Gray AT. The conjoint tendon of the latissimus dorsi and teres major: an important landmark for ultrasound-guided axillary block. *Reg Anesth Pain Med.* 2009;34:179-180.

Gray AT, Schafhalter-Zoppoth I. "Bayonet artifact" during ultrasound-guided transarterial axillary block. *Anesthesiology.* 2005;102:1291-1292.

Gelfand HJ, Ouanes JP, Lesley MR, Ko PS, Murphy JD, Suminda SM, Isaac GR, Kumar K, Wu CL. Analgesic efficacy of Ultrasound-guided regional anesthesia: meta-analysis. J Clin Anesth 2011;232:90-6

Hadžic A, Dewaele S, Gandhi K, Santos A. Volume and dose of local anesthetic necessary to block the axillary brachial plexus using ultrasound guidance. *Anesthesiology.* 2009;111:8-9.

Harper GK, Stafford MA, Hill DA. Minimum volume of local anaesthetic required to surround each of the constituent nerves of the axillary brachial plexus, using ultrasound guidance: a pilot study. *Br J Anaesth.* 2010;104:633-636.

Imasogie N, Ganapathy S, Singh S, Armstrong K, Armstrong P. A prospective, randomized, double-blind comparison of ultrasound-guided axillary brachial plexus blocks using 2 versus 4 injections. *Anesth Analg.* 2010;110:1222-1226.

Liu FC, Liou JT, Tsai YF, et al. Efficacy of ultrasound-guided axillary brachial plexus block: a comparative study with nerve stimulator-guided method. *Chang Gung Med J.* 2005;28:396-402.

Lo N, Brull R, Perlas A, et al. Evolution of ultrasound guided axillary brachial plexus blockade: retrospective analysis of 662 blocks. *Can J Anaesth.* 2008;55:408-413.

Mannion S, Capdevila X. Ultrasound guidance and success rates of axillary brachial plexus block—II. *Can J Anaesth.* 2007;54:584.

Marhofer P, Eichenberger U, Stockli S, et al. Ultrasonographic guided axillary plexus blocks with low volumes of local anaesthetics: a crossover volunteer study. *Anaesthesia.* 2010;65:266-271.

Morros C, Perez-Cuenca MD, Sala-Blanch X, Cedo F: Contribution of ultrasound guidance to the performance of the axillary brachial plexus block with multiple nerve stimulation [in Spanish]. *Rev Esp Anestesiol Reanim.* 2009;56:69-74.

O'Donnell BD, Iohom G. An estimation of the minimum effective anesthetic volume of 2% lidocaine in ultrasound-guided axillary brachial plexus block. *Anesthesiology.* 2009;111:25-29.

O'Donnell BD, Ryan H, O'Sullivan O, Iohom G. Ultrasound-guided axillary brachial plexus block with 20 milliliters local anesthetic mixture versus general anesthesia for upper limb trauma surgery: an observer-blinded, prospective, randomized, controlled trial. *Anesth Analg.* 2009;109:279-283.

Orebaugh SL, Williams BA, Vallejo M, Kentor ML. Adverse outcomes associated with stimulator-based peripheral nerve blocks with versus without ultrasound visualization. *Reg Anesth Pain Med.* 2009;34:251-255.

Perlas A, Chan VW, Simons M. Brachial plexus examination and localization using ultrasound and electrical stimulation: a volunteer study. *Anesthesiology.* 2003;99:429-435.

Perlas A, Niazi A, McCartney C, Chan V, Xu D, Abbas S. The sensitivity of motor response to nerve stimulation and paresthesia for nerve localization as evaluated by ultrasound. *Reg Anesth Pain Med.* 2006;31:445-450.

Porter JM, McCartney CJ, Chan VW. Needle placement and injection posterior to the axillary artery may predict successful infraclavicular brachial plexus block: a report of three cases. *Can J Anaesth.* 2005;52:69-73.

Remerand F, Laulan J, Couvret C, et al. Is the musculocutaneous nerve really in the coracobrachialis muscle when performing an axillary block? An ultrasound study. *Anesth Analg.* 2010;110:1729-1734.

Robards C, Clendenen S, Greengrass R. Intravascular injection during ultrasound-guided axillary block: negative aspiration can be misleading. *Anesth Analg.* 2008;107:1754-1755.

Russon K, Blanco R. Accidental intraneural injection into the musculocutaneous nerve visualized with ultrasound. *Anesth Analg.* 2007;105:1504-1505.

Russon K, Pickworth T, Harrop-Griffiths W. Upper limb blocks. *Anaesthesia.* 2010;65(Suppl 1):48-56.

Schwemmer U, Schleppers A, Markus C, Kredel M, Kirschner S, Roewer N. Operative management in axillary brachial plexus blocks: comparison of ultrasound and nerve stimulation [in German]. *Anaesthesist.* 2006;55:451-456.

Sites BD, Beach ML, Spence BC, et al. Ultrasound guidance improves the success rate of a perivascular axillary plexus block. *Acta Anaesthesiol Scand.* 2006;50:678-684.

Tedore TR, YaDeau JT, Maalouf DB, et al. Comparison of the transarterial axillary block and the ultrasound-guided infraclavicular block for upper extremity surgery: a prospective randomized trial. *Reg Anesth Pain Med.* 2009;34:361-365.

Tran de QH, Clemente A, Tran DQ, Finlayson RJ. A comparison between ultrasound-guided infraclavicular block using the "double bubble" sign and neurostimulation-guided axillary block. *Anesth Analg.* 2008;107:1075-1078.

Tran de QH, Russo G, Munoz L, Zaouter C, Finlayson RJ. A prospective, randomized comparison between ultrasound-guided supraclavicular, infraclavicular, and axillary brachial plexus blocks. *Reg Anesth Pain Med.* 2009;34:366-371.

Wong DM, Gledhill S, Thomas R, Barrington MJ. Sonographic location of the radial nerve confirmed by nerve stimulation during axillary brachial plexus blockade. *Reg Anesth Pain Med.* 2009;34:503-507.

Zetlaoui PJ, Labbe JP, Benhamou D. Ultrasound guidance for axillary plexus block does not prevent intravascular injection. *Anesthesiology.* 2008;108:761.

# 33 Ultrasound-Guided Forearm Blocks

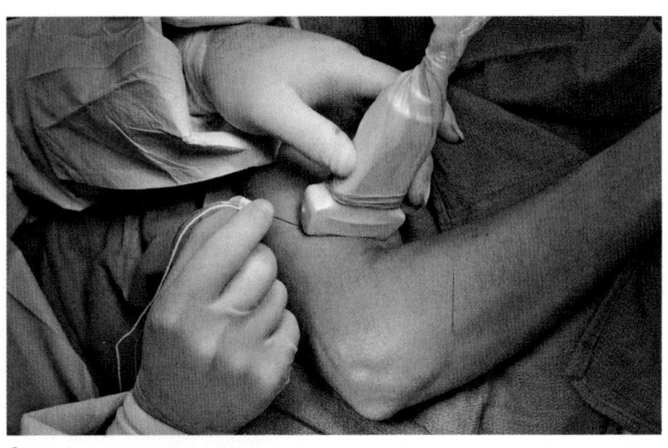

A

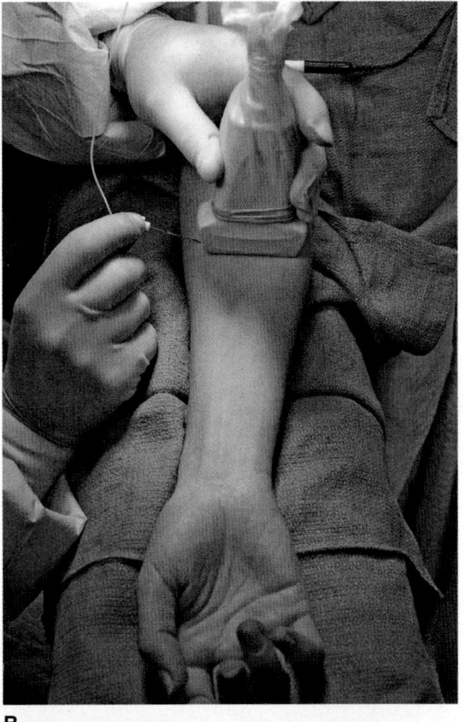

B

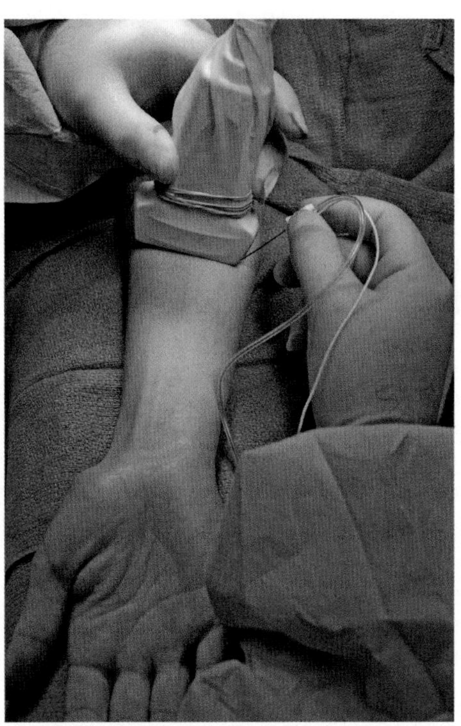

C

## BLOCK AT A GLANCE

- Indications: hand and wrist surgery
- Transducer position: transverse on the elbow and/or forearm
- Goal: injection of local anesthetic in the vicinity of individual nerves (radial, median, ulnar)
- Local anesthetic: 4–5 mL per nerve

**FIGURE 33-1.** (A) Radial nerve block above the elbow. The needle is inserted in-plane from lateral to medial direction. (B) Median nerve block at the level of the midforearm. (C) Ulnar nerve block at the level of the midforearm.

## General Considerations

Ultrasound imaging of individual nerves in the distal upper limb allows for reliable nerve blockade. The two main indications for these blocks are a stand-alone technique for hand and/or wrist surgery and as a means of rescuing or supplementing a patchy or failed proximal brachial plexus block. The main advantages of the ultrasound-guided technique over the surface-based or nerve stimulator–based techniques are the avoidance of unnecessary proximal motor and sensory blockade, that is, greater specificity. Additional advantages are avoidance of the risk of vascular puncture and a reduction in the overall volume of local anesthetic used. There are a variety of locations where a practitioner could approach each of these nerves, most of which are similar in efficacy. In this chapter, we present the approach for each nerve that we favor in our practice.

## Ultrasound Anatomy

### Radial Nerve

The radial nerve is best visualized above the lateral aspect of the elbow, lying in the fascia between the brachioradialis and the brachialis muscles (Figure 33-2). The transducer is placed transversely on the anterolateral aspect of the distal arm, 3–4 cm above the elbow crease (Figure 33-1A). The nerve appears as a hyperechoic, triangular, or oval structure with the characteristic stippled appearance of a distal peripheral nerve. The nerve divides just above the elbow crease into superficial (sensory) and deep (motor) branches. These smaller divisions of the radial nerve are more challenging to identify in the forearm; therefore, a single injection above the elbow is favored because it ensures blockade of both. The transducer can be slid up and down the axis of the arm to better appreciate the nerve within the musculature surrounding it. As the transducer is moved proximally, the nerve will be seen to travel posteriorly and closer to the humerus, to lie deep to the triceps muscles in the spiral groove (Figure 33-3).

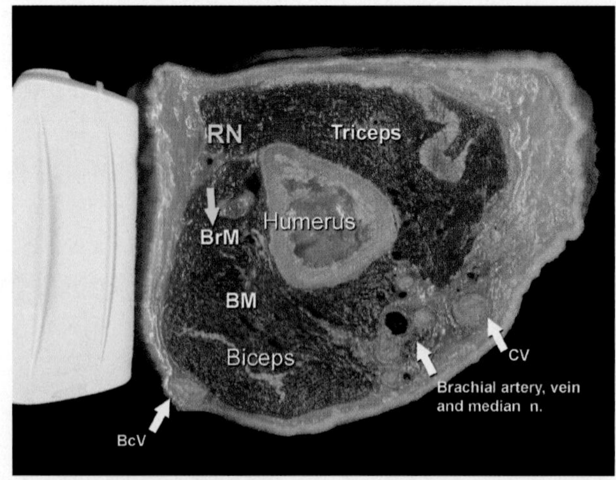


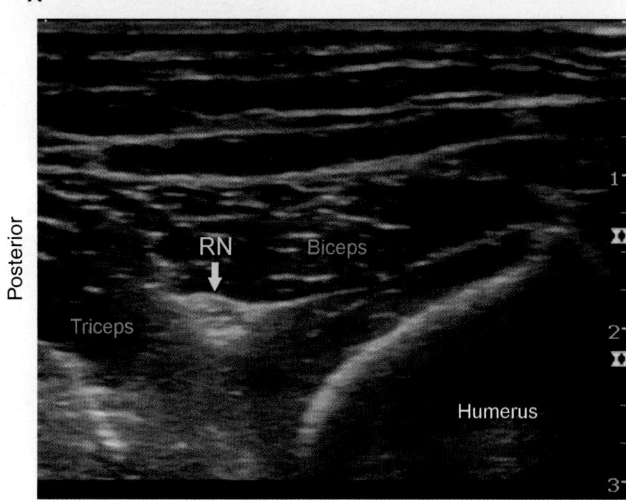


B Radial nerve, 3–4 cm above the elbow

**FIGURE 33-2.** (A) Radial nerve anatomy at the distal third of the humerus. (B) Sonoanatomy of the radial nerve at the distal humerus. Radial nerve (RN) is shown between the biceps and triceps muscles at a depth of approximately 2 cm.

### Median Nerve

The median nerve is easily imaged in the midforearm, between the flexor digitorum superficialis and flexor digitorum profundus, where the nerve typically appears as a round or oval hyperechoic structure (Figure 33-4A and B). The transducer is placed on the volar aspect of the arm in the transverse orientation and tilted back and forth until the nerve is identified (Figure 33-1B). The nerve is located in the midline of the forearm, 1–2 cm medial and deep to the pulsating radial artery. The course of the median nerve can be traced with the transducer up and down the forearm, but as it approaches the elbow or the wrist, its differentiation from adjacent tendons and connective tissue becomes more challenging.

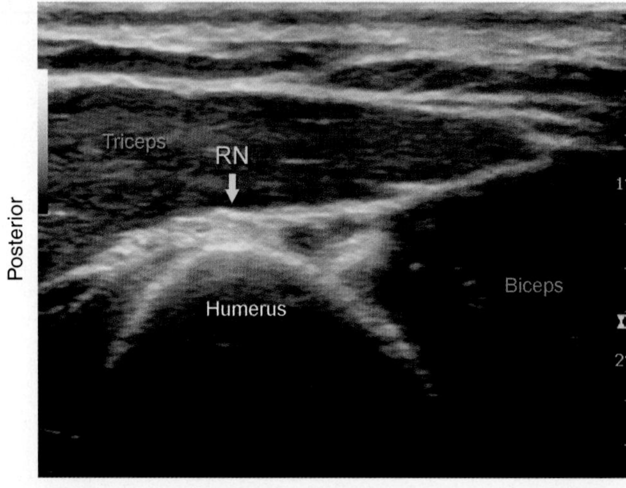


Radial nerve above the humerus

**FIGURE 33-3.** Sonoanatomy of the radial nerve in the spiral groove of the humerus. RN, radial nerve.

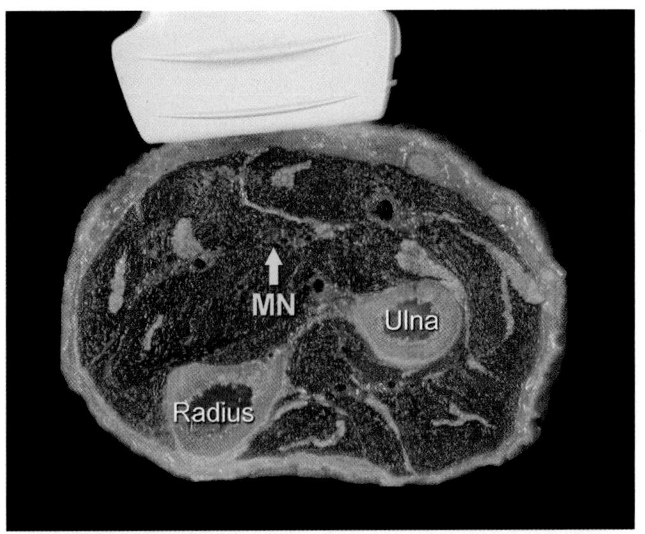


A

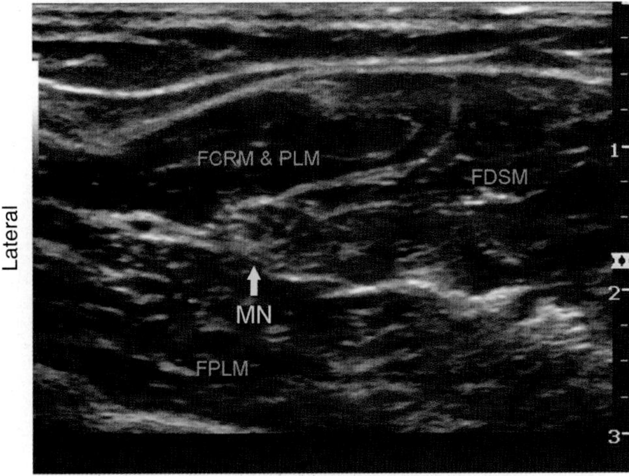


B Forearm block-median nerve

**FIGURE 33-4.** (A) Anatomy of the medianus nerve (MN) of the midforearm. (B) Sonoanatomy of the MN at the midforearm. FDSM, Flexor Digitorum Superficialis Muscle; FCRM, Flexor Carpi Radialis Muscle & PLM, Palmaris Longus Muscle; FPLM, Flexor Palmaris Longus Muscle.

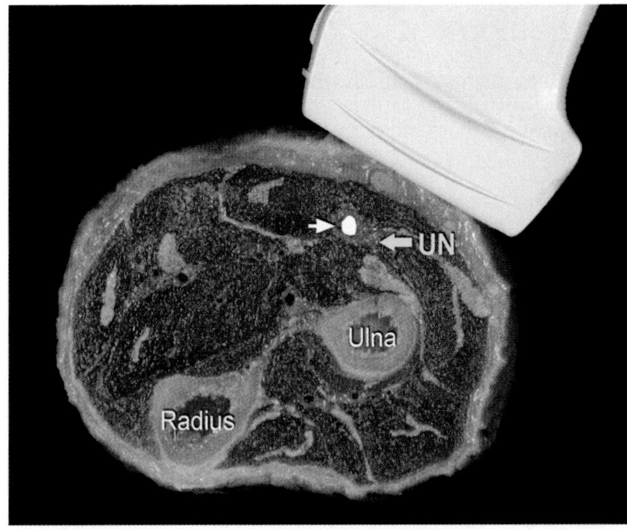


A

Lateral FDSM FCUM UA UN FDPM

B Forearm block-ulnar nerve

**FIGURE 33-5.** (A) Anatomy of the ulnar nerve at the midforearm. The ulnar nerve (UN) is closely related to the ulnar artery (UA). (B) Sonoanatomy of the ulnar nerve at the midforearm. UN is shown closely related to the UA, sandwiched between the flexor carpi ulnaris (FCUM) and flexor digitorum profundus muscles (FDPM). FDSM = Flexor Digitorum Superficialis Muscle.

## Ulnar Nerve

The ulnar nerve can be easily imaged in the midforearm, immediately medial to the ulnar artery, which acts as a useful landmark. Similar to the radial and median nerves, the ulnar nerve appears as a hyperechoic stippled structure, with a triangular to oval shape (Figure 33-5A and B). The ulnar artery and nerve separate, when the transducer is slid more proximally on the forearm, with the artery taking a more lateral and deeper course. The ulnar nerve can be traced easily proximally toward the ulnar notch, when desired, and the level of the blockade can be decided based on the desired distribution of the anesthesia as well as the ease of imaging and accessing the nerve. Sliding the transducer distally shows the nerve and artery becoming progressively shallower together as they approach the wrist where the ulnar nerve lies medial to the artery.

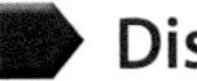

## Distribution of Blockade

As is the case with the landmark-based distal blocks, anesthetizing the radial, median, and/or ulnar nerves provides sensory anesthesia and analgesia to the respective territories of the hand and wrist. Note that the lateral cutaneous nerve of the forearm (a branch of the musculocutaneous nerve) supplies the lateral aspect of the forearm, and it may need to be blocked separately by a subcutaneous wheal distal to the elbow if lateral wrist surgery is planned. For a more comprehensive review of the innervation of the hand, see Chapter 1, Essential Regional Anesthesia Anatomy.

## Equipment

Equipment needed includes the following:

- Ultrasound machine with linear transducer (8–14 MHz), sterile sleeve, and gel
- Standard nerve block tray
- One 20-mL syringe containing local anesthetic
- A 2-in, 22–25 gauge short-bevel insulated stimulating needle
- Peripheral nerve stimulator (optional)
- Sterile gloves

### TIP

- Because these are superficial blocks of distal peripheral nerves, some practitioners choose to use a small-gauge (i.e., 25-gauge) needle. When a using small-gauge needle, however, meticulous attention should be paid to avoid an intraneural injection, which is more likely with a smaller diameter and sharp tip design.

## Landmarks and Patient Positioning

Any patient position that allows for comfortable placement of the ultrasound transducer and needle advancement is appropriate. Typically, the block is performed with the patient in the supine position. For the radial nerve block, the arm is flexed at the elbow and the hand is placed on the patient's abdomen (Figure 33-1A). This position allows for the most practical application of the transducer. The median and ulnar nerves are blocked with the arm abducted and placed on an armboard, palm facing up. (Figures 33-1 B,C)

### GOAL

The goal is to place the needle tip immediately adjacent to the nerve(s) of choice and to deposit 4–5 mL of local anesthetic in the vicinity of the nerve. It is unnecessary to completely surround the entire nerve in a doughnut pattern, although this can enhance the speed of onset of the block. As with all peripheral blocks, avoidance of resistance to injection is important to decrease the risk of an intrafascicular injection.

## Technique

### Radial Nerve

With the patient in the proper position, the skin is disinfected and the transducer positioned so as to identify the radial nerve. The needle is inserted in-plane, with the goal of traversing the biceps brachii muscle and placing the tip next to the radial nerve (Figure 33-6A). If nerve stimulation is used, a wrist or finger extension response should be elicited when the needle is in proximity to the nerve. After negative aspiration, 4–5 mL of local anesthetic is injected (Figure 33-6B). If the spread is inadequate, slight adjustments can be made and a further 2–3 mL of local anesthetic administered.

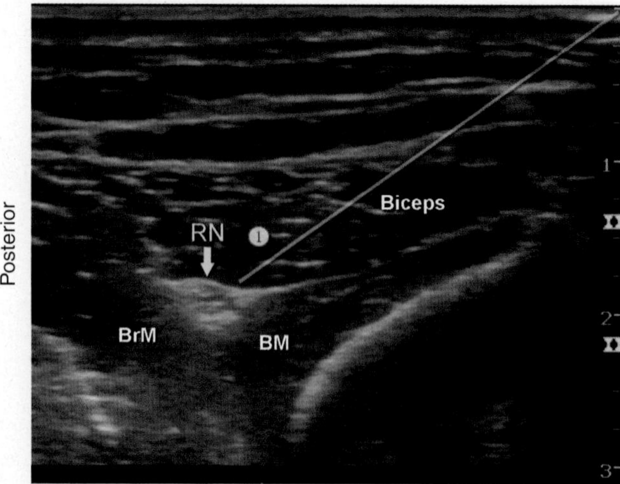


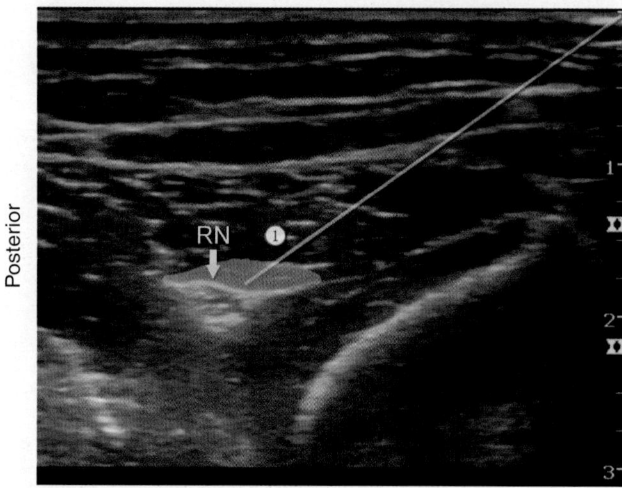


**FIGURE 33-6.** (A) Needle position to block the radial nerve (RN) at the elbow. BM - Brachialis Muscle, BrM - Brachioradialis muscle. (B) Local anesthetic (area shaded in blue) distribution to block the RN above the elbow. (1) Biceps brachii muscle.

### Median and Ulnar Nerves

With the arm abducted and the palm up, the skin of the volar forearm is disinfected and the transducer positioned transversely on the midforearm. The median nerve should be identified between the previously mentioned muscle layers.

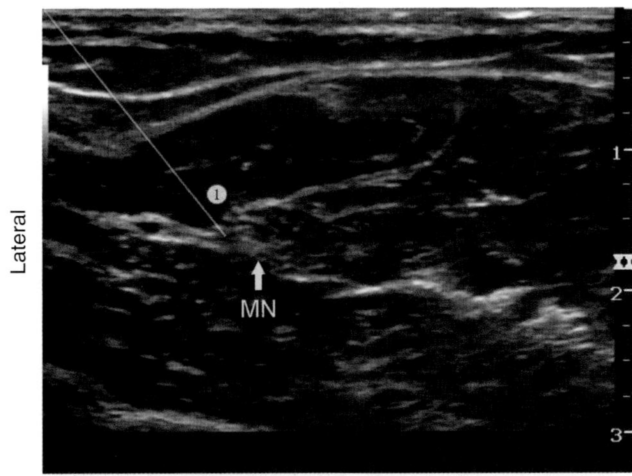


A Forearm block-median nerve

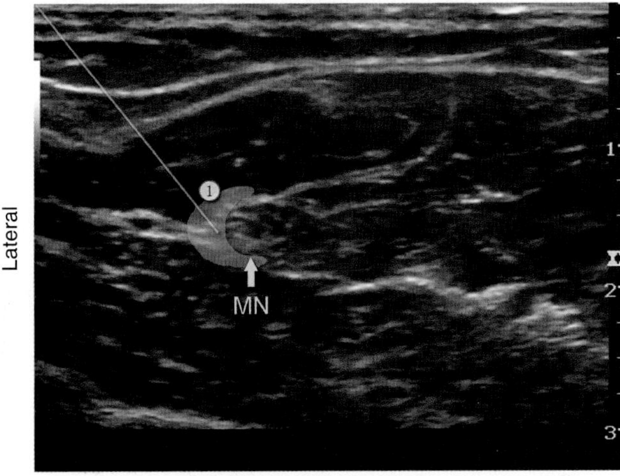


B Forearm block-median nerve

**FIGURE 33-7.** (A) Needle (1) position for the block of the median nerve (MN) at the forearm. (B) Distribution of local anesthetic for block of the MN at the forearm.

If it is not immediately visualized, the transducer should be positioned slightly more laterally and the radial artery identified, using color Doppler ultrasound. Sliding back to the midline, the nerve can be seen approximately 1–2 cm medial and 1 cm deep to the radial artery. The needle is inserted in-plane from either side of the transducer (Figure 33-7A). After negative aspiration, 4–5 mL of local anesthetic is injected (Figure 33-7B). If the spread is inadequate, slight adjustments can be made and a further 2–3 mL of local anesthetic administered.

## TIPS

- The median nerve can often "hide" in the background of the musculature. Tilting the transducer proximally or distally will bring the nerve out of the background.
    - Imaging at the level of the elbow crease readily reveals the nerve positioned medial to the brachial artery. From this location, the nerve can be traced distally.
    - When in doubt, nerve stimulation (0.5-1.0 mA) can be used to confirm localization of the correct nerve.
    - In some patients, the median and ulnar nerves often can both be anesthetized with a single skin puncture.

Then the transducer is positioned more medially until the ulnar nerve is identified. The use of color Doppler ultrasound can aid in finding the ulnar artery, which always lies lateral to the nerve at this level. The nerve should then be traced up until the artery "splits off," to minimize the likelihood of arterial puncture. The needle is inserted in-plane from either side of the transducer (the lateral side is often more ergonomic) (Figure 33-8A). After negative aspiration, 4–5 mL of local anesthetic is injected (Figure 33-8B). If the spread of

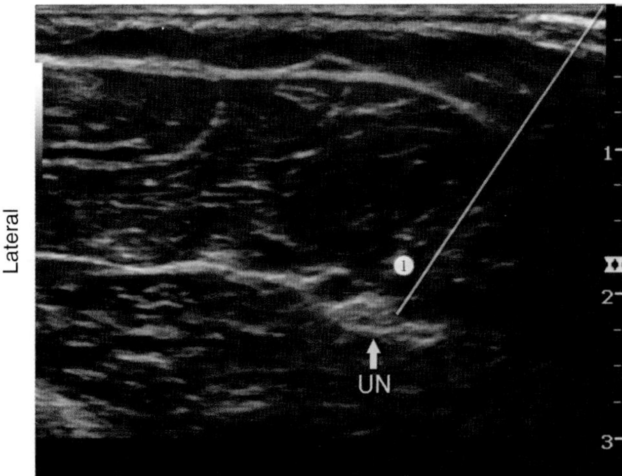


A Forearm block-ulnar nerve

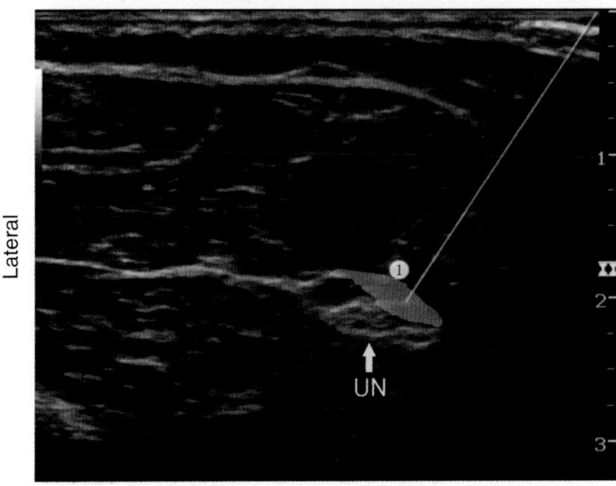


B Forearm block-ulnar nerve

**FIGURE 33-8.** (A) Needle (1) position for the block of ulnar nerve (UN) at the forearm. (B) Distribution of local anesthetic (area shaded in blue) for the block of the UN at the forearm.

the local anesthetic is inadequate, slight adjustments can be made and a further 2–3 mL administered.

## TIP

- The out-of-plane approach can also be used for all three blocks; however, we find that visualizing the needle path makes for greater consistency in placement and a lesser chance of nerve impalement.

The use of a tourniquet, either on the arm or forearm, usually requires sedation and/or additional analgesia.

## SUGGESTED READING


Eichenberger U, Stockli S, Marhofer P, et al. Minimal local anesthetic volume for peripheral nerve block: a new ultrasound-guided, nerve dimension-based method. *Reg Anesth Pain Med.* 2009;34:242-246.

Gray AT, Schafhalter-Zoppoth I. Ultrasound guidance for ulnar nerve block in the forearm. *Reg Anesth Pain Med.* 2003;28:335-339.

Lurf M, Leixnering M: Sensory block without a motor block: ultrasound-guided placement if pain catheters in forearm. Acta Anaestbesiol Scand 2010;54:257-8.

Kathirgamanathan A, French J, Foxall GL, Hardman JG, Bedforth NM. Delineation of distal ulnar nerve anatomy using ultrasound in volunteers to identify an optimum approach for neural blockade. *Eur J Anaesthesiol.* 2009;26:43-46.

McCartney CJ, Xu D, Constantinescu C, Abbas S, Chan VW. Ultrasound examination of peripheral nerves in the forearm. *Reg Anesth Pain Med.* 2007;32:434-439.

Schafhalter-Zoppoth I, Gray AT. The musculocutaneous nerve: ultrasound appearance for peripheral nerve block. *Reg Anesth Pain Med.* 2005;30:385-390.

Spence BC, Sites BD, Beach ML. Ultrasound-guided musculocutaneous nerve block: a description of a novel technique. *Reg Anesth Pain Med.* 2005;30:198-201.

# 34 Ultrasound-Guided Wrist Block

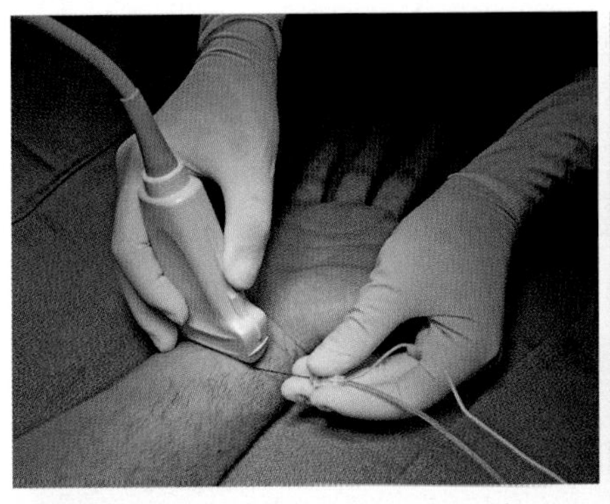
A

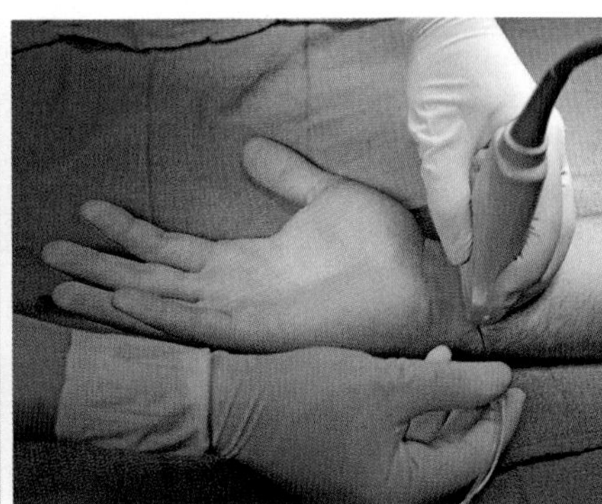
B

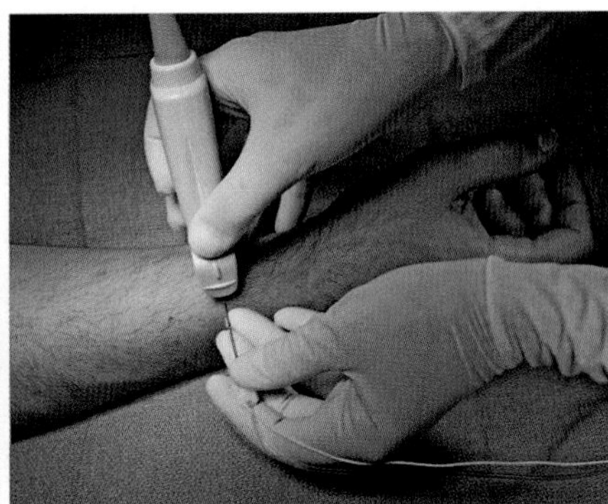
C

## BLOCK AT A GLANCE

- Indications: surgery on the hand and fingers
- Transducer position: transverse at wrist crease or distal third of the forearm
- Goal: local anesthetic injection next to medians and ulnar nerve and local anesthetic infiltration for the radial nerve
- Local anesthetic: 10–15 mL

**FIGURE 34-1.** Ultrasound-guided wrist block. Transducer and needle positions for (A) Median nerve block, (B) Ulnar nerve block, (C) Radial nerve block.

## General Considerations

The wrist block is an effective method to provide anesthesia of the hand and fingers without the arm immobility that occurs with more proximal brachial plexus blocks. Traditional wrist block technique involves advancing needles using surface landmarks toward the three nerves that supply the hand, namely the median, ulnar, and radial nerves. The ultrasound-guided approach has the advantage of direct visualization of the needle and target nerve, which may decrease the incidence of needle-related trauma. In addition, because the needle can be placed with precision immediately adjacent to the nerve, smaller volumes of local anesthetic are required for successful blockade than with a blind technique. Since the nerves are located relatively close to the surface, this is a technically easy block to perform, but knowledge of the anatomy of the soft tissues of the wrist is essential for successful blockade with minimum patient discomfort.

## Ultrasound Anatomy

Three individual nerves are involved:

### Median Nerve

The median nerve crosses the elbow medial to the brachial artery and courses toward the wrist deep to the flexor digitorum superficialis in the center of the forearm. As the muscles taper toward tendons near the wrist, the nerve assumes an increasingly superficial position until it is located beneath the flexor retinaculum in the carpal tunnel with the tendons of flexor digitorum profundus, flexor digitorum superficialis, and flexor pollicis longus. A linear transducer placed transversely at the level of the wrist crease will reveal a cluster of oval hyperechoic structures, one of which is the median nerve (Figures 34-2A and B and 34-3A and B). At this location it is easy to confuse the tendons for the nerve, and vice versa; for this reason, it is recommended that the practitioner slides the transducer 5 to 10 cm up the volar side of the forearm, leaving the tendons more distally to confirm the location of the nerve. The tendons will have disappeared on the image, leaving just muscle and the solitary median nerve, which then can be carefully traced back to the wrist, if desired. In many instances, however, it is much simpler to perform a medianus block at the midforearm, where the nerve is easier to recognize.

> **TIP**
>
> - The median nerve exhibits pronounced anisotropy. Tilting the transducer slightly will make the nerve appear alternately brighter (more contrast) or darker (less contrast) with respect to the background.

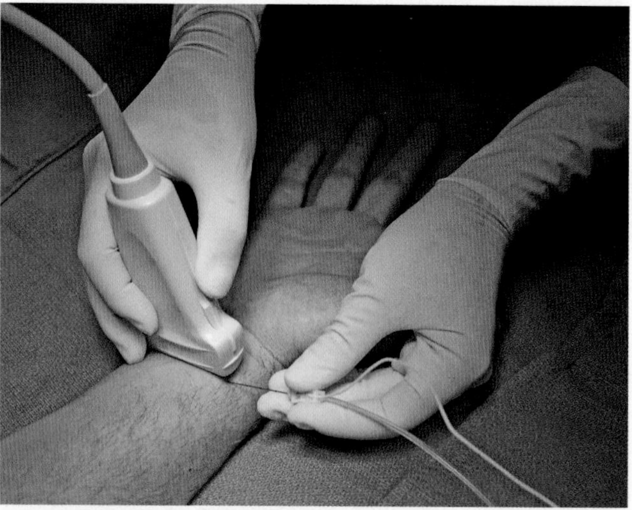

A

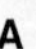

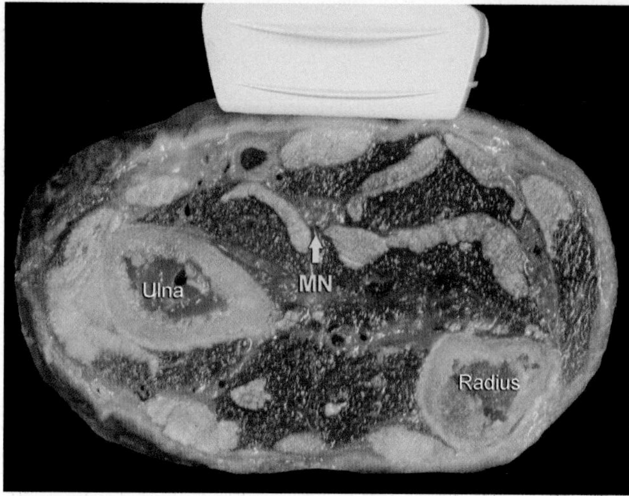


B

**FIGURE 34-2.** (A) Ultrasound-guided block of the median nerve at the wrist. (B) Cross-sectional anatomy of the median nerve (MN) at the wrist.

### Ulnar Nerve

The ulnar nerve is located medial (ulnar side) to the ulnar artery from the level of the midforearm to the wrist. This provides a useful landmark. A linear transducer placed at the level of the wrist crease will show the hyperechoic anterior surface of the ulna with shadowing behind; just lateral to the bone and very superficial will be the triangular or oval hyperechoic ulnar nerve, with the pulsating ulnar artery immediately next to it (Figures 34-4A and B and 34-5A and B). Unlike the median nerve, there are fewer structures (tendons) in the immediate vicinity that can confuse identification; however, the same confirmation scanning technique can be applied. Sliding the transducer up and down the arm helps verify that the structure is the ulnar nerve by following the course of the ulnar artery and looking for the nerve on its ulnar side.

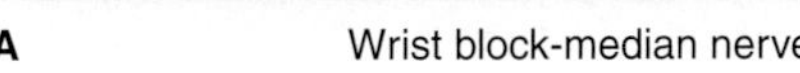


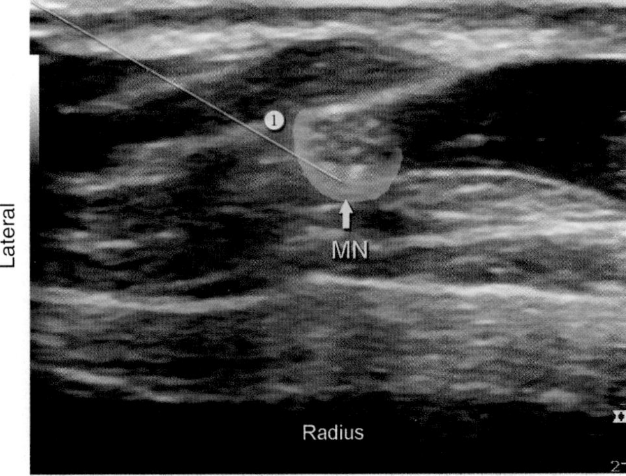


**FIGURE 34-3.** (A) Cross-sectional ultrasound image of the median nerve (MN) at the wrist. (B) Needle (1) path to reach MN at the wrist and spread of local anesthetic to block the MN.

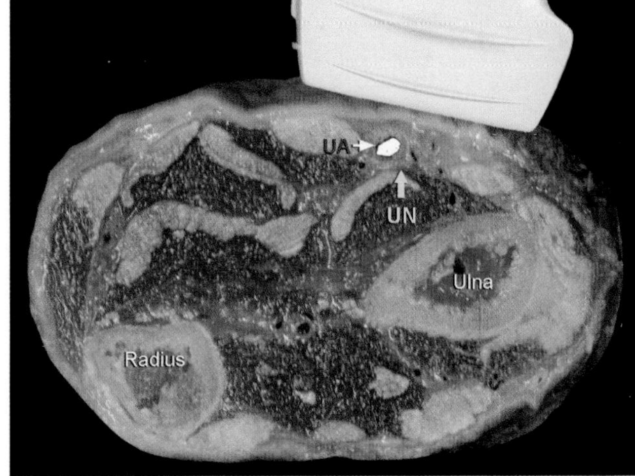


**FIGURE 34-4.** (A) Block of the ulnar nerve (UN) at the wrist. Transducer and needle position. (B) Transsectional anatomy of the UN at the wrist. UN is seen just medial to the ulnar artery (UA).

## Radial Nerve

The superficial branch of the radial nerve divides into terminal branches at the level of the wrist; for this reason, ultrasonography is not very useful for guidance for placement of the block at the level of the wrist. A subcutaneous field block around the area of the styloid process of the radius remains an easy method to perform an effective radial nerve block at the level of the wrist (refer to the wrist block in Chapter 16). However, ultrasonography can be used at the elbow level or in the midforearm. At the level of the elbow (slightly below the elbow), the nerve is easily identified as a hyperechoic oval or triangular structure in the layer between the brachialis (deep) and brachioradialis (superficial) muscles lateral to the radial artery (Figures 34-6A and B and 34-7A and B).

## Distribution of Blockade

A wrist block results in anesthesia of the entire hand. For a more comprehensive review of the distribution of each terminal nerve, please see Chapter 1, Essential Regional Anesthesia Anatomy.

## Equipment

Equipment needed includes the following:

- Ultrasound machine with linear transducer (8–14 MHz), sterile sleeve, and gel
- Standard nerve block tray (described in the equipment section)

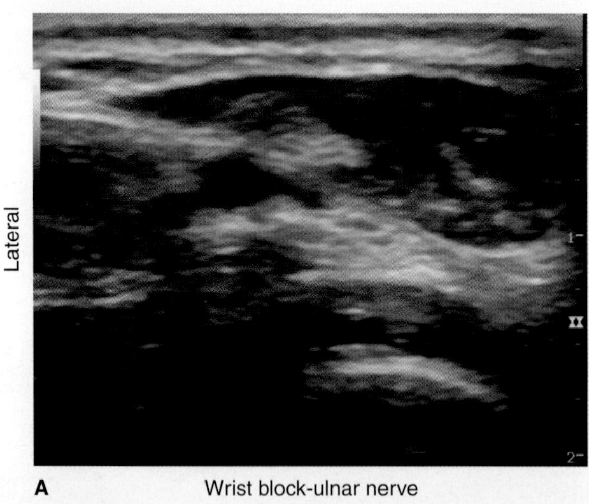


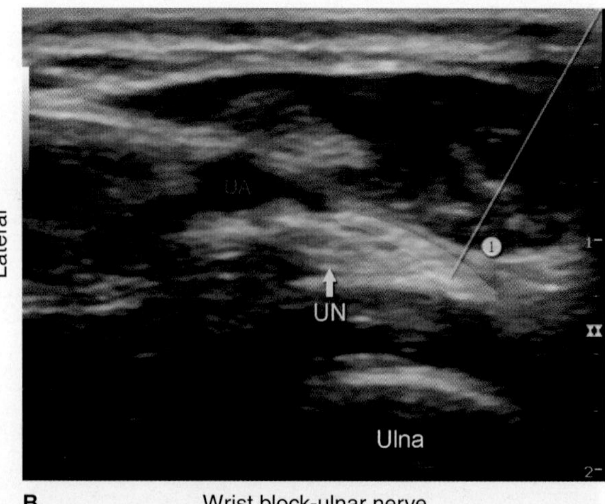


**FIGURE 34-5.** (A) Sonoanatomy of the ulnar nerve (UN) at the wrist. US, ulnar artery. (B) Needle path to reach the UN at the wrist and approximate spread of the local anesthetic (area shaded in blue) to anesthetize the UN.

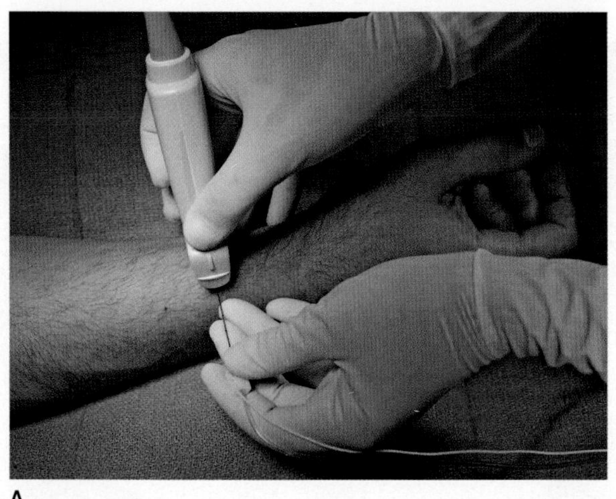


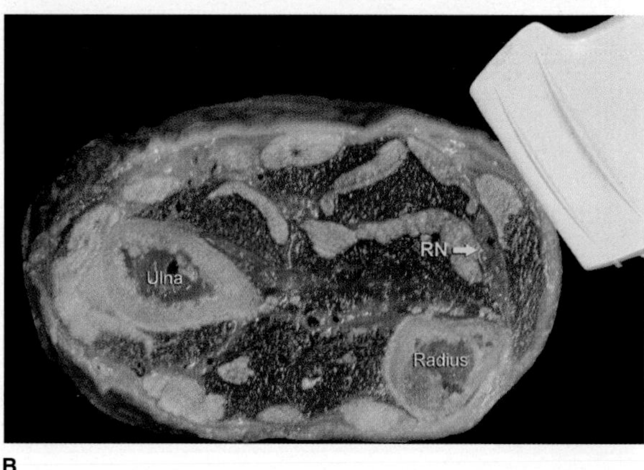


**FIGURE 34-6.** (A) Block of the radial nerve (RN) at the wrist. Transducer and needle position. (B) Cross-sectional anatomy of the RN at the wrist level. Superficial branches of the radial nerve are highly variable at this level in number, size, and depth. For that reason, block of the RN at the wrist is not an exact technique but rather infiltration of the local anesthetic in the subcutaneous tissue and underneath the superficial fascia.

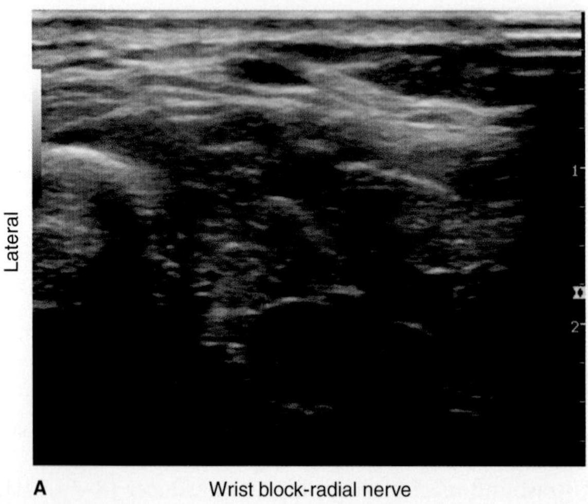


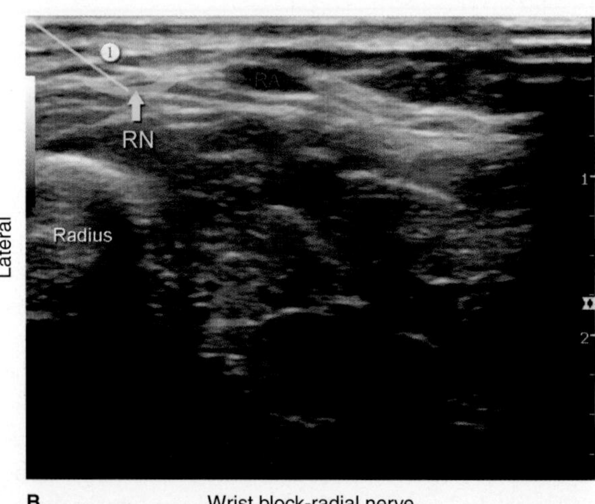


**FIGURE 34-7.** (A) Sonoanatomy of the radial nerve (RN) at the level of the wrist. (B) One branch of the RN at the wrist is shown lateral to the radial artery (RA), and the approximate needle path to reach a branch of the radial nerve is shown with an approximate spread of local anesthetic (area shaded in blue) to anesthetize it.

- One 20-mL syringe containing local anesthetic
- A 1.5-in 22- to 25-gauge needle with low-volume extension tubing
- Sterile gloves

## Landmarks and Patient Positioning

The wrist block is most easily performed with the patient in the supine position to allow for the volar surface of the wrist to be exposed. It is useful to remove splints and/or bandages on the hand to facilitate placement of the transducer and sterile preparation of the skin surface.

### GOAL

The goal is to place the needle tip immediately adjacent to each of the two/three nerves to deposit local anesthetic until its spread around the nerve is documented with ultrasound visualization.

## Technique

With the arm in the proper position, the skin is disinfected. The wrist is a "tightly packed" area that is bounded on three sides by bones. For this reason, an ultrasound-guided "wrist" block is often performed 5 to 10 cm proximal to the wrist crease where there is more room to maneuver. For each of the blocks, the needle can be inserted either in-plane or out-of-plane. Ergonomics often dictates which of these is most effective. Care must be taken when performing the ulnar and radial nerve blocks since the nerves are intimately associated with arteries. Inadvertent arterial puncture can lead to a hematoma. Successful block is predicted by the spread of local anesthetic immediately adjacent to the nerve. Multiple injections to achieve circumferential spread are usually not necessary because these nerves are small and the local anesthetic diffuses quickly into the neural tissue due to the lack of thick epineural tissues. Assuming deposition immediately adjacent to the nerve, 3 to 4 mL/nerve of local anesthetic is sufficient to ensure an effective block.

### TIP

- Always assure absence of resistance to injection to decrease the risk of intrafascicular injection.

The block dynamics and perioperative management are similar to those described in Chapter 16.

## SUGGESTED READING


Bajaj S, Pattamapaspong N, Middleton W, Teefey S: Ultrasound of the hand and wrist. J Hand Surg Am 2009;34:759-60.

Heinemeyer O, Reimers CD. Ultrasound of radial, ulnar, median and sciatic nerves in healthy subjects and patients with hereditary motor and sensory neuropathies. *Ultrasound Med Biol.* 1999:25:481-485.

Kiely PD, O'Farrell D, Riordan J, Harmon D: The use of ultrasound-guided hematoma blocks in wrist fractures. J Clin Anesth 2009;21:540-2.

Liebmann O, Price D, Mills C, et al. Feasibility of forearm ultrasonography-guided nerve blocks of the radial, ulnar, and median nerves for hand procedures in the emergency department. *Ann Emerg Med* 2006;48:558-562.

Macaire P, Singelyn F, Narchi P, Paqueron X. Ultrasound- or nerve stimulation-guided wrist blocks for carpal tunnel release: a randomized prospective comparative study. *Reg Anesth Pain Med.* 2008;33:363-368.

McCartney CJL, Xu D, Constantinescu C, et al. Ultrasound examination of peripheral nerves in the forearm. *Reg Anesth Pain Med.* 2007;32:434–439.

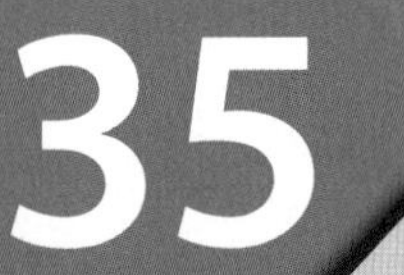


# Ultrasound-Guided Femoral Nerve Block

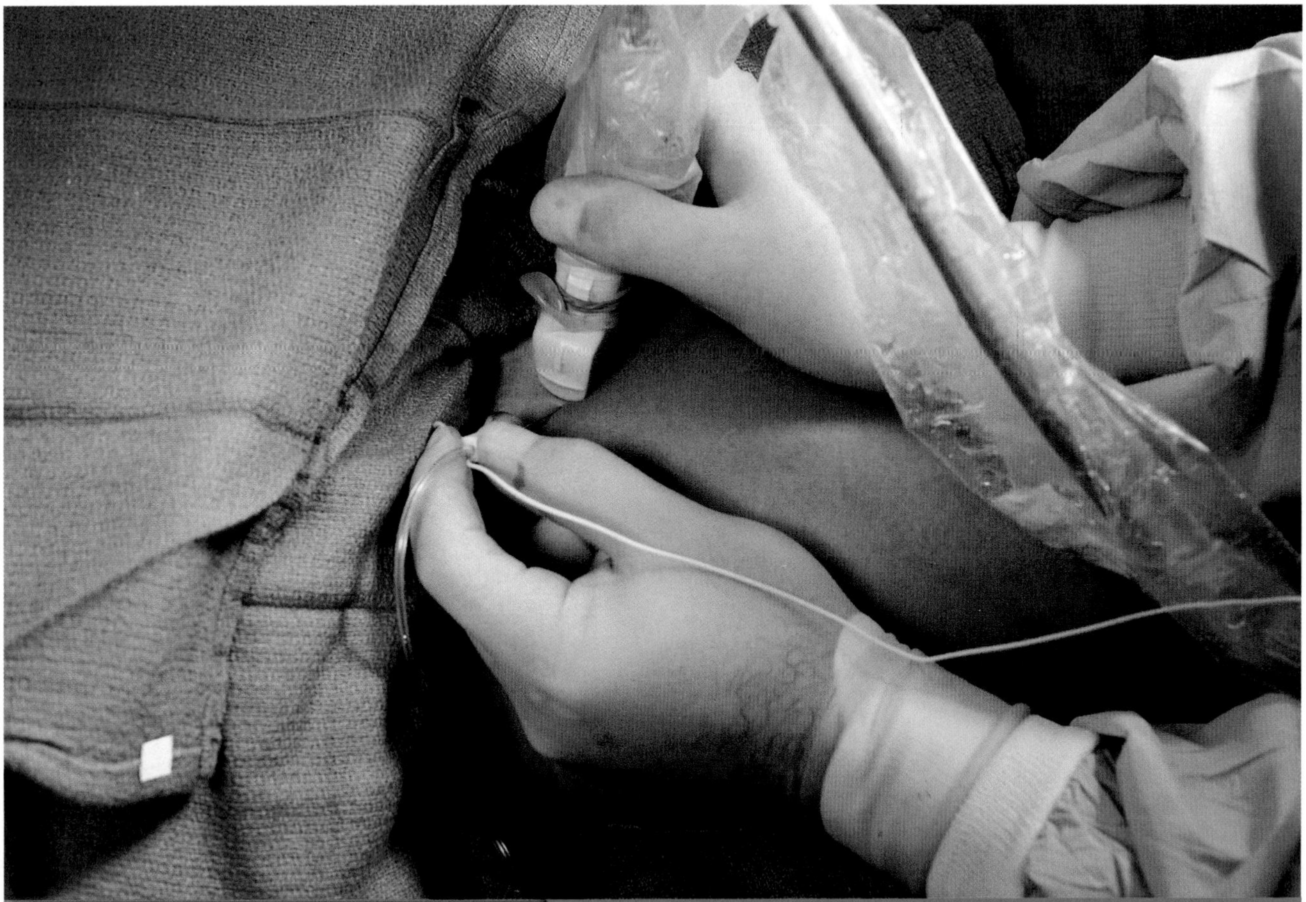

## BLOCK AT A GLANCE

- Indications: anterior thigh, femur, and knee surgery
- Transducer position: transverse, close to the femoral crease
- Goal: local anesthetic spread adjacent to the femoral nerve
- Local anesthetic: 10–20 mL

**FIGURE 35-1.** Transducer position and needle insertion using an in-plane technique to block the femoral nerve at the femoral crease.

## General Considerations

The ultrasound-guided technique of femoral nerve blockade differs from nerve stimulator or landmark-based techniques in several important aspects. Ultrasound application allows the practitioner to monitor the spread of local anesthetic and needle placement and make appropriate adjustments, should the initial spread be deemed inadequate. Also, because of the proximity to the relatively large femoral artery, ultrasound may reduce the risk of arterial puncture that often occurs with this block with the use of non-ultrasound techniques. Palpating the femoral pulse as a landmark for the block is not required with ultrasound guidance, a process that can be challenging in obese patients. Although the ability to visualize the needle and the relevant anatomy with ultrasound guidance renders nerve stimulation optional, motor response obtained during nerve stimulation often provides contributory information.

## Ultrasound Anatomy

Orientation begins with the identification of the pulsating femoral artery at the level of the inguinal crease. If it is not immediately recognized, sliding the transducer medially and laterally will bring the vessel into view eventually. Immediately lateral to the vessel, and deep to the fascia iliaca is the femoral nerve, which is typically hyperechoic and roughly triangular or oval in shape (Figure 35-2A and B). The nerve is positioned in a sulcus in the iliopsoas muscle underneath the fascia iliaca. Other structures that can be visualized are the femoral vein (medial to the artery) and occasionally the fascia lata (superficial in the subcutaneous layer). The femoral nerve typically is visualized at a depth of 2- to 4-cm.

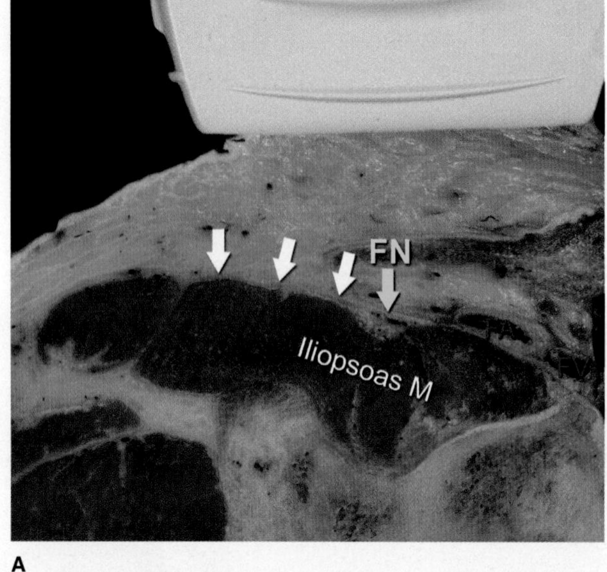


A

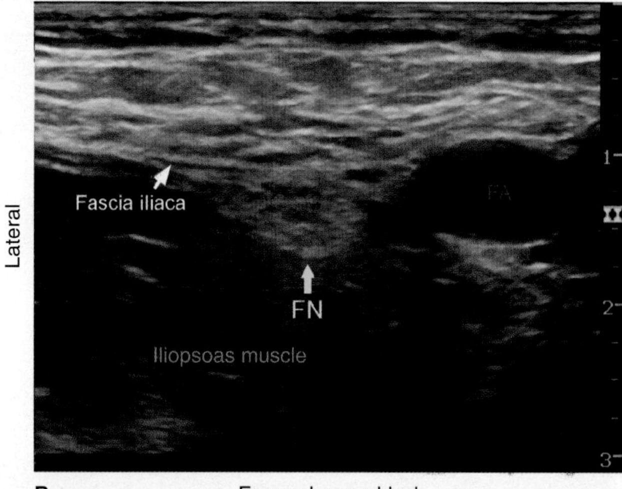


B Femoral nerve block

FIGURE 35-2. (A) Cross-sectional anatomy of the femoral nerve (FN) at the level of the femoral crease. FN is seen on the surface of the iliopsoas muscle covered by fascia iliaca. (white arrows). Femoral artery (FA) and femoral vein (FV) are seen enveloped in their own vascular fascial sheath created by one of the layers of fascia lata. (B) Sonoanatomy of the FN at the femoral triangle.

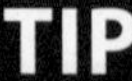

**TIP**

- Identification of the femoral nerve often is made easier by slightly tilting the transducer cranially or caudally. This adjustment helps "brighten" up the nerve and makes it appear distinct from the background.

## Distribution of Blockade

Femoral nerve block results in anesthesia of the anterior and medial thigh down to the knee (the knee included), as well as a variable strip of skin on the medial leg and foot. It also contributes branches to the articular fibers to both the hip and knee. For a more comprehensive review of the femoral nerve distribution, see Chapter 1, Essential Regional Anesthesia Anatomy.

## Equipment

Equipment needed includes the following:

- Ultrasound machine with linear transducer (8–14 MHz), sterile sleeve, and gel
- Standard nerve block tray (described in the equipment section)

- One 20-mL syringe containing local anesthetic
- A 50- to 100-mm, 22-gauge short-bevel insulated stimulating needle
- Peripheral nerve stimulator
- Sterile gloves

## Landmarks and Patient Positioning

This block typically is performed with the patient in the supine position, with the bed or table flattened to maximize operator access to the inguinal area. Although palpation of the femoral pulse is a useful landmark, it is not required because the artery should be readily visualized by placing the transducer transversely on the inguinal crease followed by slow movement laterally or medially. If nerve stimulation is used simultaneously, exposure of the thigh and patella are required to monitor the appropriate motor responses (patella twitch).

### TIP

- Exposing the inguinal region in a patient with a large abdominal pannus can be challenging. Using a wide silk tape to retract the abdomen is a useful maneuver prior to skin preparation and scanning. (Figure 35-3).

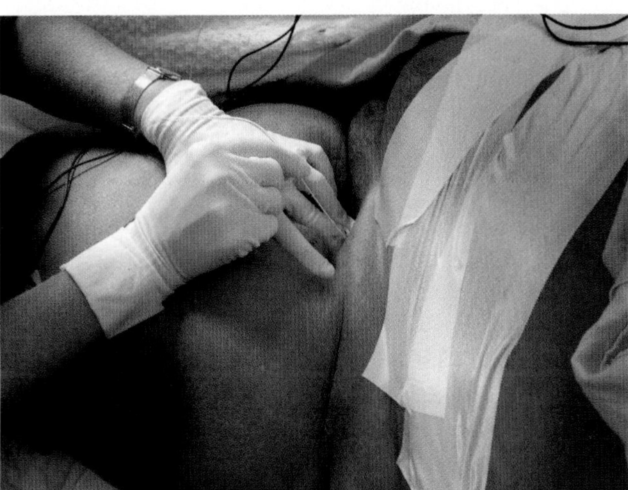

**FIGURE 35-3.** Obesity is a common problem in patients who present with an indication for femoral nerve block. Taping the adipose tissue away helps optimize the exposure to the femoral crease in patients with morbid obesity.

### GOAL

The goal is to place the needle tip immediately adjacent to the lateral aspect of the femoral nerve, either below the fascia iliaca or between the two layers of the fascia iliaca, into the wedge-shaped tissue space lateral to the femoral artery. Proper deposition of local anesthetic is confirmed by observation of the femoral nerve being lifted off of the surface of the iliopsoas muscle or of the spread of the local anesthetic above in the wedged-shaped space lateral to the artery.

## Technique

With the patient in the supine position, the skin over the femoral crease is disinfected and the transducer is positioned to identify the femoral artery and/or nerve (Figure 35-4). If the nerve is not immediately apparent lateral to the artery, tilting the transducer proximally or distally often helps to image and highlight the nerve from the rest of the iliopsoas muscle and the more superficial adipose tissue. In doing so, an effort should be made to identify the iliopsoas muscle and its fascia as well as the fascia lata because injection underneath a wrong fascial sheath may not result in spread of the local anesthetic in the desired plane. Once the femoral nerve is identified, a skin wheal of local anesthetic is made on the lateral aspect of the thigh 1 cm away from the lateral edge of the transducer. The needle is inserted in-plane in

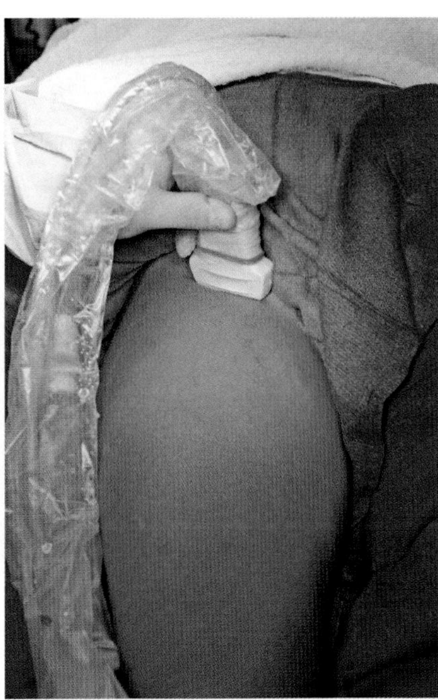

**FIGURE 35-4.** To image the femoral nerve and/or femoral vessels, the transducer is positioned transversely on the femoral crease as shown on the image.

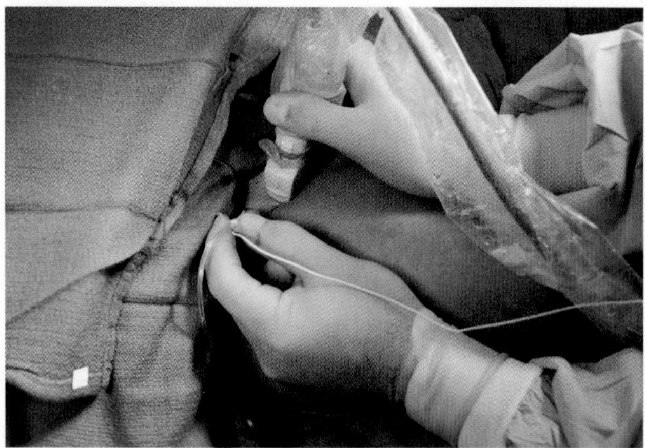

**FIGURE 35-5.** Transducer position and needle insertion using an in-plane technique to block the femoral nerve at the femoral crease.

a lateral-to-medial orientation and advanced toward the femoral nerve (Figure 35-5). If nerve stimulation is used (0.5 mA, 0.1 msec), the passage of the needle through the fascia iliaca and contact of the needle tip with the femoral nerve usually is associated with a motor response of the quadriceps muscle group. In addition, a needle passage through the fascia iliaca is often felt as a "pop" sensation. Once the needle tip is witnessed adjacent (either above, below, or lateral) to the nerve (Figure 35-6), and after careful aspiration, 1 to 2 mL of local anesthetic is injected to confirm the proper needle placement (Figure 35-7). When injection of the local anesthetic does not appear to result in a spread close to the femoral nerve, additional needle repositions and injections may be necessary.

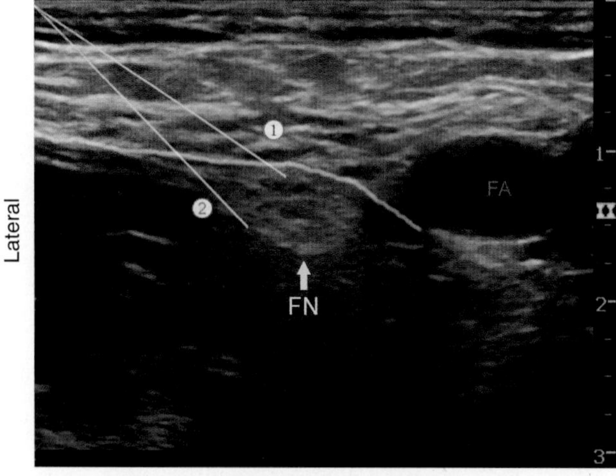


**FIGURE 35-6.** An ultrasound image of the needle path (1,2) to block the femoral nerve. Both needle positions are underneath fascia iliaca, one superficial to the femoral nerve (1) and one deeper to it (2). Either path is acceptable as long as the local anesthetic spreads within the fascia iliaca (white line) to get in contact with the femoral nerve.

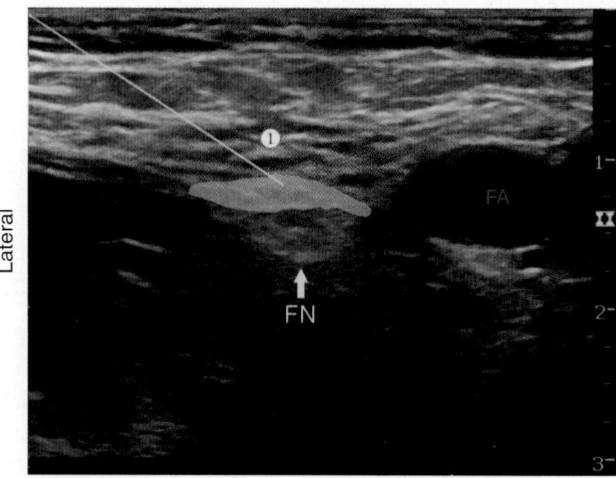


**FIGURE 35-7.** A simulated needle path (1) and spread of the local anesthetic (blue shaded area) to block the femoral nerve (FN). FA, femoral artery.

**TIPS**

- The presence of a motor response to nerve stimulation is useful but not necessary to elicit if the nerve, needle, and local anesthetic spread are well-visualized.
- Never inject against high resistance to injection because this may signal an intrafascicular needle placement.
- An out-of-plane technique can also be used. Because the needle tip may not be seen throughout the procedure, we recommend administering intermittent small boluses (0.5–1 mL) as the needle is advanced toward the nerve to indicate the location of the needle tip.
- Circumferential spread of local anesthetic around the nerve is not necessary for this block. A pool of local anesthetic immediately adjacent to either the posterolateral or the anterior aspects is sufficient.

In an adult patient, 10 to 20 mL of local anesthetic is adequate for a successful block (Figure 35-8A and B). The block dynamics and perioperative management are similar to those described in Chapter 21.

## Continuous Ultrasound-Guided Femoral Nerve Block

The goal of the continuous femoral nerve block is similar to that of the non-ultrasound-based techniques: placement of the catheter in the vicinity of the femoral nerve just deep to the fascia iliaca. The procedure consists of three phases:

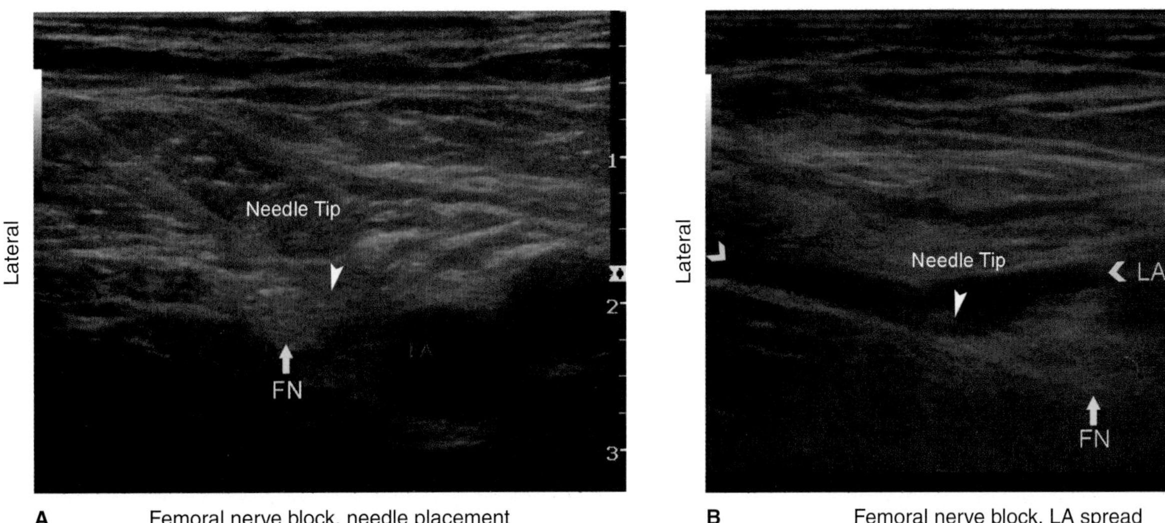


**FIGURE 35-8.** (A) An actual needle path to block the femoral nerve (FN). (B) Spread of the local anesthetic (LA) within two layers of the fascia iliaca to encircle the femoral nerve (FN). FA, femoral artery.

needle placement, catheter advancement, and securing the catheter. For the first two phases of the procedure, ultrasound can be used to ensure accuracy in most patients. The needle typically is inserted in-plane from the lateral-to-medial direction and underneath the nerve. Some clinicians prefer inserting the catheter in the longitudinal plane (inferior-to-superior), analogous to the nerve stimulation-guided technique. No data exist on whether or not one technique is superior to the other. However, the in-line approach from the lateral-to-medial has worked very well in our practice, and it is our preference because it is simpler when using ultrasound guidance.

## TIP

- Both stimulating and nonstimulating catheters can be used, although for simplicity we prefer nonstimulating catheters for this indication.

The needle is advanced until the tip is adjacent to the nerve. Proper placement of the needle can be confirmed by obtaining a motor response of the quadriceps/patella, at which point 5 mL of local anesthetic is injected. This small dose of local anesthetic serves to ensure adequate distribution of the local anesthetic, as well as to make the advancement of the catheter easier. This first phase of the procedure does not significantly differ from the single-injection technique. The second phase of the procedure involves maintaining the needle in the proper position and inserting the catheter 2 to 4 cm into the space surrounding the femoral nerve (Figure 35-9). Insertion of the catheter can be accomplished by either a single operator or with a helper. Catheter position is observed on ultrasound as the catheter is being inserted and/or with an injection through the catheter to document its proper location.

The catheter is secured by either taping it to the skin or tunneling. Preference of one technique over the other varies among clinicians, although no data exist on which one is a more secure method. The decision regarding which

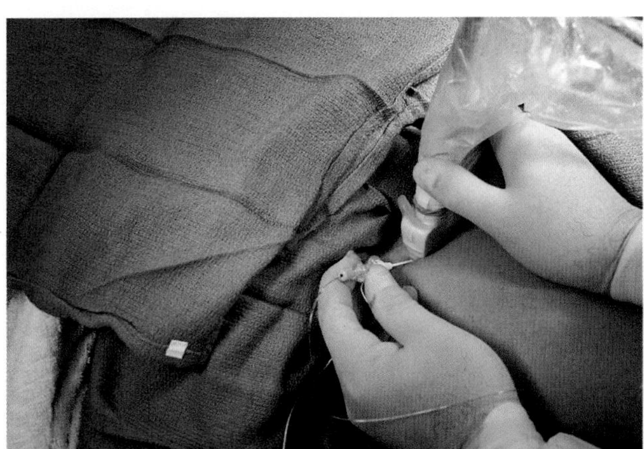

**FIGURE 35-9.** Continuous femoral nerve block. Needle is seen inserted in-plane approaching the nerve from lateral to medial, although it would seem intuitive that a longitudinal insertion of the needle would have advantages with regard to the catheter placement. The technique demonstrated here is simpler and routinely used in our practice with consistent success. The catheter should be inserted 2–4 cm past the needle tip.

method to use could be based on the patient's age (no tunneling for younger patients: less mobile skin, avoidance of posttunneling scar formation), duration of the catheter therapy, and anatomy. In general, the inguinal area is quite mobile and the femoral nerve is not particularly deep, two factors that predispose to catheter dislodgment. The more lateral the starting point for needle insertion for the continuous femoral nerve block, the longer the catheter will be within the iliacus muscle, which may help prevent dislodgment because muscle tends to stabilize a catheter better than adipose tissue. Our empirical infusion regimen for femoral nerve block in an adult patient is ropivacaine 0.2% at a 5 mL/hour infusion rate and a 5 mL/hour patient-controlled bolus.

# ULTRASOUND-GUIDED FEMORAL NERVE BLOCK

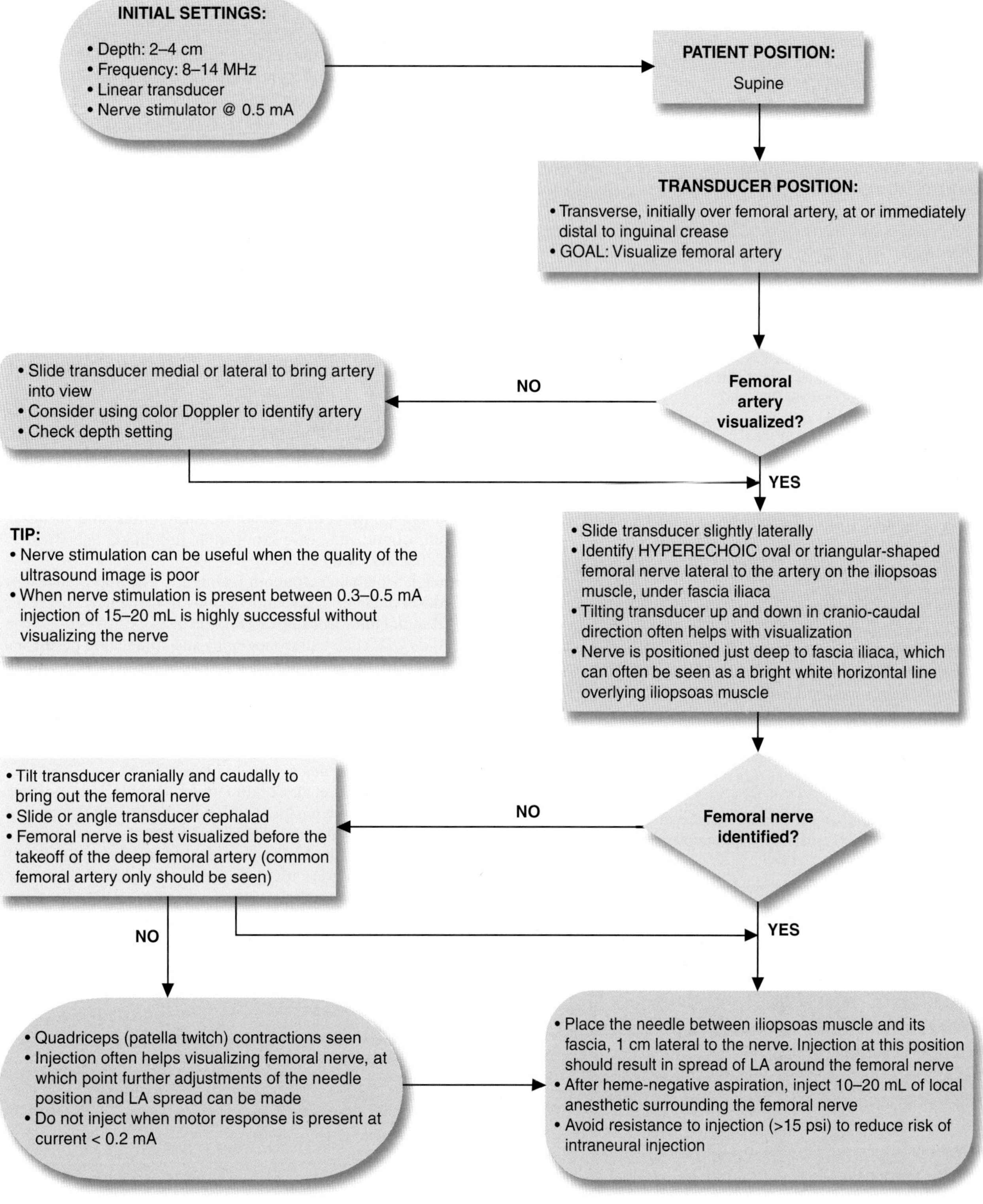

## SUGGESTED READING

Bech B, et al. The successful use of peripheral nerve blocks for femoral amputation. *Acta Anaesthesiol Scand.* 2009;53(2):257-260.

Bodner G, et al. Ultrasound of the lateral femoral cutaneous nerve: normal findings in a cadaver and in volunteers. *Reg Anesth Pain Med.* 2009;34(3):265-268.

Casati A, et al. Effects of ultrasound guidance on the minimum effective anaesthetic volume required to block the femoral nerve. *Br J Anaesth.* 2007;98(6):823-827.

Errando CL. Ultrasound-guided femoral nerve block: catheter insertion in a girl with skeletal abnormalities [in Spanish]. *Rev Esp Anestesiol Reanim.* 2009;56(3):197-198.

Forget P. Bad needles can't do good blocks. *Reg Anesth Pain Med.* 2009;34(6):603.

Fredrickson M. "Oblique" needle-probe alignment to facilitate ultrasound-guided femoral catheter placement. *Reg Anesth Pain Med.* 2008;33(4):383-384.

Fredrickson MJ, Danesh-Clough TK. Ambulatory continuous femoral analgesia for major knee surgery: a randomised study of ultrasound-guided femoral catheter placement. *Anaesth Intensive Care.* 2009;37(5):758-766.

Fredrickson MJ, Kilfoyle DH, Neurological complication analysis of 1000 ultrasound guided peripheral nerve blocks for elective orthopaedic surgery: a prospective study. *Anaesthesia.* 2009;64(8):836-844.

Gurnaney H, Kraemer F, Ganesh A. Ultrasound and nerve stimulation to identify an abnormal location of the femoral nerve. *Reg Anesth Pain Med.* 2009;34(6):615.

Helayel PE, et al. Ultrasound-guided sciatic-femoral block for revision of the amputation stump. Case report. *Rev Bras Anestesiol* 2008;58(5):482-4, 480-2.

Hotta K, et al. Ultrasound-guided combined femoral nerve and lateral femoral cutaneous nerve blocks for femur neck fracture surgery—case report [in Japanese]. *Masui.* 2008;57(7):892-894.

Ito H, et al. Ultrasound-guided femoral nerve block [in Japanese]. *Masui.* 2008;57(5):575-579.

Koscielniak-Nielsen ZJ, Rasmussen H, Hesselbjerg L. Long-axis ultrasound imaging of the nerves and advancement of perineural catheters under direct vision: a preliminary report of four cases. *Reg Anesth Pain Med.* 2008;33(5):477-482.

Lang SA. Ultrasound and the femoral three-in-one nerve block: weak methodology and inappropriate conclusions. *Anesth Analg.* 1998;86(5):1147-1148.

Marhofer P, et al. Fifteen years of ultrasound guidance in regional anaesthesia: Part 2-recent developments in block techniques. *Br J Anaesth.* 2010;104(6):673-683.

Marhofer P, et al. Ultrasonographic guidance improves sensory block and onset time of three-in-one blocks. *Anesth Analg.* 1997;85(4):854-857.

Mariano ER, et al. Ultrasound guidance versus electrical stimulation for femoral perineural catheter insertion. *J Ultrasound Med.* 2009;28(11):1453-1460.

Murray JM, Derbyshire S, Shields MO. Lower limb blocks. *Anaesthesia.* 2010;65(Suppl 1):57-66.

Niazi AU, et al. Methods to ease placement of stimulating catheters during in-plane ultrasound-guided femoral nerve block. *Reg Anesth Pain Med.* 2009;34(4):380-381.

Oberndorfer U, et al. Ultrasonographic guidance for sciatic and femoral nerve blocks in children. *Br J Anaesth.* 2007;98(6): 797-801.

O'Donnell BD, Mannion S. Ultrasound-guided femoral nerve block, the safest way to proceed? *Reg Anesth Pain Med.* 2006;31(4):387-388.

Reid N, et al. Use of ultrasound to facilitate accurate femoral nerve block in the emergency department. *Emerg Med Australas.* 2009;21(2):124-130.

Salinas FV. Ultrasound and review of evidence for lower extremity peripheral nerve blocks. *Reg Anesth Pain Med.* 2010;35 (2 Suppl):S16-25.

Schafhalter-Zoppoth I, Moriggl B. Aspects of femoral nerve block. *Reg Anesth Pain Med.* 2006;31(1):92-93.

Sites BD, et al. A single injection ultrasound-assisted femoral nerve block provides side effect-sparing analgesia when compared with intrathecal morphine in patients undergoing total knee arthroplasty. *Anesth Analg.* 2004;99(5):1539-1543.

Sites BD, et al. A comparison of sensory and motor loss after a femoral nerve block conducted with ultrasound versus ultrasound and nerve stimulation. *Reg Anesth Pain Med.* 2009;34(5):508-513.

Soong J, Schafhalter-Zoppoth I, Gray AT. The importance of transducer angle to ultrasound visibility of the femoral nerve. *Reg Anesth Pain Med.* 2005;30(5):505.

Tran de QH, et al. Ultrasonography and stimulating perineural catheters for nerve blocks: a review of the evidence. *Can J Anaesth.* 2008;55(7):447-457.

Tsui B, Suresh S. Ultrasound imaging for regional anesthesia in infants, children, and adolescents: a review of current literature and its application in the practice of extremity and trunk blocks. *Anesthesiology.* 2010;112(2):473-492.

Villegas Duque A, et al. Continuous femoral block for postoperative analgesia in a patient with poliomyelitis [in Spanish]. *Rev Esp Anestesiol Reanim.* 2010;57(2):123-124.

Wang AZ, et al. Ultrasound-guided continuous femoral nerve block for analgesia after total knee arthroplasty: catheter perpendicular to the nerve versus catheter parallel to the nerve. *Reg Anesth Pain Med.* 2010;35(2):127-131.

# 36 Ultrasound-Guided Fascia Iliaca Block

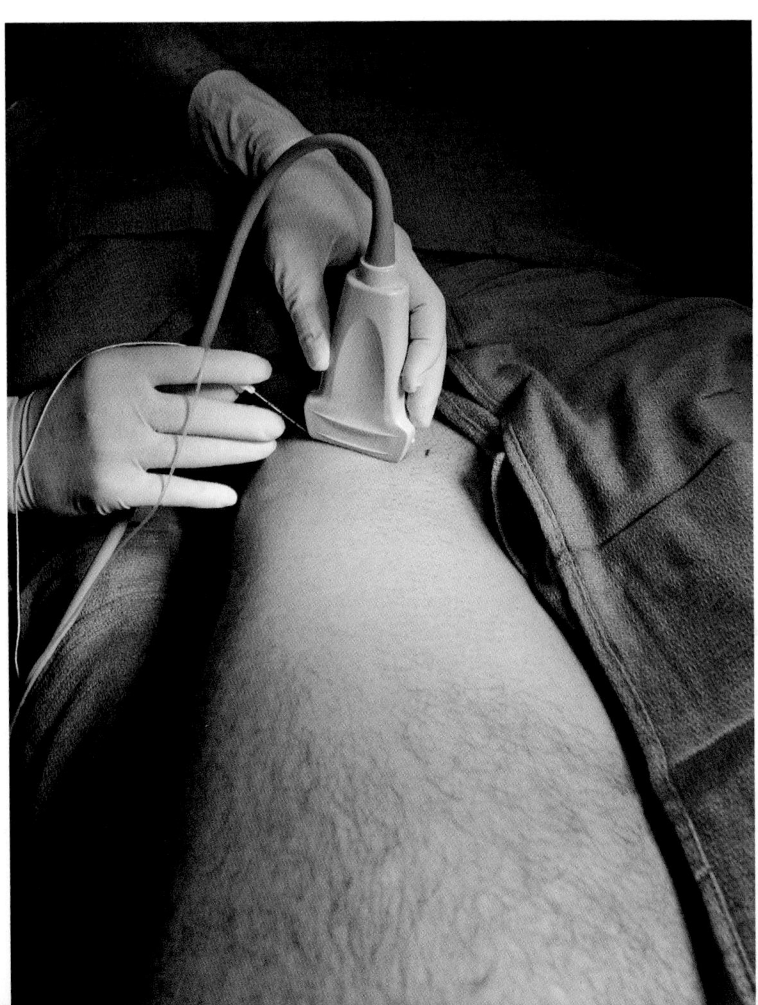

## BLOCK AT A GLANCE

- Indications: anterior thigh and knee surgery, analgesia following hip and knee procedures
- Transducer position: transverse, close to the femoral crease and lateral to the femoral artery (blue dot)
- Goal: medial-lateral spread of local anesthetic underneath fascia iliaca
- Local anesthetic: 30–40 mL of dilute local anesthetic (e.g., 0.2% ropivacaine)

**FIGURE 36-1.** Needle insertion for the fascia iliaca block. The blue dot indicates the position of the femoral artery.

## General Considerations

Fascia iliaca block is a low-tech alternative to a femoral nerve or a lumbar plexus block. The mechanism behind this block is that the femoral and lateral femoral cutaneous nerves lie under the iliacus fascia. Therefore, a sufficient volume of local anesthetic deposited beneath the fascia iliaca, even if placed some distance from the nerves, has the potential to spread underneath the fascia and reach these nerves. Traditionally, it was believed that the local anesthetic could also spread underneath fascia iliaca proximally toward the lumbosacral plexus; however, this has not been demonstrated consistently. The non-ultrasound technique involved placement of the needle at the lateral third of the distance from the anterior superior iliac spine and the pubic tubercle, using a "double-pop" technique as the needle passes through fascia lata and fascia iliaca. However, block success with this "feel" technique is sporadic because false "pops" can occur. The ultrasound-guided technique is essentially the same; however, monitoring of the needle placement and local anesthetic delivery assures deposition of the local anesthetic into the correct plane.

## Ultrasound Anatomy

The fascia iliaca is located anterior to the iliacus muscle (on its surface) within the pelvis. It is bound superolaterally by the iliac crest and medially merges with the fascia overlying the psoas muscle. Both the femoral nerve and the lateral cutaneous nerve of the thigh lie under the iliacus fascia in their intrapelvic course. Anatomic orientation begins in the same manner as with the femoral block: with identification of the femoral artery at the level of the inguinal crease. If it is not immediately visible, sliding the transducer medially and laterally will eventually bring the vessel into view. Immediately lateral and deep to the femoral artery and vein is a large hypoechoic structure, the iliopsoas muscle (Figure 36-2). It is covered by a thin layer of connective tissue fascia, which can be seen separating the muscle from the subcutaneous tissue superficial to it. The hyperechoic femoral nerve should be seen wedged between the iliopsoas muscle and the fascia iliaca, lateral to the femoral artery. The fascia lata (superficial in the subcutaneous layer) is more superficial and may have more then one layer. Moving the transducer laterally several centimeters brings into view the sartorius muscle covered by its own fascia as well as the fascia iliaca. Further lateral movement of the transducer reveals the anterior superior iliac spine (Figure 36-2). Additional anatomical detail can be seen in cross sectional anatomy in Section 7. Since the anatomy is essentially identical, it is not repeated here.

**TIP**

- The transducer should be placed at the level of the femoral crease and oriented parallel to the crease.

## Distribution of Blockade

The distribution of anesthesia and analgesia that is accomplished with the fascia iliaca block depends on the extent of the local anesthetic spread and the nerves blocked. Blockade of the femoral nerve results in anesthesia of the anterior and medial thigh (down to and including the knee) and anesthesia of a variable strip of skin on the medial leg and foot. The femoral nerve also contributes to articular fibers to both the hip and knee. The lateral femoral cutaneous nerve confers cutaneous innervation to the anterolateral thigh. For a more comprehensive review of the femoral and lateral femoral cutaneous nerves and lumbar plexus nerve distribution, refer to Chapter 01, Essential Regional Anesthesia Anatomy.

## Equipment

Equipment needed is:

- Ultrasound machine with linear transducer (6–14 MHz), sterile sleeve, and gel

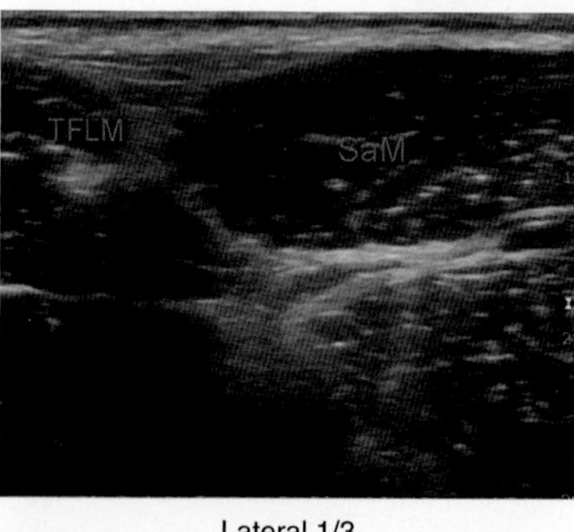


Lateral 1/3

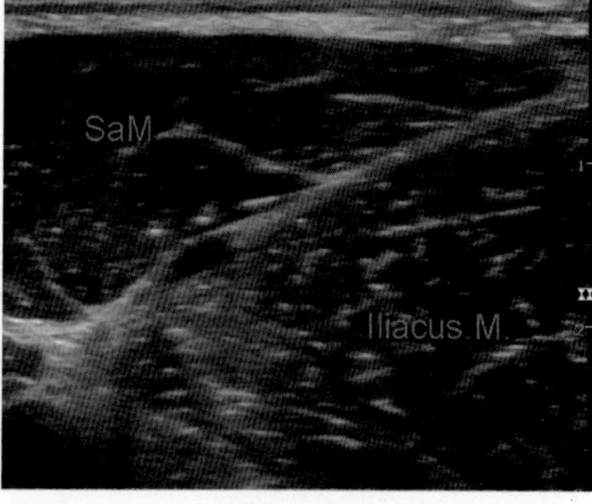


Middle 1/3

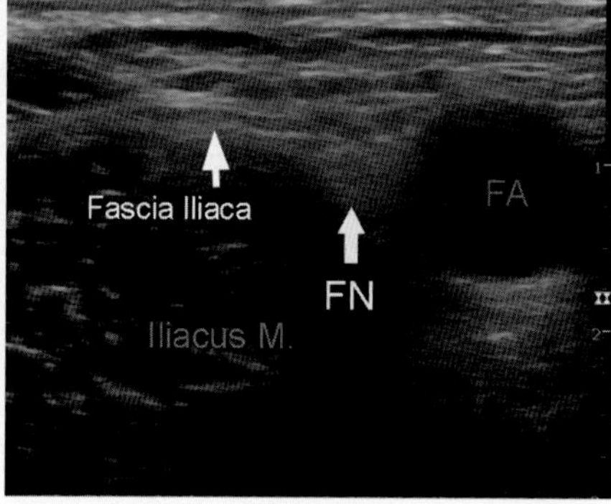


Medial 1/3

**FIGURE 36-2.** A panoramic view of ultrasound anatomy of the femoral (inguinal) crease area. From lateral to medial shown are tensor fascia lata muscle (TFLM), sartorius muscle (SaM), Iliac muscle, fascia iliaca, femoral nerve (FN), and femoral artery (FA). The lateral, middle and medial 1/3s are derived by dividing the line between the FA and anterior-superior iliac spine in three equal 1/3 sections.

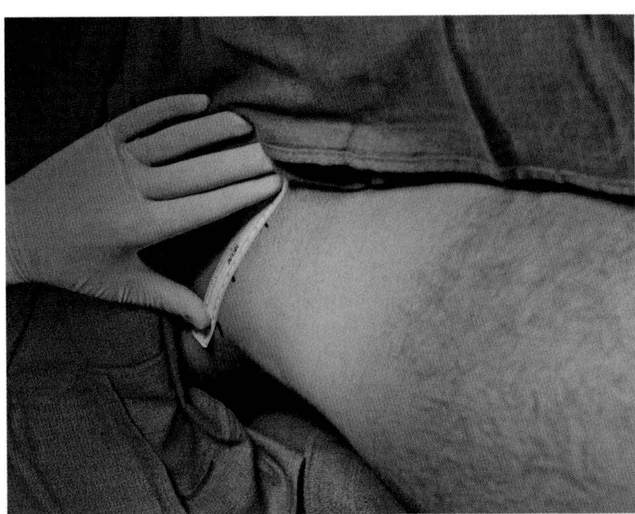

**FIGURE 36-3.** The ruler is positioned to divide the distance between the femoral artery and anterior superior spine in 3 equal parts as described in Figure 36-2.

- Standard nerve block tray (described in the equipment section)
- Two 20-mL syringes containing local anesthetic
- 80- to 100-mm, 22-gauge needle (short bevel aids in feeling the fascial "pops")
- Sterile gloves

## Landmarks and Patient Positioning

This block is typically performed with the patient in the supine position, with the bed or table flattened to maximize access to the inguinal area (Figure 36-3). Although palpation of a femoral pulse is a useful landmark, it is not required because the artery is quickly visualized by placement of the transducer transversely on the inguinal crease, followed by slow movement laterally or medially.

## GOAL

The goal is to place the needle tip under the fascia iliaca approximately at a lateral third of the line connecting anterior superior iliac spine to the pubic tubercle (injection is made several centimeters lateral to the femoral artery) and to deposit a relatively large volume (30–40 mL) of local anesthetic until its spread laterally toward the iliac spine and medially toward the femoral nerve is documented with ultrasound visualization.

## Technique

With the patient in the proper position, the skin is disinfected and the transducer positioned to identify the

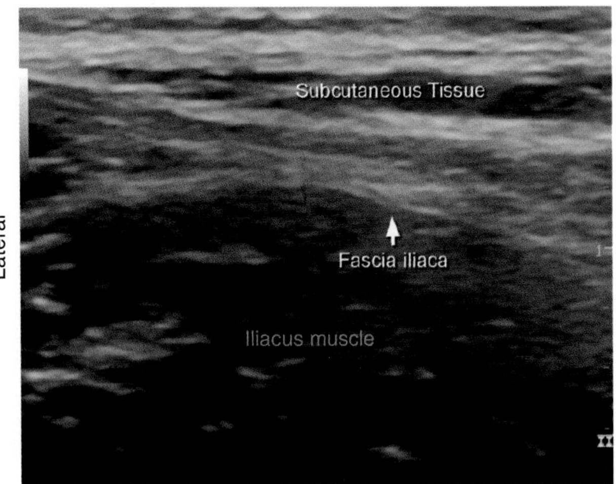


**FIGURE 36-4.** Magnified image of the fascia iliaca.

femoral artery and the iliopsoas muscle and fascia iliaca. The transducer is moved laterally until the sartorius muscle is identified. After a skin wheal is made, the needle is inserted in-plane (Figure 36-1). As the needle passes through fascia iliaca the fascia is first seen indented by the needle. As the needle eventually pierces through the fascia, pop may be felt and the fascia may be seen to "snap" back on the ultrasound image. After negative aspiration, 1 to 2 mL of local anesthetic is injected to confirm the proper injection plane between the fascia (Figure 36-4) and the iliopsoas muscle (Figure 36-5A, B, and C). If local anesthetic spread occurs above the fascia or within the substance of the muscle itself, additional needle repositions and injections may be necessary. A proper injection will result in the separation of the fascia iliaca by the local anesthetic in the medial-lateral direction from the point of injection as described. If the spread is deemed inadequate, additional injections laterally or medially to the original needle insertion or injection can be made to facilitate the medial-lateral spread.

## TIPS

- The fascia iliaca block is a large-volume block. Its success depends on the spread of local anesthetic along a connective tissue plane. For this reason, 30 to 40 mL of injectate is necessary to accomplish the block.
- The spread of the local anesthetic is monitored with ultrasonography. If the pattern of the spread is not adequate (e.g., the local is forming a collection in one location and not "layering out"), injection is stopped and needle repositioned before continuing. Additional injections may be made to assure adequate spread.

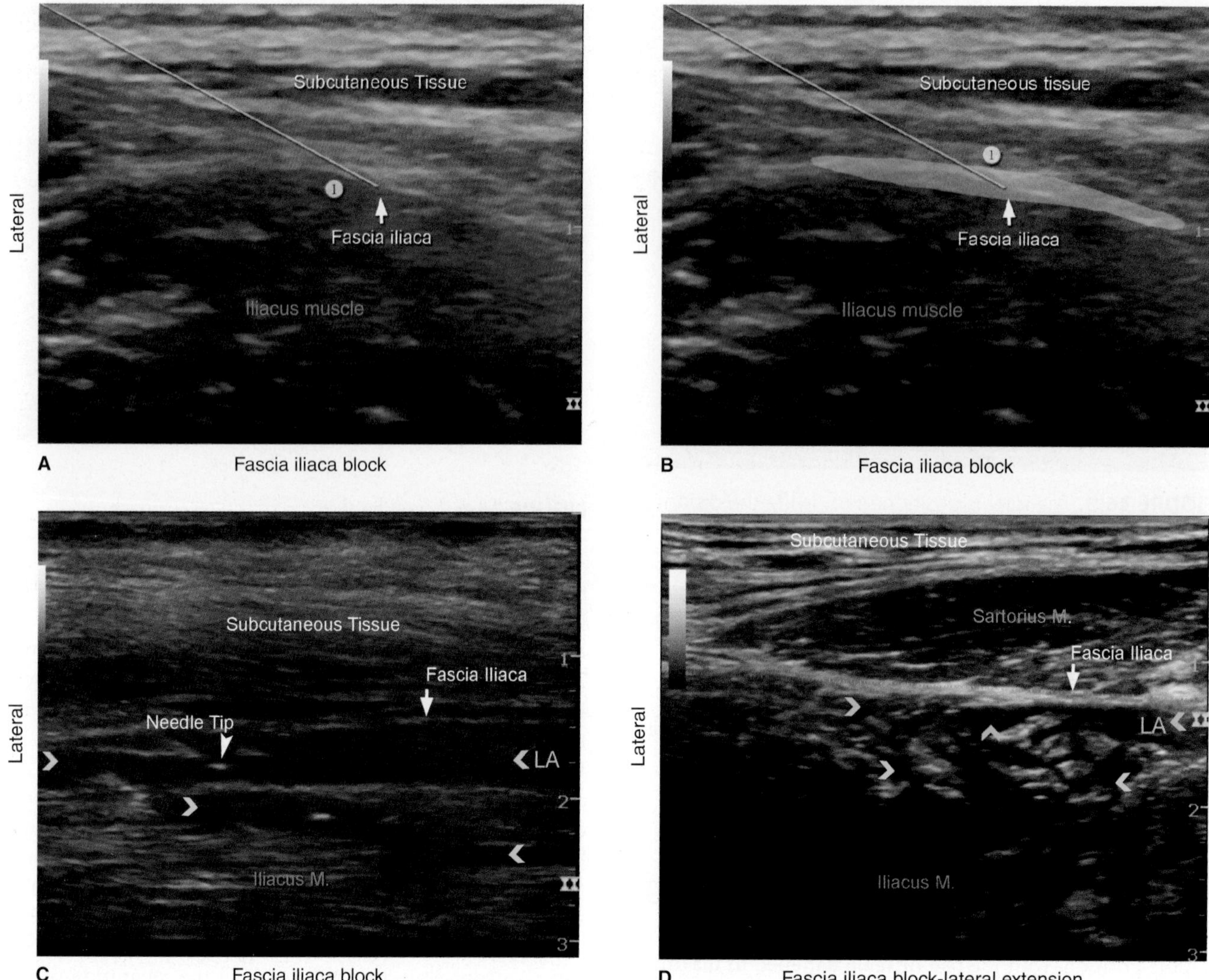


**FIGURE 36-5.** (A) Path of the needle for the fascia iliaca block. The needle ❶ is shown underneath the fascia iliaca lateral to the femoral artery (not seen) but not too deep to be lodged into the iliac muscle. (B) A simulated spread (area shaded in blue) of the local anesthetic to accomplish a fascia iliaca block. (C) Spread of the local anesthetic (LA) under the fascia iliaca. Some local anesthetic is also seen deep within the iliacus muscle (yellow arrows). When this occurs, the needle should be pulled back more superficially. (D) Extension of the LA laterally underneath the sartorius muscle. Some LA fills the adipose tissue between fascia iliaca and iliacus muscle (yellow arrows).

In an adult patient, between 30 and 40 mL of local anesthetic is usually required for successful blockade. The success of the block is best predicted by documenting the spread of the local anesthetic toward the femoral nerve medially and underneath the sartorius muscle laterally. In obese patients, an out of plane technique may be favored. The block should result in blockade of the femoral in all instances (100%) and lateral femoral nerve (80%-100%). Block of anterior branch of the obturator nerve is unreliable with fascia iliaca block. When required, this nerve should be blocked as described in Chapter 37.

# ULTRASOUND-GUIDED FASCIA ILIACA BLOCK

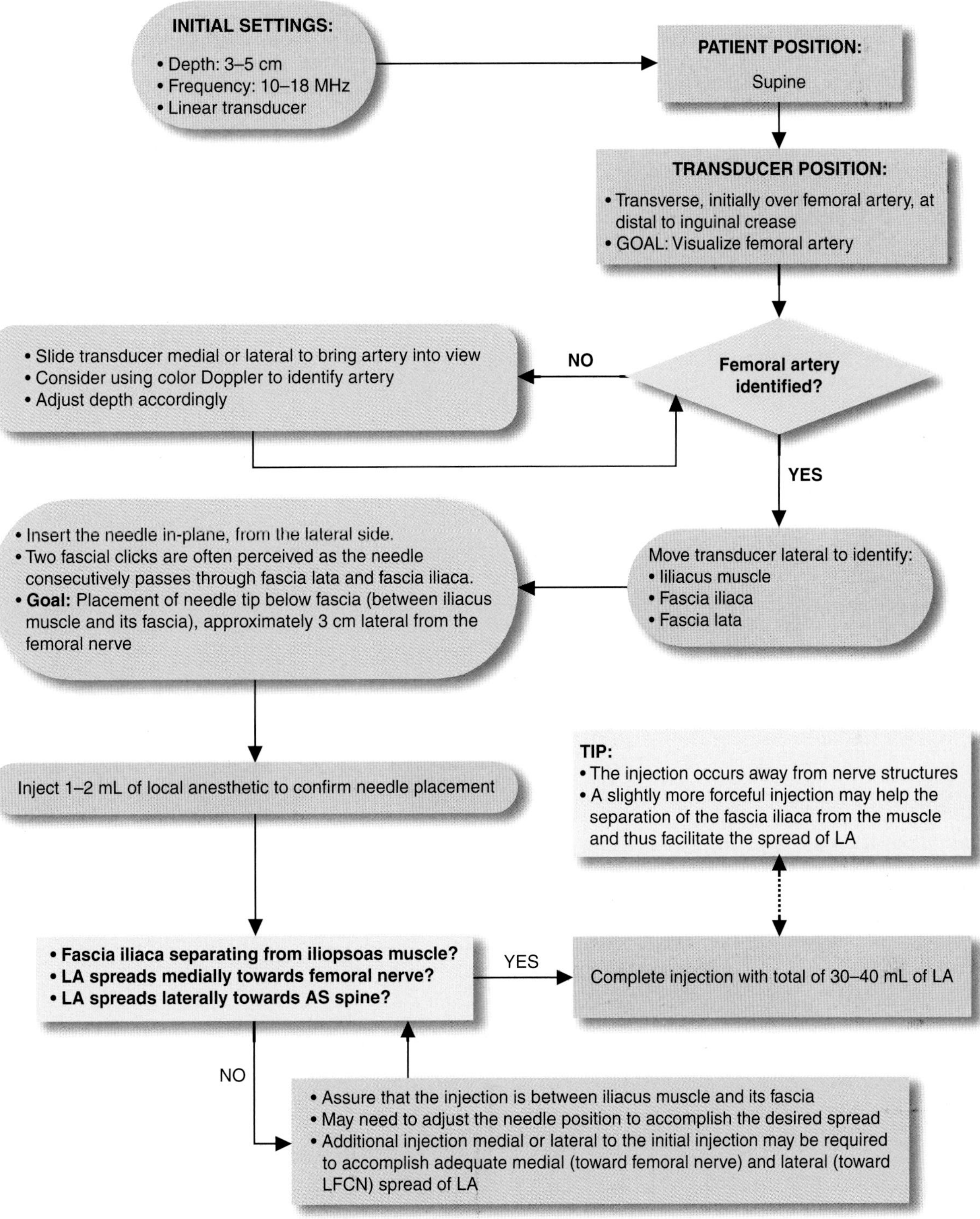

## SUGGESTED READING

Dolan J, Williams A, Murney E, Smith M, Kenny GN. Ultrasound guided fascia iliaca block: a comparison with the loss of resistance technique. *Reg Anesth Pain Med.* 2008;33:526-531.

Foss NB, Kristensen BB, Bundgaard M, et al. Fascia iliaca compartment blockade for acute pain control in hip fracture patients: a randomized, placebo-controlled study. *Anesthesiology.* 2007;106:773-778.

Hebbard P, Ivanusic J, Sha S. Ultrasound-guided supra-inguinal fascia iliaca block: a cadaveric evaluation of a novel approach. *Anaesthesia.* 2011;66:300-305.

Minville V, Gozlan C, Asehnoune K, et al. Fascia-iliaca compartment block for femoral bone fracture in prehospital medicine in a 6-yr-old child. *Eur J Anaesthesiol.* 2006;23:715-716.

Mouzopolous G, Vasiliadis G, Lasanianos N, et al. Fascia iliaca block prophylaxis for hip fracture patients at risk for delirium: a randomized placebo-controlled study. *J Orthop Traumatol.* 2009;10:127-133.

Swenson JD, Bay N, Loose E, et al. Outpatient management of continuous peripheral nerve catheters placed using ultrasound guidance: an experience in 620 patients. *Anesth Analg.* 2006;103:1436-1443.

Wambold D, Carter C, Rosenberg AD. The fascia iliaca block for postoperative pain relief after knee surgery. *Pain Pract.* 2001;1:274-277.

Yun MJ, Kim YH, Han MK, et al. Analgesia before a spinal block for femoral neck fracture: fascia iliaca compartment block. *Acta Anaesthesiol Scand.* 2009;53:1282-1287.

# 37 Ultrasound-Guided Obturator Nerve Block

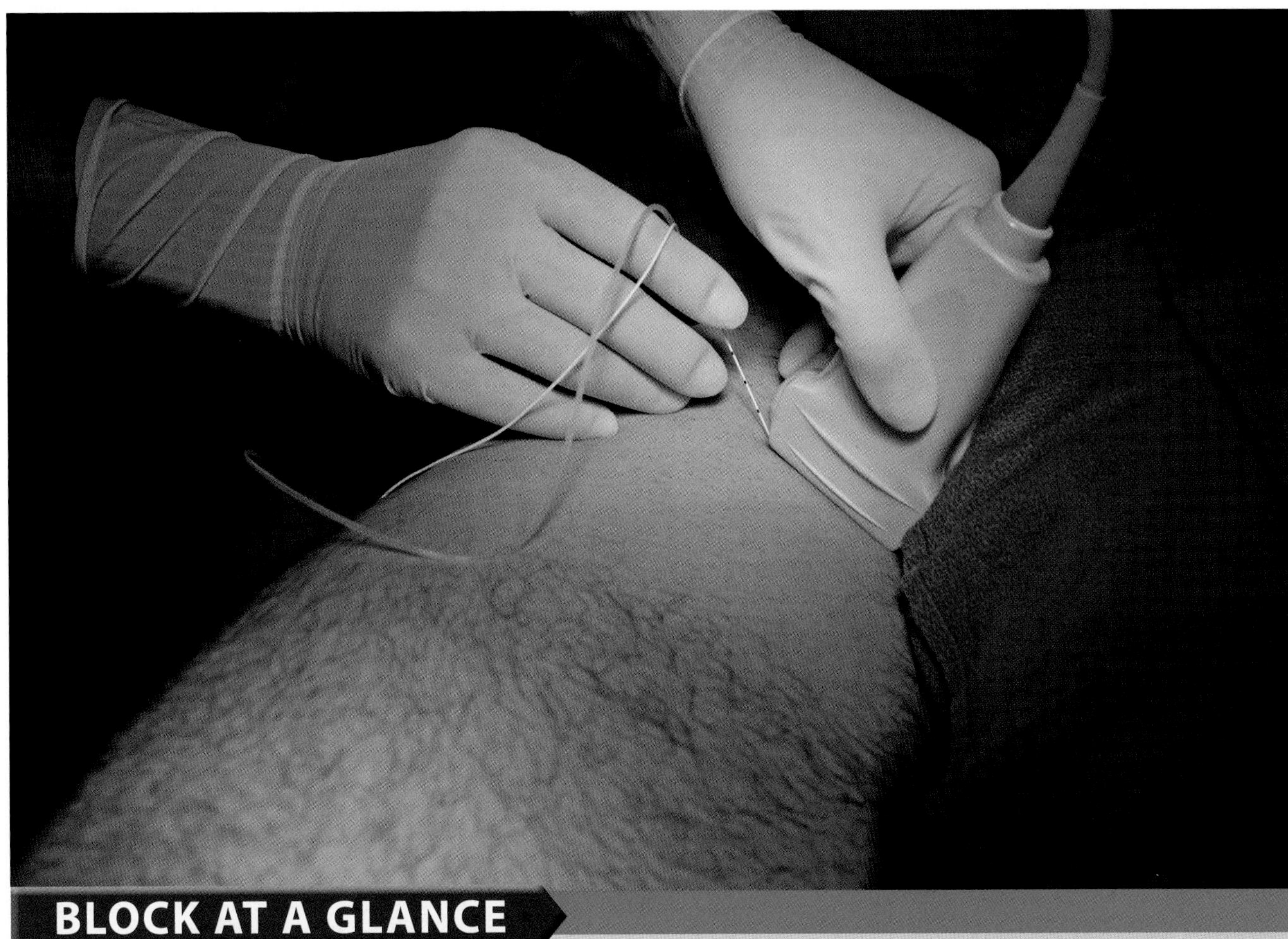

## BLOCK AT A GLANCE

- Indications: Relief of painful adductor muscle contractions, to prevent adduction of thigh during transurethral bladder surgery, additional analgesia after major knee surgery
- Transducer position: Medial aspect of thigh
- Goal: Local anesthetic spread in the interfascial muscle plane in which the nerves lie or around the anterior and posterior branches of the obturator nerve
- Local anesthetic: 5–10 mL around each interfascial space or branches of obturator nerve

**FIGURE 37-1.** Needle insertion using an in-plane technique to accomplish an obturator nerve block.

## General Considerations

There is renewed interest in obturator nerve block because of the recognition that the obturator nerve is spared after a "3-in-1 block" and yet can be easier accomplished using ultrasound guidance. In some patients, the quality of postoperative analgesia is improved after knee surgery when an obturator nerve block is added to a femoral nerve block. However, a routine use of the obturator block does not result in improved analgesia in all patients having knee surgery. For this reason, obturator block is used selectively.

Ultrasound-guided obturator nerve block is simpler to perform, more reliable, and associated with patient discomfort when compared with surface landmark-based techniques.

There are two approaches to performing ultrasound-guided obturator nerve block. The interfascial injection technique relies on injecting local anesthetic solution into the fascial planes that contain the branches of the obturator nerve. With this technique, it is not important to identify the branches of obturator nerve on the sonogram but rather to identify the adductor muscles and the fascial boundaries within which the nerves lie. This is similar in concept to other fascial plane blocks (e.g. transversus abdominis plane block [TAP]) where local anesthetic solution is injected between the internal oblique and transverse abdominis muscles without the need to indentify the nerves. Alternatively, the branches of the obturator nerve can be visualized with ultrasound imaging and blocked after eliciting a motor response.

## Anatomy

The obturator nerve forms in the lumbar plexus from the anterior primary rami of L2-L4 roots and descends to the pelvis in the psoas muscle. In most individuals, the nerve divides into an anterior branch and posterior branch before exiting the pelvis through the obturator foramen. In the thigh, at the level of the femoral crease, the *anterior branch* is located between the fascia of pectineus and adductor brevis muscles. The anterior branch lies further caudad between the pectineus and adductor brevis muscles. The anterior branch provides motor fibers to the adductor muscles and cutaneous branches to the medial aspect of the thigh. The anterior branch has a great variability in the extent of sensory innervation of the medial thigh. The *posterior branch* lies between the fascial planes of the adductor brevis and adductor magnus muscles (Figures 37-2 and 37-3). The posterior branch

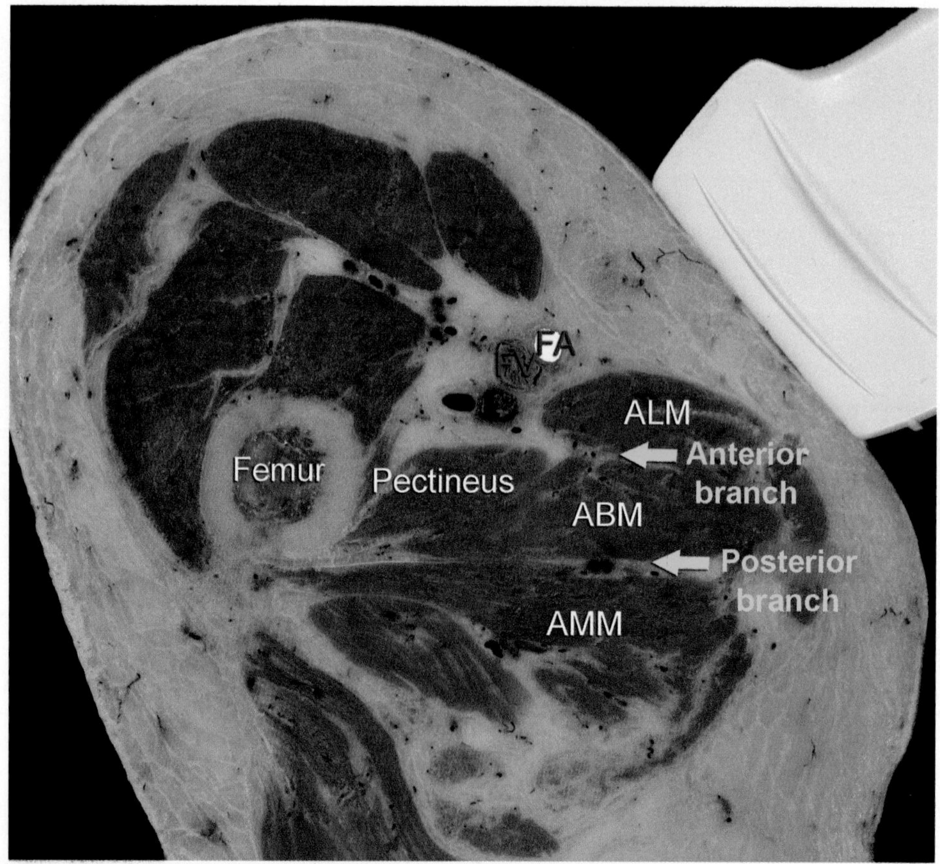


**FIGURE 37-2.** Cross-sectional anatomy of relevance to the obturator nerve block. Shown are femoral vessels (FV, FA), pectineus muscle, adductor longus (ALM), adductor brevis (ABM), and adductor magnus (AMM) muscles. The anterior branch of the obturator nerve is seen between ALM and ABM, whereas the posterior branch is seen between ABM and AMM.

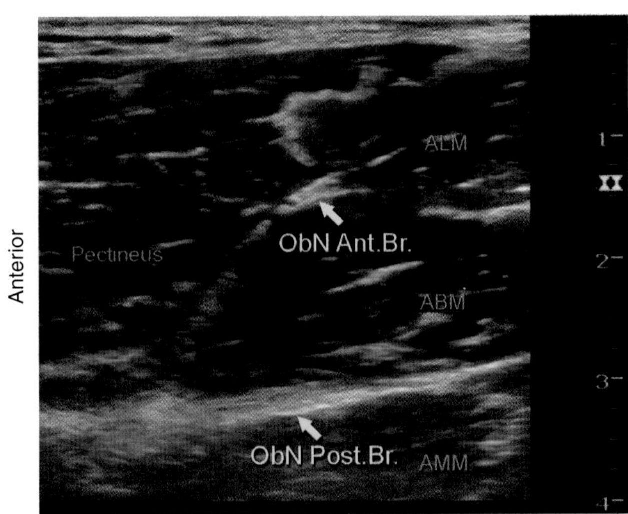


**FIGURE 37-3.** Anterior branch (Ant. Br.) of the obturator nerve (ObN) is seen between the adductor longus (ALM) and the adductor brevis (ABM), whereas the posterior branch (Post. Br.) is seen between the ABM and the adductor magnus (AMM).

is primarily a motor nerve for the adductors of the thigh; however it also may provide articular branches to the medial aspect of the knee joint. The articular branches to the hip joint usually arise from the obturator nerve proximal to its division and only occasionally from the individual branches (Figure 37-4).

## TIP

- A psoas compartment (lumbar plexus) block is required to reliably block the articular branches of the obturator nerve to the hip joint because they usually depart proximal to where obturator nerve block is performed.

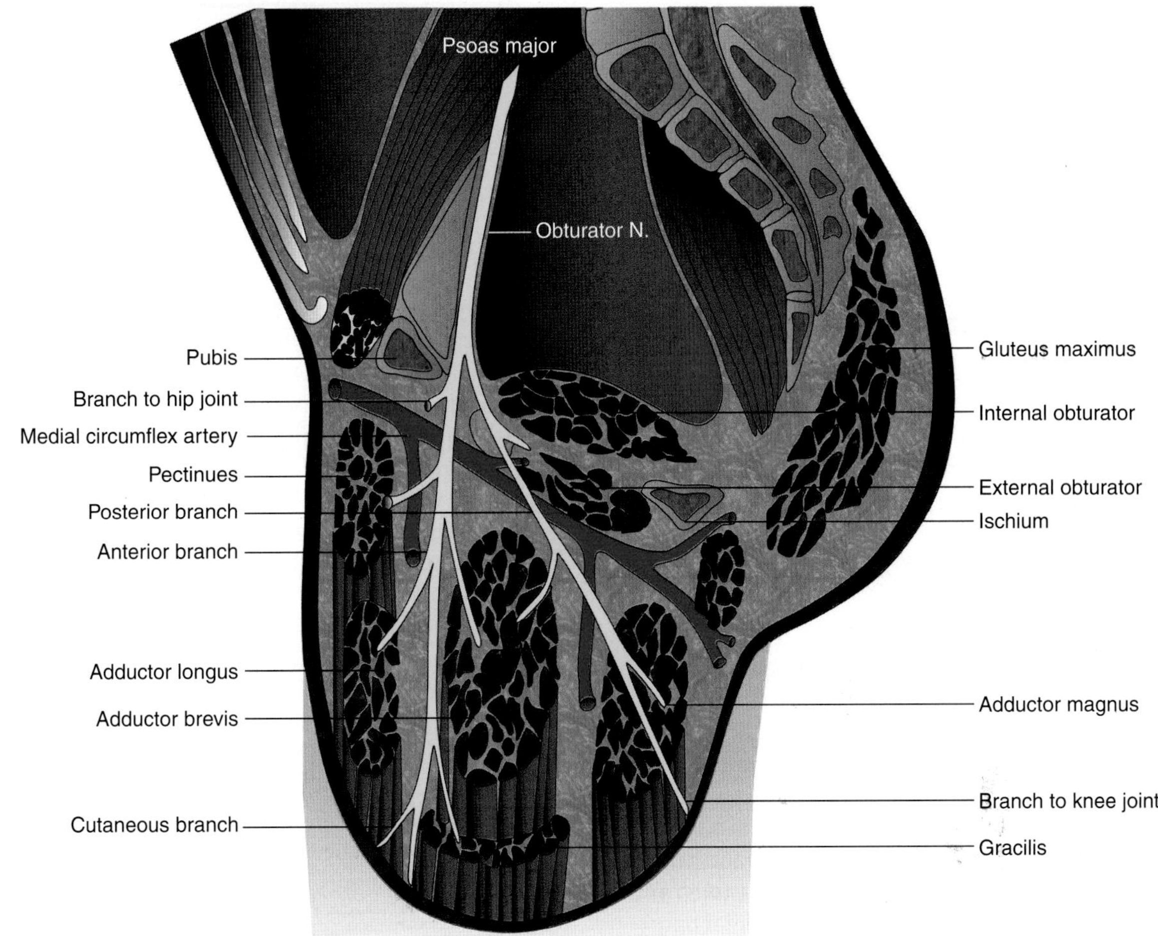


**FIGURE 37-4.** The course and divisions of the obturator nerve and their relationship to the adductor muscles.

## Distribution of Blockade

Because there is great variability in the cutaneous innervation to the medial thigh, demonstrated weakness or absence of adductor muscle strength is the best method of documenting a successful obturator nerve block, rather than a decreased skin sensation in the expected territory. However, the adductor muscles of the thigh may have co-innervation from the femoral nerve (pectineus) and sciatic nerve (adductor magnus). For this reason, complete loss of adductor muscle strength is also uncommon despite a successful obturator nerve block.

### TIP

- A simple method of assessing adductor muscle strength (motor block) is to instruct the patient to adduct the blocked leg from an abducted position against resistance. Weakness or inability to adduct the leg indicates a successful obturator nerve block.

## Equipment

Equipment needed includes the following:

- Ultrasound machine with linear (or curved) transducer (5–13 MHz), sterile sleeve, and gel
- Standard block tray
- A 20-mL syringe containing local anesthetic solution
- A 10-cm, 21–22 gauge short-bevel insulated needle
- Peripheral nerve stimulator (optional)
- Sterile gloves

## Landmarks and Patient Positioning

With the patient supine, the thigh is slightly abducted and laterally rotated. The block can be performed either at the level of femoral (inguinal) crease medial to the femoral vein or 1 to 3 cm inferior to the inguinal crease on the medial aspect (adductor compartment) of the thigh (Figure 37-5).

### GOAL

The goal of the interfascial injection technique for blocking the obturator nerve is to inject local anesthetic solution into the interfascial space between the pectineus and adductor brevis muscles to block the *anterior* branch and the adductor brevis and adductor magnus muscles to block the *posterior* branch. When using ultrasound guidance with nerve stimulation, the anterior and posterior branches of the of obturator nerve are identified and stimulated to elicit a motor response prior to injecting local anesthetic solution around each branch.

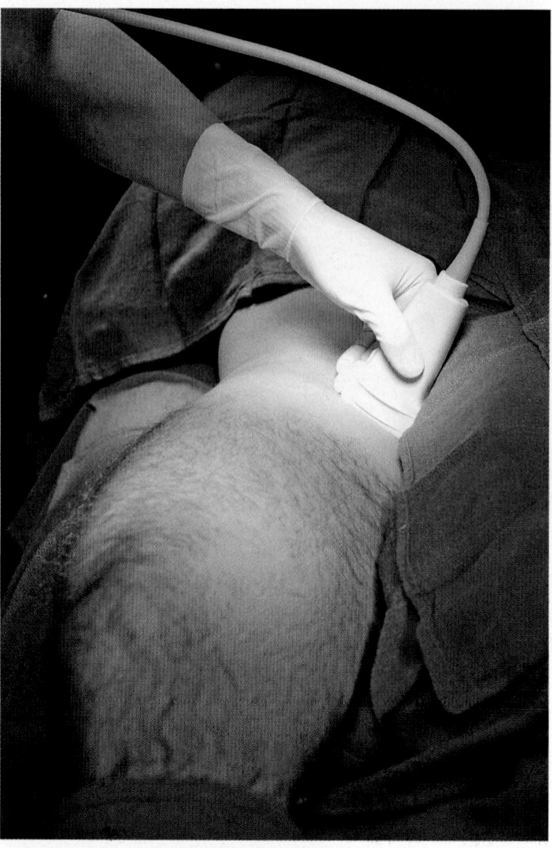

**FIGURE 37-5.** A transducer position to image the obturator nerve. The transducer is positioned medial to the femoral artery slightly below the femoral crease.

## Technique

The *interfascial* approach is performed at the level of the femoral crease. With this technique, it is important to identify the adductor muscles and their fascial planes in which the individual nerves are enveloped.

With the patient supine, the leg is slightly abducted and externally rotated. The ultrasound transducer is placed to visualize the femoral vessels. The transducer is advanced medially along the crease to identify the adductor muscles and their fasciae. The anterior branch is sandwiched between the pectineus and adductor brevis muscles, whereas the posterior branch is located the fascial plane between the adductor brevis and adductor magnus muscles. The block needle is advanced to initially position the needle tip between the pectineus and adductor brevis at the junction of middle and posterior third of their fascial interface (Figure 37-6). At this point, 5 to 10 mL of local anesthetic solution is injected. The needle is advanced further to position the needle tip between the adductor brevis and adductor magnus muscles, and 5 to 10 mL of local anesthetic is injected (Figure 37-6B). It is important for the local anesthetic solution to spread into the interfascial space and not be injected into the muscles. Correct injection of

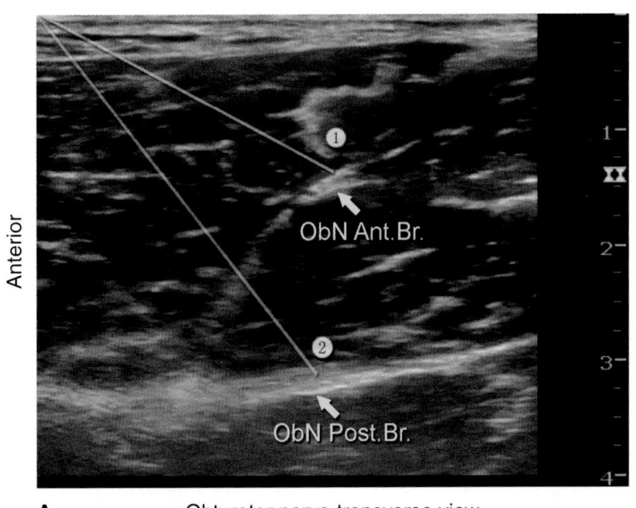


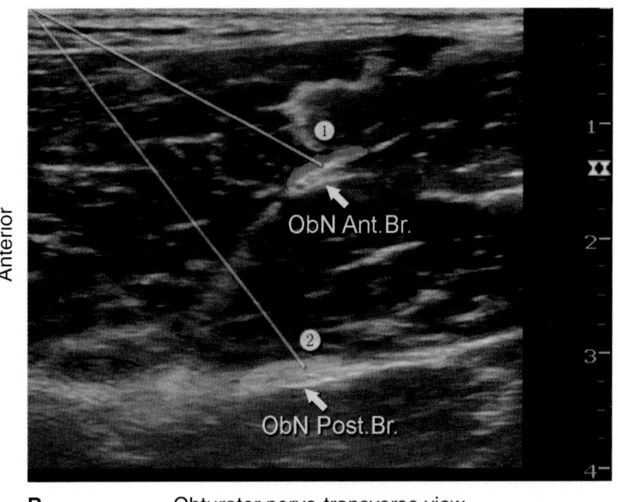


**FIGURE 37-6.** (A) Needle paths required to reach the anterior branch ❶ and the posterior branch ❷ of the obturator nerve (ObN). (B) Simulated dispersion of the local anesthetic to block the anterior ❶ and posterior ❷ branches of the obturator nerve. In both examples, an in-plane needle insertion is used.

local anesthetic solution into the interfascial space results in accumulation of the injectate between target muscles. The needle may have to be repositioned to allow for precise interfascial injection.

Alternatively, the cross-sectional image of branches of the obturator nerve can be obtained by scanning 1 to 3 cm distal to the inguinal crease on the medial aspect of thigh. The nerves appear as hyperechoic, flat, lip-shaped structures invested in the fascia of adductor muscles. The anterior branch is located between the adductor longus and adductor brevis muscles, whereas the posterior branch is between the adductor brevis and adductor magnus muscles. An insulated block needle attached to the nerve stimulator is advanced toward the nerve either in an out-of-plane or in-plane trajectory. After eliciting the contraction of the adductor muscles, 5 to 7 mL of local anesthetic is injected around each branch of the obturator nerve (Figure 37-6B).

## TIPS

- The usual precautions to prevent intravascular injection should be taken because this is a highly vascular area (standard monitoring, adding epinephrine to local anesthetic solution, fractionating the dose, maintaining verbal contact with patient).
- When nerve stimulation is used, adduction of the thigh can be obtained without proper nerve identification. This is due to direct muscle or muscle branch stimulation with currents >1.0 mA. Decreasing the current intensity helps distinguish between nerve versus direct muscle stimulation.
- It is not necessary to optimize motor response to a predetermined nerve stimulator current; the role of nerve stimulation is simply to confirm that a structure is indeed a nerve.

## ULTRASOUND-GUIDED OBTURATOR BLOCK

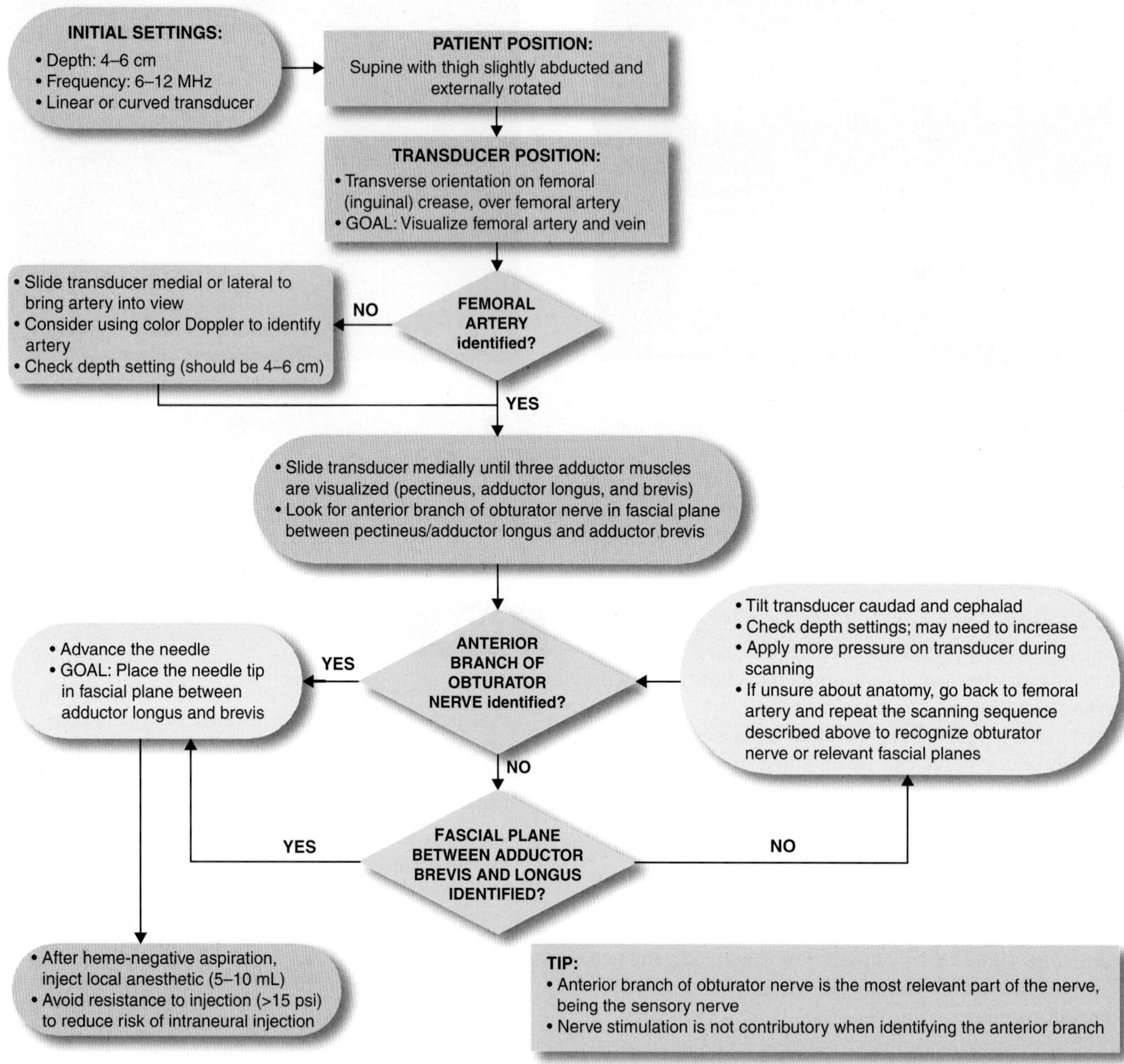

## SUGGESTED READING

Akkaya T, Ozturk E, Comert A, et al. Ultrasound-guided obturator nerve block: a sonoanatomic study of a new methodologic approach. *Anesth Analg.* 2009;108(3):1037-1041.

Anagnostopoulou S, Kostopanagiotou G, Paraskeuopoulos T, Chantzi C, Lolis E, Saranteas T. Anatomic variations of the obturator nerve in the inguinal region: implications in conventional and ultrasound regional anesthesia techniques. *Reg Anesth Pain Med.* 2009;34:33-39.

Bouaziz H, Vial F, Jochum D, et al. An evaluation of the cutaneous distribution after obturator nerve block. *Anesth Analg.* 2002;94:445-449.

Macalou D, Trueck S, Meuret P, et al. Postoperative analgesia after total knee replacement: the effect of an obturator nerve block added to the femoral 3-in-1 nerve block. *Anesth Analg.* 2004;99:251-254.

Marhofer P, Harrop-Griffiths W, Willschke H, Kirchmair L: Fifteen years of ultrasound guidance in regional anaesthesia: Part 2-recent developments in block techniques. *Br J Anaesth* 2010; 104:673-83.

McNamee DA, Parks L, Milligan KR. Post-operative analgesia following total knee replacement: an evaluation of the addition of an obturator nerve block to combined femoral and sciatic nerve block. *Acta Anaesthesiol Scand.* 2002;46:95-99.

Sakura S, Hara K, Ota J, Tadenuma S: Ultrasound-guided peripheral nerve blocks for anterior cruciate ligament reconstruction: effect of obturator nerve block during and after surgery. *J Anesth* 2010;24:411-7.

Sinha SK, Abrams JH, Houle T, Weller R. Ultrasound guided obturator nerve block: an interfascial injection approach without nerve stimulation. *Reg Anesth Pain Med.* 2009;34(3):261-264.

Snaith R, Dolan J: Ultrasound-guided interfascial injection for peripheral obturator nerve block in the thigh. *Reg Anesth Pain Med* 2010;35:314-5.

Soong J, Schafhalter-Zoppoth I, Gray AT. Sonographic imaging of the obturator nerve for regional block. *Reg Anesth Pain Med.* 2007;32:146-151.

# 38 Ultrasound-Guided Saphenous Nerve Block

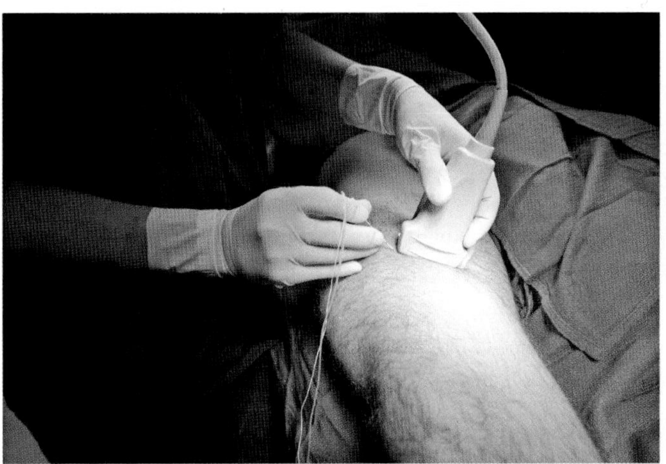

A

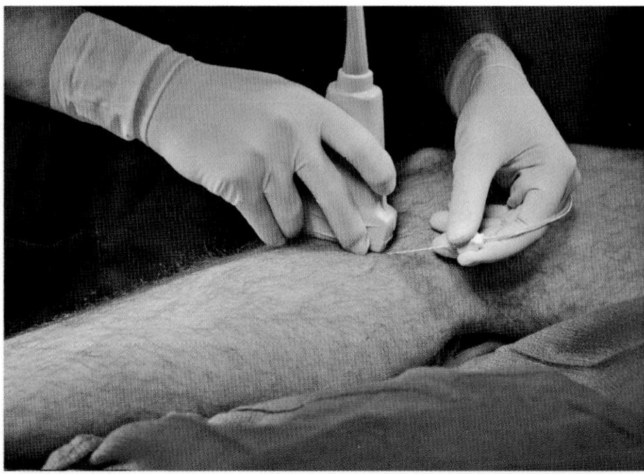

B

## BLOCK AT A GLANCE

- Indications: saphenous vein stripping or harvesting, supplementation for medial foot/ankle surgery in combination with a sciatic nerve block
- Transducer position: transverse on anteromedial mid thigh or below the knee at the level of the tibial tuberosity, depending on the approach chosen (proximal/distal).
- Goal: local anesthetic spread lateral to the femoral artery and deep to the sartorius muscle or more distal, below the knee, adjacent to the saphenous vein.
- Local anesthetic: 5–10 mL

**FIGURE 38-1.** Needle insertion to block the saphenous nerve at the level of the mid thigh (A) or below the knee (B).

## General Considerations

The saphenous nerve is the terminal sensory branch of the femoral nerve. It supplies innervation to the medial aspect of the leg down to the ankle and foot. Blockade of the nerve can be sufficient for superficial procedures in this area; however, it is most useful as a supplement to a sciatic block for foot and ankle procedures that involve the superficial structures in medial territory. The use of ultrasound guidance has improved the success rates of the saphenous blocks, compared with field blocks below the knee and blind transsartorial approaches. The ultrasound-guided techniques described here are relatively simple, quick to perform, and fairly reproducible.

## Ultrasound Anatomy

The sartorius muscle forms a "roof" over the adductor canal in the lower half of the thigh in its descent laterally-to-medially across the anterior thigh. The muscle appears as an oval shape beneath the subcutaneous layer of adipose tissue. Often, the femoral artery, which passes beneath the muscle, can also be palpated. The sides of the triangular canal are formed by the vastus medialis laterally and adductor longus or magnus medially (depending on how proximal or distal the scan is). The saphenous nerve is infrequently seen on the ultrasound image; however, sometimes it is visualized as a small round hyperechoic structure medial to the artery. A femoral vein accompanies the artery and saphenous nerve, which are all typically visualized at 2 to 3 cm depth. When attempting to identify the saphenous nerve on ultrasound image, the following anatomic considerations should be kept in mind:

- Above the knee: The saphenous nerve pierces the fascia lata between the tendons of the sartorius and gracilis muscles before becoming a subcutaneous nerve.
- The saphenous nerve also may surface between the sartorius and vastus medialis muscles. (Figure 38-2 A, B, and C).

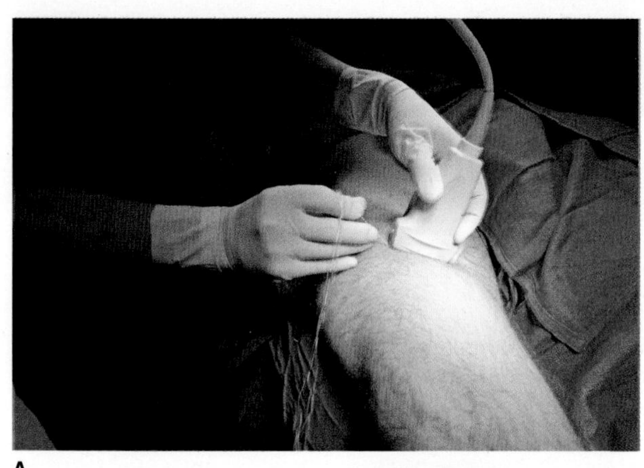

A

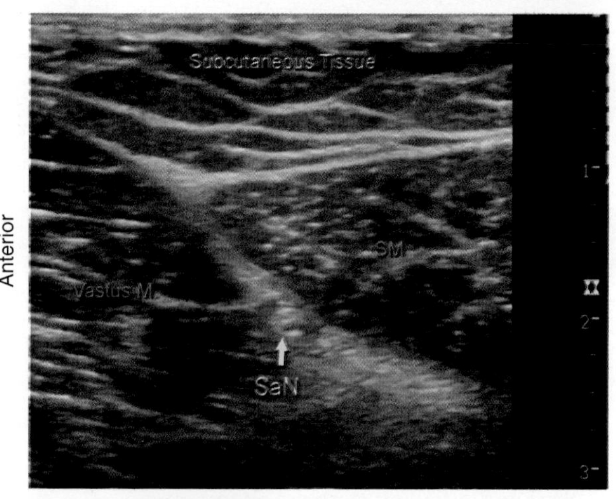


B Saphenous nerve block above knee

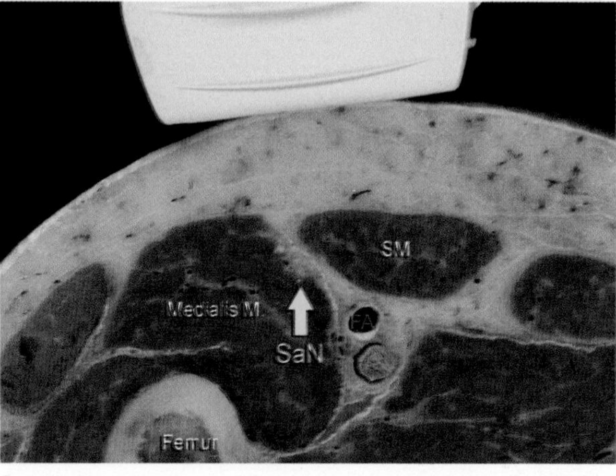


C

**FIGURE 38-2.** (A) Transducer and needle position for a saphenous nerve block at the level of the midthigh. (B) Ultrasound anatomy demonstrating saphenous nerve (SaN) in the tissue plane between the sartorius muscle (SM) and vastus medialis muscle. (C) Cross-sectional anatomy of the saphenous nerve at the level of the thigh. Saphenous nerve is shown positioned between the SM and the vastus medialis muscle. In this example the sartorius nerve is positioned superficially to the femoral artery (FA) and vein (unlabeled oval structure posterior to the FA).

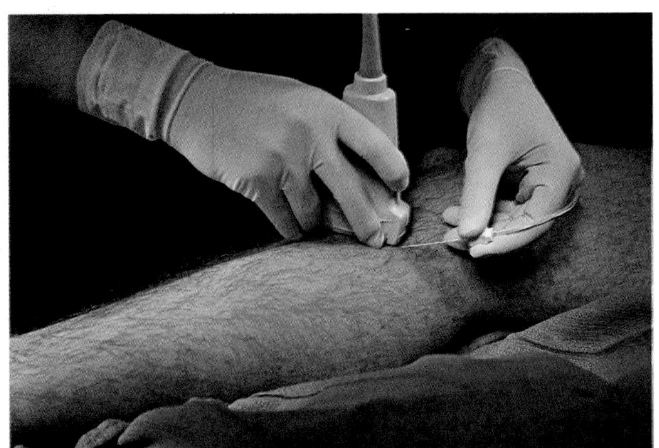

A

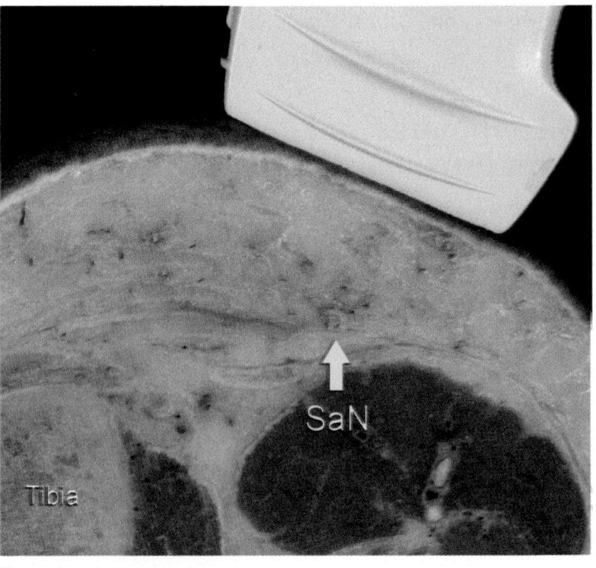


B

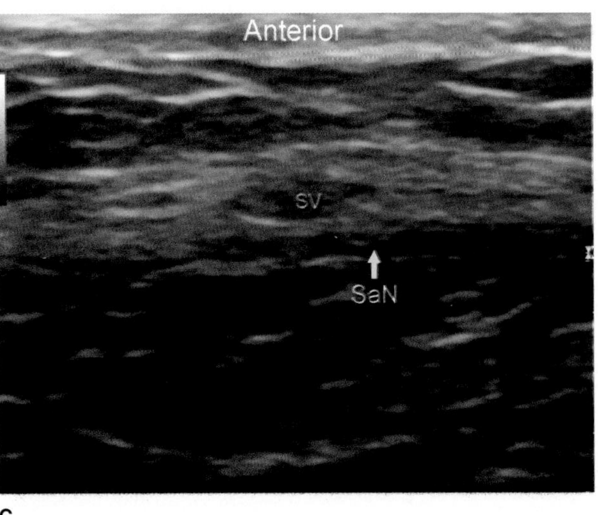


C

**FIGURE 38-3.** (A) Ultrasound transducer and needle insertion technique to block the saphenous nerve (SaN) at the level of the tibial tuberosity. (B) Cross-sectional anatomy of the SaN at the level of the tibial tuberosity. (C) Ultrasound image of the saphenous nerve (SaN) at the level below the knee. SaN is seen in the immediate vicinity of the saphenous vein (SV). Transducer should be applied lightly to avoid compression of the saphenous vein (SV) because the vein serves as an important landmark for technique.

- Below the knee, the nerve passes along the tibial side of the leg, adjacent to the great saphenous vein subcutaneously (Figure 38-3A, B, and C).
- At the ankle, a branch of the nerve is located medially next to the subcutaneously positioned saphenous vein.

## Distribution of Blockade

Saphenous nerve block results in anesthesia of a variable strip of skin on the medial leg and foot. For a more comprehensive review of the femoral and saphenous nerve distributions, see Chapter 1. Of note, although saphenous nerve is a strictly sensory block, an injection of the local anesthetic in the adductor canal can result in the partial motor block of the vastus medialis. For this reason, caution must be excercised when advising patients regarding the safety of unsupported ambulation after proximal saphenous block.

## Equipment

Equipment needed is as follows:

- Ultrasound machine with linear transducer (8–14 MHz), sterile sleeve, and gel
- Standard nerve block tray (described in Chapter 3)
- One 10-mL syringe containing local anesthetic
- A 50-mm, 22-gauge short-bevel needle

- Peripheral nerve stimulator to elicit sensory sensation.
- Sterile gloves

## Landmarks and Patient Positioning for Proximal Approach

The patient is placed in any position that allows for comfortable placement of the ultrasound transducer and needle advancement. Although prone and lateral approaches are possible, this block typically is performed with the patient in the supine position, with the thigh abducted and externally rotated to allow access to the medial thigh (Figure 38-2A). If difficulty confirming the sartorius muscle is encountered, exposure of the entire thigh in order to scan down from the anterosuperior iliac spine is useful.

## GOAL

The goal is to place the needle tip just medial to the femoral artery, below the sartorius muscle, and to deposit 5 to 10 mL of local anesthetic until its spread around the artery is confirmed with ultrasound visualization. Block of the nerve at other, more distal and superficial locations consists of a simple subcutaneous infiltration of the tissues in the immediate vicinity of the nerve but can be done under ultrasound guidance.

## Technique

With the patient in the proper position, the skin is disinfected and the transducer is placed anteromedially, approximately mid thigh position or somewhat lower. If the artery is not immediately obvious, several maneuvers to identify it can be used, including color Doppler scanning to trace the femoral artery caudally from the inguinal crease. Once the femoral artery is identified, the needle is inserted in-plane in a lateral-to-medial orientation, and advanced toward the femoral artery (Figure 38-4A). If nerve stimulation is used (0.5 mA, 0.1 msec), the passage of the needle through the sartorius and/or adductor muscles and into the adductor canal is usually associated with the patient reporting a paresthesia in the saphenous nerve distribution. Once the needle tip is visualized medial to the artery and after careful aspiration, 1 to 2 mL of local anesthetic is injected to confirm the proper injection site (Figure 38-4B). When injection of the local anesthetic does not appear to result in its spread beside the femoral artery, additional needle repositions and injections may be necessary.

## TIPS

- An out-of-plane technique can also be used through the belly of the sartorius muscle. Because the needle tip may not be seen throughout the procedure, small boluses of local anesthetic are administered (0.5–1 mL) as the needle is advanced toward the adductor canal, to confirm the location of the needle tip.
- Visualization of the nerve is *not* necessary for this block; the saphenous nerve is not always well imaged. Administration of 5 to 10 mL of local anesthetic next to the artery should suffice without confirming the nerve position.

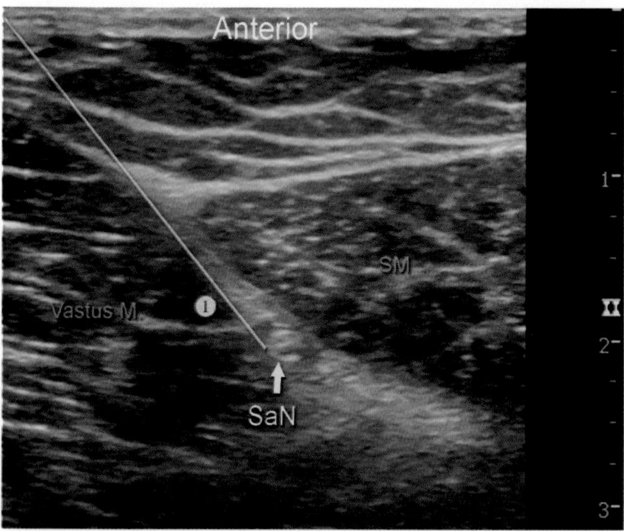


A Saphenous nerve block above knee: Needle insertion

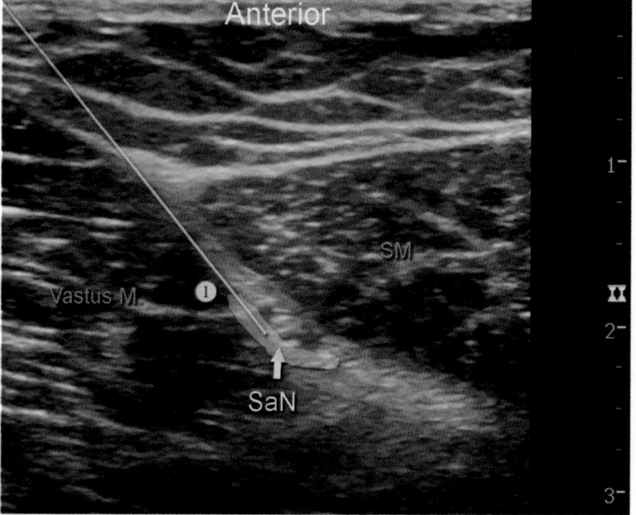


B Saphenous nerve block above knee: Injection

**FIGURE 38-4.** (A) Simulated needle path ❶ to reach the saphenous nerve (SaN) at the level of the midthigh. (B) Simulated needle path ❶ and the distribution of the local anesthetic (area shaded in blue) to anesthetize the SaN at the midthigh level. SM, sartorius muscle; Vastus M, vastus medialus muscle. Femoral artery is not well seen in this image; it is positioned immediately posterior to SaN.

In an adult patient, usually 5 to 10 mL of local anesthetic is adequate for successful blockade. Because the saphenous nerve is a purely sensory nerve, high concentrations of local anesthetic are not required and in fact may delay patient ambulation should local anesthetic spread to one of the motor branches of the femoral nerve serving the quadriceps muscle.

**TIP**

- The nerve to the vastus medialis muscle also lies in the adductor canal (in its proximal portion). Practitioners should be aware of this and the potential for partial quadriceps weakness following this approach to the saphenous nerve block. Patient education and assistance with ambulation should be encouraged.

## ULTRASOUND-GUIDED SAPHENOUS NERVE BLOCK

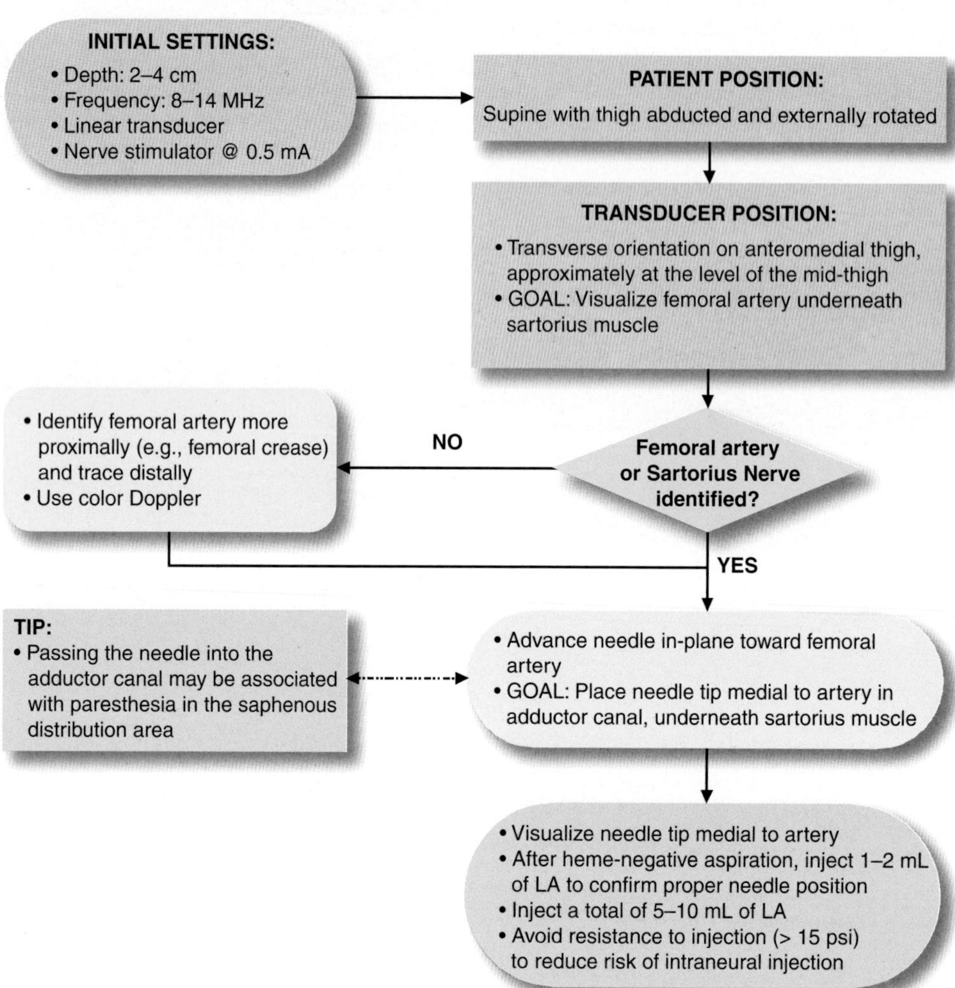

## SUGGESTED READING

Davis JJ, Bond TS, Swenson JD. Adductor canal block: more than just the saphenous nerve? Reg Anesth Pain Med. 2009;34:618-619.

Gray AT, Collins AB. Ultrasound-guided saphenous nerve block. *Reg Anesth Pain Med.* 2003;28:148.

Horn JL, Pitsch T, Salinas F, Benninger B. Anatomic basis to the ultrasound-guided approach for saphenous nerve blockade. *Reg Anesth Pain Med.* 2009;34:486-489.

Kirkpatrick JD, Sites BD, Antonakakis JG. Preliminary experience with a new approach to performing an ultrasound-guided saphenous nerve block in the mid- to proximal femur. *Reg Anesth Pain Med.* 2010;35:222-223.

Krombach J, Gray AT. Sonography for saphenous nerve block near the adductor canal. *Reg Anesth Pain Med.* 2007;32:369-370.

Lundblad M, Kapral S, Marhofer P, et al. Ultrasound-guided infrapatellar nerve block in human volunteers: description of a novel technique. *Br J Anaesth.* 2006;97:710-714.

Manickam B, Perlas A, Duggan E, Brull R, Chan VW, Ramlogan R. Feasibility and efficacy of ultrasound-guided block of the saphenous nerve in the adductor canal. *Reg Anesth Pain Med.* 2009;34:578-580.

Miller BR. Ultrasound-guided proximal tibial paravenous saphenous nerve block in pediatric patients. *Paediatr Anaesth.* 2010;20:1059-1060

Saranteas T, Anagnostis G, Paraskeuopoulos T, Koulalis D, Kokkalis Z, Nakou M, Anagnostopoulou S, Kostopanagiotou G. Anatomy and clinical implications of the ultrasound-guided subsartorial saphenous nerve block. *Reg Anesth Pain Med.* 2011;36:399-402.

Tsai PB, Karnwal A, Kakazu C, Tokhner V, Julka IS. Efficacy of an ultrasound-guided subsartorial approach to saphenous nerve block: a case series. *Can J Anaesth.* 2010;57:683-688.

Tsui BC, Ozelsel T. Ultrasound-guided transsartorial perifemoral artery approach for saphenous nerve block. *Reg Anesth Pain Med.* 2009;34:177-178.

# 39 Ultrasound-Guided Sciatic Block

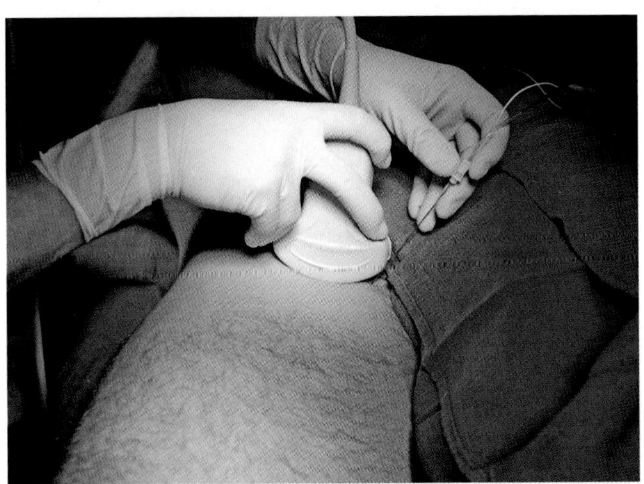

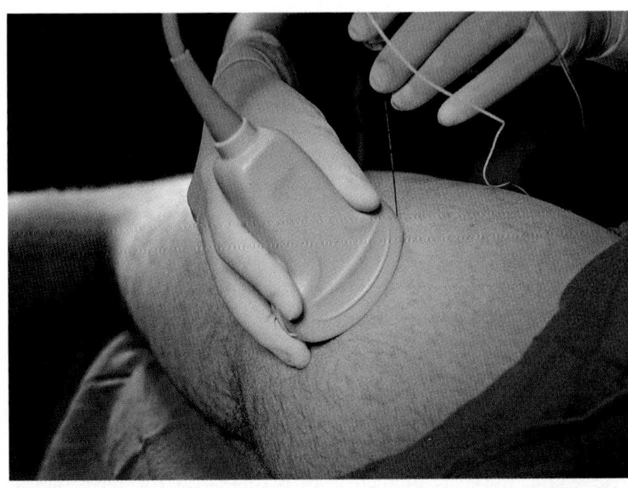

## BLOCK AT A GLANCE

- Indications: foot and ankle surgery; analgesia following knee surgery
- Transducer position:

  ANTERIOR APPROACH: transverse on the proximal medial thigh

  TRANSGLUTEAL APPROACH: transverse on the posterior buttock, between the ischial tuberosity and greater trochanter
- Goal: local anesthetic spread adjacent to the sciatic nerve
- Local anesthetic: 15–20 mL

**FIGURE 39.1-1.** (A) Needle insertion to block the sciatic nerve using an anterior approach. Note that a curved (phased array) lower frequency transducer is used either in-plane (shown) or out-of-plane needle insertion can be used. (B) Transgluteal approach to sciatic block; patient position, transducer (curved) placement and needle insertion.

# PART 1: ANTERIOR APPROACH

## General Considerations

The anterior approach to sciatic block can be useful in patients who cannot be positioned in the lateral position due to pain, trauma, presence of external fixation devices interfering with positioning, and other issues. It also may be well-suited to patients who require postoperative blocks for analgesia following a total knee arthroplasty. Ultrasonography adds the benefit of no requirement for the palpation of a femoral pulse or the use of geometry for identification of the skin puncture point. In addition, using the ultrasound-guided approach should reduce the risk of puncture of the femoral artery as compared with the landmark-based approach. The actual scanning and needle insertion are performed on the anteromedial aspect of the proximal thigh, rather than the anterior surface, and may require a slight abduction and external rotation of the thigh. This block is not well suited to insertion of catheters because a large needle must traverse several muscles (causing pain and possibly hematomas), an awkward catheter location (medial thigh), and catheter insertion at approximately perpendicular angle to the sciatic nerve is difficult.

## Ultrasound Anatomy

The sciatic nerve is imaged approximately at the level of the minor trochanter. At this location, a curved transducer placed over the anteromedial aspect of the thigh will reveal the musculature of all three fascial compartments of the thigh: anterior, medial, and posterior (Figures 39.1-2 and 39.1-3). Beneath the superficial sartorius muscle is the femoral artery, and deep and medial to this vessel is the profunda femoris artery. Both of these can be identified with color Doppler ultrasound for orientation. The femur is easily seen as a hyperechoic rim with the corresponding shadow beneath the vastus intermedius. Medial to the femur is the body of the adductor magnus muscle, separated by the fascial plane(s) of the hamstrings muscles. The sciatic nerve is visualized as a hyperechoic, slightly flattened oval structure sandwiched between these two muscle planes. The nerve is typically visualized at a depth of 6 to 8 cm (Figure 39.1-3).

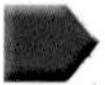

## Distribution of Blockade

Sciatic nerve block results in anesthesia of the posterior aspect of the knee, hamstrings muscles, and entire lower limb below the knee, both motor and sensory, with the exception of skin on the medial leg and foot (saphenous nerve). The skin of the posterior aspect of the thigh is supplied by the posterior cutaneous nerve of the thigh, which has its origin from the sciatic nerve more proximal than the anterior approach. It is, therefore, not blocked by the anterior approach. Practically, however, the lack of anesthesia in its distribution is of little clinical consequence. For a more comprehensive review of the sciatic nerve distribution, see Chapter 1.

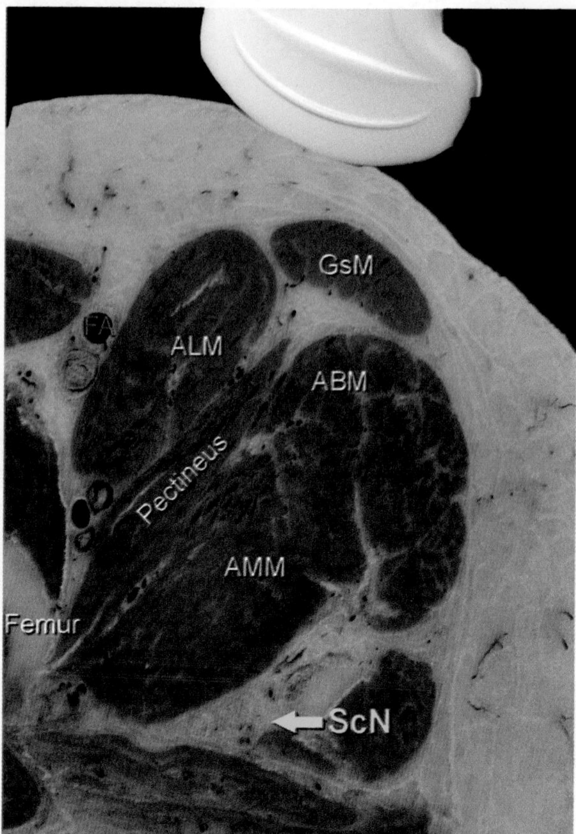


**FIGURE 39.1-2.** Cross- sectional anatomy of the sciatic nerve (ScN). Shown are femoral artery (FA), adductor longus muscle (ALM), pectineus muscle, adductor magnus muscle (AMM), adductor brevis muscle (ABM), gracilis muscle (GsM), and the femur. The sciatic nerve is seen posterior to the AMM.

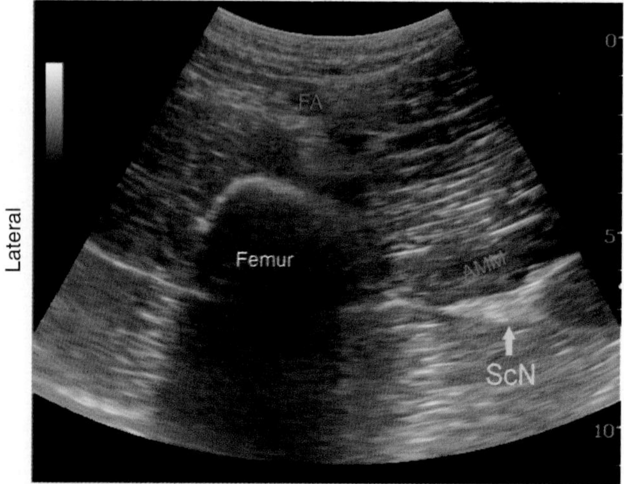


**FIGURE 39.1-3.** Ultrasound anatomy of the sciatic nerve. From superficial to deep; femoral artery (FA) and femur laterally, adductor magnus muscle (AMM) and sciatic nerve (ScN) laterally. The sciatic nerve is typically located at a depth of 6 to 8 cm.

## Equipment

Equipment needed is as follows:

- Ultrasound machine with curved (phased array) transducer (2–8 MHz), sterile sleeve, and gel
- Standard nerve block tray (described in the equipment section)
- One 20-mL syringe containing local anesthetic
- A 100-mm, 21 to 22 gauge short-bevel insulated stimulating needle
- Peripheral nerve stimulator
- Sterile gloves

## Landmarks and Patient Positioning

Anterior approach to sciatic nerve block is performed with the patient in the supine position. The hip is abducted to facilitate transducer and needle placement (Figure 39.1-4 and 39.1-5). When feasible, the hip and knee should be somewhat flexed to facilitate exposure. If nerve stimulation is to be used at the same time (recommended), exposure of the calf and foot are required to observe motor responses. In either case, it is useful to expose the entire thigh to appreciate the distance from the groin to knee.

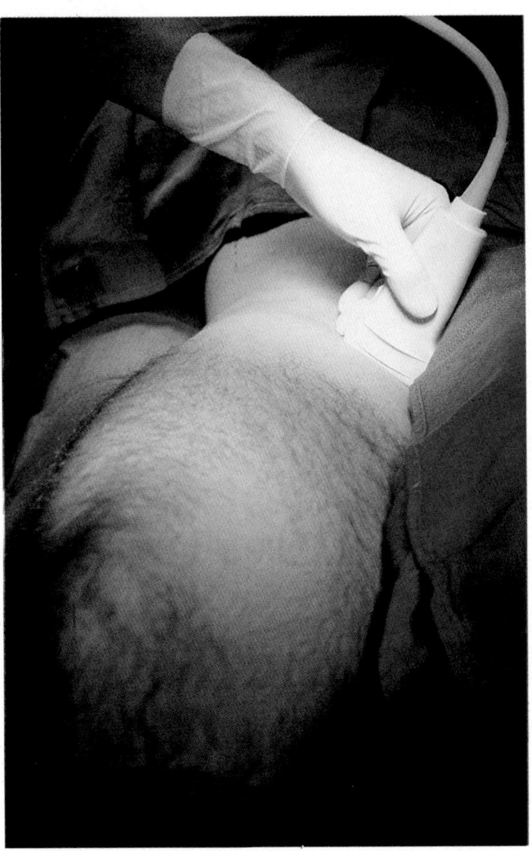

**FIGURE 39.1-4.** Transducer position to visualize the sciatic nerve through the anterior approach.

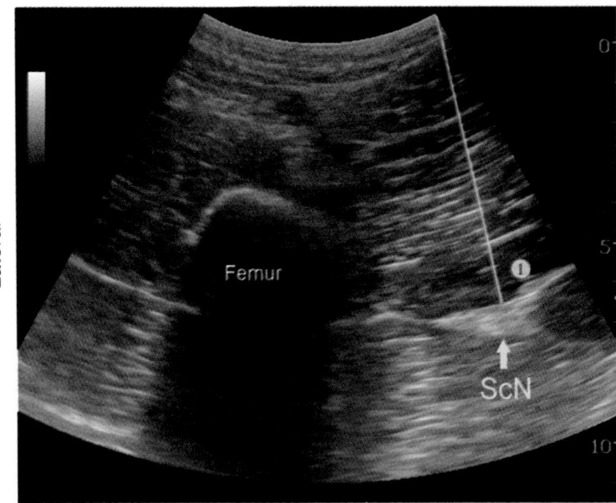


**FIGURE 39.1-5.** A simulated needle path using an out of plane technique to reach the sciatic nerve (ScN) through the anterior approach.

## GOAL

The goal is to place the needle tip immediately adjacent to the sciatic nerve, between the adductor muscles and biceps femoris muscle, and deposit 15 to 20 mL of local anesthetic until spread around the nerve is documented.

## Technique

With the patient in the proper position, the skin is disinfected and the transducer positioned so as to identify the sciatic nerve. If the nerve is not immediately apparent, sliding and tilting the transducer proximally or distally can be useful to improve the contrast and bring the nerve "out" of the background from the musculature. Finally, if the patient is able to dorsiflex and/or plantar flex the ankle, this maneuver often causes the nerve to rotate or otherwise move within the muscular planes, facilitating identification. Once identified, the needle is inserted in-plane or out of plane (more common in our program) from the medial aspect of the thigh and advanced toward the sciatic nerve (Figure 39.1-5). If nerve stimulation is used (1.0 mA, 0.1 msec), the contact of the needle tip with the sciatic nerve is usually associated with a motor response of the calf or foot. Once the needle tip is deemed to be in the proper position, 1 to 2 mL of local anesthetic is injected to confirm the adequate distribution of injectate. Such injection helps delineate the sciatic nerve within its intramuscular tunnel, but it may displace the sciatic nerve away from the needle. Improper spread of the local anesthetic or nerve displacement may require an additional advancement of the needle. When injection of the local anesthetic does not appear to result in a spread around the sciatic nerve, additional needle repositions and injections are necessary.

## TIP

- Insertion of the needle in an out-of-plane manner with hydro-dissection/localization is often a more logical method to accomplish this block.

In an adult patient, 15 to 20 mL of local anesthetic is usually adequate for successful blockade (Figure 39.1-6). Although a single injection of such volume of local anesthetic suffices, it may be beneficial to inject two to three smaller aliquots at different locations to assure the spread of the local anesthetic solution around the sciatic nerve. The block dynamics and perioperative management are similar to those described in the nerve stimulator technique section, Chapter 19.

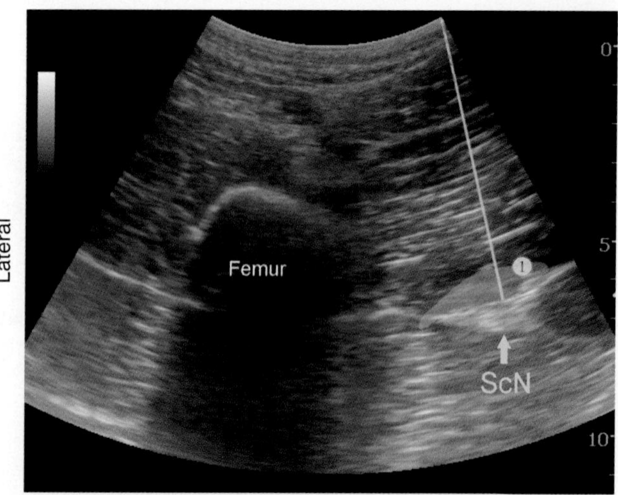


**FIGURE 39.1-6.** Simulated needle path using an out-of-plane technique with local anesthetic ❶ and proper distribution of local anesthetic to anesthetize the sciatic nerve (ScN).

# ULTRASOUND-GUIDED ANTERIOR SCIATIC NERVE BLOCK

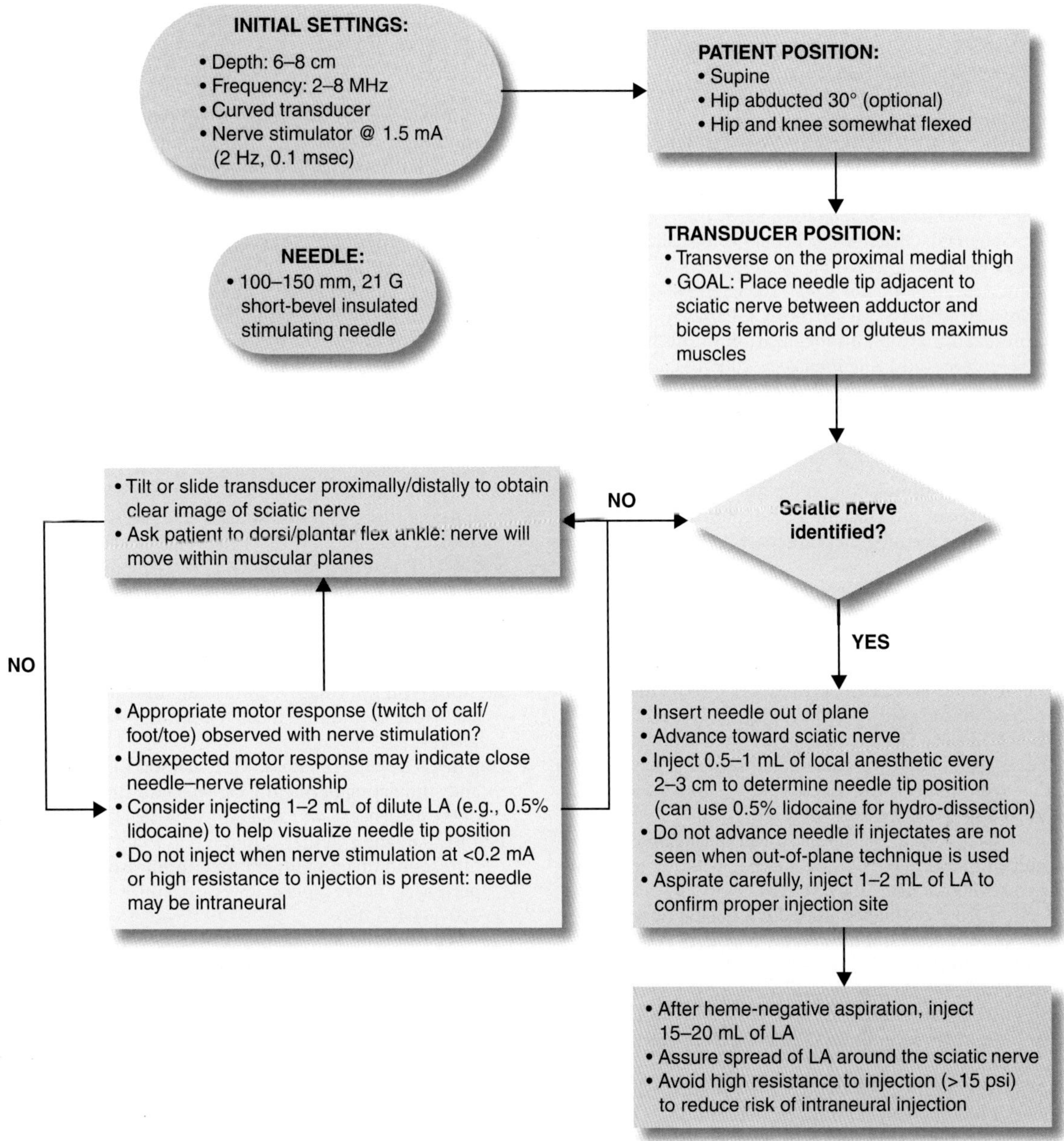

## SUGGESTED READING


Abbas S, Brull R. Ultrasound-guided sciatic nerve block: description of a new approach at the subgluteal space. *Br J Anaesth.* 2007;99:445-446.

Barrington MJ, Lai SL, Briggs CA, Ivanusic JJ, Gledhill SR. Ultrasound-guided midthigh sciatic nerve block-a clinical and anatomical study. *Reg Anesth Pain Med.* 2008;33:369-376.

Bruhn J, Moayeri N, Groen GJ, et al. Soft tissue landmark for ultrasound identification of the sciatic nerve in the infragluteal region: the tendon of the long head of the biceps femoris muscle. *Acta Anaesthesiol Scand.* 2009; 53: 921-5

Bruhn J, Van Geffen GJ, Gielen MJ, Scheffer GJ. Visualization of the course of the sciatic nerve in adult volunteers by ultrasonography. *Acta Anaesthesiol Scand.* 2008;52:1298-1302.

Chan VW, Nova H, Abbas S, McCartney CJ, Perlas A, Xu DQ. Ultrasound examination and localization of the sciatic nerve: a volunteer study. *Anesthesiology.* 2006;104:309-314.

Chantzi C, Saranteas T, Zogogiannis J, Alevizou N, Dimitriou V. Ultrasound examination of the sciatic nerve at the anterior thigh in obese patients. *Acta Anaesthesiol Scand.* 2007;51:132.

Danelli G, Ghisi D, Fanelli A, et al. The effects of ultrasound guidance and neurostimulation on the minimum effective anesthetic volume of mepivacaine 1.5% required to block the sciatic nerve using the subgluteal approach. *Anesth Analg.* 2009;109:1674-1678.

Danelli G, Ghisi D, Ortu A. Ultrasound and regional anesthesia technique: are there really ultrasound guidance technical limits in sciatic nerve blocks? *Reg Anesth Pain Med.* 2008;33:281-282.

Domingo-Triado V, Selfa S, Martinez F, et al. Ultrasound guidance for lateral midfemoral sciatic nerve block: a prospective, comparative, randomized study. *Anesth Analg.* 2007;104:1270-1274.

Fredrickson MJ, Kilfoyle DH. Neurological complication analysis of 1000 ultrasound guided peripheral nerve blocks for elective orthopaedic surgery: a prospective study. *Anaesthesia.* 2009;64:836-844.

Gnaho A, Eyrieux S, Gentili M. Cardiac arrest during an ultrasound-guided sciatic nerve block combined with nerve stimulation. *Reg Anesth Pain Med.* 2009;34:278.

Gray AT, Collins AB, Schafhalter-Zoppoth I. Sciatic nerve block in a child: a sonographic approach. *Anesth Analg.* 2003;97:1300-1302.

Hamilton PD, Pearce CJ, Pinney SJ, Calder JD. Sciatic nerve blockade: a survey of orthopaedic foot and ankle specialists in North America and the United Kingdom. *Foot Ankle Int.* 2009;30:1196-1201.

Karmakar MK, Kwok WH, Ho AM, Tsang K, Chui PT, Gin T. Ultrasound-guided sciatic nerve block: description of a new approach at the subgluteal space. *Br J Anaesth.* 2007;98:390-395.

Latzke D, Marhofer P, Zeitlinger M, et al. Minimal local anaesthetic volumes for sciatic nerve block: evaluation of ED 99 in volunteers. *Br J Anaesth.* 2010;104:239-244.

Marhofer P, Harrop-Griffiths W, Willschke H, Kirchmair L. Fifteen years of ultrasound guidance in regional anaesthesia: Part 2-recent developments in block techniques. *Br J Anaesth.* 2010;104:673-683.

Murray JM, Derbyshire S, Shields MO. Lower limb blocks. *Anaesthesia.* 2010;65(Suppl 1):57-66.

Oberndorfer U, Marhofer P, Bosenberg A, et al. Ultrasonographic guidance for sciatic and femoral nerve blocks in children. *Br J Anaesth.* 2007;98:797-801.

Ota J, Sakura S, Hara K, Saito Y. Ultrasound-guided anterior approach to sciatic nerve block: a comparison with the posterior approach. *Anesth Analg.* 2009;108:660-665.

Pham Dang C, Gourand D. Ultrasound imaging of the sciatic nerve in the lateral midfemoral approach. *Reg Anesth Pain Med.* 2009;34:281-282.

Salinas FV. Ultrasound and review of evidence for lower extremity peripheral nerve blocks. *Reg Anesth Pain Med.* 2010;35:S16-25.

Saranteas T. Limitations in ultrasound imaging techniques in anesthesia: obesity and muscle atrophy? *Anesth Analg.* 2009;109:993-994.

Saranteas T, Chantzi C, Paraskeuopoulos T, et al. Imaging in anesthesia: the role of 4 MHz to 7 MHz sector array ultrasound probe in the identification of the sciatic nerve at different anatomic locations. *Reg Anesth Pain Med.* 2007;32:537-538.

Saranteas T, Chantzi C, Zogogiannis J, et al. Lateral sciatic nerve examination and localization at the mid-femoral level: an imaging study with ultrasound. *Acta Anaesthesiol Scand.* 2007;51:387-388.

Saranteas T, Kostopanagiotou G, Paraskeuopoulos T, Vamvasakis E, Chantzi C, Anagnostopoulou S. Ultrasound examination of the sciatic nerve at two different locations in the lateral thigh: a new approach of identification validated by anatomic preparation. *Acta Anaesthesiol Scand.* 2007;51:780-781.

Sites BD, Neal JM, Chan V. Ultrasound in regional anesthesia: where should the "focus" be set? *Reg Anesth Pain Med.* 2009;34:531-533.

Tran de QH, Munoz L, Russo G, Finlayson RJ. Ultrasonography and stimulating perineural catheters for nerve blocks: a review of the evidence. *Can J Anaesth.* 2008;55:447-457.

Tsui BC, Dillane D, Pillay J, Ramji AK, Walji AH. Cadaveric ultrasound imaging for training in ultrasound-guided peripheral nerve blocks: lower extremity. *Can J Anaesth.* 2007;54:475-480.

Tsui BC, Finucane BT. The importance of ultrasound landmarks: a "traceback" approach using the popliteal blood vessels for identification of the sciatic nerve. *Reg Anesth Pain Med.* 2006;31:481-482.

Tsui BC, Ozelsel TJ. Ultrasound-guided anterior sciatic nerve block using a longitudinal approach: "expanding the view." *Reg Anesth Pain Med.* 2008;33:275-276.

van Geffen GJ, Bruhn J, Gielen M. Ultrasound-guided continuous sciatic nerve blocks in two children with venous malformations in the lower limb. *Can J Anaesth.* 2007;54:952-953.

van Geffen GJ, Gielen M. Ultrasound-guided subgluteal sciatic nerve blocks with stimulating catheters in children: a descriptive study. *Anesth Analg.* 2006;103:328-333.

# PART 2: TRANSGLUTEAL AND SUBGLUTEAL APPROACH

## General Considerations

The use of ultrasonographic guidance greatly expanded the options that practitioners have for accomplishing the block of the sciatic nerve because the nerve can be imaged at several convenient levels. With the transgluteal approach, the needle is inserted just distal deep to the gluteus maximus muscle to reach the sciatic nerve. The sciatic nerve at the gluteal crease is readily identified in a predictable anatomic arrangement, between two osseous landmarks (*ischial tuberosity* and the *greater trochanter*) and beneath a well-defined muscle plane. The use of ultrasound visualization decreases the need for the geometry and measurements that are required for the classic landmark-based approaches. With the subgluteal approach, the nerve simply reached a few centimeters distally, just below the level of the subgluteal crease where imaging is not interfered by the bones. The preference of one approach over the other is made based on the patient's anatomic characteristics and personal preference.

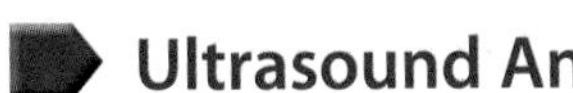

## Ultrasound Anatomy

At this transgluteal level, the sciatic nerve is visualized in the short axis between the two hyperechoic bony prominences of the ischial tuberosity and the greater trochanter of the femur (Figure 39.2-1 and 39.2-2). The gluteus maximus muscle is seen as the most superficial muscular layer bridging the two osseous structures, typically several centimeters thick. The sciatic nerve is located immediately deep to the gluteus muscles, superficial to the quadratus femoris muscle. Often, it is slightly closer to the ischial tuberosity (medial) aspect than the greater trochanter (lateral). At this location in the thigh, it is seen as an oval or roughly triangular hyperechoic structure. At the subgluteal level, however, the sciatic nerve is positioned deep to the long head of the biceps muscle and the posterior surface of the adductor magnus.

## Distribution of Blockade

Sciatic nerve block results in anesthesia of the entire lower limb below the knee, both motor and sensory blockade, with the exception of a variable strip of skin on the medial leg and foot, which is the territory of the saphenous nerve, a branch of the femoral nerve. In addition, both the transgluteal and subgluteal approaches provide motor blockade of the hamstring muscles. The skin of the posterior aspect of the thigh however, is supplied by the posterior cutaneous nerve of the thigh, which has its origin from the sciatic nerve more proximal than the subgluteal approach. It is, therefore, unreliably anesthetized with subgluteal block; however, it is of relatively

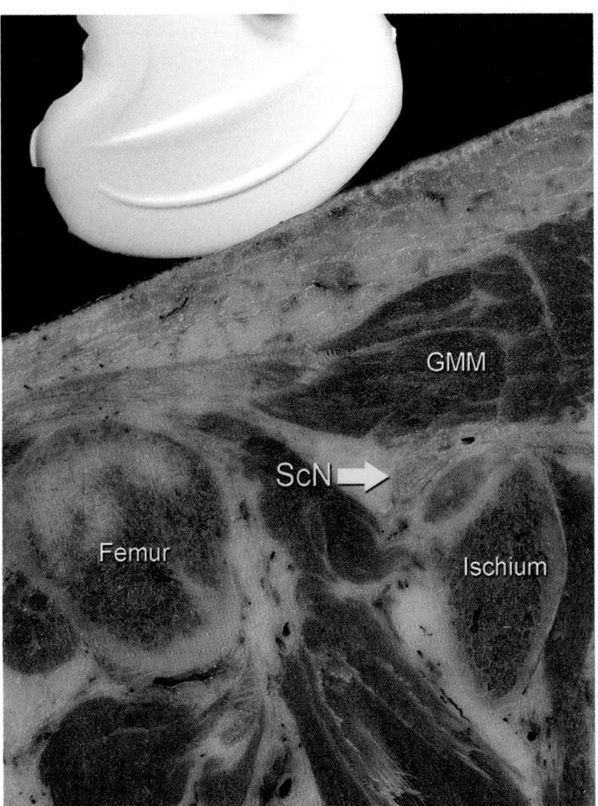


**FIGURE 39.2-1.** Transsectional anatomy of the sciatic nerve at the transgluteal level. Sciatic nerve (ScN) is seen between the greater trochanter of the femur and the ischium tuberosity, just below the gluteus maximus (GMM) muscle.

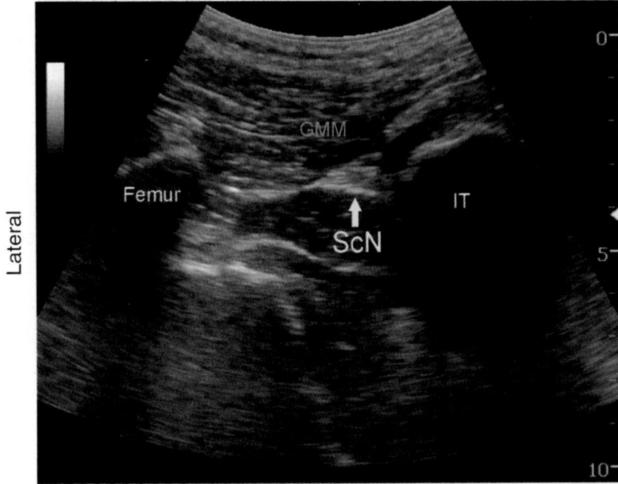


Sciatic nerve block-posterior approach

**FIGURE 39.2-2.** An ultrasound image demonstrating the sonoanatomy of the sciatic nerve (ScN). The ScN often assumes an ovoid or triangular shape and it is positioned underneath the gluteus muscle (GMM) between the ischium tuberosity (IT) and femur.

little clinical importance. For a more comprehensive review of the sciatic nerve distribution, see Chapter 1, Essential Regional Anesthesia Anatomy.

## Equipment

Equipment needed is as follows:

- Ultrasound machine with curved (phase array) transducer (2–8 MHz), sterile sleeve, and gel
- Standard nerve block tray (described in the equipment section)
- One 20-mL syringe containing local anesthetic
- A 100-mm, 21 to 22-gauge short-bevel insulated stimulating needle
- Peripheral nerve stimulator
- Sterile gloves

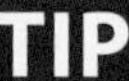

### TIP

- Although a linear transducer occasionally can be used for smaller size patients for this block, the curved transducer permits the operator to visualize a wider field, including the osseous landmarks. The ischial tuberosity and greater trochanter are rarely seen on the same image when using a linear transducer.

## Landmarks and Patient Positioning

Any patient position that allows for comfortable placement of the ultrasound transducer and needle advancement is appropriate. Typically for either the transgluteal or subgluteal block, this involves placing the patient in a position between the lateral decubitus and prone position (Figures 39.2-3 and 39.2-4). The legs are flexed in the hip and knee. When nerve stimulation is used simultaneously (suggested), exposure of the hamstrings, calf, and foot is required to detect and interpret motor responses. The round osseous prominences of the greater trochanter and ischial tuberosity are palpated and, if desired, marked with a skin marker. Scanning is begun in the depression between the two bones.

### GOAL

The goal is to place the needle tip adjacent to the sciatic nerve, below the fascial plane of the gluteus muscles (thus, transgluteal technique) and to deposit 15 to 20 mL of local anesthetic until its spread around the nerve is documented.

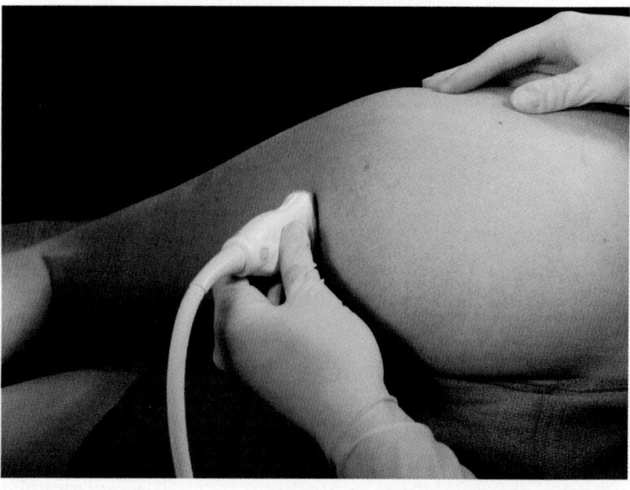

**FIGURE 39.2-3.** Patient position and transducer application for subgluteal approach to sciatic block..

## Technique

The description of the technique in this chapter will focus primarily on the transgluteal approach. However, since the subgluteal approach is performed just a few centimeters more distal and it is technically easier, the reader can easily perform either approach by using general guidelines provided and referring to Figure 39.2-3, Figure 39.2-4, and algorithms at the end of the chapter. With the patient in the described position, the skin is disinfected and the transducer is positioned so as to identify the sciatic nerve (Figure 39.2-4). If the nerve is not immediately apparent, tilting the transducer proximally or distally can help improve the contrast and bring the nerve "out" of the background of the musculature. Often, the nerve is much better imaged *after* the injection

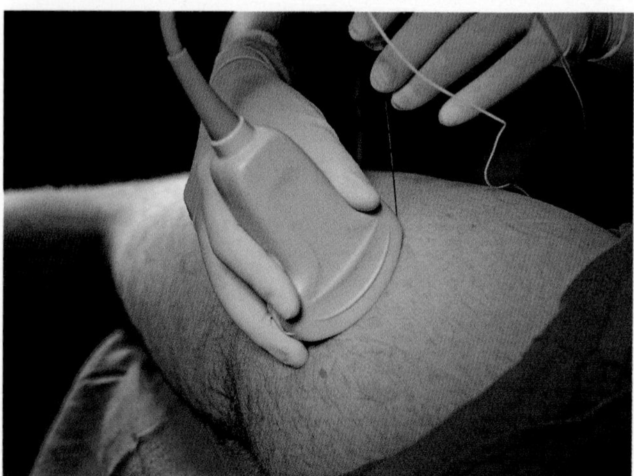

**FIGURE 39.2-4.** Transgluteal approach to sciatic block; patient position, transducer (curved) placement and needle insertion.

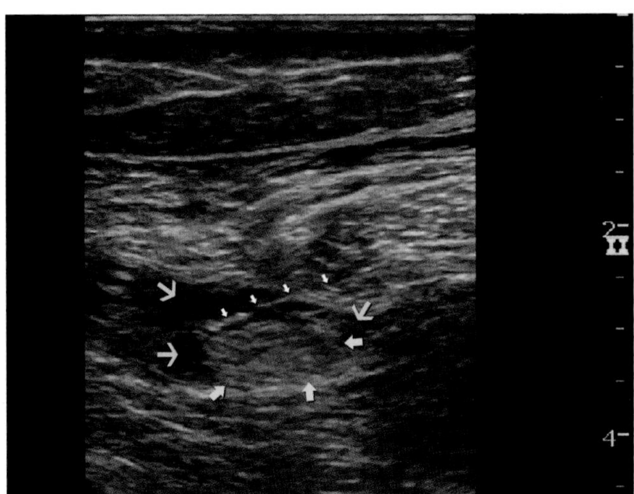

**FIGURE 39.2-5.** Sciatic nerve (yellow arrows) as seen in the subgluteal position (linear transducer), needle path (white arrows) and local anesthetic (turquoise arrows) in the intramuscular tunnel surrounding the sciatic nerve.

of local anesthetic (Figure 39.2-5). Alternatively, sliding the transducer slightly proximally or distally can improve the quality of the image and allow for better visualization. Once identified, the needle is inserted in-plane, typically from the lateral aspect of the transducer and advanced toward the sciatic nerve. If nerve stimulation is used (1.0 mA, 0.1 msec), the passage of the needle through the anterior fascial plane of the gluteus muscles often is associated with a motor response of the calf or foot. Once the needle tip is positioned adjacent to the nerve (Figure 39.2-6A) and after careful aspiration to rule out an intravascular needle placement, 1 to 2 mL of local anesthetic is injected to document the proper injection site. Such injection often displaces the sciatic nerve away from the needle; therefore, an additional advancement of the needle 1 to 2 mm toward the nerve may be necessary to ensure the proper spread of the local anesthetic. When injection of the local anesthetic does not appear to result in a spread around the sciatic nerve, additional needle repositions and injections may be necessary. Assuring the absence of high resistance to injection is of utmost importance because the needle tip is difficult to visualize on ultrasound due to the steep angle and depth of the needle placement.

## TIPS

- Never inject against high resistance to injection (>15 psi) because this may signal an intraneural injection.
- The ability to distinguish the sciatic nerve from its soft tissue surroundings often is improved after the injection of local anesthetic; this can be used as a marker to confirm the proper identification of the nerve when injection begins.

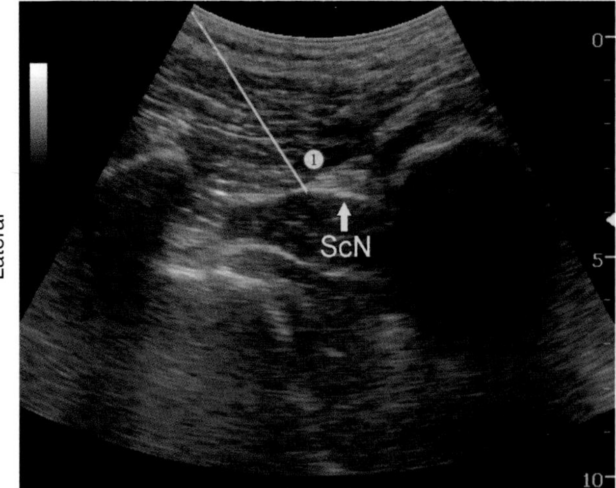


A Sciatic nerve block-posterior approach

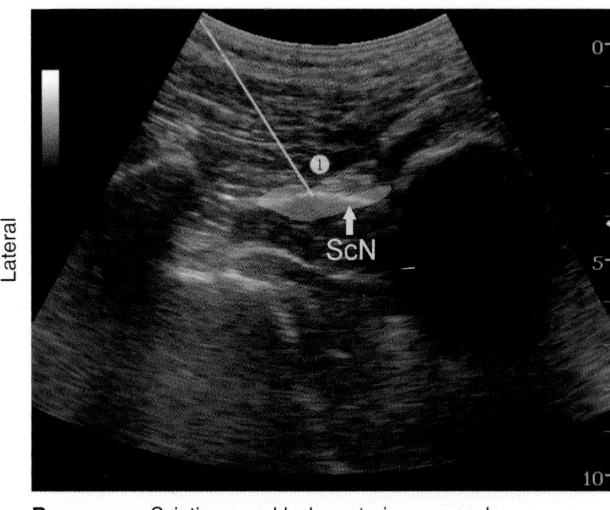


B Sciatic nerve block-posterior approach

**FIGURE 39.2-6.** (A) Ultrasound image demonstrating the simulated needle path to reach the sciatic nerve (ScN) using an in-plane technique in transgluteal approach. The simulated needle (1) is shown transversing the gluteus muscle with its tip positioned at the lateral aspect of the sciatic nerve. (B) Needle path and distribution of local anesthetic (blue shaded area) to block the ScN through the transgluteal approach.

In an adult patient, 15 to 20 mL of local anesthetic is usually adequate for successful blockade of sciatic nerve (Figure 39.2-6). Although a single injection of such volumes of local anesthetic suffices, it may be beneficial to inject two to three smaller aliquots at different locations to ensure the spread of the local anesthetic solution around the sciatic nerve. The block dynamics and perioperative management are similar to those described in Chapter 19.

## Continuous Ultrasound-Guided Subgluteal Sciatic Block

The goal of the continuous sciatic block is similar to the non-ultrasound-based techniques: to place the catheter in the vicinity of the sciatic nerve between the gluteus maximus and quadratus femoris muscles. The procedure consists of three phases: needle placement, catheter advancement, and securing the catheter. For the first two phases of the procedure, ultrasound visualization can be used to ensure accuracy in most patients. The needle typically is inserted in-plane from the lateral to medial direction and underneath the fascia to enter the subgluteal space.

Advancement of the needle until the tip is adjacent to the nerve and deep to the gluteus maximus fascia should ensure appropriate catheter location. Proper placement of the needle also can be confirmed by obtaining a motor response of the calf or foot at which point, 4 to 5 mL of local anesthetic is injected. This small dose of local anesthetic serves to ensure adequate distribution of the local anesthetic as well as to make the advancement of the catheter easier. This first phase of the procedure does not significantly differ from the single-injection technique. The second phase of the procedure involves maintaining the needle in the proper position and inserting the catheter 3 to 5 cm beyond the needle tip into the subgluteal space in the vicinity of the sciatic nerve. Insertion of the catheter requires an assistant when it is done under ultrasound guidance. Alternatively, the catheter can be inserted using a longitudinal view. With this approach, after successful imaging of the sciatic nerve in the cross-sectional view, the transducer is rotated 90° so that the sciatic nerve is visualized in the longitudinal view. However, this approach requires significantly greater ultrasound imaging skills.

The catheter is secured by either taping it to the skin or tunneling. A common infusion strategy includes ropivacaine 0.2% at 5 mL/minute with a patient-controlled bolus of 5 mL/hour.

# ULTRASOUND-GUIDED SCIATIC NERVE BLOCK (TRANSGLUTEAL LOCATION)

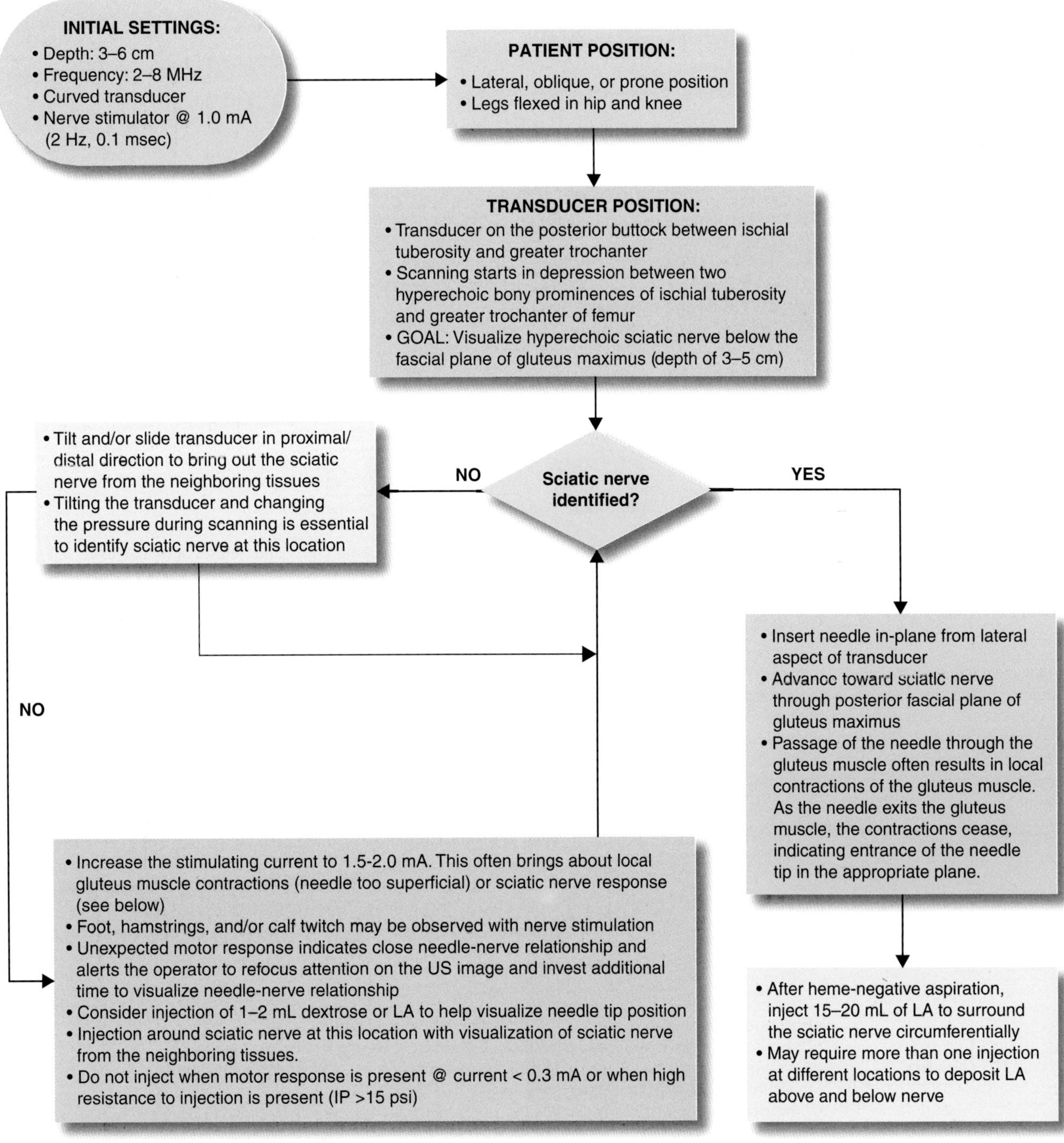

# ULTRASOUND-GUIDED SCIATIC NERVE BLOCK (SUBGLUTEAL LOCATION)

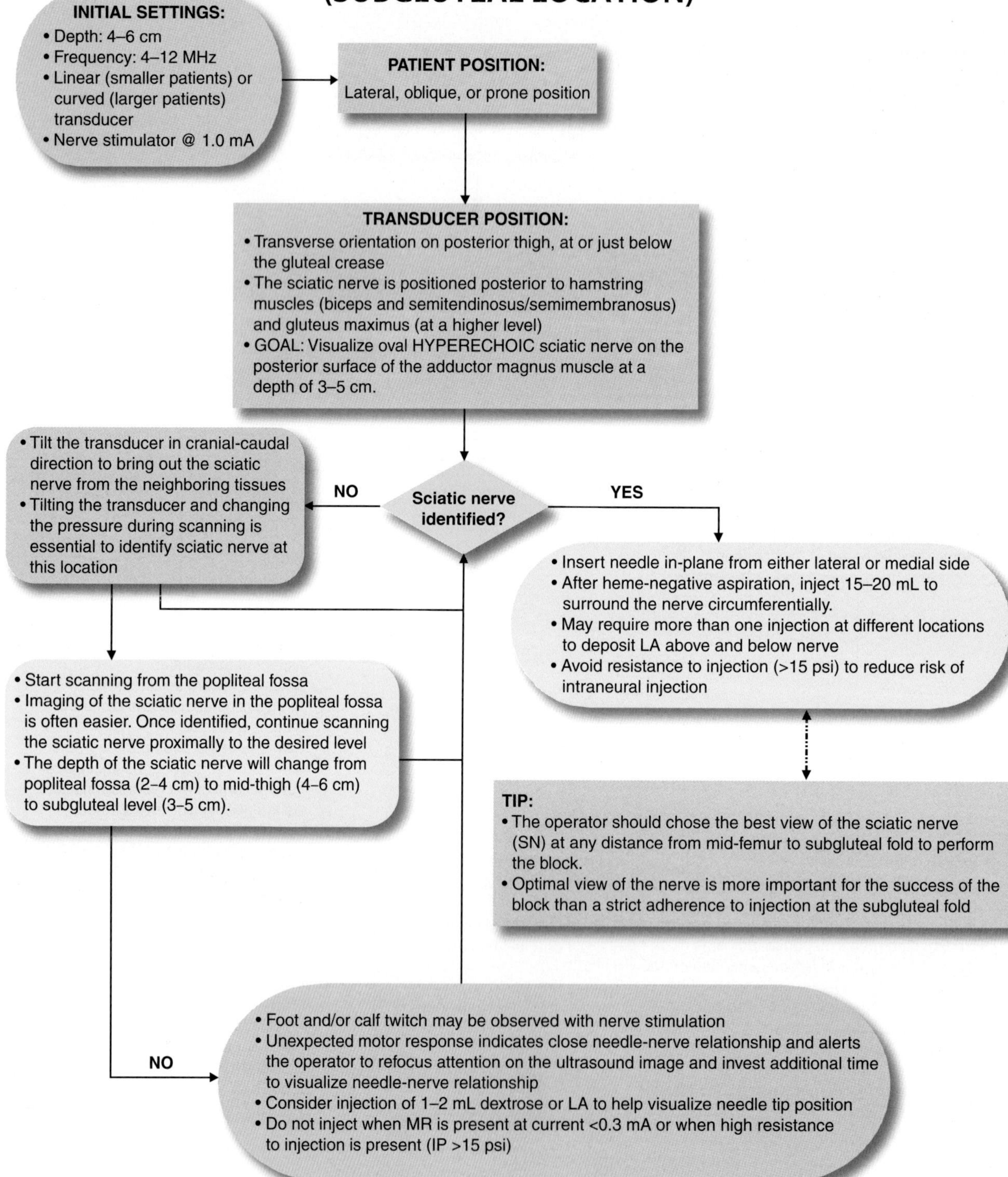

## SUGGESTED READING


Abbas S, Brull R. Ultrasound-guided sciatic nerve block: description of a new approach at the subgluteal space. *Br J Anaesth.* 2007;99:445-446.

Barrington MJ, Lai SL, Briggs CA, Ivanusic JJ, Gledhill SR. Ultrasound-guided midthigh sciatic nerve block-a clinical and anatomical study. *Reg Anesth Pain Med.* 2008;33:369-376.

Bruhn J, Moayeri N, Groen GJ, et al. Soft tissue landmark for ultrasound identification of the sciatic nerve in the infragluteal region: the tendon of the long head of the biceps femoris muscle. *Acta Anaesthesiol Scand.* 2009;53:921-925.

Bruhn J, Van Geffen GJ, Gielen MJ, Scheffer GJ. Visualization of the course of the sciatic nerve in adult volunteers by ultrasonography. *Acta Anaesthesiol Scand.* 2008;52:1298-1302.

Chan VW, Nova H, Abbas S, McCartney CJ, Perlas A, Xu DQ. Ultrasound examination and localization of the sciatic nerve: a volunteer study. *Anesthesiology.* 2006;104:309-314.

Chantzi C, Saranteas T, Zogogiannis J, Alevizou N, Dimitriou V. Ultrasound examination of the sciatic nerve at the anterior thigh in obese patients. *Acta Anaesthesiol Scand.* 2007;51:132.

Danelli G, Ghisi D, Fanelli A, et al. The effects of ultrasound guidance and neurostimulation on the minimum effective anesthetic volume of mepivacaine 1.5% required to block the sciatic nerve using the subgluteal approach. *Anesth Analg.* 2009;109:1674-1678.

Danelli G, Ghisi D, Ortu A. Ultrasound and regional anesthesia technique: are there really ultrasound guidance technical limits in sciatic nerve blocks? *Reg Anesth Pain Med.* 2008;33:281-282.

Domingo-Triado V, Selfa S, Martinez F, et al. Ultrasound guidance for lateral midfemoral sciatic nerve block: a prospective, comparative, randomized study. *Anesth Analg.* 2007;104:1270-1274.

Fredrickson MJ, Kilfoyle DH. Neurological complication analysis of 1000 ultrasound guided peripheral nerve blocks for elective orthopaedic surgery: a prospective study. *Anaesthesia.* 2009;64:836-844.

Gnaho A, Eyrieux S, Gentili M. Cardiac arrest during an ultrasound-guided sciatic nerve block combined with nerve stimulation. *Reg Anesth Pain Med.* 2009;34:278.

Gray AT, Collins AB, Schafhalter-Zoppoth I. Sciatic nerve block in a child: a sonographic approach. *Anesth Analg.* 2003;97:1300-1302.

Hamilton PD, Pearce CJ, Pinney SJ, Calder JD. Sciatic nerve blockade: a survey of orthopaedic foot and ankle specialists in North America and the United Kingdom. *Foot Ankle Int.* 2009;30:1196-1201.

Karmakar MK, Kwok WH, Ho AM, Tsang K, Chui PT, Gin T. Ultrasound-guided sciatic nerve block: description of a new approach at the subgluteal space. *Br J Anaesth.* 2007;98:390-395.

Latzke D, Marhofer P, Zeitlinger M, et al. Minimal local anaesthetic volumes for sciatic nerve block: evaluation of ED 99 in volunteers. *Br J Anaesth.* 2010;104:239-244.

Latzke D, Marhofer P, Zeitlinger M, Machata A, Neumann F, Lackner E, Kettner SC: Minimal local anaesthetic volumes for sciatic nerve block: evaluation of ED 99 in volunteers. Br J Anaesth 2010; 104: 239-44

Marhofer P, Harrop-Griffiths W, Willschke H, Kirchmair L. Fifteen years of ultrasound guidance in regional anaesthesia: Part 2-recent developments in block techniques. *Br J Anaesth.* 2010;104:673-683.

Marhofer P, Harrop-Griffiths W, Willschke H, Kirchmair L: Fifteen years of ultrasound guidance in regional anaesthesia: Part 2-recent developments in block techniques. Br J Anaesth 2010; 104: 673-83

Murray JM, Derbyshire S, Shields MO. Lower limb blocks. *Anaesthesia.* 2010;65(Suppl 1):57-66.

Murray JM, Derbyshire S, Shields MO: Lower limb blocks. Anaesthesia 2010; 65 Suppl 1: 57-66

Oberndorfer U, Marhofer P, Bosenberg A, et al. Ultrasonographic guidance for sciatic and femoral nerve blocks in children. *Br J Anaesth.* 2007;98:797-801.

Ota J, Sakura S, Hara K, Saito Y. Ultrasound-guided anterior approach to sciatic nerve block: a comparison with the posterior approach. *Anesth Analg.* 2009;108:660-665.

Pham Dang C, Gourand D. Ultrasound imaging of the sciatic nerve in the lateral midfemoral approach. *Reg Anesth Pain Med.* 2009;34:281-282.

Salinas FV. Ultrasound and review of evidence for lower extremity peripheral nerve blocks. *Reg Anesth Pain Med.* 2010;35:S16-25.

Salinas FV: Ultrasound and review of evidence for lower extremity peripheral nerve blocks. Reg Anesth Pain Med 2010; 35: S16-25

Salinas FV: Ultrasound and review of evidence for lower extremity peripheral nerve blocks. Reg Anesth Pain Med 2010; 35: S16-25

Saranteas T. Limitations in ultrasound imaging techniques in anesthesia: obesity and muscle atrophy? *Anesth Analg.* 2009;109:993-994.

Saranteas T, Chantzi C, Paraskeuopoulos T, et al. Imaging in anesthesia: the role of 4 MHz to 7 MHz sector array ultrasound probe in the identification of the sciatic nerve at different anatomic locations. *Reg Anesth Pain Med.* 2007;32:537-538.

Saranteas T, Chantzi C, Zogogiannis J, et al. Lateral sciatic nerve examination and localization at the mid-femoral level: an imaging study with ultrasound. *Acta Anaesthesiol Scand.* 2007;51:387-388.

Saranteas T, Kostopanagiotou G, Paraskeuopoulos T, Vamvasakis E, Chantzi C, Anagnostopoulou S. Ultrasound examination of the sciatic nerve at two different locations in the lateral thigh: a new approach of identification validated by anatomic preparation. *Acta Anaesthesiol Scand.* 2007;51:780-781.

Sites BD, Neal JM, Chan V. Ultrasound in regional anesthesia: where should the "focus" be set? *Reg Anesth Pain Med.* 2009;34:531-533.

Tran de QH, Munoz L, Russo G, Finlayson RJ. Ultrasonography and stimulating perineural catheters for nerve blocks: a review of the evidence. *Can J Anaesth.* 2008;55:447-457.

Tsui BC, Dillane D, Pillay J, Ramji AK, Walji AH. Cadaveric ultrasound imaging for training in ultrasound-guided peripheral nerve blocks: lower extremity. *Can J Anaesth.* 2007;54:475-480.

Tsui BC, Finucane BT. The importance of ultrasound landmarks: a "traceback" approach using the popliteal blood vessels for identification of the sciatic nerve. *Reg Anesth Pain Med.* 2006;31:481-482.

Tsui BC, Ozelsel TJ. Ultrasound-guided anterior sciatic nerve block using a longitudinal approach: "expanding the view." *Reg Anesth Pain Med.* 2008;33:275-276.

van Geffen GJ, Bruhn J, Gielen M. Ultrasound-guided continuous sciatic nerve blocks in two children with venous malformations in the lower limb. *Can J Anaesth.* 2007;54:952-953.

van Geffen GJ, Gielen M. Ultrasound-guided subgluteal sciatic nerve blocks with stimulating catheters in children: a descriptive study. *Anesth Analg.* 2006;103:328-333.

# 40 Ultrasound-Guided Popliteal Sciatic Block

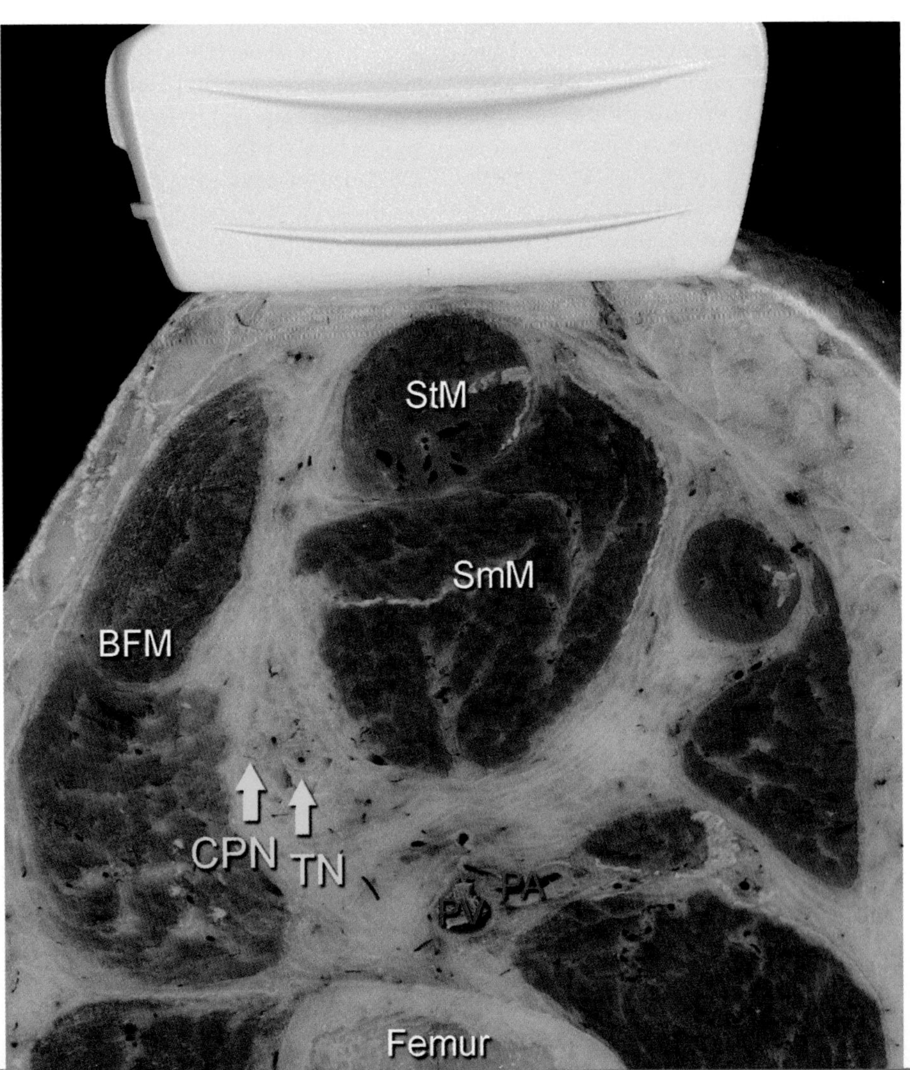


## BLOCK AT A GLANCE

- Indications: foot and ankle surgery; analgesia following knee surgery
- Transducer position: transverse on the lateral aspect of thigh or over popliteal fossa
- Goal: local anesthetic spread surrounding the sciatic nerve within epineural sheath
- Local anesthetic: 20–30 mL

**FIGURE 40-1.** Cross-sectional anatomy of the sciatic nerve in the popliteal fossa. Shown are common peroneal nerve (CPN), tibial nerve (TN), popliteal artery (PA), popliteal vein (PV), femur, biceps femoris (BFM), semimembranosus (SmM) and semitendinosus (StM) muscles.

## General Considerations

Performance of a sciatic block above the popliteal fossa benefits from ultrasound guidance in several ways. The anatomy of the sciatic nerve as it approaches the popliteal fossa can be variable, and the division into the tibial nerve (TN) and common peroneal nerve (CPN) occurs at a variable distance from the crease. Knowledge of the location of the TPN and CPN in relation to each other is beneficial in ensuring the anesthesia of both divisions of the sciatic nerve. Moreover, with nerve stimulator–based techniques, larger volumes (e.g., >40 mL) of local anesthetic often are required to increase the chance of block success and rapid onset. A reduction in local anesthetic volume can be achieved with ultrasound guidance because the injection can be halted once adequate spread is documented. The two approaches to the popliteal sciatic block common in our practice are the lateral approach with patient in supine (more commonly, oblique position) and the posterior approach (Figure 40-2). It should be noted that with the lateral approach, the resulting ultrasound image is identical to the image in the posterior approach. Both are discussed in this chapter. Only the patient position and needle path differ between the two approaches; the rest of the technique details are essentially the same.

## Ultrasound Anatomy

With the posterior and the lateral approaches, the transducer position is identical; thus the sonographic anatomy appears the same. However, note that although the image appears the same, there is a 180° difference in patient orientation. Beginning with the transducer in the transverse position at the popliteal crease, the popliteal artery is identified, aided with the color Doppler ultrasound when necessary, at a depth of approximately 3 to 4 cm. The popliteal vein accompanies the artery. On either side of the artery are the biceps femoris muscles (lateral) and the semimembranosus and semitendinosus muscles (medial). Superficial (i.e., toward the skin surface) and lateral to the artery is the tibial nerve, seen as a hyperechoic, oval, or round structure with a stippled or honeycomb pattern on the interior (Figure 40-3A and B). If difficulty in identifying the nerve is encountered, the patient can be asked to dorsiflex and plantar flex the ankle, which makes the nerve rotate or move in relation to its surroundings. Once the tibial nerve is identified, an attempt can be made to visualize the common peroneal nerve, which is located even more superficial and lateral to the tibial nerve. The transducer should be slid proximally until the tibial and peroneal nerves are visualized coming together to form the sciatic nerve before its division. (Figure 40-4A and B). This junction usually occurs at a distance between 5 and 10 cm from the popliteal crease but this may occur very close to the crease or (less commonly) more proximally in the thigh. As the transducer is moved proximally, the popliteal vessels move anteriorly (i.e., deeper) and therefore become less visible. Adjustments in depth, gain, and direction of the ultrasound beam should be made to keep the nerve visible at all times. The sciatic nerve typically is visualized at a depth of 2 to 4 cm.

**TIP**

- In our practice, most popliteal blocks are with the patient in the oblique position using either posterior or lateral approach.

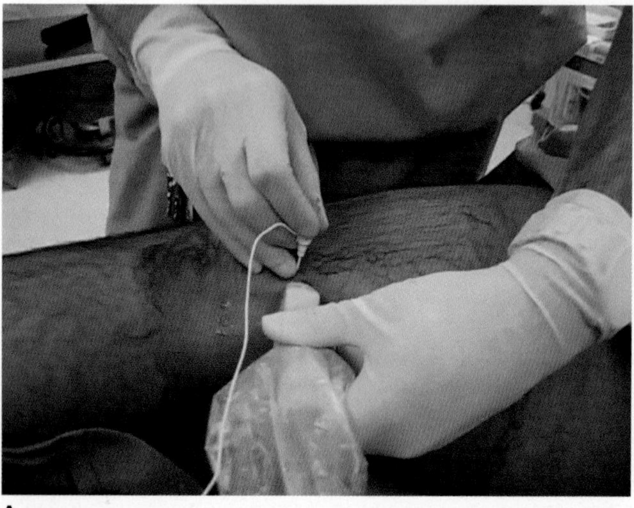

A

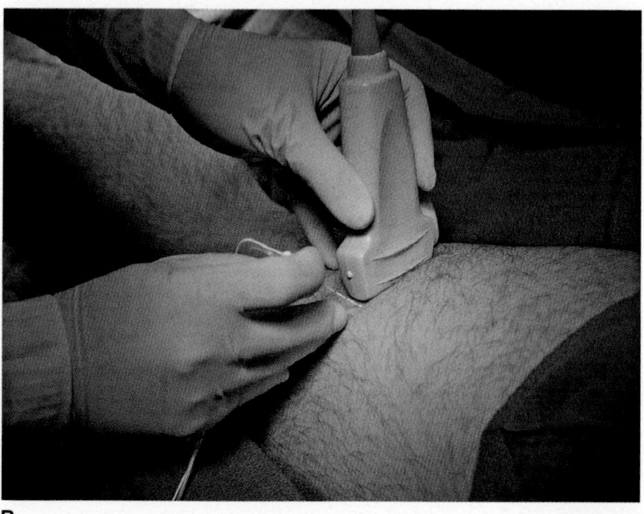

B

**FIGURE 40-2.** Posterior approach to ultrasound-guided popliteal sciatic block can be performed with the patient in the oblique position (A) or with the patient prone (B).

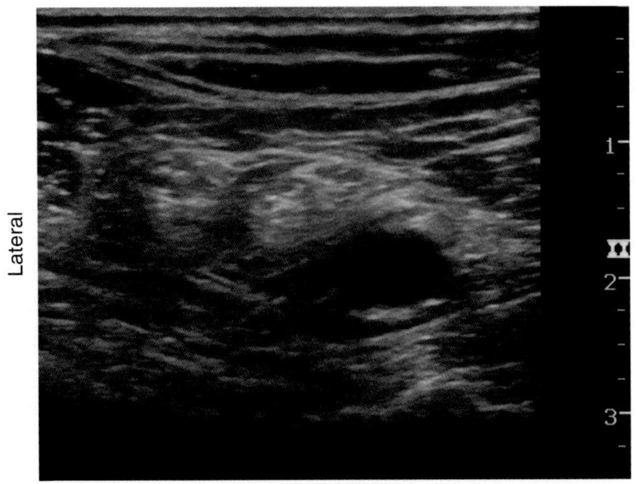


A Common peroneal and tibial nerve-3 cm above popliteal crease

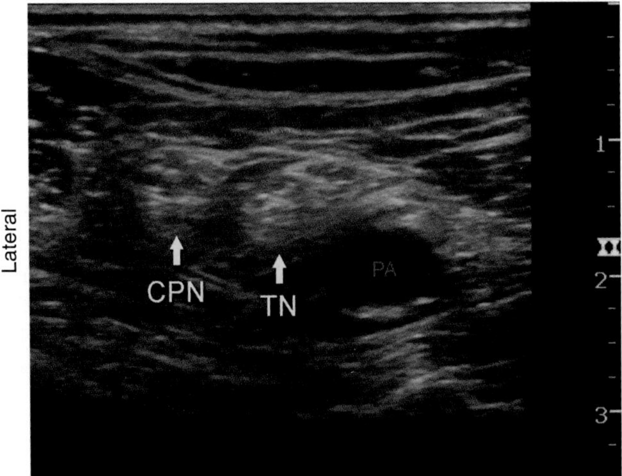


B Common peroneal and tibial nerve-3 cm above popliteal crease, labeled

**FIGURE 40-3.** (A) The sonoanatomy of the sciatic nerve at the popliteal fossa. The two main divisions of the sciatic nerve, tibial (TN) and common peroneal nerves (CPN), are seen immediately lateral and superficial to the popliteal artery, respectively. (B) Sonoanatomy of the popliteal fossa with the structures labeled. TN and CPN are lateral and superficial to PA. Images 40-3A and B were taken at 5 cm above the popliteal fossa crease where the TN and CPN have just started diverging.

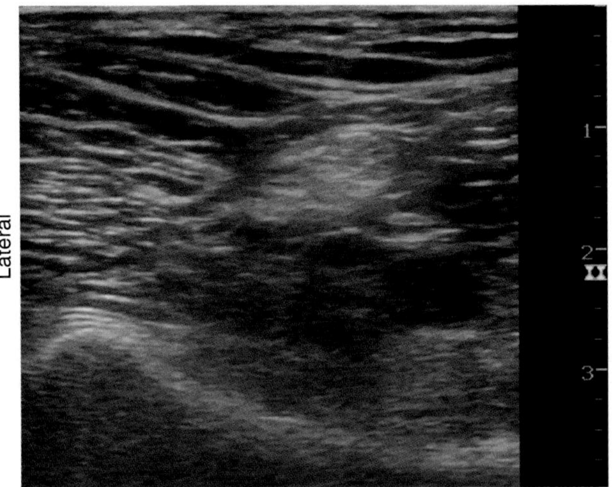


A Popliteal sciatic nerve block

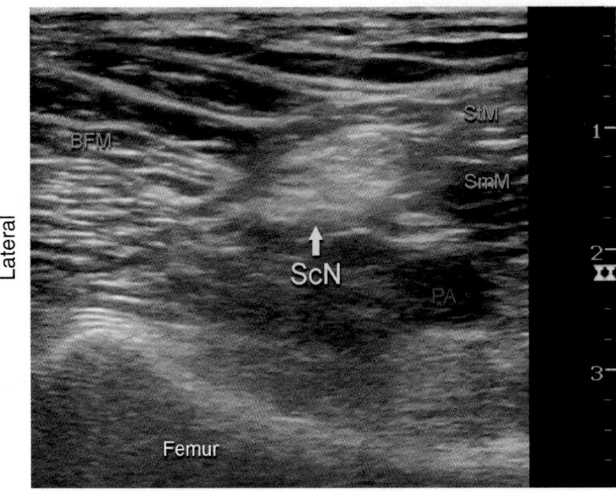


B Popliteal sciatic nerve block, labeled

**FIGURE 40-4.** (A) Sonoanatomy of the sciatic nerve (ScN) before its division. (B) Sonoanatomy of the popliteal fossa with the structures labeled. Shown are ScN, superior and lateral to the popliteal artery (PA), positioned between bicep femoris (BFM) and semimembranosus (SmM) and semitendinosus (StM) muscles.

## Distribution of Blockade

Sciatic nerve block results in anesthesia of the entire lower limb below the knee, both motor and sensory, with the exception of a variable strip of skin on the medial leg and foot, which is the territory of the saphenous nerve, a branch of the femoral nerve. The motor fibers to the hamstring muscles are spared; however, sensory fibers to the posterior aspect of the knee are still blocked. For a more comprehensive review of the sciatic nerve distribution, see Chapter 1, Essential Regional Anesthesia Anatomy.

## Equipment

The following equipment is needed:

- Ultrasound machine with linear transducer (8–12 MHz), sterile sleeve, and gel (rarely, in a very obese patient, a curved transducer might be needed)
- Standard nerve block tray (described in the equipment section, Chapter 3)
- Two 20-mL syringes containing local anesthetic
- 50- to 100-mm, 21- to 22-gauge short-bevel insulated stimulating needle
- Peripheral nerve stimulator
- Sterile gloves

## Lateral Approach

### Landmarks and Patient Positioning

This block is performed with the patient in the supine or oblique (more convenient) position. Sufficient space must be made to accommodate the transducer beneath the knee and thigh. This can be accomplished either by resting the foot on an elevated footrest or flexing the knee while an assistant stabilizes the foot and ankle on the bed (Figure 40-5). If nerve stimulation is used at the same time, exposure of the calf and foot are required to observe motor responses.

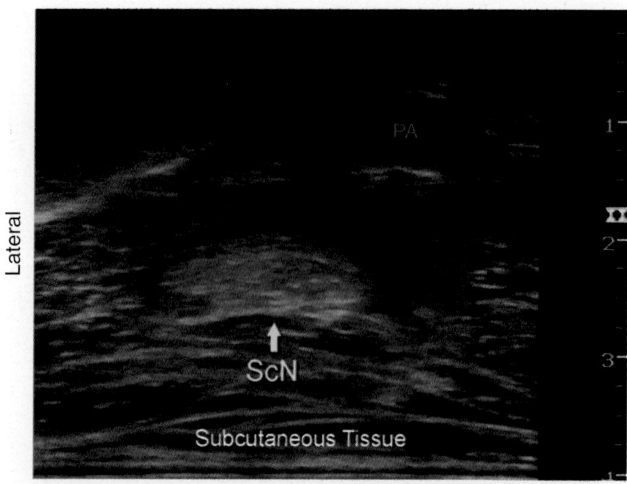


Popliteal sciatic nerve block-lateral approach

**FIGURE 40-6.** Sonoanatomy of the popliteal fossa imaged with the transducer positioned as in Figure 40-5. The image appears inverted compared to the image in the lateral/oblique position.

**GOAL**

**The goal is to inject the local anesthetic within the common epineurium that envelops the TN and CPN. Alternatively, separate blocks of TN and CPN can be made.**

### Technique

With the patient in the proper position, the skin is disinfected and the transducer positioned to identify the sciatic nerve (Figure 40-5). If the nerve is not immediately apparent, tilting the transducer proximally or distally can help improve the contrast and bring the nerve "out" of the background (Figure 40-6). Alternatively, sliding the transducer slightly proximally or distally may improve the quality of the image and allow for better visualization. Once identified, a skin wheal is made on the lateral aspect of the thigh 2 to 3 cm above the lateral edge of the transducer. Then the needle is inserted in-plane in a horizontal orientation from the lateral aspect of the thigh and advanced toward the sciatic nerve (Figure 40-7). If nerve stimulation is used (0.5 mA, 0.1 msec), the contact of the needle tip with the sciatic nerve usually is associated with a motor response of the calf or foot. Once the needle tip is witnessed adjacent to the nerve, and after careful aspiration, 1 to 2 mL of local anesthetic is injected to confirm the proper injection site. Such injection should result in

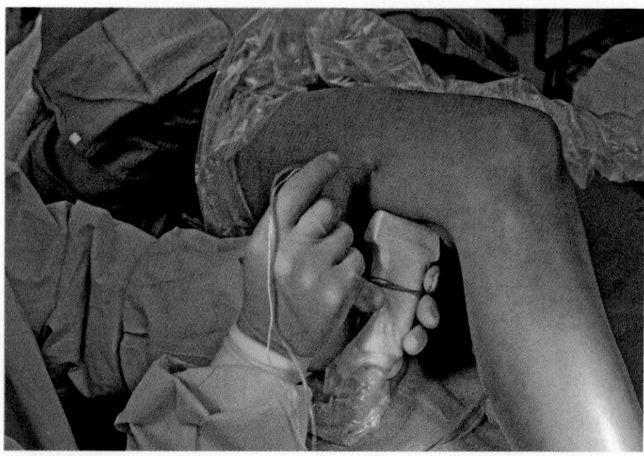

**FIGURE 40-5.** Needle insertion technique to block the sciatic nerve in the popliteal fossa using lateral approach with patient in the supine position.

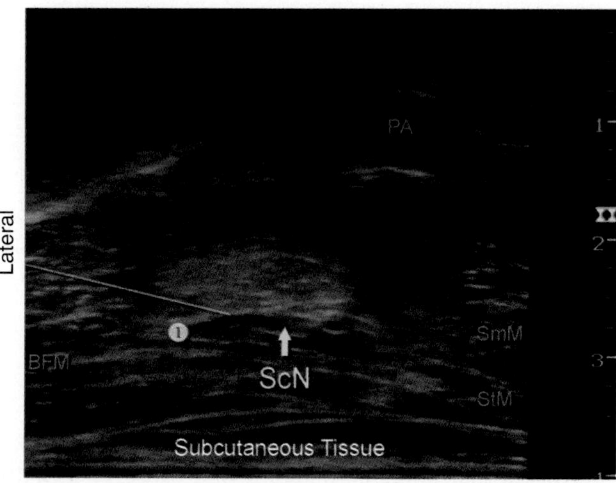


Popliteal sciatic nerve block-lateral approach

**FIGURE 40-7.** Simulated needle path and the proper needle tip placement to block the sciatic nerve (ScN) through the lateral approach. BFM - Biceps femoris muscle, SmM - Semimembranosus muscle. StM - Semitendinosus muscle, PA- Popliteal artery.

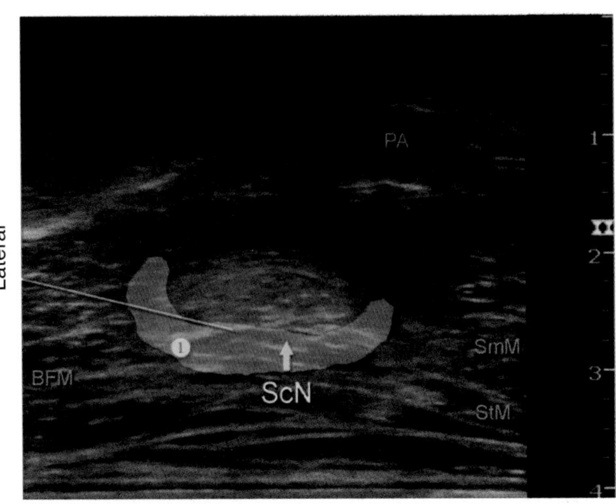


**FIGURE 40-8.** Simulated needle path and local anesthetic distribution to block the sciatic nerve in the popliteal fossa using the lateral approach.

distribution of the local anesthetic within the epineural sheath, and often, separation of the TN and CPN. When injection of the local anesthetic does not appear to result in a spread around the sciatic nerve (Figure 40-8), additional needle repositions and injections may be necessary. When injecting into the epineurium, correct injection is recognized as local anesthetic spread proximally and distally to the site of the injection around both divisions of the nerve. This typically results in separation of TN and CPN during and after the injection.

## TIPS

- To improve the visualization of the needle, a skin puncture site 2 to 3 cm lateral to the transducer will reduce the acuity of the angle with respect to the ultrasound beam, Figure 40-5.
- The presence of a motor response to nerve stimulation is useful but not necessary to elicit if the nerve, needle, and local anesthetic spread are well visualized.
- Never inject against high resistance to injection because this may signal an intraneural injection (IP must be < 15 psi).

Although a single injection of local may suffice, it may be beneficial to inject two to three smaller aliquots at different locations to ensure the spread of the local anesthetic solution around the sciatic nerve. The block dynamics and perioperative management are similar to those described in Chapter 20.

## Posterior Approach

### Landmarks and Patient Positioning

This block is performed with the patient in the prone or oblique position with the legs slightly abducted. A small footrest is useful to facilitate identification of a motor response if nerve stimulation is used. Also, it relaxes the hamstring tendons, making transducer placement and manipulation easier.

### Technique

With the patient in the proper position, the skin is disinfected and the transducer positioned to identify the sciatic nerve (Figure 40-2). Similar maneuvers as described for the lateral approach can be made to better visualize the nerve. Once identified, a skin wheal is made immediately lateral or medial to the transducer. Then the needle is inserted in plane and advanced toward the sciatic nerve (Figures 40-9 and 40-10). If nerve stimulation is used (0.5 mA, 0.1 msec), the contact of the needle tip with the sciatic nerve often is associated with a motor response of the calf or foot. Once the needle tip is confirmed to be adjacent to the nerve, the syringe is gently aspirated and the local anesthetic deposited. Needle repositioning and injection of smaller aliquots is frequently required to ensure adequate circumferential spread of the local anesthetic (Figure 40-11).

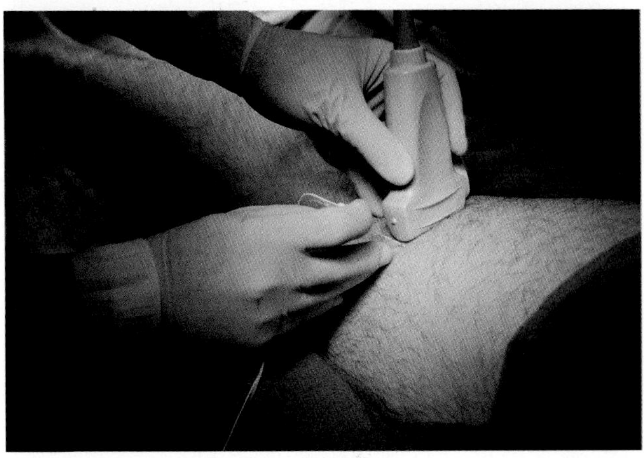

**FIGURE 40-9.** Transducer position and in-plane needle insertion to block the sciatic nerve at the popliteal fossa with patient in prone position.

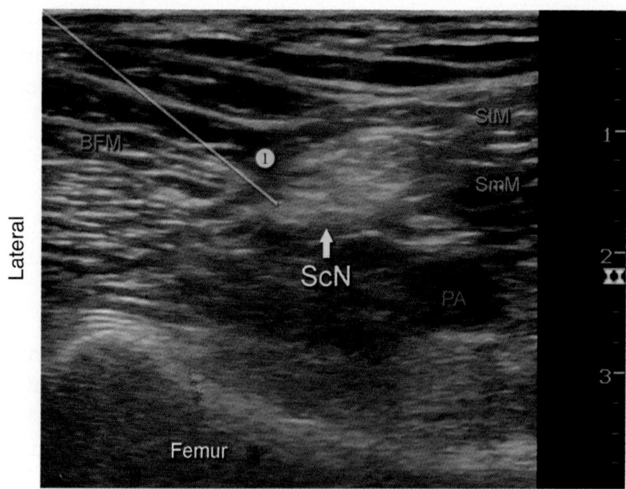


**FIGURE 40-10.** Simulated needle path to reach the sciatic nerve in the popliteal fossa through the posterior approach. The sciatic nerve (ScN) is seen in the adipose tissue of the popliteal fossa between bicep femoris muscle (BFM) laterally and the semitendinosus and semimembranosus muscles medially (Stm, SmM).

## TIP

- In the posterior approach to popliteal block, either an in-plane or out-of-plane technique can be used. While the in-plane approach is the most common at NYSORA, the advantage of the out-of-plane approach is that the path of the needle is through skin and adipose tissue rather than the muscles.

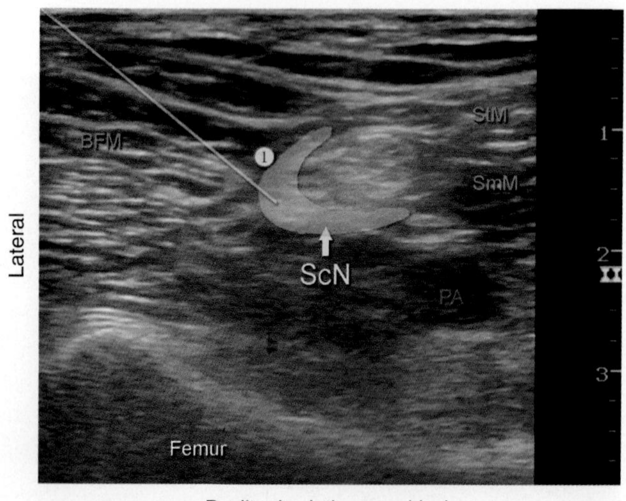


**FIGURE 40-11.** Simulated needle insertion path, needle tip position, and distribution of local anesthetic (area shaded in blue) to anesthetize the sciatic nerve.

## Continuous Ultrasound-Guided Popliteal Sciatic Block

The goal of the continuous popliteal sciatic block is to place the catheter in the vicinity of the sciatic nerve within the popliteal fossa. The procedure consists of three phases: needle placement, catheter advancement, and securing the catheter. For the first two phases of the procedure, ultrasound can be used to ensure accuracy in most patients. Typically, the needle is inserted in the same manner as described for the single-shot blocks. An in-plane approach, however, is favored in our practice for the catheter technique because it allows for monitoring of the catheter placement (Figure 40-12).

Proper placement of the needle can be confirmed by obtaining a motor response of the calf or foot, at which point 4 to 5 mL of local anesthetic is injected. This small dose of local anesthetic can make advancement of the catheter easier. The second phase of the procedure involves maintaining the needle in the proper position and inserting the catheter 2 to 4 cm into the space surrounding the sciatic nerve. Insertion of the catheter can be accomplished by either a single operator or with an assistant. Proper position of the catheter is assured by an injection through the catheter and confirming the location and distribution of the injectate and/or monitoring catheter insertion on ultrasound real-time.

The catheter is secured by either taping it to the skin or tunneling. There is no agreement among clinicians regarding what constitutes the ideal catheter securing system. Some clinicians prefer one method over the other. However, the decision regarding which method to use could be based on the patient's age, duration of the catheter therapy, and anatomy. The lateral approach may have some advantage

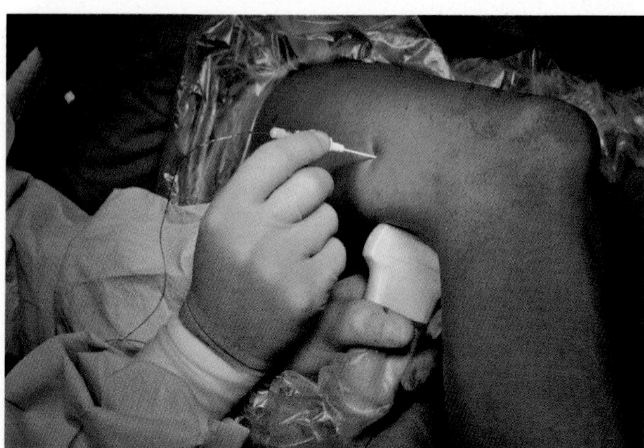

**FIGURE 40-12.** Continuous sciatic block in the popliteal fossa using a lateral approach with patient in the supine position. The needle is positioned within the epineural sheath of the sciatic nerve. After an injection of a small volume of local anesthetic to confirm the needle position a catheter is inserted 2–4 cm past the needle tip. Pre-loading the catheter is useful in facilitating the procedure.

over the prone approach with regard to catheter placement. First, the biceps femoris muscle tends to stabilize the catheter and decrease the chance of dislodgment, compared with the subcutaneous tissue of the popliteal fossa in the prone approach. Second, if the knee is to be flexed and extended, the side of the thigh is less mobile than the back of the knee. Finally, access to the catheter site is more convenient with the lateral approach compared with the prone approach. A commonly suggested starting infusion regimen is to infuse ropivacaine 0.2% at 5 mL/hour with a patient-delivered bolus of 5 mL every 60 minutes.

# ULTRASOUND-GUIDED POPLITEAL SCIATIC BLOCK

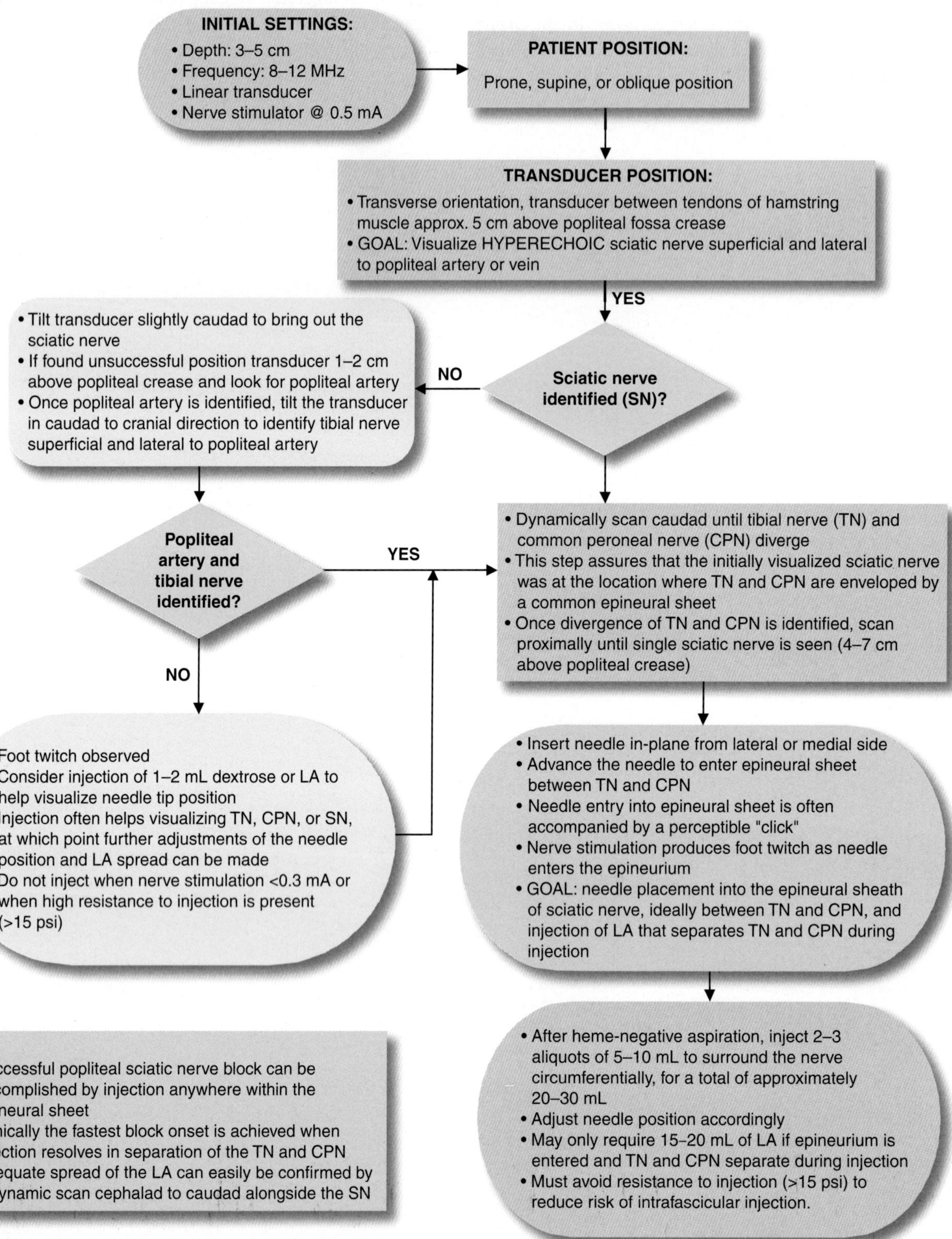

## SUGGESTED READING


Aguirre J, Perinola L, Borgeat A: Ultrasound-guided evaluation of the local anesthetic spread parameters required for a rapid surgical popliteal sciatic nerve block. *Reg Anesth Pain Med.* 2011; 36:308–309.

Aguirre J, Ruland P, Ekatodramis G, Borgeat A. Ultrasound versus neurostimulation for popliteal block: another vain effort to show a non existing clinical relevant difference. *Anaesth Intensive Care.* 2009;37:665–666.

Aguirre J, Valentin Neudorfer C, Ekatodramis G, Borgeat A. Ultrasound guidance for sciatic nerve block at the popliteal fossa should be compared with the best motor response and the lowest current clinically used in neurostimulation technique. *Reg Anesth Pain Med.* 2009;34:182–183.

Barrington MJ, Lai SL, Briggs CA, Ivanusic JJ, Gledhill SR. Ultrasound-guided midthigh sciatic nerve block-a clinical and anatomical study. *Reg Anesth Pain Med.* 2008;33:369–376.

Bendtsen TF, Nielsen TD, Rohde CV, Kibak K, Linde F: Ultrasound guidance improves a continuous popliteal sciatic nerve block when compared with nerve stimulation. *Reg Anesth Pain Med.* 2011;36: 181–184.

Bruhn J, Van Geffen GJ, Gielen MJ, Scheffer GJ. Visualization of the course of the sciatic nerve in adult volunteers by ultrasonography. *Acta Anaesthesiol Scand.* 2008;52:1298–1302.

Brull R, Macfarlane AJ, Parrington SJ, Koshkin A, Chan VW: Is circumfrential injection advantageous for ultrasound-guided popliteal sciatic nerve block?: A proof-of-concept study. *Reg Anesth Pain Med.* 2011;36:266–270

Buys MJ, Arndt CD, Vagh F, Hoard A, Gerstein N. Ultrasound-guided sciatic nerve block in the popliteal fossa using a lateral approach: onset time comparing separate tibial and common peroneal nerve injections versus injecting proximal to the bifurcation. *Anesth Analg.* 2010;110:635–637.

Chin KJ, Perlas A, Brull R, Chan VW. Ultrasound guidance is advantageous in popliteal nerve blockade. *Anesth Analg.* 2008;107:2094–2095.

Clendenen SR, York JE, Wang RD, Greengrass RA. Three-dimensional ultrasound-assisted popliteal catheter placement revealing aberrant anatomy: implications for block failure. *Acta Anaesthesiol Scand.* 2008;52:1429–1431.

Compere V, Cornet C, Fourdrinier V, et al. Thigh abscess as a complication of continuous popliteal sciatic nerve block. *Br J Anaesth.* 2005;95:255–256.

Danelli G, Fanelli A, Ghisi D, et al. Ultrasound vs nerve stimulation multiple injection technique for posterior popliteal sciatic nerve block. *Anaesthesia.* 2009;64:638–642.

Dufour E, Quennesson P, Van Robais AL, et al. Combined ultrasound and neurostimulation guidance for popliteal sciatic nerve block: a prospective, randomized comparison with neurostimulation alone. *Anesth Analg.* 2008;106:1553–1558.

Eisenberg JA, Calligaro KD, Kolakowski S, et al. Is balloon angioplasty of peri-anastomotic stenoses of failing peripheral arterial bypasses worthwhile? *Vasc Endovascular Surg.* 2009;43:346–351.

Eurin M, Beloeil H, Zetlaoui PJ. A medial approach for a continuous sciatic block in the popliteal fossa [in French]. *Can J Anaesth.* 2006;53:1165–1166.

Gray AT, Huczko EL, Schafhalter-Zoppoth I. Lateral popliteal nerve block with ultrasound guidance. *Reg Anesth Pain Med.* 2004;29:507–509.

Gurkan Y, Sarisoy HT, Caglayan C, Solak M, Toker K. "Figure of four" position improves the visibility of the sciatic nerve in the popliteal fossa. *Agri.* 2009;21:149–154.

Huntoon MA, Huntoon EA, Obray JB, Lamer TJ. Feasibility of ultrasound-guided percutaneous placement of peripheral nerve stimulation electrodes in a cadaver model: part one, lower extremity. *Reg Anesth Pain Med.* 2008;33:551–557.

Ilfeld BM, Sandhu NS, Loland VJ, Madison SJ, Suresh PJ, Mariano ER, Bishop ML, Schwartz AK, Lee DK: Ultrasound-guided (needle-in-plane) perineural catheter insertion: the effect of catheter-insertion distance on postoperative analgesia. *Reg Anesth Pain Med.* 2011;36:261–265.

Jang SH, Lee H, Han SH. Common peroneal nerve compression by a popliteal venous aneurysm. *Am J Phys Med Rehabil.* 2009;88:947–950.

Khabiri B, Arbona F, Norton J. "Gapped supine" position for ultrasound guided lateral popliteal fossa block of the sciatic nerve. *Anesth Analg.* 2007;105:1519.

Koscielniak-Nielsen ZJ, Rasmussen H, Hesselbjerg L. Long-axis ultrasound imaging of the nerves and advancement of perineural catheters under direct vision: a preliminary report of four cases. *Reg Anesth Pain Med.* 2008;33:477–482.

Mariano ER, Cheng GS, Choy LP, et al. Electrical stimulation versus ultrasound guidance for popliteal-sciatic perineural catheter insertion: a randomized controlled trial. *Reg Anesth Pain Med.* 2009;34:480–485.

Mariano ER, Loland VJ, Sandhu NS, Bishop ML, Lee DK, Schwartz AK, Girard PJ, Ferguson EJ, Ilfeld BM: Comparative efficacy of ultrasound-guided and stimulating popliteal-sciatic perineural catheters for postoperative analgesia. *Can J. Anaesth.* 2010;10: 919–926.

Minville V, Zetlaoui PJ, Fessenmeyer C, Benhamou D. Ultrasound guidance for difficult lateral popliteal catheter insertion in a patient with peripheral vascular disease. *Reg Anesth Pain Med.* 2004;29:368–370.

Morau D, Levy F, Bringuier S, Biboulet P, Choquet O, Kassim M, Bernard N, Capdevilla X: Ultrasound-guided evaluation of the local anesthetic spread parameters required for a rapid surgical popliteal sciatic nerve block. *Reg Anesth Pain Med.* 2010;35: 559–564.

Orebaugh SL, Bigeleisen PE, Kentor ML. Impact of a regional anesthesia rotation on ultrasonographic identification of anatomic structures by anesthesiology residents. *Acta Anaesthesiol Scand.* 2009;53:364–368.

Orebaugh SL, Williams BA, Vallejo M, Kentor ML. Adverse outcomes associated with stimulator-based peripheral nerve blocks with versus without ultrasound visualization. *Reg Anesth Pain Med.* 2009;34:251–255.

Perkins JM. Standard varicose vein surgery. *Phlebology.* 2009; 24(Suppl 1):34–41.

Perlas A, Brull R, Chan VW, McCartney CJ, Nuica A, Abbas S. Ultrasound guidance improves the success of sciatic nerve block at the popliteal fossa. *Reg Anesth Pain Med.* 2008;33:259–265.

Perlas A, Chan VW, Brull R. Several "correct" approaches to nerve stimulator-guided popliteal fossa block. *Reg Anesth Pain Med.* 2009;34:624–625.

Prasad A, Perlas A, Ramlogan R, Brull R, Chan V: Ultrasound-guided popliteal block distal to sciatic nerve bifurcation shortens onset time: a prospective randomized double-blind study. *Re Anesth Pain Med.* 2010;35:267–271.

Robards C, Hadžić A, Somasundaram L, et al. Intraneural injection with low-current stimulation during popliteal sciatic nerve block. *Anesth Analg.* 2009;109:673–677.

Sala Blanch X, Lopez AM, Carazo J, et al. Intraneural injection during nerve stimulator-guided sciatic nerve block at the popliteal fossa. *Br J Anaesth.* 2009;102:855–861.

Sinha A, Chan VW. Ultrasound imaging for popliteal sciatic nerve block. *Reg Anesth Pain Med.* 2004;29:130–134.

Sit M, Higgs JB. Non-popliteal synovial rupture. *J Clin Rheumatol.* 2009;15:185–189.

Sites BD, Gallagher J, Sparks M. Ultrasound-guided popliteal block demonstrates an atypical motor response to nerve stimulation in 2 patients with diabetes mellitus. *Reg Anesth Pain Med.* 2003;28:479–482.

Sites BD, Gallagher JD, Tomek I, Cheung Y, Beach ML. The use of magnetic resonance imaging to evaluate the accuracy of a handheld ultrasound machine in localizing the sciatic nerve in the popliteal fossa. *Reg Anesth Pain Med.* 2004;29:413–416.

Tsui BC, Finucane BT. The importance of ultrasound landmarks: a "traceback" approach using the popliteal blood vessels for identification of the sciatic nerve. *Reg Anesth Pain Med.* 2006;31:481–482.

Tuveri M, Borsezio V, Argiolas R, Medas F, Tuveri A. Ultrasonographic venous anatomy at the popliteal fossa in relation to tibial nerve course in normal and varicose limbs. *Chir Ital.* 2009;61:171–177.

van Geffen GJ, van den Broek E, Braak GJ, Giele JL, Gielen MJ, Scheffer GJ. A prospective randomised controlled trial of ultrasound guided versus nerve stimulation guided distal sciatic nerve block at the popliteal fossa. *Anaesth Intensive Care.* 2009;37:32–37.

Verelst P, van Zundert A: Ultrasound-guided popliteal block shortens onset time compared to prebifurcation sciatic block. *Reg Anesth Pain Med.* 2010;35:565–566.

# 41 Ultrasound-Guided Ankle Block

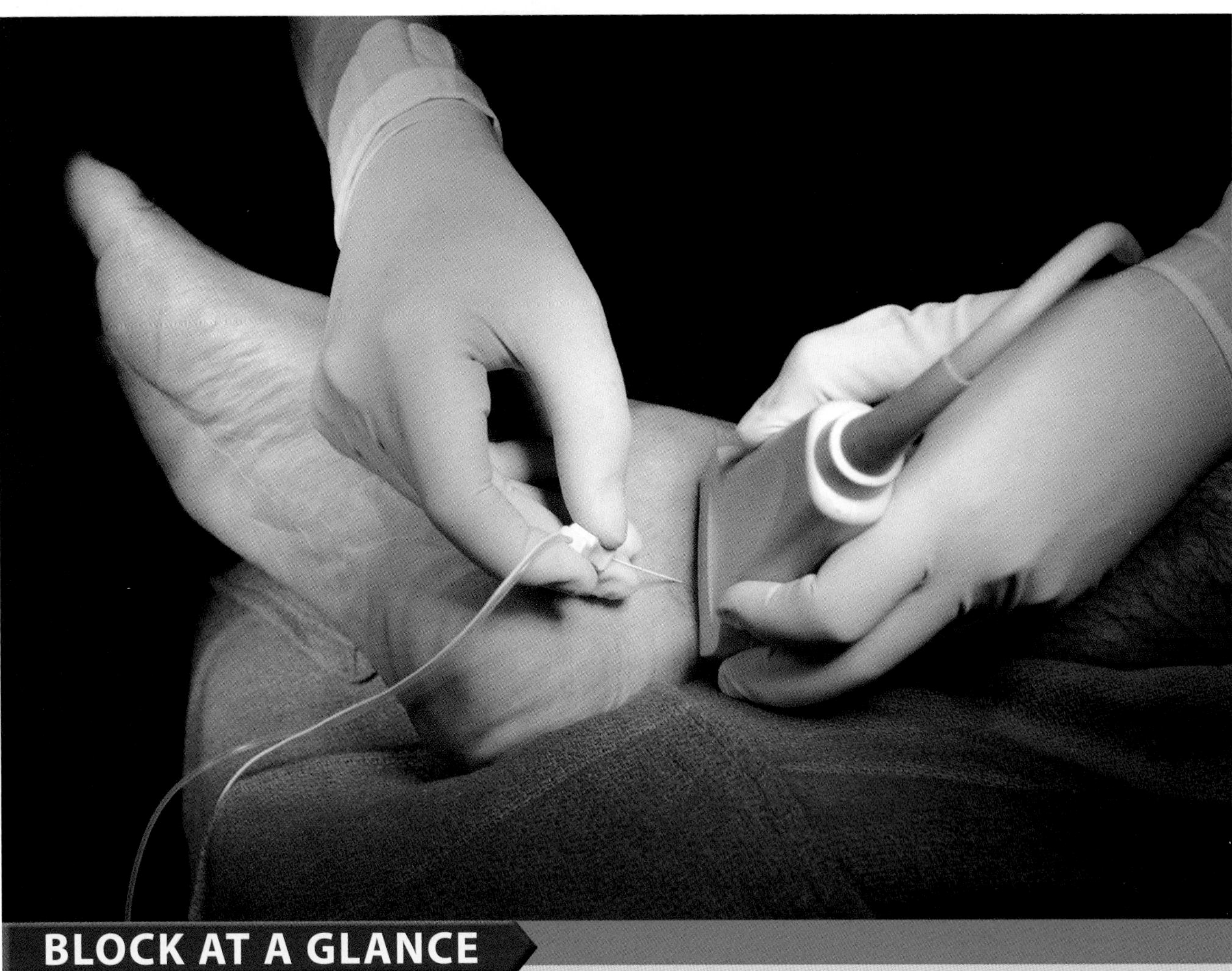

## BLOCK AT A GLANCE

- Indications: surgery on the foot and toes
- Transducer position: about the ankle and depends on the nerve to be blocked
- Goal: local anesthetic spread surrounding each individual nerve
- Local anesthetic: 3-10 mL per nerve

**FIGURE 41-1.** Block of the posterior tibial nerve using an out-of-plane technique.

## General Considerations

Using an ultrasound-guided technique affords a practitioner the ability to reduce the volume of local anesthetic required for ankle blockade. Because the nerves involved are located relatively close to the surface, ankle blocks are easy to perform technically; however, knowledge of the anatomy of the ankle is essential to ensure success.

## Ultrasound Anatomy

Ankle block involves anesthetizing five separate nerves: 2 deep nerves and 3 superficial nerves. The 2 deep nerves are tibial (TN) and deep peroneal nerve (DPN). The superficial nerves are superficial peroneal, sural and saphenous. All nerves except saphenous nerve are terminal branches of the sciatic nerve; saphenous nerve is a cutaneous extension of the femoral nerve.

### Tibial Nerve

The tibial nerve is the largest of the five nerves at the ankle level and provides innervation to the heel and sole of the foot. With a linear transducer placed transversely at (or just proximal to) the level of the medial malleolus, the nerve can be seen immediately posterior to the posterior tibial artery (Figures 41-1, 41-2, and 41-3A and B). Color Doppler can be very useful in depicting the posterior tibial artery when it is not readily apparent. The nerve typically appears hyperechoic with dark stippling. A useful mnemonic for the relevant structures in the vicinity is **T**om, **D**ick **AN**d **H**arry, which refers to, from anterior to posterior, the **t**ibialis anterior tendon, flexor **d**igitorum longus tendon, **a**rtery/**n**erve/vein, and flexor **h**allucis longus tendon. These tendons can resemble the nerve in appearance, which can be confusing. The nerve's intimate relationship with the artery should be kept in mind to avoid misidentification.

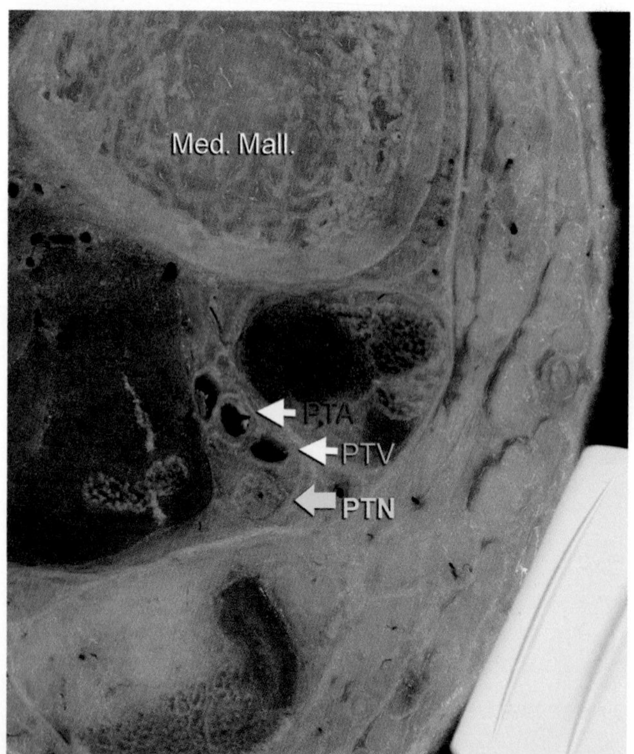


**FIGURE 41-2.** Cross-sectional anatomy of the posterior tibial nerve at the level of the ankle. Shown are posterior tibial artery (PTA) and vein (PTV) behind the medial malleolus (Med. Mall.) The posterior tibial nerve (PTN) is just posterior and superficial to the posterior tibial vessels.

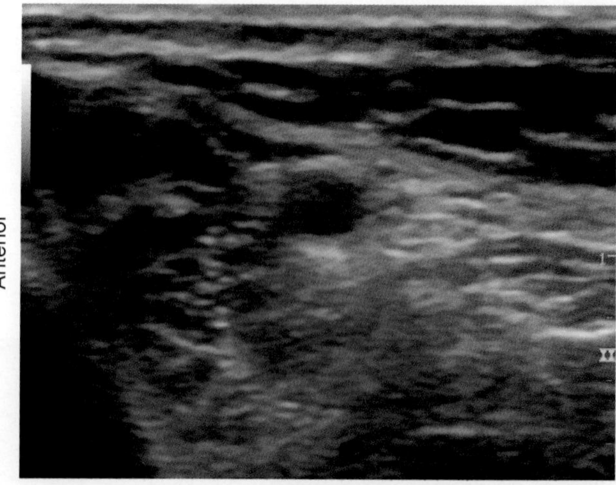


A Ankle block-posterior tibial nerve

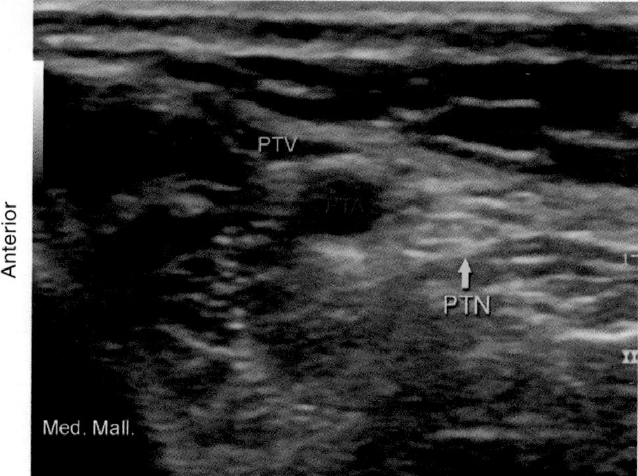


B Ankle block-posterior tibial nerve

**FIGURE 41-3.** (A) Ultrasound image of the posterior tibial nerve. (B) Posterior tibial nerve (PTN) is seen posterior to the posterior tibial artery (PTA). Med. Mall., medial malleolus; PTV, posterior tibial vein.

### Deep Peroneal Nerve

This branch of the common peroneal nerve innervates the web space between the first and second toes. As it approaches the ankle, the nerve crosses the anterior tibial artery from a medial to lateral position. A transducer placed in the transverse orientation at the level of the extensor retinaculum will

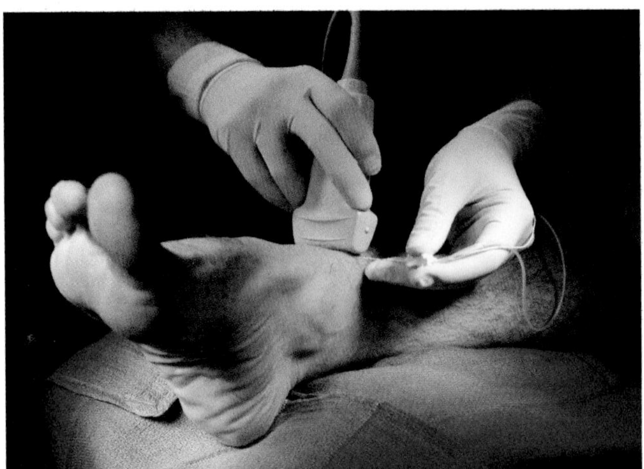

**FIGURE 41-4.** Deep peroneal nerve block: the transducer position and needle insertion to block the deep peroneal nerve at the level of the ankle.

show the nerve lying immediately lateral to the artery, on the surface of the tibia (Figures 41-4, 41-5, and 41-6A, B). The nerve usually appears hyperechoic, but it is small and often difficult to distinguish from the surrounding tissue.

**TIP**

- The deep peroneal nerve is often difficult to distinguish from neighboring tissues. Once local anesthetic injection begins next to the artery, the nerve becomes easier to distinguish from the surrounding tissue.

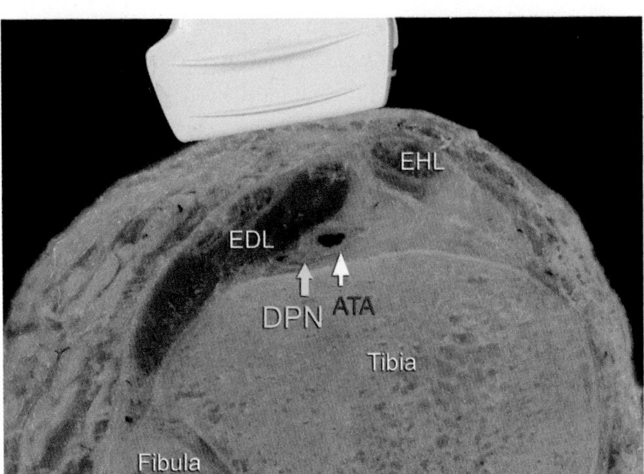


**FIGURE 41-5.** Cross-sectional anatomy of the deep peroneal nerve at the level of the ankle. The deep peroneal nerve is located just lateral to anterior tibial artery (ATA) and between the extensor digitorum longus (EDL) and tibia. Note the proximity of the extensor hallucis longus (EHL) that can serve as an important landmark. DPN, deep peroneal nerve.

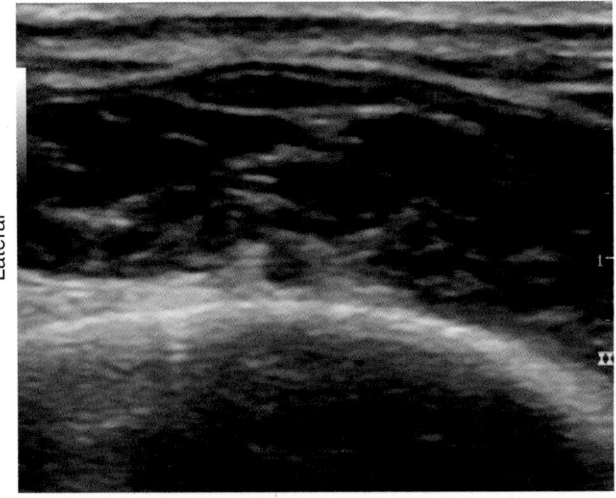


A Ankle block-deep peroneal nerve

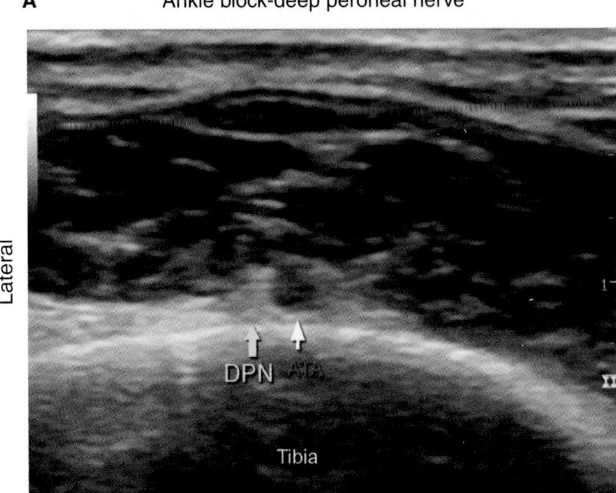


B Ankle block-deep peroneal nerve

**FIGURE 41-6.** (A) Ultrasound image of the deep peroneal nerve (DPN) is seen at the surface of the tibia just lateral to the anterior tibial artery (ATA). (B) Ultrasound anatomy of the DPN at the level of the ankle with the structures labeled.

## Superficial Peroneal Nerve

The superficial peroneal nerve innervates the dorsum of the foot. It emerges to lie superficial to the fascia 10 to 20 cm above the ankle joint on the anterolateral surface of the leg. A transducer placed transversely on the leg, approximately 5 cm proximal and anterior to the lateral malleolus, will identify the hyperechoic nerve lying in the subcutaneous tissue immediately superficial to the fascia (Figures 41-7, 41-8, and 41-9A and B). If the nerve is not readily apparent, the transducer can be traced proximally on the leg until, at the lateral aspect, the extensor digitorum longus and peroneus longus muscles can be seen with a prominent groove between them leading to the fibula (Figure 41-10A and B). The superficial peroneal nerve is located in this intermuscular septum, just deep to the fascia. Once it is identified at this more proximal location, it can be traced distally to the ankle. Because the superficial nerves are rather small, their identification with ultrasound is not always possible in a busy clinical environment.

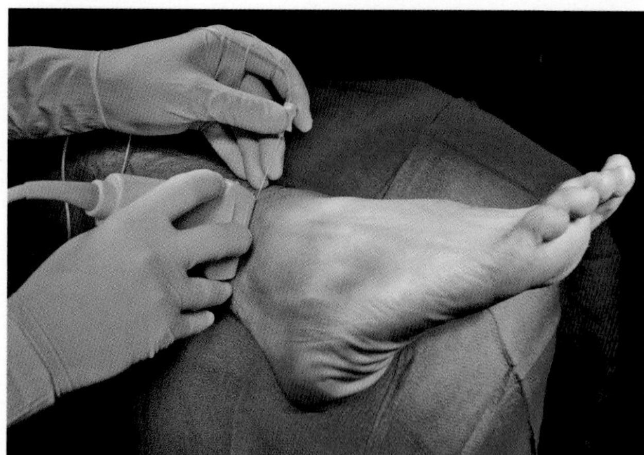

**FIGURE 41-7.** Transducer position and needle insertion to block the superficial peroneal nerve.

## TIP

- The use of a small-gauge needle is recommended to decrease the patient discomfort.

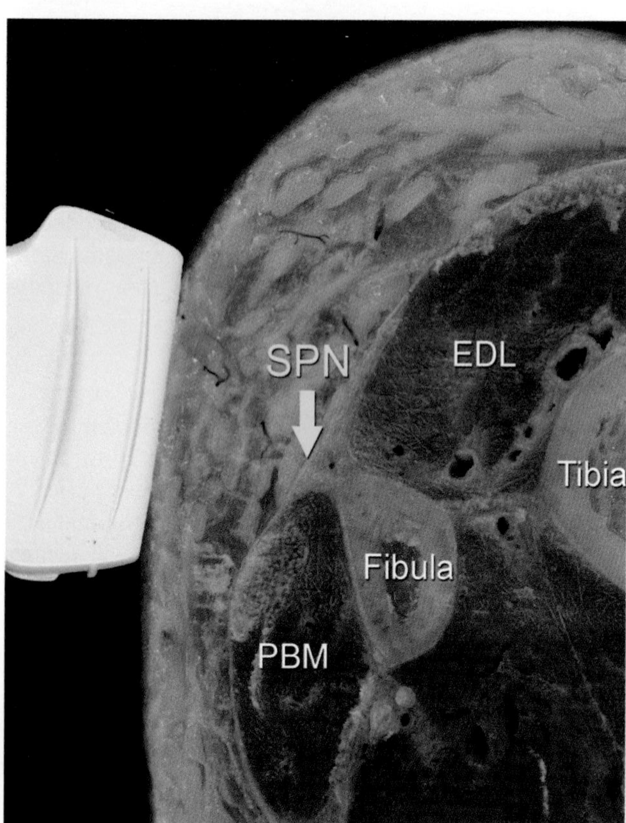


**FIGURE 41-8.** Cross-sectional anatomy of the superficial peroneal nerve (SPN). EDL, extensor digitorum longus muscle; PBM, peroneus brevis muscle.

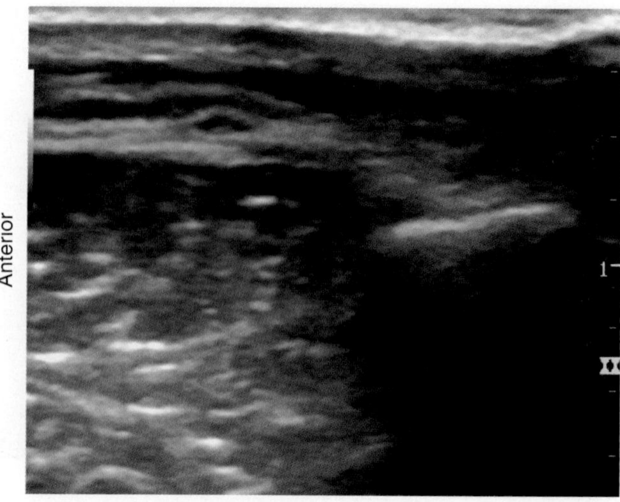


A Ankle block-superficial peroneal nerve

B Ankle block-superficial peroneal nerve

**FIGURE 41-9.** (A) Ultrasound anatomy of the superficial peroneal nerve (SPN). (B) Ultrasound anatomy of the superficial peroneal nerve with structures labeled. PBM, peroneus brevis muscle.

## Sural Nerve

The sural nerve innervates the lateral margin of the foot and ankle. Proximal to the lateral malleolus, the sural nerve can be visualized as a small hyperechoic structure that is intimately associated with the small saphenous vein (Figures 41-11, 41-12, and 41-13A, B). A calf tourniquet can be used to increase the size of the vein, aiding in identification of the nerve.

## Saphenous Nerve

The saphenous nerve innervates the medial malleolus and a variable portion of the medial aspect of the leg below the knee. The nerve travels down the medial leg alongside the saphenous vein. Because it is a small nerve, it is best visualized 10–15 cm proximal to the medial malleolus, using

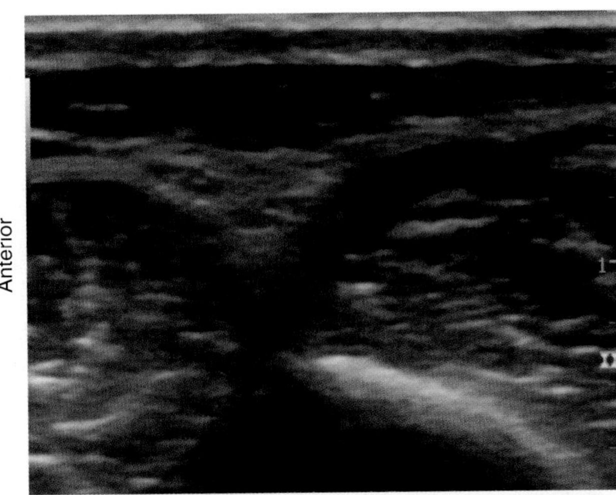


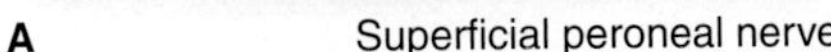


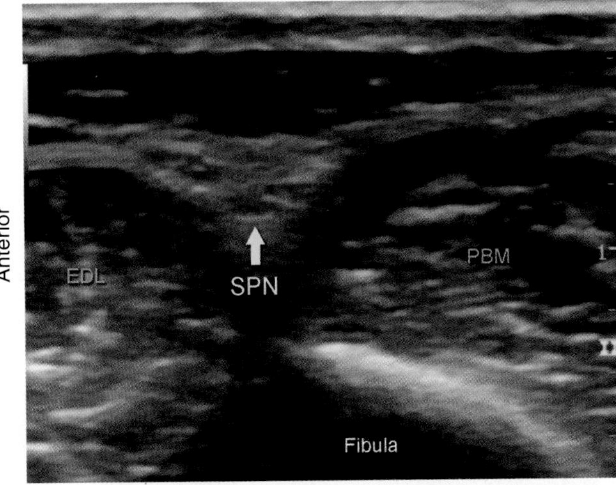


**FIGURE 41-10.** (A) Ultrasound anatomy of the superficial peroneal nerve. (B) Ultrasound anatomy of the nerve with structures labeled. EDL, extensor digitorum longus muscle; PBM, peroneus brevis muscle; SPN, superficial peroneal nerve.

the saphenous vein as a landmark (Figures 41-14, 41-15, and 41-16A, B). A proximal calf tourniquet can be used to assist in increasing the size of the vein. The nerve appears as a small hyperechoic structure.

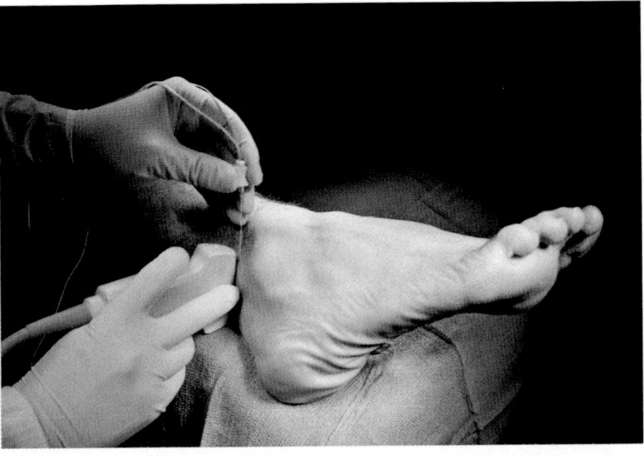

**FIGURE 41-11.** Transducer position and needle insertion to block the sural nerve.

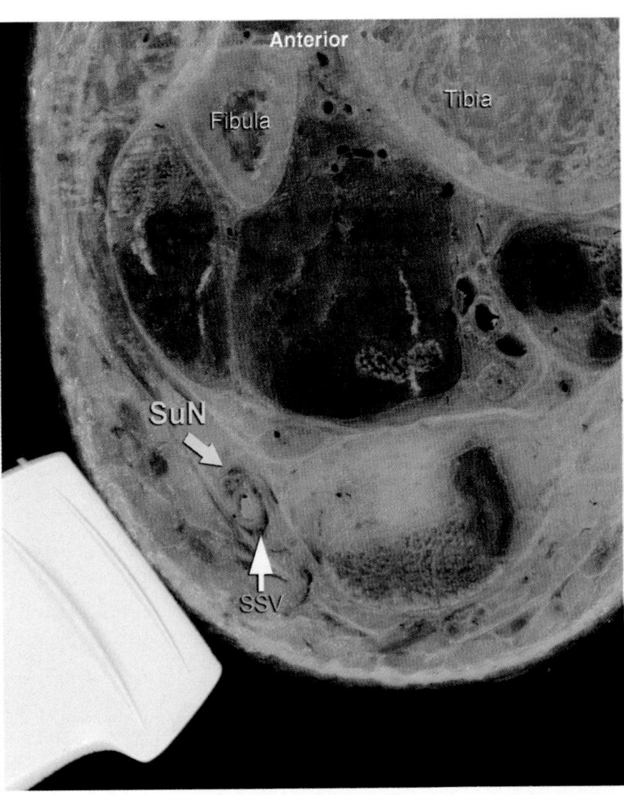


**FIGURE 41-12.** Cross-sectional anatomy of the sural nerve at the level of the ankle. Shown is sural nerve (SuN) in the immediate vicinity of the small saphenous vein (SSV).

## TIP

- When using veins as landmarks, use as little pressure as possible on the transducer to permit the veins to fill.

## Distribution of Blockade

An ankle block results in anesthesia of the entire foot. For a more comprehensive review of the distribution of each nerve, see Chapter 1.

## Equipment

Equipment needed is as follows:

- Ultrasound machine with linear transducer (8–18 MHz), sterile sleeve, and gel
- Standard nerve block tray (described in the equipment section)

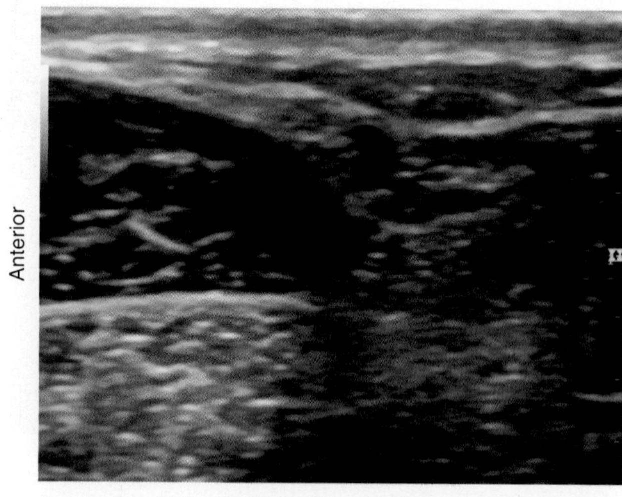


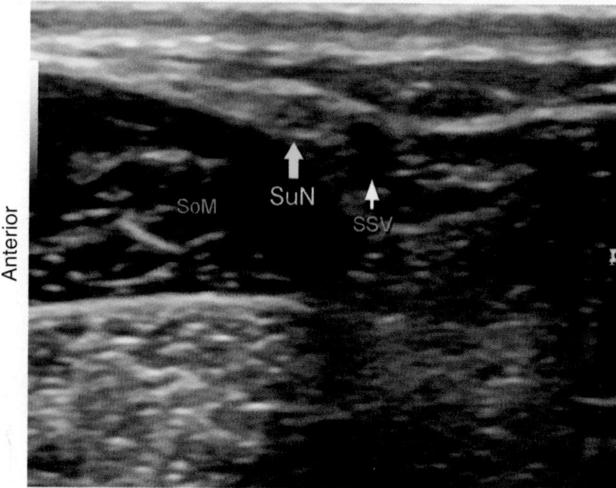


**FIGURE 41-13.** (A) Ultrasound anatomy of the sural nerve (SuN). The SuN is seen immediately anterior to the small saphenous vein (SSV). (B) The ultrasound anatomy of the SuN with the structures labeled. SoM, soleus muscle.

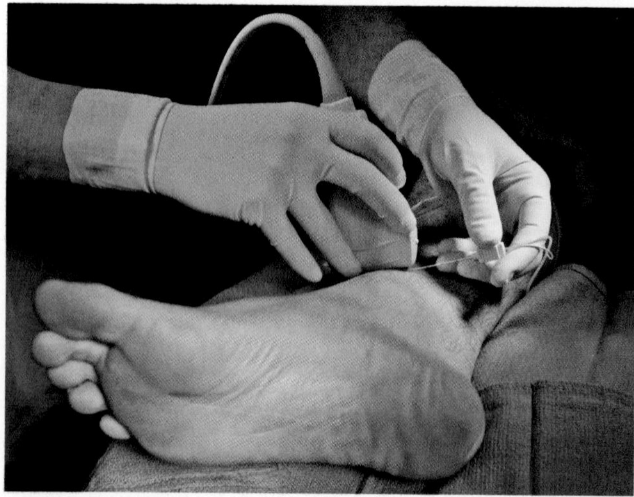

**FIGURE 41-14.** Transducer position and needle position to block the saphenous nerve.

## GOAL

**The goal is to place the needle tip immediately adjacent to each of the five nerves and deposit local anesthetic until the spread around each nerve is documented.**

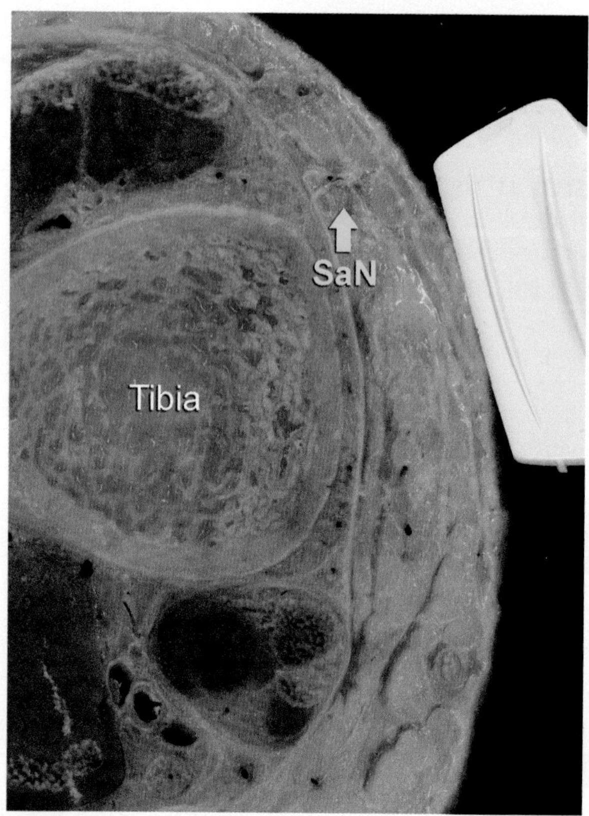


**FIGURE 41-15.** Cross-sectional anatomy of the saphenous nerve (SaN) at the level of the ankle.

- Three 10 mL syringes containing local anesthetic
- A 1.5-in 22- to 25-gauge needle with low-volume extension tubing *or* a control syringe
- Sterile gloves

## Landmarks and Patient Positioning

The block is usually performed with the patient in the supine position. A footrest underneath the calf facilitates access to the ankle, especially for the tibial and sural nerve blocks. An assistant is helpful to maintain internal or external rotation of the leg, as needed.

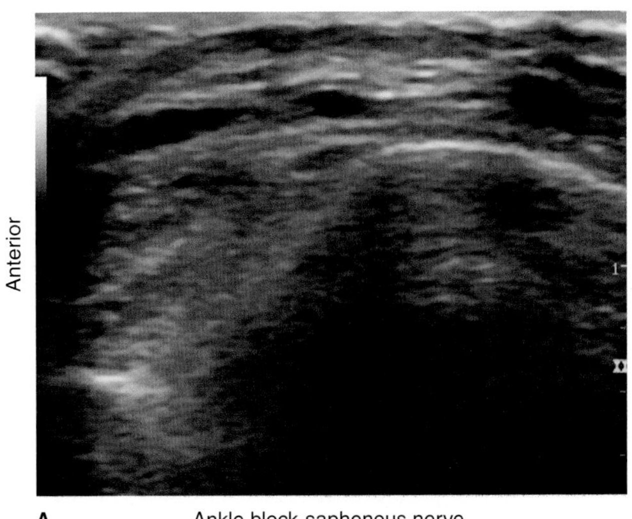


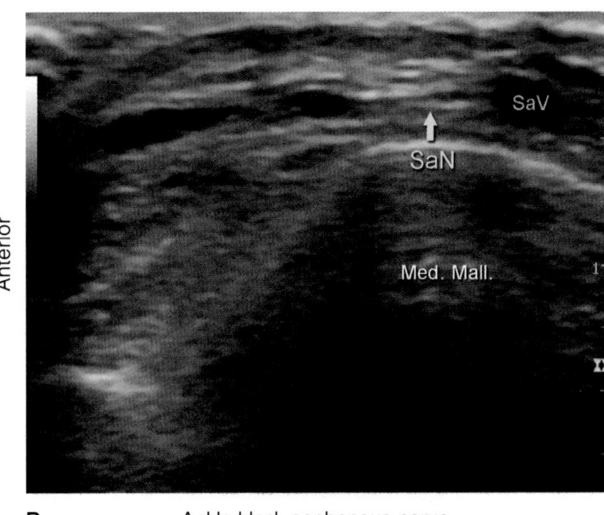


**FIGURE 41-16.** (A) Ultrasound anatomy of the saphenous nerve (SaN) at the level of the ankle. The SaN is seen just anterior to the small saphenous vein (SaV). (B) Ultrasound anatomy of the saphenous nerve with the structures labeled.

## Technique

With the patient in the proper position, the skin is disinfected. For each of the blocks, the needle can be inserted either in-plane or out-of-plane. Ergonomics often dictates which of these is the most effective. Successful block is predicted by the spread of local anesthetic immediately adjacent to the nerve; redirection to achieve circumferential spread is not necessary because these nerves are small and the local anesthetic diffuses quickly into the neural tissue. Assuming deposition immediately adjacent to the nerve, 3 to 5 mL of local anesthetic per nerve is typically required to ensure an effective block.

### TIP

- Never inject against high resistance to injection (IP >15 psi) because it may signal an intraneural injection.

The block dynamics and perioperative management are similar to those described in Chapter 22.

## SUGGESTED READING

Antonakakis JG, Scalzo DC, Jorgenson AS, et al. Ultrasound does not improve the success rate of a deep peroneal nerve block at the ankle. *Reg Anesth Pain Med.* 2010;35:217-221.

Benzon HT, Sekhadia M, Benzon HA, et al. Ultrasound-assisted and evoked motor response stimulation of the deep peroneal nerve. *Anesth Analg.* 2009;109:2022-2024.

Canella C, Demondion X, Guillin R, et al. Anatomic study of the superficial peroneal nerve using sonography. *AJR Am J Roentgenol.* 2009;193:174-179.

Redborg KE, Antonakakis JG, Beach ML, Chinn CD, Sites BD. Ultrasound improves the success rate of a tibial nerve block at the ankle. *Reg Anesth Pain Med.* 2009;34:256-260.

Redborg KE, Sites BD, Chinn CD, et al. Ultrasound improves the success rate of a sural nerve block at the ankle. *Reg Anesth Pain Med.* 2009;34:24-28.

Snaith R, Dolan J. Ultrasound-guided superficial peroneal nerve block for foot surgery. *AJR Am J Roentgenol.* 2010;194:W538.

# 42 Common Ultrasound-Guided Truncal and Cutaneous Blocks

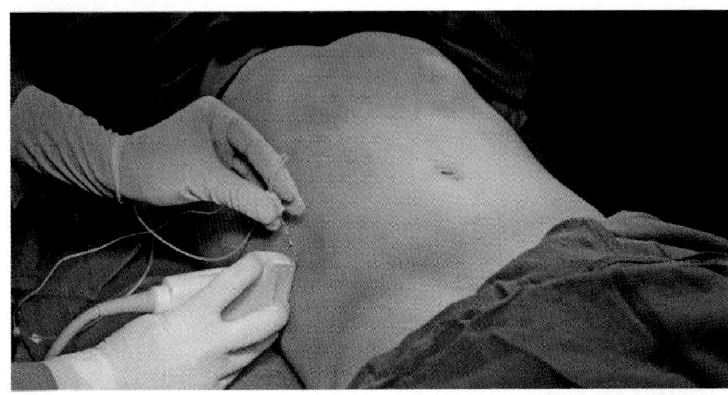

A

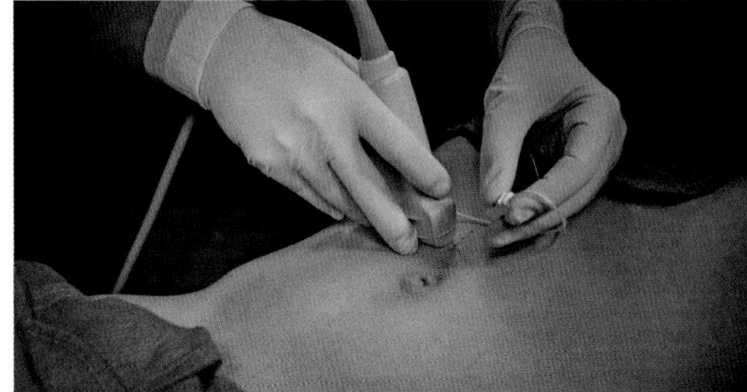

C

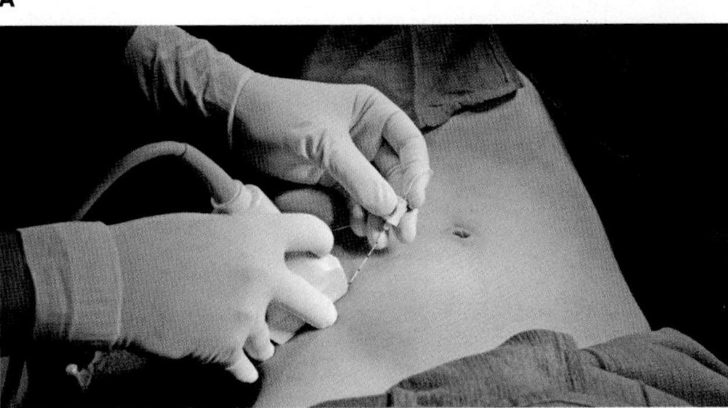

B

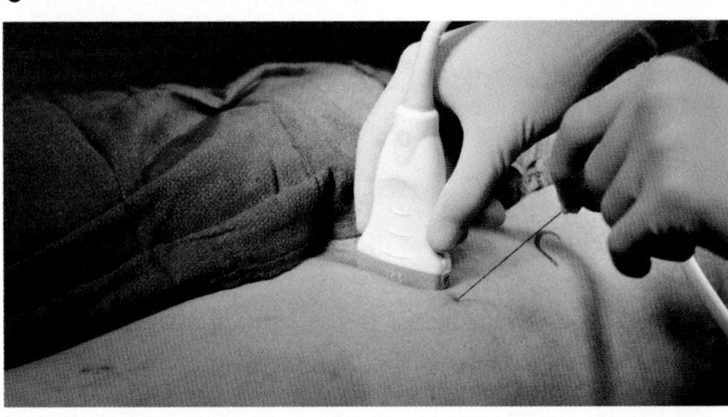

D

## BLOCK AT A GLANCE

### A - TRANSVERSUS ABDOMINIS PLANE (TAP)

- Indications: postoperative analgesia for laparotomy, appendectomy, laparoscopic surgery, abdominoplasty, and cesarean delivery; as an alternative to epidural anesthesia for operations on the abdominal wall
- Transducer position: transverse on the abdomen, at the anterior axillary line, between the costal margin and the iliac crest
- Goal: local anesthetic spread between the transversus abdominis and internal oblique muscle planes
- Local anesthetic: 20-30 mL of 0.25% ropivacaine per side (adults)

### B - ILIOHYPOGASTRIC AND ILIOINGUINAL NERVE

- Indications: anesthesia and postoperative analgesia for inguinal hernia repair and other inguinal surgery; analgesia following suprapubic incision
- Transducer position: oblique on abdomen, on a line joining the anterior superior iliac spine (ASIS) with the umbilicus
- Goal: local anesthetic spread between the transversus abdominis and internal oblique muscle planes, in the vicinity of the two nerves
- Local anesthetic: 10 mL per side (adults); 0.15 mL/kg per side (children)

### C - RECTUS SHEATH

- Indications: postoperative analgesia for umbilical hernia repair and other umbilical surgery
- Transducer position: transverse on abdomen, immediately lateral to umbilicus
- Goal: local anesthetic spread between rectus muscle and posterior rectus sheath
- Local anesthetic: 10 mL per side (adults); 0.1 mL/kg per side (children)

### D - LATERAL FEMORAL CUTANEOUS NERVE

- Indications: postoperative analgesia for hip surgery, meralgia paresthetica, and muscle biopsy of the proximal lateral thigh
- Transducer position: transverse, immediately inferior to the anterior superior iliac spine (ASIS); the lateral edge of sartorius (SaM) muscle should be visualized with ultrasound (US)
- Goal: local anesthetic spread between the tensor fascia latae (TFL) and the sartorius muscle
- Local anesthetic: 5–10 mL (adults)

**FIGURE 42.1-1.** (A) Transducer position and needle insertion to accomplish a transverse abdominal plane block. (B) Transducer position and needle insertion to accomplish iliohypogastric and ilioinguinal nerve blocks. (C) Transducer position and needle insertion to accomplish rectus sheath block. (D) Transducer position and needle insertion to accomplish a lateral femoral cutaneous nerve (LFCN) block.

# PART 1: ULTRASOUND-GUIDED TRANSVERSUS ABDOMINIS PLANE BLOCK

## General Considerations

The ultrasound-guided transversus abdominis plane block, or TAP has become a commonly used regional anesthesia technique for a variety of indications. It is largely devoid of complications and can be performed time-efficiently, either at the beginning or the end of surgery for use as postoperative analgesia. Similar to ilioinguinal and iliohypogastric nerve blocks, the method relies on guiding the needle with ultrasound to the plane between the transversus abdominis and internal oblique muscles, to block the anterior rami of the lower six thoracic nerves (T7-T12) and the first lumbar nerve (L1). Injection of local anesthetic within the TAP potentially can provide unilateral analgesia to the skin, muscles, and parietal peritoneum of the anterior abdominal wall from T7 to L1, although in clinical practice, the extent of the block is variable.

## Ultrasound Anatomy

The anterior abdominal wall (skin, muscles, and parietal peritoneum) is innervated by the anterior rami of the lower six thoracic nerves (T7-T12) and the first lumbar nerve (L1). Terminal branches of these somatic nerves course through the lateral abdominal wall within a plane between the internal oblique and transversus abdominis muscles. This intermuscular plane is called the transversus abdominis plane. Injection of local anesthetic within the TAP can result in unilateral analgesia to the skin, muscles, and parietal peritoneum of the anterior abdominal wall. The exact cephalad-caudad spread and extent of anesthesia and analgesia obtained with the TAP block is variable. This subject is not well researched; the actual coverage is likely dependent on the technique details, place of needle insertion (lateral-medial) and volume of local anesthetic injected. Additionally, the patient's anatomical characteristics may also influence the spread of the injected solutions.

Imaging of the abdominal wall between the costal margin and the iliac crest reveals three muscle layers, separated by a hyperechoic fascia: the outermost external oblique (EOM), the internal oblique (IOM), and the transversus abdominis muscles (TAM) (Figures 42.1-2 and 42.1-3). Immediately below this last muscle is the transversalis fascia, followed by the peritoneum and the intestines below, which can be recognized as moving structures because of peristalsis. The nerves of the abdominal wall are not visualized consistently, although this is not necessary to accomplish a block.

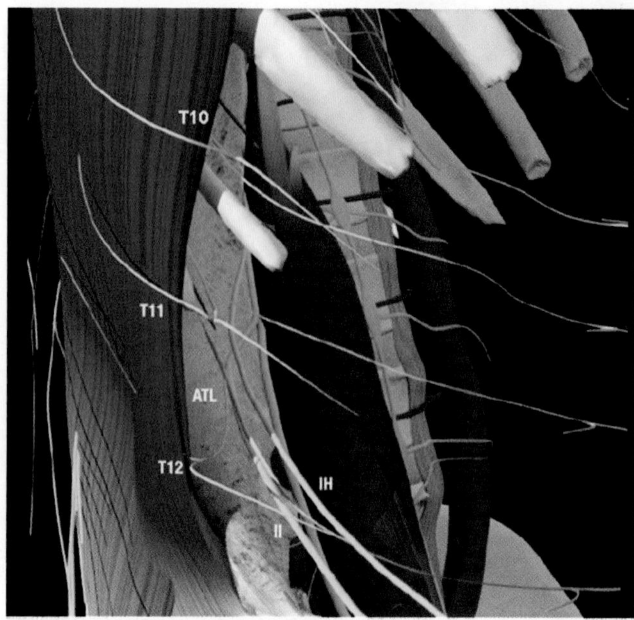


**FIGURE 42.1-2.** Innervation of the anterior and lateral abdominal wall. IH, iliohypogastric nerve; IL, ilioinguinal nerve.

**TIP**

- Obese patients have a large subcutaneous layer of fat that can make positive identification of the three muscle layers challenging. A rule of thumb is that the internal oblique muscle is always the "thickest" layer, and the transversus abdominis is the "thinnest."

## Distribution of Blockade

The exact distribution of abdominal wall anesthesia following a TAP block has not been well documented or entirely agreed on by practitioners. The most fervent proponents of

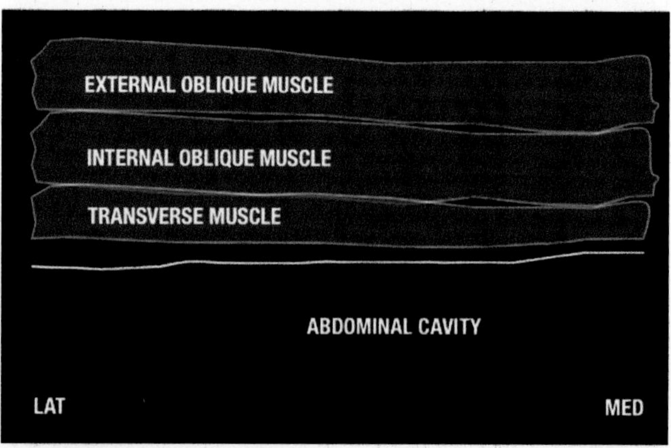


**FIGURE 42.1-3.** Schematic representation of the abdominal wall muscles.

TAP technique maintain that reliable blockade of dermatomes T10-L1 can be achieved with moderate volumes of local anesthetic (e.g., 20–25 mL). Claims of blockade up to T7 after single injection of large volume have been made, but these results are not consistently reproduced in clinical practice. In our practice, some TAP blocks have resulted in complete anesthesia for inguinal herniorrhaphy; at other times, the results have been less consistent. Additional research is indicated to clarify the spread of anesthesia and factors that influence it.

## Equipment

Equipment needed is as follows:

- Ultrasound machine with linear transducer (6–18 MHz), sterile sleeve, and gel (in very obese patients, and when a more posterior approach is used, a curved transducer might be needed)
- Standard nerve block tray
- Two 20-mL syringes containing local anesthetic
- A 50- to 100-mm, 20- to 21-gauge needle
- Sterile gloves

## Landmarks and Patient Positioning

This block typically is performed with the patient in the supine position. The iliac crest and costal margin should be palpated and the space between them in the mid-axillary line (usually 8–10 cm) identified as the initial transducer location. The block is almost always performed under general anesthesia in pediatric patients; a common option for adults as well.

### GOAL

**The goal is to place the needle tip in the plane between the IOM and the TAM, to deposit local anesthetic between the muscle layers, and confirm the proper spread of the injectate under ultrasound guidance.**

## Technique

With the patient supine, the skin is disinfected and the transducer placed on the skin (Figure 42.1-4). The three muscle layers should be identified (Figures 42.1-5A and B). Sliding the transducer slightly cephalad or caudad will aid the identification. Once the transverse abdominal plane is identified, a skin wheal is made 2 to 3 cm medial to the medial aspect of the transducer, and the needle is inserted in-plane in a medial to lateral orientation (Figures 42.1-1A and 42.1-6). The needle is guided through the subcutaneous tissue, EOM, and IOM. A "pop" may be felt as the needle tip enters the plane between the two muscles. After gentle aspiration, 1 to 2 mL of local anesthetic is injected to

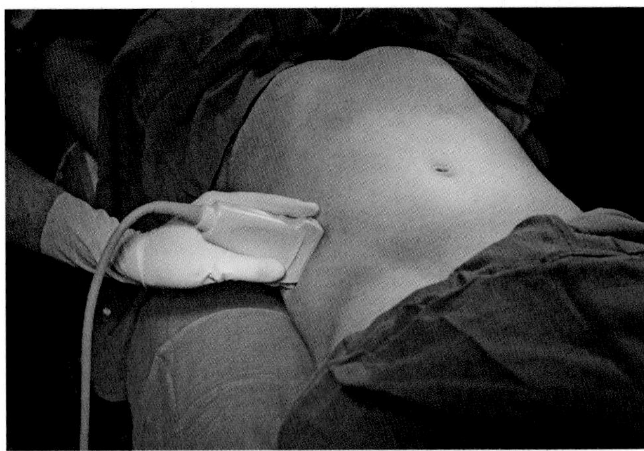

**FIGURE 42.1-4.** Transducer position in the transverse abdominal, at the anterior axillary line, between the costal margin and the iliac crest.

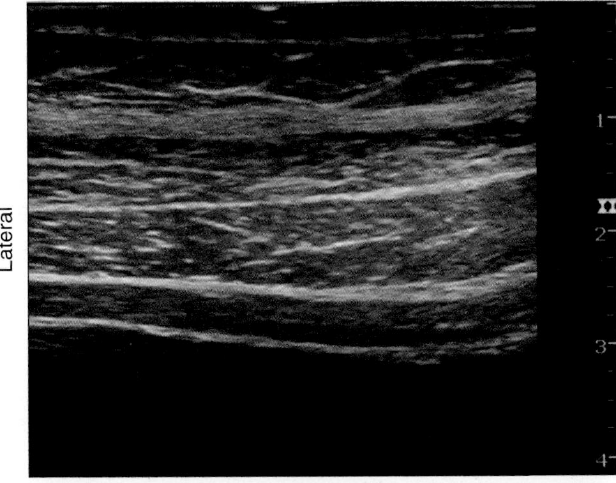


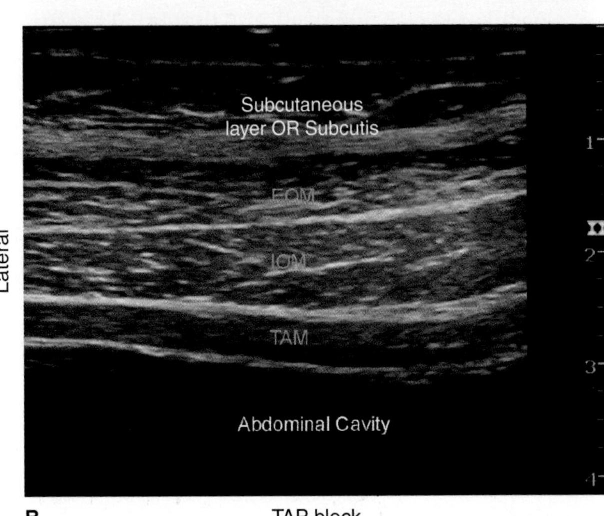


**FIGURE 42.1-5.** (A) Ultrasound anatomy of the abdominal wall layers. (B) Labeled ultrasound anatomy of the abdominal wall layers, EOM, external oblique muscle; IOM, internal oblique muscle; TAM, transverse abdominis muscle.

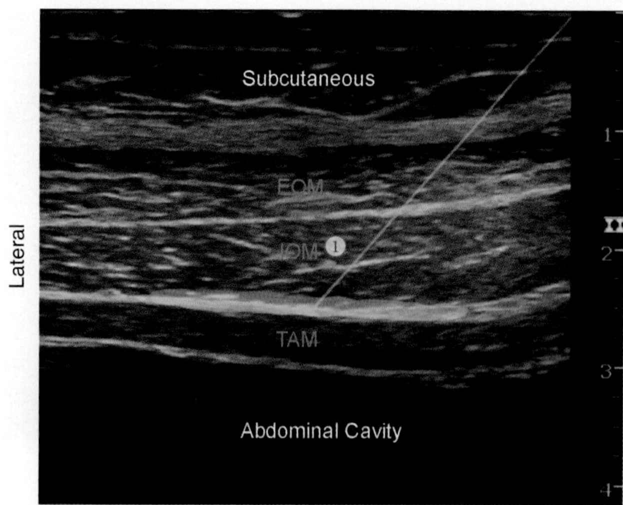


**FIGURE 42.1-6.** Simulated needle insertion (1) and distribution of LA (blue shaded area) to accomplish transversus abdominis plane (TAP) block. Shown are the external oblique muscle (EOM), internal oblique muscle (IOM), and the transverse abdominal muscle (TAM). Needle tip is positioned in the tissue sheath between IOM and TAM.

verify the location of the needle tip (Figure 42.1-6). When injection of the local anesthetic appears to be intramuscular, the needle is advanced or withdrawn carefully 1 to 2 mm and another bolus is administered. This gesture is repeated until the correct plane is achieved.

## TIP

- An out-of-plane technique is more useful in obese patients. Because the needle tip may not be seen throughout the procedure, we recommend administering intermittent small boluses (0.5–1 mL) as the needle is advanced through the internal oblique muscle to confirm the position of the needle tip.

In an adult patient, 20 mL of local anesthetic per side is usually sufficient for successful blockade. We most commonly use ropivacaine 0.25%. In children, a volume of 0.4 mL/kg per side is adequate for effective analgesia when using ultrasound guidance.

## SUGGESTED READING

Abrahams MS, Horn JL, Noles LM, Aziz MF: Evidence-based medicine: ultrasound guidance for truncal blocks. *Reg Anesth Pain Med* 2010;35:S36-42.

Belavy D, Cowlishaw PJ, Howes M, Phillips F. Ultrasound-guided transversus abdominis plane block for analgesia after Caesarean delivery. *Br J Anaesth*. 2009;103:726-730.

Carney J, McDonnell JG, Ochana A, et al. The transversus abdominis plane block provides effective postoperative analgesia in patients undergoing total abdominal hysterectomy. *Anesth Analg*. 2008;107(6):2056.

Chiono J, Bernard N, Bringuier S, Biboulet P, Choquet O, Morau D, Capdevilla X: The ultrasound-guided transversus abdominis plane block for anterior iliac crest bone graft postoperative pain relief: a prospective descriptive study. *Reg Anesth Pain Med* 2010;35:(6)520-524.

Finnerty O, Carney J, McDonnell JG: Trunk blocks for abdominal surgery. *Anaesthesia* 2010; 65 Suppl 1:76-83.

Griffiths JD, Middle JV, Barron FA, Grant SJ, Popham PA, Royse CF: Transversus abdominis plane block does not provide additional benefit to multimodal analgesia in gynecological cancer surgery. *Anesth Analg* 2010;111(3):797-801.

Hebbard P. Subcostal transversus abdominis plane block under ultrasound guidance. *Anesth Analg*. 2008;106(2):674.

Hebbard P, Fujiwara Y, Shibata Y, Royse C. Ultrasound-guided transversus abdominis plane (TAP) block. *Anaesth Intensive Care*. 2007;35:616-617.

Hebbard PD, Royse CF: Lack of efficacy with transversus abdominis plane block: is it the technique, the end points, or the statistics? *Reg Anesth Pain Med* 2010;35:324.

Heil JW, Ilfeld BM, Loland VJ, Sandhu NS, Mariano ER: Ultrasound-guided transversus abdominis plane catheters and ambulatory perineural infusion for outpatient inguinal hernia repair. *Reg Anesth Pain Med* 2010;35(6):556-558.

Kanazi GE, Aouad MT, Abdallah FW, Khatib MI, Adham AM, Harfoush DW, Siddik-Sayyid SM: The Analgesic Efficacy of Subarachnoid Morphine in Comparison with Ultrasound-Guided Transversus Abdominis Plane Block After Cesarean Delivery: A Randomized Controlled Trial. *Anesth Analg* 2010;111:475-481.

Lancaster P, Chadwick M. Liver trauma secondary to ultrasound-guided transversus abdominis plane block. *Br J Anaesth*. 2010;104:509-510.

Lee TH, Barrington MJ, Tran TM, Wong D, Hebbard PD. Comparison of extent of sensory block following posterior and subcostal approaches to ultrasound-guided transversus abdominis plane block. *Anaesth Intensive Care*. 2010; 38:452-460.

McDonnell JG, Curley G, Carney J, et al. The analgesic efficacy of transversus abdominis plane block after cesarean delivery: a randomized controlled trial. *Anesth Analg*. 2008;106(1):186.

McDonnell JG, O'Donnell B, Curley G, et al. The analgesic efficacy of transversus abdominis plane block after abdominal surgery: a prospective randomized controlled trial. *Anesth Analg*. 2007;104(1):193.

McDonnell JG, O'Donnell BD, Farrell T, et al. Transversus abdominis plane block: a cadaveric and radiological evaluation. *Reg Anesth Pain Med*. 2007;32(5):399.

Mukhtar K, Khattak I: Transversus abdominis plane block for renal transplant recipients. *Br J Anaesth* 2010;104:663-664.

Niraj G, Kelkar A, Fox AJ. Application of the transversus abdominis plane block in the intensive care unit. *Anaesth Intensive Care*. 2009;37:650-652.

O'Connor K, Renfrew C: Subcostal transversus abdominis plane block. *Anaesthesia* 2010;65:91-92.

Petersen PL, Mathiesen O, Torup H, Dahl JB. The transversus abdominis plane block: a valuable option for postoperative analgesia? A topical review. *Acta Anaesthesiol Scand*. 2010;54:529-535.

Rafi AN. Abdominal field block: a new approach via the lumbar triangle. *Anaesthesia*. 2001;56(10):1024.

Rozen WM, Tran TM, Ashton MW, et al. Refining the course of the thoracolumbar nerves: a new understanding of the

innervation of the anterior abdominal wall. *Clin Anat.* 2008;21(4):325.
Shibata Y, Sato Y, Fujiwara Y, et al. Transversus abdominis plane block. *Anesth Analg.* 2007;105(3):883; author reply 883.
Suresh S, Chan VW. Ultrasound guided transversus abdominis plane block in infants, children and adolescents: a simple procedural guide for their performance. *Paediatr Anaesth.* 2009;19:296-299.
Tran TM, Ivanusic JJ, Hebbard P, et al. Determination of spread of injectate after ultrasound-guided transversus abdominis plane block: a cadaveric study. *Br J Anaesth.* 2009;102(1):123.
Walker G: Transversus abdominis plane block: a note of caution! *Br J Anaesth* 2010;104:265.
Walter EJ, Smith P, Albertyn R, et al. Ultrasound imaging for transversus abdominis blocks. *Anaesthesia.* 2008;63(2):211.

# PART 2: ULTRASOUND-GUIDED ILIOHYPOGASTRIC AND ILIOINGUINAL NERVE BLOCKS

## General Considerations

Ilioinguinal and iliohypogastric nerves are contained in a well-defined tissue plane between the transversus abdominis and internal oblique muscles. The ability to easily image the musculature of the abdominal wall makes blocking these two nerves much more exact than the "feel-based" blind technique.

## Ultrasound Anatomy

Imaging of the abdominal wall medial and superior to the ASIS reveals three muscle layers, separated by hyperechoic fascia: the outermost external oblique (EOM), the internal oblique (IOM), and the transversus abdominis muscles (TAM) (Figures 42.2-1A and B). Immediately below transversus abdominus muscle is the fascia transversalis, located just above the peritoneum and the abdominal cavity below, easily recognized as moving structures due to peristalsis. The hyperechoic osseous prominence of the anterior-superior iliac spine (ASIS) is a useful landmark which can be used as a reference, and is seen on the lateral side of the US image in Figure 42.2-1. The iliohypogastric and ilioinguinal nerves pierce the TAM above the ilium and lie in the plane between the TAM and the IOM. They are often seen side by side or up to 1 cm apart, and they typically appear as hypoechoic ovals. Use of color Doppler may be useful to identify the deep circumflex iliac artery, which lies adjacent to the nerves in the same plane as an additional landmark useful in identifying the nerves.

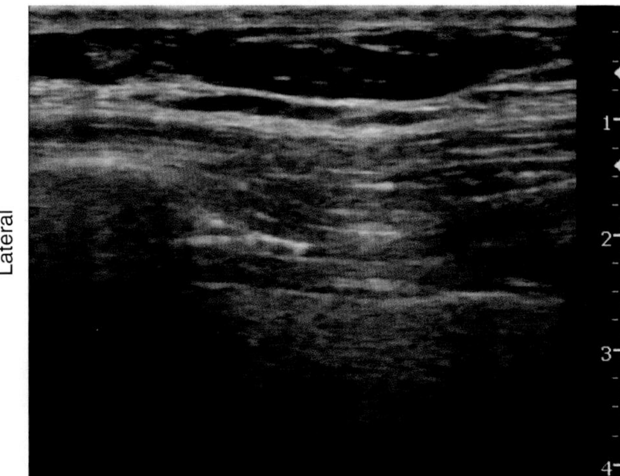


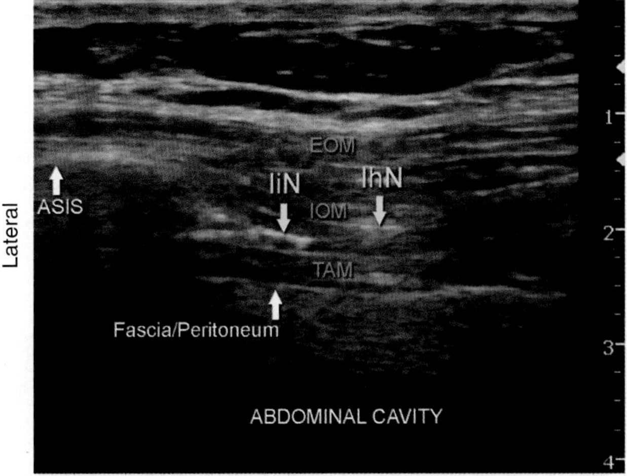


**FIGURE 42.2-1.** (A) Ultrasound anatomy of the iliohypogastric and ilioinguinal nerve. (B) Labeled ultrasound anatomy of the iliohypogastric and ilioinguinal nerve, ASIS, anterior superior iliac spine; EOM, external oblique muscle; IOM, internal oblique muscle; TAM, transverse abdominal muscle; IiN, ilioinguinal nerve; IhN, iliohypogastric nerve.

## Distribution of Blockade

Block of the iliohypogastric and ilioinguinal nerves results in anesthesia of the hypogastric region, the inguinal crease, the upper medial thigh, the mons pubis, part of the labia, the root of the penis, and the anterior part of the scrotum. There is considerable variation in sensory distribution between individuals.

## Equipment

Equipment needed is as follows:

- Ultrasound machine with linear transducer (6–18 MHz), sterile sleeve, and gel
- Standard nerve block tray
- Syringe(s) with 20 mL of local anesthetic
- 50-100 mm, 21-22 gauge needle
- Sterile gloves

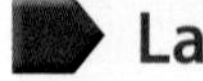

## Landmarks and Patient Positioning

The block of the iliohypogastric and ilioinguinal nerves is done in supine position. Palpation of the ASIS provides the initial landmark for transducer placment. This block is often performed under general anesthesia, particularly in pediatric patients.

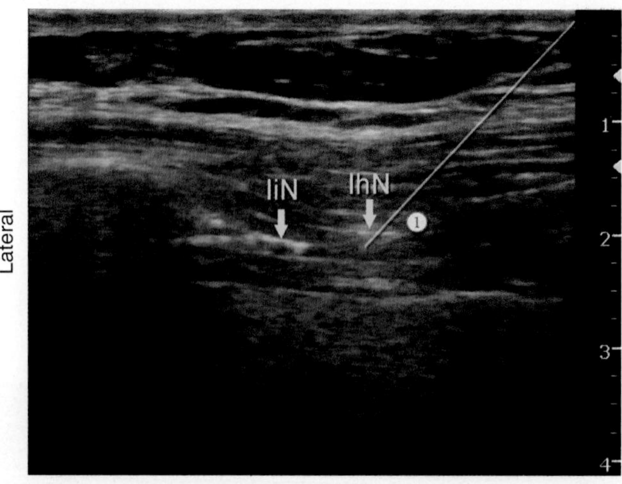


**FIGURE 42.2-3.** Simulated needle path (1) to reach the ilioinguinal (IiN) and iliohypogastric (IhN) nerves.

## GOAL

The goal is to place the needle tip in the plane between the IOM and the TAM, and deposit local anesthetic between the muscle layers.

## Technique

With the patient supine, the skin is disinfected and the transducer placed medial to the ASIS, oriented on a line joining the ASIS with the umbilicus (Figure 42.2-2). The three muscle layers should be identified. The nerves should appear as hypoechoic ovals between the IOM and TAM muscles. Moving the transducer slightly cephalad or caudad to trace the nerves can be useful. In addition, color Doppler may be used to attempt to visualize the deep circumflex iliac artery. A skin wheal is made on the medial aspect of the transducer, and the needle is inserted in-plane in a medial to lateral orientation, through the subcutaneous tissue, EOM, and IOM, and is advanced toward the ilioinguinal and iliohypogastric nerves (Figure 42.1-1B and Figure 42.2-3). A pop may be felt as the needle tip enters the plane between the muscles. After

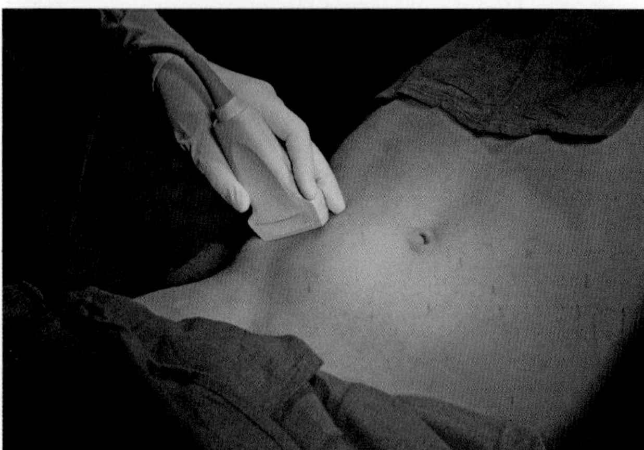

**FIGURE 42.2-2.** Transducer position to image the ilioinguinal (IiN) and iliohypogastric nerves (IhN). The transducer is positioned in the immediate vicinity of the anterior superior iliac spine (ASIS).

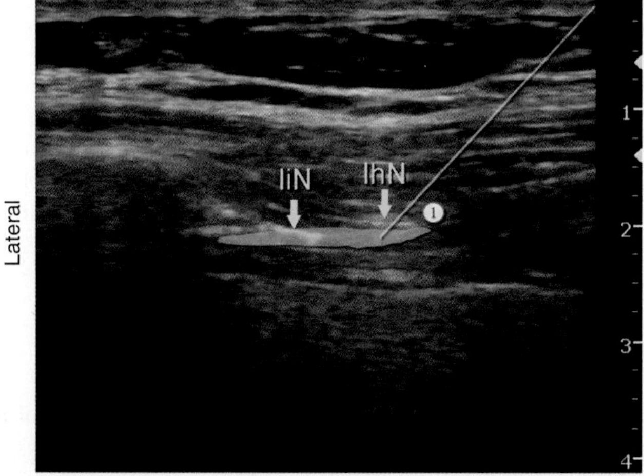


**FIGURE 42.2-4.** Simulated needle path (1) and spread of local anesthetic (area shaded in blue) to anesthetize the ilioinguinal and iliohypogastric nerves.

gentle aspiration, 1 to 2 mL of local anesthetic is injected to confirm the needle tip position (Figure 42.2-4). When injection of the local anesthetic appears to be intramuscular, the needle is advanced or withdrawn carefully 1 to 2 mm and another bolus is administered. This is repeated until the correct needle position is achieved. The block can be done either with in-plane or out-of-plane needle insertion.

## TIP

- An out-of-plane technique may be a better option in obese patients. Because the needle tip may not always be seen throughout the procedure, we recommend administering intermittent small boluses (0.5–1 mL) as the needle is advanced through the internal oblique muscle, confirming the position of the needle tip.

In an adult patient, 10 mL of local anesthetic per side is usually sufficient for successful blockade. In children, a volume of 0.15 mL/kg per side (ropivacaine 0.5%) is adequate for effective analgesia when using ultrasound guidance.

## SUGGESTED READING

Aveline C, Le Hetet H, Le Roux A, Vautier P, Cognet F, Vinet E, Tison C, Bonnet F: Comparison between ultrasound-guided transversus abdominis plane and conventional ilioinguinal/iliohypogastric nerve block for day-case open inguinal hernia repair. *Br J Anaesth* 2011;106:380-6.

Eichenberger U, Greher M, Kirchmair L, Curatolo M, Morggl B: Ultrasound-guided blocks of the ilioinguinal and iliohypogastric nerve: accuracy of a select new technique confirmaed by anatomical dissection. *Br J Anaesth* 2006;97:238-431.

Ford S, Dosani M, Robinson AJ, Campbell GC, Ansermino JM, Lim J, Lauder GR: Defining the reliability of sonoanatomy idenification by novices in ultrasound-guided pediatric ilioinguinal and iliohypogastric nerve blockade. *Anesth Analg* 2009;109:1793-8.

Gofeld M, Christakis M: Sonographically guided ilioinguinal nerve block. *J Ultrasound Med* 2006;25:1571-5.

Gucev G, Yasui GM, Chang TY, Lee J: Bilateral ultrasound-guided continuous ilioinguinal-iliohypogastic block for pain relief after cesarean delivery. *Anesth Analg* 2008;106:1220-2.

Mei W, Jin C, Feng L, Zhang Y, Luo A, Zhang C, Tian Y: Case report: bilateral ultrasound-guided transversus abdominis plane block combined with ilioinguinal-iliohypogastric nerve block for cesarean delivery anesthesia. *Anesth Analg* 2011;113:143-7.

Weintraud M, Lundlab M, Kettner SC, Willschke H, Kapral S, Lonnqvist PA, Koppatz K, Turnheim K, Bsenberg A, Marhofer P: Ultrasound versus landmark-based technique for ilioinguinal-iliohypogastric nerve blockade in children: the implication on plasma levels of ropivacaine. *Anesth Analg* 2009;108:1488-92.

# PART 3: ULTRASOUND-GUIDED RECTUS SHEATH BLOCK

## General Considerations

The rectus sheath block is a useful technique for umbilical surgery, particularly in pediatric patients. Ultrasound guidance allows for a greater reliability in administering local anesthetic in the correct plane and decreasing the potential for complications. The placement of the needle is in the proximity to the peritoneum and the epigastric arteries. Guiding the needle under ultrasound guidance to the posterior rectus sheath rather than relying on "pops," such as in the traditional, non-ultrasound techniques, makes this block more reproducible and reduces the risk of inadvertent peritoneal and vascular punctures.

## Ultrasound Anatomy

The rectus abdominis muscle is oval shaped, positioned under the superficial fascia of the abdomen. Laterally, the aponeurosis of the external oblique, internal oblique and transversus abdominis muscles split to form two lamellae that surround the muscle anteriorly and posteriorly (forming the rectus sheath), before rejoining again in the midline to insert on the linea alba (Figures 42.3-1A and B). The 9th, 10th, and 11th intercostal nerves are located in the space between the rectus abdominis muscle and its posterior rectus sheath, although they are usually difficult to depict sonographically. Color Doppler reveals small epigastric arteries in the same plane. Deep to the rectus sheath is preperitoneal fat, peritoneum, and abdominal content (bowel), which can usually be observed moving with peristalsis.

## Distribution of Blockade

Blockade of the nerves of the rectus sheath results in anesthesia of the periumbilical area (spinal dermatomes 9, 10, and 11). It is a rather specific, limited region of blockade, hence its specific indications.

## Equipment

Equipment needed is as follows:

- Ultrasound machine with linear transducer (6–18 MHz), sterile sleeve, and gel
- Standard nerve block tray
- 20-mL syringe containing local anesthetic
- 50-100 mm, 22-gauge short-bevel needle
- Sterile gloves

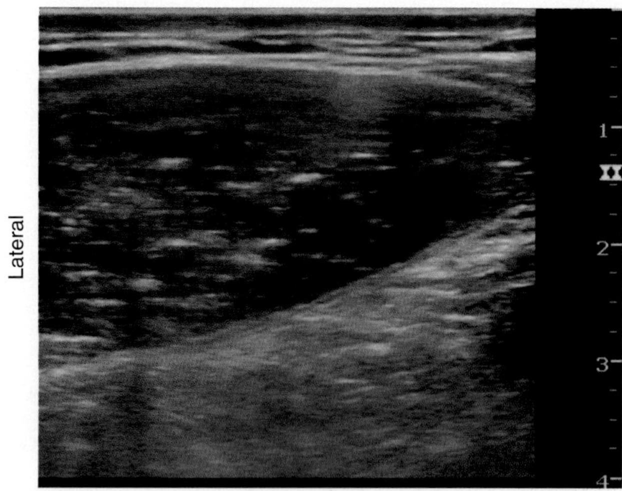


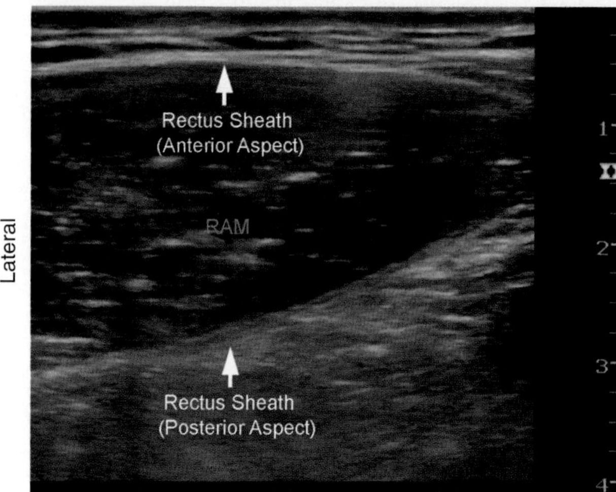


**FIGURE 42.3-1.** (A) Ultrasound anatomy of the rectus abdominis sheath. (B) Labeled Ultrasound anatomy of the rectus abdominis sheath. RAM, rectus abdominis muscle.

## Landmarks and Patient Positioning

Typically this block is performed in the supine position.

## GOAL

The goal is to place the needle tip just posterior to the rectus muscle but anterior to the posterior rectus sheath. Once the needle tip is positioned correctly, local anesthetic is deposited between the muscle and posterior rectus sheath, and correct spread is confirmed on ultrasound. An additional aliquot of local anesthetic is injected just posterior to the sheath.

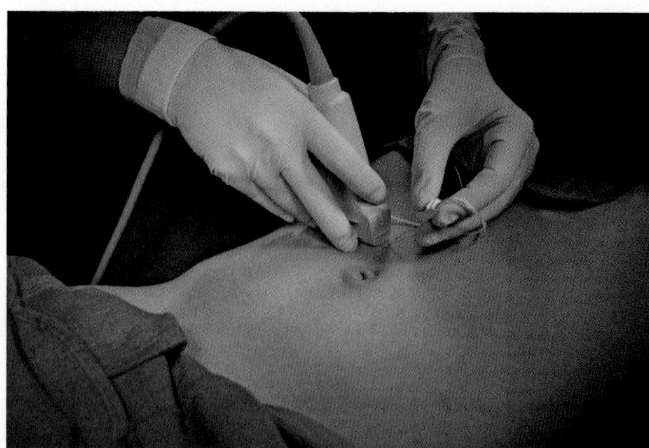

**FIGURE 42.3-2.** Transducer position and needle insertion to accomplish rectus sheath block.

## Technique

With the patient in supine position, the skin is disinfected and the transducer placed at the level of the umbilicus immediately lateral, in transverse position (Figure 42.3-2). Color Doppler can be used to identify the epigastric arteries so that their puncture can be avoided. The needle is inserted in-plane in a medial to lateral orientation, through the subcutaneous tissue, to pearce through the anterior rectus sheath (Figure 42.3-3). Out-of-plane technique is also suitable and often preferred in obese patients. The needle is further advanced through the body of the muscle until the tip rests on the posterior rectus sheath. After negative aspiration, 1 to 2 mL of local anesthetic is injected to verify needle tip location (Figure 42.3-4). When injection of the local anesthetic appears to be intramuscular, the needle is advanced

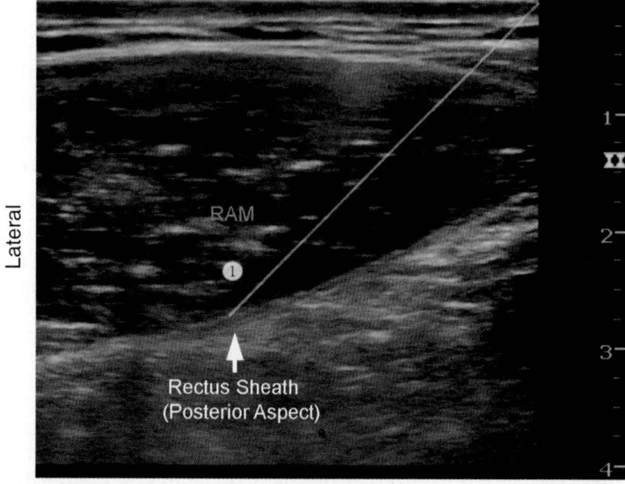


**FIGURE 42.3-3.** Simulated needle path (1) to accomplish the rectus sheath block. Needle tip is positioned between the posterior aspect of the rectus abdominis muscle (RAM) and the rectus sheath (posterior aspect).

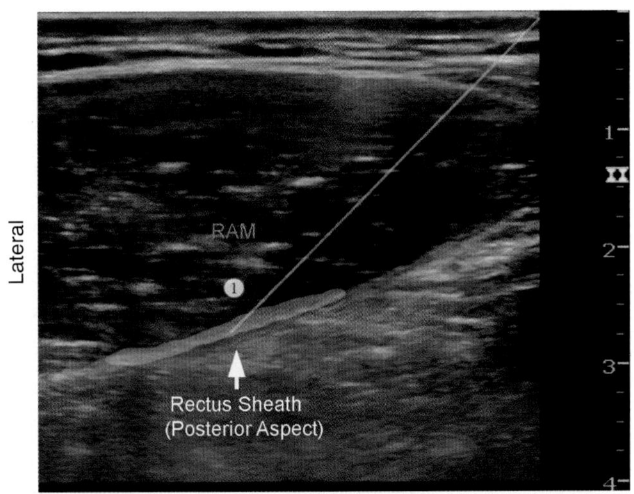


**FIGURE 42.3-4.** Simulated needle path (1) and spread of local anesthetic (blue shaded area) to accomplish the rectus sheath block. Local anesthetic should spread just underneath and within the posterior aspect of the rectus sheath. RAM, rectus abdominis muscle.

1 to 2 mm and its position is checked by injection of another aliquot of local anesthetic. This is repeated until the correct needle position is achieved. When a large volume of local anesthetic is planned (e.g. in combining billateral TAP and rectus abdominis sheath blocks), the described "hydrodisection" for the purpose of localization of the needle tip can be done using 0.9% saline or chlorprocaine to decrease the total mass of the more toxic, longer acting local anesthetic.

## TIP

- An out-of-plane technique can also be used directly through the belly of the rectus muscle. Because the needle tip may not always be seen throughout the procedure, small boluses of local anesthetic are injected as the needle is advanced toward the posterior rectus sheath, confirming the correct position of the needle tip.

In an adult patient, 10 mL of local anesthetic (e.g., 0.5% ropivacaine) per side is usually sufficient for successful blockade. In children, a volume of 0.1 mL/kg per side is adequate for effective analgesia.

## SUGGESTED READING

Abrahams MS, Horn JL, Noles LM, Aziz MF. Evidence-based medicine: ultrasound guidance for truncal blocks. *Reg Anesth Pain Med.* 2010;35:S36-42.

Dolan J, Lucie P, Geary T, Smith M, Kenny GN. The rectus sheath block: accuracy of local anesthetic placement by trainee anesthesiologists using loss of resistance or ultrasound guidance. *Reg Anesth Pain Med.* 2009;34:247-250.

Dolan J, Smith M. Visualization of bowel adherent to the peritoneum before rectus sheath block: another indication for the use of ultrasound in regional anesthesia. *Reg Anesth Pain Med.* 2009;34:280-281.

Husain NK, Ravalia A. Ultrasound-guided ilio-inguinal and rectus sheath nerve blocks. *Anaesthesia.* 2006;61:1126.

Kato J, Ueda K, Kondo Y, Aono M, Gokan D, Shimizu M, Ogawa S: Does ultrasound-guided rectus sheath block reduce adbominal pain in patients with postherpetic neuralgia? *Anesth Analg* 2011;112:(3)740-741.

Phua DS, Phoo JW, Koay CK. The ultrasound-guided rectus sheath block as an anaesthetic in adult paraumbilical hernia repair. *Anaesth Intensive Care.* 2009;37:499-500.

Sandeman DJ, Dilley AV. Ultrasound-guided rectus sheath block and catheter placement. *ANZ J Surg.* 2008;78:621-623.

Shido A, Imamachi N, Doi K, Sakura S, Saito Y: Continuous local anesthetic infusion through ultrasound-guided rectus sheath catheters. *Can J Anaesth* 2010;57:1046-1047.

Tanaka M, Azuma S, Hasegawa Y, et al. Case of inguinal hernia repair with transversus abdominis plane block and rectus sheath block [in Japanese]. *Masui.* 2009;58:1306-1309.

Willschke H, Bosenberg A, Marhofer P, et al. Ultrasonography-guided rectus sheath block in paediatric anaesthesia—a new approach to an old technique. *Br J Anaesth.* 2006;97:244-249.

# PART 4: ULTRASOUND-GUIDED LATERAL FEMORAL CUTANEOUS NERVE BLOCK

##  General Considerations

The lateral femoral cutaneous nerve (LFCN) divides into approximately two to five branches innervating the lateral and upper aspects of the thigh. Many studies have described how the variable anatomy of the lateral femoral cutaneous nerve makes it challenging to perform an effective landmark-based technique block. Ultrasound guidance, however, allows more accurate needle insertion into the appropriate fascial plane where lateral femoral cutaneous nerve passes through, allowing for a higher success rate.

## Ultrasound Anatomy

The lateral femoral cutaneous nerve typically is located between the tensor fasciae latae (TFLM) and sartorius (SaM) muscles, 1 to 2 cm medial and inferior to the anterior superior iliac spine (ASIS) and 0.5 to 1.0 cm deep to the skin surface (Figure 42.4-1). Ultrasound imaging of the lateral femoral cutaneous nerve yields an oval hypoechoic structure in cross-sectional view. The lateral edge of the sartorius muscle is a useful landmark, and as such, it can be relied on throughout the procedure. (Figures 42.4-2A and B). The LFCN branches sometimes may be seen across the anterior margin of the TFL.

##  Distribution of Blockade

Block of the lateral femoral cutaneous nerve provides anesthesia or analgesia in the anterolateral thigh. There is a large variation in the area of sensory coverage among individuals because of the highly variable course of LFCN and its branches.

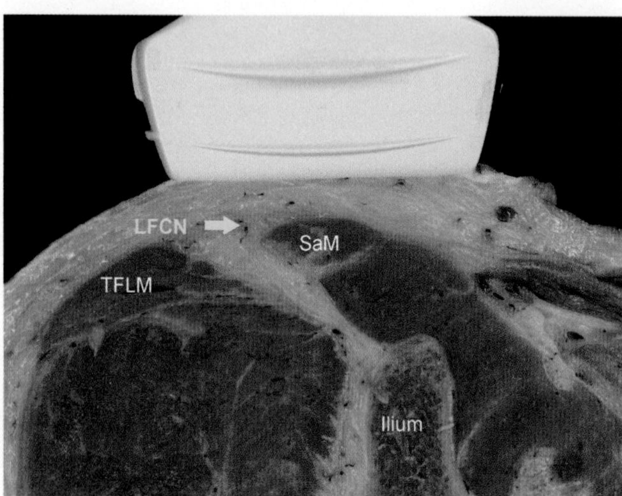


**FIGURE 42.4-1.** Cross-sectional anatomy of the lateral femoral cutaneous nerve (LFCN). Shown are LFCN, sartorius muscle (SaM), and tensor fascia latae muscle (TFLM).

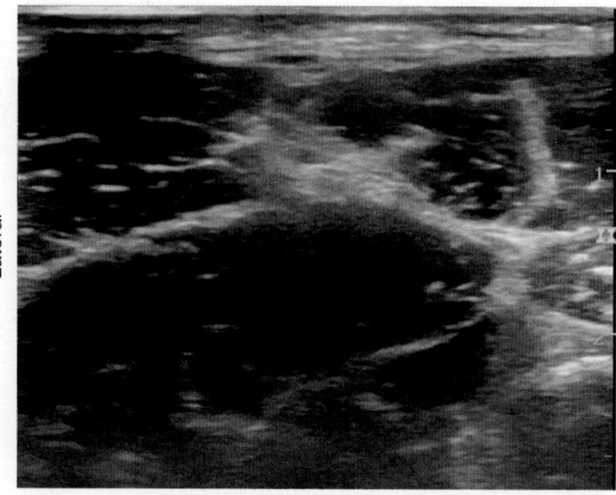


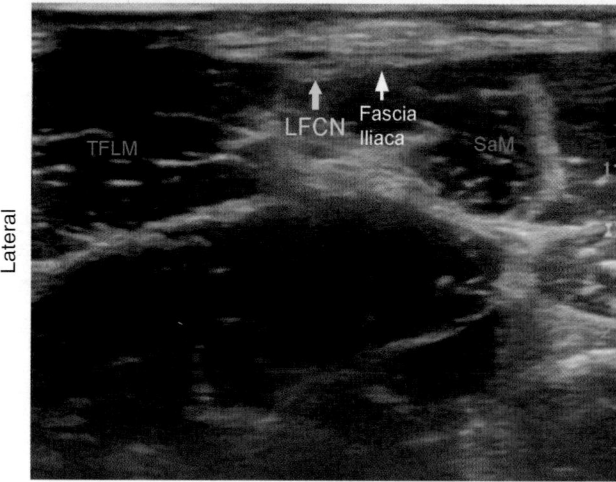


**FIGURE 42.4-2.** (A) Ultrasound anatomy of the lateral femoral cutaneous nerve (LFCN). (B) Labeled ultrasound anatomy of the LFCN.

##  Equipment

Equipment needed is as follows:

- Ultrasound machine with linear transducer (6–18 MHz), sterile sleeve, and gel
- Standard nerve block tray
- Syringe(s) with 10 mL of local anesthetic (LA)
- 50-mm, 22- to 24-gauge needle
- Sterile gloves

##  Landmarks and Patient Positioning

Block of the lateral femoral cutaneous nerve is performed with the patient in the supine or lateral position. Palpation of the anterior-superior spine provides the initial landmark for transducer placement; the transducer is first positioned at 2 cm inferior and medial to the ASIS and adjusted accordingly. Typically, the nerve is identified slightly more distally in its course. If nerve stimulator is used, precise identification of the LFCN may be confirmed by eliciting a tingling sensation on the lateral side of the thigh.

## GOAL

The goal is to inject local anesthetic in the plane between the tensor fasciae latae and the sartorius muscle, typically 1 to 2 cm medial and inferior to the anterior-superior iliac spine.

## Technique

With the patient supine, the skin is disinfected and the transducer placed immediately inferior to the ASIS, parallel to the inguinal ligament (Figure 42.4-3). The tensor fasciae latae and the sartorius muscle should be identified. The nerve should appear as a small hypoechoic oval structure between the tensor fasciae latae and the sartorius muscle in a short-axis view. A skin wheal is then made on the lateral aspect of the transducer, and the needle is inserted in-plane in a lateral to medial orientation, through the subcutaneous tissue and the tensor fasciae latae muscle (Figure 42.4-4A). A pop may be felt as the needle tip enters the plane between the tensor fascia latae and sartorius muscles. After gentle aspiration, 1 to 2 mL of LA is injected to verify the needle tip position. When the injection of the LA appears to be intramuscular, the needle is withdrawn or advanced 1 to 2 mm and another bolus is administered. This is repeated until the correct position is achieved by visualizing the spread of the LA in the described plane between the tensor fasciae latae and sartorius muscles (Figure 42.4-4B).

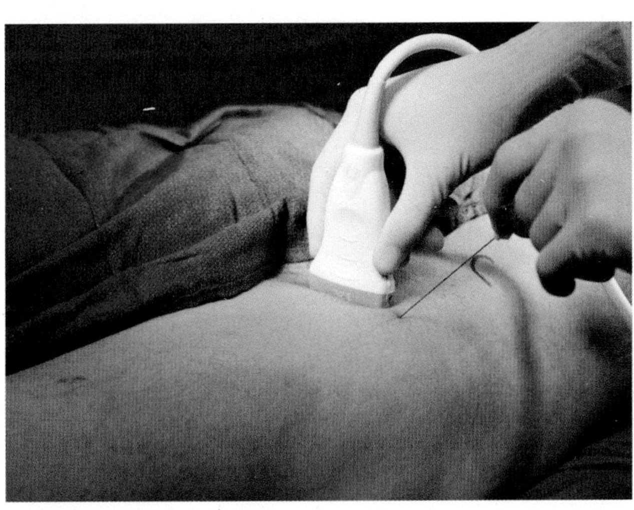

**FIGURE 42.4-3.** Transducer position and needle insertion to accomplish a lateral femoral cutaneous nerve (LFCN) block.

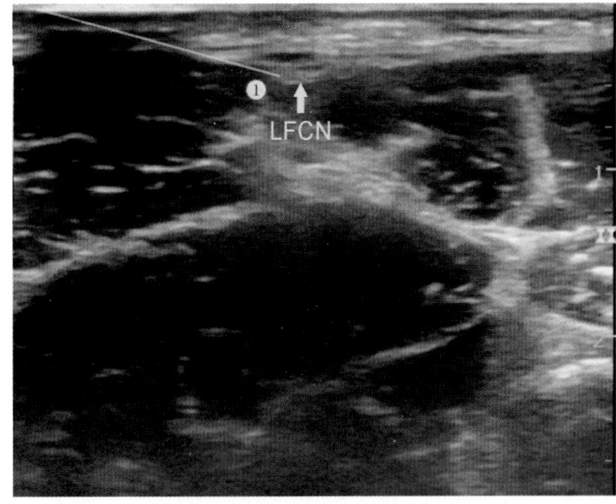


A Lateral femoral cutaneous nerve

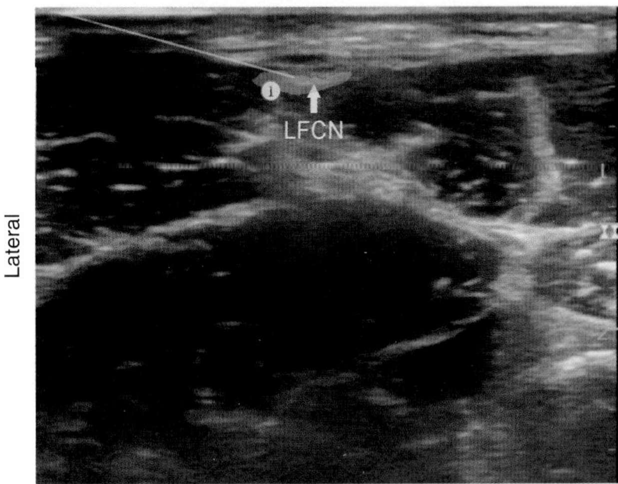


B Lateral femoral cutaneous nerve

**FIGURE 42.4-4.** (A) Simulated needle path (1) to block the LCFN. (B) Simulated needle path (1) and local anesthetic spread (area shaded in blue) to anesthetize the LFCN.

## TIP

- An out-of-plane technique can also be used for this nerve block. Because the needle tip may not be seen throughout the procedure, small boluses of local anesthetic (0.5–1 mL) are injected as the needle is advanced, to confirm the exact position.

In an adult patient, 5 to 10 mL of LA is usually sufficient for successful blockade. In children, a volume of 0.15 mL/kg per side is adequate for effective analgesia.

## SUGGESTED READING

Bodner G, Bernathova M, Galiano K, Putz D, Martinoli C, Felfernig M. Ultrasound of the lateral femoral cutaneous nerve: normal findings in a cadaver and in volunteers. *Reg Anesth Pain Med.* 2009;34(3):265-268.

Carai A, Fenu G, Sechi E, Crotti FM, Montella A. Anatomical variability of the lateral femoral cutaneous nerve: findings from a surgical series. *Clin Anat.* 2009;22(3):365-370.

Damarey B, Demondion X, Boutry N, Kim HJ, Wavreille G, Cotten A. Sonographic assessment of the lateral femoral cutaneous nerve. *J Clin Ultrasound.* 2009;37(2):89-95.

Hara K, Sakura S, Shido A: Ultrasound-guided lateral femoral cutaneous nerve block: comparison of two techiques. *Anaesth Intensive Care* 2011;39:69-72.

Hebbard P, Ivanusic J, Sha S. Ultrasound-guided supra-inguinal fascia iliaca block: a cadaveric evaluation of a novel approach. *Anaesthesia.* 2011;66(4):300-305.

Hurdle MF, Weingarten TN, Crisostomo RA, Psimos C, Smith J. Ultrasound-guided blockade of the lateral femoral cutaneous nerve: technical description and review of 10 cases. *Arch Phys Med Rehabil.* 2007;88(10):1362-1364.

Ng I, Vaghadia H, Choi PT, Helmy N. Ultrasound imaging accurately identifies the lateral femoral cutaneous nerve. *Anesth Analg.* 2008;107(3):1070-1074.

Ropars M, Morandi X, Huten D, Thomazeau H, Berton E, Darnault P. Anatomical study of the lateral femoral cutaneous nerve with special reference to minimally invasive anterior approach for total hip replacement. *Surg Radiol Anat.* 2009;31(3):199-204.

Sürücü HS, Tanyeli E, Sargon MF, Karahan ST. An anatomic study of the lateral femoral cutaneous nerve. *Surg Radiol Anat.* 1997;19(5):307-310.

Tumber PS, Bhatia A, Chan VW: Ultrasound-guided lateral femoral cutaneous nerve block for meralgia paresthetica. *Anesth Analg* 2008;106:1021-1022.

# Ultrasound-Guided Neuraxial and Perineuraxial Blocks

# 43 Introduction

*Manoj Karmakar and Catherine Vandepitte*

Central neuraxial blocks (CNBs), which include spinal, epidural, combined spinal epidural (CSE), and caudal epidural injections, are commonly practiced regional anesthesia techniques in the perioperative period, for obstetric anesthesia and analgesia, as well as for managing chronic pain.[1] Traditionally, CNBs are performed using surface anatomic landmarks, operator tactile sensation (loss of resistance) during needle advancement, and/or visualizing the free flow of cerebrospinal fluid. Although anatomic landmarks are fortuitous because spinous processes provide a relatively reliable surface landmark in many patients, they are not always easily recognized or reliable signs in patients with obesity,[2] edema, underlying spinal deformity, or after back surgery. Even in the absence of spine abnormalities, data suggest that a clinical estimate of a specific intervertebral space based on the surface anatomy may not be accurate in many patients.[3,4] In other words, a clinical estimate of an intervertebral space often results in needle placement one or two spinal levels higher than intended.[3,5,6] This estimation error has been attributed as a cause of injury of the conus medullaris or spinal cord after spinal anesthesia.[5,7] The difficulty of identifying the correct level is particularly present in patients with obesity and when accessing intervertebral space in the upper spinal levels.[3,5,7] Therefore, the Tuffier's line, a surface anatomic landmark that is used ubiquitously during CNB, is not a consistent landmark.[6] Moreover, because of the blind nature of the landmark-based techniques, it is not possible for the operator to predict the ease or difficulty of needle placement prior to skin puncture. In a study of 300 spinal anesthetics, 15% of attempts were judged to be technically difficult, and 10% required more than five attempts.[8] In another study including 202 patients who were under 50 years of age, failed CNB was reported in 5% of cases.[9] Thus the need to establish a more reliable method to identify the spinal levels and needle advancement toward the neuraxis continues to inspire clinical and imaging studies.

Although a number of surface-based landmarks and nerve stimulation–guided peripheral nerve block techniques are well established, localization and blockade of the deeper positioned peripheral nerves and plexi remain largely "blind" procedures (e.g., lumbar plexus block, sciatic block, and infraclavicular block). This is particularly true with nerve block procedures where nerve stimulation is not easily accomplished due to the specifics of the anatomy (e.g., deep position) and where the goal of the procedure is to place the needle in a certain anatomical space, rather than localize the nerves that are not easily accessible to nerve stimulation (e.g., intercostals blocks, paravertebral blocks, and fascia iliaca blocks). Consequently, significant research efforts have focused on improving the current techniques of blockade and establishing more reliable surface landmarks and needle orientation procedures.[10–12] Due to the nature of the surface-based procedures and inherent difficulty with electrolocalization of deeply positioned peripheral nerves, many of these procedures are not used commonly and are confined to a few practices where substantial expertise is available. The introduction of ultrasound guidance in regional anesthesia has sparked a renewed interest in these procedures.[13,14] Ultrasound can be used to depict the location and spatial relationship (e.g., depth) of the osseous landmarks to help estimate both the correct site as well as the depth of needle insertion.

Imaging of the deep structures as well as structures that are concealed by osseous processes requires considerable skill and dexterity. In addition, needle visualization and needle–nerve interface can be challenging because of interference with the osseous structures and depth of the needle placement. Given these limitations and a close relationship of the nerve structures to the centroneuroaxis, questions have been raised about the overall safety of ultrasound-guided neuraxial blocks, lumbar plexus and paravertebral blocks if taught as a standard practice. At the time of this publication, ultrasound-guided blocks for the purpose of neuraxial anesthesia, and perineuraxially located nerves and plexi are not well-established. These advanced ultrasound-guided or ultrasound-assisted block techniques are currently practiced only by experts who have spent considerable time mastering ultrasound anatomy. Often, even the most experienced privately admit that ultrasound-guided centroneuraxial blocks are not practical as a routine practice. For example, in our practice most centroneuraxial blocks are done without ultrasound guidance, whereas ultrasound is being increasingly used for lumbar plexus and paraveretebral blocks. For this reason and to avoid imparting a false impression that these are standard techniques, we have opted to discuss them within the context of ultrasound anatomy, rather than as well-established procedures. An informed reader then can make use of the presented anatomical, pharmacological and technical information to devise own techniques and/or make decisions regarding the applicability of ultrasound in these techniques in his/her own practice.

## REFERENCES


1. Cook TM, Counsell D, Wildsmith JA. Major complications of central neuraxial block: report on the Third National Audit Project of the Royal College of Anaesthetists. *Br J Anaesth.* 2009;102(2):179-190.
2. Stiffler KA, Jwayyed S, Wilber ST, Robinson A. The use of ultrasound to identify pertinent landmarks for lumbar puncture. *Am J Emerg Med.* 2007;25(3):331-334.
3. Broadbent CR, Maxwell WB, Ferrie R, Wilson DJ, Gawne-Cain M, Russell R. Ability of anaesthetists to identify a marked lumbar interspace. *Anaesthesia.* 2000;55(11):1122-1126.
4. Furness G, Reilly MP, Kuchi S. An evaluation of ultrasound imaging for identification of lumbar intervertebral level. *Anaesthesia.* 2002;57(3):277-280.
5. Holmaas G, Frederiksen D, Ulvik A, Vingsnes SO, Ostgaard G, Nordli H. Identification of thoracic intervertebral spaces by means of surface anatomy: a magnetic resonance imaging study. *Acta Anaesthesiol Scand.* 2006;50(3):368-373.
6. Reynolds F. Damage to the conus medullaris following spinal anaesthesia. *Anaesthesia.* 2001;56(3):238-247.
7. Hamandi K, Mottershead J, Lewis T, Ormerod IC, Ferguson IT. Irreversible damage to the spinal cord following spinal anesthesia. *Neurology.* 2002;59(4):624-626.
8. Tarkkila P, Huhtala J, Salminen U. Difficulties in spinal needle use. Insertion characteristics and failure rates associated with 25-, 27- and 29-gauge Quincke-type spinal needles. *Anaesthesia.* 1994;49(8):723-725.
9. Seeberger MD, Lang ML, Drewe J, Schneider M, Hauser E, Hruby J. Comparison of spinal and epidural anesthesia for patients younger than 50 years of age. *Anesth Analg.* 1994;78(4):667-673.
10. Boezaart AP, Lucas SD, Elliot CE. Paravertebral block: cervical, thoracic, lumbar, and sacral [review]. *Curr Opin Anaesthesiol.* 2009; 22(5):637-643.
11. Capdevila X, Coimbra C, Choquet, O. Approaches to the lumbar plexus; success, risks, and outcome [review]. *Reg Anesth Pain Med.* 2005;30(2):150-162.
12. Capdevila X, Macaire P, Dadure C, et al. Continuous psoas compartment block for postoperative analgesia after total hip arthroplasty: new landmarks, technical guidelines, and clinical evaluation. *Anesth Analg.* 2002;94(6):1606-1613.
13. Seki S, Yamauchi M, Kawamura M, Namiki A, Sato Y, Fujiwara Y. Technical advantages of ultrasound-guided obturator nerve block compared with the nerve stimulating technique [in Japanese]. *Masui.* 2010;59(6):686-690.
14. Salinas FV. Ultrasound and review of evidence for lower extremity peripheral nerve blocks [review]. *Reg Anesth Pain Med.* 2010;35(2 Suppl):S16-25.

# Spinal Sonography and Considerations for Ultrasound-Guided Central Neuraxial Blockade

*Wing Hong Kwok and Manoj Karmakar*

##  Introduction

Ultrasound scanning (US) can offer several advantages when used to guide placement of the needle for centroneuraxial blocks (CNBs). It is noninvasive, safe, simple to use, can be performed expeditiously, provides real-time images, is devoid from adverse effects, and it may be beneficial in patients with abnormal or variant spinal anatomy. When used for chronic pain interventions, US also eliminates or reduces exposure to radiation. In expert hands, the use of US for epidural needle insertion was shown to reduce the number of puncture attempts,[1–4] improve the success rate of epidural access on the first attempt,[2] reduce the need to puncture multiple levels,[2–4] and improve patient comfort during the procedure.[3] These advantages led the National Institute of Clinical Excellence (NICE) in the United Kingdom to recommend the routine use of ultrasound for epidural blocks.[5] Incorporating these recommendations into clinical practice, however, has met significant obstacles. As one example, a recent survey of anesthesiologists in the United Kingdom showed that >90% of respondents were not trained in the use of US to image the epidural space.[6] In this chapter, we describe techniques of US imaging of the spine, the relevant sonoanatomy, and practical considerations for using US-guided CNB and nerve blocks close to the centroneuroaxis.

## 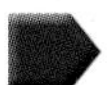 Historical Background

Bogin and Stulin were probably the first to report using US for central neuraxial interventional procedures.[7] In 1971, they described using US to perform lumbar puncture.[7] Porter and colleagues, in 1978, used US to image the lumbar spine and measure the diameter of the spinal canal in diagnostic radiology.[8] Cork and colleagues were the first group of anesthesiologists to use US to locate the landmarks relevant for epidural anesthesia.[9] Thereafter, US was used mostly to preview the spinal anatomy and measure the distances from the skin to the lamina and epidural space before epidural puncture.[10,11] More recently, Grau and coworkers, from Heidelberg in Germany, conducted a series of studies, significantly contributing to the current understanding of spinal sonography.[1–4,12–15] These investigators described a two-operator technique consisting of real-time US visualization of neuraxial space using a paramedian sagittal axis and insertion of the needle through the midline to accomplish a combined spinal-epidural block.[4] The quality of the US image at the time, however, was substantially inferior to that of today's equipment, thus hindering acceptance and further research in this area. Recent improvements in US technology and image clarity have allowed for much greater clarity during imaging of the spine and neuraxial structures.[16,17]

## 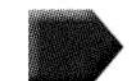 Ultrasound Imaging of the Spine

### Basic Considerations

Because the spine is located at a depth, US imaging of the spine typically requires the use of low-frequency ultrasound (5-2 MHz) and curved array transducers. Low-frequency US provides good penetration but unfortunately, it lacks the spatial resolution at the depth (5–7 cm) at which the neuraxial structures are located. The osseous framework of the spine, which envelops the neuraxial structures, reflects much of the incident US signal before it reaches the spinal canal, presenting additional challenges in obtaining good quality images. Recent improvements in US technology, the greater image processing capabilities of US machines, the availability of compound imaging, and the development of new scanning protocols have improved the ability to image the neuraxial space significantly. As a result, today it is possible to reasonably accurately delineate the neuraxial anatomy relevant for CNB. Also of note is that technology once only available in the high-end, cart-based U.S. systems is now available in portable US devices, making them even more practical for spinal sonography and US-guided CNB applications.

### Ultrasound Scan Planes

Although anatomic planes have already been described elsewhere in this text, the importance of understanding them for imaging of the neuraxial space dictates another, more detailed review. There are three anatomical planes: median, transverse, and coronal (Figure 44-1). The *median* plane is a longitudinal plane that passes through the midline bisecting the body into equal right and left halves. The *sagittal* plane is

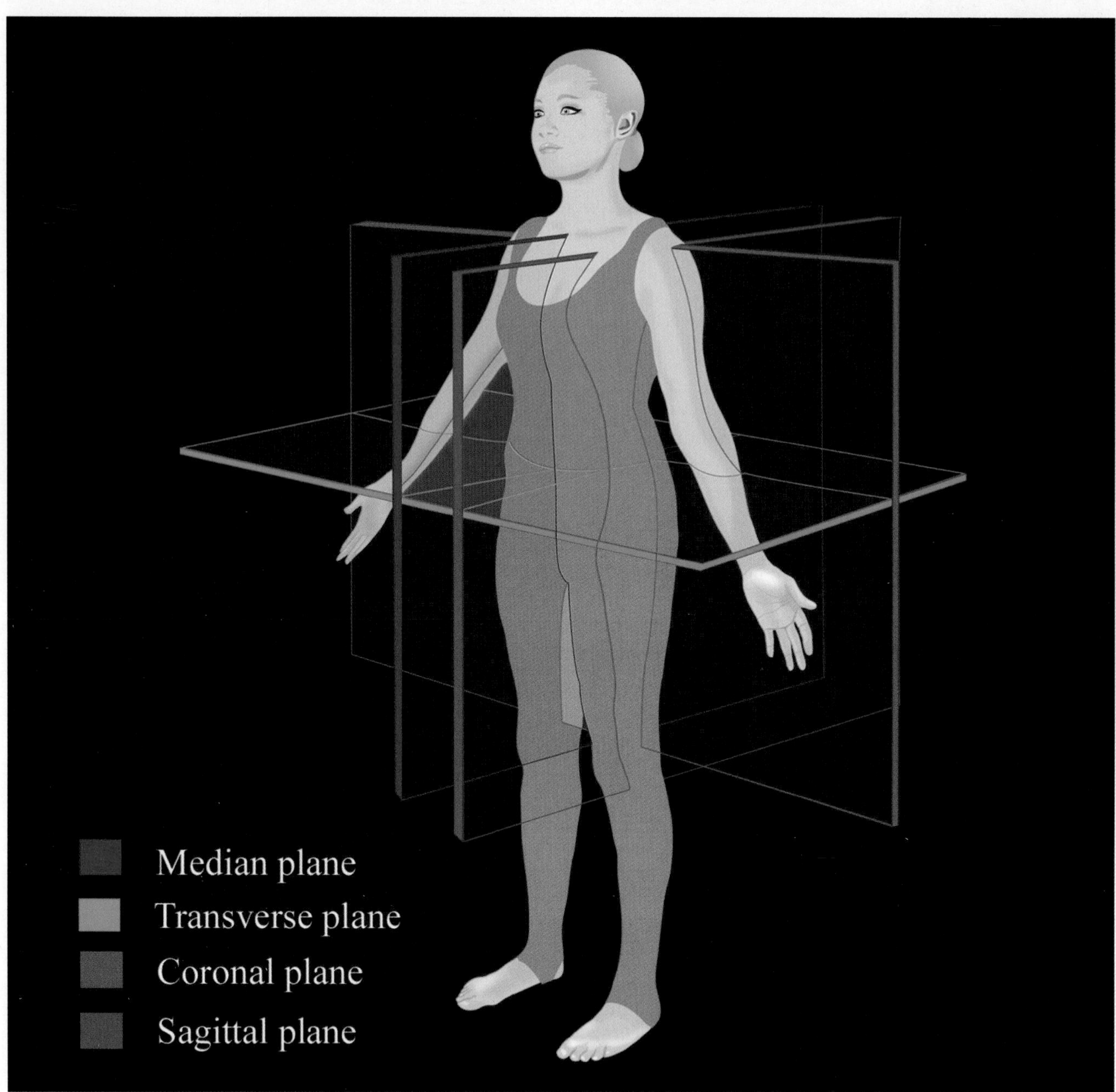


**FIGURE 44-1.** Anatomic planes of the body.

a longitudinal plane that is parallel to the median plane and perpendicular to the ground. Therefore, the median plane also can be defined as the sagittal plane that is exactly in the middle of the body (median sagittal plane). The *transverse* plane, also known as the axial or horizontal plane, is parallel to the ground. The *coronal* plane, also known as the frontal plane, is perpendicular to the ground. A US scan of the spine can be performed in the transverse (transverse scan) or longitudinal (sagittal scan) axis with the patient in the sitting, lateral decubitus, or prone position. The two scanning planes complement each other during a US examination of the spine. A sagittal scan can be performed through the midline (median sagittal scan) or through a paramedian (paramedian sagittal scan) plane. Grau et al suggested a paramedian sagittal plane to visualize the neuraxial structures.[12] The US visibility of neuraxial structures can be further improved when the spine is imaged in the paramedian oblique sagittal. During a paramedian oblique sagittal scan (PMOSS), the transducer is positioned 2 to 3 cm lateral to the midline (paramedian) in the sagittal axis and it is also tilted slightly medially, that is, toward the midline (Figure 44-2). The purpose of the medial tilt is to ensure that the US signal

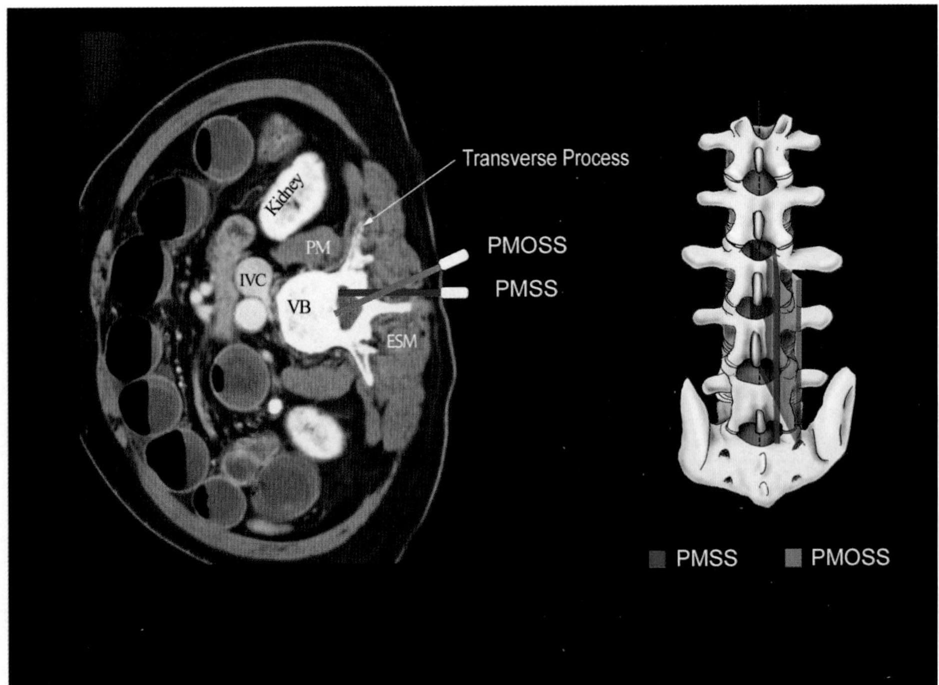


**FIGURE 44-2.** Paramedian sagittal scan (PMSS) of the lumbar spine. The PMSS is represented by the red color and the paramedian oblique sagittal axis of scan (PMOSS) is represented by the blue color. Note how the plane of imaging during a PMOSS is tilted slightly medially. This is done to ensure that most of the ultrasound energy enters the spinal canal through the widest part of the interlaminar space. ICV, inferior vena cava; VB, vertebral body; PM, psoas muscle; ESM, erector spinae muscle.

enters the spinal canal through the widest part of the interlaminar space and not the lateral sulcus of the canal.

## Sonoanatomy of the Spine

Detailed knowledge of the vertebral anatomy is essential to understand the sonoanatomy of the spine. Unfortunately, cross-sectional anatomy texts describe the anatomy of the spine in traditional orthogonal planes, that is, the transverse, sagittal, and coronal planes. This often results in difficulty interpreting the spinal sonoanatomy because US imaging is generally performed in an *arbitrary* or intermediary plane by tilting, sliding, and rotating the transducer. Moreover, currently there are limited data on spinal sonography or on how to interpret US images of the spine.

Several anatomic models recently became available that can be used to learn musculoskeletal US imaging techniques (human volunteers), the sonoanatomy relevant for peripheral nerve blocks (human volunteers or cadavers), and the required interventional skills (tissue mimicking phantoms, fresh cadavers). However, few models or tools are available to learn and practice spinal sonoanatomy or the interventional skills required for US-guided CNB. Karmakar and colleagues recently described the use of a "water-based spine phantom" (Figure 44-3A) to study the osseous anatomy of the lumbosacral spine[16,18] and a "pig carcass phantom" model[19] (Figure 44-4A) to practice the hand-eye coordination skills required to perform US-guided CNB.[19] Computer-generated anatomic reconstruction from the Visible Human Project data set that corresponds to the US scan planes is another useful way of studying the sonoanatomy of the spine. Multiplanar three-dimensional (3D) reconstruction from a high-resolution 3D computed tomography (CT) data set of the spine can be used to study and validate the sonographic appearance of the various osseous elements of the spine (Figure 44-5).

## Water-Based Spine Phantom

The *water-based spine phantom*[18] is based on a model described previously by Greher and colleagues to study the osseous anatomy of relevance to US-guided lumbar facet nerve block.[20] The model is prepared by immersing a commercially available lumbosacral spine model in a water bath. A low-frequency curved array transducer submerged into water is used to scan in the transverse and sagittal axes (Figure 44-3A). Each osseous element of the spine produces a "characteristic" sonographic pattern. The ability

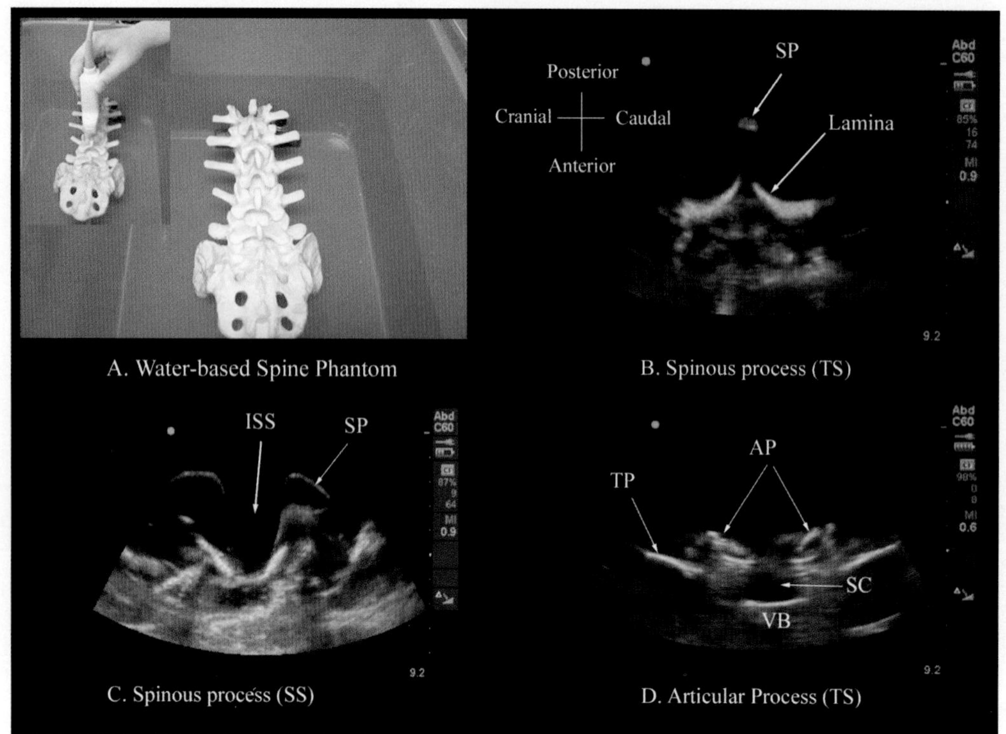


**FIGURE 44-3.** (A) The water-based spine phantom and sonograms of the spinous process in the (B) transverse and (C) midsagittal or median axes, and (D) a scan through the interspinous space. SP, spinous process; ISS, interspinous space; TP, transverse process; AP, articular process; SC, spinal canal; VB, vertebral body; TS, transverse scan; SS, sagittal scan.

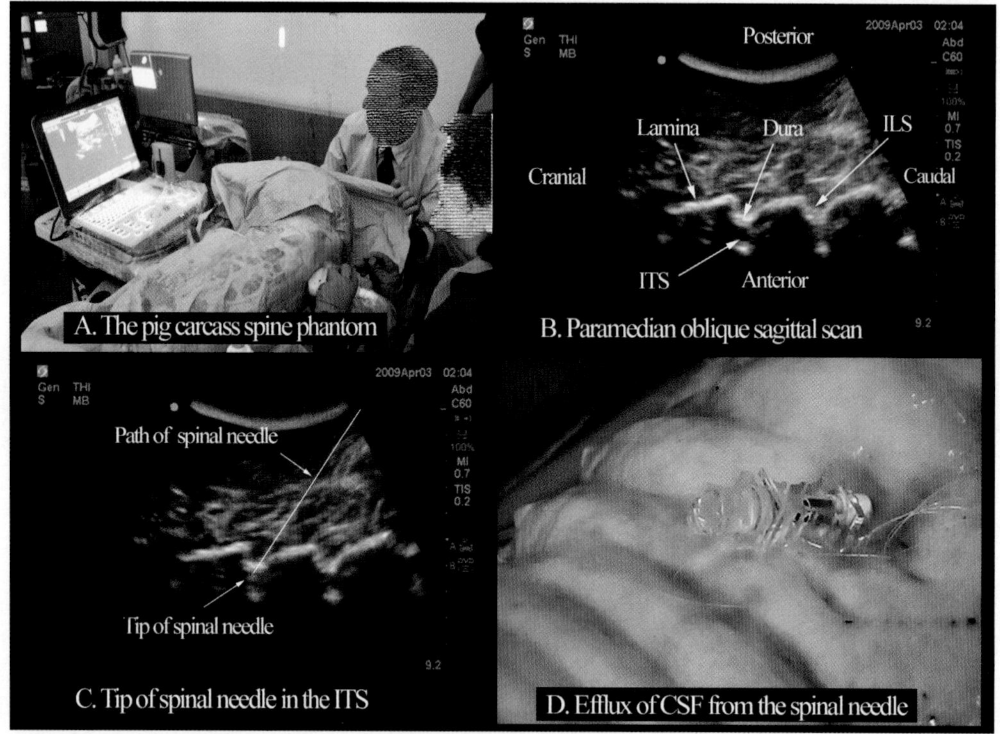


**FIGURE 44-4.** The "Pig carcass spine phantom" (A) being used to practice central neuraxial blocks at a workshop, (B) paramedian oblique sagittal sonogram of the lumbar spine, (C) sonogram showing the tip of a spinal needle in the ITS (intrathecal space), (D) picture showing the efflux of cerebrospinal fluid (CSF) from the hub of a spinal needle that has been inserted into the ITS. ILS, interlaminar space.

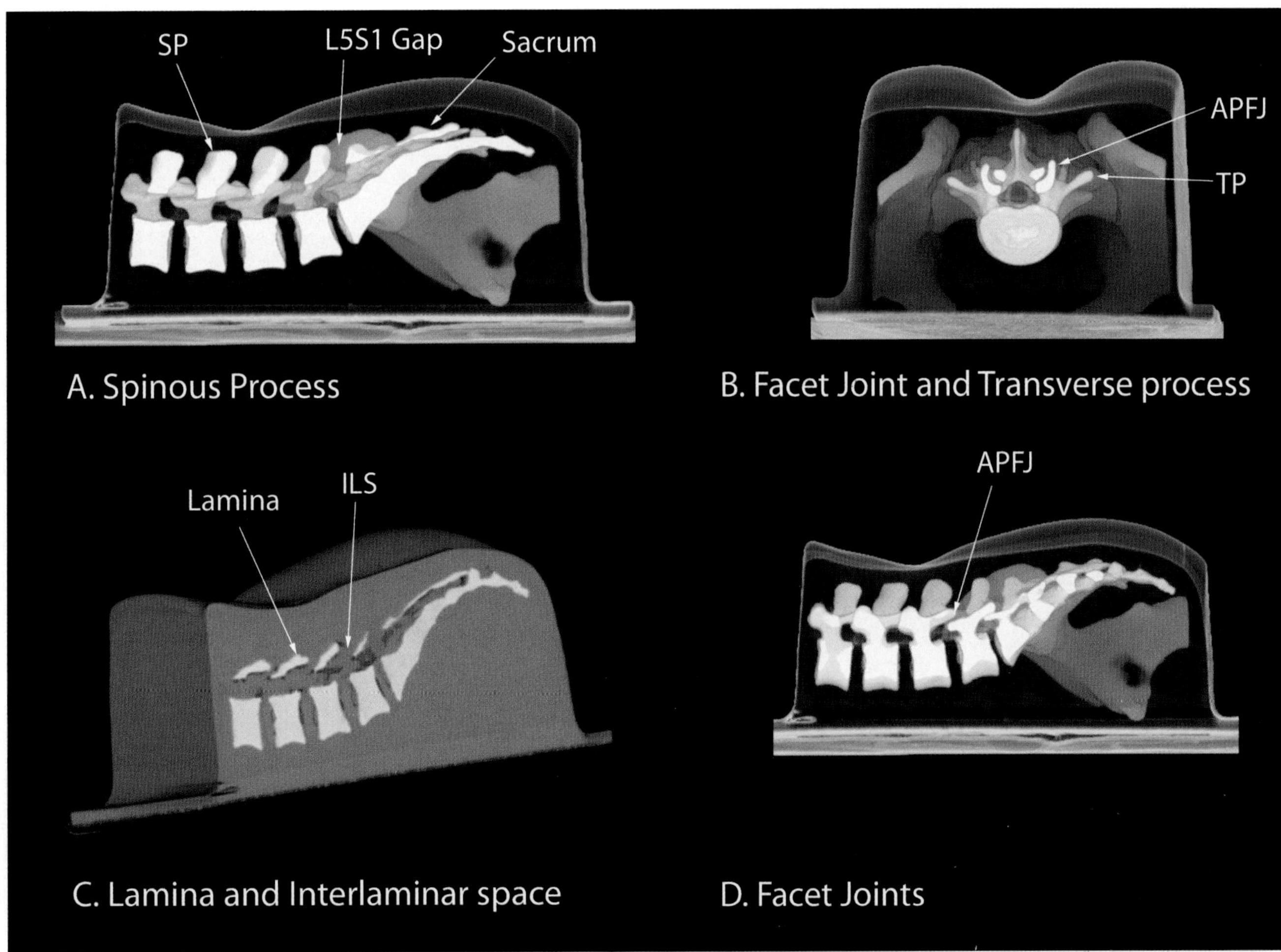


**FIGURE 44-5.** Three-dimensional reconstruction of high-resolution computed tomography scan data set from a lumbar training phantom (CIRS Model 034, CIRS Inc., Norfolk, VA, USA). (A) Median sagittal scan of the spinous process (SP), (B) transverse interspinous view of the articular process (AP), transverse process (TP), and facet joint (FJ), (C) paramedian oblique sagittal scan showing the lamina and interlaminar space (ILS), and (D) paramedian sagittal scan at the level of the articular processes. ISS, interspinous space.

to recognize these sonographic patterns is an important step toward understanding the sonoanatomy of the spine. Representative US images of the spinous process, lamina, articular processes, and the transverse process from the water-based spine phantom are presented in Figures 44-3 and 44-6. The advantage of this water-based spine phantom is that water produces an anechoic (black) background against which the hyperechoic reflections from the bone are clearly visualized. The water-based spine phantom allows a see-through real-time visual validation of the sonographic appearance of a given osseous element by performing the scan with a marker (e.g., a needle) in contact with it (Figure 44-6A). The described model is also inexpensive, easily prepared, requires little time to set up, and can be used repeatedly without deteriorating or decomposing, as animal tissue-based phantoms do.

## Ultrasound Imaging of the Lumbar Spine

### Sagittal Scan

The patient is positioned in the sitting, lateral, or prone position with the lumbosacral spine maximally flexed. The transducer is placed 1 to 2 cm lateral to the spinous process (i.e., in the paramedian sagittal plane) at the lower back with its orientation marker directed cranially. A slight tilt medially during the scan is assumed to insonate in a *paramedian oblique sagittal* plane. First, the sacrum is identified as a flat hyperechoic structure with a large acoustic shadow anteriorly (Figure 44-7). When the transducer is slid in a cranial direction, a gap is seen between the sacrum and the lamina of the L5 vertebra, which is the L5-S1 interlaminar space,

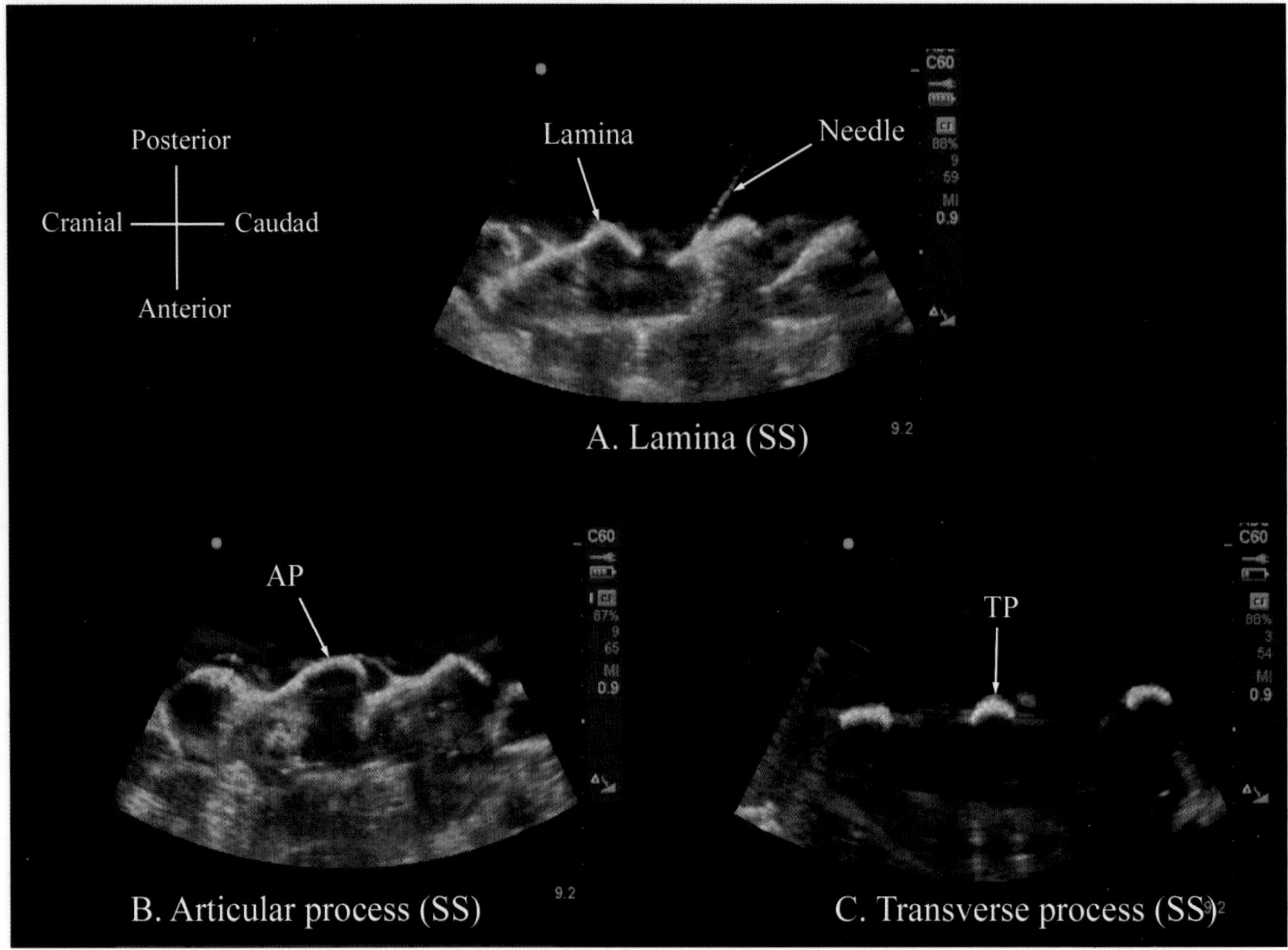


**FIGURE 44-6.** Paramedian sagittal sonogram of the (A) lamina, (B) articular process, and (C) transverse process from the water-based spine phantom. Note the needle in contact with the lamina in (A), a method that was used to validate the sonographic appearance of the osseous elements in the phantom.

also referred to as the L5-S1gap (Figure 44-7).[16,17,21] The L3-4 and L4-5 interlaminar spaces can now be located by counting upward (Figure 44-8).[16,17] The erector spinae muscles are hypoechoic and lie superficial to the laminae. The lamina appears hyperechoic and is the first osseous structure visualized (Figure 44-8). Because bone impedes the penetration of US, there is an acoustic shadow anterior to each lamina. The sonographic appearance of the lamina produces a pattern that resembles the head and neck of a horse, which Karmakar and colleagues referred to as the "horse head sign" (Figures 44-5C, 44-6A, and 44-8).[16] The interlaminar space is the gap between the adjoining lamina and is the "acoustic window" through which the neuraxial structures are visualized within the spinal canal. The ligamentum flavum appears as a hyperechoic band across adjacent lamina). The posterior dura is the next hyperechoic structure anterior to the ligamentum flavum, and the epidural space is the hypoechoic area (a few millimeters wide) between the ligamentum flavum and the posterior dura. The thecal sac with the cerebrospinal fluid is the anechoic space anterior to the posterior dura (Figure 44-8). The cauda equina, which is located within the thecal sac, often is seen as multiple horizontal, hyperechoic shadows within the anechoic thecal sac. Pulsations of the cauda equina are identified in some patients.[16,17] The anterior dura also is hyperechoic, but it is not always easy to differentiate it from the posterior longitudinal ligament and the vertebral body because they are of similar echogenicity (isoechoic) and especially closely related. Often, what results is a single, composite, hyperechoic reflection anteriorly that we refer to as the "anterior complex" (Figure 44-8).[16,17] If the transducer slides medially, that is, to the median sagittal plane, the tips of the spinous processes of the L3-L5 vertebra, which appear as crescent-shaped structures, are seen (Figures 44-3C, 44-5A, and 44-9).[16] The acoustic window between the spinous processes in the median plane is narrow and may prevent clear visualization of the neuraxial structures within the spinal canal. In contrast, if the transducer is moved slightly laterally from the paramedian sagittal plane at the level of the lamina, the articular processes of the vertebra are seen. The articular processes appear as one continuous,

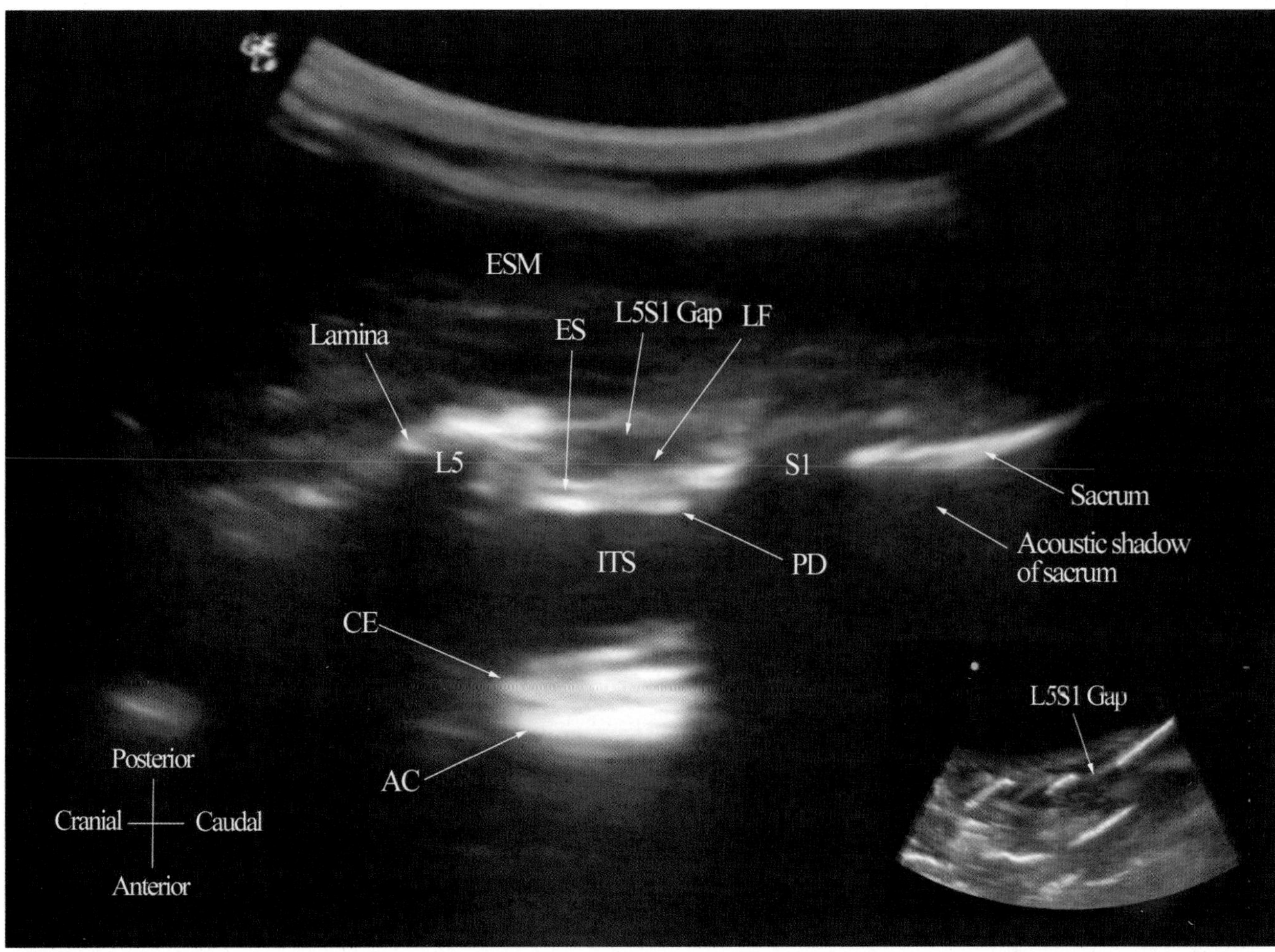


**FIGURE 44-7.** Paramedian sagittal sonogram of the lumbosacral junction. The posterior surface of the sacrum is identified as a flat hyperechoic structure with a large acoustic shadow anterior to it. The dip or gap between the sacrum and the lamina of L5 is the L5-S1 intervertebral space or the L5-S1 gap. ESM, erector spinae muscle; ES, epidural space; LF, ligamentum flavum; PD, posterior dura; ITS, intrathecal space; CE, cauda equina; and AC, anterior complex.

hyperechoic wavy line with no intervening gaps (Figures 44-5D, 44-6B, and 44-10), as seen at the level of the lamina.[16] The articular processes in a sagittal sonogram produce a sonographic pattern that resembles multiple camel humps, which are referred to as the "camel hump sign" (Figures 44-6B and 44-10). A sagittal scan lateral to the articular processes brings the transverse processes of the L3-L5 vertebrae into view. The transverse processes are recognized by their crescent-shaped hyperechoic reflections with their concavity facing anteriorly and an acoustic shadow anterior to them (Figures 44-6C and 44-11).[22] This produces a sonographic pattern that we refer to as the "trident sign" because of its resemblance to the trident (Latin *tridens* or *tridentis*) that is often associated with Poseidon, the god of the sea in Greek mythology, and the Trishula of the Hindu god Shiva (Figure 44-11).[22]

## Transverse Scan

For a transverse scan of the lumbar spine, the US transducer is positioned over the spinous process (transverse spinous process view) with the patient in the sitting or lateral position. On a transverse sonogram, the spinous process and the lamina on either side are seen as a hyperechoic reflection anterior to which there is a dark acoustic shadow that completely obscures the underlying spinal canal and thus the neuraxial structures (Figures 44-3B and 44-12). Therefore, this view is not suitable for imaging of the neuraxial structures but can be useful for identifying the midline when the spinous processes cannot be palpated (e.g., in obese patients). However, if the transducer is slid slightly cranially or caudally, it may be possible to perform a transverse scan through the interspinous space (transverse interspinous view) (Figures 44-3D, 44-5D, and 44-13).[16,23] It is important to tilt the transducer slightly cranially or caudally to align the US beam to the interspinous space and optimize the US image. In the transverse interspinous view, the posterior dura, thecal sac, and the anterior complex can be visualized (from a posterior to anterior direction) within the spinal canal in the midline and the articular processes, and the transverse processes are visualized laterally (Figure 44-13).[16,23]

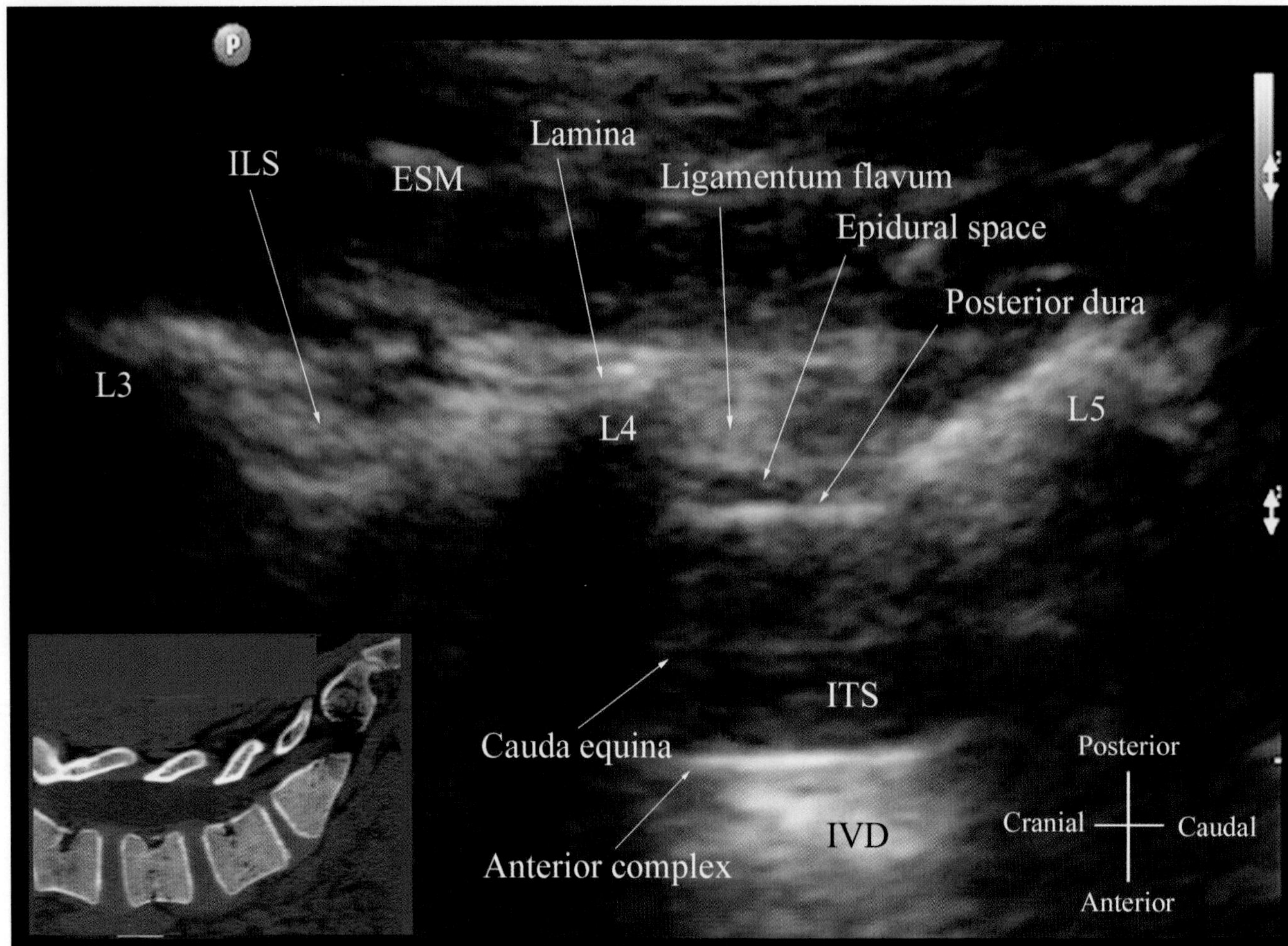


**FIGURE 44-8.** Paramedian oblique sagittal sonogram of the lumbar spine at the level of the lamina showing the L3-4 and L4-5 interlaminar spaces. Note the hypoechoic epidural space (few millimeters wide) between the hyperechoic ligamentum flavum and the posterior dura. The intrathecal space is the anechoic space between the posterior dura and the anterior complex in the sonogram. The cauda equina nerve fibers are also seen as hyperechoic longitudinal structures within the thecal sac. The hyperechoic reflections seen in front of the anterior complex are from the intervertebral disc (IVD). Picture in the inset shows a corresponding computed tomography (CT) scan of the lumbosacral spine in the same anatomic plane as the ultrasound scan. The CT slice was reconstructed from a three-dimensional CT data set from the author's archive. ESM, erector spinae muscle; ILS, interlaminar space; LF, ligamentum flavum; ES, epidural space; PD, posterior dura; CE, cauda equina; ITS, intrathecal space; AC, anterior complex; IVD, intervertebral disc; L3, lamina of L3 vertebra; L4, lamina of L4 vertebra; L5, lamina of L5 vertebra.

The ligamentum flavum is rarely visualized in the transverse interspinous view, possibly due to anisotropy caused by the arch-like attachment of the ligamentum flavum to the lamina. The epidural space is also less frequently visualized in the transverse interspinous scan than in the PMOSS. The transverse interspinous view can be used to examine for rotational deformities of the vertebra, such as in scoliosis. Normally, both the lamina and the articular processes on either side are located symmetrically (Figures 44-3D, 44-5D, and 44-13). However, if there is asymmetry, then a rotational deformity of the vertebral column[24] should be suspected and the operator can anticipate a potentially difficult CNB.

## Ultrasound Imaging of the Thoracic Spine

US imaging of the thoracic spine is more challenging than imaging the lumbar spine; the ability to visualize the neuraxial structures with US may vary with the level at which the imaging is performed. Regardless of the level at which the scan is performed, the thoracic spine is probably best imaged with the patient in the sitting position. In the lower thoracic region (T9-12), the sonographic appearance of the neuraxial structures is comparable to that in the lumbar region because of comparable vertebral anatomy

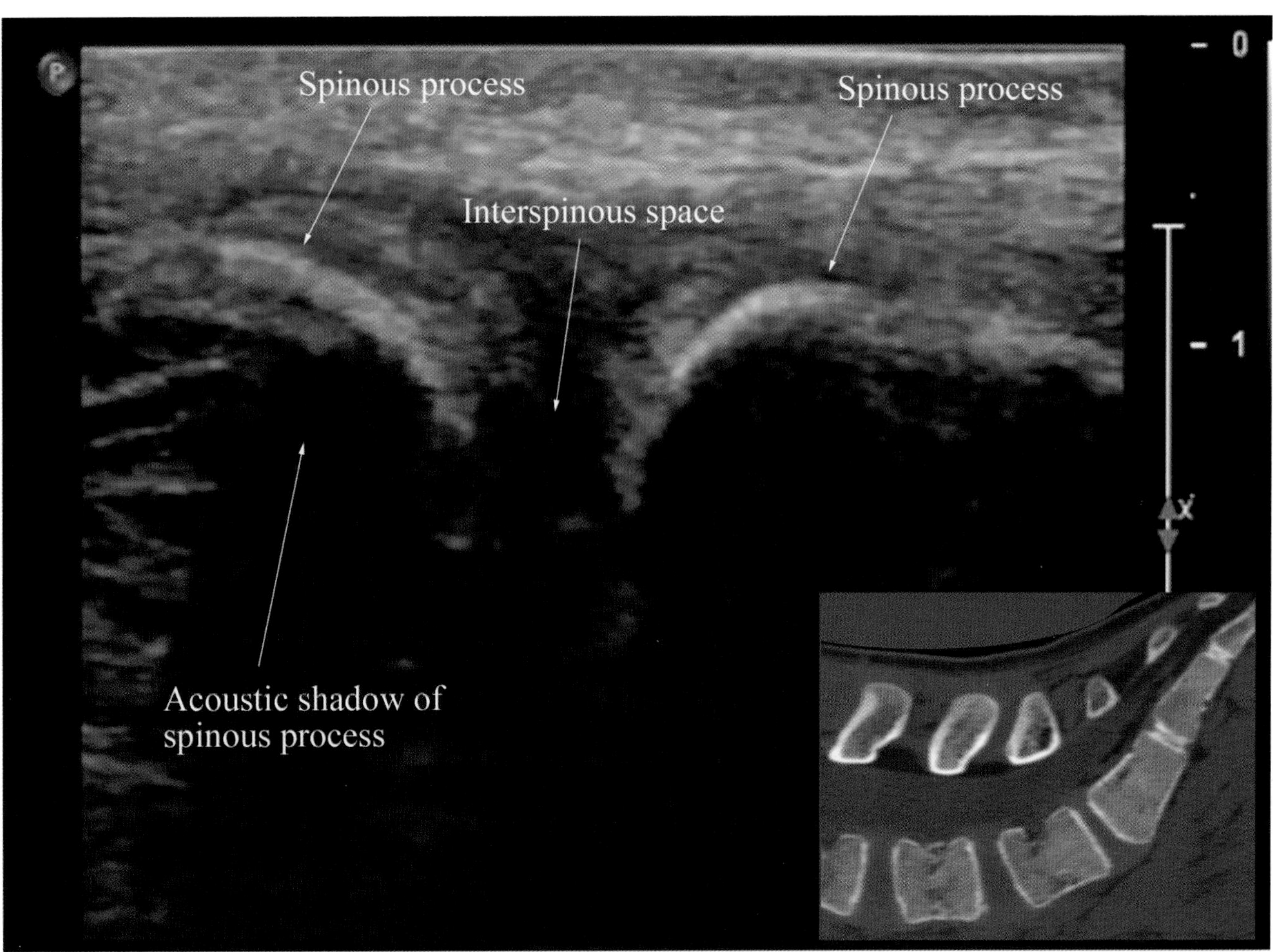


**FIGURE 44-9.** Median sagittal sonogram of the lumbar spine showing the crescent shaped hyperechoic reflections of the spinous processes. Note the narrow interspinous space in the midline. Picture in the inset shows a corresponding computed tomography (CT) scan of the lumbosacral spine through the median plane. The CT slice was reconstructed from a three-dimensional CT data set from the author's archive.

(Figure 44-14). However, the acute angulation of the spinous processes and the narrow interspinous and interlaminar spaces in the midthoracic region results in a narrow acoustic window with limited visibility of the underlying neuraxial anatomy (Figure 44-15). In the only published report describing US imaging of the thoracic spine, Grau and colleagues[13] performed US imaging of the thoracic spine at the T5-6 level in young volunteers and correlated findings with matching magnetic resonance imaging (MRI) images. They reported that the transverse axis produced the best images of the neuraxial structures. Epidural space, however, was best visualized in the paramedian scans.[13] Regardless, US was limited in being able to delineate the epidural space or the spinal cord but was better than MRI in demonstrating the posterior dura.[13] The transverse interspinous view, however, is almost impossible to obtain in the midthoracic region, and therefore the transverse scan provides little useful information for CNB other than to help identify the midline. In contrast, PMOSS, despite the narrow acoustic window, provides more useful information relevant for CNB. The laminae are seen as flat hyperechoic structures with acoustic shadowing anteriorly, and the posterior dura is consistently visualized in the acoustic window (Figures 44-14 and 44-15). However, the epidural space, spinal cord, central canal, and the anterior complex are difficult to delineate in the midthoracic region (Figure 44-15).

## Ultrasound Imaging of the Sacrum

Usually, US imaging of the sacrum is performed to identify the sonoanatomy relevant for a caudal epidural injection.[25] Because the sacrum is a superficial structure, a high-frequency linear array transducer can be used for the scan.[16,25] The patient is positioned in the lateral or prone position with a pillow under the abdomen to flex the lumbosacral spine.

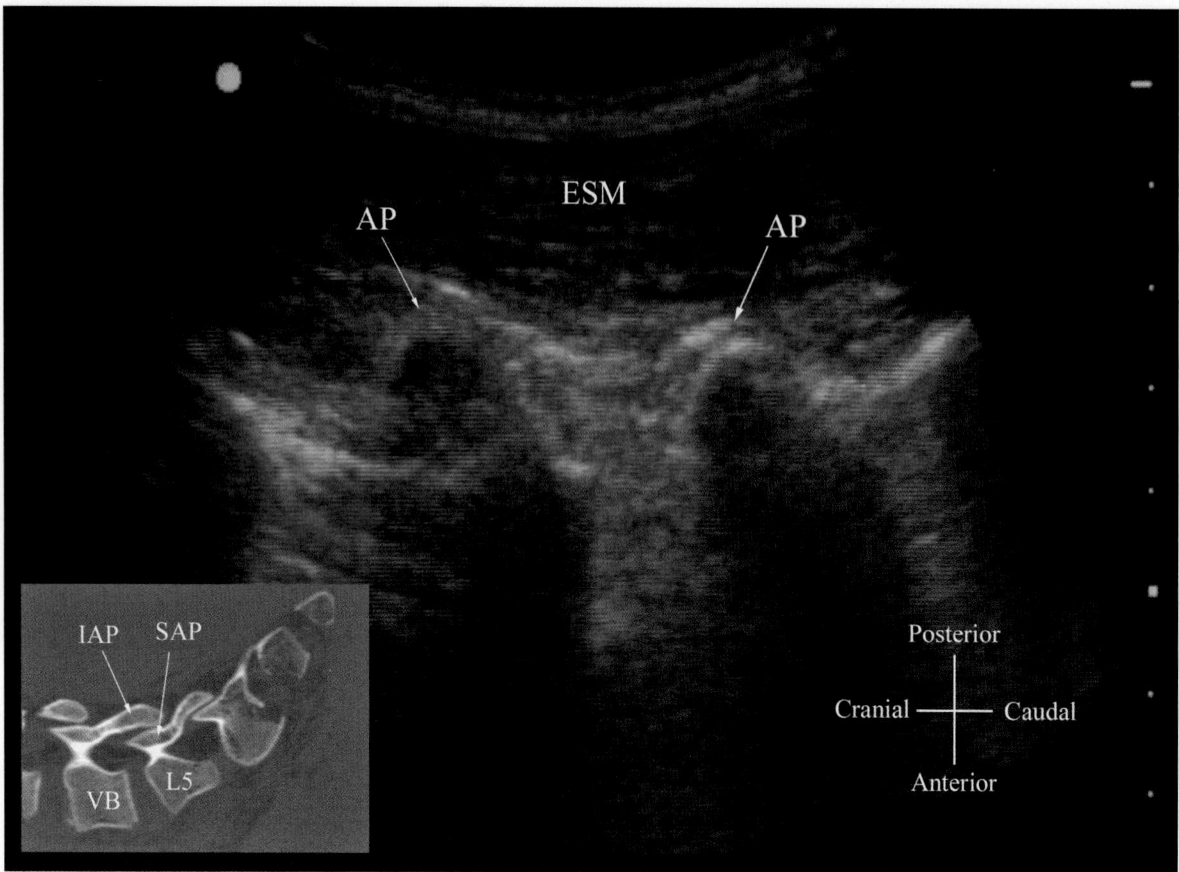


**FIGURE 44-10.** Paramedian sagittal sonogram of the lumbar spine at the level of the articular process (AP) of the vertebra. Note the "camel hump" appearance of the articular processes. Picture in the inset shows a corresponding computed tomography (CT) scan of the lumbosacral spine at the level of the articular processes. The CT slice was reconstructed from a three-dimensional CT data set from the author's archive. ESM, erector spinae muscle; IAP, inferior articular process; SAP, superior articular process.

The caudal epidural space is the continuation of the lumbar epidural space and commonly accessed via the sacral hiatus. The sacral hiatus is located at the distal end of the sacrum, and its lateral margins are formed by the two sacral cornua covered by the sacrococcygeal ligament. On a transverse sonogram of the sacrum at the level of the sacral hiatus, the sacral cornua are seen as two hyperechoic reversed U-shaped structures, one on either side of the midline (Figure 44-16).[16,25] Connecting the two sacral cornua, and deep to the skin and subcutaneous tissue, is a hyperechoic band, the sacrococcygeal ligament.[16,25] Anterior to the sacrococcygeal ligament is another hyperechoic linear structure, which represents the posterior surface of the sacrum. The hypoechoic space between the sacrococcygeal ligament and the bony posterior surface of the sacrum is the caudal epidural space. The two sacral cornua and the posterior surface of the sacrum produce a pattern on the sonogram that we refer to as the "frog eye sign" because of its resemblance to the eyes of a frog (Figure 44-16).[16] On a sagittal sonogram of the sacrum at the level of the sacral cornua, the sacrococcygeal ligament, the base of sacrum, and the caudal canal are also clearly visualized (Figure 44-17).[16]

## Technical Aspects of Ultrasound-Guided Central Neuraxial Blocks

"USG CNB can be performed as an off-line or in-line technique. Off-line technique involves performing a prepuncture scan (scout scan) to preview the spinal anatomy, determine the optimal site, depth and trajectory for needle insertion before performing a traditional spinal or epidural injection.[26,27] In contrast, an in-line technique involves performing a real-time USG CNB by a single[17] or two[4] operators." Real-time US-guided CNB demands a high degree of manual dexterity and hand–eye coordination. Therefore, the operator should have sound knowledge of the basics of US, be familiar with the sonoanatomy of the spine and scanning techniques, and have the necessary interventional skills before attempting a real-time US-guided CNB. At this

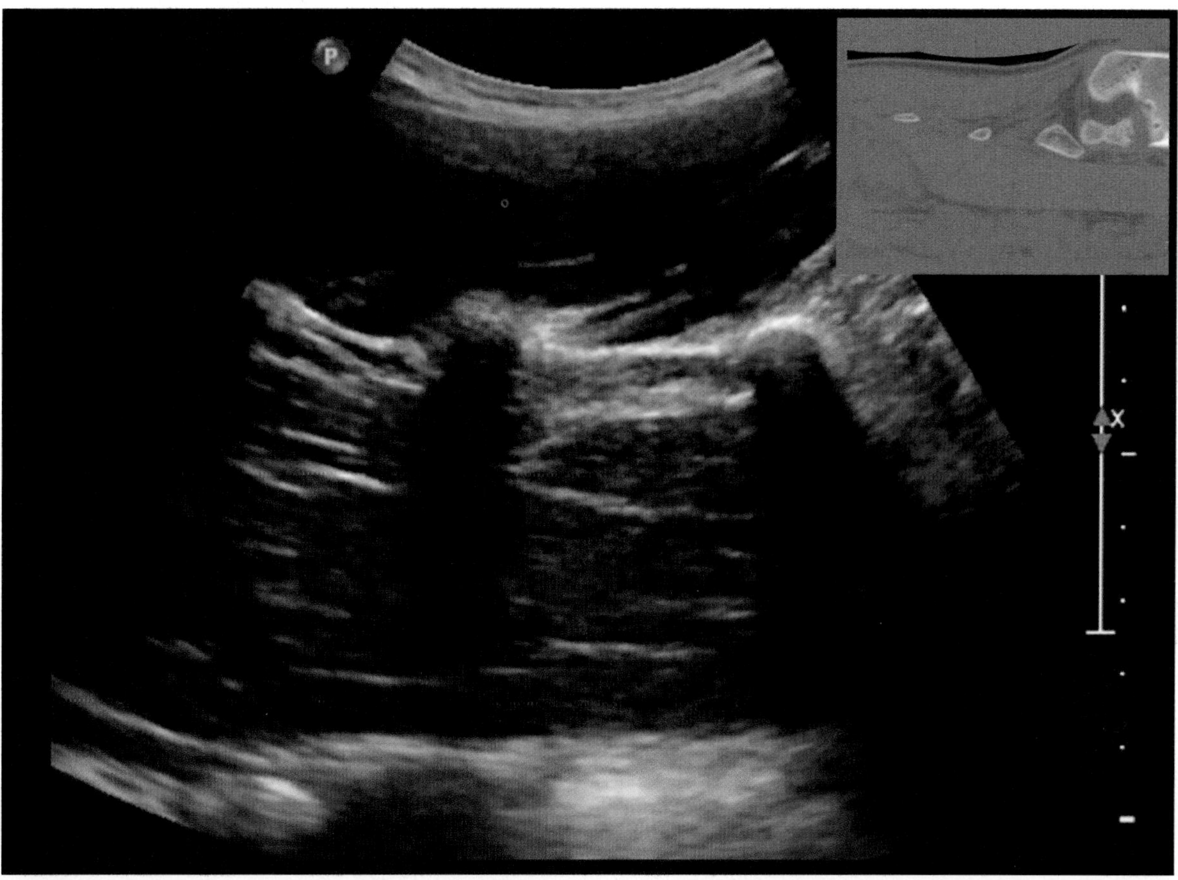


**FIGURE 44-11**. Paramedian sagittal sonogram of the lumbar spine at the level of the transverse processes (TPs). Note the hyperechoic reflections of the TPs with their acoustic shadow that produces the "trident sign." The psoas muscle is seen in the acoustic window between the transverse processes and is recognized by its typical hypoechoic and striated appearance. Part of the lumbar plexus is also seen as a hyperechoic shadow in the posterior part of the psoas muscle between the transverse processes of L4 and L5 vertebra. Picture in the inset shows a corresponding computed tomography (CT) scan of the lumbosacral spine at the level of the transverse processes. The CT slice was reconstructed from a three-dimensional CT data set from the author's archive.

time, there are no data on the safety of the US gel if it is introduced into the meninges or the nervous tissues during US-guided regional anesthesia procedures. Therefore, it is difficult to make recommendations; although some clinicians have resorted to using a sterile normal saline solution applied using sterile swabs as an alternative coupling agent to keep the skin moist under the footprint of the transducer.[17]

## TIPS

- The use of saline instead of US gel results in a slight deterioration of the quality of the US image compared with that obtained during the scout scan. This can be compensated for by manually adjusting the overall gain and compression settings.
- While preparing the US transducer, a thin layer of sterile US gel is applied onto the footprint of the transducer and covered with a sterile transparent dressing, making sure no air is trapped between the footprint and the dressing. The transducer and its cable are then covered with a sterile plastic sleeve.
- All of these additional steps that go into preparing the equipment during an US-guided CNB may increase the potential for infection via contamination. Therefore, strict asepsis must be maintained, and we recommend that local protocols be established for US-guided CNB.
- Several custom covers for use in regional anesthesia recently were introduced and make a significant improvement over the improvised techniques of covering the transducer.

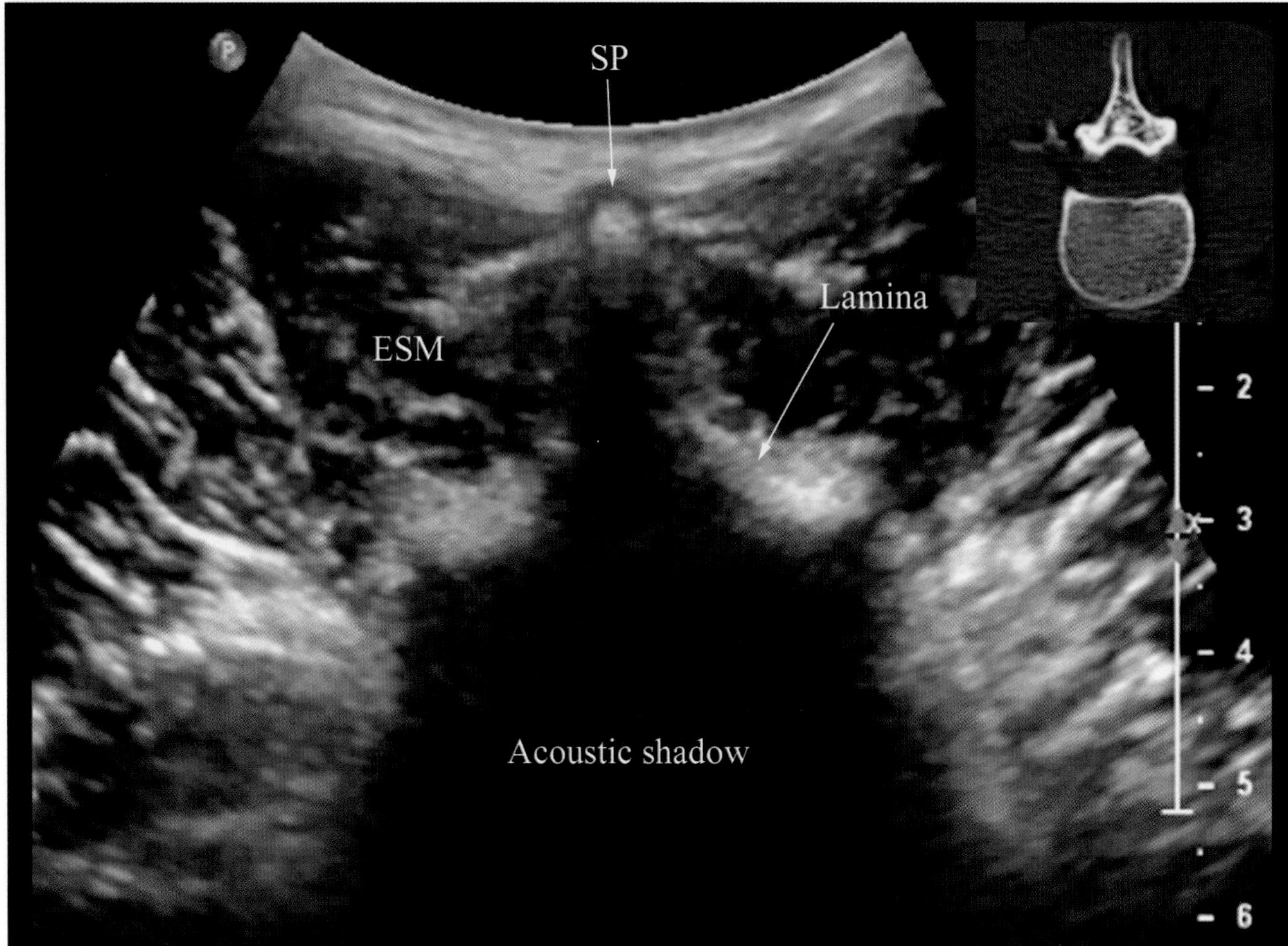


**FIGURE 44-12.** Transverse sonogram of the lumbar spine with the transducer positioned directly over the spinous process (i.e., transverse spinous process view). Note the acoustic shadow of the spinous process and lamina that completely obscures the spinal canal and the neuraxial structures. Picture in the inset shows a corresponding computed tomography (CT) scan of the lumbar vertebra. The CT slice was reconstructed from a three-dimensional CT data set from the author's archive. SP, spinous process; ESM, erector spinae muscle.

## Spinal Injection

There are limited data in the published medical literature on the use of US for spinal (intrathecal) injections,[28,29] although US has been reported to guide lumbar punctures by radiologists[30] and emergency physicians.[31] Most available data are anecdotal case reports.[28,29,32–34] Yeo and French, in 1999, were the first to describe the successful use of US to assist spinal injection in a patient with abnormal spinal anatomy.[34] They used US to locate the vertebral midline in a parturient with severe scoliosis with Harrington rods in situ.[34] Yamauchi and colleagues describe using US to preview the neuraxial anatomy and measure the distance from the skin to the dura in a postlaminectomy patient before the intrathecal injection was performed under X-ray guidance.[33] Costello and Balki described using US to facilitate spinal injection by locating the L5-S1 gap in a parturient with poliomyelitis and previous Harrington rod instrumentation of the spine.[28] Prasad and colleagues report using US to assist spinal injection in a patient with obesity, scoliosis, and multiple previous back surgeries with instrumentation.[29] More recently, Chin and colleagues[32] described real-time US-guided spinal anesthesia in two patients with abnormal spinal anatomy (one had lumbar scoliosis and the other had undergone spinal fusion surgery at the L2-3 level).

## Lumbar Epidural Injection

US imaging can be used to preview the underlying spinal anatomy[2–4] or to guide the Tuohy needle in real time[17] during a lumbar epidural access. Moreover, real-time US guidance for epidural access can be performed by a single[17] or two[4] operators. In the latter technique, described by Grau and colleagues[4] for combined spinal epidural anesthesia, one operator performs the US scan via the paramedian axis while the other carries the needle insertion through the midline approach using a "loss-of-resistance" technique.[4] Using

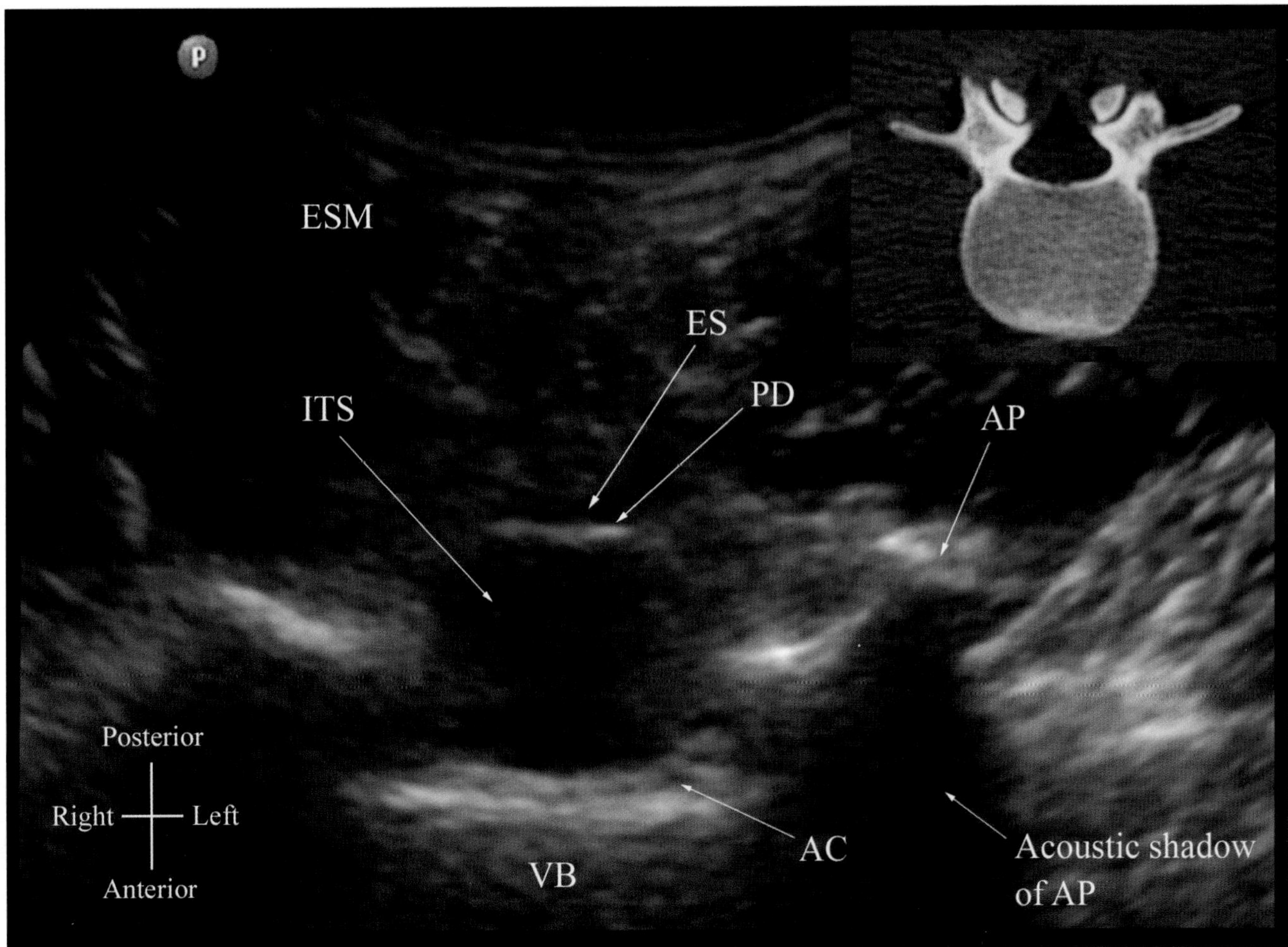


**FIGURE 44-13.** Transverse sonogram of the lumbar spine with the transducer positioned such that the ultrasound beam is insonated through the interspinous space (i.e., transverse interspinous view). The epidural space, posterior dura, intrathecal space, and the anterior complex are visible in the midline, and the articular process (AP) is visible laterally on either side of the midline. Note how the articular processes on either side are symmetrically located. Picture in the inset shows a corresponding computed tomography (CT) scan of the lumbar vertebra. The CT slice was reconstructed from a three-dimensional CT data set from the author's archive. ESM, erector spinae muscle; ES, epidural space; PD, posterior dura; ITS, intrathecal space; AC, anterior complex; VB, vertebral body.

this approach, Grau and colleagues reported the ability to visualize the advancing epidural needle despite different axes of the US scan and needle insertion.[4] They were able to visualize the dural puncture in all patients, as well as dural tenting in a few cases, during the needle-through-needle spinal puncture.[4]

Karmakar and colleagues recently described a technique of real-time, US guided epidural injection in conjunction with loss of resistance (LOR) to saline.[17] The epidural access was performed by a single operator, and the epidural needle was inserted in the plane of the US beam via the paramedian axis.[17] Generally, it is possible to visualize the advancing epidural needle in real time until it engages in the ligamentum flavum.[17] The need for a second operator to perform the LOR can be circumvented by using a spring-loaded syringe (e.g., Episure AutoDetect syringe, Indigo Orb, Inc., Irvine, CA, USA), with an internal compression spring that applies constant pressure on the plunger (Figure 44-18).[17] Anterior displacement of the posterior dura and widening of the posterior epidural space are the most frequently visualized changes within the spinal canal. Compression of the thecal sac can be seen occasionally.[17] These ultrasonographic signs of a correct epidural injection were previously described in children.[35] The neuraxial changes that occur within the spinal canal following the "loss of resistance" to saline may have clinical significance.[17] Despite the ability to use real-time US for establishing epidural access, visualization of an indwelling epidural catheter in adults proved to be more challenging. Occasionally, anterior displacement of the posterior dura and widening of the posterior epidural space after an epidural bolus injection via the catheter can be observed and can be used as a surrogate marker of the

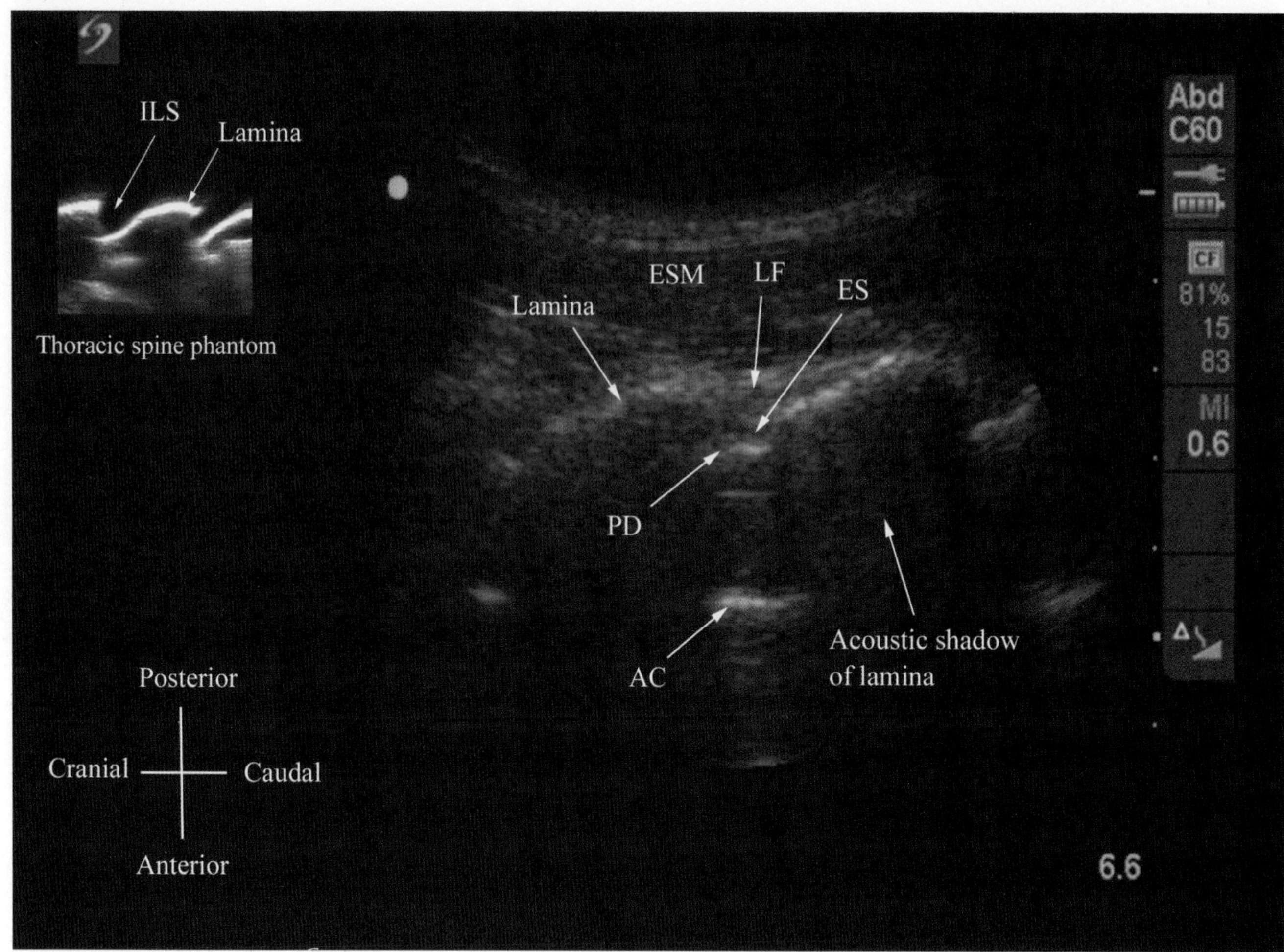


**FIGURE 44-14.** Paramedian oblique sagittal sonogram of the lower-thoracic spine. Note the narrow acoustic window through which the ligamentum flavum (LF), posterior dura (PD), epidural space (ES), and anterior complex (AC) are visible. Picture in the inset shows a sagittal sonogram of the thoracic spine from the water-based spine phantom. ILS, interlaminar space.

location of the catheter tip. Grau and colleagues postulated that this may be related to the small diameter and poor echogenicity of conventional epidural catheters.[15] It remains to be seen whether or not the imminent development of echogenic needles and catheters will have an impact on the ability to visualize epidurally placed catheters.

## Thoracic Epidural Injection

There are no published data on USG thoracic epidural blocks. This lack may be due to the poor US visibility of the neuraxial structures in the thoracic region compared with the lumbar region (see previous section) and the associated technical difficulties. However, despite the narrow acoustic window, the lamina, the interlaminar space, and the posterior dura are visualized consistently when using the paramedian axis (Figures 44-14 and 44-15). The epidural space is more difficult to delineate, but it also is best visualized in a paramedian scan.[13] As a result, a US-assisted technique can be used to perform thoracic epidural catheterization via the paramedian window. In this approach, the patient is positioned in the sitting position and a PMOSS is performed at the desired thoracic level with the orientation marker of the transducer directed cranially. Under strict aseptic precautions (described previously) the Tuohy needle is inserted via the paramedian axis in real time and in the plane of the US beam. The needle is advanced steadily until it contacts the lamina or enters the interlaminar space. At this point, the US transducer is removed and a traditional loss of resistance to saline technique is used to access the epidural space. Because the lamina is relatively superficial in

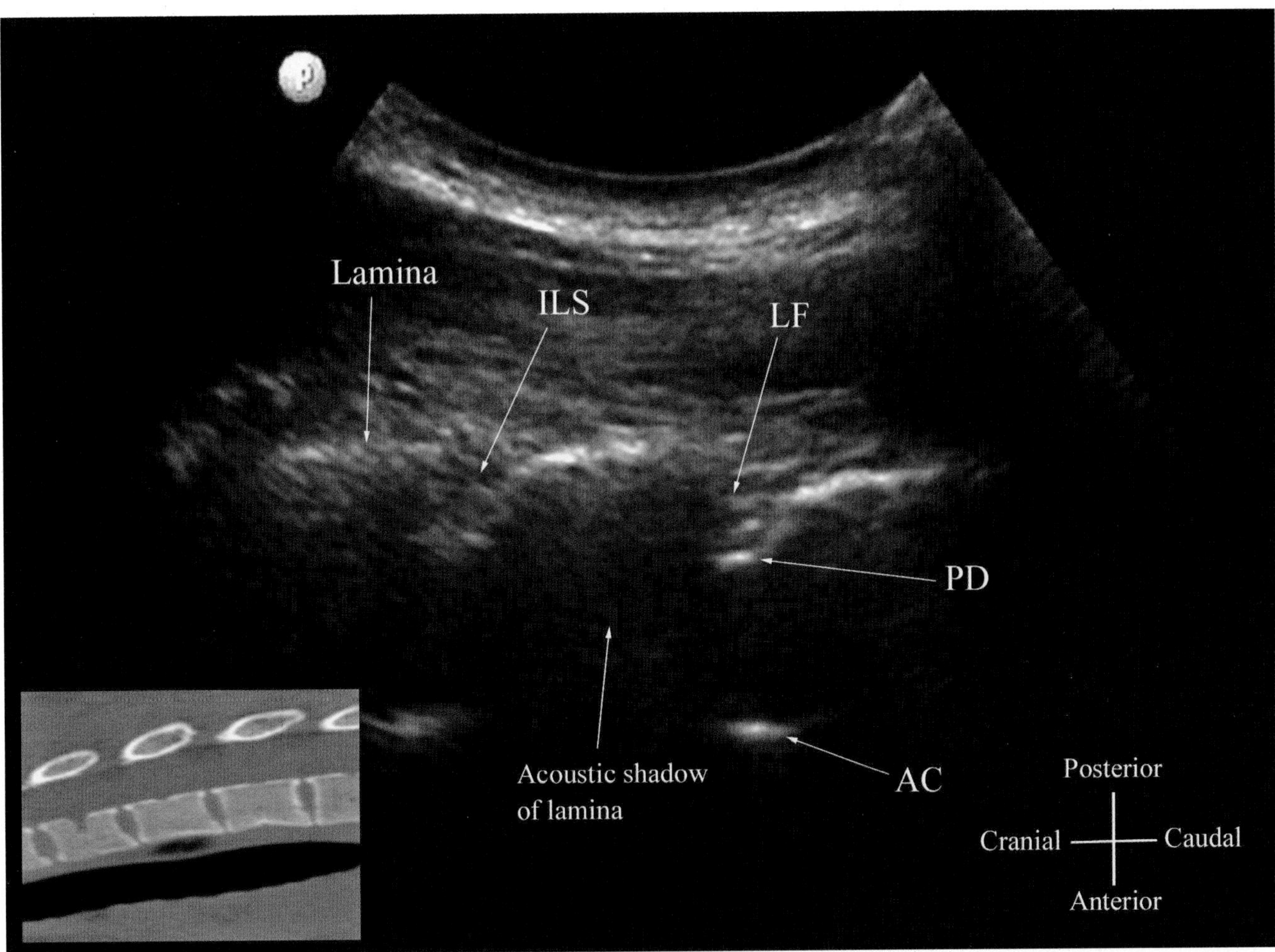


**FIGURE 44-15.** Paramedian oblique sagittal sonogram of the midthoracic spine. The posterior dura (PD) and the anterior complex (AC) are visible through the narrow acoustic window. Picture in the inset shows a corresponding computed tomography (CT) scan of the midthoracic spine. The CT slice was reconstructed from a three-dimensional CT data set from the author's archive. ILS, interlaminar space; LF, ligamentum flavum.

the thoracic region, it is possible to visualize the advancing Tuohy needle in real time. Preliminary experience with this approach indicates that US may improve the likelihood of thoracic epidural access on the first attempt. However, more research to compare the US-assisted technique as described with the traditional approach is necessary before more definitive recommendations on the utility and safety of US for this indication can be made.

## Caudal Epidural Injection

For an USG caudal epidural injection, a transverse (Figure 44-16) or sagittal (Figure 44-17) scan is performed at the level of the sacral hiatus. Because the sacral hiatus is a superficial structure, a high-frequency (13-6 MHz) linear array transducer is used for the scan as described previously. The needle can be inserted in the short (out-of-plane) or long axis (in-plane). For a long-axis needle insertion, a sagittal scan is performed and the passage of the block needle through the sacrococcygeal ligament into the sacral canal is visualized in real time (Figure 44-19). However, because the sacrum impedes the travel of the US, there is a large acoustic shadow anteriorly, which makes it impossible to visualize the tip of the needle or the spread of the injectate within the sacral canal. An inadvertent intravascular injection, which reportedly occurs in 5 to 9% of procedures, cannot be detected using US. As a result, the clinician still should factor in traditional clinical signs such as the "pop" or "give" as the needle traverses the sacrococcygeal ligament, ease of injection, absence of subcutaneous swelling, "whoosh test," nerve stimulation, or assessing the clinical effects of the injected drug to confirm the correct needle placement. Chen and colleagues reported a 100% success rate in placing a caudal needle under US guidance as confirmed by contrast fluoroscopy.[25] This report is encouraging, considering that even in experienced hands, failure to place a needle in the caudal epidural

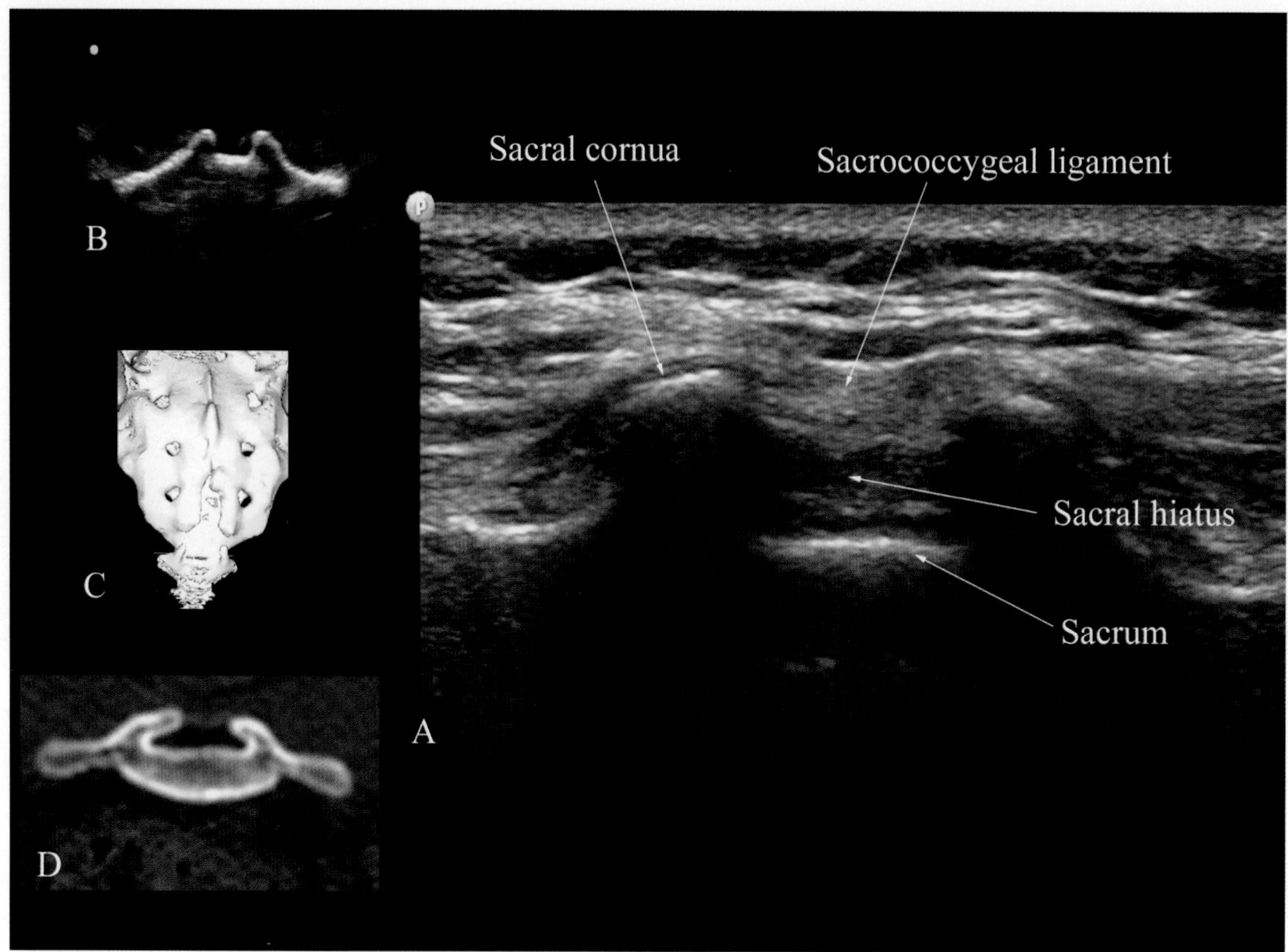


**FIGURE 44-16.** Transverse sonogram of the sacrum at the level of the sacral hiatus. Note the two sacral cornua and the hyperechoic sacrococcygeal ligament that extends between the two sacral cornua. The hypoechoic space between the sacrococcygeal ligament and the posterior surface of the sacrum is the sacral hiatus. Figures in the inset (B) shows the sacral cornua from the water-based spine phantom, (C) shows a three-dimensional (3D) reconstructed image of the sacrum at the level of the sacral hiatus from a 3D CT data set from the author's archive, and (D) shows a transverse CT slice of the sacrum at the level of the sacral cornua.

space successfully is as high as 25%.[25,36] More recently, Chen and colleagues[37] described using US imaging as a screening tool during caudal epidural injections.[37] In their cohort of patients, the mean diameter of the sacral canal at the sacral hiatus was 5.3 + 2 mm and the distance between the sacral cornua (bilateral) was 9.7 + 1.9 mm.[37] These researchers also identified that the presence of sonographic features such as a closed sacral hiatus and a sacral canal diameter of around 1.5 mm are associated with a greater probability for failure.[37] Based on the published data, it can be concluded that US guidance, despite its limitation, can be useful as an adjunct tool for caudal epidural needle placement and has the potential to improve technical outcomes and minimize failure rates and exposure to radiation in the chronic pain setting, and therefore it deserves further investigation.

## Clinical Utility of Ultrasound for Central Neuraxial Blocks

Outcome data on the use of US for CNB are limited and have primarily focused on the lumbar region. Most studies to date evaluated the utility of an out-of-plane prepuncture US scan or scout scan. A scout scan allows the operator to identify the midline[23] and accurately determine the interspace for needle insertion,[16,17,21] which are useful in patients in whom anatomic landmarks are difficult to palpate, such as in those with obesity,[1,38] edema of the back, or abnormal anatomy (scoliosis,[1,39] postlaminectomy surgery,[33] or spinal instrumentation).[28,29,34] It also allows the operator to preview the neuraxial anatomy,[2-4,17,40] identify asymptomatic spinal abnormalities such as in spina bifida,[41] predict the depth to

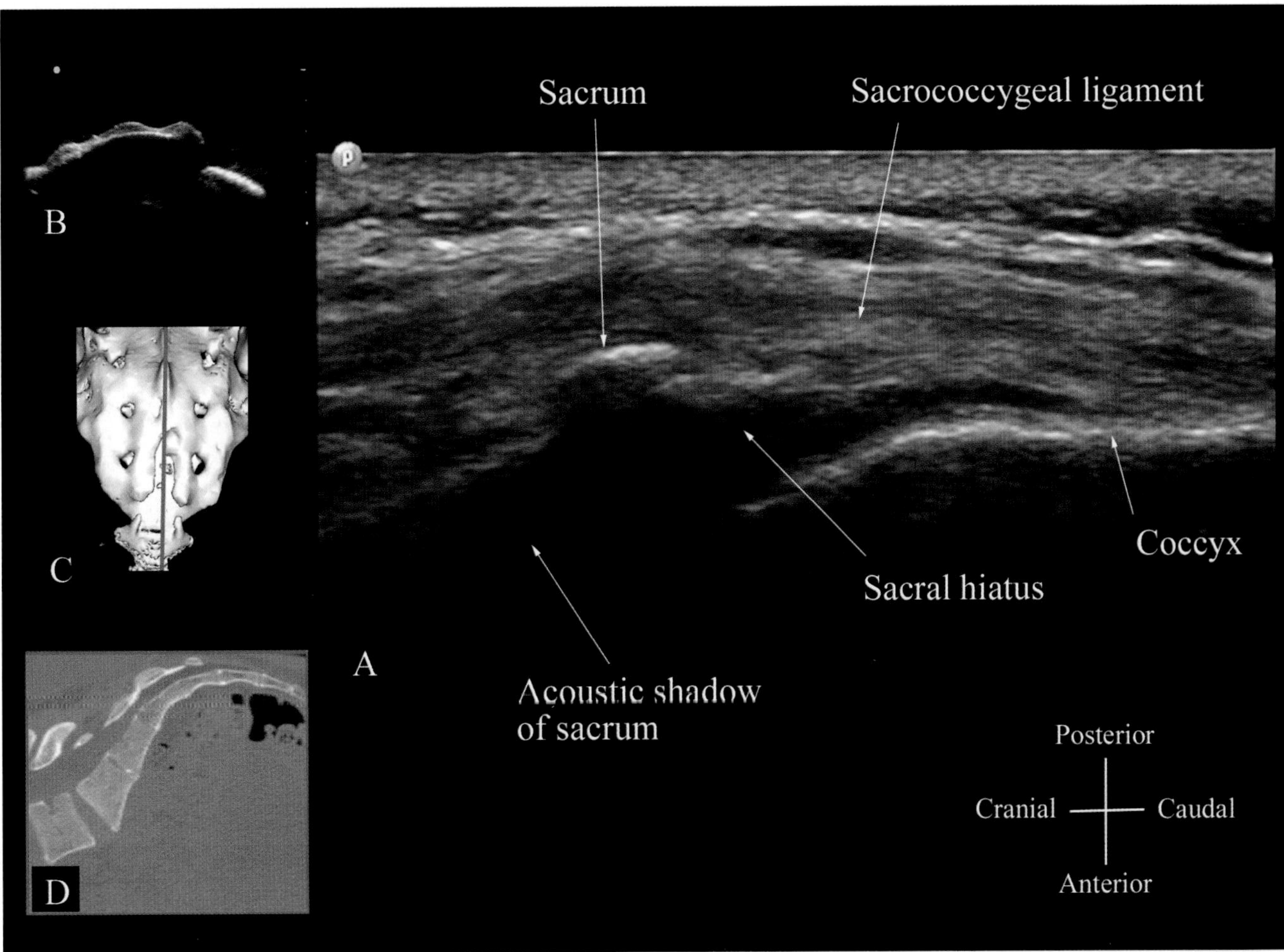


**FIGURE 44-17.** Sagittal sonogram of the sacrum at the level of the sacral hiatus. Note the hyperechoic sacrococcygeal ligament that extends from the sacrum to the coccyx and the acoustic shadow of the sacrum that completely obscures the sacral canal. Figures in the inset: (B) shows the sacral hiatus from the water-based spine phantom, (C) shows a three-dimensional (3D) reconstructed image of the sacrum at the level of the sacral hiatus from a 3D CT data set from the author's archive, and (D) shows a sagittal CT slice of the sacrum at the level of the sacral cornua.

the epidural space,[2,3,9,10] particularly in obese patients,[26] identify ligamentum flavum defects,[42] and determine the optimal site and trajectory for needle insertion.[3,15] Cumulative evidence suggests that a US examination performed before the epidural puncture improves the success rate of epidural access on the first attempt,[2] reduces the number of puncture attempts[1–4] or the need to puncture multiple levels,[2–4] and also improves patient comfort during the procedure.[3] A scan can be useful in patients with presumed difficult epidural access, such as in those with a history of difficult epidural access, obesity, and kyphosis or scoliosis of the lumbar spine.[1] When used for obstetric epidural anesthesia, US guidance was reported to improve the quality of analgesia, reduce side effects, and improve patient satisfaction.[1,4] A scout scan may also improve the learning curve of students for epidural blocks in parturients.[14] Currently, there are limited data on the utility of real-time US guidance for epidural access,[4,17] although the preliminary reports indicate it may improve technical outcomes.[4]

## Education and Training

Learning US-guided CNB techniques takes time and patience. Regardless of the technique used, US-guided CNB and, in particular, real-time US-guided CNB, are advanced techniques and are by far the most difficult USG interventions. Likewise, peri-centroneuraxial blocks, such as lumbar plexus and paravertebral blocks, also demand a high degree of manual dexterity, hand–eye coordination, and an ability to conceptualize two-dimensional information into a 3D image. Therefore, before attempting to perform a US-guided CNB or peri-centroneuraxial blocks, the operator should have knowledge of the basics of US, be familiar with the sonoanatomy of the spine and lumbar plexus, and have the necessary interventional skills. It is advisable to start by attending a course or workshop tailored for this purpose where the operator can learn the basic scanning techniques, spinal sonoanatomy, and the interventional skills. More experience in spinal sonography can also be acquired by scanning human volunteers.[43]

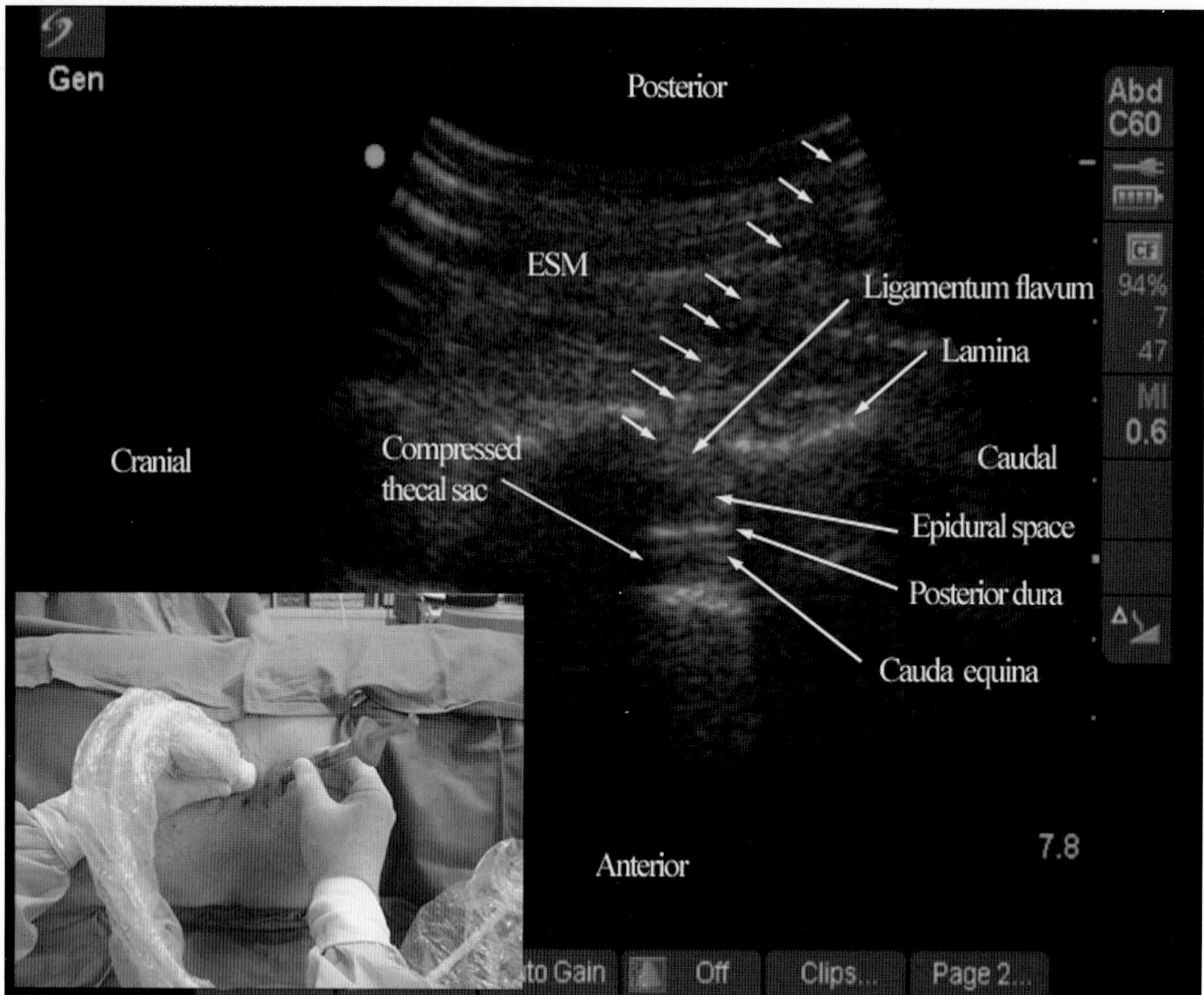


**FIGURE 44-18.** Paramedian oblique sagittal sonogram of the lumbar spine showing the sonographic changes within the spinal canal after the "loss of resistance" to saline. Note the anterior displacement of the posterior dura, widening of the posterior epidural space, and compression of the thecal sac. The cauda equina nerve roots are also now better visualized within the compressed thecal sac in this patient. Picture in the inset shows how the Episure AutoDetect syringe was used to circumvent the need for a third hand for the "loss of resistance."

Today, there are several models (phantoms) for practicing US-guided central neuraxial interventions. The "water-based spine phantom"[18] is useful for learning the osseous anatomy of the spine, but it is not a good model for learning US-guided spinal interventions because it lacks tissue mimicking properties. Spinal and paraspinal sonography is often taught at workshops, but they are not suitable for practicing actual techniques. Fresh cadaver courses are available, and they allow participants to study the neuraxial sonoanatomy and practice US-guided CNB with realistic haptic feedback, but they may be limited by the quality of the US images. However, such courses are uncommon and conducted in anatomy departments with the cadavers in a position that rarely mimics what is practiced in the operating room. Anesthetized pigs can also be used, but animal ethics approval is required and, for the organizers, a license from the local health department to conduct such workshops. They entail infectious precautions, and religious beliefs may preclude its use as a model. Moreover, such workshops are conducted in designated animal laboratories that are typically small and not suited to accommodate large groups of participants. To circumvent some of these problems, the group at the Chinese University Hong Kong recently introduced the "pig carcass spine phantom," (Figure 44-4),[19] an excellent model that can be used in conference venues and provides excellent tactile and visual feedback.[19] The limitation of the "pig carcass spine phantom" is that it is a decapitated model and there is loss of cerebrospinal fluid during the preparation process. This presentation results in air artifacts and loss of contrast within the spinal canal during

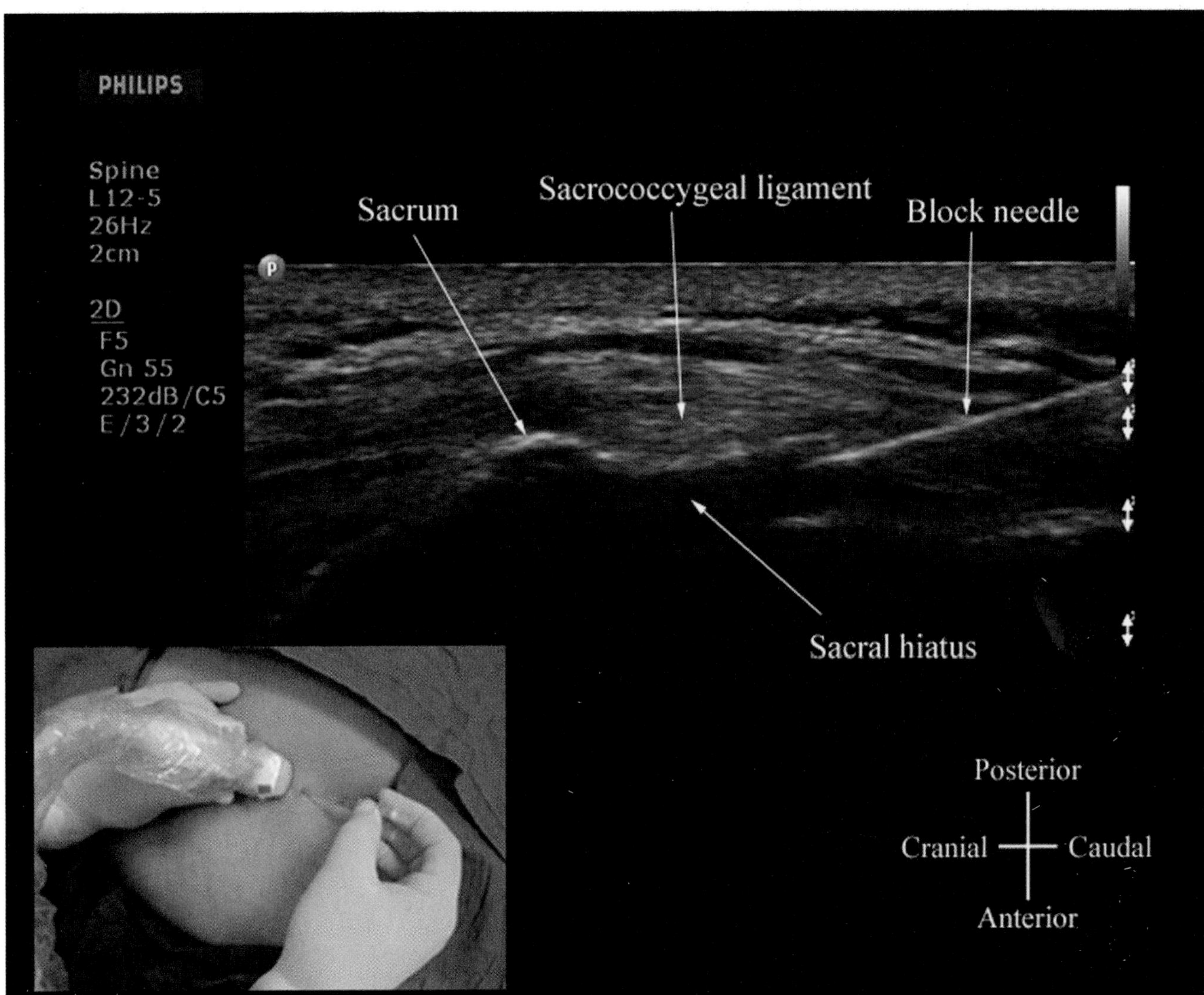


**FIGURE 44-19.** Sagittal sonogram of the sacrum at the level of the sacral hiatus during a real-time ultrasound-guided caudal epidural injection. Note the hyperechoic sacrococcygeal ligament and the block needle that has been inserted in the plane (in-plane) of the ultrasound beam. Picture in the inset shows the position and orientation of the transducer and the direction in which the block needle was inserted.

spinal sonography unless the thecal sac is cannulated at its cranial end and continuously irrigated with fluid (normal saline), a process that requires surgical dissection to isolate the thecal sac. Therefore, an "in vitro" model that can facilitate the learning of the scanning techniques and the hand–eye coordination skills required for real-time US-guided CNB is highly desirable. A low-cost gelatin-based US phantom of the lumbosacral spine recently was proposed.[44] However, the gelatin phantom is soft in consistency, lacks tissue-mimicking echogenic properties, does not provide a haptic feedback, is easily contaminated with mold and bacteria, and needle track marks limit its usefulness,[44] all of which preclude its extended use. Karmakar and colleagues recently developed a "gelatin-agar spine phantom" that overcomes some of the drawbacks of the gelatin-based spine phantom. It is mechanically stable, has a tissue-like texture and echogenicity, needle track marks are less of a problem, and it can be used over extended periods of time to study the osseous anatomy of the lumbosacral spine and to practice the hand–eye coordination skills required to perform US-guided CNB.[45]

Once the basic skills are attained, it is best to start by performing US-guided spinal injections, under supervision, before progressing to performing epidural blocks. Real-time US-guided epidurals can be technically challenging, even for an experienced operator. If there is no experience in US-guided CNB locally, it is advisable to visit a center where such interventions are practiced. At this time, there is no knowledge of the length of the learning curve for US-guided CNB or how many such interventions are needed to become proficient in performing real-time US-guided CNB. Further research in this area is warranted.

## Conclusion

US-guided CNB is a promising alternative to traditional landmark-based techniques. It is noninvasive, safe, simple to use, can be quickly performed, does not involve exposure to radiation, provides real-time images, and is free from adverse effects. Experienced sonographers are able to visualize neuraxial structures with satisfactory clarity using US, and the understanding of spinal sonoanatomy continues to be clarified. A scout scan allows the operator to preview the spinal anatomy, identify the midline, locate a given intervertebral level, accurately predict the depth to the epidural space, and determine the optimal site and trajectory for needle insertion. Use of US also improves the success rate of epidural access on the first attempt, reduces the number of puncture attempts or the need to puncture multiple levels, and improves patient comfort during the procedure. It is an excellent teaching tool for demonstrating the anatomy of the spine and improves the learning curve of epidural blocks in parturients. US guidance also may allow the use of CNB in patients who in the past may have been considered unsuitable for such procedures due to abnormal spinal anatomy. However, US guidance for CNB is still in its early stages of development, and evidence to support its use is sparse. The initial experience suggests that US-guided CNB is technically demanding, and, therefore, unlikely to replace traditional methods of performing CNB in the near future because traditional methods are well established as simple, safe, and effective in most patients. We envision that as US technology continues to improve and as more anesthesiologists embrace it and acquire the skills necessary to perform US-guided interventions, US-guided CNB may become the standard of care in the future.

## REFERENCES


1. Grau T, Leipold RW, Conradi R, Martin E. Ultrasound control for presumed difficult epidural puncture. *Acta Anaesthesiol Scand.* 2001;45(6):766-771.
2. Grau T, Leipold RW, Conradi R, Martin E, Motsch J. Ultrasound imaging facilitates localization of the epidural space during combined spinal and epidural anesthesia. *Reg Anesth Pain Med.* 2001;26(1):64-67.
3. Grau T, Leipold RW, Conradi R, Martin E, Motsch J. Efficacy of ultrasound imaging in obstetric epidural anesthesia. *J Clin Anesth.* 2002;14(3):169-175.
4. Grau T, Leipold RW, Fatehi S, Martin E, Motsch J. Real-time ultrasonic observation of combined spinal-epidural anaesthesia. *Eur J Anaesthesiology.* 2004;21(1):25-31.
5. National Institute for Health and Clinical Excellence (NICE). Ultrasound Guided Epidural Catheterization of the Epidural Space: Understanding NICE Guidance. January 2008. http://guidance.nice.org.uk/IPG249/Guidance/pdf/English
6. Mathieu S, Dalgleish DJ. A survey of local opinion of NICE guidance on the use of ultrasound in the insertion of epidural catheters. *Anaesthesia.* 2008;63(10):1146-1147.
7. Bogin IN, Stulin ID. Application of the method of 2-dimensional echospondylography for determining landmarks in lumbar punctures. *Zh Nevropatol Psikhiatr Im S S Korsakova.* 1971;71:1810-1811.
8. Porter RW, Wicks M, Ottewell D. Measurement of the spinal canal by diagnostic ultrasound. *J Bone Joint Surg Br.* 1978;60-B(4):481-484.
9. Cork RC, Kryc JJ, Vaughan RW. Ultrasonic localization of the lumbar epidural space. *Anesthesiology.* 1980;52(6):513-516.
10. Currie JM. Measurement of the depth to the extradural space using ultrasound. *Br J Anaesth.* 1984;56(4):345-347.
11. Wallace DH, Currie JM, Gilstrap LC, Santos R. Indirect sonographic guidance for epidural anesthesia in obese pregnant patients. *Reg Anesth.* 1992;17(4):233-236.
12. Grau T, Leipold RW, Horter J, Conradi R, Martin EO, Motsch J. Paramedian access to the epidural space: the optimum window for ultrasound imaging. *J Clin Anesth.* 2001;13(3): 213-217.
13. Grau T, Leipold RW, Delorme S, Martin E, Motsch J. Ultrasound imaging of the thoracic epidural space. *Reg Anesth Pain Med.* 2002;27(2):200-206.
14. Grau T, Bartusseck E, Conradi R, Martin E, Motsch J. Ultrasound imaging improves learning curves in obstetric epidural anesthesia: a preliminary study. *Can J Anaesth.* 2003;50(10):1047-1050.
15. Grau T. The evaluation of ultrasound imaging for neuraxial anesthesia. *Can J Anaesth.* 2003;50(6):R1-R8.
16. Karmakar MK. Ultrasound for central neuraxial blocks. *Techniques Reg Anesth Pain Manage.* 2009;13(3):161-170.
17. Karmakar MK, Li X, Ho AM, Kwok WH, Chui PT. Real-time ultrasound-guided paramedian epidural access: evaluation of a novel in-plane technique. *Br J Anaesth.* 2009;102(6):845-854.
18. Karmakar MK, Li X, Kwok WH, Ho AM, Ngan Kee WD. The "water-based-spine-phantom"—a small step towards learning the basics of spinal sonography. *Br J Anaesth.* Available at: http://bja.oxfordjournals.org/cgi/qa-display/short/brjana_el;4114.
19. Kwok WH, Chui PT, Karmakar MK. Pig carcass spine phantom—a model to learn ultrasound guided neuraxial interventions. *Reg Anesth Pain Med.* 2010;35(5):472-473.
20. Greher M, Scharbert G, Kamolz LP et al. Ultrasound-guided lumbar facet nerve block: a sonoanatomic study of a new methodologic approach. *Anesthesiology.* 2004;100(5):1242-1248.
21. Furness G, Reilly MP, Kuchi S. An evaluation of ultrasound imaging for identification of lumbar intervertebral level. *Anaesthesia.* 2002;57(3):277-280.
22. Karmakar MK, Ho AM, Li X, Kwok WH, Tsang K, Kee WD. Ultrasound-guided lumbar plexus block through the acoustic window of the lumbar ultrasound trident. *Br J Anaesth.* 2008;100(4):533-537.
23. Carvalho JC. Ultrasound-facilitated epidurals and spinals in obstetrics. *Anesthesiol Clin.* 2008;26(1):145-158.
24. Suzuki S, Yamamuro T, Shikata J, Shimizu K, Iida H. Ultrasound measurement of vertebral rotation in idiopathic scoliosis. *J Bone Joint Surg Br.* 1989;71(2):252-255.
25. Chen CP, Tang SF, Hsu TC, et al. Ultrasound guidance in caudal epidural needle placement. *Anesthesiology.* 2004;101(1):181-184.
26. Balki M, Lee Y, Halpern S, Carvalho JC. Ultrasound imaging of the lumbar spine in the transverse plane: the correlation between estimated and actual depth to the epidural space in obese parturients. *Anesth Analg.* 2009;108(6):1876-1881.
27. Chin KJ, Perlas A, Singh M, et al. An ultrasound-assisted approach facilitates spinal anesthesia for total joint arthroplasty. *Can J Anaesth.* 2009;56(9):643-650.
28. Costello JF, Balki M. Cesarean delivery under ultrasound-guided spinal anesthesia [corrected] in a parturient with poliomyelitis and Harrington instrumentation. *Can J Anaesth.* 2008;55(9):606-611.
29. Prasad GA, Tumber PS, Lupu CM. Ultrasound guided spinal anesthesia. *Can J Anaesth.* 2008;55(10):716-717.

30. Coley BD, Shiels WE, Hogan MJ. Diagnostic and interventional ultrasonography in neonatal and infant lumbar puncture. *Pediatr Radiol.* 2001;31(6):399-402.
31. Peterson MA, Abele J. Bedside ultrasound for difficult lumbar puncture. *J Emerg Med.* 2005;28(2):197-200.
32. Chin KJ, Chan VW, Ramlogan R, Perlas A. Real-time ultrasound-guided spinal anesthesia in patients with a challenging spinal anatomy: two case reports. *Acta Anaesthesiol Scand.* 2010;54(2):252-255.
33. Yamauchi M, Honma E, Mimura M, Yamamoto H, Takahashi E, Namiki A. Identification of the lumbar intervertebral level using ultrasound imaging in a post-laminectomy patient. *J Anesth.* 2006;20(3):231-233.
34. Yeo ST, French R. Combined spinal-epidural in the obstetric patient with Harrington rods assisted by ultrasonography. *Br J Anaesth.* 1999;83(4):670-672.
35. Rapp HJ, Folger A, Grau T. Ultrasound-guided epidural catheter insertion in children. *Anesth Analg.* 2005;101(2):333-339.
36. Tsui BC, Tarkkila P, Gupta S, Kearney R. Confirmation of caudal needle placement using nerve stimulation. *Anesthesiology.* 1999;91(2):374-378.
37. Chen CP, Wong AM, Hsu CC, et al. Ultrasound as a screening tool for proceeding with caudal epidural injections. *Arch Phys Med Rehabil.* 2010;91(3):358-363.
38. Stiffler KA, Jwayyed S, Wilber ST, Robinson A. The use of ultrasound to identify pertinent landmarks for lumbar puncture. *Am J Emerg Med.* 2007;25(3):331-334.
39. McLeod A, Roche A, Fennelly M. Case series: Ultrasonography may assist epidural insertion in scoliosis patients. *Can J Anaesth.* 2005;52(7):717-720.
40. Arzola C, Davies S, Rofaeel A, Carvalho JC. Ultrasound using the transverse approach to the lumbar spine provides reliable landmarks for labor epidurals. *Anesth Analg.* 2007;104(5):1188-1192.
41. Asakura Y, Kandatsu N, Hashimoto A, Kamiya M, Akashi M, Komatsu T. Ultrasound-guided neuroaxial anesthesia: accurate diagnosis of spina bifida occulta by ultrasonography. *J Anesth.* 2009;23(2):312-313.
42. Lee Y, Tanaka M, Carvalho JC. Sonoanatomy of the lumbar spine in patients with previous unintentional dural punctures during labor epidurals. *Reg Anesth Pain Med.* 2008;33(3):266-270.
43. Margarido CB, Arzola C, Balki M, Carvalho JC. Anesthesiologists' learning curves for ultrasound assessment of the lumbar spine. *Can J Anaesth.* 2010;57(2):120-126.
44. Bellingham GA, Peng PWH. A low-cost ultrasound phantom of the lumbosacral spine. *Reg Anesth Pain Med.* 2010;35(3):290-293.
45. Li JW, Karmakar MK, LI X, Kwok WH, Ngan Kee WD. The "Gelatin-agar Lumbosacral Spine Phantom"—a simple model for learning the basic skills required to perform real-time sonographically guided central neuraxial blocks. *J Ultrasound Med.* 2011 Feb;30(2):263-72.

# Sonography of Thoracic Paravertebral Space and Considerations for Ultrasound-Guided Thoracic Paravertebral Block

*Catherine Vandepitte, Tatjana Stopar Pintaric, and Philippe E. Gautier*

Thoracic paravertebral block (PVB) is a well-established technique for perioperative analgesia in patients having thoracic, chest wall, or breast surgery or for pain management with rib fractures. Ultrasound guidance can be used to help identify the paravertebral space (PVS) and needle placement, and to monitor the spread of the local anesthetic. Importantly, interference of the closely related osseous structures with ultrasound imaging and the proximity of the highly vulnerable neuraxial structures make it imperative that all well-described technique precautions are exercised, regardless of the ultrasound imaging. In this chapter, we describe general principles of thoracic PVB, rather than propose a cookbook with specific techniques and step-by-step directions. The reader is advised to use the anatomic information and techniques presented here to devise an approach in line with own clinical experience.

## Anatomy and General Considerations

Thoracic PVB is accomplished by an injection of local anaesthetic into the PVS, which contains thoracic spinal nerves with their branches, as well as the sympathetic trunk. Anatomically, the PVS is a wedge-shaped area positioned between the heads and necks of the ribs (Figure 45-1). Its posterior wall is formed by the superior *costotransverse ligament*, the anterolateral wall is the *parietal pleura* with the endothoracic fascia, and the medial wall is the lateral surface of the *vertebral body* and intervertebral disk.[1] The PVS medially communicates with the epidural space via the intervertebral foramen inferiorly and superiorly across the head and neck of the ribs.[2–5] Consequently, injection of local anesthetic into the PVS space often results in unilateral (or bilateral) epidural anesthesia. The cephalad limit of the PVS is not defined, whereas the caudad limit is at the origin of the psoas muscle at L1.[6] Likewise, the PVS space communicates with the intercostal spaces laterally, leading to the spread of the local anesthetic into the intercostals sulcus and resultant intercostal blockade as part of the mechanism of action (Figure 45-2).

## Transverse In-line Technique

Similar to techniques not using ultrasound guidance, the patient can be positioned in the sitting or lateral decubitus position with the site of surgical interest uppermost. Either a linear or phased array (curved) transducer can be used however, latter may be used only in slim patients. A high-frequency (10–12 MHz) transducer is used to obtain images in the axial (transverse) plane at the selected level, with the transducer positioned just lateral to the spinous process (Figure 45-3). For most patients, the depth of field is set about 3 cm to start scanning. The transverse processes and ribs are visualized as hyperechoic structures with acoustic shadowing below them (Figure 45-3). Once the transverse processes and ribs are identified, the transducer is moved slightly caudad into the intercostal space between adjacent ribs to identify the thoracic PVS and the adjoining intercostal space. The PVS appears as a wedge-shaped hypoechoic layer demarcated by the hyperechoic reflections of the pleura below and the internal intercostal membrane above (Figure 45-3). The hyperechoic line of the pleura and underlying hyperechoic air artifacts move with respiration. The goal of the technique is to insert the needle into the PVS and inject local anesthetic, resulting in downward displacement of the pleura, indicating proper spread of the local anesthetic (Figure 45-3).

Although ultrasound-guided thoracic PVB is essentially a superficial, simple technique, visualization of the needle and its tip and control of its path at all times are essential to avoid inadvertent pleural puncture or entry into the intervertebral foramen. For this reason, in-plane

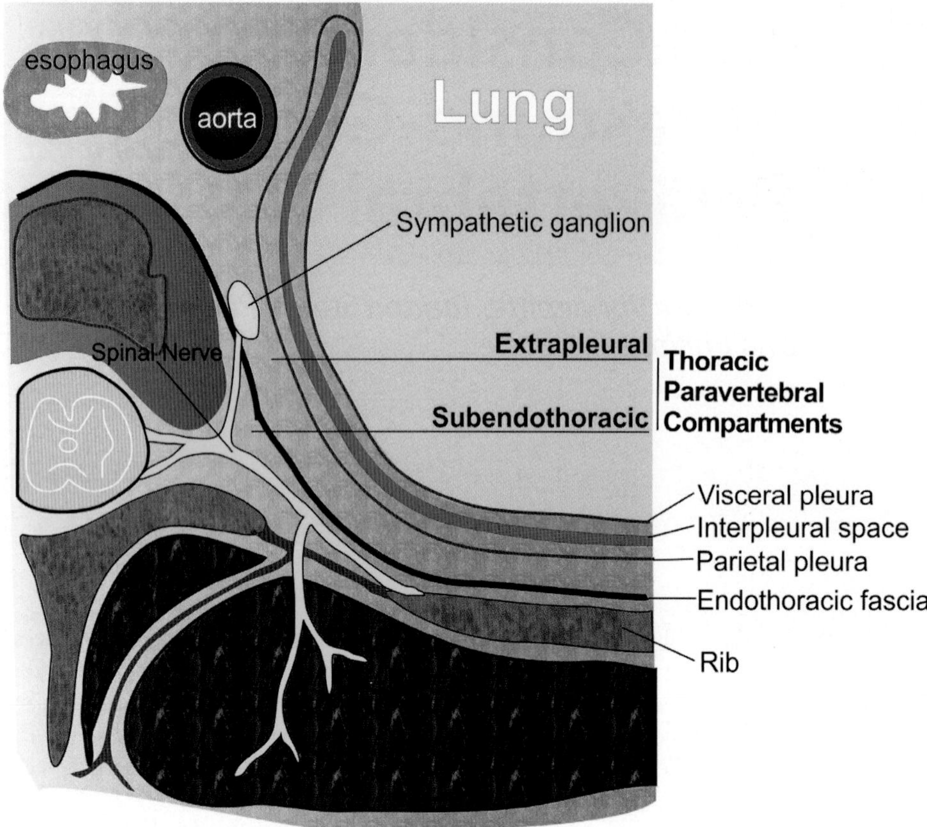


**FIGURE 45-1.** A schematic representation of the thoracic paravertebral space and its structures of relevance to paravertebral block.

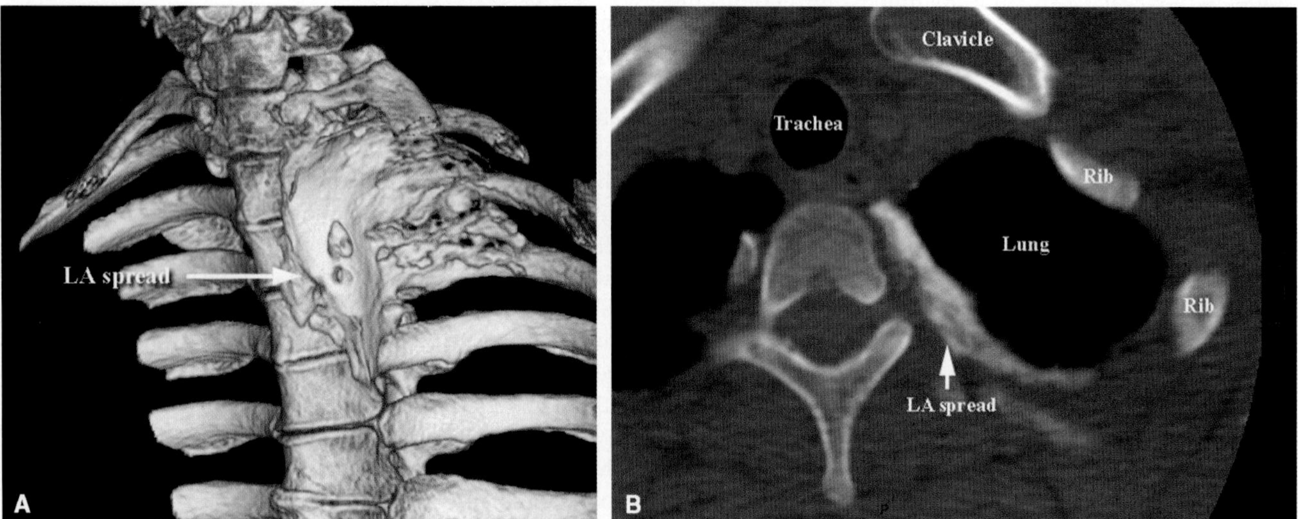


**FIGURE 45-2.** (A) Three-dimensional magnetic resonance reconstruction image of the spread of local anesthetic (5 mL) within the paravertebral space. (B) A computed topography image of the local anesthetic (LA) spread in the thoracic paravertebral space. The contrast is seen spreading in the medial to lateral and anterior to posterior direction underneath the parietal pleura.

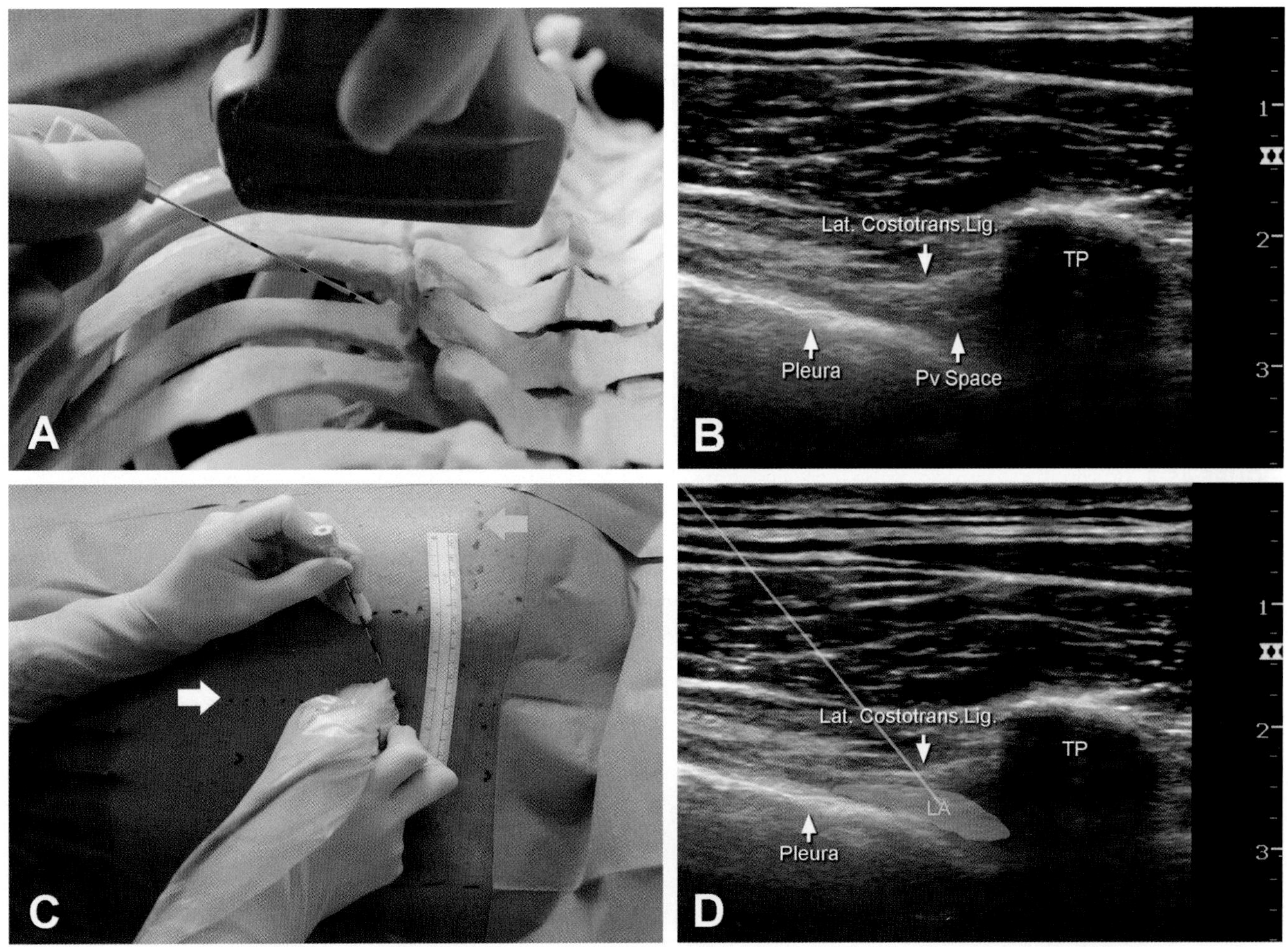


**FIGURE 45-3.** An ultrasound-guided thoracic paravertebral block. (A) Transducer position and needle orientation. (B) Corresponding ultrasound image. (C) Patient is in oblique lateral position. The outlined surface landmarks are: (>) = spinous processes; gray arrow = left scapula; white arrow = paramedian line 3 cm (transverse processes). (D) Needle insertion path and correct injection of local anesthetic. TP = transverse process.

needle insertion with direction towards the centroneuraxis is probably best avoided in obese patients. Insertion of a catheter through the needle placed in the PVS carries a risk of catheter (mis)placement into the epidural or mediastinal space, or through the pleura into the thoracic cavity (Figure 45-4).[7]

Several recommendations are suggested to decrease the risk of potential complications with ultrasound-guided thoracic PVB:

- In-plane advancement of the needle should be reserved only for patients who image well; visualization of the needle path at all times is crucial to reduce the risk of needle entry in unwanted locations (pleura, neuraxial space).
- Orienting the bevel of the Tuohy needle tip away from the pleura may reduce the risk of penetrating the pleura.
- A pop often is felt as the needle penetrates the internal intercostal membrane, alerting the operator of the needle position in the PVS.
- Aspiration for blood should always be carried out before injection.
- Local anesthetic (15–20 mL) is injected *slowly* in small increments, avoiding forceful high-pressure injection to reduce the risk of bilateral epidural spread.

## Longitudinal out-of-plane technique

Out-of-plane ultrasound-guided thoracic paravertebral block is the most common approach to PVB in our practice (Figure 45-5). We feel that this technique is inherently safer then in-line techniques as the needle path is not towards the neuraxis. In addition, this technique is analogous to the

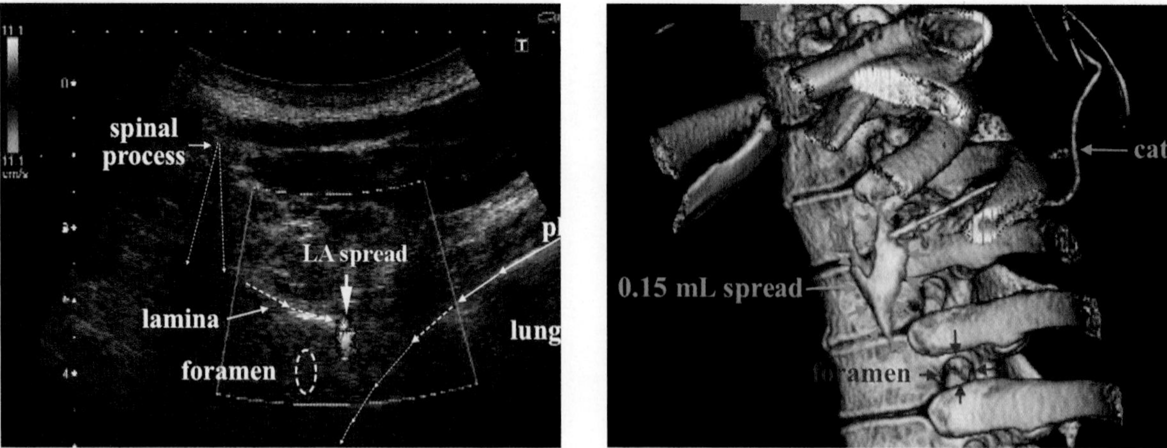


**FIGURE 45-4.** (A) Ultrasound image of the local anesthetic (LA) spread during a thoracic paravertebral block. (B) A three-dimensional magnetic resonance image demonstrating catheter insertion into the thoracic paravertebral space and injection of a small amount of local anesthetic.

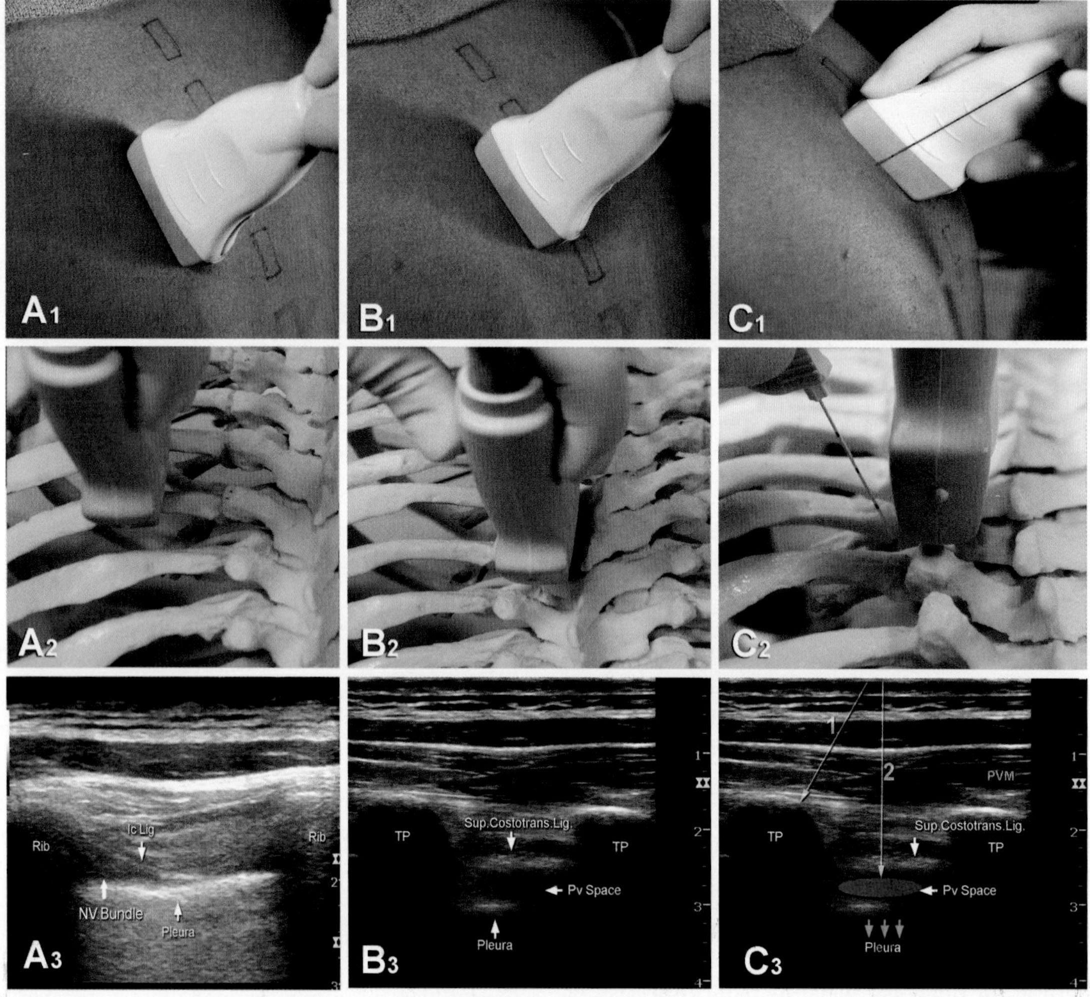


**FIGURE 45-5.** Longitudinal, out-of-plane approach to thoracic paravertebral block. The transducer is first placed 5-6 cm lateral to the spinous processes to identify ribs, parietal pleura and intercostal spaces (A1-A3). The transducer is then moved progressively medially to identify transverse processes (B1-B3). Transverse processes (TP) appear square and deeper then ribs (round, superficial). The needle is inserted out-of-plane to contact the TP (C1-C2 and C3, line 1) and then walked off the TP (C3, line 2) inferior or superior to TP to enter the paravertebral space and injection local anesthetic (blue). Proper injection displaces the pleura (blue arrows). PVM - paravertebral muscles.

true-and-tried surface-based techniques, except that with ultrasound-guided technique, transverse processes can be more accurately identified. The best strategy is to start the scanning process 5-10 cm laterally to identify the rounded ribs and parietal pleura underneath. The transducer is then moved progressively more medially until transverse processes are identified as more squared structured and deeper to the ribs. Too medial transducer placement will yield image of the laminae, at which point the transducer is moved slightly laterally to image transverse processes. Once the transverse processes are identified, a needle is inserted out-of-plane to contact the transfer process and then, walk off the transfer process 1-1.5 cm deeper to inject local anesthetic. While the position of the needle tip may not be seen with this technique, an injection of the local anesthetic will result in displacement of the parietal pleura. The process is then repeated for each desired level. In our opinion, a pragmatic needle insertion 1-1.5 cm past the transverse may be safer then using spread of the injected to displace the pleura as the end-point.

## REFERENCES


1. Bouzinac A, Delbos A, Mazieres M, Rontes O: Ultrasound-guided bilateral paravertebral thoracic block in an obese patient. *Ann Fr Anesth* 2010;30:162-163.
2. Cowie B, McGlade D, Ivanusic J, Barrington MJ: Ultrasound-guided thoracic paravertebral blockade: a cadaveric study. *Anesth Analg* 2010;110:1735-1739.
3. Eason MJ, Wyatt R. Paravertebral thoracic block—a reappraisal. *Anaesthesia.* 1979;34:638-642.
4. Karmakar MK, Chui PT, Joynt GM, Ho AM. Thoracic paravertebral block for management of pain associated with multiple fractured ribs in patients with concomitant lumbar spinal trauma. *Reg Anesth Pain Med.* 2001;26:169-173.
5. Lonnqvist PA, Hildingsson U. The caudal boundary of the thoracic paravertebral space. A study in human cadavers. *Anaesthesia.* 1992;47(12):1051.
6. Luyet C, Eichenberger1 U, Greif1 R, et al. Ultrasound-guided paravertebral puncture and placement of catheters in human cadavers: an imaging study. *Br J Anaesth.* 2009;102 (4): 534-539.
7. Luyet C, Herrmann G, Ross S, Vogt A, Greif R, Moriggl B, Eichenberger U: Ultrasound-guided thoracic paravertebral punture and placement of catheters in human cadavers. *Br J Anaesth* 2011;106:246-254.
8. Moorthy SS, Dierdorf SF, Yaw PB. Influence of volume on the spread of local anesthetic–methylene blue solution after injection for intercostal block. *Anesth Analg.* 1992;75:389-391.
9. Mowbray A, Wong KK. Low volume intercostal injection. A comparative study in patients and cadavers. *Anaesthesia.* 1988;43:633-634.
10. Mowbray A, Wong KK, Murray JM. Intercostal catheterisation. An alternative approach to the paravertebral space. *Anaesthesia.* 1987;42:958-961.
11. Renes SH, Bruhn J, Gielen MJ, Scheffer GJ, van Geffen GJ: In-plane ultrasound-guided thoracic paravertebral block: a preliminary report of 36 cases with radiologic confirmation of catheter position. *Reg Anesth Pain Med* 2010;35:212-6.
12. SC OR, Donnell BO, Cuffe T, Harmon DC, Fraher JP, Shorten G: Thoracic paravertebral block using real-time ultrasound guidance. *Anesth Analg* 2010;110:248-251.

# Ultrasound of the Lumbar Paravertebral Space and Considerations for Lumbar Plexus Block

*Manoj Karmakar and Catherine Vandepitte*

## Introduction

Lumbar plexus block (LPB) traditionally is performed using surface anatomic landmarks to identify the site for needle insertion and eliciting quadriceps muscle contraction in response to nerve electro-localization, as described in the nerve stimulator–guided chapter. The main challenges in accomplishing LPB relate to the depth at which the lumbar plexus is located and the size of the plexus, which requires a large volume of local anesthetic for success. Due to the deep anatomic location of the lumbar plexus, small errors in landmark estimation or angle miscalculations during needle advancement can result in needle placement away from the plexus or at unwanted locations. Therefore, monitoring of the needle path and final needle tip placement should increase the precision of the needle placement and the delivery of the local anesthetic. Although computed tomography and fluoroscopy can be used to increase the precision during LPB, these technologies are impractical in the busy operating room environment, costly, and associated with radiation exposure. It is only logical, then, that ultrasound-guided LPB is of interest because of the ever-increasing availability of portable machines and the improvement in the quality of the images obtained.[1,2]

## Anatomy and Sonoanatomy

Lumbar plexus block, also known as psoas compartment block, comprises an injection of local anesthetic in the fascial plane within the posterior aspect of the psoas major muscle. Because the roots of the lumbar plexus are located in this plane, an injection of a sufficient volume of local anesthetic in the postero-medial compartment of the psoas muscle results in block of the majority of the plexus (femoral nerve, lateral femoral cutaneous nerve, and the obturator nerve). The anterior boundary of the fascial plane that contains the lumbar plexus is formed by the fascia between the anterior two thirds of the compartment of the psoas muscle that originates from the anterolateral aspect of the vertebral body and the posterior one third of the muscle that originates from the anterior aspect of the transverse processes. This arrangement explains why the transverse processes are closely related to the plexus and therefore are used as the main landmark during LPB.

A scan for the LPB can be performed in the transverse or longitudinal axes. The ultrasound transducer is positioned 3 to 4 cm lateral to the lumbar spine for either orientation. The following settings usually are used to start the scanning:

- Abdominal preset
- Depth: 11–12 cm
- Frequency: 4–8 MHz
- Tissue harmonic imaging and compound imaging functions engaged where available
- Adjustment of the overall gain and time-gain compensation

## Longitudinal Scan Anatomy

Regardless of the technique, the operator first should identify the transverse processes on a longitudinal sonogram (Figure 46-1). One technique is to first identify the flat surface of the sacrum and then scan proximally until the intervertebral

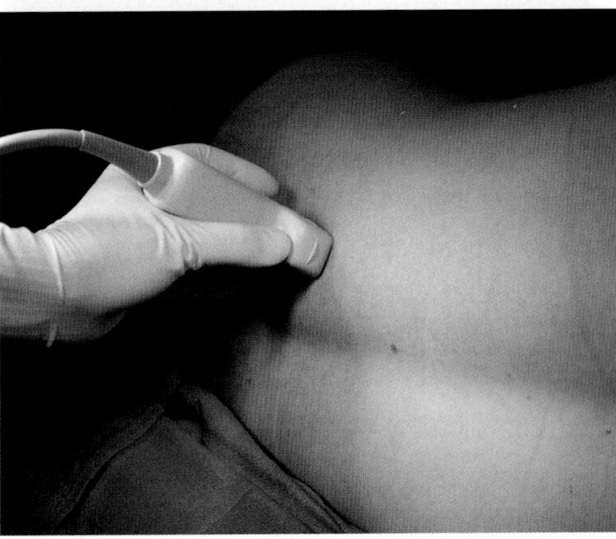

**FIGURE 46-1.** Transducer position (curved transducer, longitudinal view) to image the central neuroaxis, transverse processes, and estimate the needle and depth to the lumbar plexus using a longitudinal view.

space between L5 and S1 is recognized as an interruption of the sacral line continuity. Once the operator identifies the transverse process of L5, the transverse process of the other lumbar vertebrae are easily identified by a dynamic cephalad scan in ascending order. The acoustic shadow of the transverse process has a characteristic appearance, often referred to as a "trident sign" (Figure 46-2A). Once the transverse processes are recognized, the psoas muscle is imaged through the acoustic window of the transverse processes. The psoas muscle appears as a combination of longitudinal hyperechoic striations within a typical hypoechoic muscle appearance just deep to the transverse processes (Figure 46-2B). Although some of the hyperechoic striations may appear particularly intense and mislead the operator to interpret them as roots of lumbar plexus, the identification of the roots in a longitudinal scan is not reliable without nerve stimulation. This unreliability is partly due to the fact that intramuscular connective tissue (e.g., septa, tendons) within the psoas muscle are thick and may be indistinguishable from the nerve roots at such a deep location. As the transducer is moved progressively cephalad, the lower pole of the kidney often comes into view as low as L2-L4 in some patients (Figure 46-3A and B).

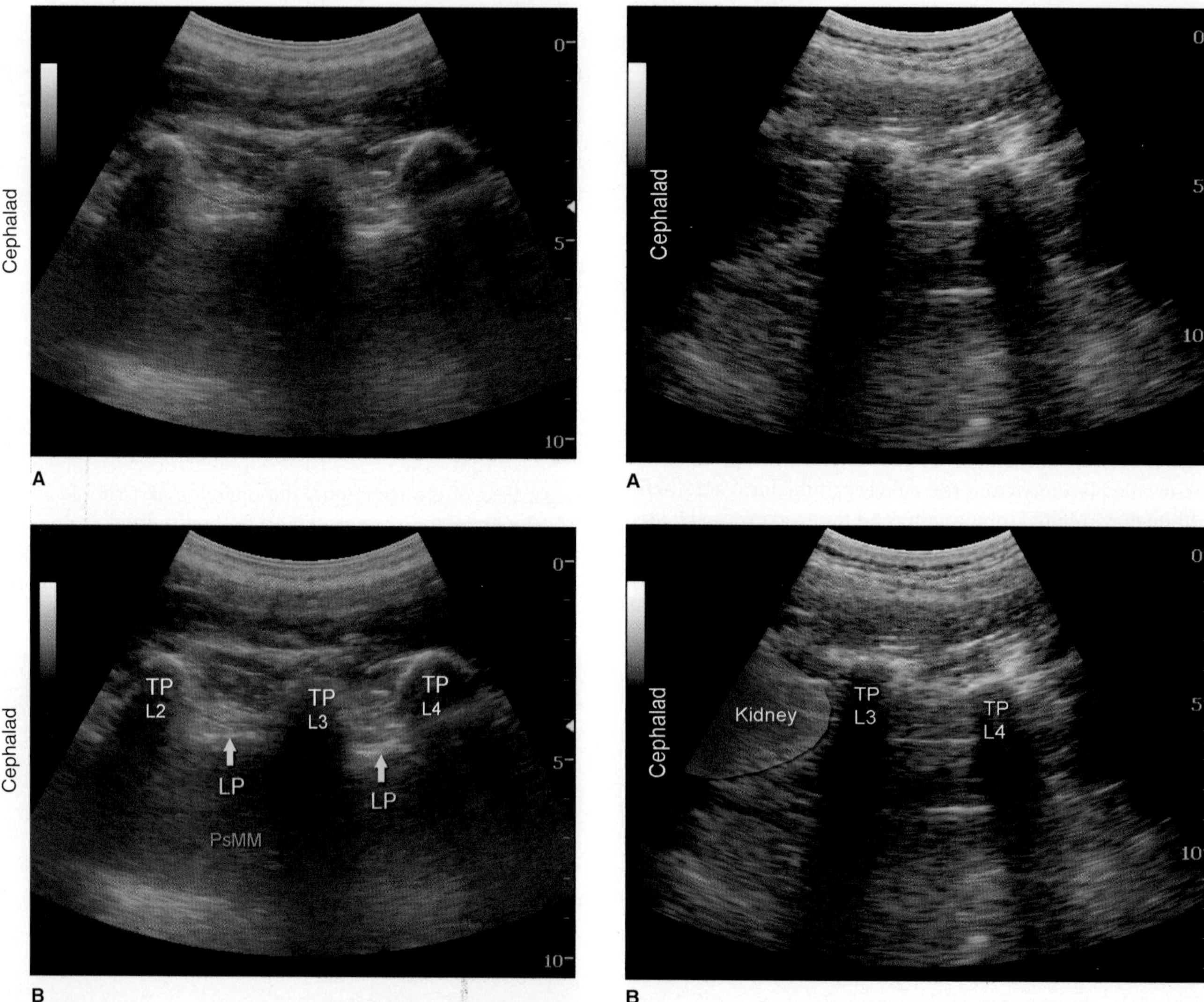


**FIGURE 46-2.** (A) Ultrasound anatomy of the lumbar paravertebral space demonstrating transverse processes at a depth of approximately 3 cm. Lower frequency, curved transducer is used optimize imaging at the deep location and obtain a greater angular view, respectively. (B) Labeled ultrasound anatomy of the lumbar paravertebral space with structures labeled. TP, transverse process; LP, lumbar plexus roots (most likely); PsMM, psoas major muscle.

**FIGURE 46-3.** (A) Ultrasound image of the lumbar paravertebral space at the L2-L3 level demonstrating the lower pole of the kidney on the left-hand side of the image at approximately 5 cm depth. (B) Labeled ultrasound image of the lumbar paravertebral space at L2-L3 level demonstrating the lower pole of the kidney on the left-hand side of the image at approximately 5 cm depth. TP, transverse process.

## Transverse Scan Anatomy

Kirchmair and colleagues were among the first to describe the sonoanatomy of relevance for LPB.[3] They reported the ability to accurately guide a needle to the posterior part of the psoas muscle, where the roots of the lumbar plexus are located, using ultrasound guidance in cadavers.[4,5] Since, significant advances in ultrasound technology have taken place, allowing for much improved image quality, which have allowed Karmakar and colleagues to devise an alternative approach to the lumbar plexus using ultrasonographic identification of the transverse processes as the guide.[6] With this scanning technique, the transducer is positioned 4 to 5 cm lateral to the lumbar spinous process at the L3-L4 level and directed slightly medially to assume a *transverse oblique* orientation (Figure 46-4). This approach allows imaging of the lumbar paravertebral region with the erector spinae muscle, transverse process, the psoas major muscle, quadrates lumborum, and the anterolateral surface of the vertebral body (Figure 46-5A, B, and C). In the transverse oblique view, the inferior vena cava (IVC), on the right-sided scan, or the aorta, on the left-sided scan, also can be seen and provide additional information on the location of the psoas muscle, which is positioned superficial to these vessels. In this view, the psoas muscle appears slightly hypoechoic with multiple hyperechogenic striations within. The lower pole of the kidney can often be seen, when scanning at the L2-L4 level, as an oval structure that ascends and descends with respirations (Figure 46-6). The key to obtaining adequate images of the psoas muscle and lumbar plexus with the transverse oblique scan is to insonate between two adjacent transverse processes. This scanning method avoids acoustic shadow of the transverse processes, which obscures the underlying psoas muscle and the intervertebral foramen (angle between the transverse process and vertebral body) and allows visualization of the articular process of the facet joint (APFJ) as well. Because the intervertebral foramen is located at the angle between the APFJ and vertebral body, lumbar nerve roots often can be depicted.

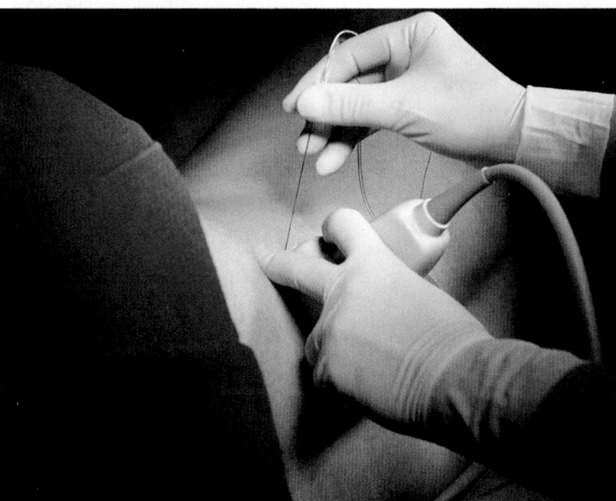

**FIGURE 46-4.** Patient position (lateral decubitus position) transducer (curved, linear array) placement and the needle insertion angle to block the lumbar plexus using oblique transverse view.

## Techniques of Ultrasound-Guided Lumbar Plexus Block

Kirchmair and colleagues suggested a *paramedial sagittal scan technique* with transverse scan to delineate the psoas major muscle at the L3-L5 level with the patient in the lateral position. Once a satisfactory image is obtained, the needle is inserted in-plane medial to the transducer approximately 4 cm lateral to the midline. Then the needle is advanced toward the posterior part of the lumbar plexus until the correct position is confirmed by obtaining a quadriceps motor response to nerve stimulation (1.5–2.0 mA). Needle–nerve contact and distribution of the local anesthetic is not always well seen, although lumbar plexus roots may be better visualized after the injection. Injection, dosing, and monitoring principles are the same as with the nerve stimulator–guided technique.

More recently, Karmakar and colleagues described the "trident sign technique," which uses an easily recognizable ultrasonographic landmark, transverse processes, and an out-of-plane needle insertion. The trident sign technique derives its name from the characteristic ultrasonographic appearance of the transverse processes (*trident*) to estimate the depth and location of the lumbar plexus. After application of ultrasound gel to the skin over the lumbar paravertebral region, the ultrasound transducer is positioned approximately 3 to 4 cm lateral and parallel to the lumbar spine to produce a longitudinal scan of the lumbar paravertebral region (Figure 46-7). Then the transducer is moved caudally, while still maintaining the same orientation, until the sacrum and the L5 transverse process become visible (Figure 46-8). The lumbar transverse processes are identified by their hyperechoic reflections and acoustic shadowing beneath which is typical of bone. Once the L5 transverse process is visible, the transducer is moved cephalad gradually, to identify the L3-L4 level. The goal of the technique is to guide the needle through the acoustic window between the transverse processes (between the "teeth of the trident") of L3-L4 or L2-L3 into the posterior part of the psoas major muscle containing the roots of the lumbar plexus (Figure 46-2B). After obtaining ipsilateral quadriceps muscle contractions, the block is carried out using the previously described injection and pharmacology considerations (Figures 46-9 and 46-10).

A paramedial scan also can be used with an in-plane needle approach. In this technique, an insulated needle is inserted in-plane from the caudal end (Figure 46-4) of the transducer while maintaining the view of the transverse processes. Again, the goal is to pass the needle and inject local anesthetic with a real-time visualization of the needle path and injection into the posterior part of the psoas muscle (Figure 46-5).

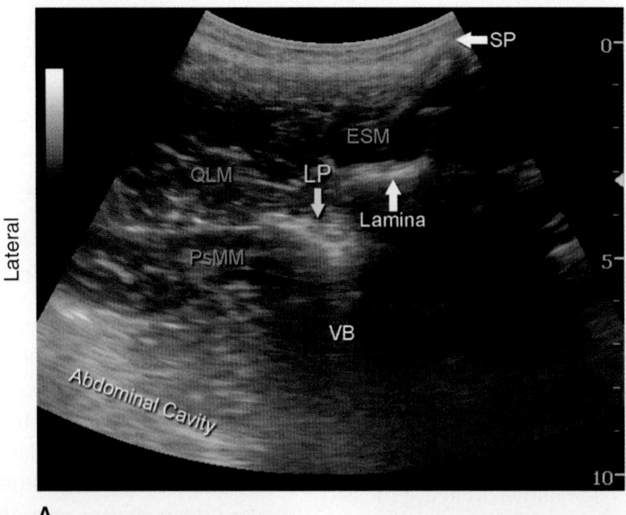


A

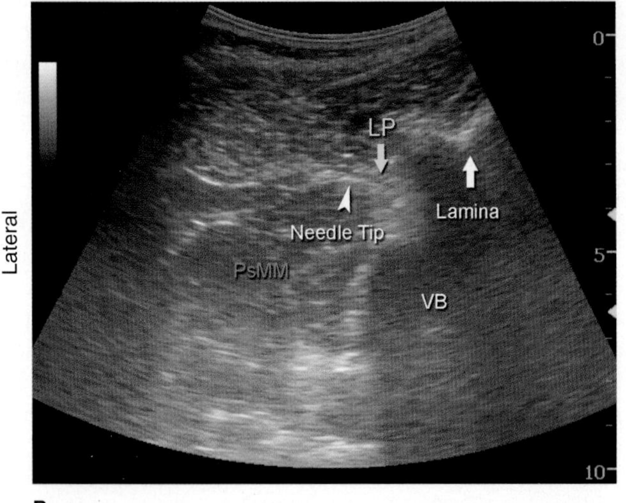


B

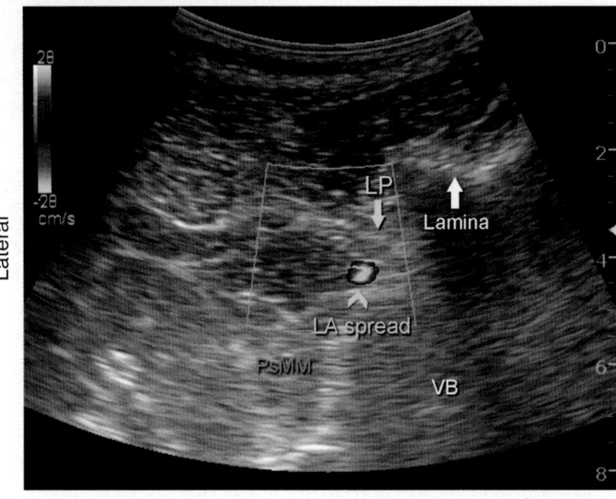


C

**FIGURE 46-5.** (A) Ultrasound anatomy of the lumbar paravertebral space using transverse oblique view. SP, spinal process; ESM, erectors spinae muscle; QLM, quadratus lumborum muscle; PsMM, psoas major muscle; VB, vertebral body. The lumbar plexus root is seen just below the lamina as it exits the interlaminar space and enters into the posterior medial aspect of the PsMM. (B) Needle path in ultrasound-guided lumbar plexus block using transverse oblique view. LP, lumbar plexus; PsMM, psoas major muscle; VB, vertebral body. (C) Spread of the local anesthetic solution with lumbar plexus block injection. Due to the deep location of the plexus, spread of the local anesthetic may not always be well seen. Color Doppler imaging can be used to help determine the location of the injectate.

In summary, ultrasound-guided LPB is a technically advanced procedure. Experience with ultrasound anatomy and less technically challenging nerve regional anesthesia techniques are useful to ensure success and safety. Although the use of ultrasound in LPB is not widely accepted, in expert hands, ultrasound guidance can increase the accuracy and possibly safety, by providing information on the location, arrangement, and depth of the osseous and muscular tissues of importance in LPB. It should be kept in mind that the dorsal branch of the lumbar artery is closely related to the transverse processes and the posterior part of the psoas muscle. Considering the rich vascularity of the lumbar paravertebral area, the use of smaller gauge needles and avoidance of this block in patients on anticoagulants is prudent. Injections into this area should be carried out without excessive force because high-injection pressure can lead to unwanted epidural spread and/or rapid intravascular injection.[7] Lumbar plexus block in patients with obesity or advanced age can be more challenging. Aging is associated with a reduction in skeletal muscle mass (sarcopenia) and replacement of the muscle mass by adipose tissue, leading to changes in ultrasound absorption and scattering.

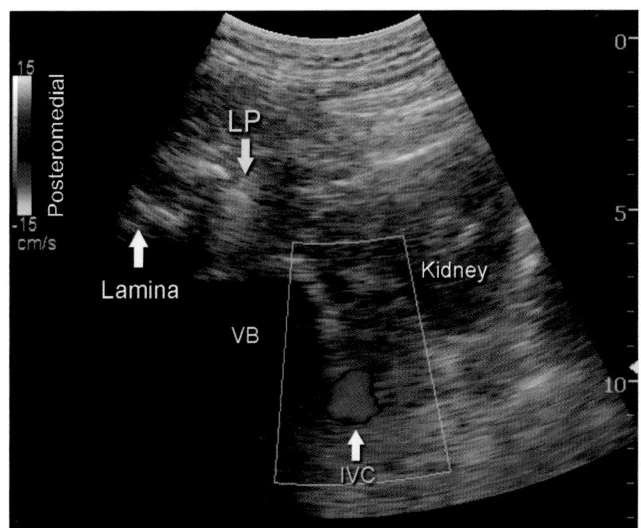


**FIGURE 46-6.** Ultrasound image of the lumbar paravertebral space demonstrating the complex anatomy of the region. LP, lumbar plexus; VB, vertebral body. Power Doppler ultrasound is capturing the flow in the inferior vena cava (IVC). The right kidney is also visualized.

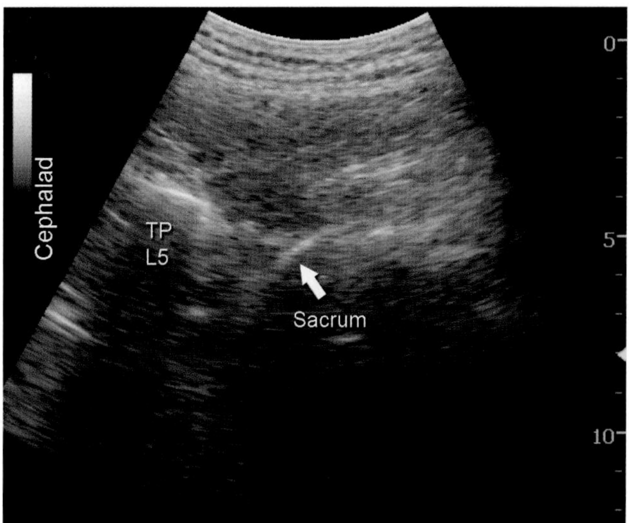


**FIGURE 46-8.** Transverse image of lumbar paravertebral space demonstrating sacrum and transverse process (TP) of L5. Starting the scanning process from the sacral area and progressing cephalad allows the identity of the individual transverse processes (levels). As the transducer is moved cephalad and the surface of the sacrum disappears, the next osseous structure that appears is the transverse process (TP) of L5.

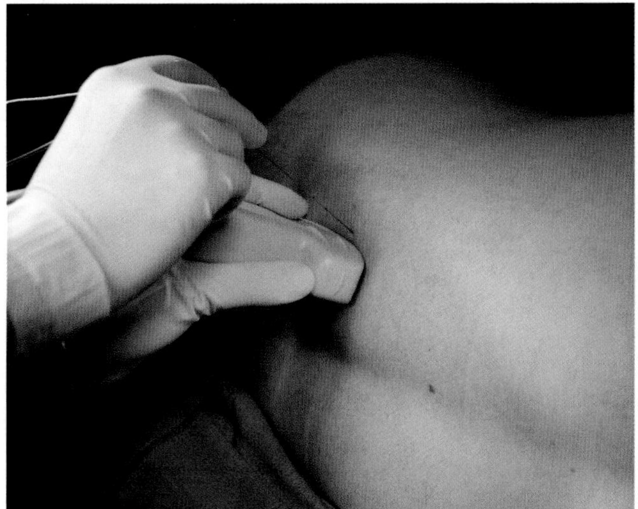

**FIGURE 46-7.** Transducer position (curved, phased array) and the needle insertion plane to accomplish ultrasound-guided lumbar plexus block in the longitudinal view and an out-of-plane needle insertion.

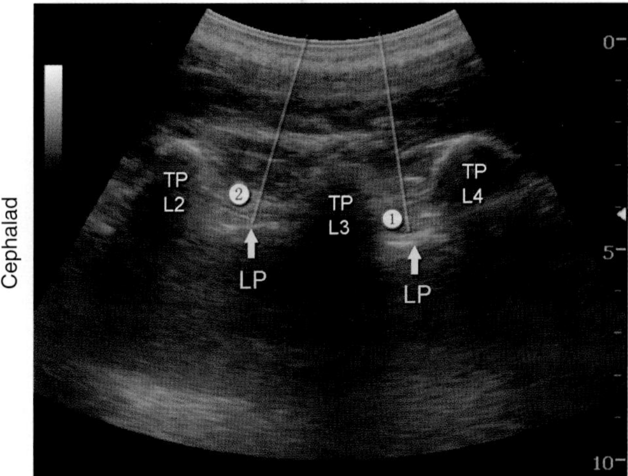


**FIGURE 46-9.** Simulated needle insertion paths (1,2) to inject local anesthetics at two different levels to accomplish a lumbar plexus (LP) block. Needles (1 and 2) are seen lodged about 2 cm deeper and between the transverse processes (TPs) using an out-of-plane technique.

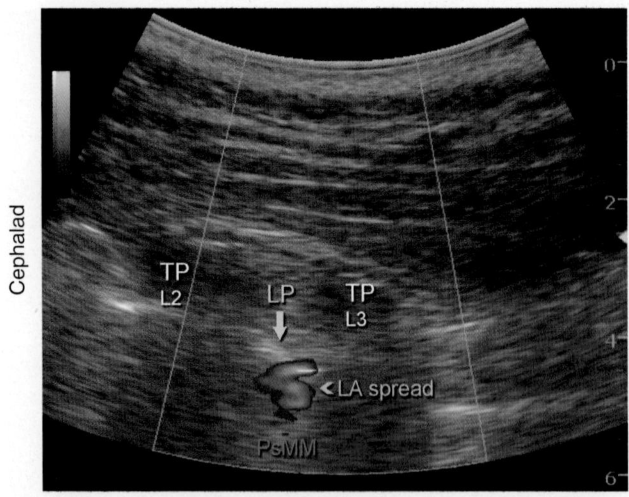


Lumbar paravetebral block-injecting LA

**FIGURE 46-10.** Local anesthetic (LA) disposition during injection of local anesthetic into the psoas muscle and the L2-L3 level. The spread of LA is often not well seen using two-dimensional imaging. LP, lumbar plexus; TP, transverse process.

## REFERENCES

1. Doi, K., S. Sakura, and K. Hara, A modified posterior approach to lumbar plexus block using a transverse ultrasound image and an approach from the lateral border of the transducer. *Anaesth Intensive Care*, 2010;38:213-214.
2. Ilfeld, B.M., V.J. Loland, and E.R. Mariano, Prepuncture ultrasound imaging to predict transverse process and lumbar plexus depth for psoas compartment block and perineural catheter insertion: a prospective, observational study. *Anesth Analg*, 2010;110:1725-1728.
3. Kirchmair L, Entner T, Wissel J, Moriggl B, Kapral S, Mitterschiffthaler G. A study of the paravertebral anatomy for ultrasound-guided posterior lumbar plexus block. *Anesth Analg*. 2001;93:477-481.
4. Kirchmair L, Entner T, Kapral S, Mitterschiffthaler G. Ultrasound guidance for the psoas compartment block: an imaging study. *Anesth Analg*. 2002;94:706-710.
5. Farny J, Drolet P, Girard M. Anatomy of the posterior approach to the lumbar plexus block. *Can J Anaesth*. 1994;41:480-485.
6. Karmakar MK, Ho AM-H, Li X, Kwok WH, Tsang K, Ngan Kee WD. Ultrasound-guided lumbar plexus block through the acoustic window of the lumbar ultrasound trident. *Br J Anaesth*. 2008;100(4):533-537.
7. Gadsden JC, Lindenmuth DM, Hadžić A, Xu D, Somasundarum L, Flisinski KA. Lumbar plexus block using high-pressure injection leads to contralateral and epidural spread. *Anesthesiology*. 2008;109(4):683-688.

SECTION 7

# Atlas of Ultrasound-Guided Anatomy

# LIST OF ABBREVIATIONS

APLT Abductor Pollicis Longus Tendon
A Artery
AA Axillary Artery
ABM Adductor Brevis Muscle
Acc Accessory
AcP Accessory Process
ALM Adductor Longus Muscle
AMM Adductor Magnus Muscle
AN Axillary Nerve
Ant. Anterior
ASeM Anterior Serratus Muscle
ASIS Anterior Superior Iliac Spine
ASM Anterior Scalene Muscle
ATA Anterior Tibial Artery
ATT Anterior Tibialis Tendon
AV Axillary Vein
BA Brachial Artery
BcV Basilic Vein
BFM Biceps Femoris Muscle
BM Brachialis Muscle
BP Brachial Plexus
Br. Branch
BrM Brachioradialis Muscle
C Cervical
CA Carotid Artery
CBM Coracobrachialis Muscle
Cl Clavicle
CP Cervical Plexus
CPN Common Peroneal Nerve
Cut Cutaneous
CV Cephalic Vein
DGA Descending Genicular Artery
DPN Deep Peroneal Nerve
DSA Dorsal Scapular Artery
DSN Dorsal Scapular Nerve
ECRLM Extensor Carpi Radialis Longus Muscle
ECUM Extensor Carpi Ulnaris Muscle
EDL Extensor Digitorum Longus
EDT Extensor Digitorum Tendons
EDM Extensor Digitorum Muscle
EHL Extensor Hallucis Longus
EIM Extensor Indicis Muscle
EOM External Oblique Muscle
EPLM Extensor Pollicis Longus Muscle
EPLT Extensor Pollicis Longus Tendon
ESM Erector Spinae Muscle
Ext External
FA Femoral Artery
FCRM Flexor Carpi Radialis Muscle
FCRT Flexor Carpi Radialis Tendon
FCUM Flexor Carpi Ulnaris Muscle
FDPM Flexor Digitorum Profundus Muscle
FDSM Flexor Digitorum Superficialis Muscle
FPLM Flexor Pollicis Longus Muscle
FPLT Flexor Pollicis Longus Tendon
GlA Gluteal Artery
Glu Gluteal
GMM Gluteus Maximus Muscle
GON Greater Occipital Nerve
GsM Gracilis Muscle
IA Iliac Artery
Ic Intercostal
Ing. Inguinal
IcM Intercostal Muscle
IhN Iliohypogastric Nerve
IiN Ilioinguinal Nerve
IJV Internal Jugular Vein
Inf. Inferior
Int. Internal
IObCM Inferior Oblique Capitis Muscle
IOM Internal Oblique Muscle
IPA Internal Pudendal Artery
IpM Iliopsoas Muscle
IT Ischial Tuberosity
IvD Intervertebral Disc
IvF Intervertebral Foramen
LAbCN Lateral Antebrachial Cutaneous Nerve
Lat. Lateral
LC Lateral Cord
LtDM Latissimus Dorsi Muscle
LDM Longissimus Dorsi Muscle
LFCN Lateral Femoral Cutaneous Nerve
Lig. Ligament
Long. Longitudinal
LP Lumbar Plexus
LsCM Longissimus Capitis Muscle

| | |
|---|---|
| LThN | Long Thoracic Nerve |
| MAbCN | Medial Antebrachial Cutaneous Nerve |
| Mall. | Malleolus |
| MaP | Mammillary process |
| MBCN | Medial Branchial Cutaneous Nerve |
| MC | Medial Cord |
| MCN | Musculocutaneous Nerve |
| Med. | Medial |
| MfM | Multifidus Muscle |
| Mid | Middle |
| MN | Median Nerve |
| MSA | Medial Superficial Artery |
| MSM | Middle Scalene Muscle |
| N. | Nerve |
| Nv. | Neurovascular |
| ObN | Obturator Nerve |
| PA | Popliteal Artery |
| PAbCN | Posterior Antebrachial Cutaneous Nerve |
| PBM | Peroneus Brevis Muscle |
| PC | Posterior Cord |
| PCHA | Posterior Cirrcumflex Humeral Artery |
| PFA | Profunda Femoris Artery |
| PhN | Phrenic Nerve |
| PIA | Posterior Interosseous Artery |
| PIN | Posterior Interossesous Nerve |
| PLM | Palmaris Longus Muscle |
| PLM | Peroneus (Fibularis) Longus Muscle |
| PLT | Palmaris Longus Tendon |
| PMaM | Pectoralis Major Muscle |
| PMiM | Pectoralis Minor Muscle |
| Post. | Posterior |
| PQM | Pronator Quadratus Muscle |
| PrTM | Pronator Teres Muscle |
| PsMM | Psoas Major Muscle |
| PTA | Posterior Tibial Artery |
| PTM | Peroneus Tertius Muscle |
| PuN | Pudendal Nerve |
| PuT | Pubic Tubercle |
| Pv | Paravertebral |
| QFM | Quadriceps Femoris Muscle |
| QLM | Quadratus Lumborum Muscle |
| RAM | Rectus Abdominis Muscle |
| RAN | Rectus Abdominis Nerve |
| RFM | Rectus Femoris Muscle |
| RhM | Rhomboid Muscle |
| RN | Radial Nerve |
| SaM | Sartorius Muscle |
| SaN | Saphenous Nerve |
| SaV | Great Saphenous Vein |
| SbsN | Subscapular Nerve |
| ScA | Subclavian Artery |
| SCM | Sternocleidomastoid Muscle |
| ScN | Sciatic Nerve |
| SePSM | Serratus Posterior Superior Muscle |
| SG | Stellate Ganglion |
| SmM | Semimembranosus Muscle |
| SoM | Soleus Muscle |
| SP | Spinous Process |
| SPaBr | Superfical Palmar Branch |
| SpC | Spinal Canal |
| SPN | Superficial Peroneal Nerve |
| SpsA | Suprascapular Artery |
| SpsM | Supraspinatus Muscle |
| SpsN | Suprascapular Nerve |
| SsCM | Semispinalis Capitis Muscle |
| SSV | Small Saphenous Vein |
| StM | Semitendinosus Muscle |
| SUCA | Superior Ulnar Collateral Artery |
| SuN | Sural Nerve |
| Sup. | Superior |
| SV | Superficial Veins |
| TAM | Transverse Abdominis Muscle |
| TCT | Thyrocervical Trunk |
| TF | Transversalis Fascia |
| TFLM | Tensor Fascia Latae Muscle |
| Th | Thyroid |
| TMaM | Teres Major Muscle |
| TN | Tibial Nerve |
| TP | Transverse Process |
| Tr | Trunk |
| Trans | Transverse |
| TrM | Trapezius Muscle |
| UA | Ulnar Artery |
| UN | Ulnar Nerve |
| VA | Vertebral Artery |
| Vas. | Vastus |
| VB | Vertebral Body |

## Greater Occipital Nerve, Transverse View

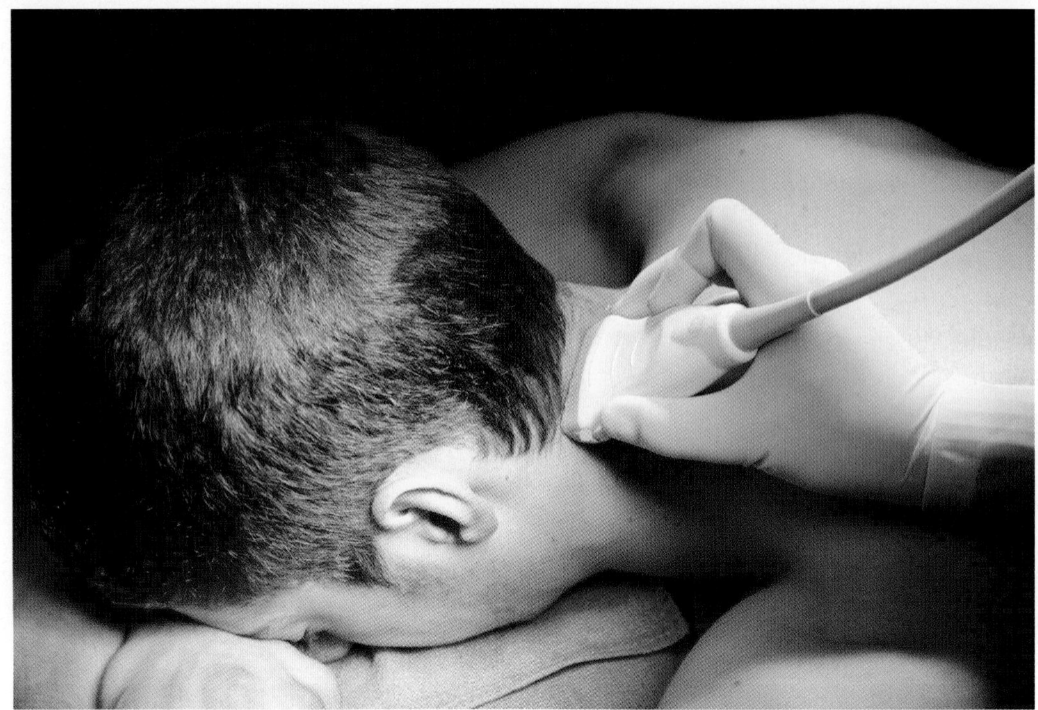

**FIGURE 7.1.1A** Ultrasound transducer position to image the greater occipital nerve in transverse view.

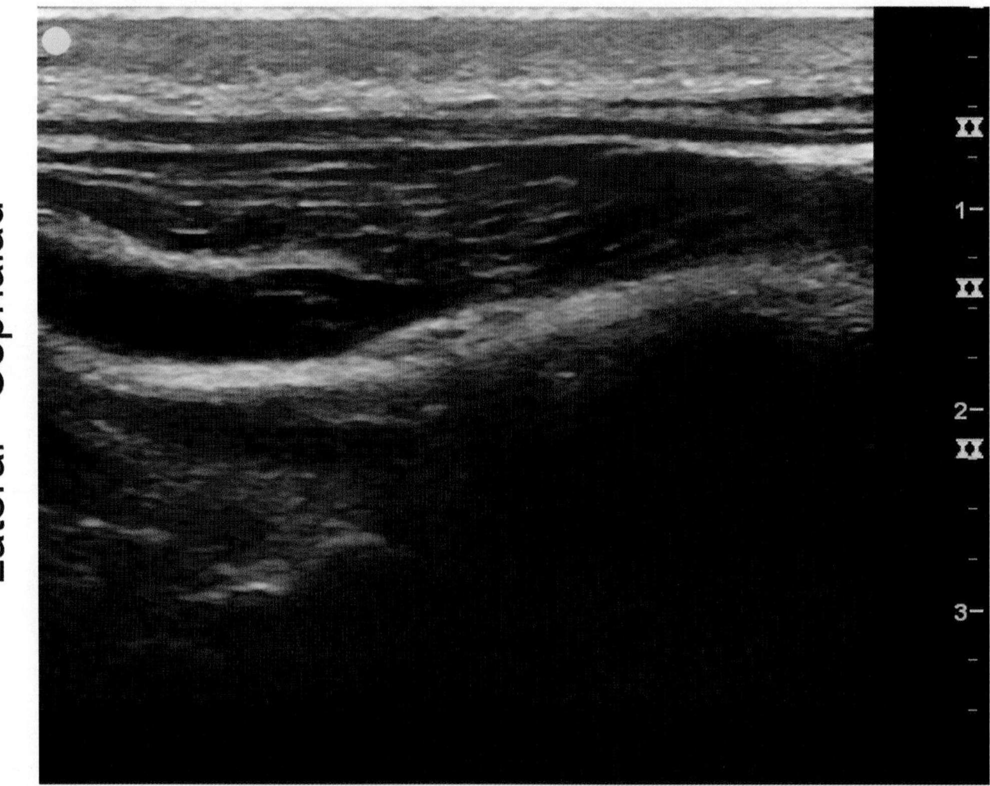


**FIGURE 7.1.1B** Ultrasound image of greater occipital nerve in transverse view.

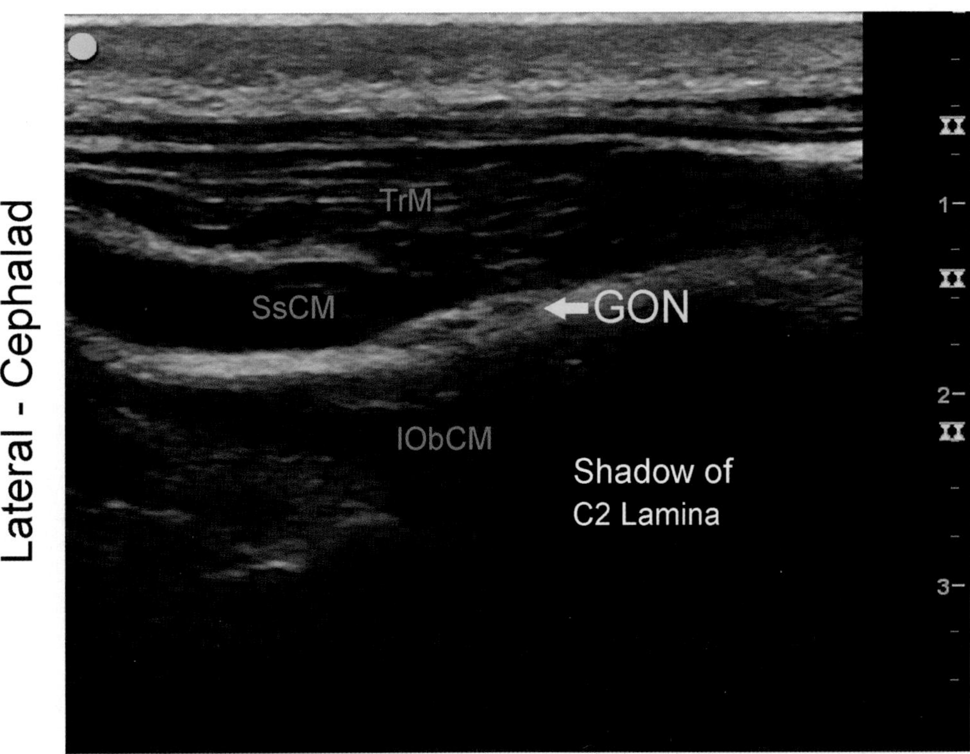


**FIGURE 7.1.1C** Labeled ultrasound image of greater occipital nerve, transverse view.

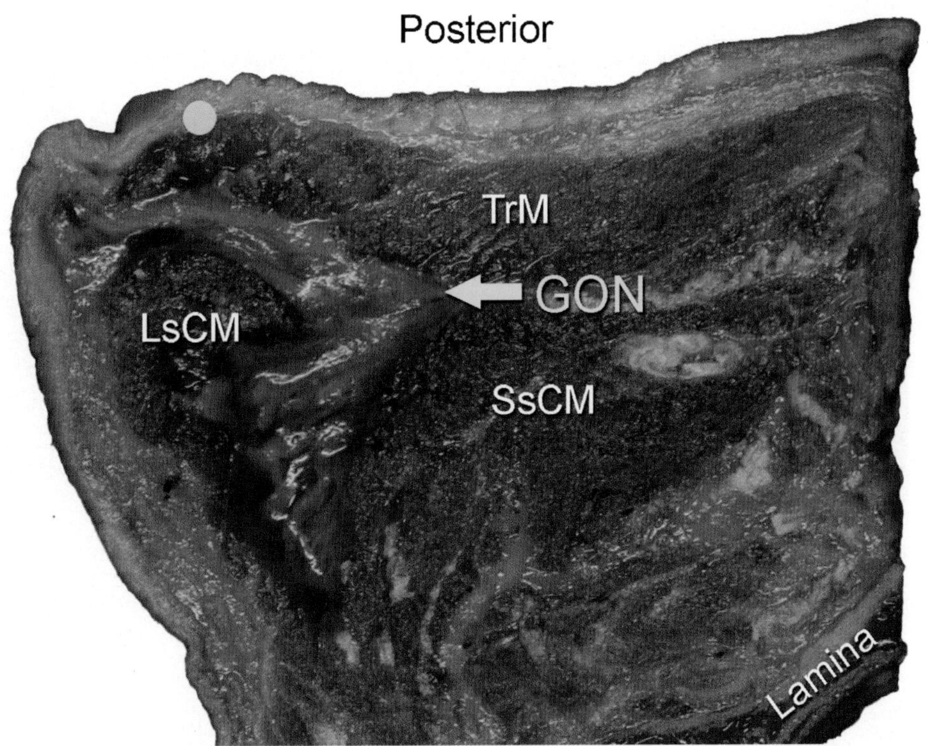


**FIGURE 7.1.1D** Labeled cross-sectional anatomy of greater occipital nerve, transverse view.

**Abbreviations:** TrM, Trapezius Muscle; SsCM, Semispinalis Capitis Muscle; IObCM, Inferior Oblique Capitis Muscle; GON, Greater Occipital Nerve; LsCM, Longissimus Capitis Muscle.

# Greater Occipital Nerve, Longitudinal View

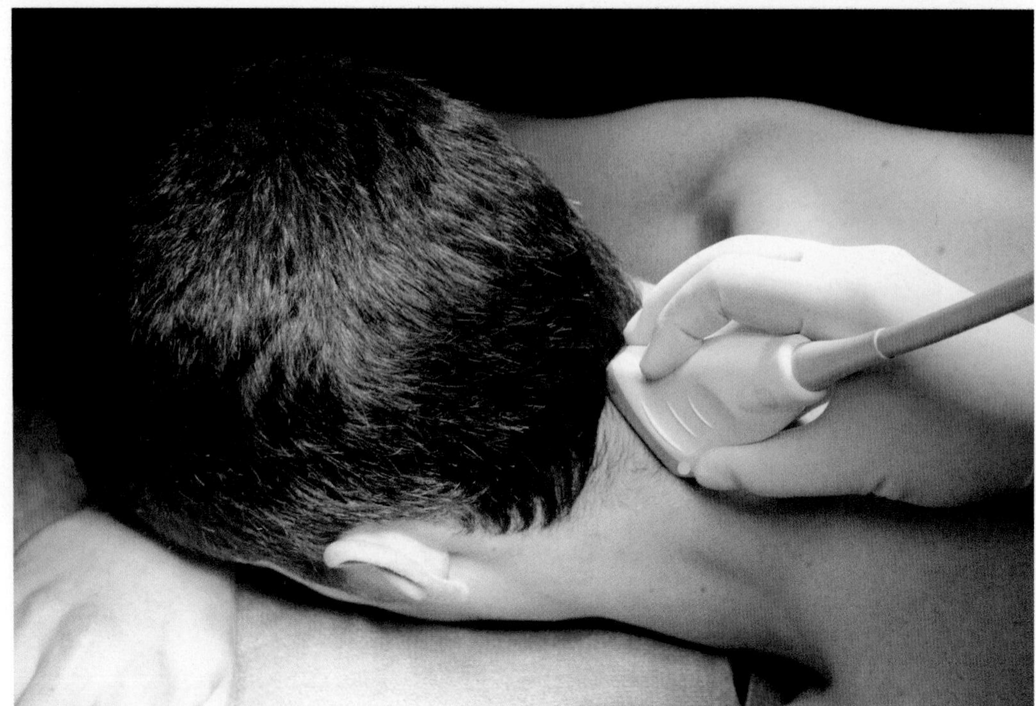

**FIGURE 7.1.2A** Ultrasound transducer position to image the greater occipital nerve, longitudinal view.

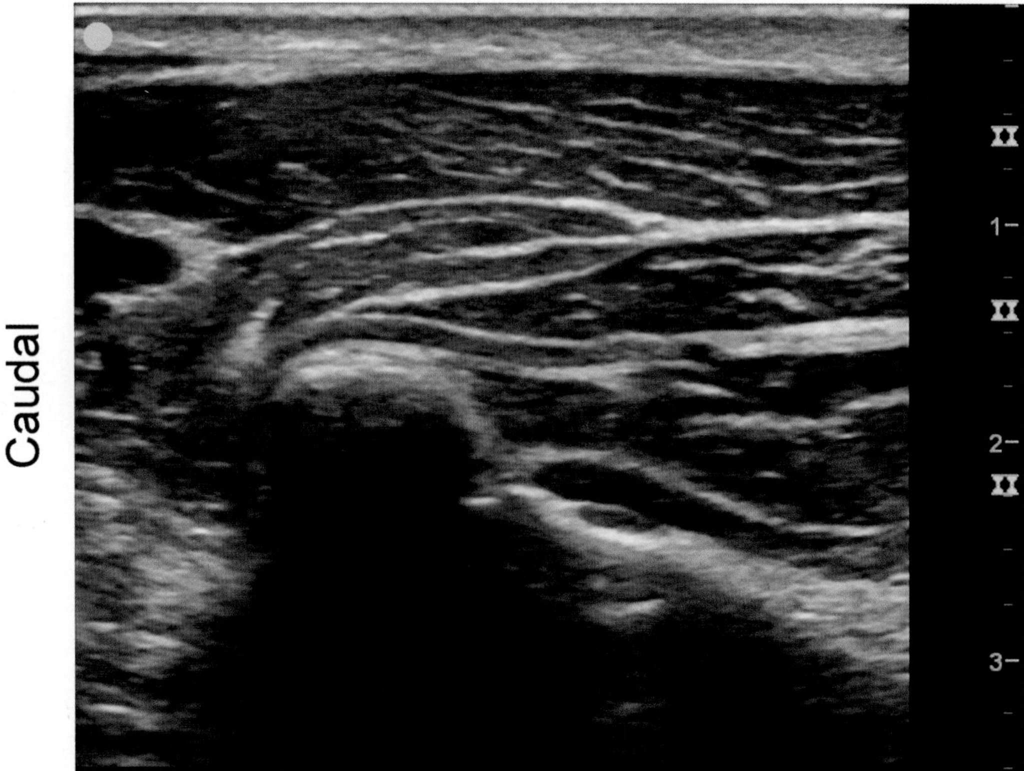


**FIGURE 7.1.2B** Ultrasound image of greater occipital nerve, longitudinal view.

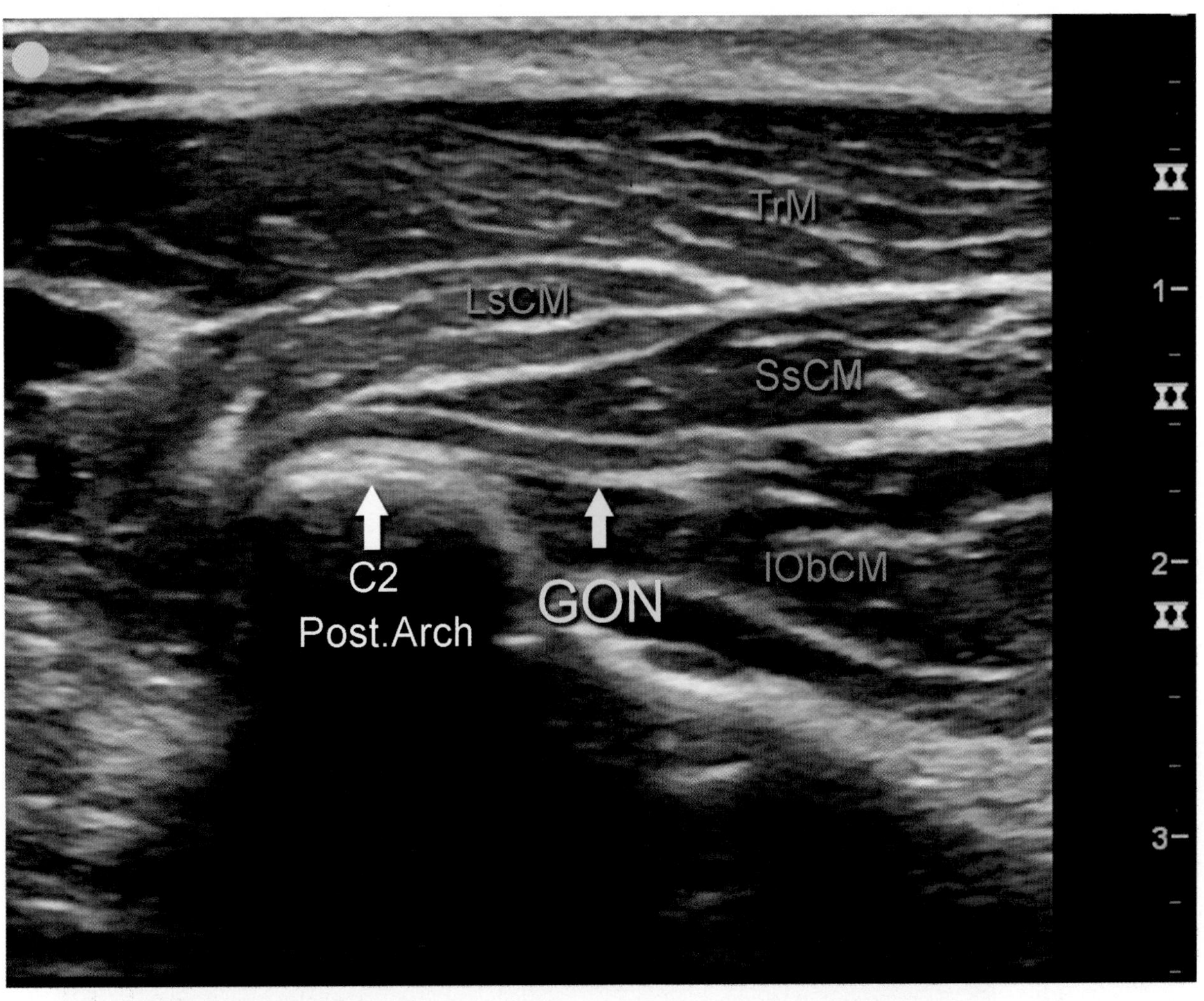


**FIGURE 7.1.2C** Labeled ultrasound image of greater occipital nerve, longitudinal view.

**Abbreviations:** TrM, Trapezius Muscle; SsCM, Semispinalis Capitis Muscle; IObCM, Inferior Oblique Capitis Muscle; GON, Greater Occipital Nerve; LsCM, Longissimus Capitis Muscle.

## Mandibular Nerve

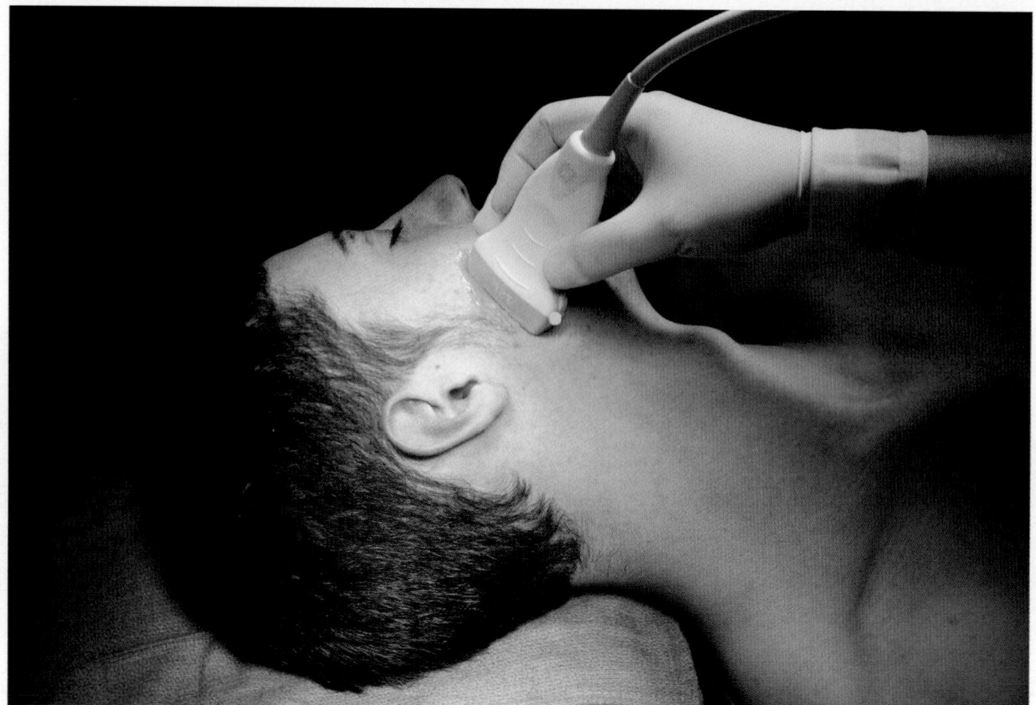

**FIGURE 7.2.1A** Ultrasound transducer position to image the mandibular nerve.

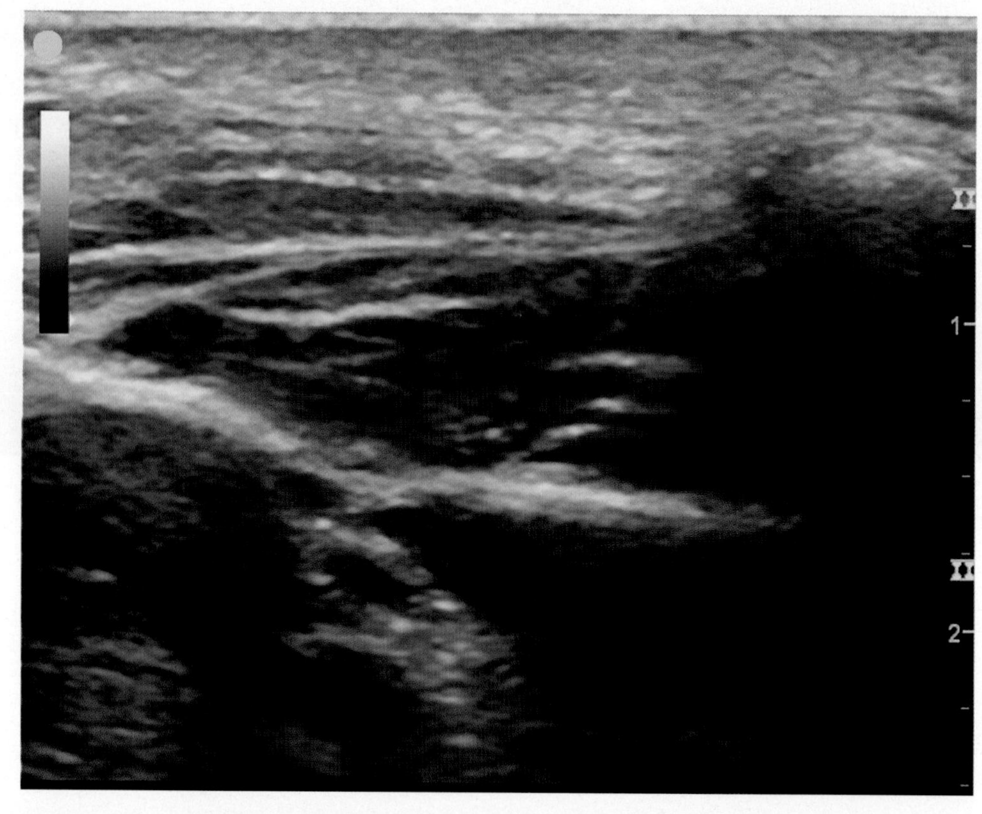


**FIGURE 7.2.1B** Ultrasound image of mandibular nerve.

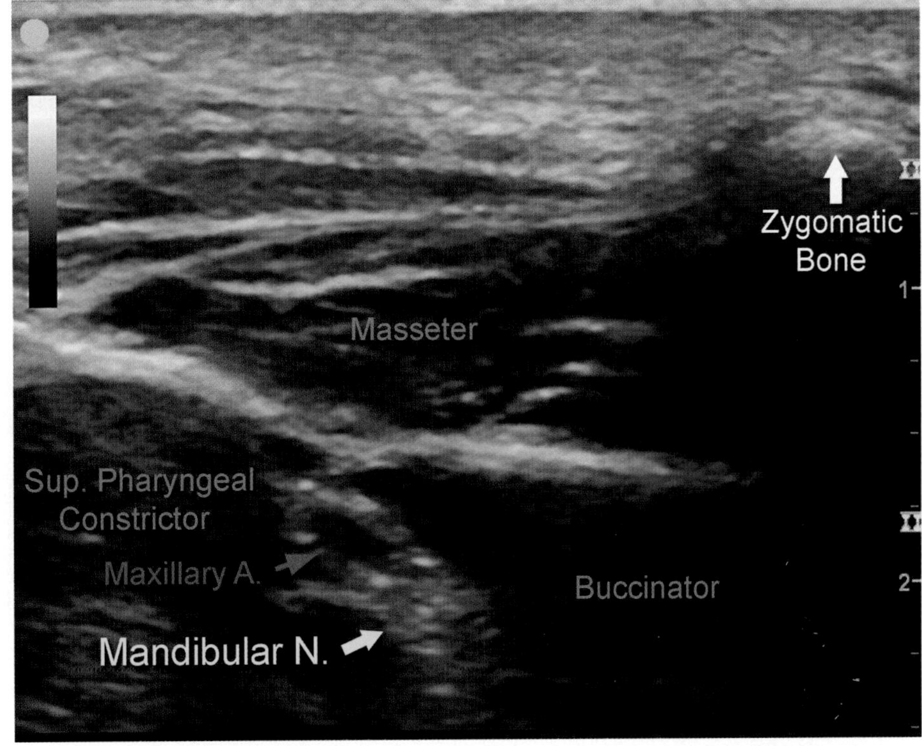


**FIGURE 7.2.1C** Labeled ultrasound image of mandibular nerve.

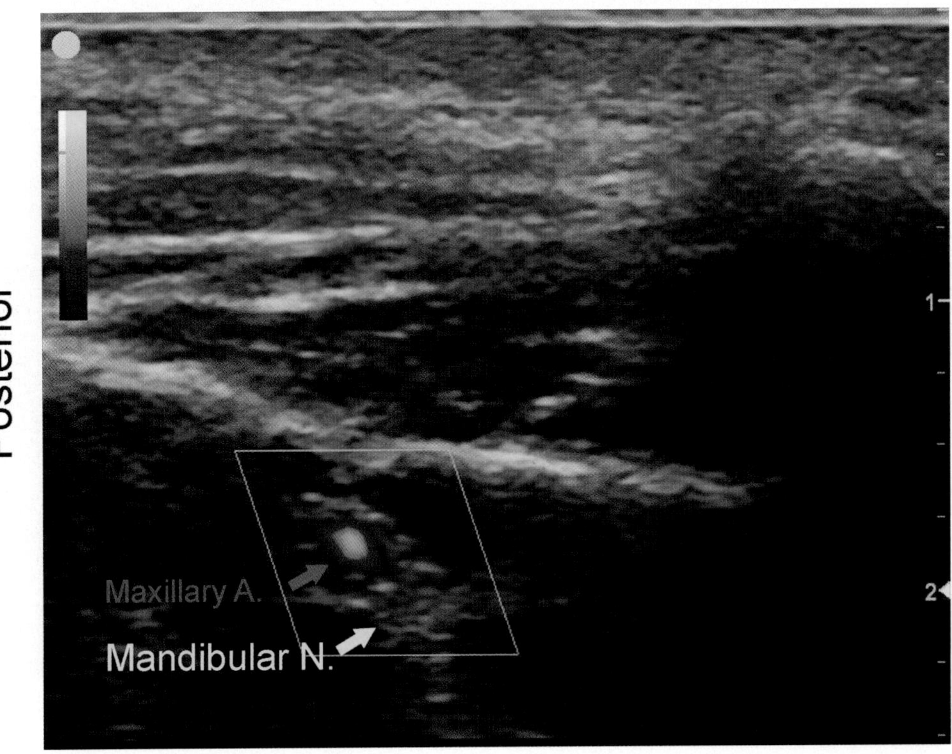


**FIGURE 7.2.1D** Labeled ultrasound image of mandibular nerve with color Doppler.

# Maxillary Nerve

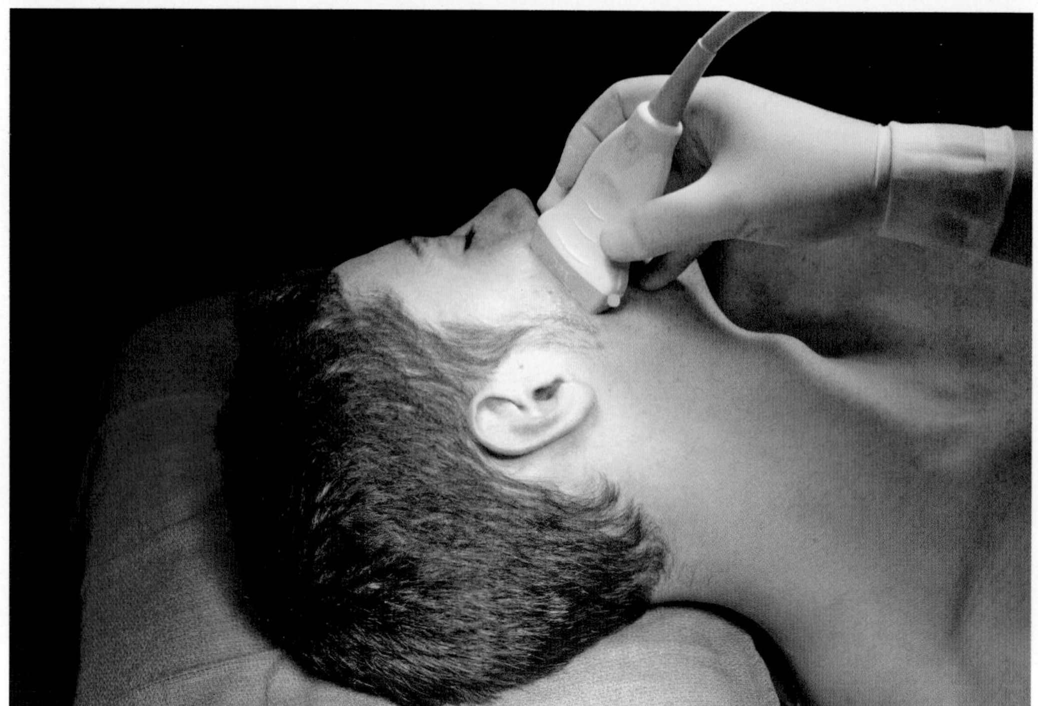

**FIGURE 7.3.1A** Ultrasound transducer position to image the maxillary nerve.

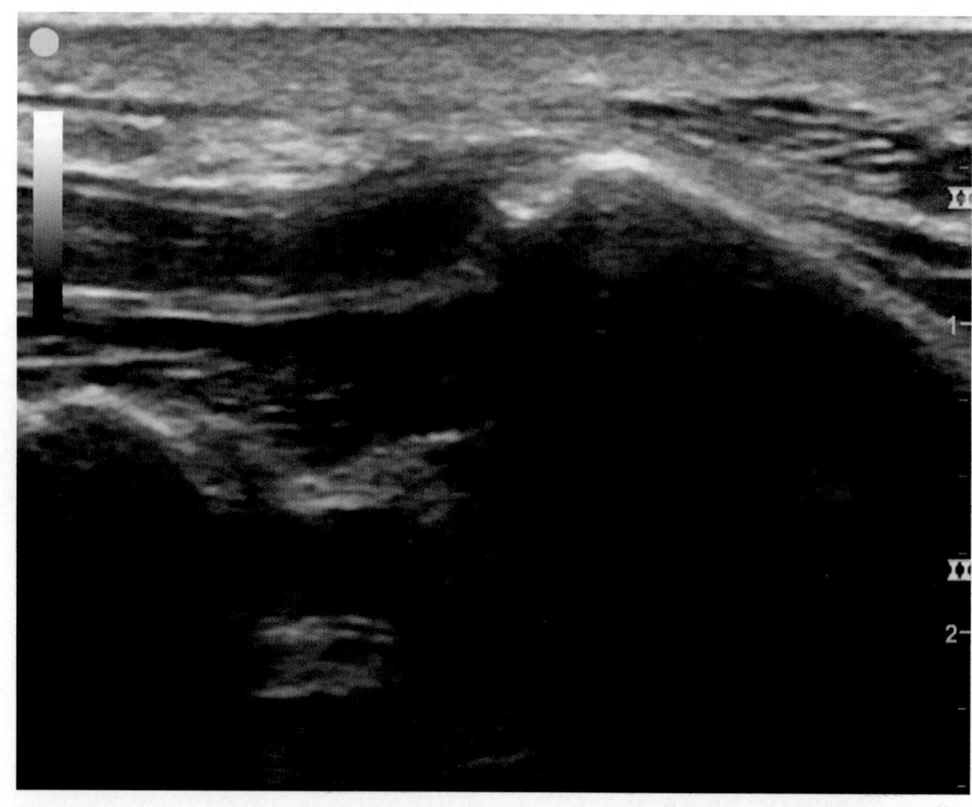


**FIGURE 7.3.1B** Ultrasound image of maxillary nerve.

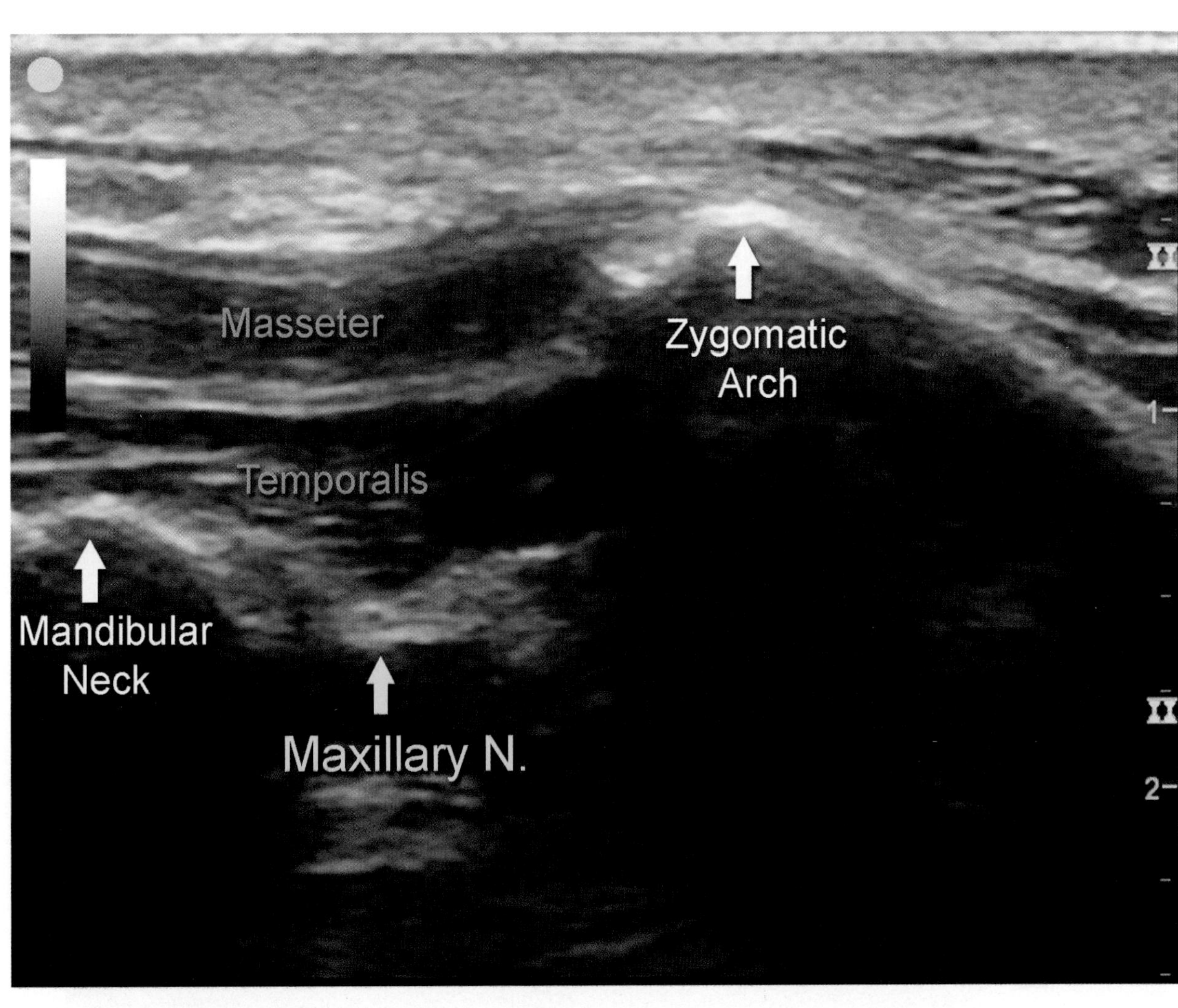


**FIGURE 7.3.1C** Labeled ultrasound anatomy of maxillary nerve, transverse view.

# Long Thoracic Nerve

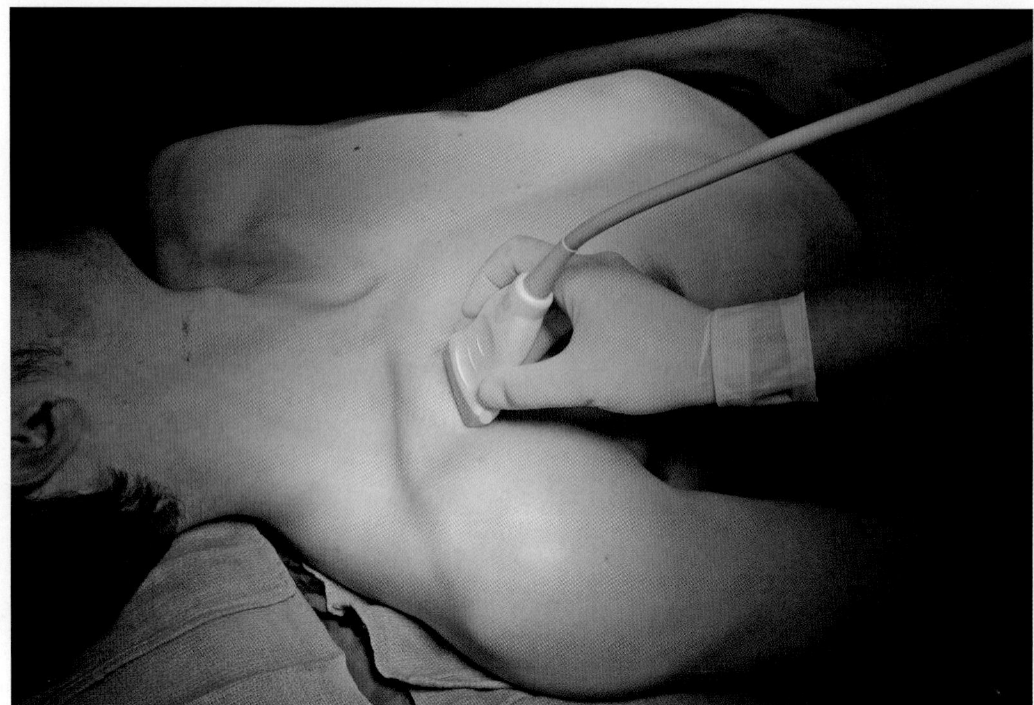

**FIGURE 7.4.1A** Ultrasound transducer position to image the long thoracic nerve.

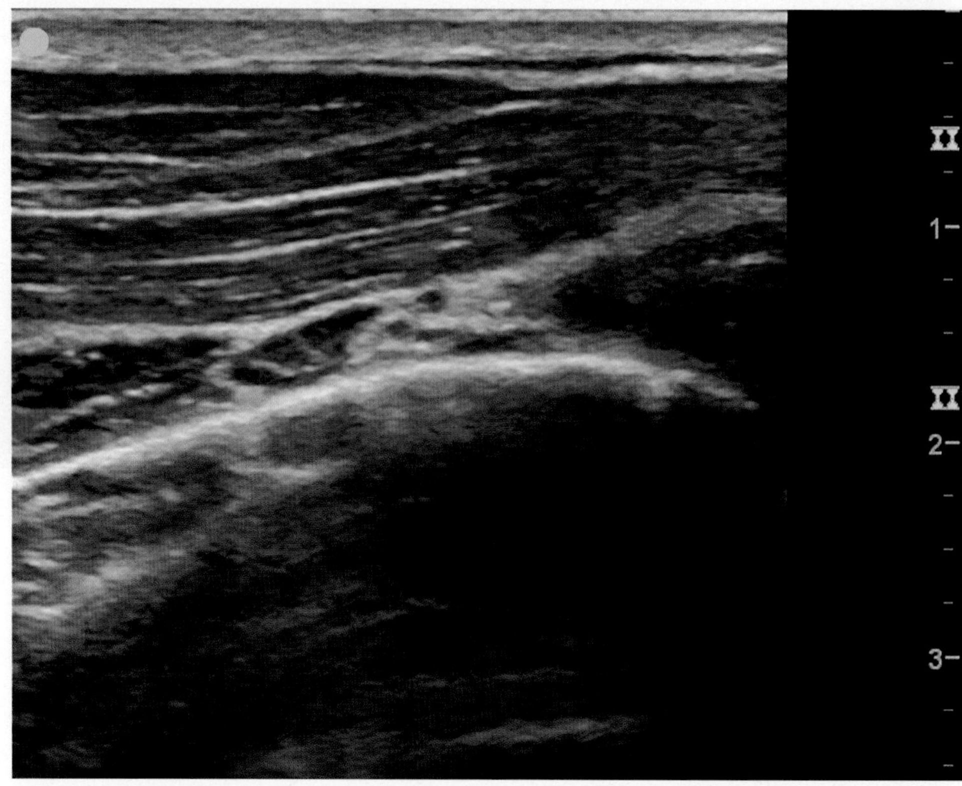


**FIGURE 7.4.1B** Ultrasound image of long thoracic nerve.

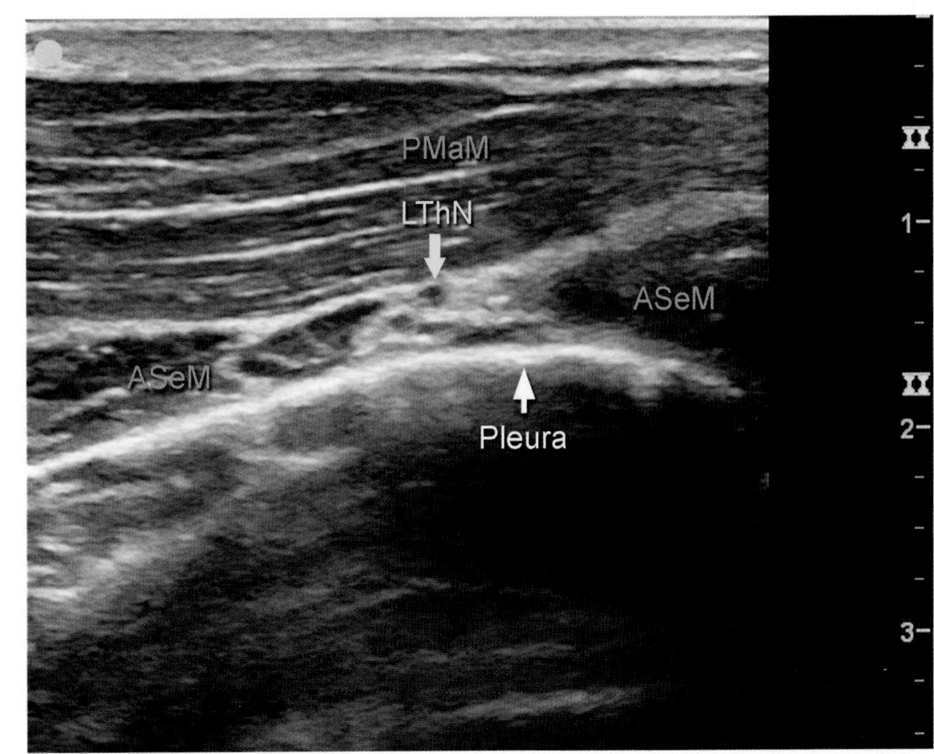


**FIGURE 7.4.1C** Labeled ultrasound image of long thoracic nerve.

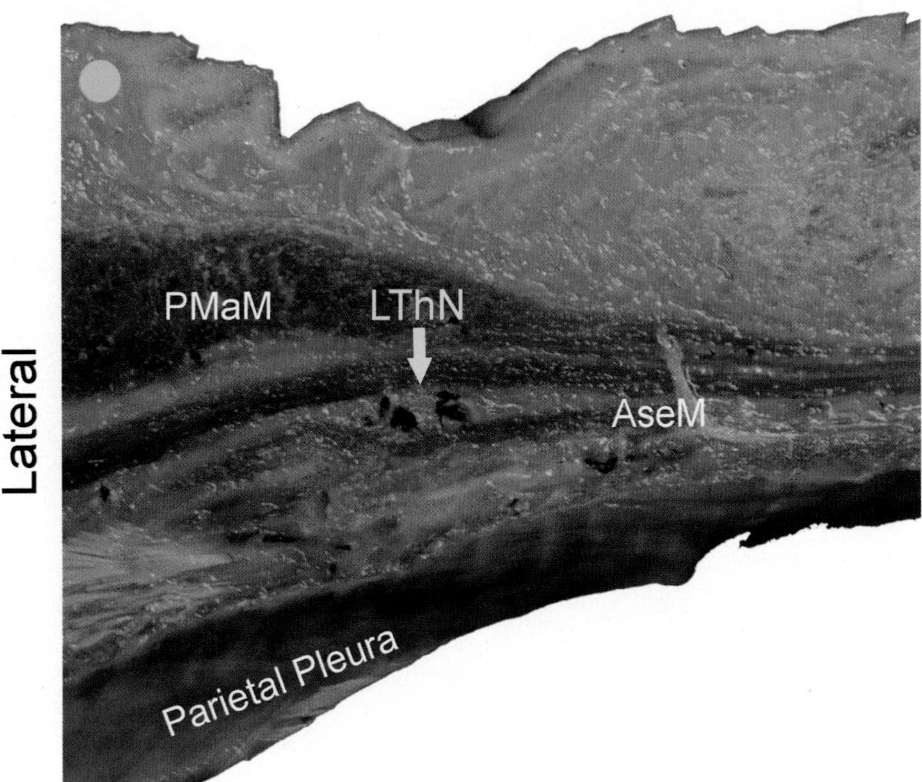


**FIGURE 7.4.1D** Labeled cross-sectional anatomy of long thoracic nerve.

**Abbreviations:** AseM, Anterior Serratus Muscle; LThN, Long Thoracic Nerve; PMaM, Pectoralis Major Muscle.

## Suprascapular Artery and Nerve

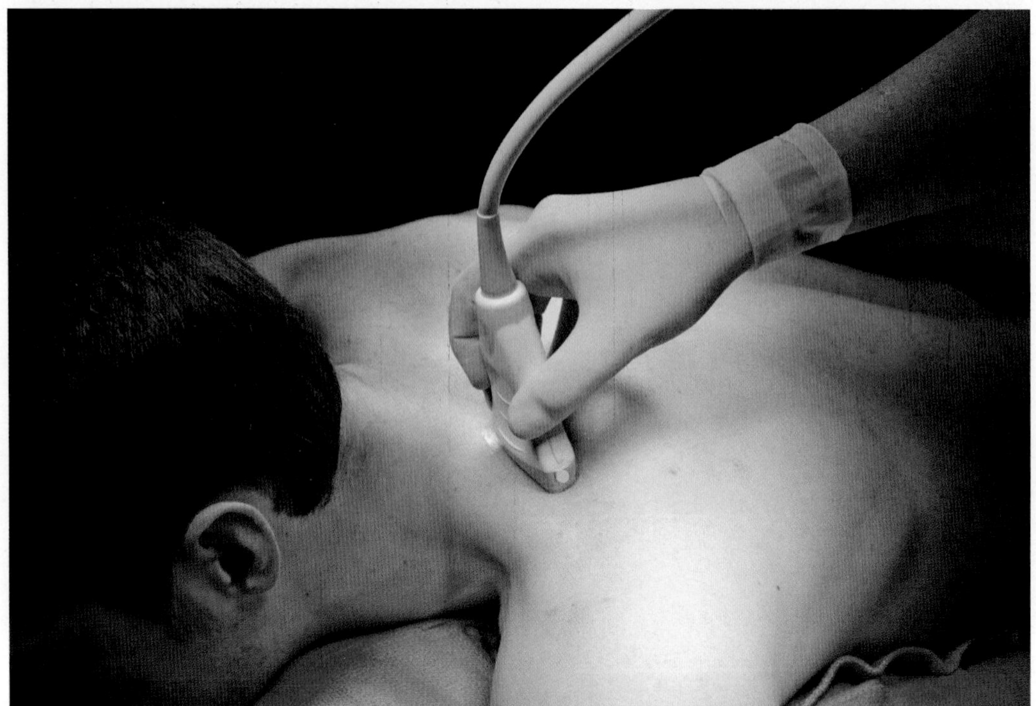

**FIGURE 7.5.1A** Ultrasound transducer position to image the suprascapular artery and nerve.

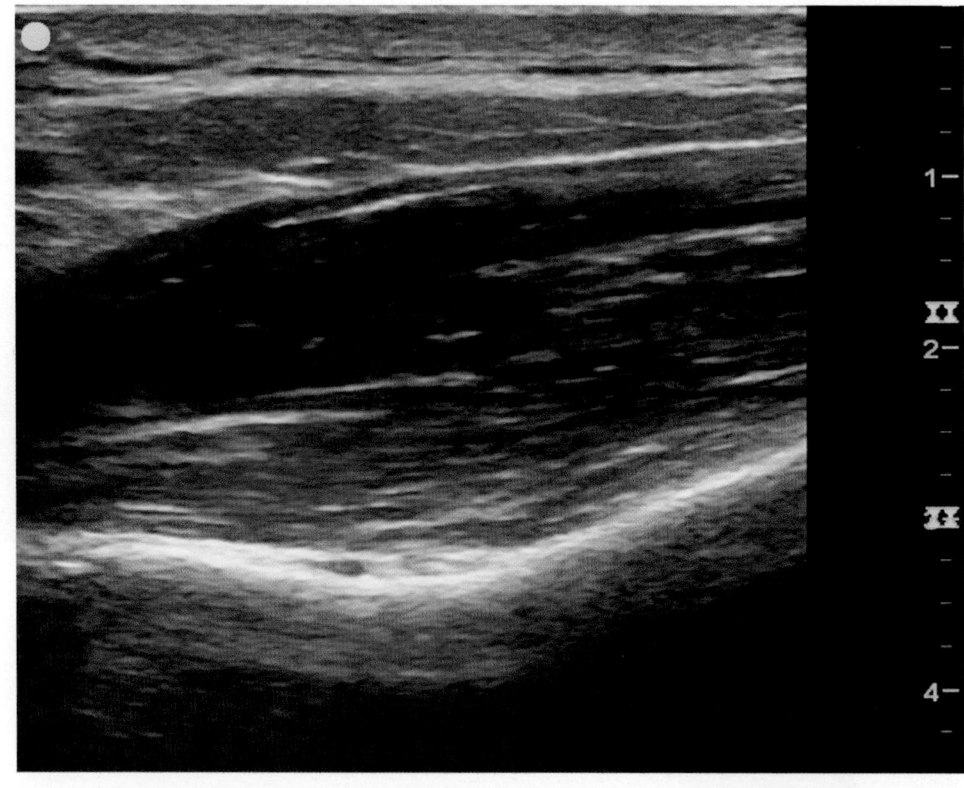


**FIGURE 7.5.1B** Ultrasound image of suprascapular artery and nerve.

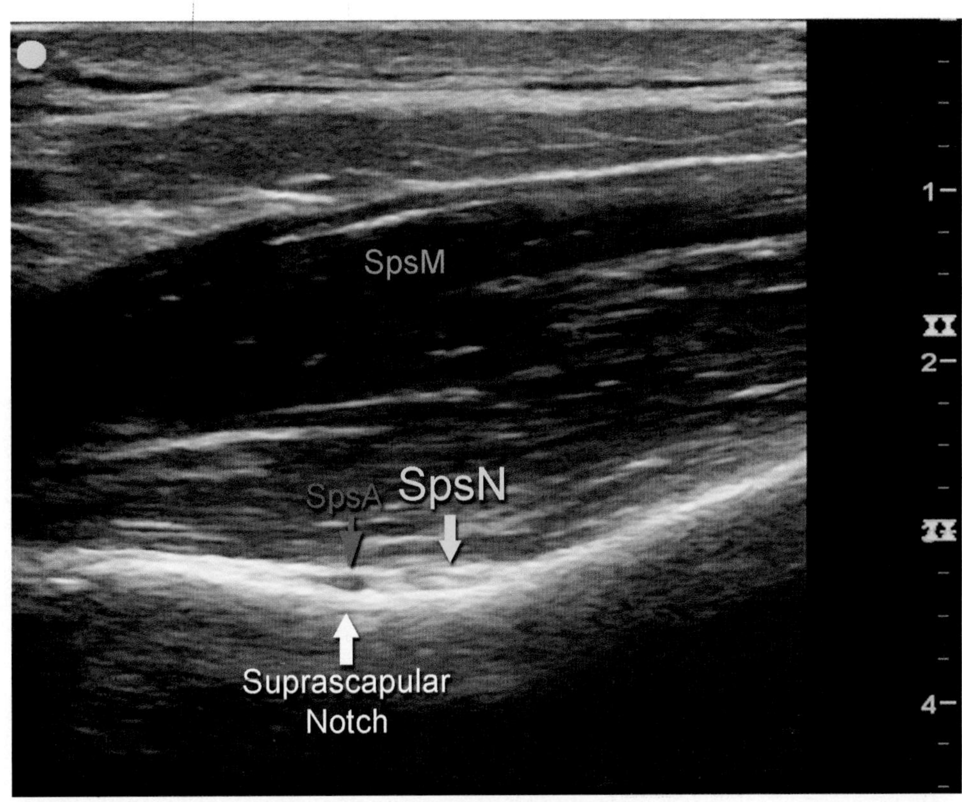


**FIGURE 7.5.1C** Labeled ultrasound image of suprascapular artery and nerve.

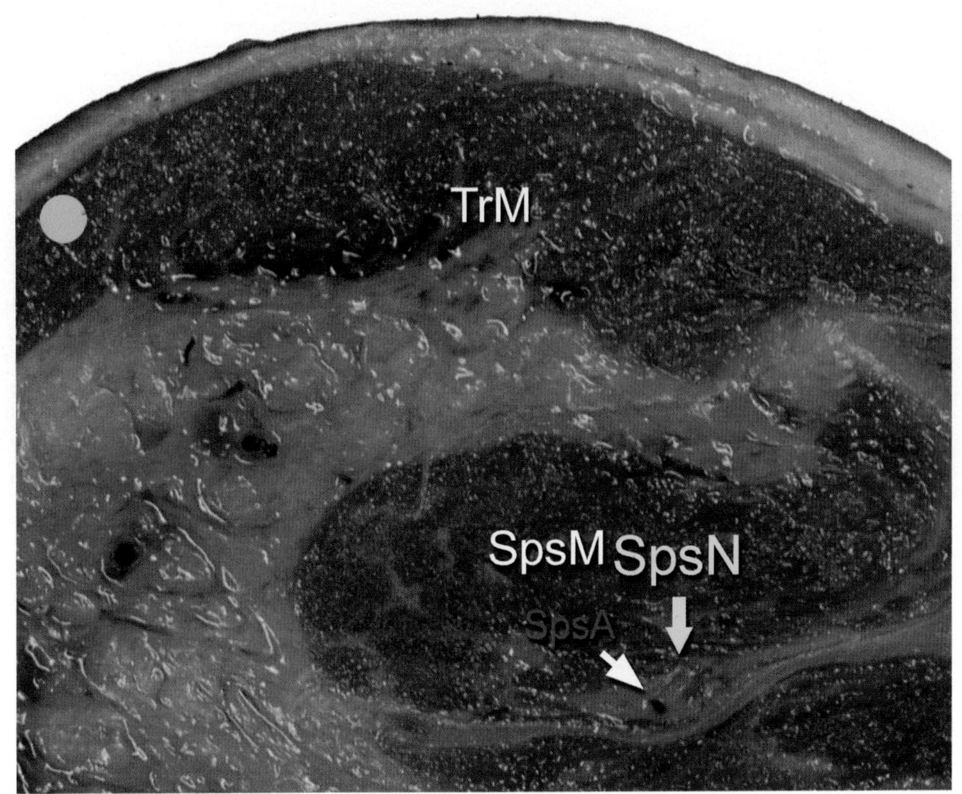


**FIGURE 7.5.1D**

**Abbreviations:** SpsN, Suprascapular Nerve; SpsM, Supraspinatus Muscle; SpsA, Suprascapular Artery.

## Suprascapular Artery and Nerve (Continued)

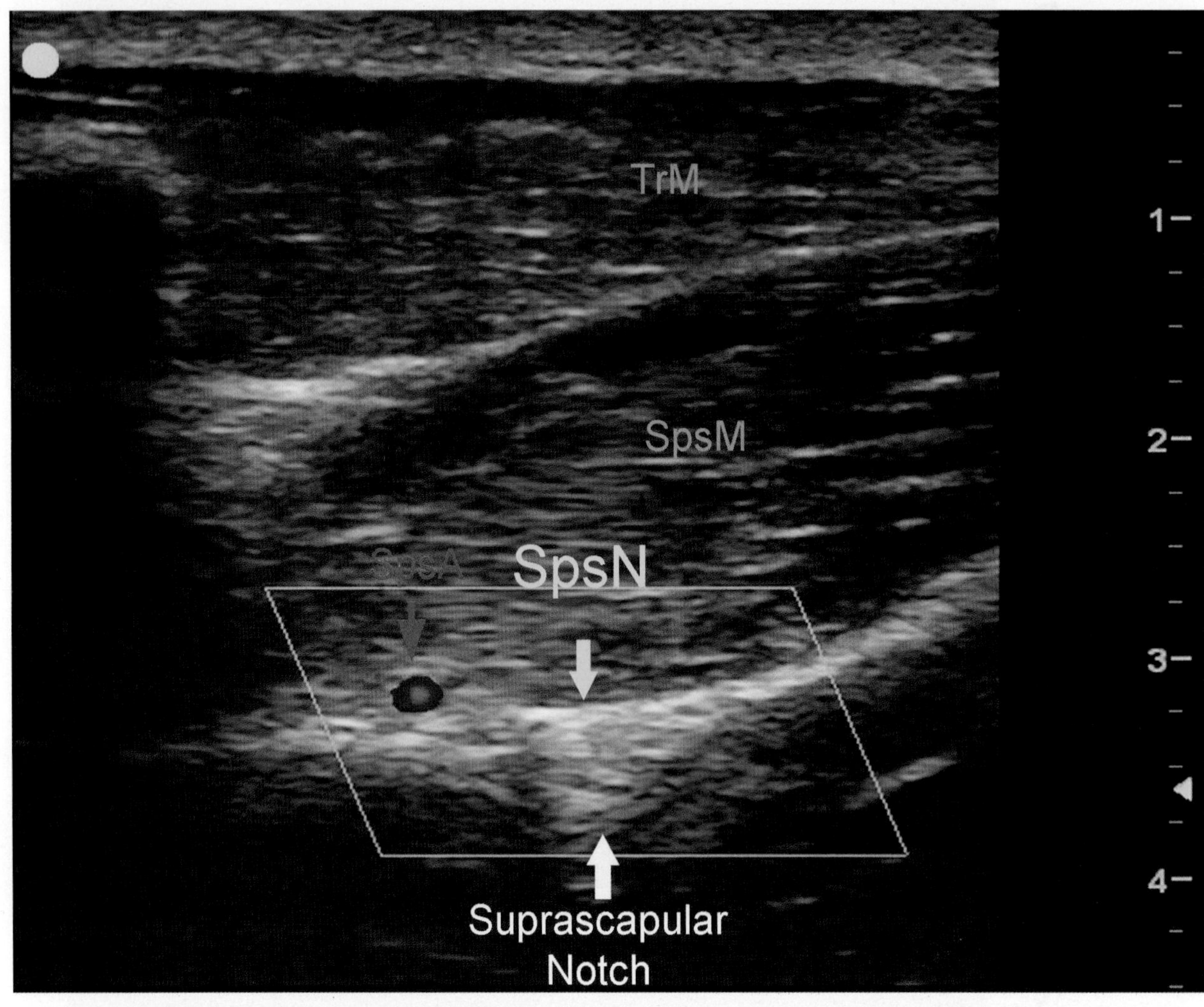


**FIGURE 7.5.1D** Labeled ultrasound image of suprascapular artery and nerve with color flow Doppler.

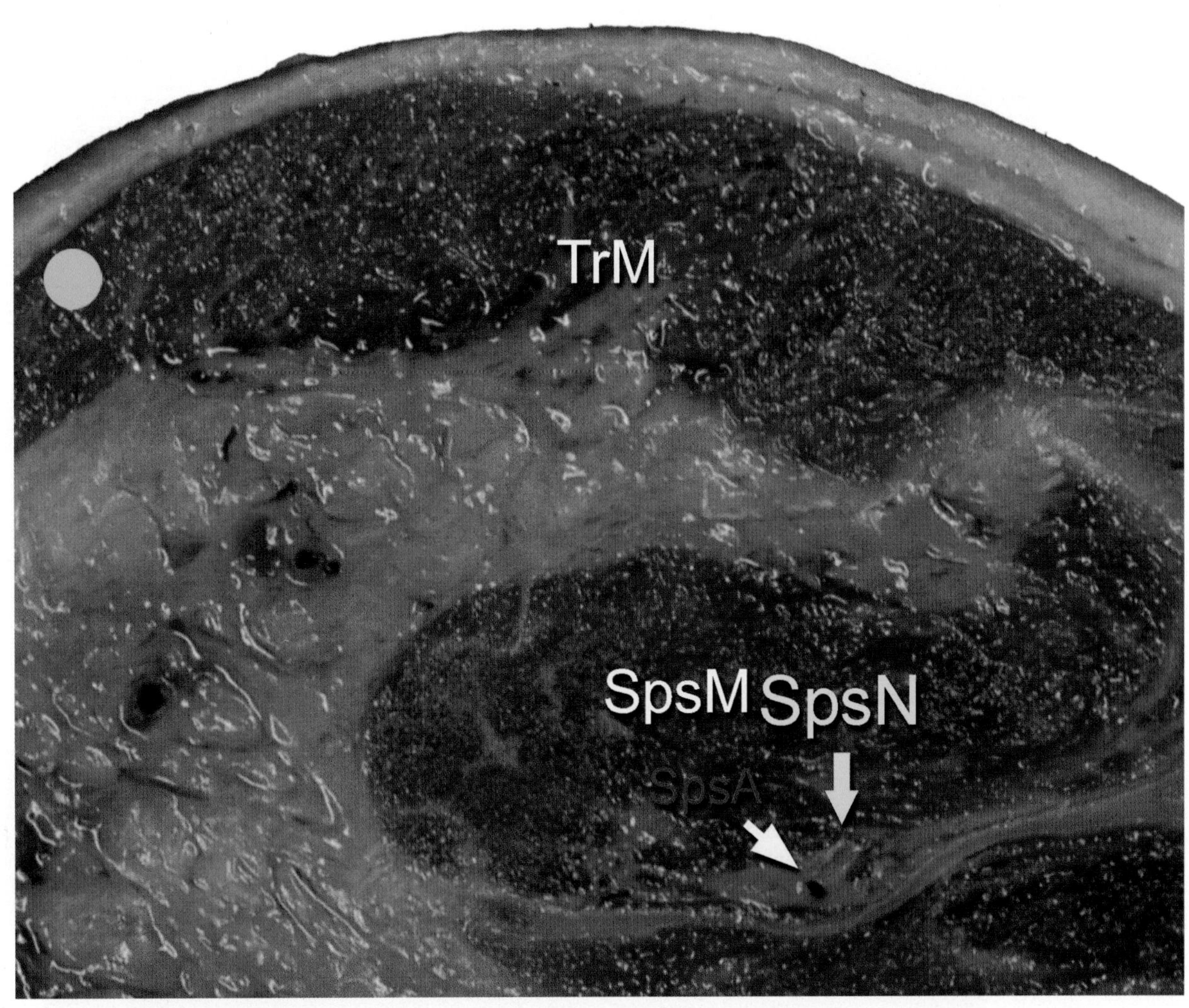


**FIGURE 7.5.1E** Labeled cross-sectional anatomy of suprascapular artery and nerve.

**Abbreviations:** SpsN, Suprascapular Nerve; SpsM, Supraspinatus Muscle, SpsA, Suprascapular Artery; TrM, Trapezius Muscle.

## Suprascapular Nerve, Longitudinal View

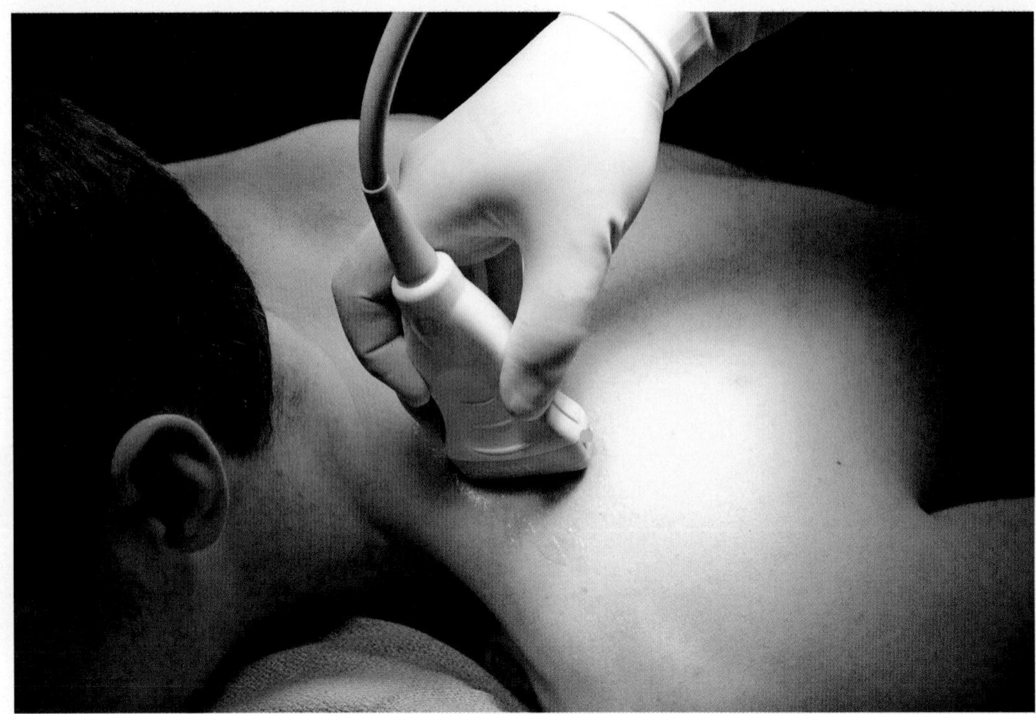

**FIGURE 7.5.2A** Ultrasound transducer position to image the suprascapular nerve, longitudinal view.

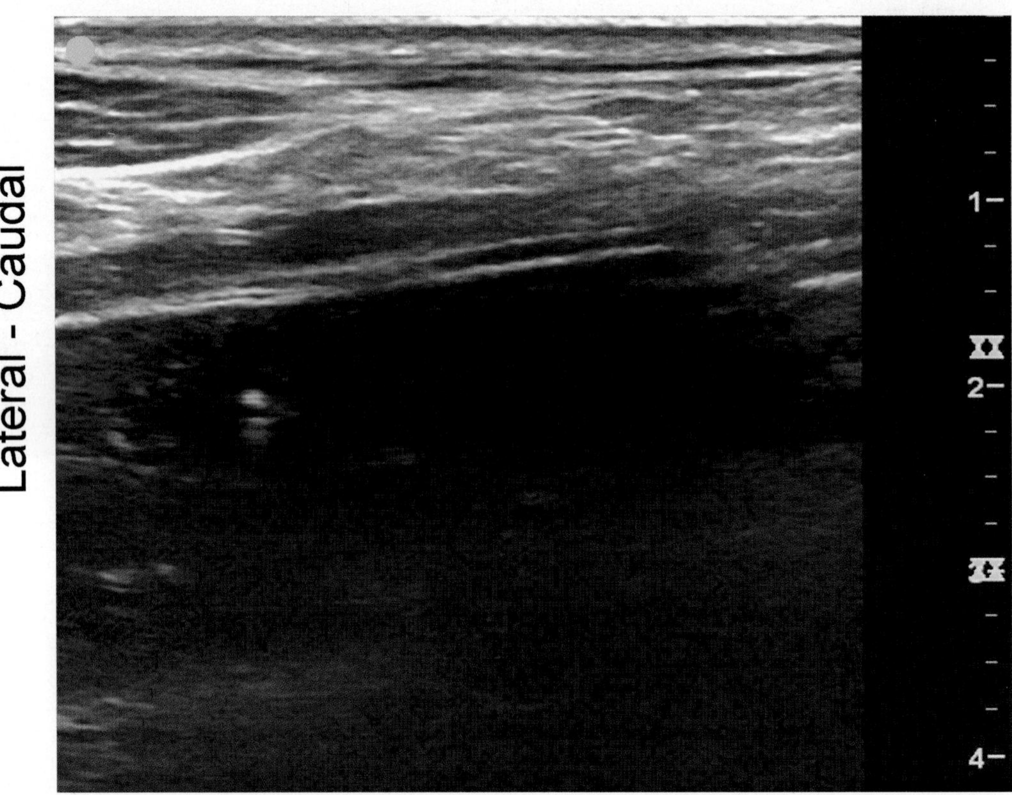


**FIGURE 7.5.2B** Ultrasound image of suprascapular nerve, longitudinal view.

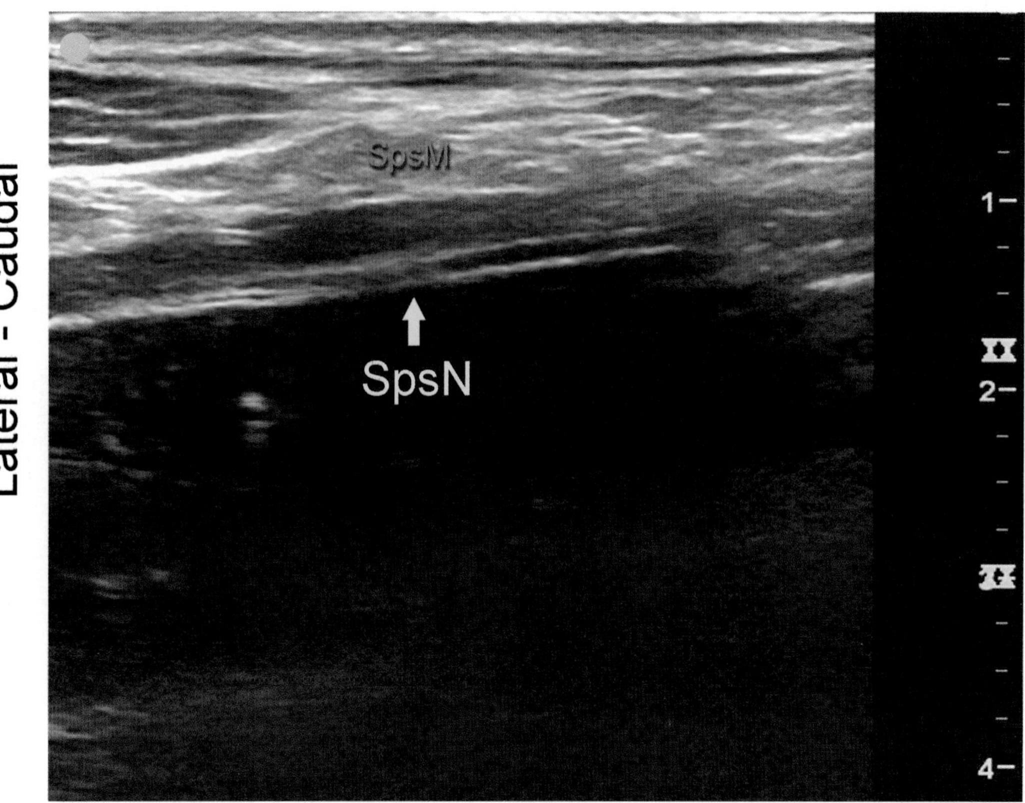


**FIGURE 7.5.2C** Labeled ultrasound image of suprascapular nerve, longitudinal view.

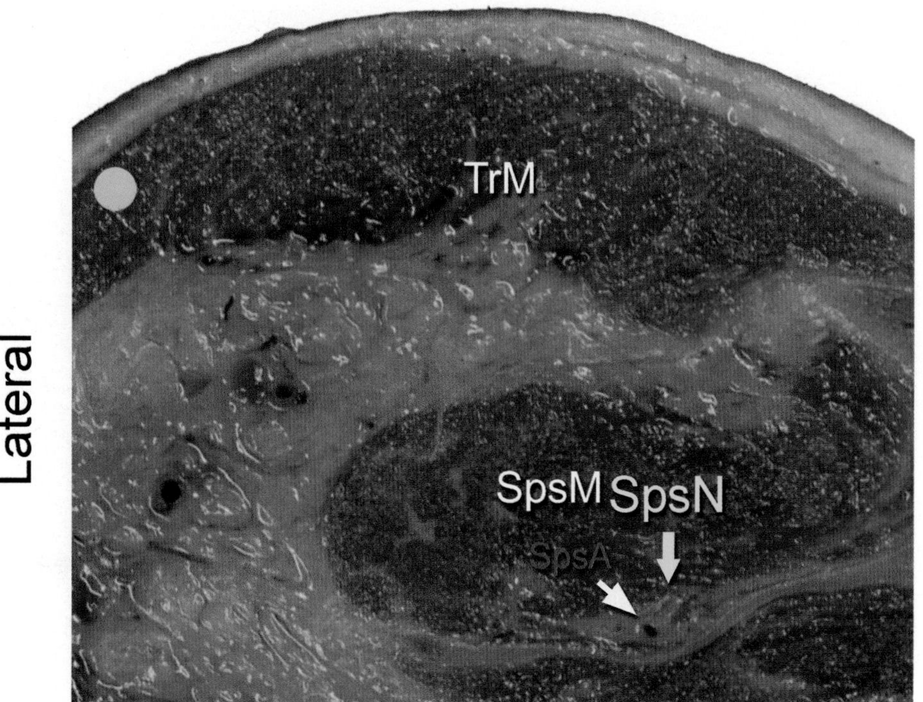


**FIGURE 7.5.2D**

**Abbreviations:** SpsN, Suprascapular Nerve; SpsM, Suprascapular Muscle; TrM, Trapezius Muscle.

# Dorsal Scapular Nerve

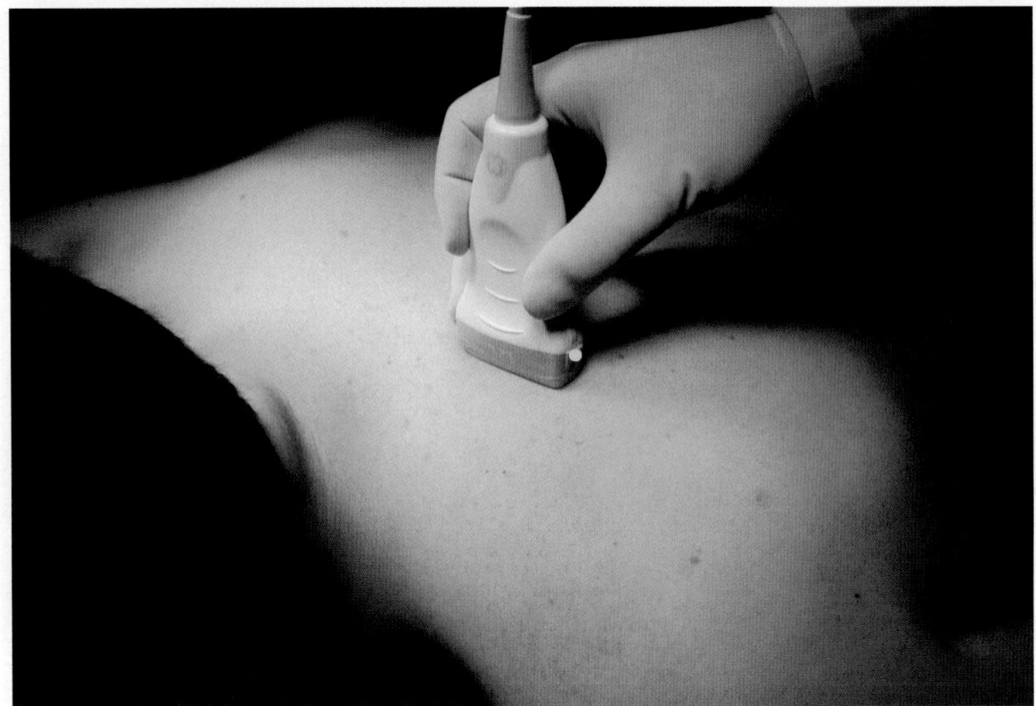

**FIGURE 7.6.1A** Ultrasound transducer position to image the dorsal scapular nerve.

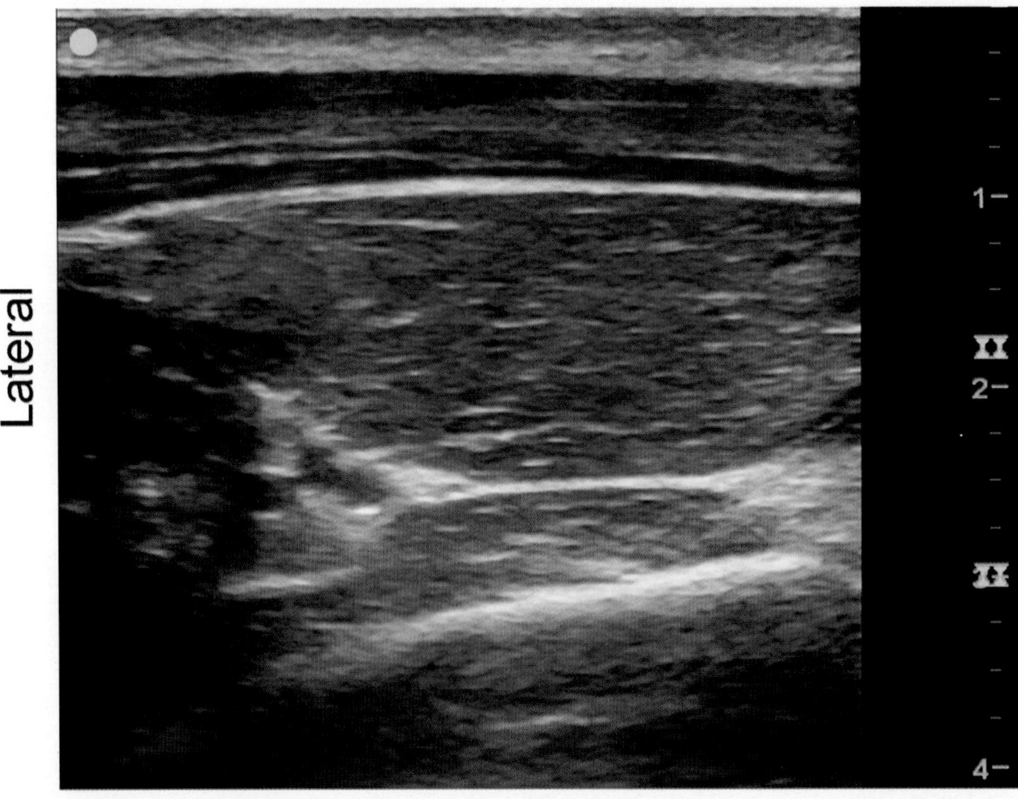


**FIGURE 7.6.1B** Ultrasound image of dorsal scapular nerve.

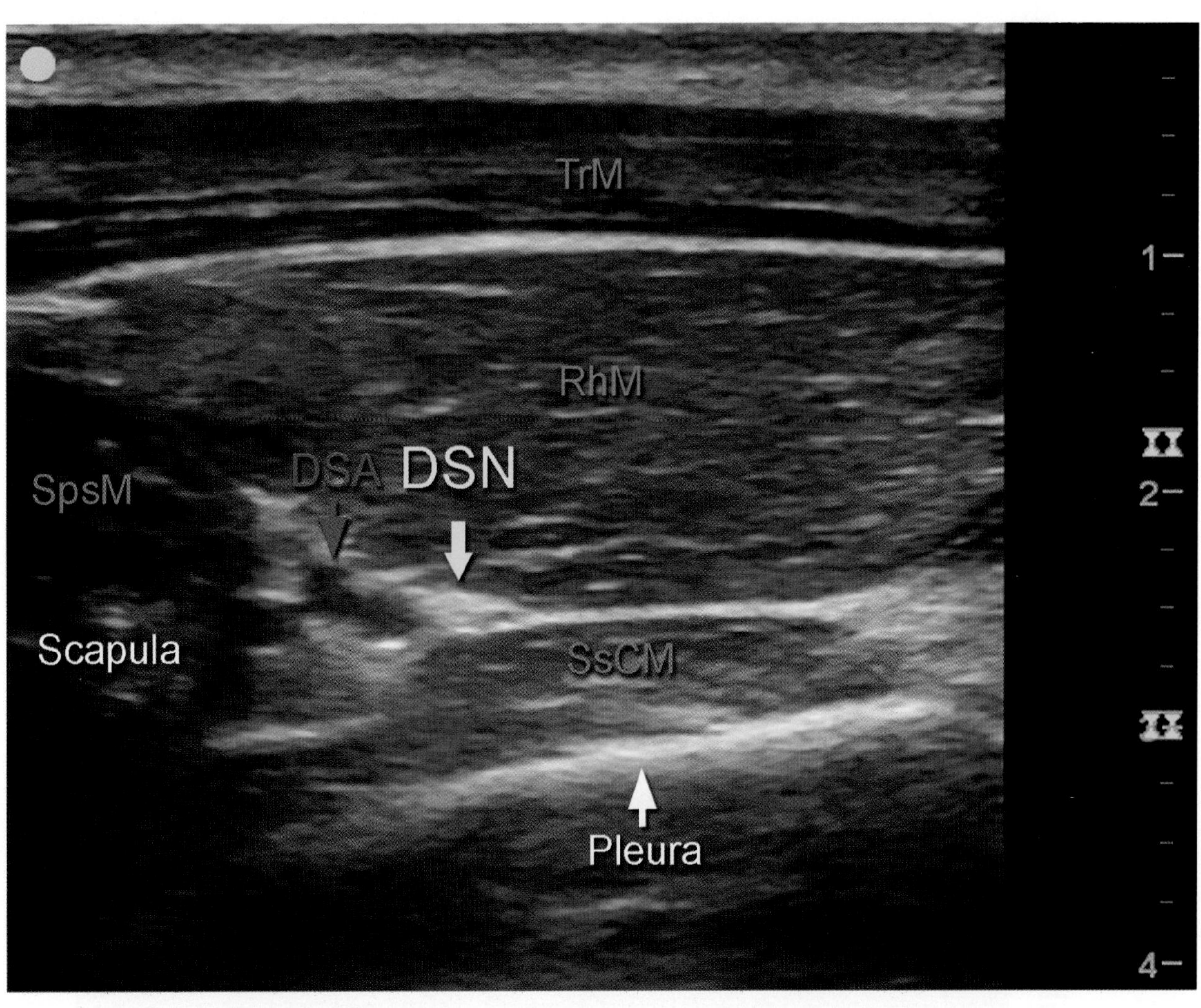


**FIGURE 7.6.1C** Labeled ultrasound image of dorsal scapular nerve.

**Abbreviations:** DSN, dorsal scapular nerve; DSA, dorsal scapular artery; SsCM, Semispinalis Capitis Muscle; RhM, Rhomboids Muscle; TrM, Trapezius Muscle.

# Intercostal Space, High Thoracic Level

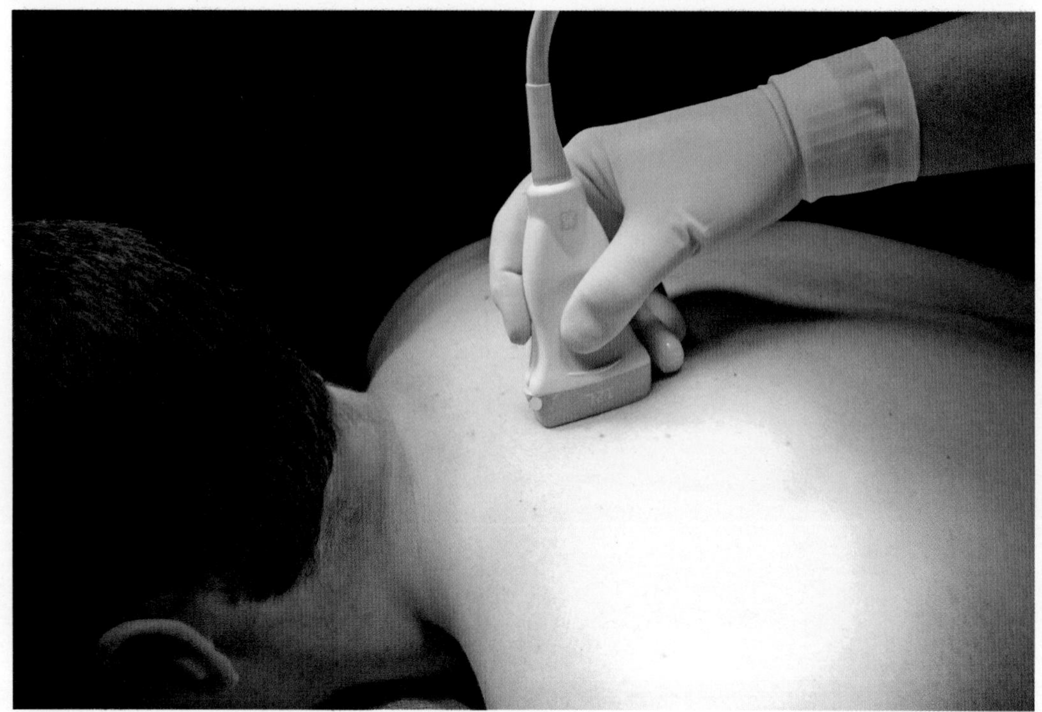

**FIGURE 7.7.1A** Ultrasound transducer position to image the intercostal space at the high thoracic level.

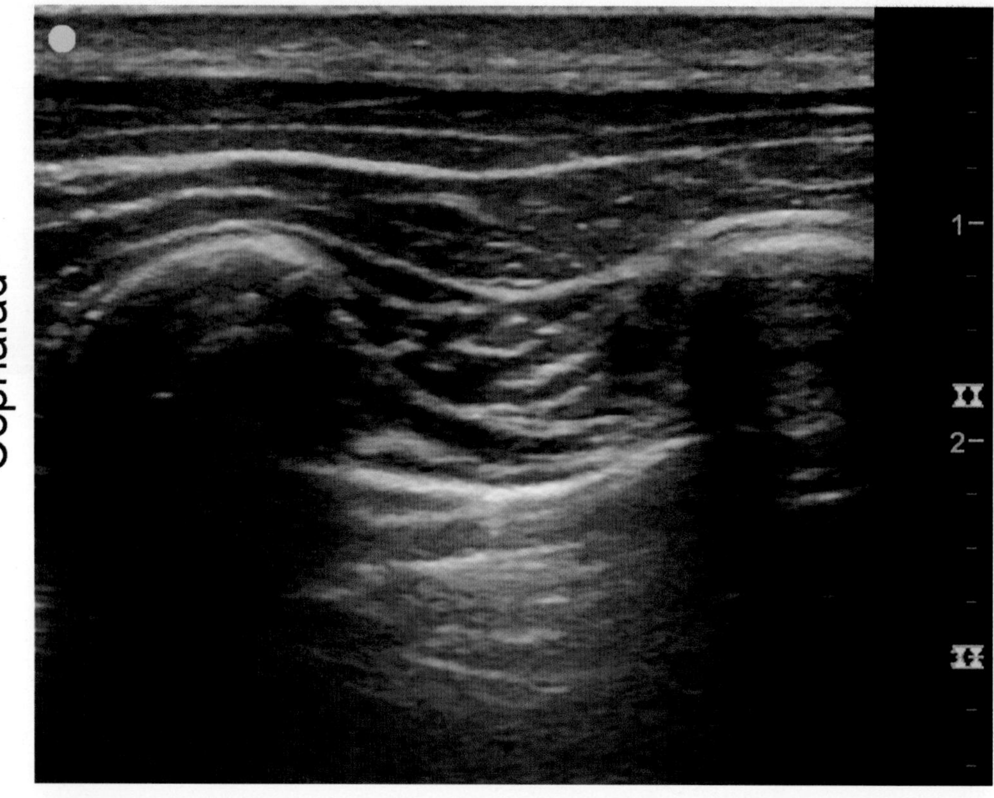


**FIGURE 7.7.1B** Ultrasound image of the intercostal space at the high thoracic level.

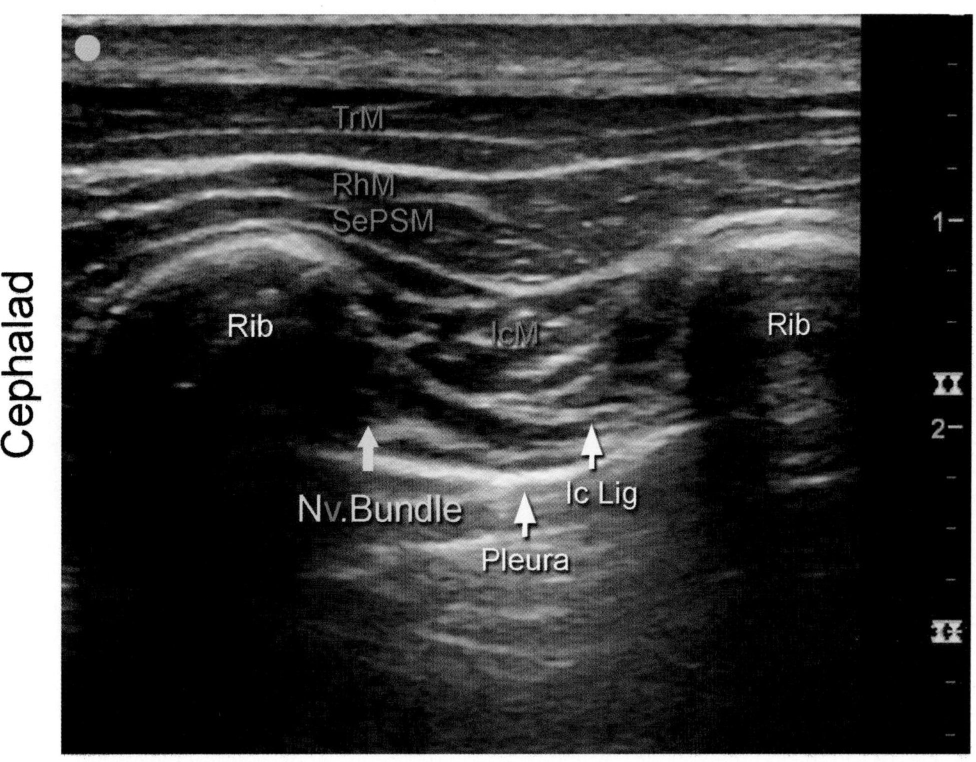


**FIGURE 7.7.1C** Labeled ultrasound image of the intercostal space at the high thoracic level.

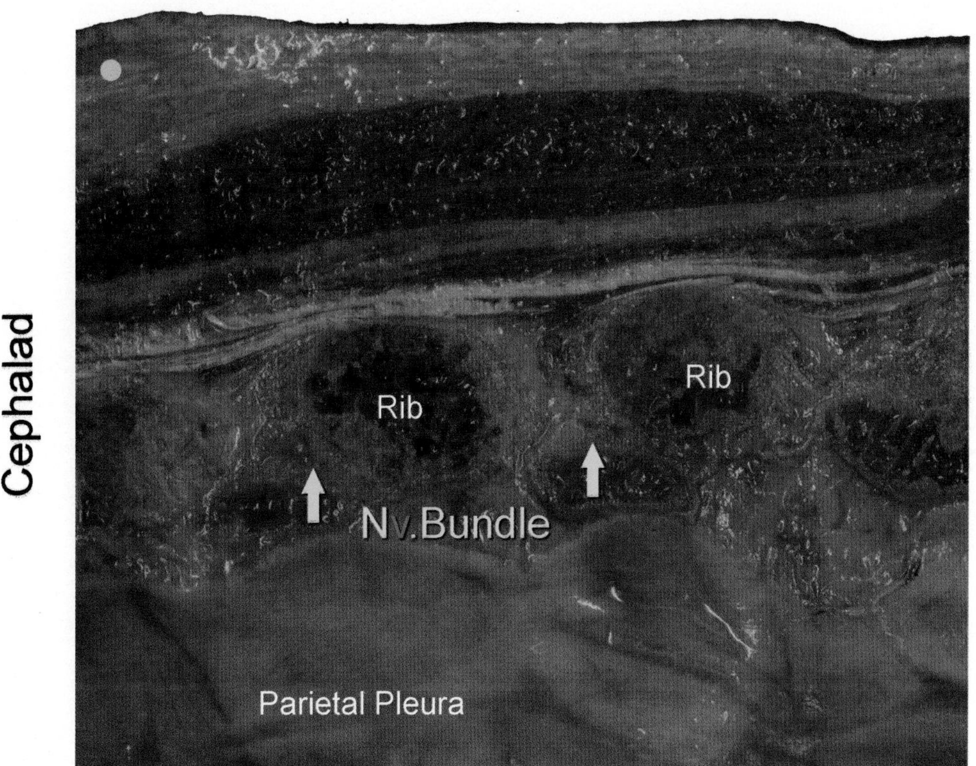


**FIGURE 7.7.1D** Labeled cross-sectional anatomy of intercostal space, at the high thoracic level.

**Abbreviations:** TrM, Trapezius Muscle; RhM, Rhomboid Muscle; SePSM, Serratus Posterior Superior Muscle; IcM, Intercostal Muscle; Ic Lig - Intercostal Ligament; Nv, Neurovascular.

# Interscalene Brachial Plexus, Transverse View, C5 Level

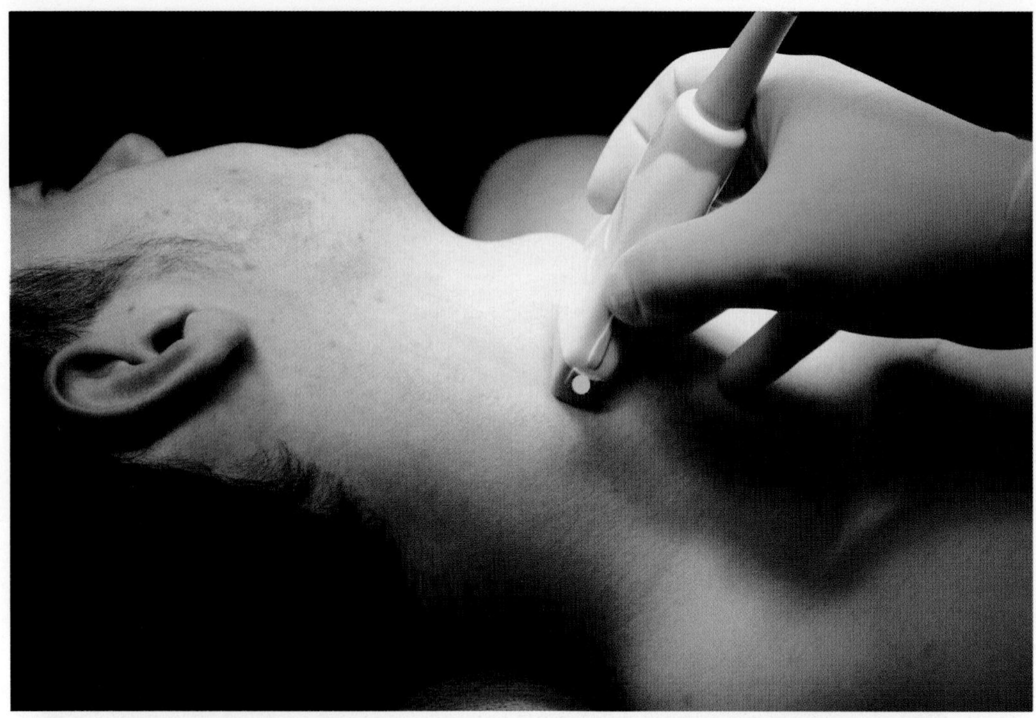

**FIGURE 7.8.1A** Ultrasound transducer position to image the interscalene brachial plexus, transverse view.

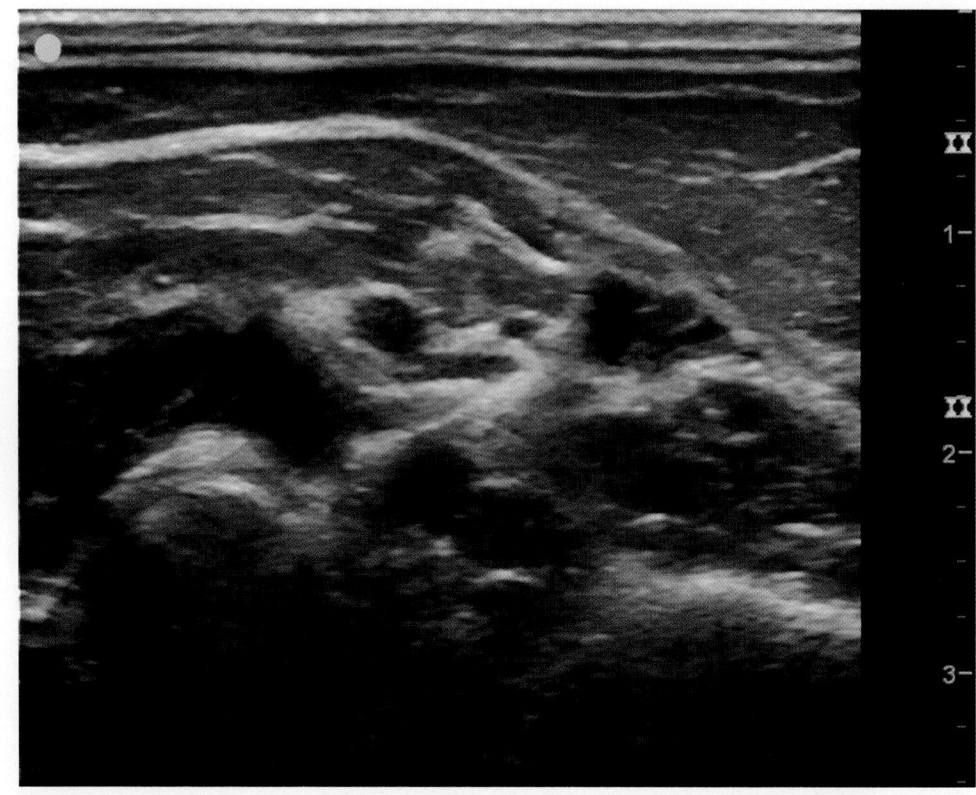


**FIGURE 7.8.1B** Ultrasound image of the interscalene brachial plexus, transverse view.

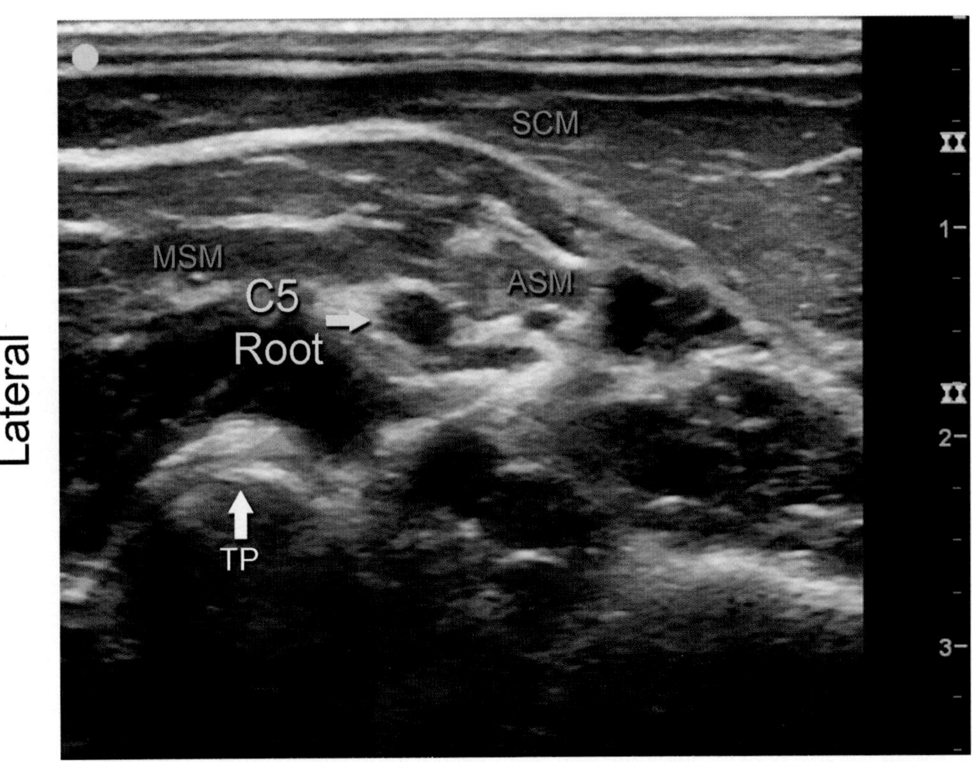


**FIGURE 7.8.1C** Labeled ultrasound image of the interscalene brachial plexus, transverse view.

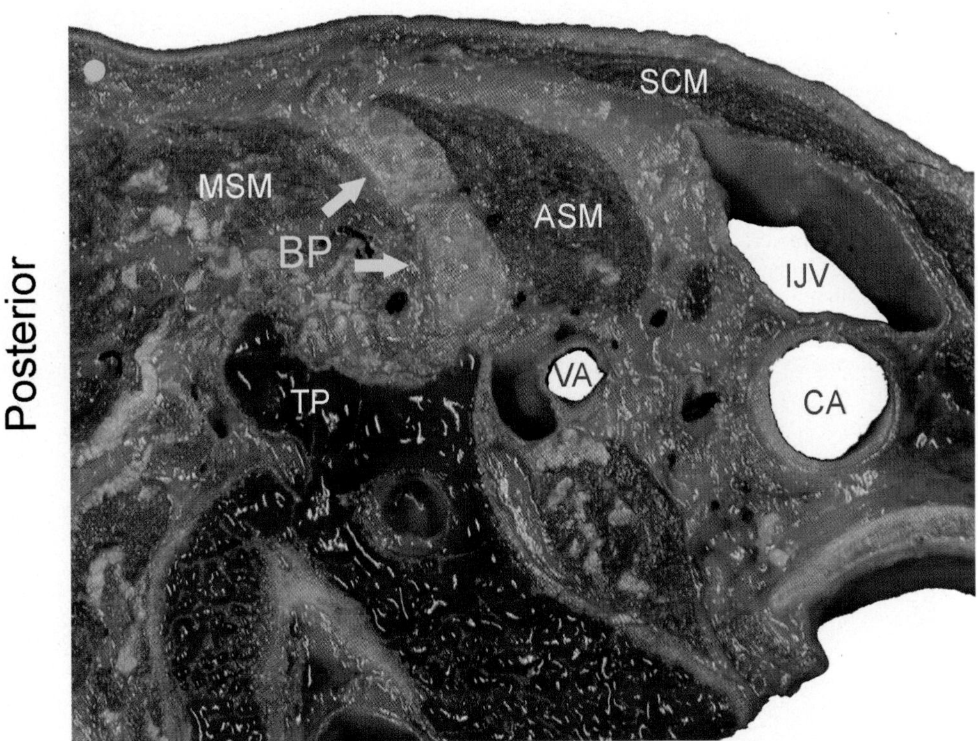


**FIGURE 7.8.1D** Labeled cross-sectional anatomy of the interscalene brachial plexus.

**Abbreviations:** SCM, sternocleidomastoid muscle; ASM, anterior scalene muscle; MSM, middle scalene muscle; TP, transverse process.

## Interscalene Brachial Plexus, Longitudinal View

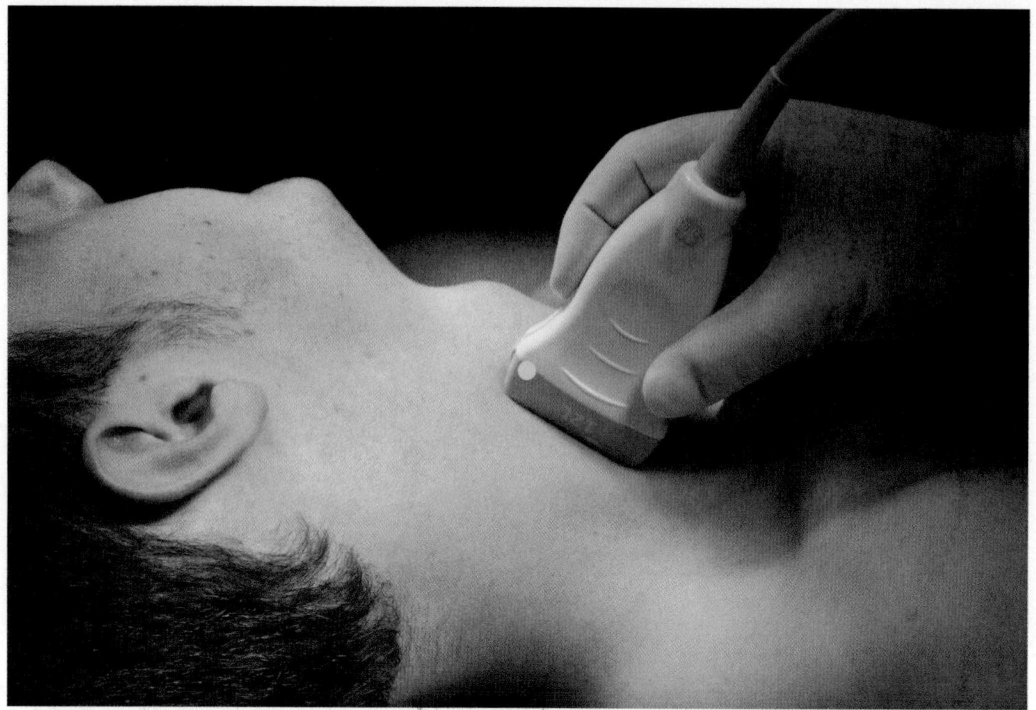

**FIGURE 7.8.2A** Ultrasound transducer position to image the interscalene brachial plexus, longitudinal view.

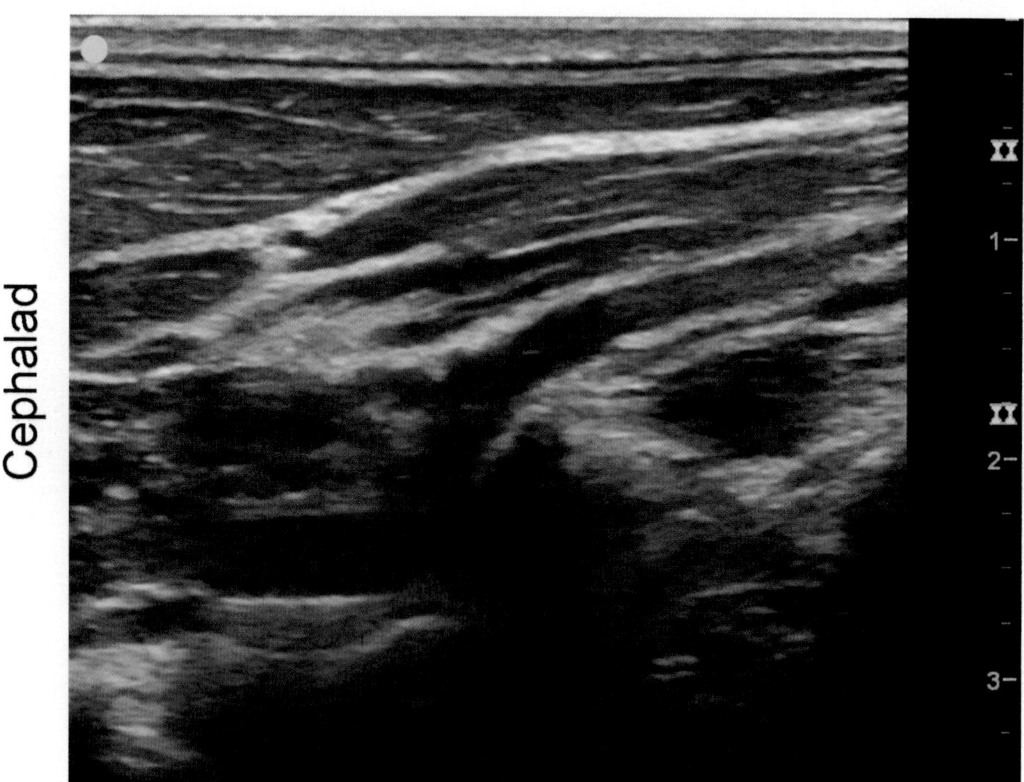


**FIGURE 7.8.2B** Ultrasound image of the interscalene brachial plexus, longitudinal view.

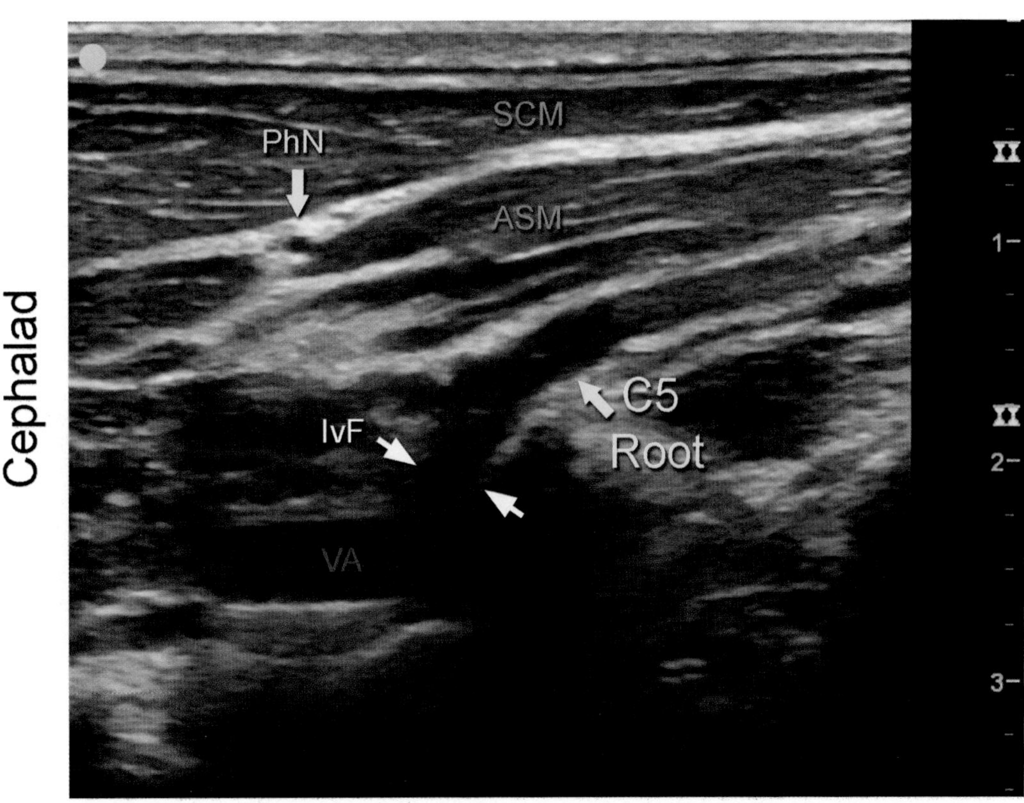


**FIGURE 7.8.2C** Labeled ultrasound image of the interscalene brachial plexus, longitudinal view.

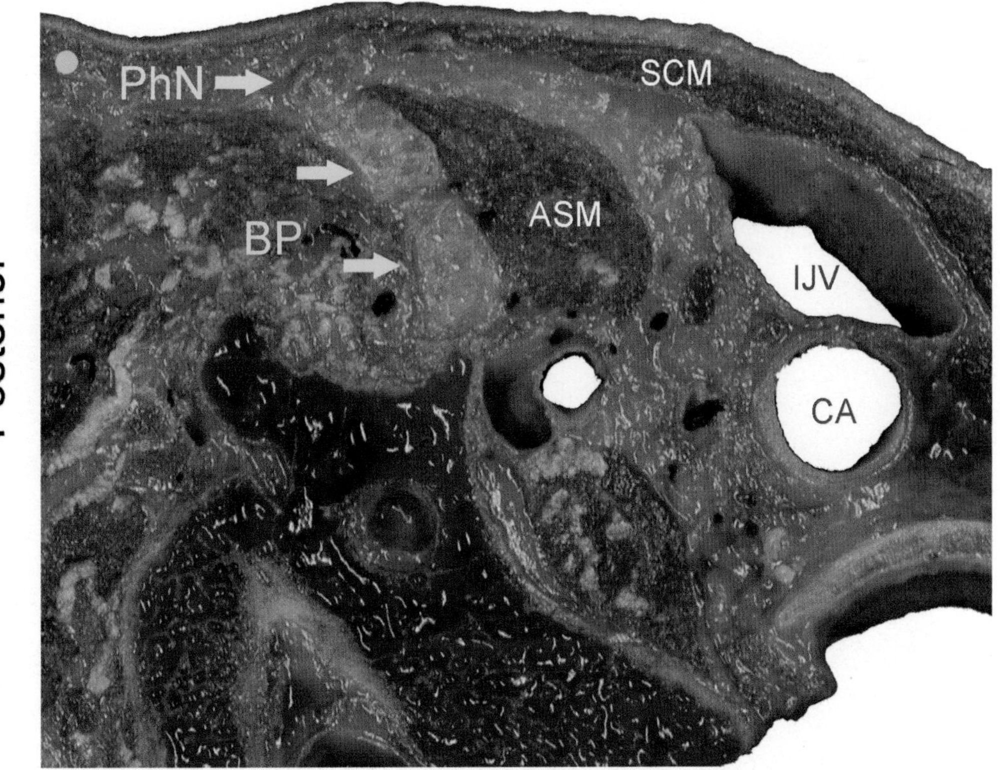


**FIGURE 7.8.2D**

**Abbreviations:** SCM, sternocleidomastoid muscle; ASM, anterior scalene muscle; MSM, middle scalene muscle; TP, transverse process; PhN, Phrenic nerve; IvF, Intervertebral Foramen; VA, vertebral artery.

## Phrenic Nerve at the Interscalene Level

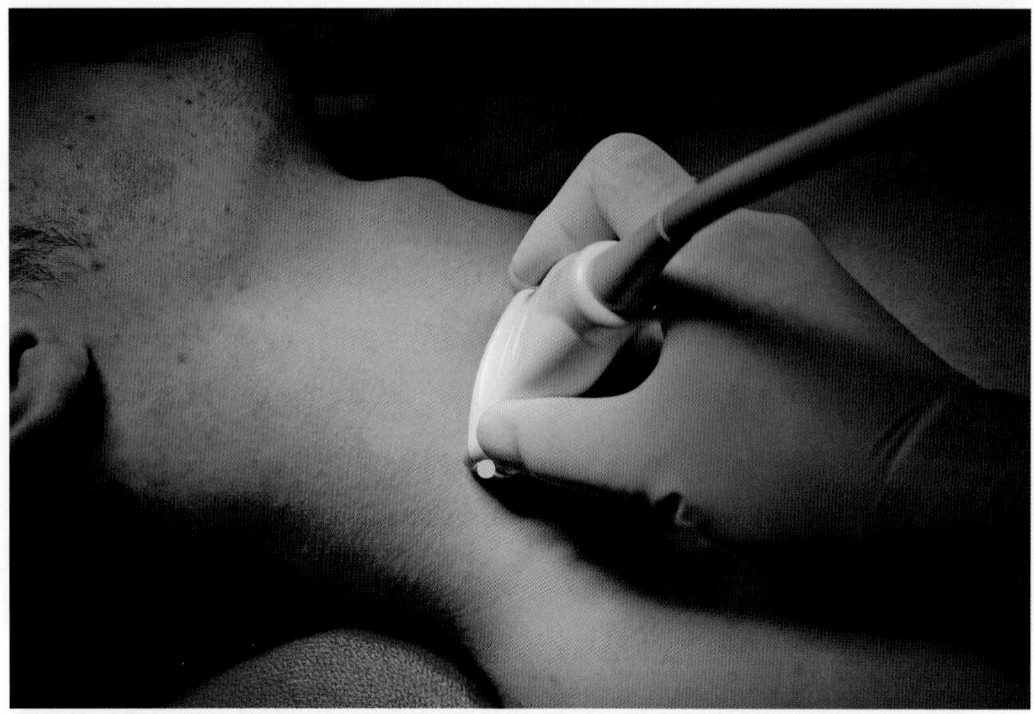

**FIGURE 7.9.1A** Ultrasound transducer position to image the phrenic nerve at the interscalene level.

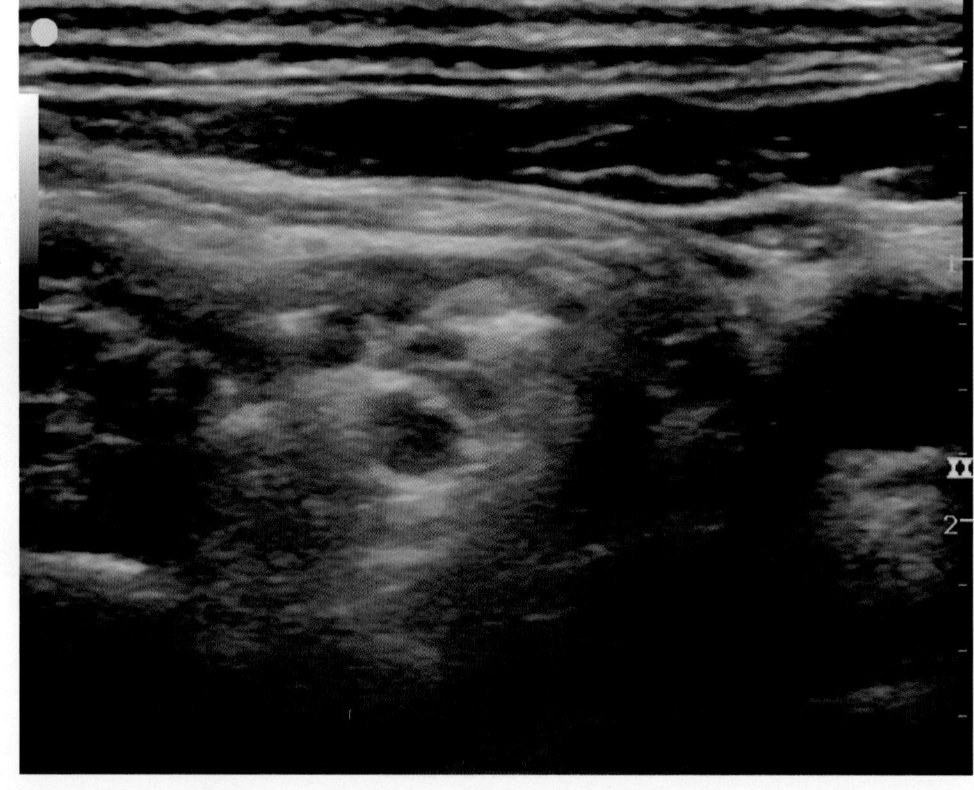


**FIGURE 7.9.1B** Ultrasound image of the phrenic nerve.

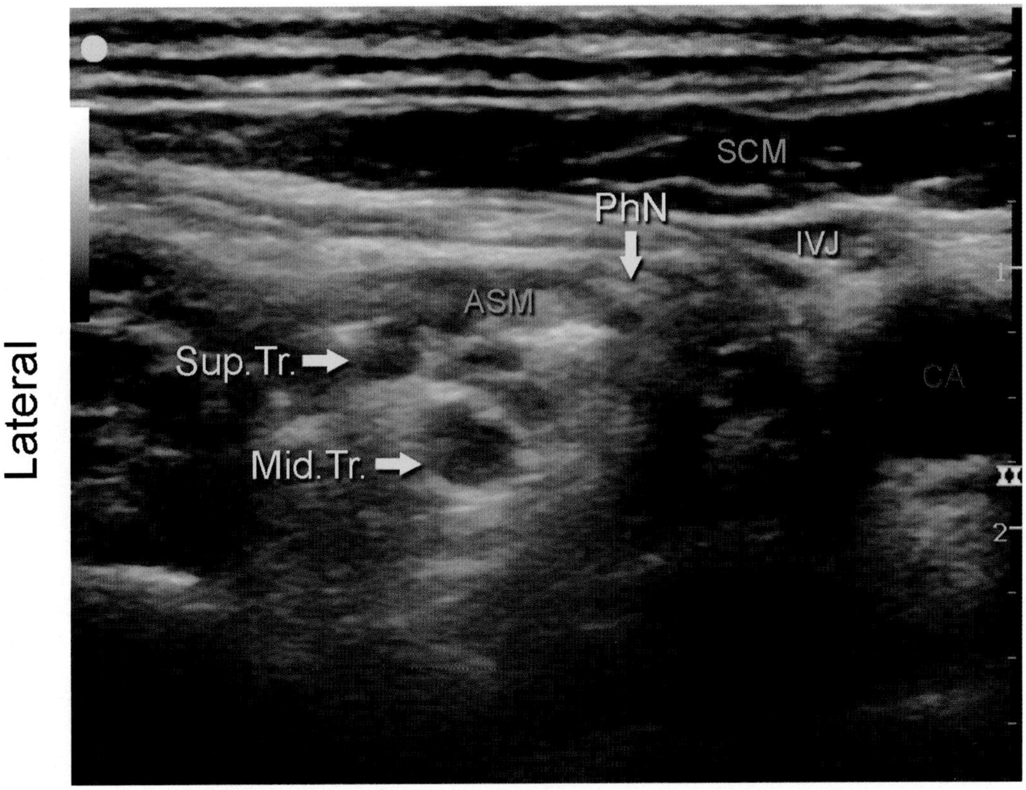

**FIGURE 7.9.1C** Labeled ultrasound image of the phrenic nerve.

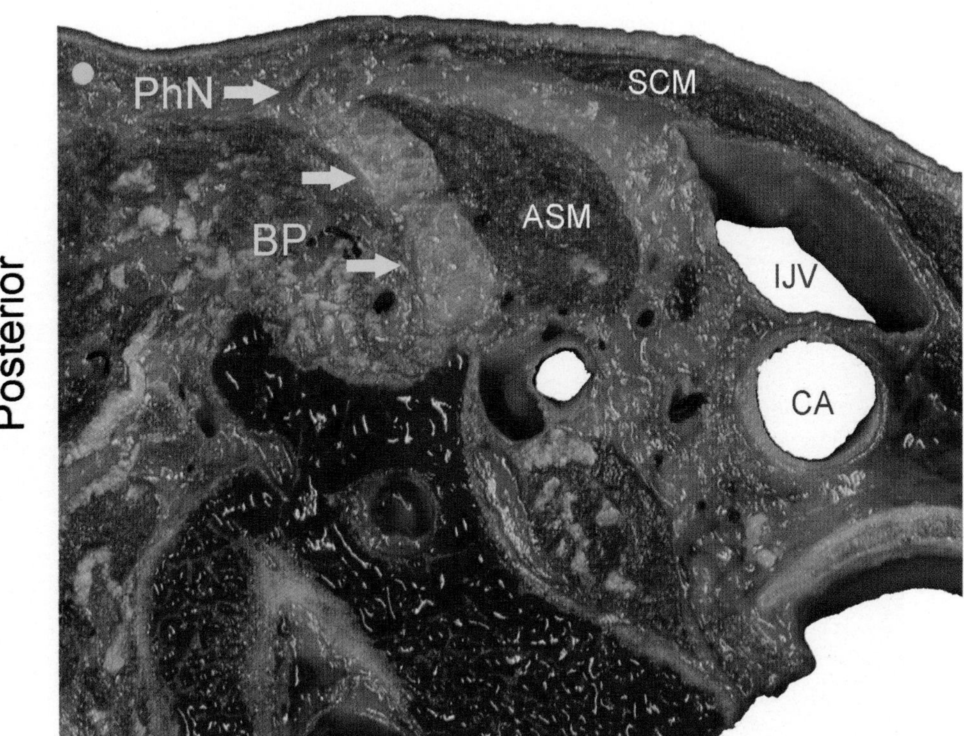


**FIGURE 7.9.1D** Labeled cross-sectional anatomy of the phrenic nerve.

**Abbreviations:** SCM, sternocleidomastoid muscle; IVJ, internal jugular vein; ASM, anterior scalene muscle; CA, carotid artery; PhN, Phrenic nerve; Sup. Tr. , Superior Trunk; Mid. Tr., Middle trunk; BP, Brachial Plexus.

# Accessory Phrenic Nerve

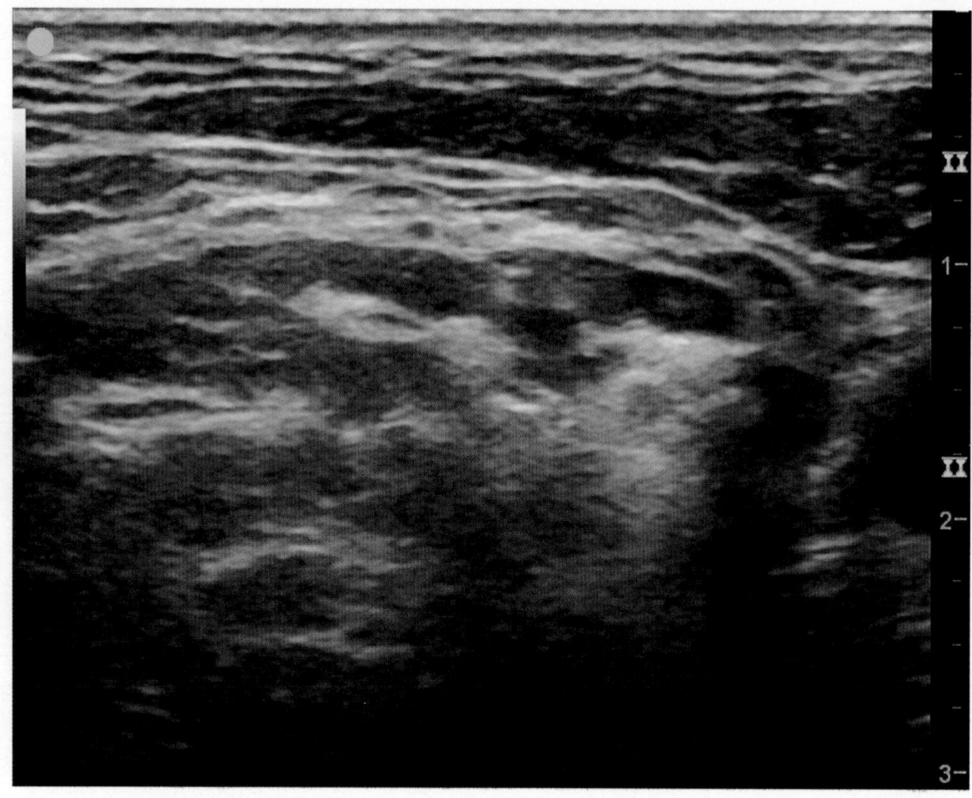


**FIGURE 7.9.2A** Ultrasound image of the accessory phrenic nerve.

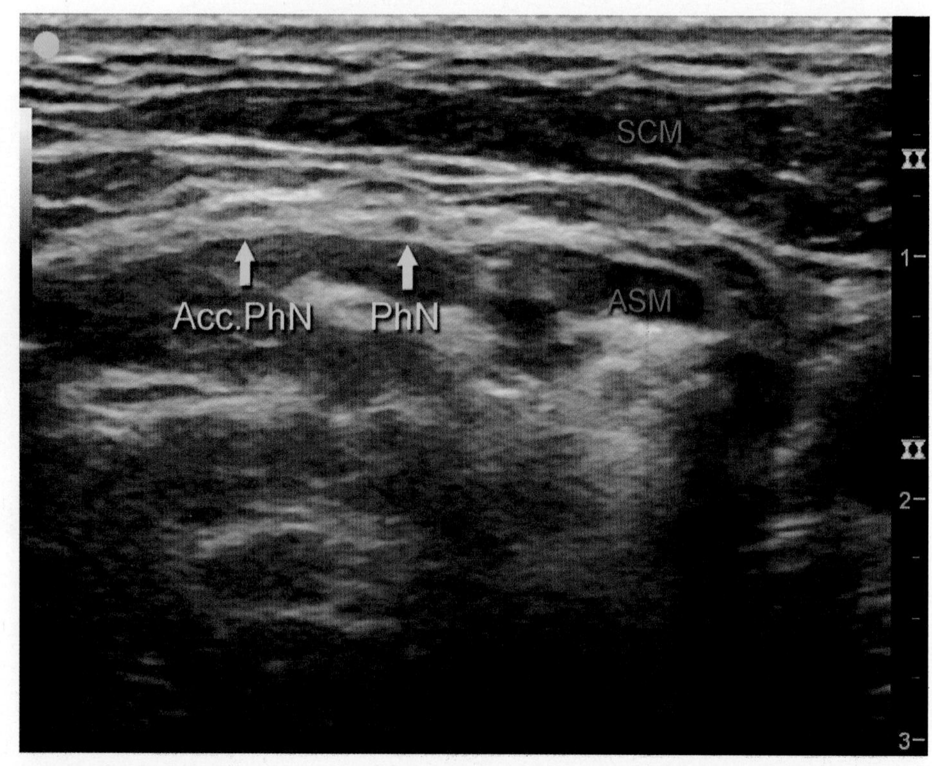


**FIGURE 7.9.2B** Labeled ultrasound image of the accessory phrenic nerve.

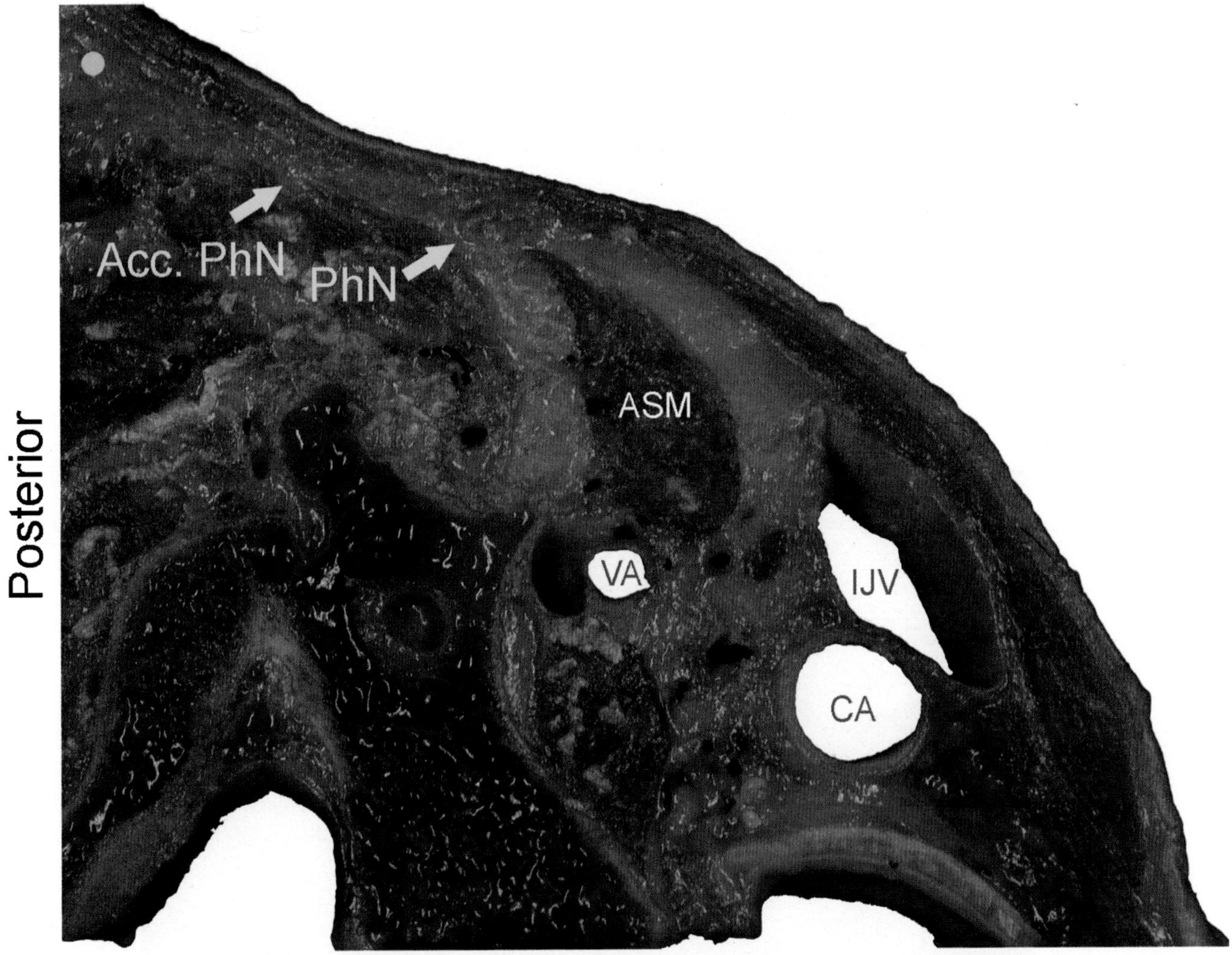

**FIGURE 7.9.2C** Labeled cross-sectional anatomy of the accessory phrenic nerve.

**Abbreviations:** SCM, sternocleidomastoid muscle; IVJ, internal jugular vein; ASM, anterior scalene muscle; CA, carotid artery; PhN, Phrenic nerve; Acc. PhN, Accessory Phrenic Nerve; VA, vertebral artery.

# Ansa Cervicalis and Phrenic Nerve, Transverse View

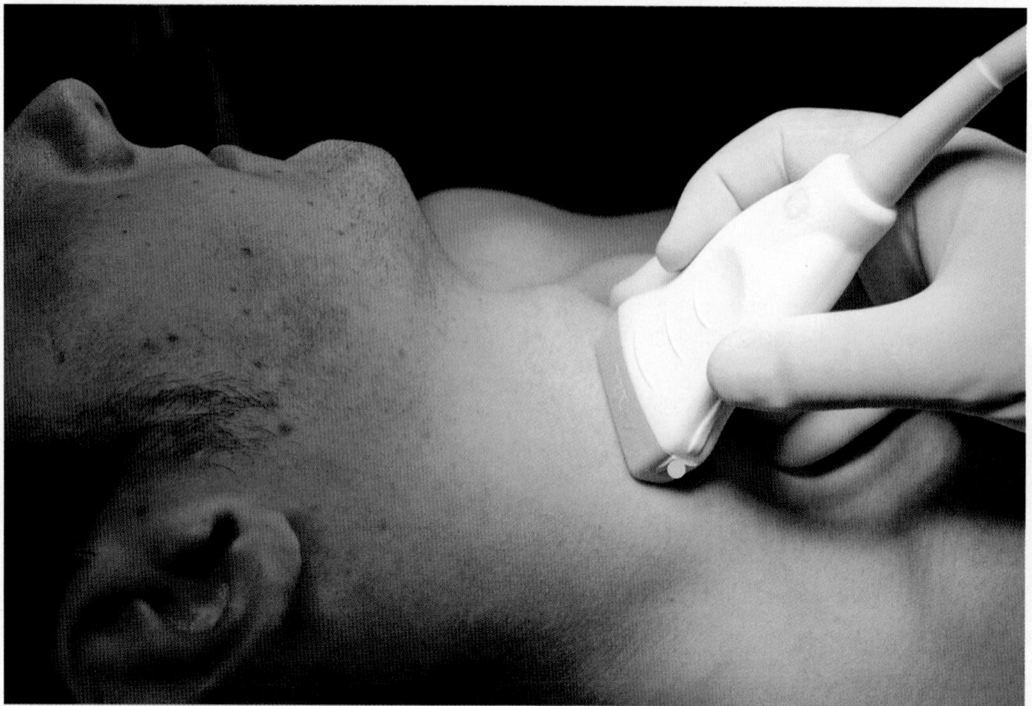

**FIGURE 7.10.1A** Ultrasound transducer position to image the ansa cervicalis and phrenic nerve, transverse view.

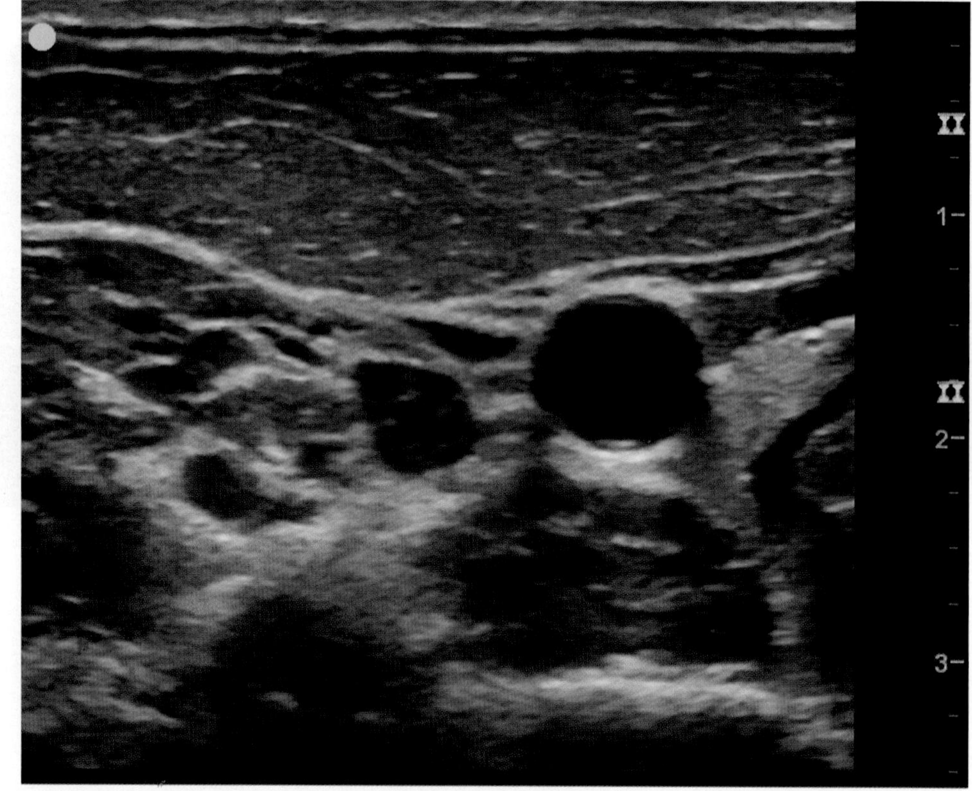


**7.10.1B** Ultrasound image of the ansa cervicalis and phrenic nerve, transverse view.

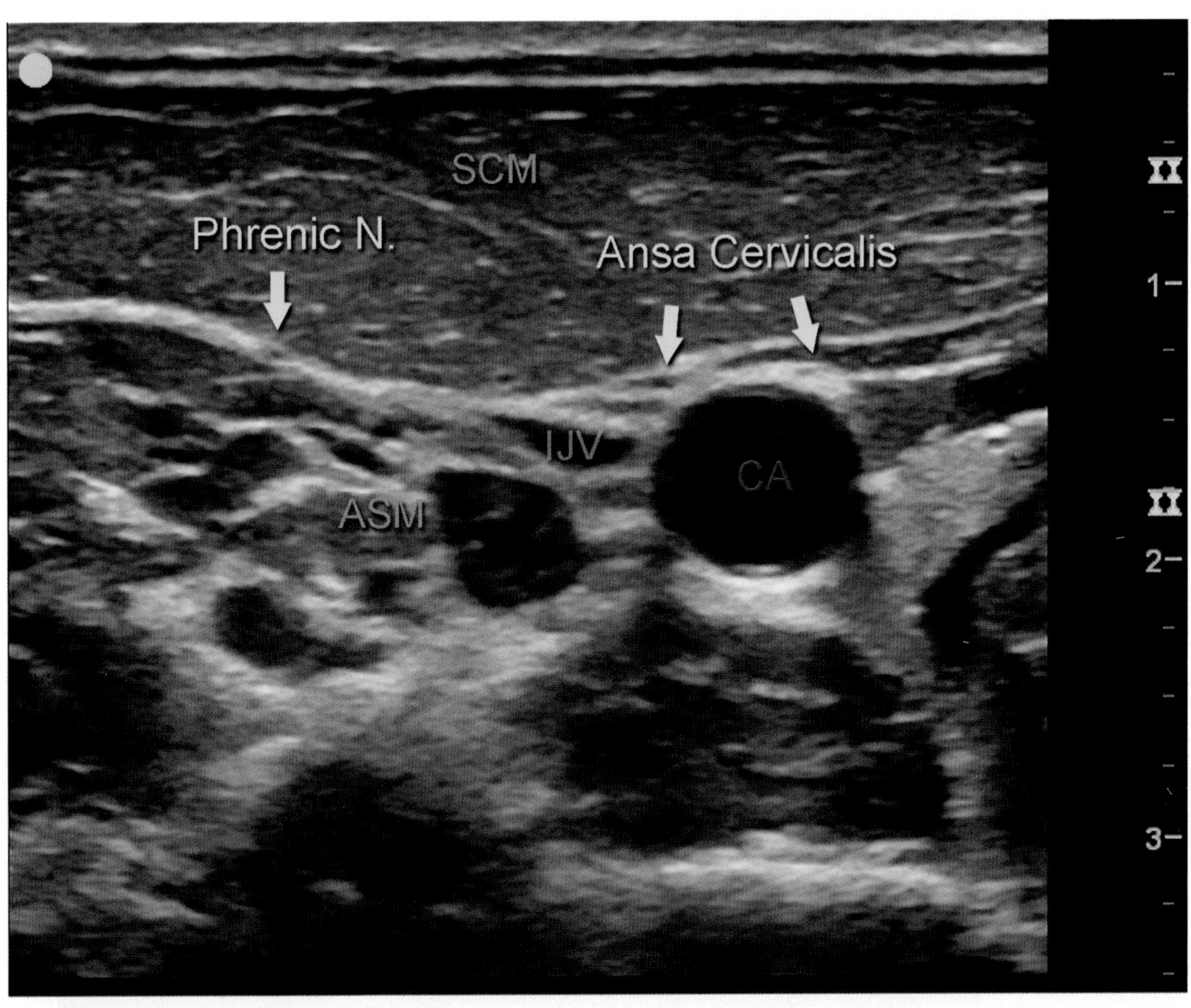


**FIGURE 7.10.1C** Labeled ultrasound image of the ansa cervicalis and phrenic nerve, transverse view.

**Abbreviations:** SCM, sternocleidomastoid muscle; IVJ, internal jugular vein; ASM, anterior scalene muscle; CA, carotid artery.

## Vagus Nerve

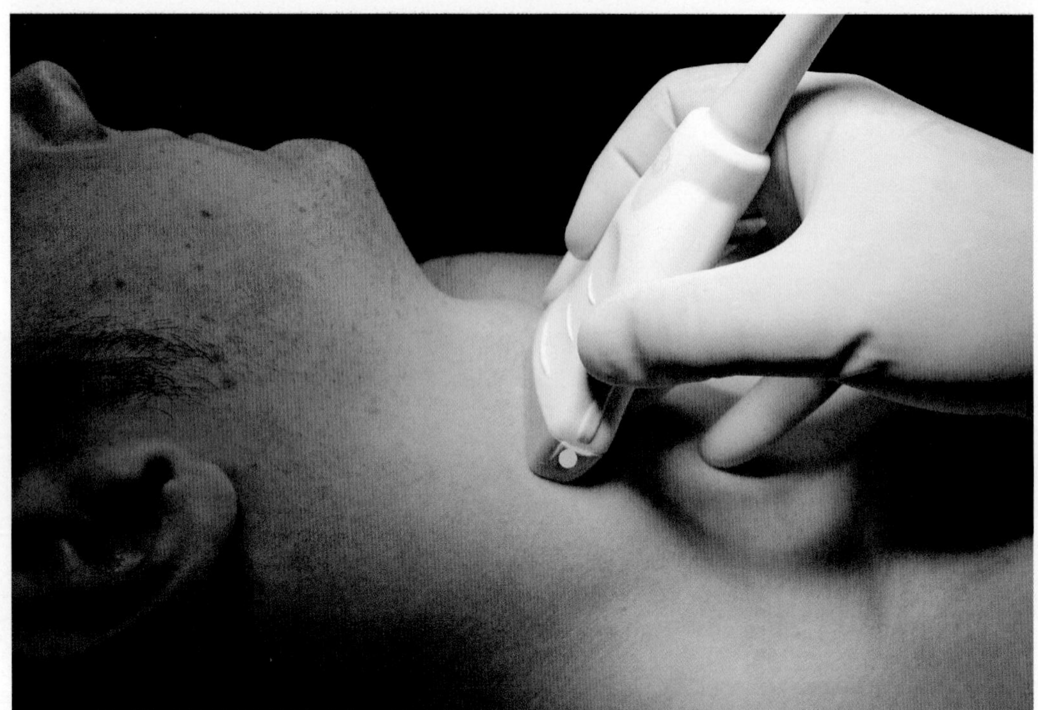

**FIGURE 7.11.1A** Ultrasound transducer position to image the vagus nerve.

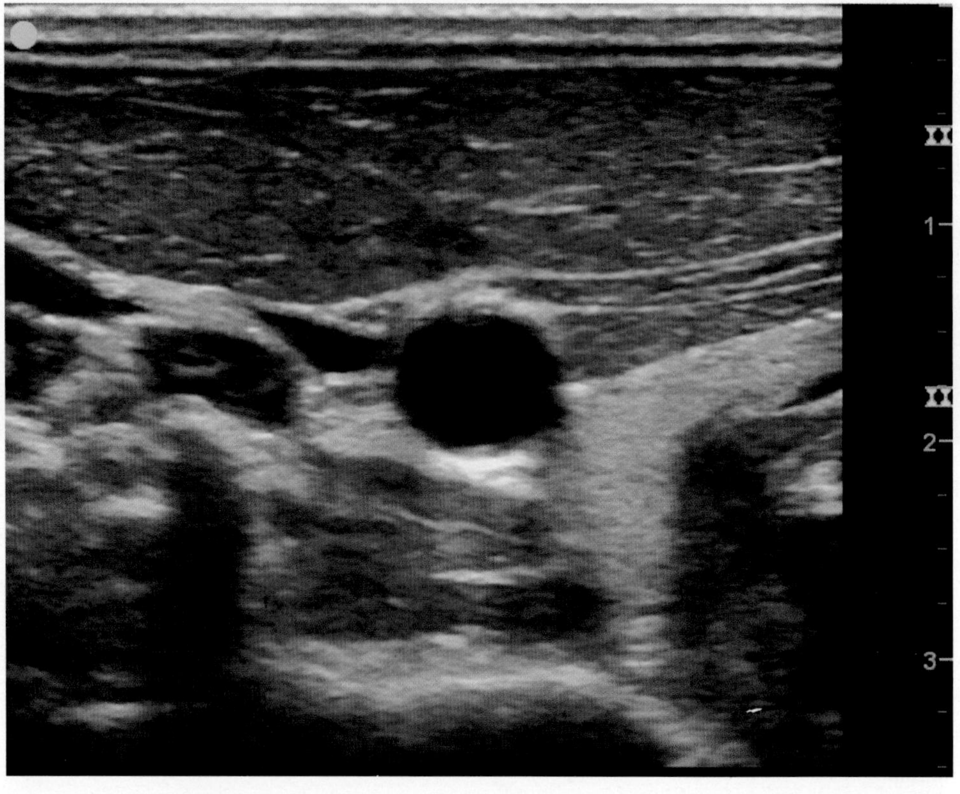


**FIGURE 7.11.1B** Ultrasound image of the vagus nerve.

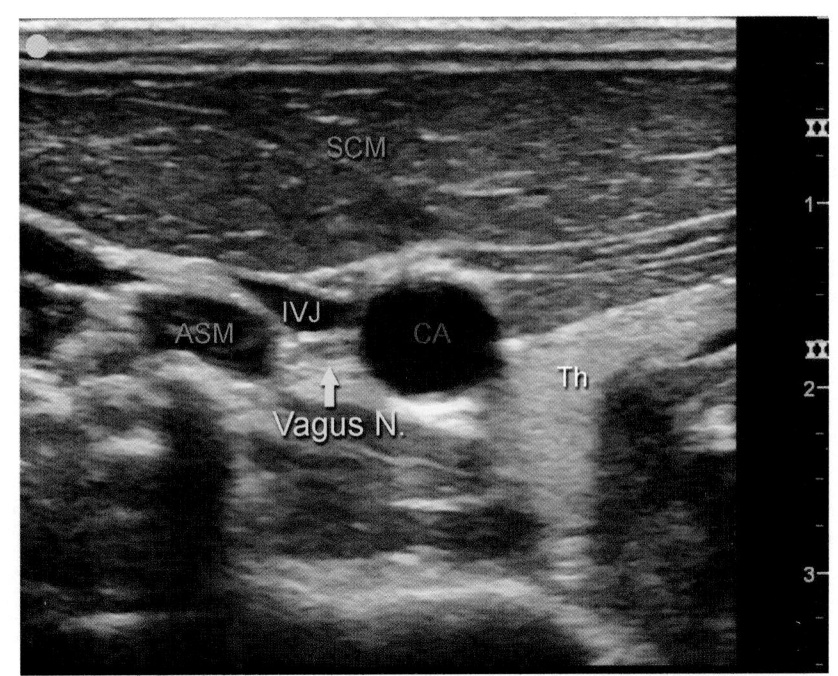


**FIGURE 7.11.1C** Labeled ultrasound image of the vagus nerve.

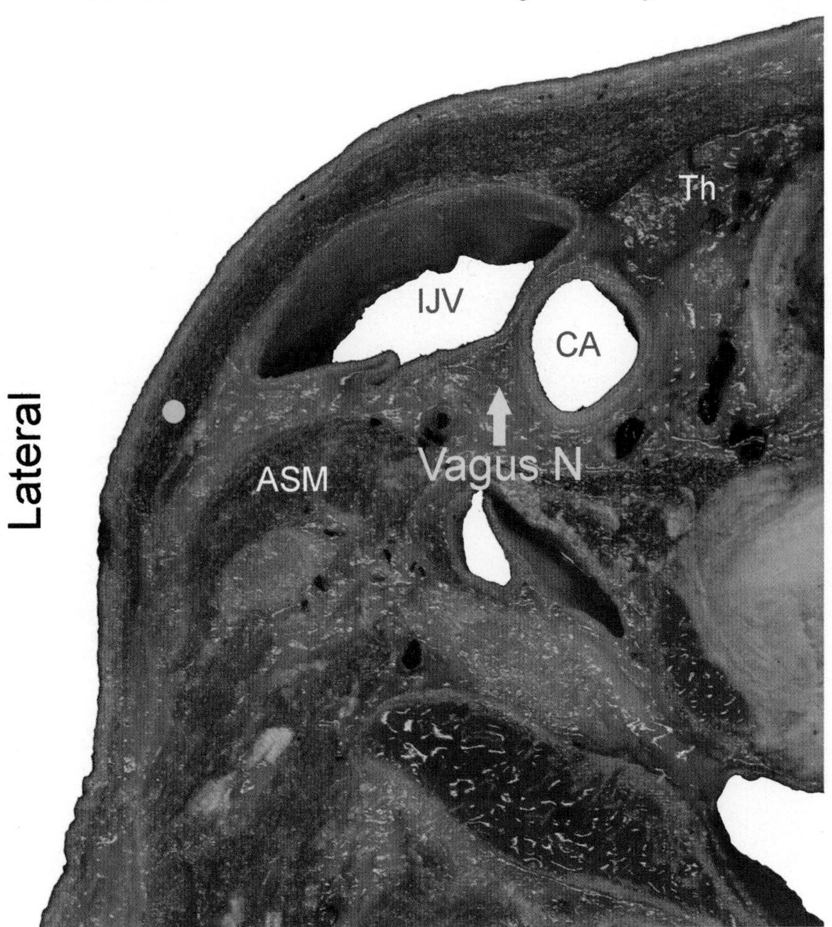


**FIGURE 7.11.1D** Labeled cross-sectional anatomy of the vagus nerve.

**Abbreviations:** SCM, sternocleidomastoid muscle; IVJ, internal jugular vein; ASM, anterior scalene muscle; CA, carotid artery; Th, Thyroid.

## Stellate Ganglion

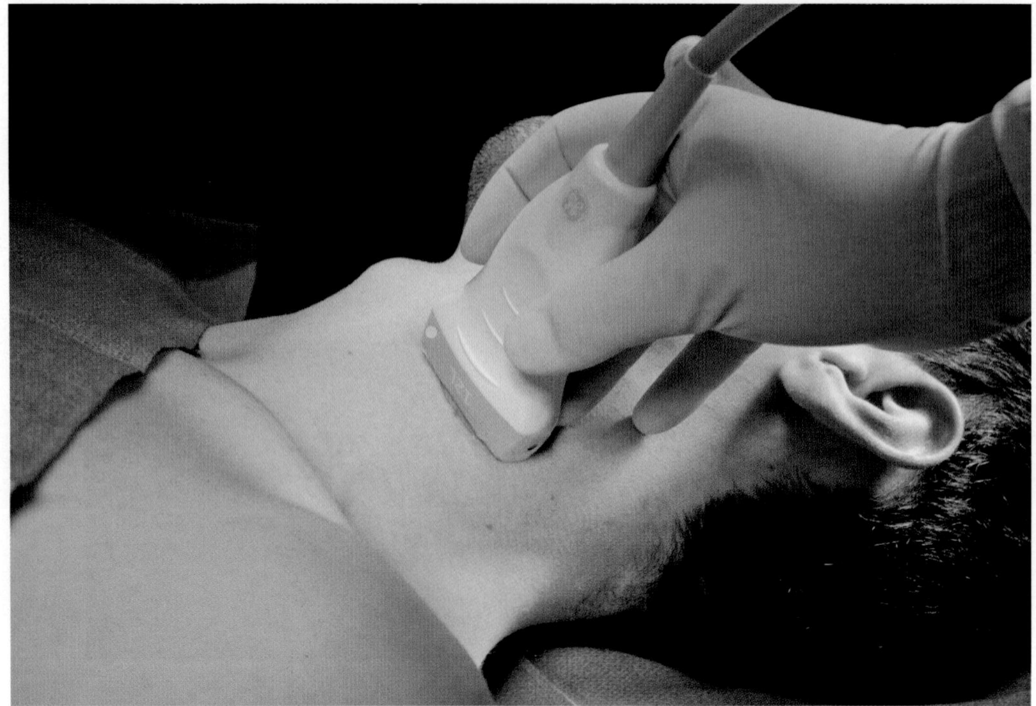

**FIGURE 7.12.1A** Ultrasound transducer position to image the stellate ganglion.

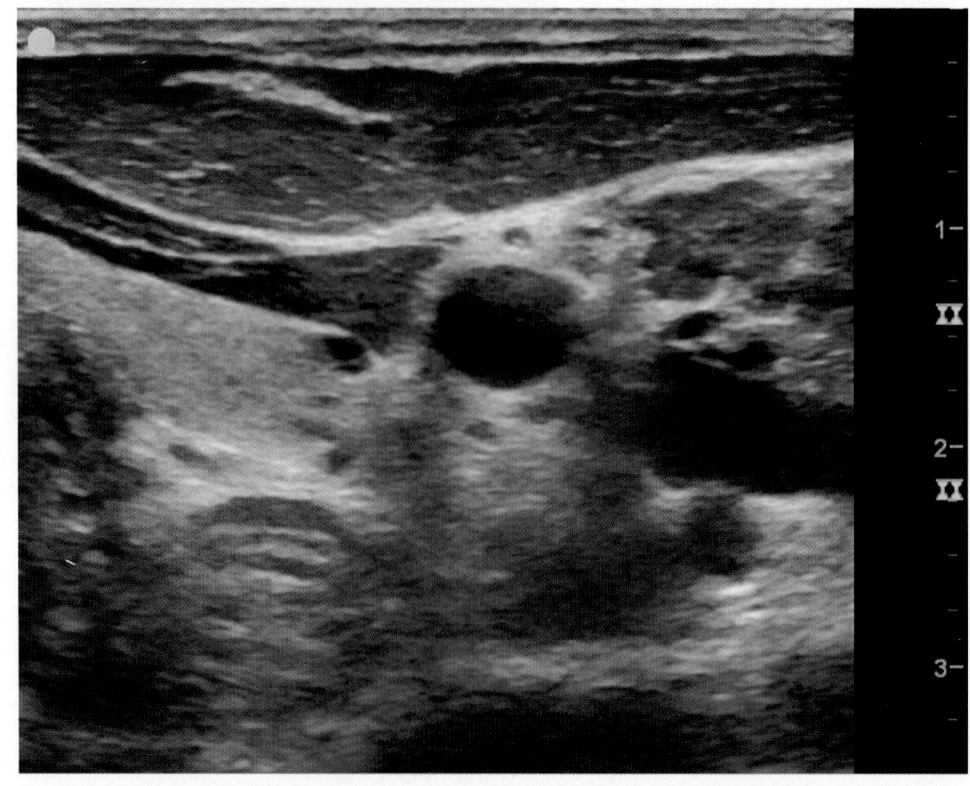


**FIGURE 7.12.1B** Ultrasound image of the stellate ganglion.

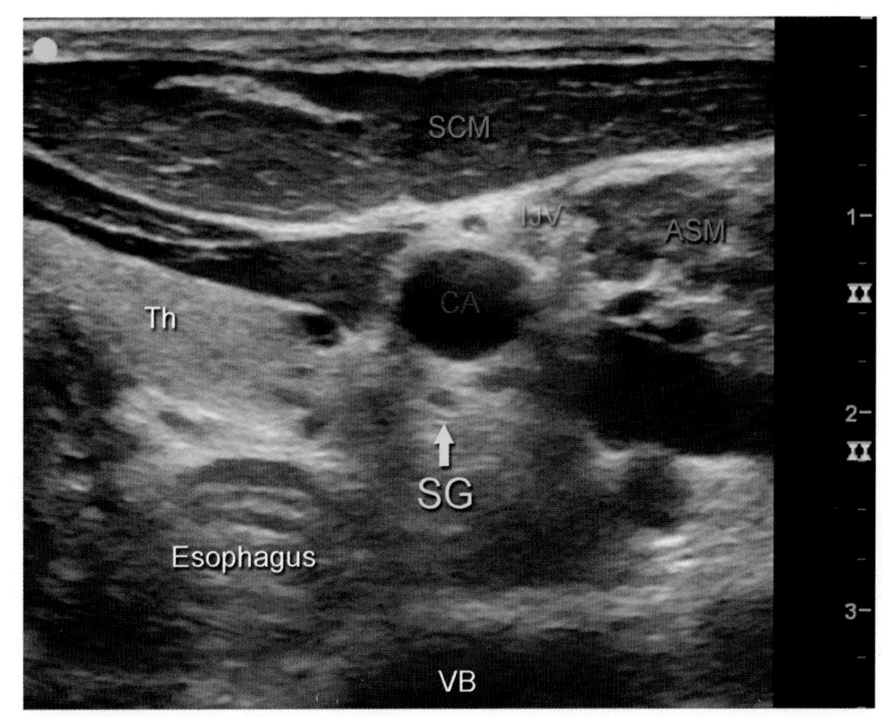


**FIGURE 7.12.1C** Labeled Ultrasound image of the stellate ganglion.

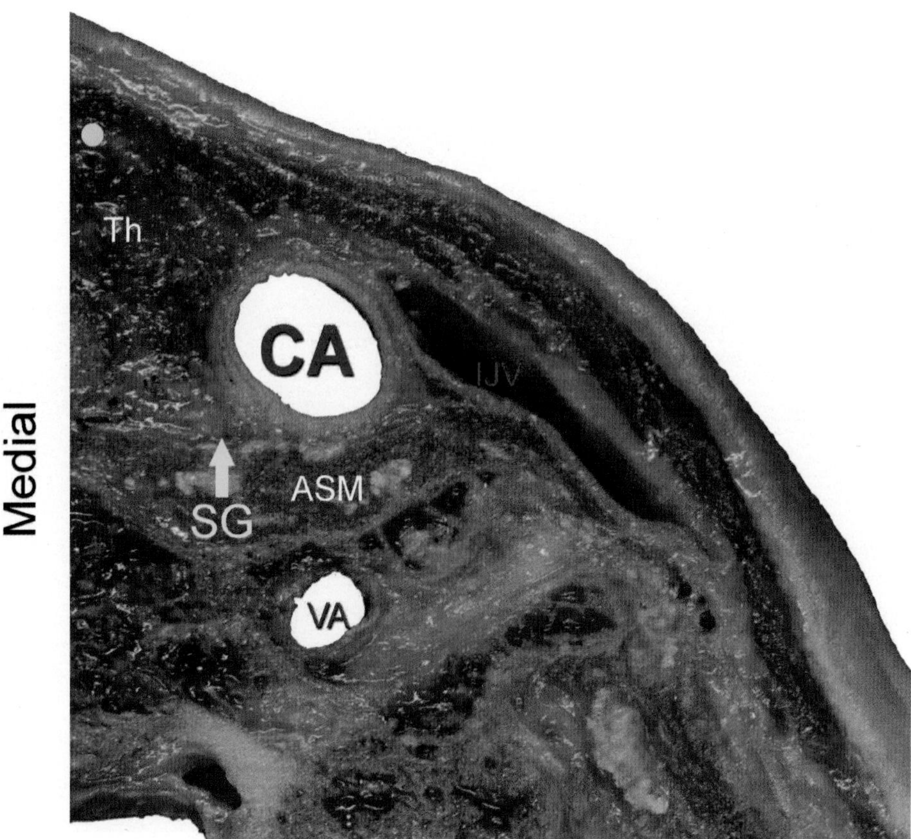


**FIGURE 7.12.1D** Labeled cross-sectional anatomy of the stellate ganglion.

**Abbreviations:** SCM, sternocleidomastoid muscle; IVJ, internal jugular vein; ASM, anterior scalene muscle; CA, carotid artery; VA, vertebral artery; SG, Stellate Ganglion; Th, Thyroid; VB, Vertebral body.

## Vertebral Artery, Transverse View

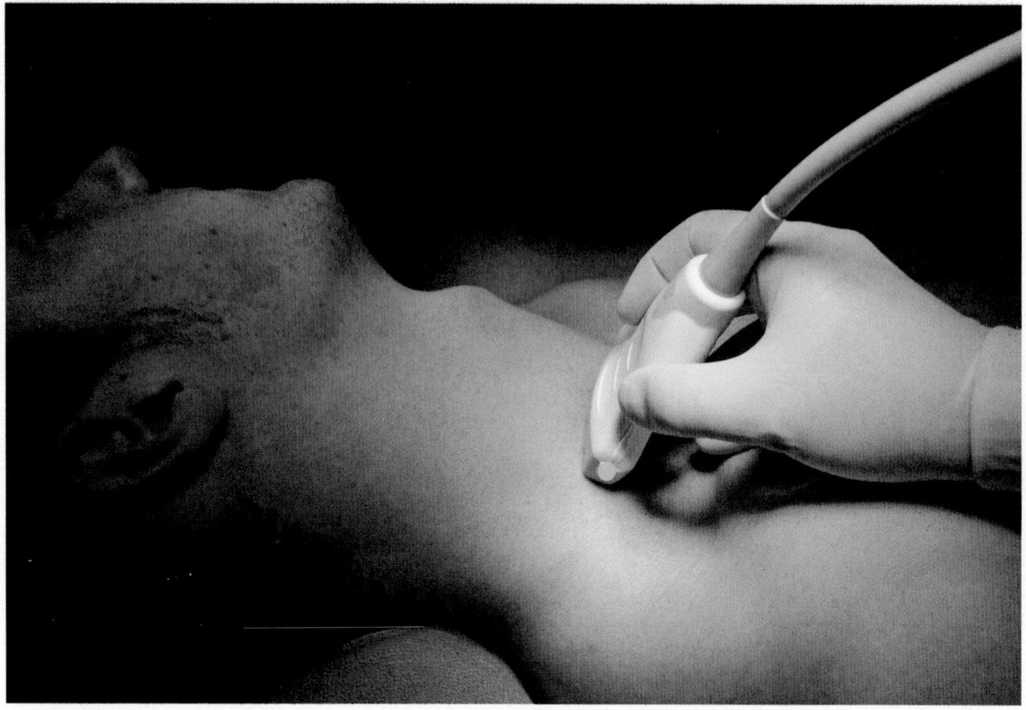

**FIGURE 7.13.1A** Ultrasound transducer position to image the vertebral artery, transverse view.

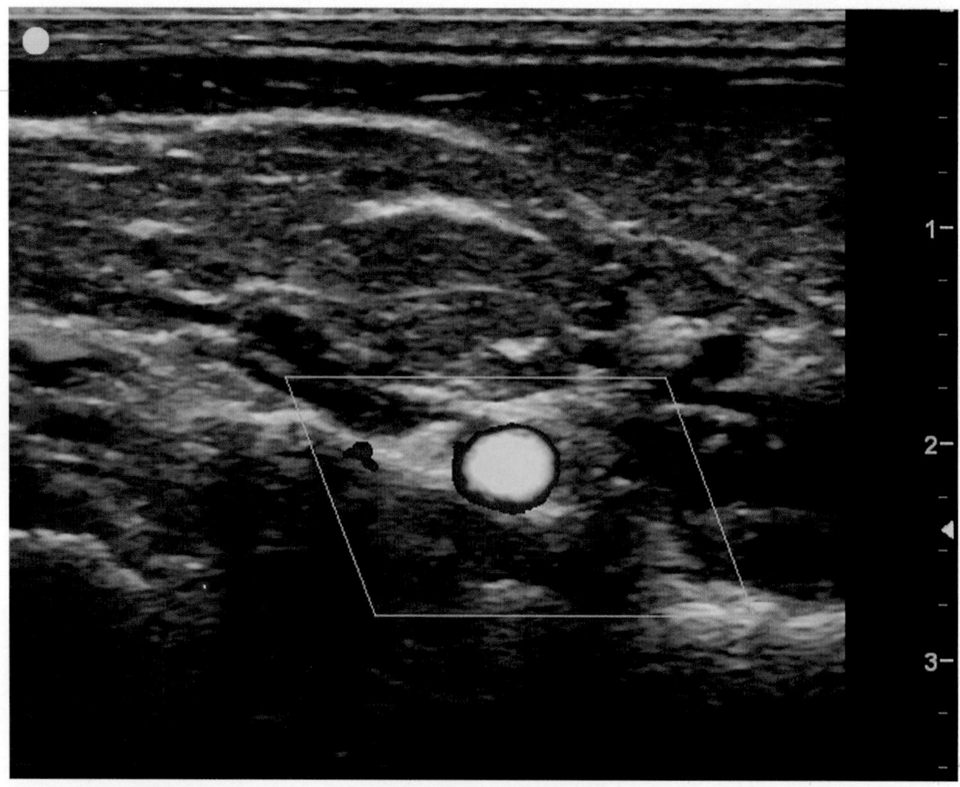


**FIGURE 7.13.1B** Ultrasound image of the vertebral artery, transverse view.

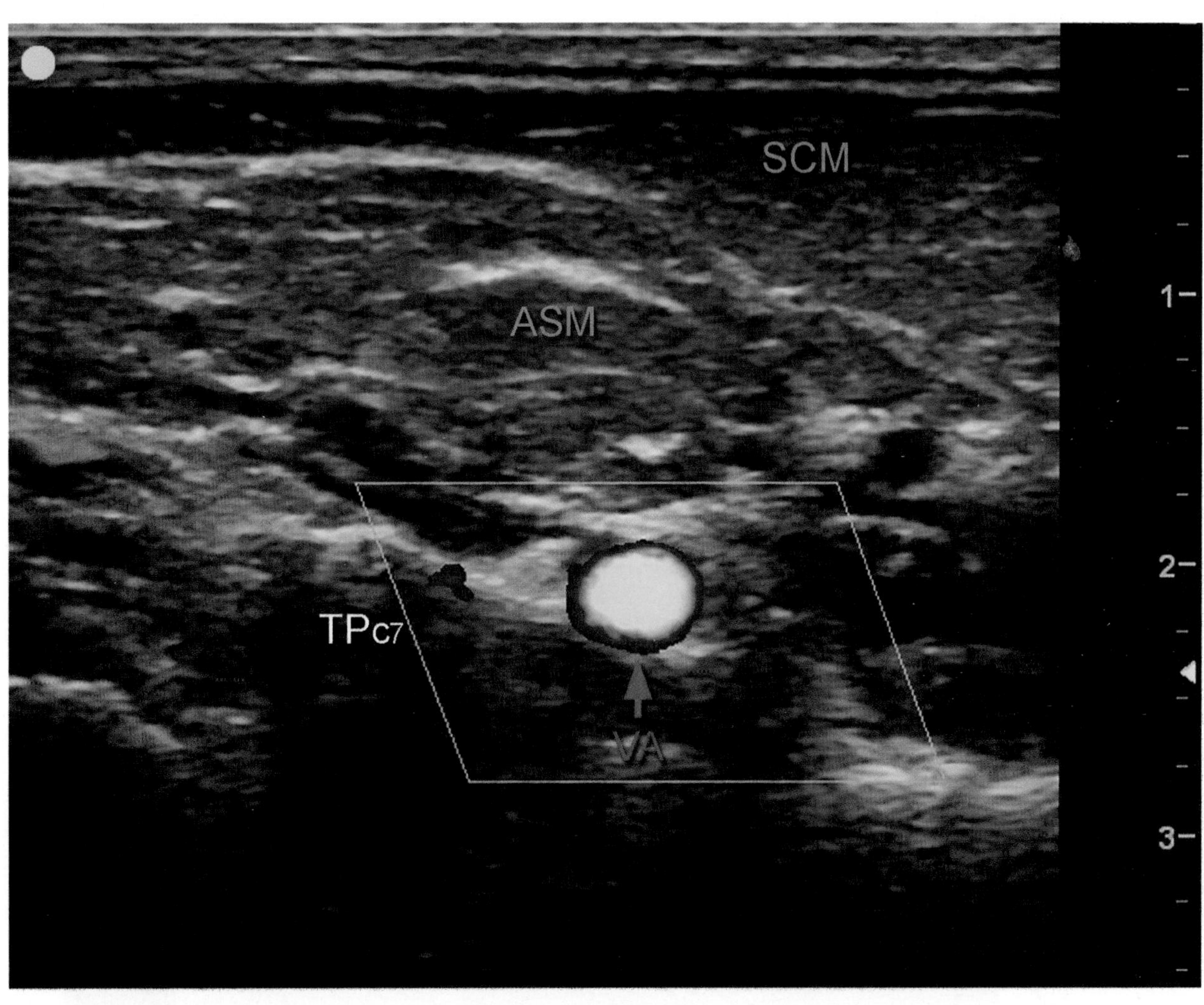


**FIGURE 7.13.1C** Labeled ultrasound image of the vertebral artery and muscles, transverse view.

**Abbreviations:** SCM, sternocleidomastoid muscle; ASM, anterior scalene muscle; VA, vertebral artery; TP, transverse process.

# Vertebral Artery, Longitudinal View

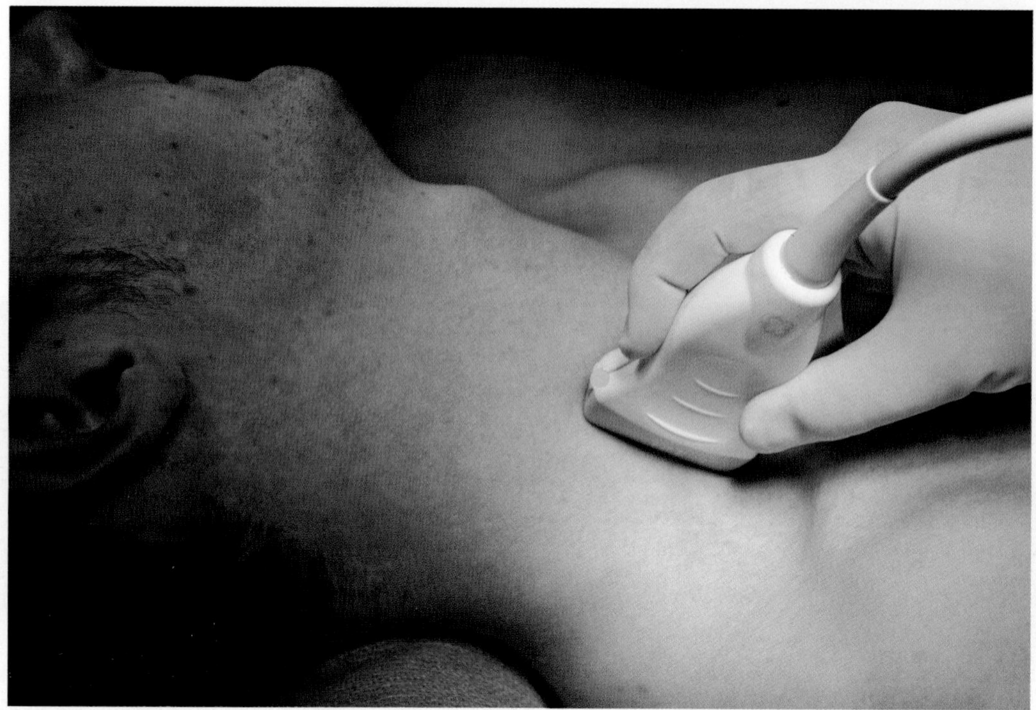

**FIGURE 7.13.2A** Ultrasound transducer position to image the vertebral artery, longitudinal view.

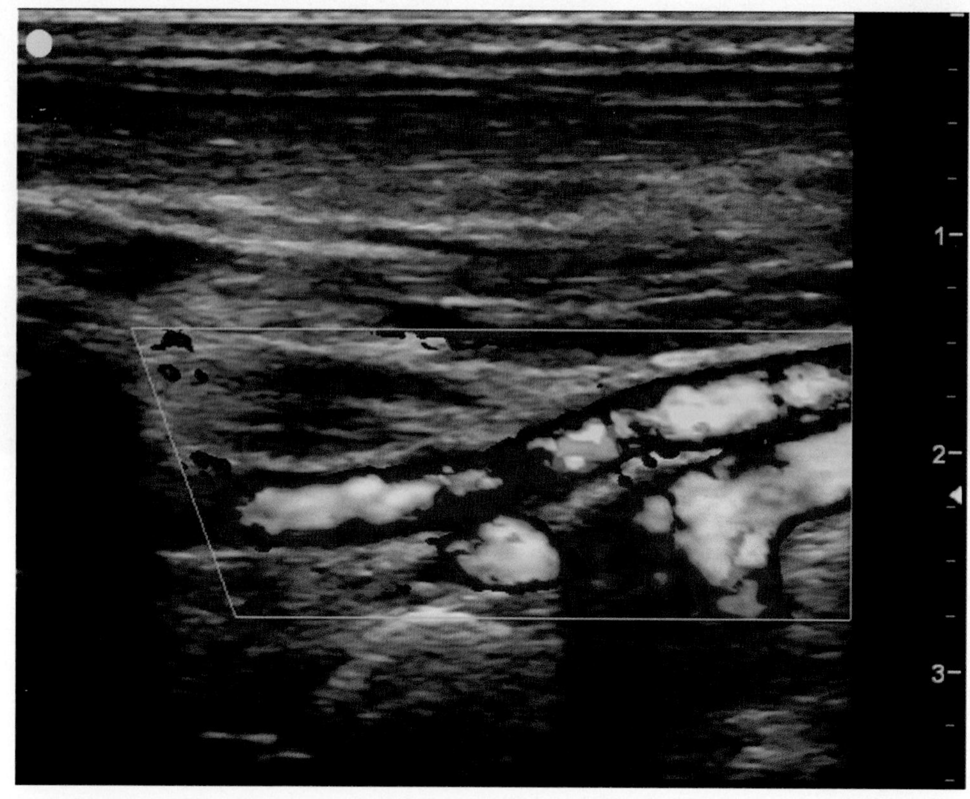


**FIGURE 7.13.2B** Ultrasound image of the vertebral artery, longitudinal view.

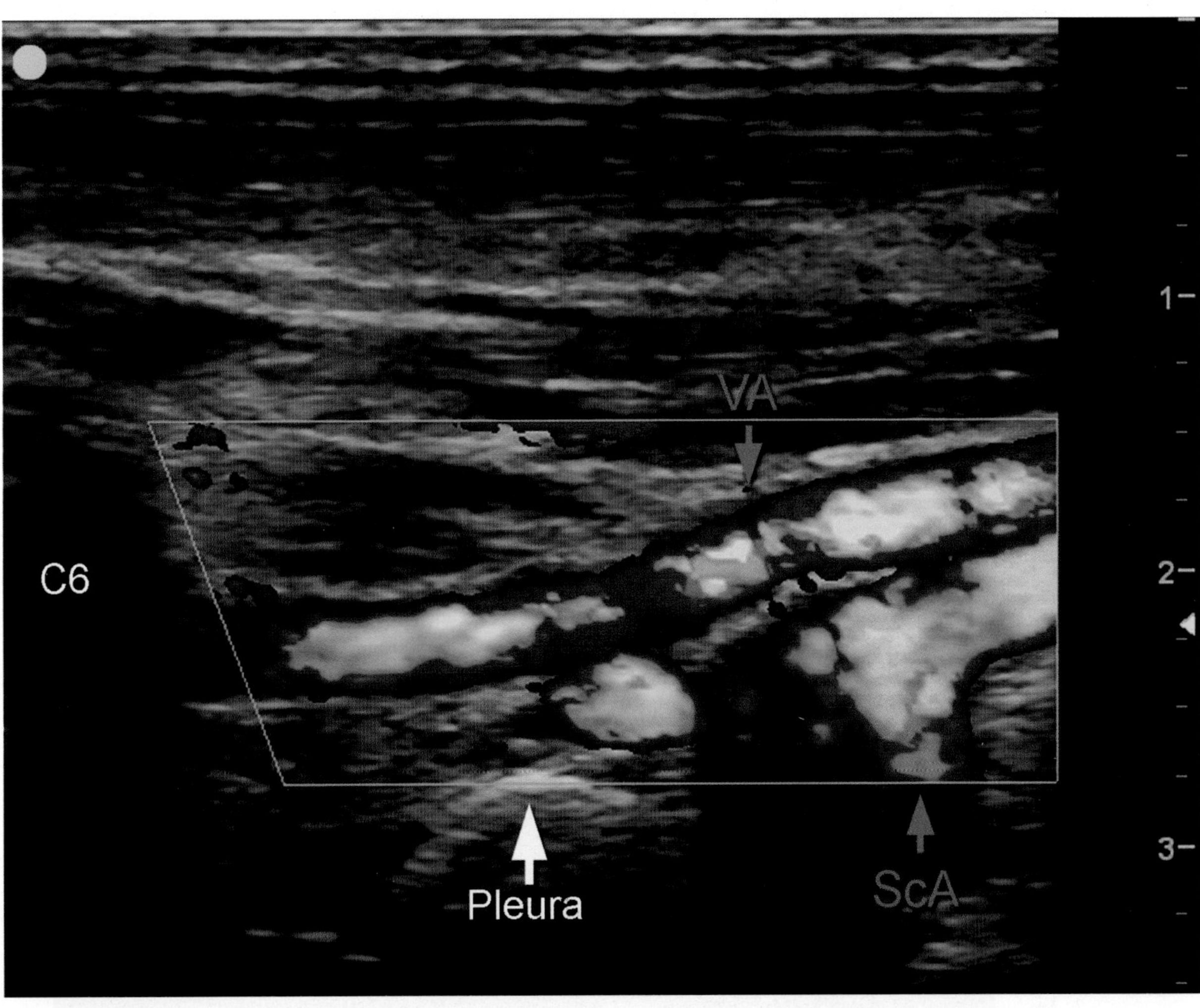


**FIGURE 7.13.2C** Labeled ultrasound image of the vertebral artery, longitudinal view.

**Abbreviations:** VA, vertebral artery; ScA, Subclavian Artery.

## Supraclavicular Brachial Plexus

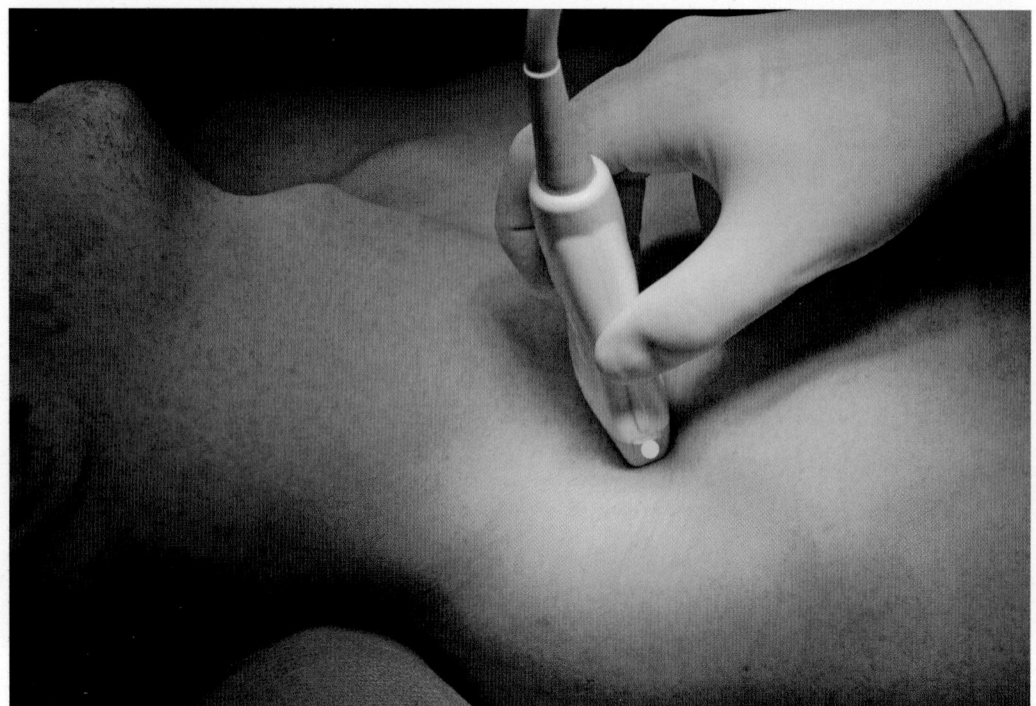

**FIGURE 7.14.1A** Ultrasound transducer position to image the supraclavicular brachial plexus.

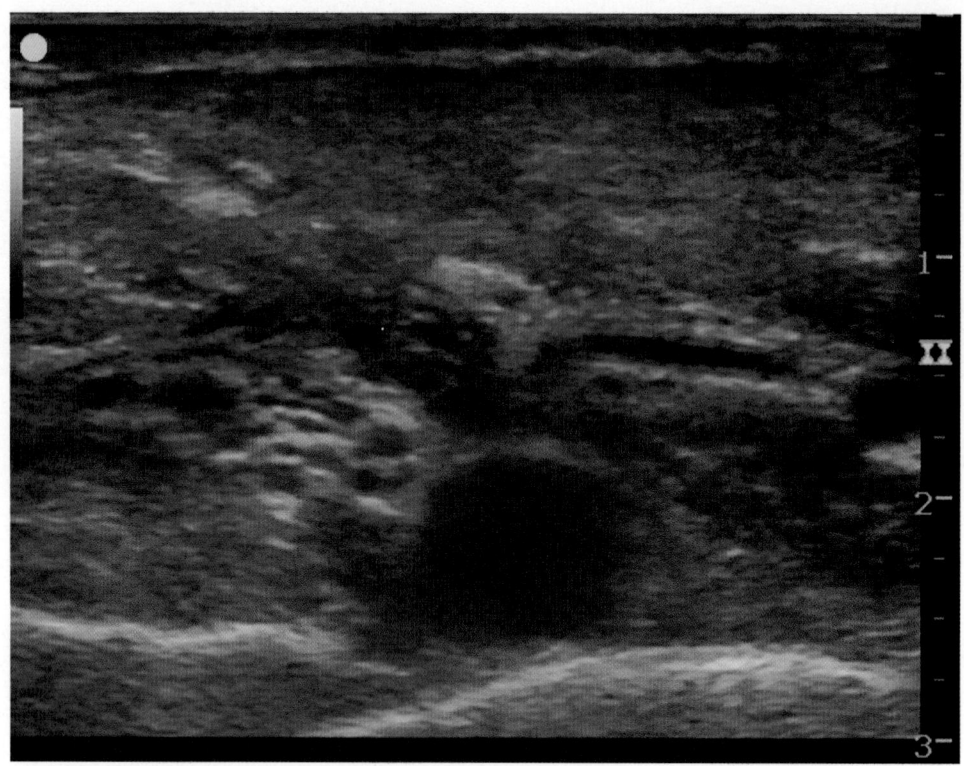


**FIGURE 7.14.1B** Ultrasound image of the supraclavicular brachial plexus.

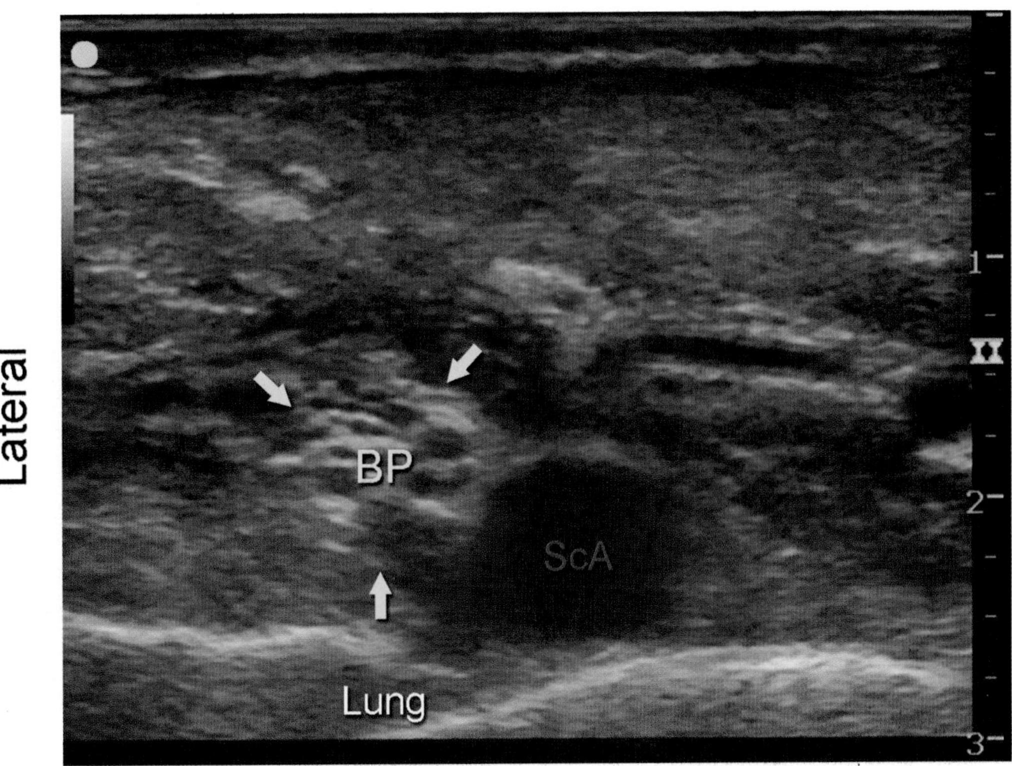


**FIGURE 7.14.1C** Labeled ultrasound image of the supraclavicular brachial plexus.

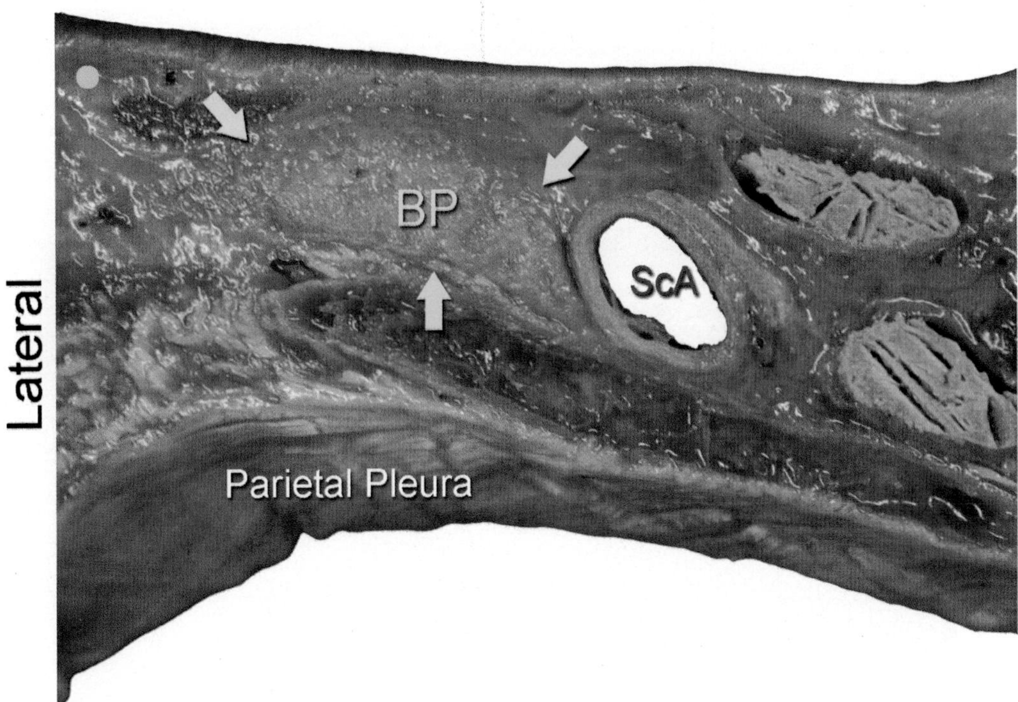


**FIGURE 7.14.1D** Labeled cross-sectional anatomy of the supraclavicular brachial plexus.

**Abbreviations:** BP, Brachial Plexus; ScA, Subclavian Artery.

## Subclavian Artery, Dorsal Scapular Artery, and Brachial Plexus

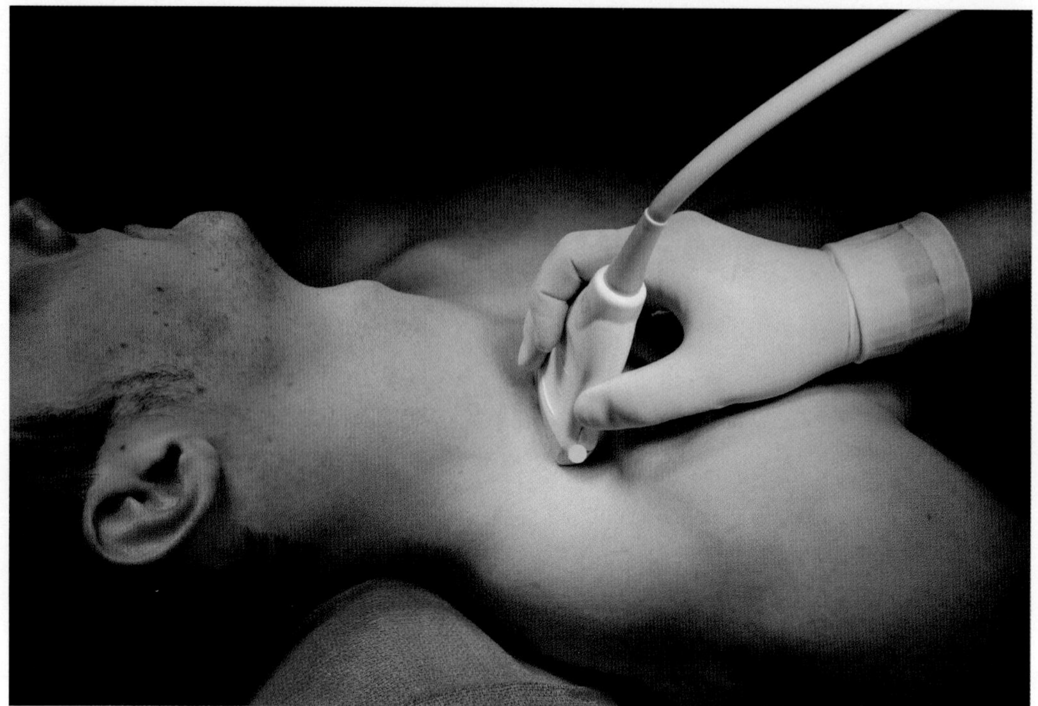

**FIGURE 7.14.2A** Ultrasound transducer position to image the subclavian artery.

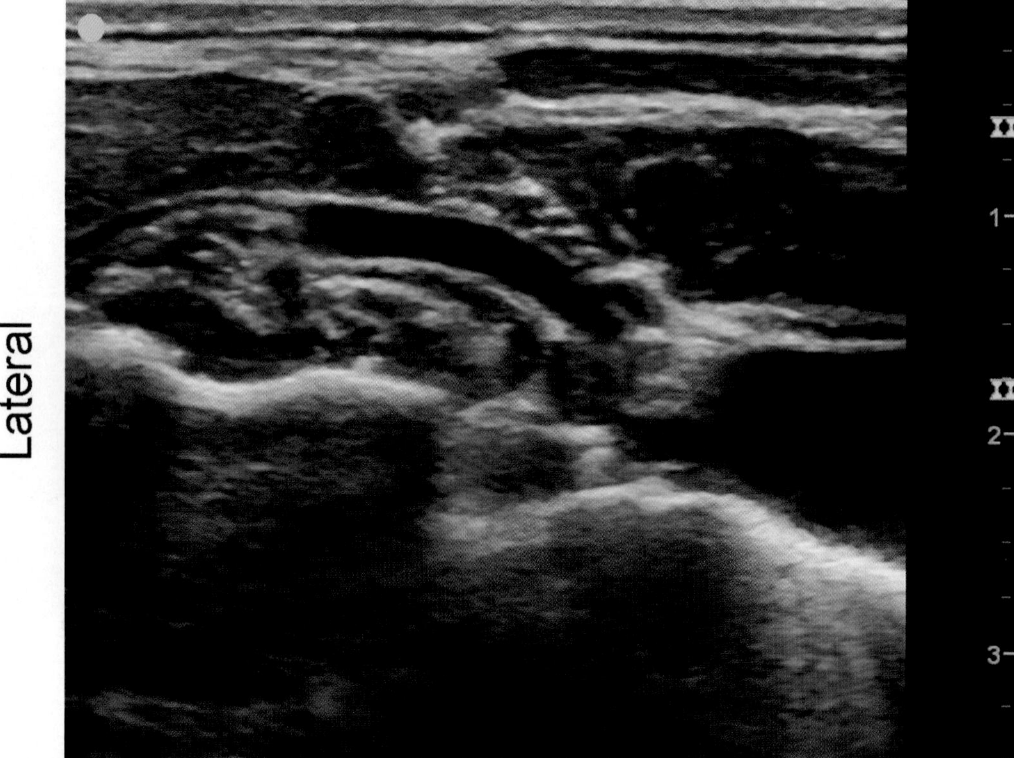


**FIGURE 7.14.2B** Ultrasound image of the subclavian artery and supraclavicular brachial plexus.

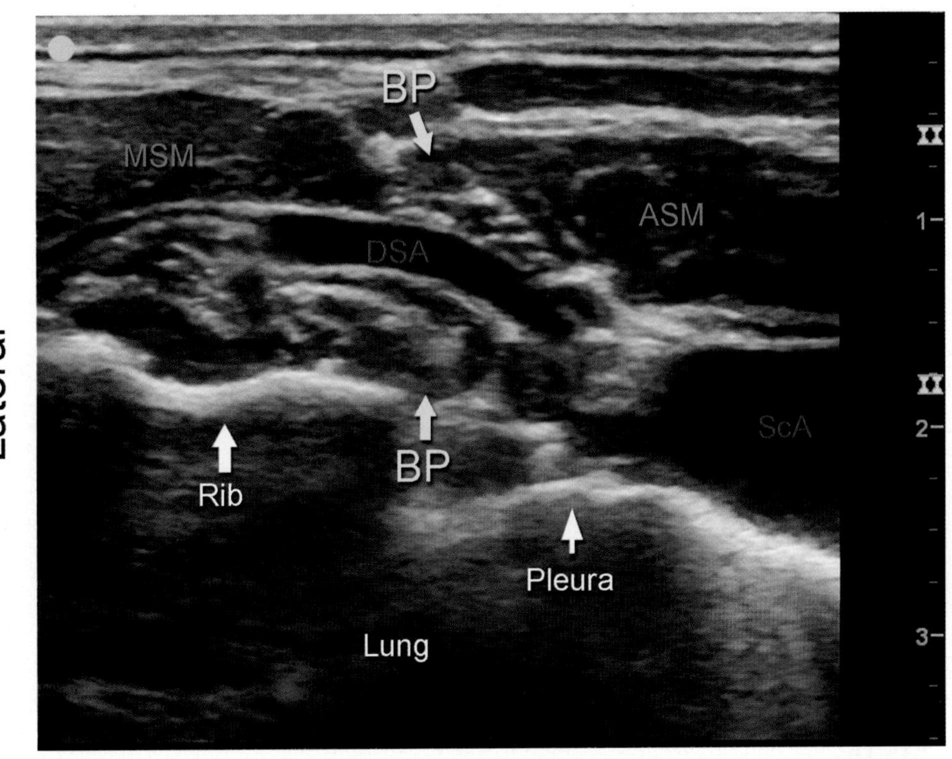


**FIGURE 7.14.2C** Labeled ultrasound image of the dorsal scapular artery and supraclavicular brachial plexus.

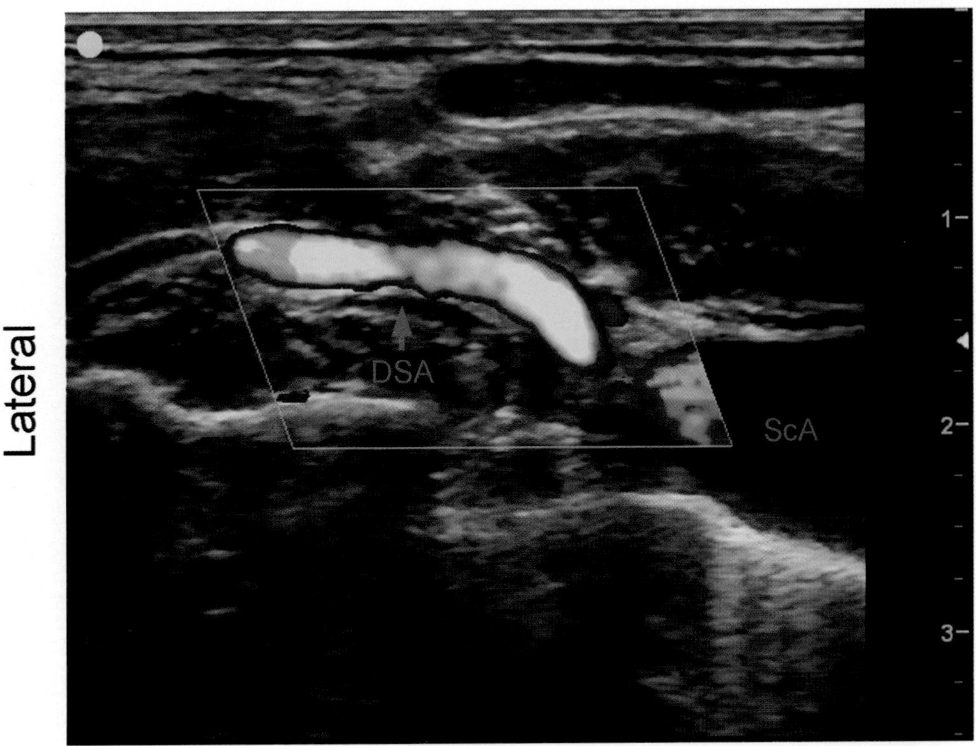


**FIGURE 7.14.2D** Labeled ultrasound image of the subclavian artery and dorsal scapular artery.

**Abbreviations:** BP, Brachial Plexus; ASM, Anterior Scalene Muscle; MSM, Middle Scalene Muscle; ScA, Subclavian Artery, DSA, Dorsal Scapular Artery.

## Infraclavicular Brachial Plexus, Transverse View

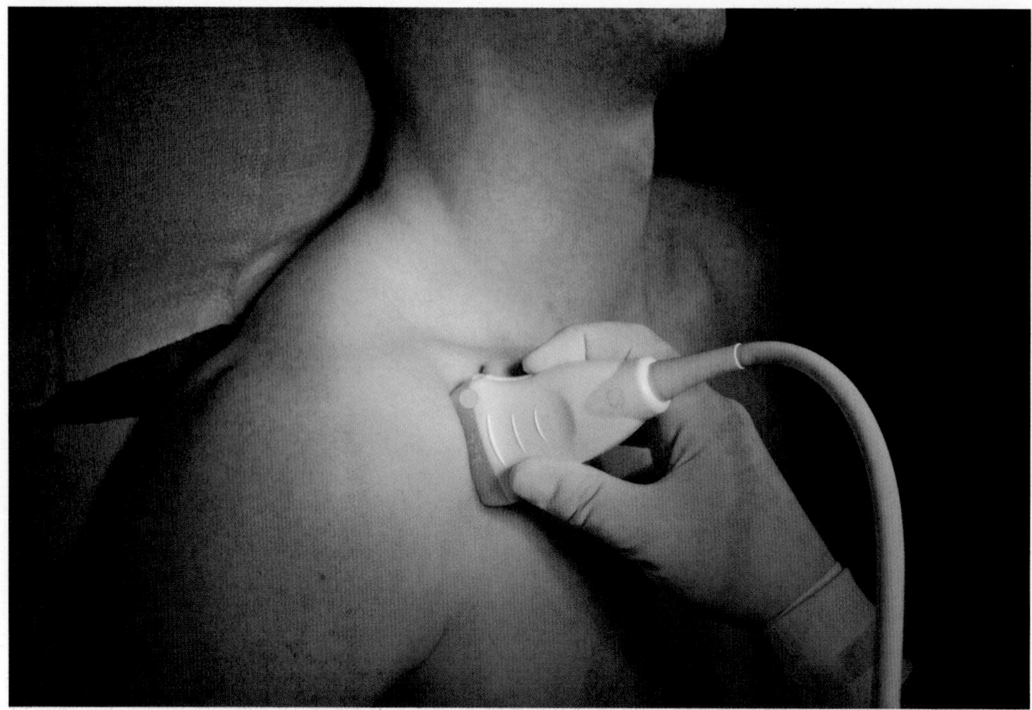

**FIGURE 7.15.1A** Ultrasound transducer position to image the infraclavicular brachial plexus, transverse view.

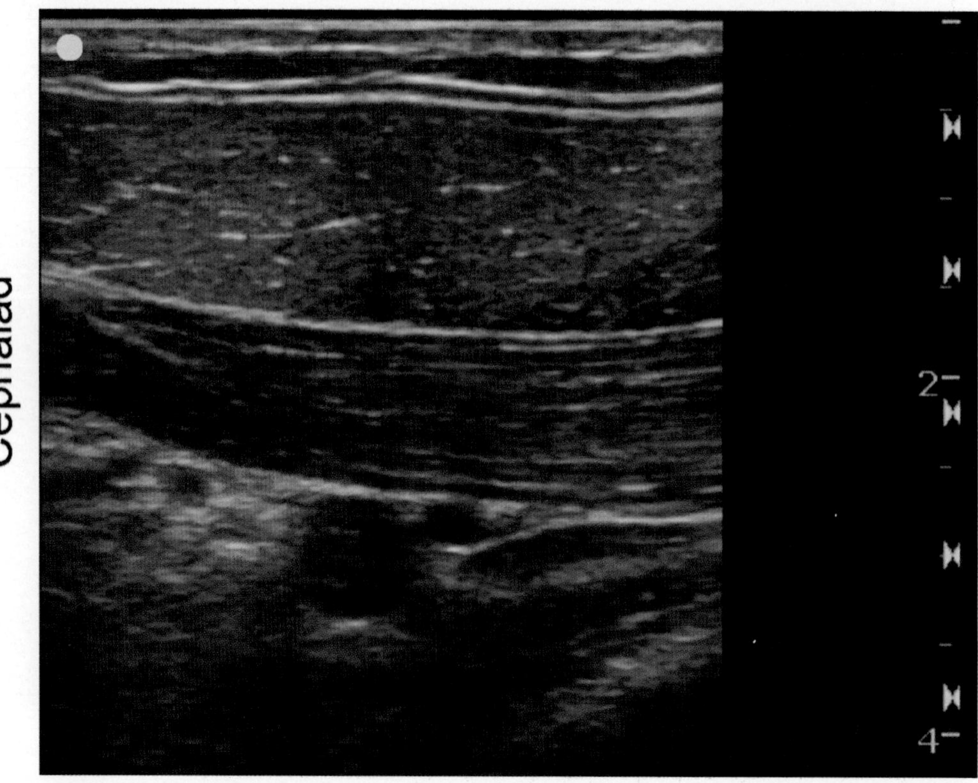


**FIGURE 7.15.1B** Ultrasound image of the lateral and posterior cords of the brachial plexus, transverse view.

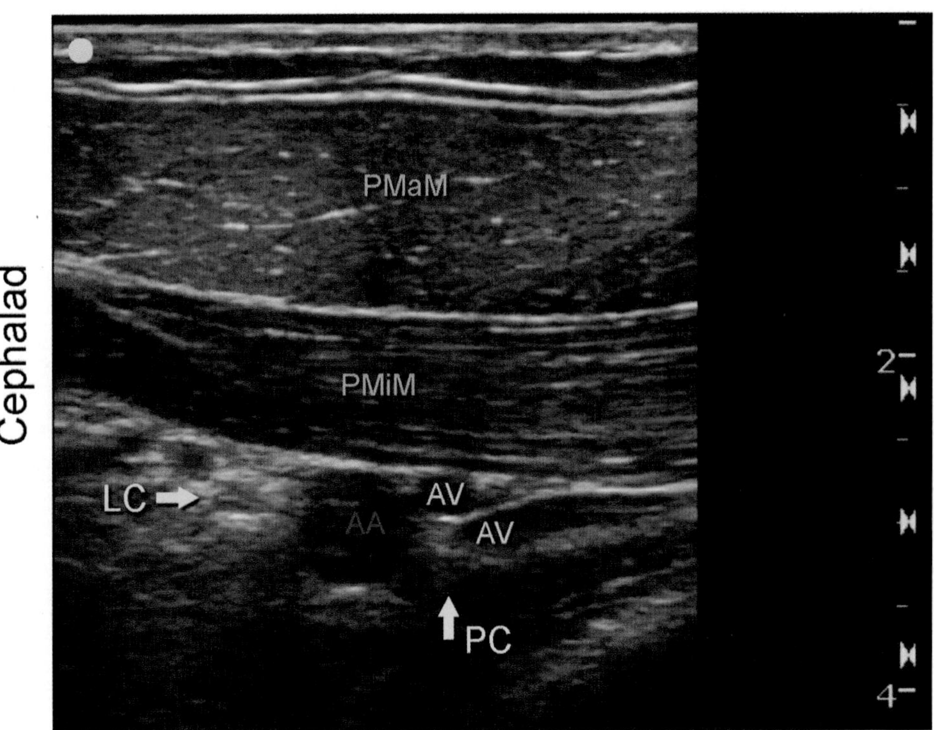


**FIGURE 7.15.1C** Labeled ultrasound image of the lateral and posterior cords of the brachial plexus, transverse view.

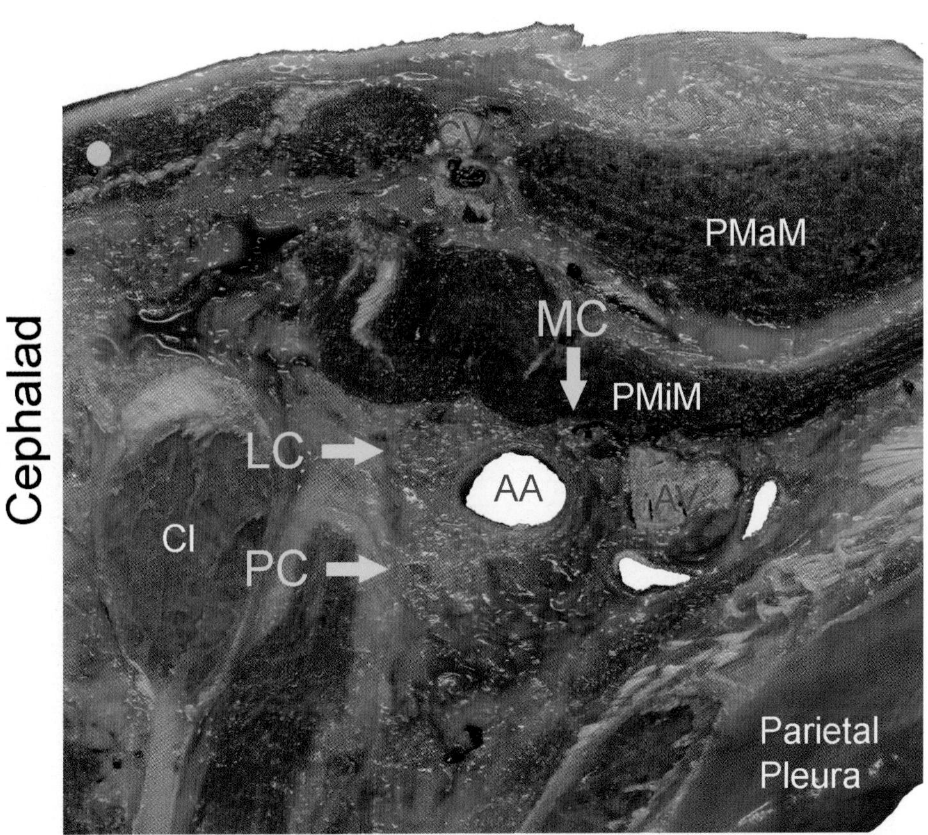


**FIGURE 7.15.1D** Labeled cross-sectional anatomy of the infraclavicular brachial plexus.

**Abbreviations:** PMaM, Pectoralis Major Muscle; PMiM, Pectoralis Minor Muscle; AA, Axillary Artery; AV, Axillary vein; PC, Posterior Cord; LC, Lateral Cord; MC, Medial Cord; Cl, Clavicle.

# Infraclavicular Brachial Plexus Lateral and Posterior Cords, Longitudinal View

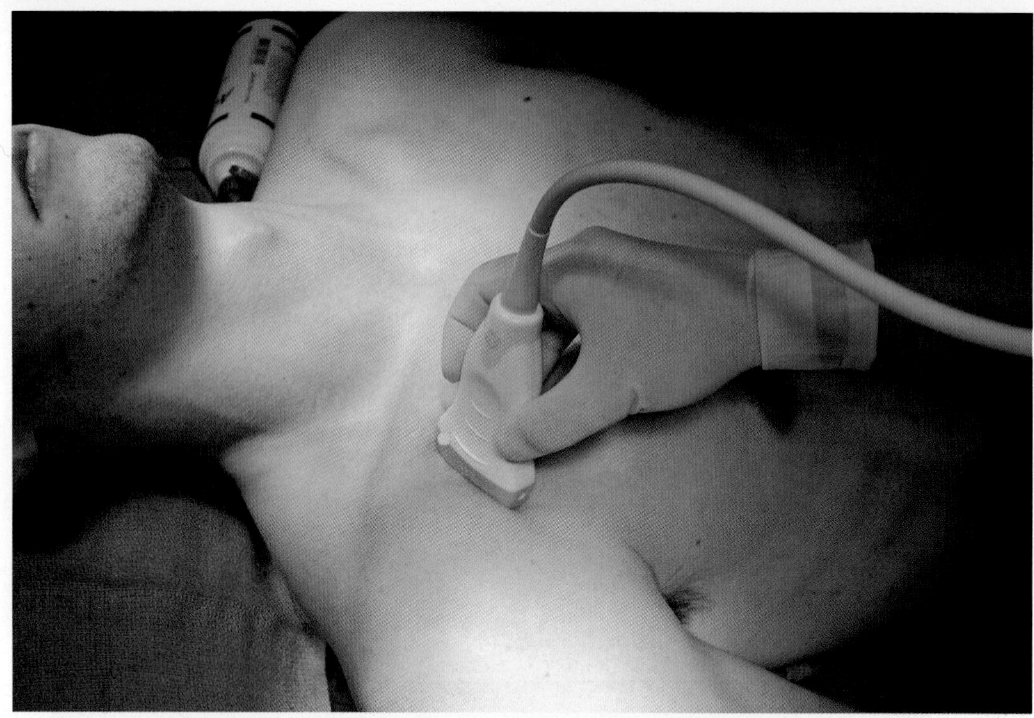

**FIGURE 7.15.2A** Ultrasound transducer position to image the infraclavicular brachial plexus lateral and posterior cords, longitudinal view.

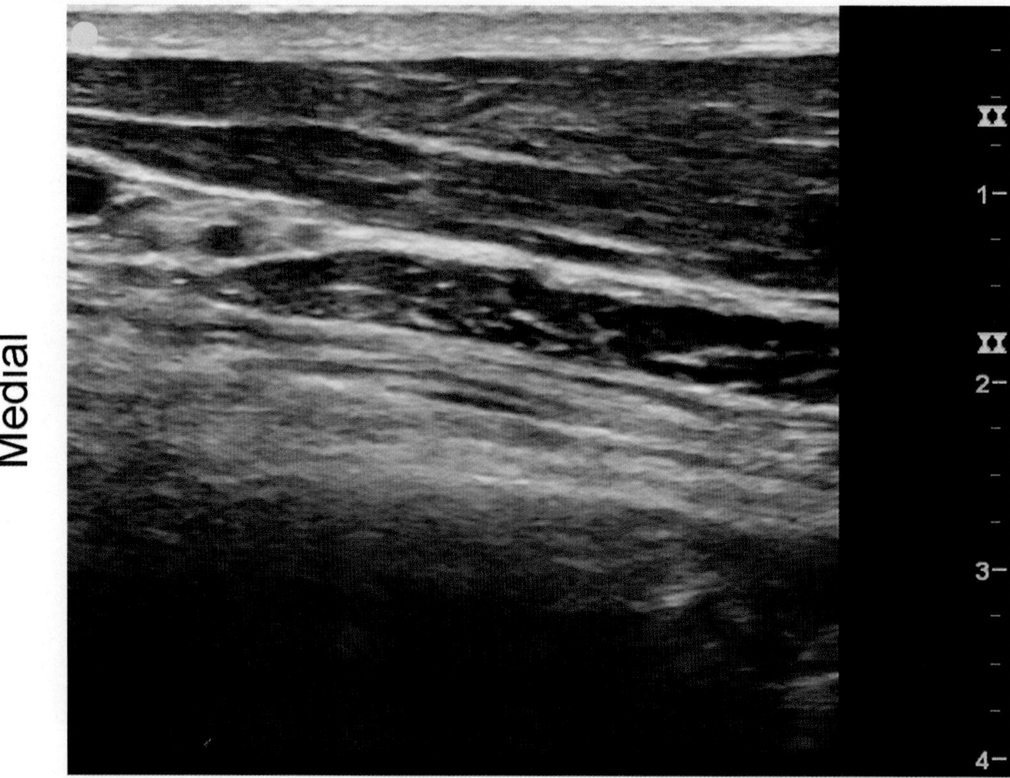


**FIGURE 7.15.2B** Ultrasound image of the infraclavicular brachial plexus lateral and posterior cords, longitudinal view.

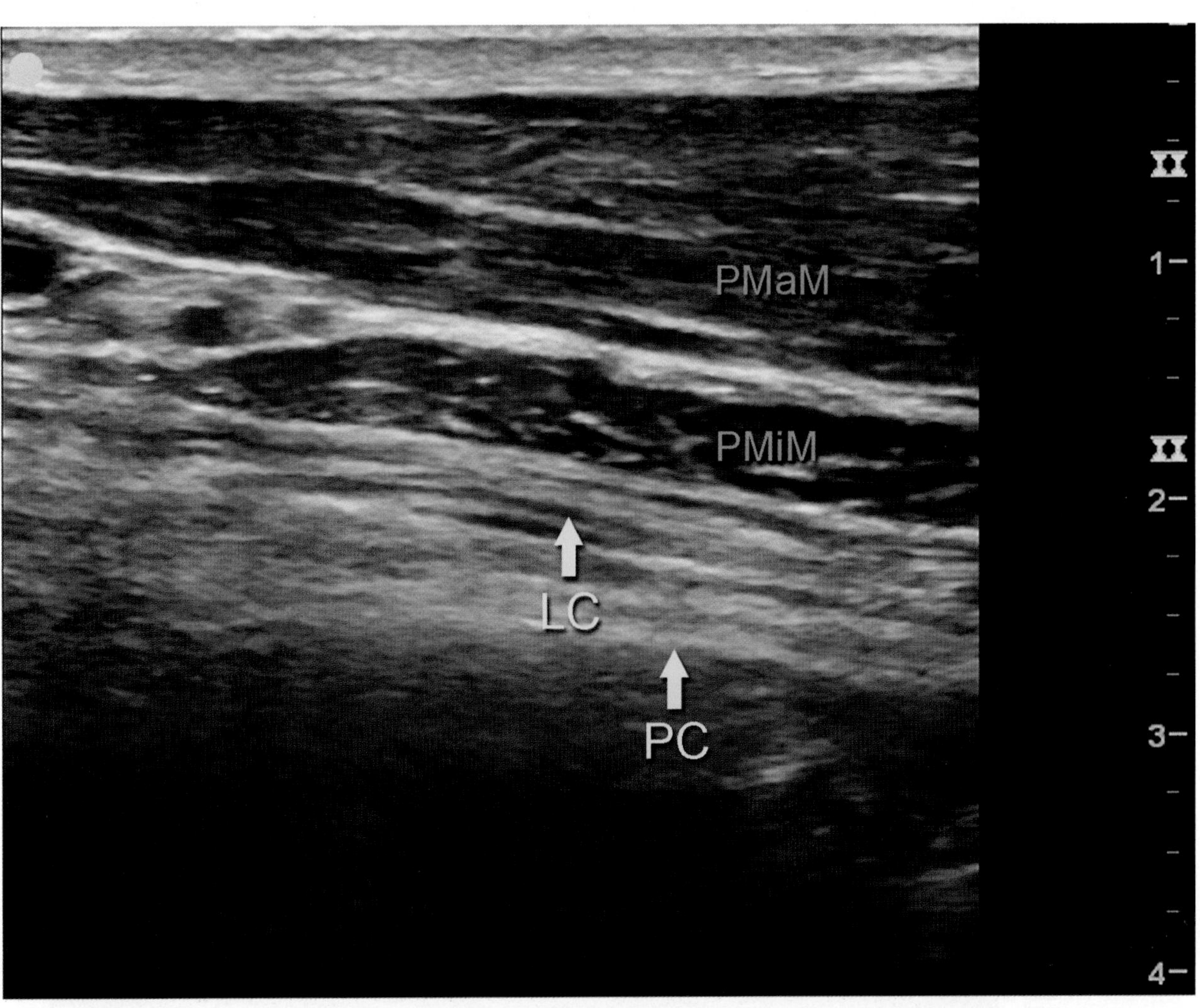


**FIGURE 7.15.2C** Labeled ultrasound image of the infraclavicular brachial plexus lateral and posterior cords, longitudinal view.

**Abbreviations:** PMaM, Pectoralis Major Muscle; PMiM, Pectoralis Minor Muscle; LC, Lateral Cord; PC, Posterior Cord.

## Infraclavicular Brachial Plexus Medial Cord, Transverse View

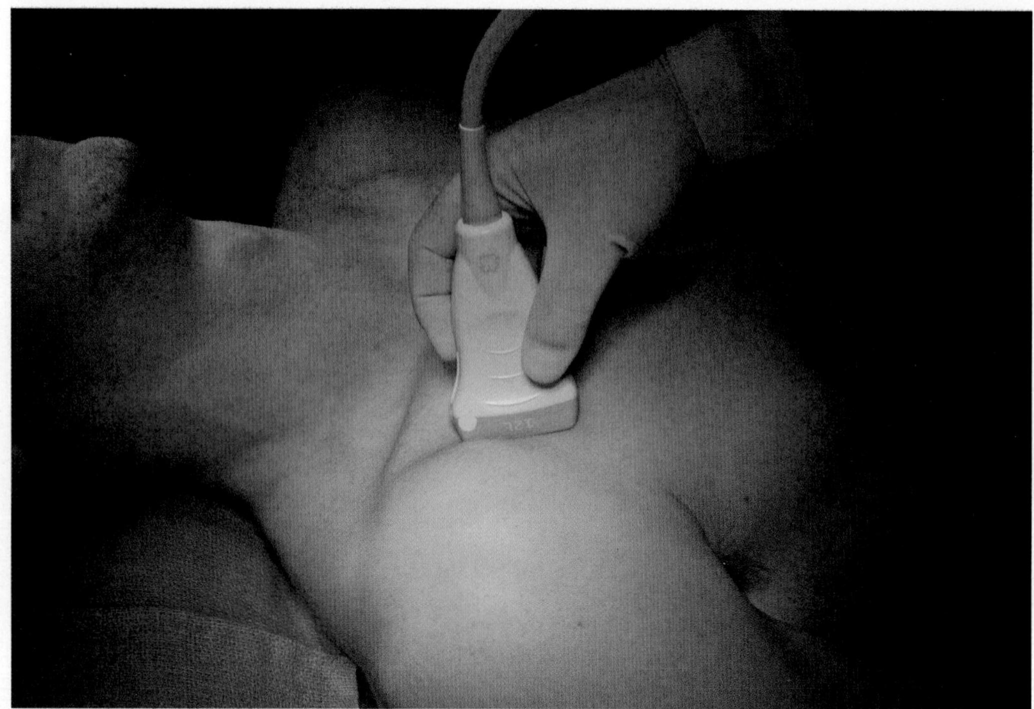

**FIGURE 7.15.3A** Ultrasound transducer position to image the infraclavicular brachial plexus medial cord, transverse view.

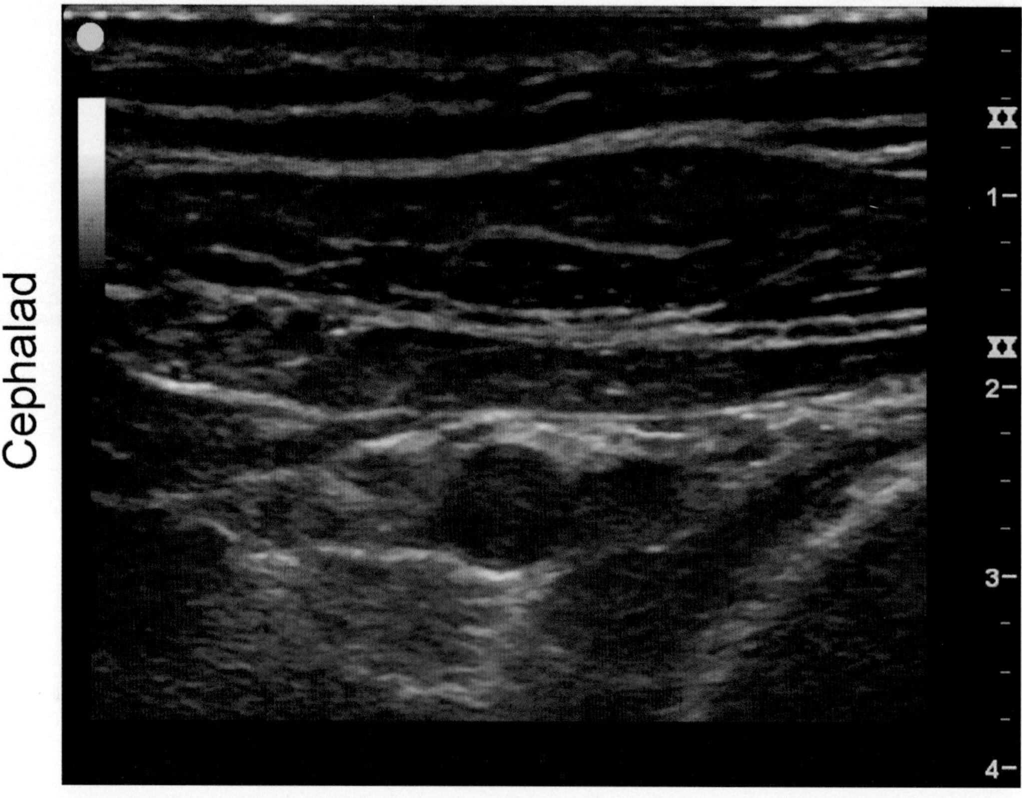


**FIGURE 7.15.3B** Ultrasound image of the infraclavicular brachial plexus medial cord, transverse view.

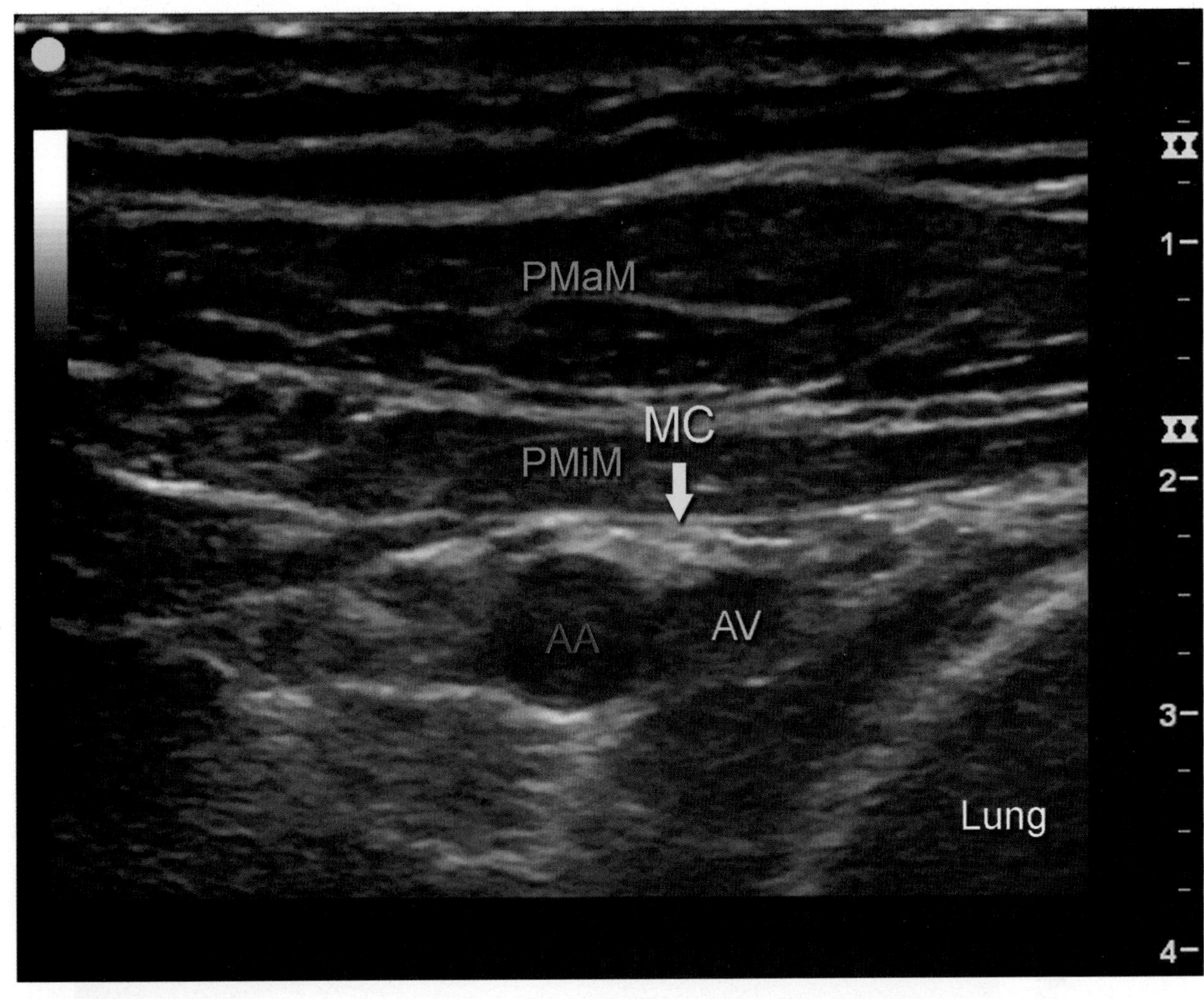


**FIGURE 7.15.3C** Labeled ultrasound image of the infraclavicular brachial plexus medial cord, transverse view.

**Abbreviations:** PMaM, Pectoralis Major Muscle; PMiM, Pectoralis Minor Muscle; MC, Medial Cord; AA, Axillary Artery; AV, Axillary Vein.

# Infraclavicular Brachial Plexus Medial Cord, Longitudinal View

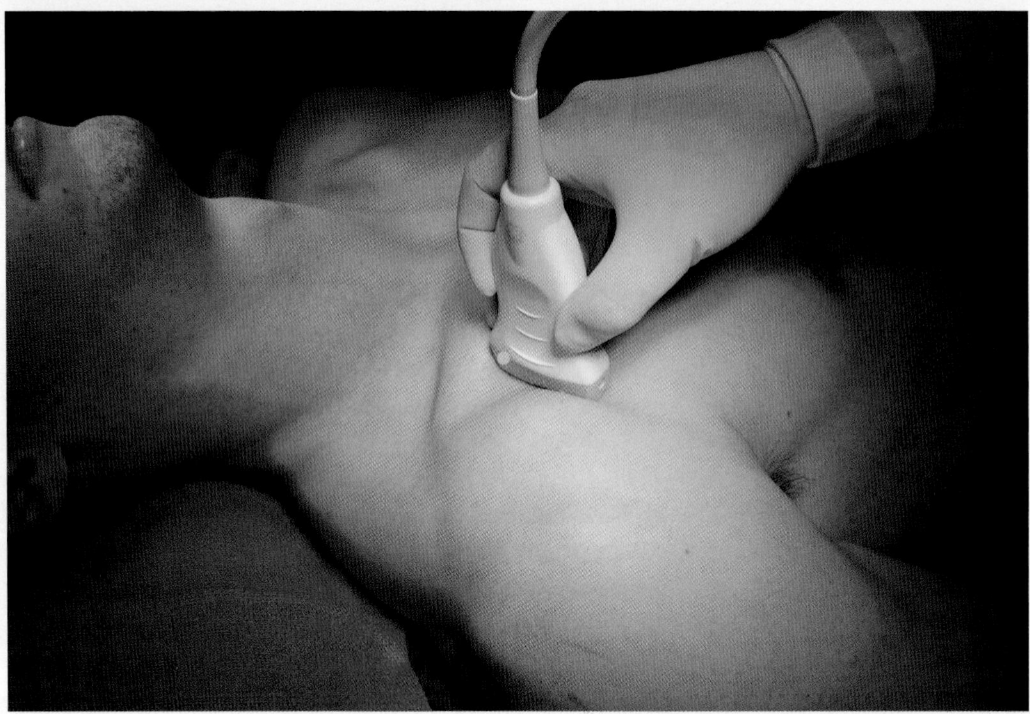

**FIGURE 7.15.4A** Ultrasound transducer position to image the infraclavicular brachial plexus medial cord, longitudinal view.

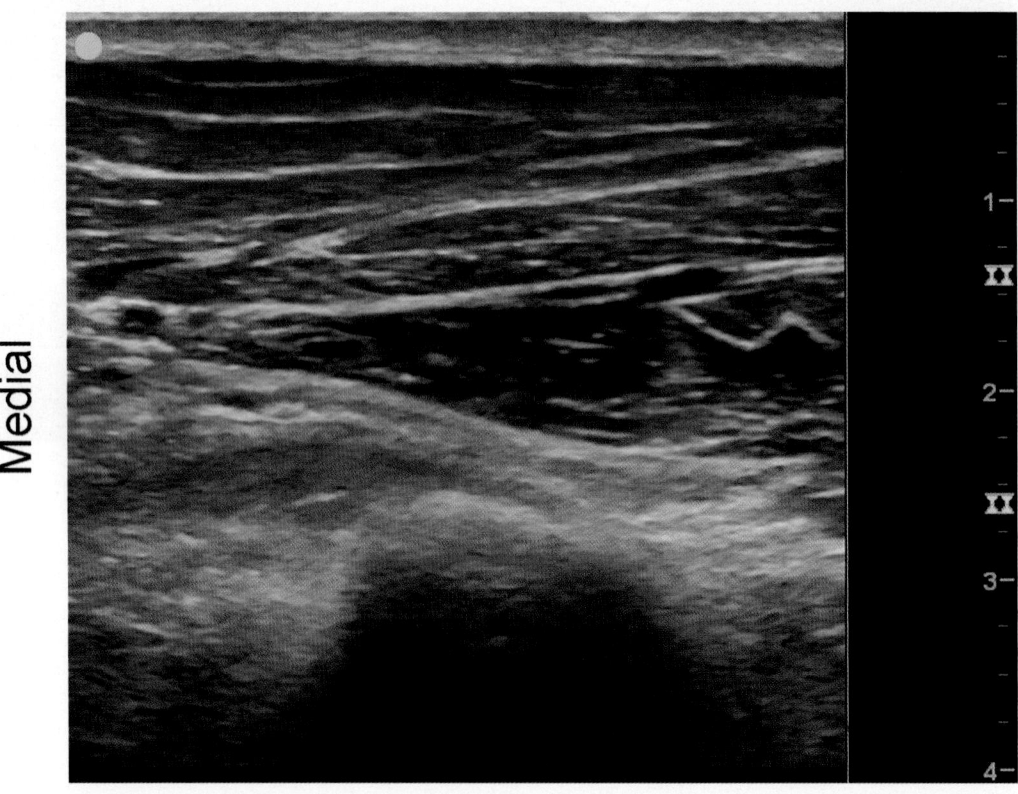


**FIGURE 7.15.4B** Ultrasound image of the infraclavicular brachial plexus medial cord, longitudinal view.

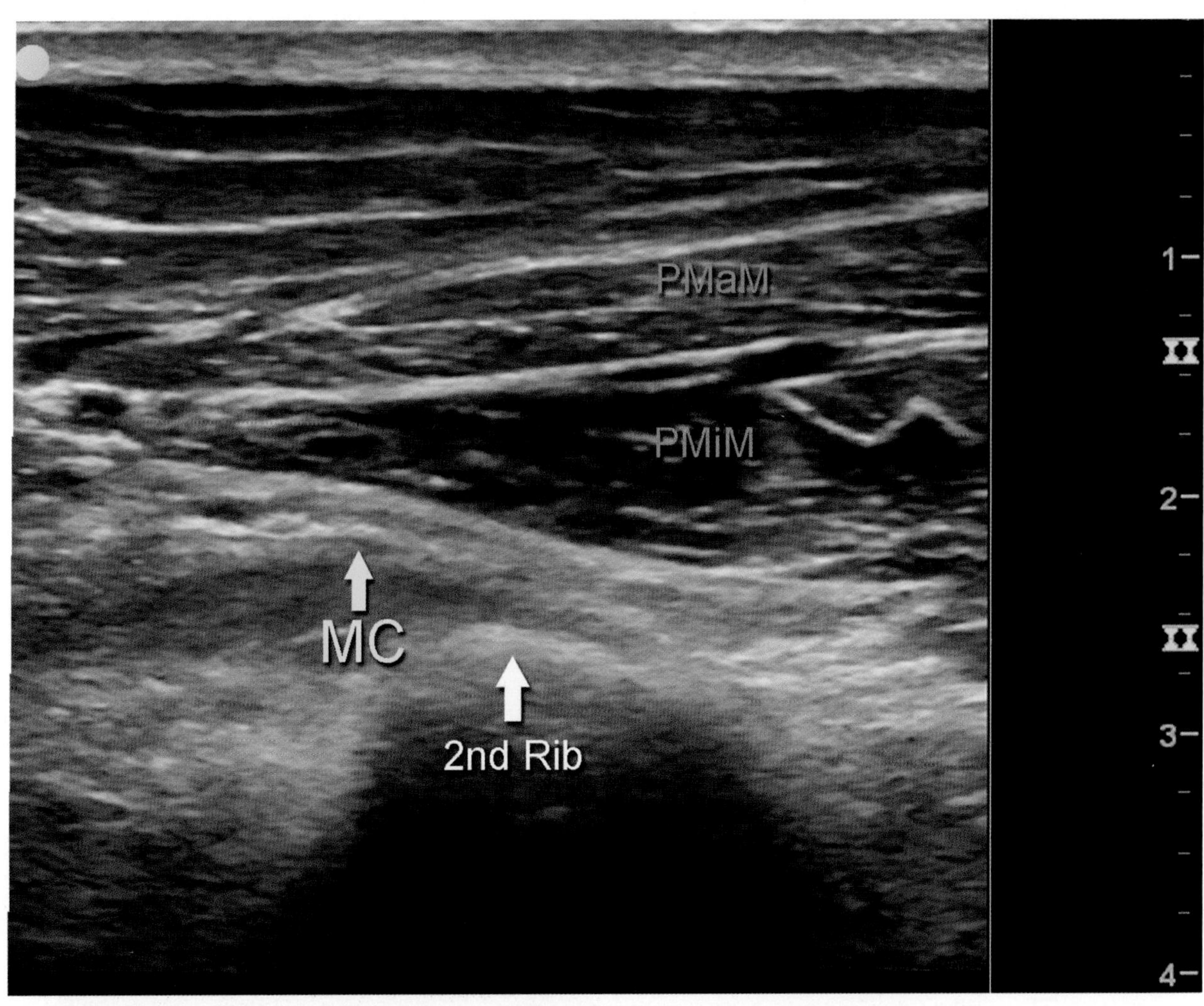


**FIGURE 7.15.4C** Labeled ultrasound image of the infraclavicular brachial plexus medial cord, longitudinal view.

**Abbreviations:** PMaM, Pectoralis Major Muscle; PMiM, Pectoralis Minor Muscle; MC, Medial Cord.

## Axillary Nerve

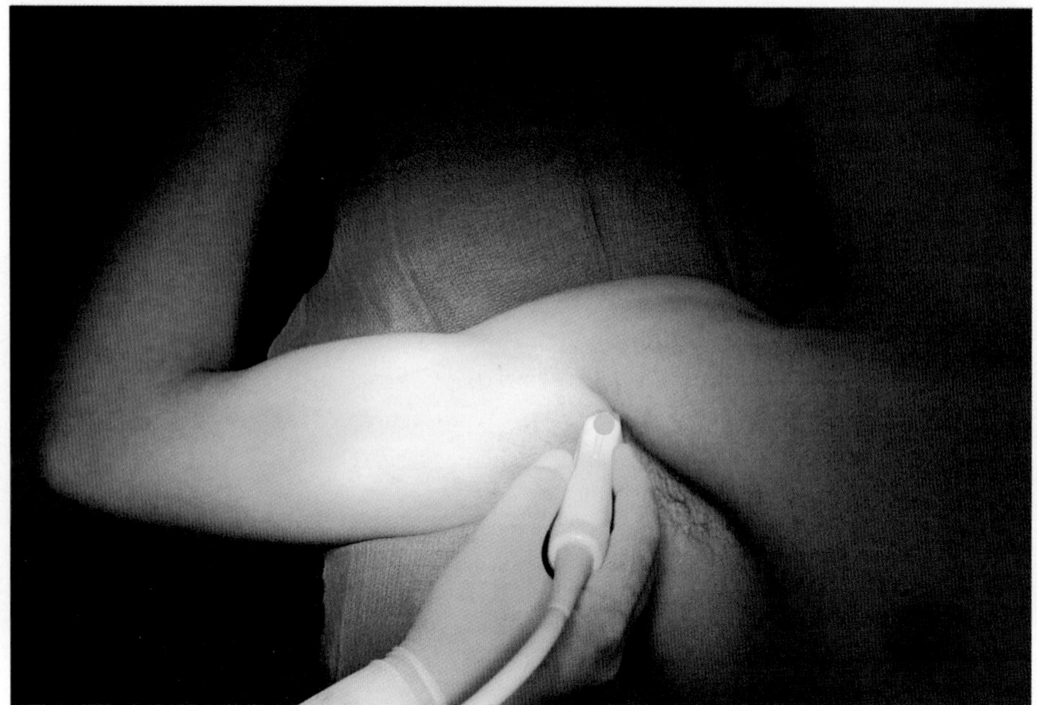

**FIGURE 7.16.1A** Ultrasound transducer position to image the axillary nerve.

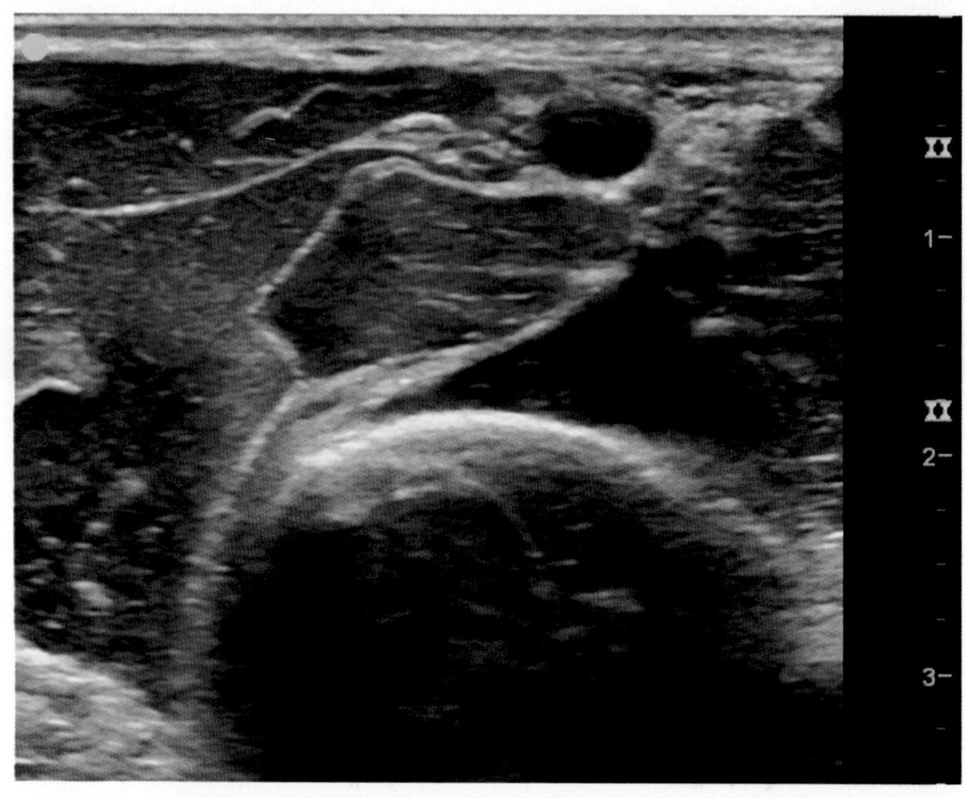


**FIGURE 7.16.1B** Ultrasound image of the axillary nerve.

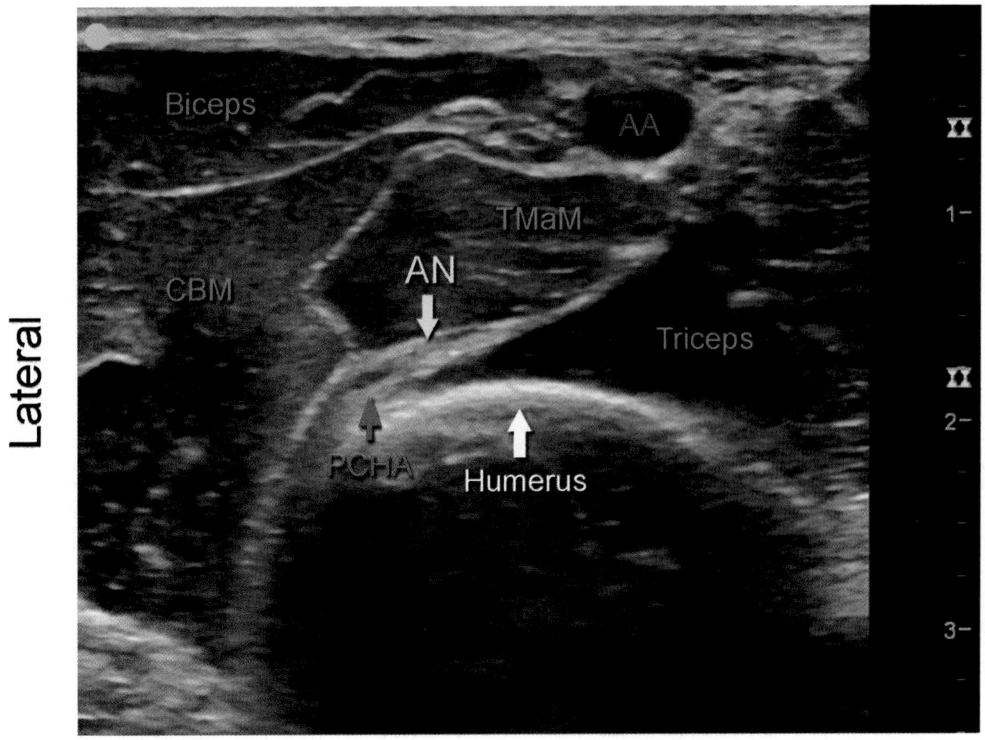

**FIGURE 7.16.1C** Labeled ultrasound image of the axillary nerve.

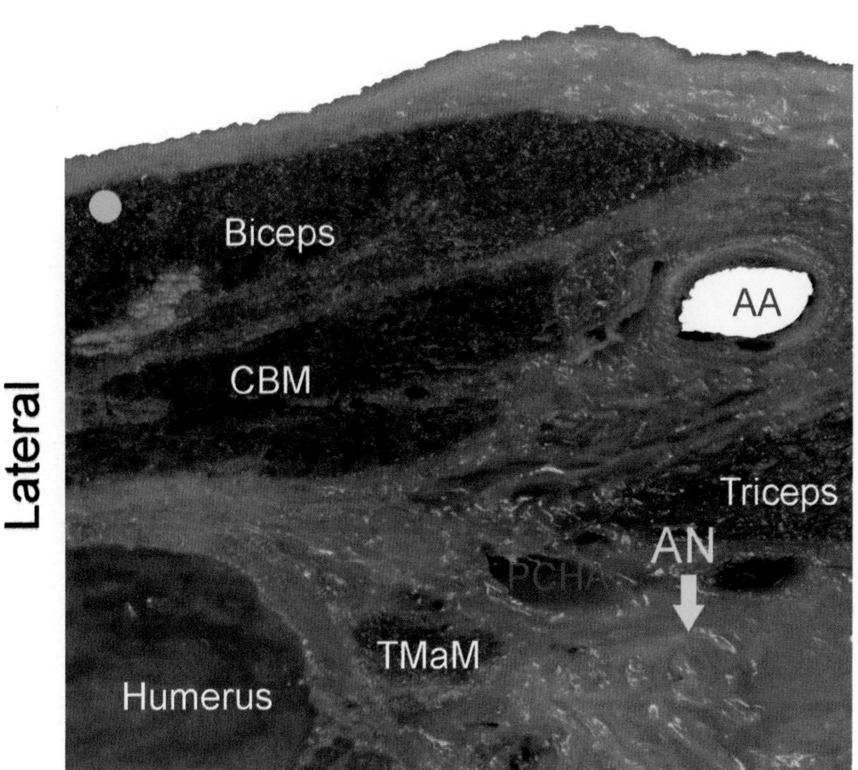


**FIGURE 7.16.1D** Labeled cross-sectional anatomy of the axillary nerve.

**Abbreviations:** AA, Axillary Artery; TMaM, Teres Major Muscle; AN, Axillary Nerve; CBM, Coracobrachialis Muscle; PCHA, Posterior Circumflex Humeral Artery.

# Axilla: Median, Ulnar, Radial, and Musculocutaneous Nerves

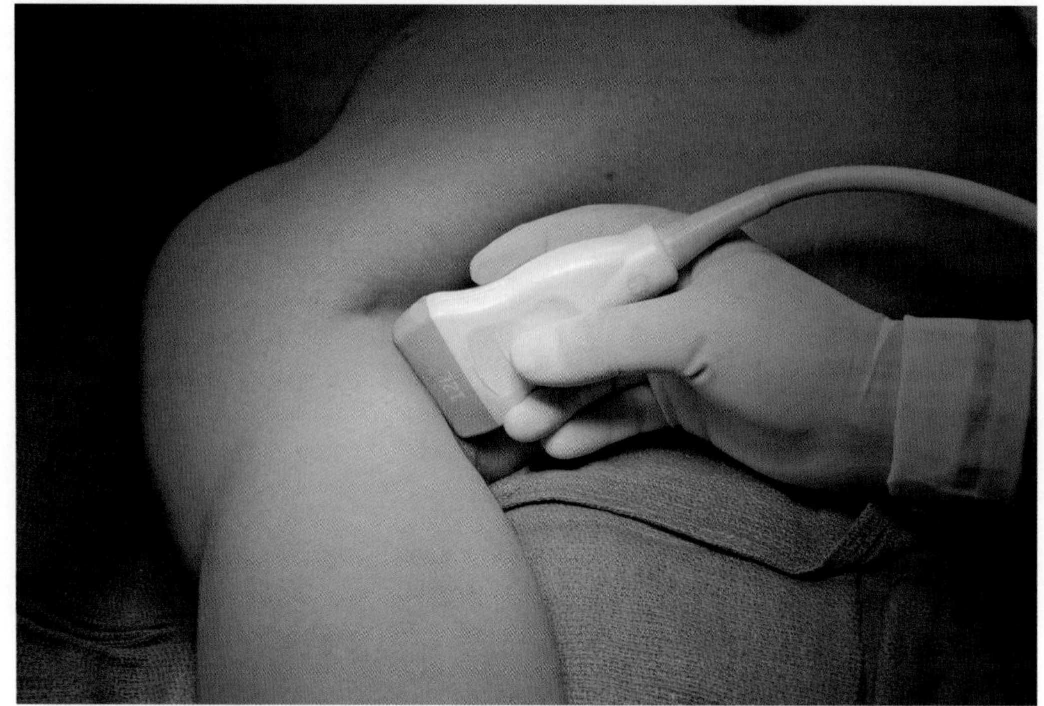

**FIGURE 7.17.1A** Ultrasound transducer position to image the axilla: median, ulnar, radial, and musculocutaneous nerves.

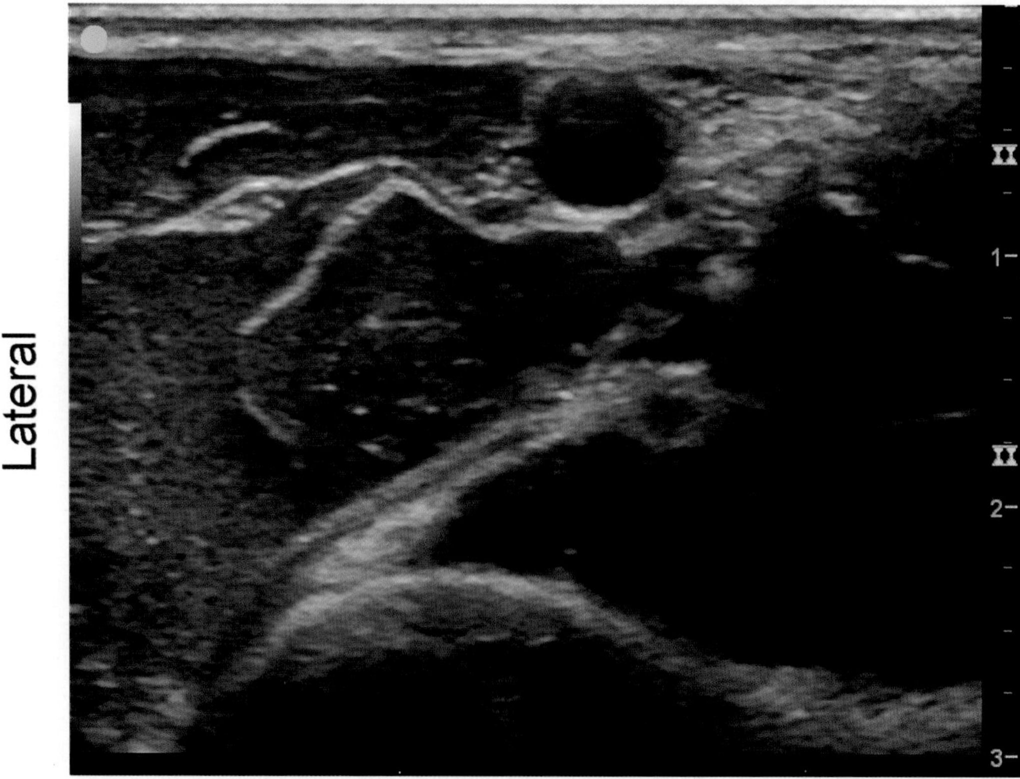


**FIGURE 7.17.1B** Ultrasound image of the axilla: median, ulnar, radial, and musculocutaneous nerves.

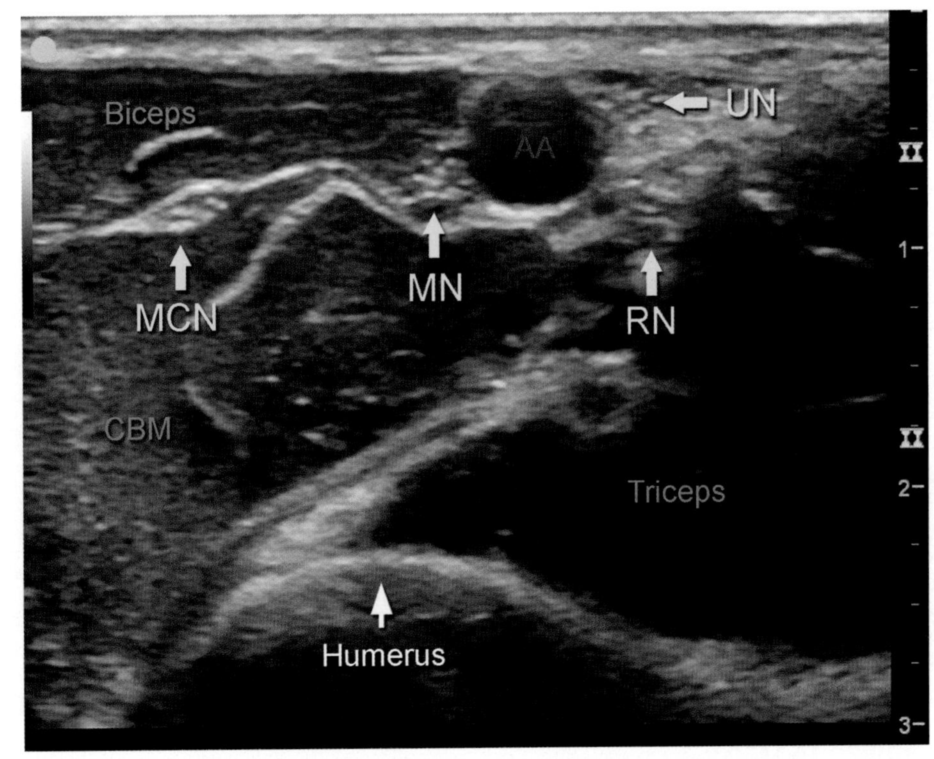


**FIGURE 7.17.1C** Labeled ultrasound image of the axilla: median, ulnar, radial, and musculocutaneous nerves.

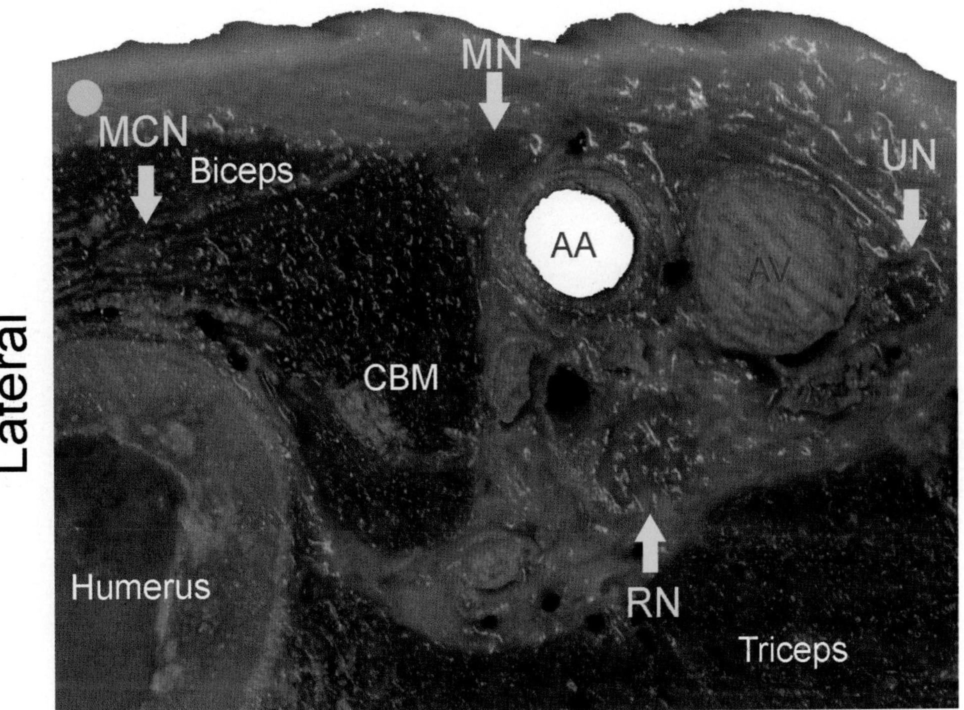


**FIGURE 7.17.1D** Labeled cross-sectional anatomy of the axilla: median, ulnar, radial, and musculocutaneous nerves.

**Abbreviations:** UN, Ulnary Nerve; MN, Median Nerve; RN, Radial Nerve; MCN, Musculocutaneous Nerve; AA, Axillary Nerve; CBM, Coracobrachialis Muscle; AV, Axillary Vein.

# Axilla: Musculocutaneous Nerve

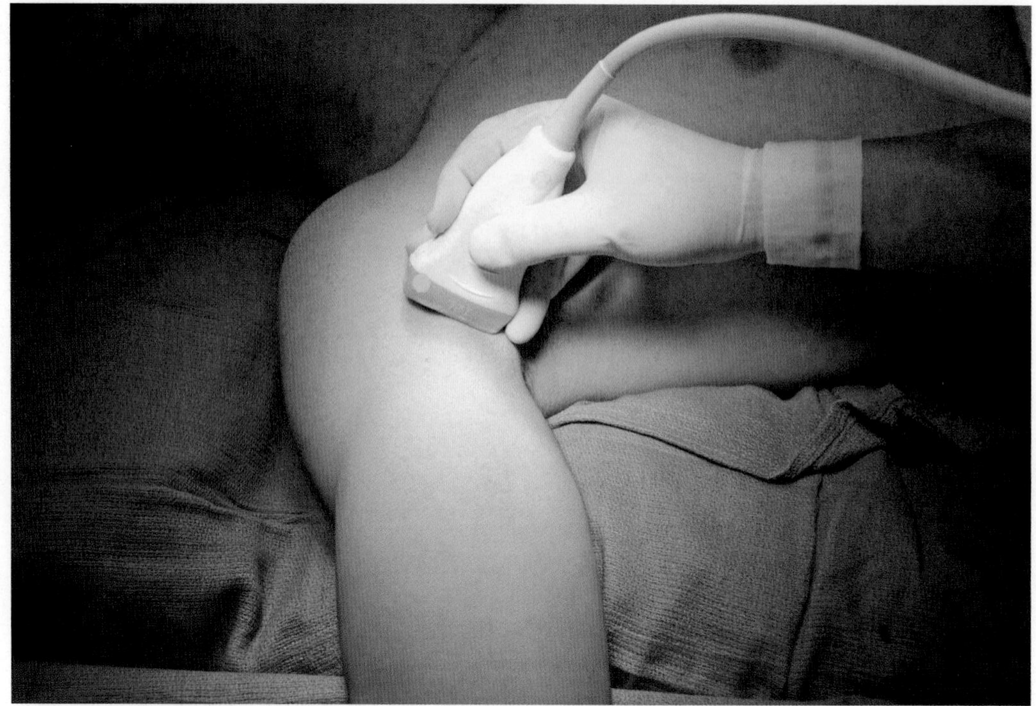

**FIGURE 7.18.1A** Ultrasound transducer position to image the axilla: musculocutaneous nerve.

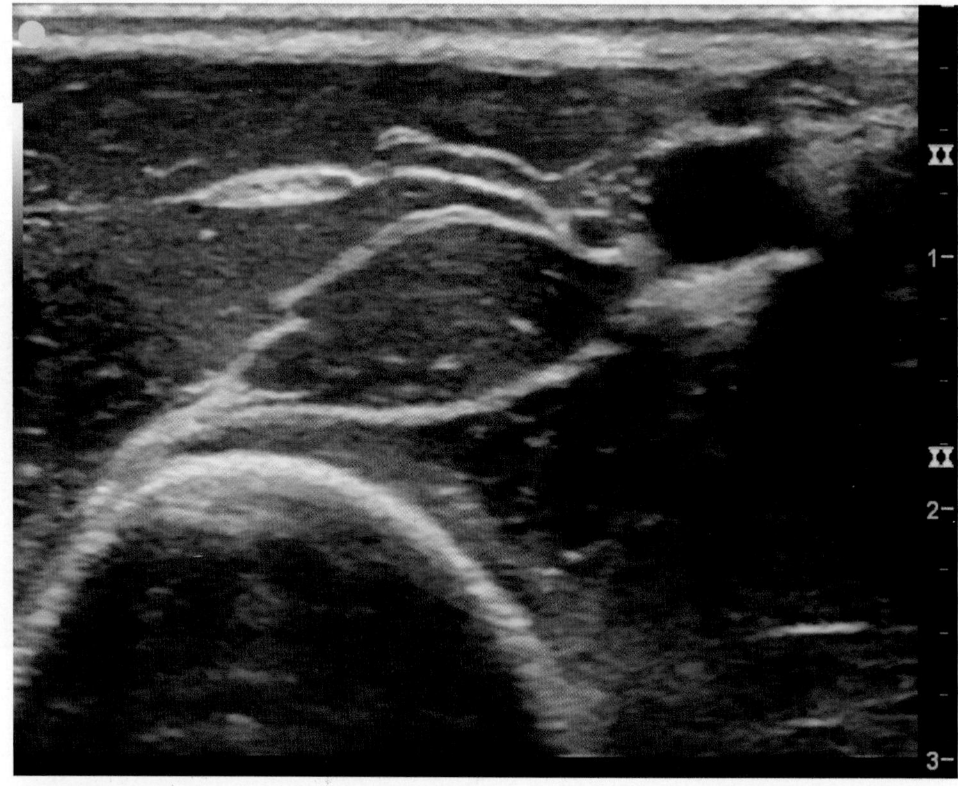


**FIGURE 7.18.1B** Ultrasound image of the axilla: musculocutaneous nerve.

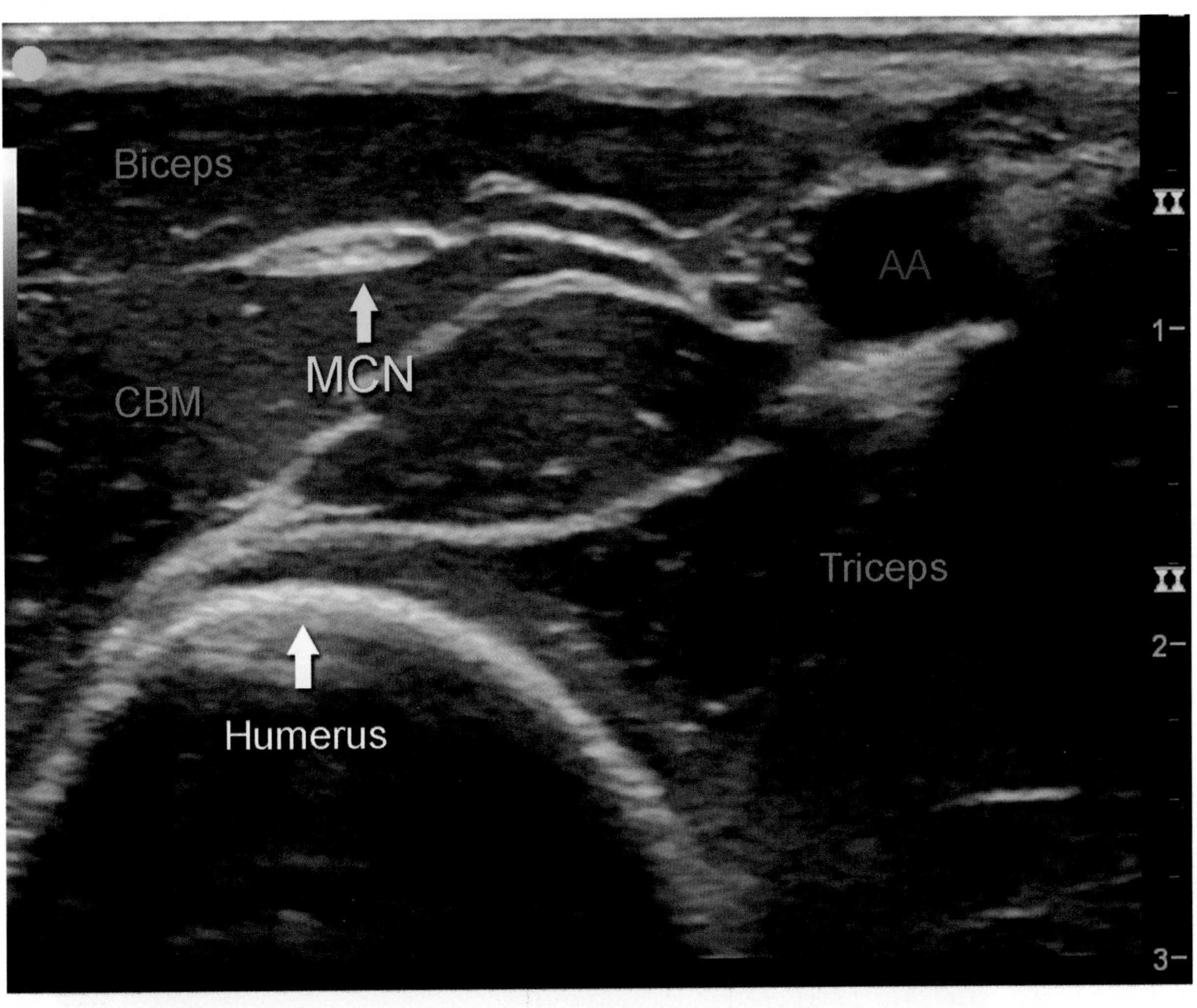


**FIGURE 7.18.1C** Labeled ultrasound image of the axilla: musculocutaneous nerve.

**Abbreviations:** MCN, Musculocutaneous Nerve; AA, Axillary Nerve; CBM, Coracobrachialis Muscle; AV.

# Axilla: Ulnar Nerve

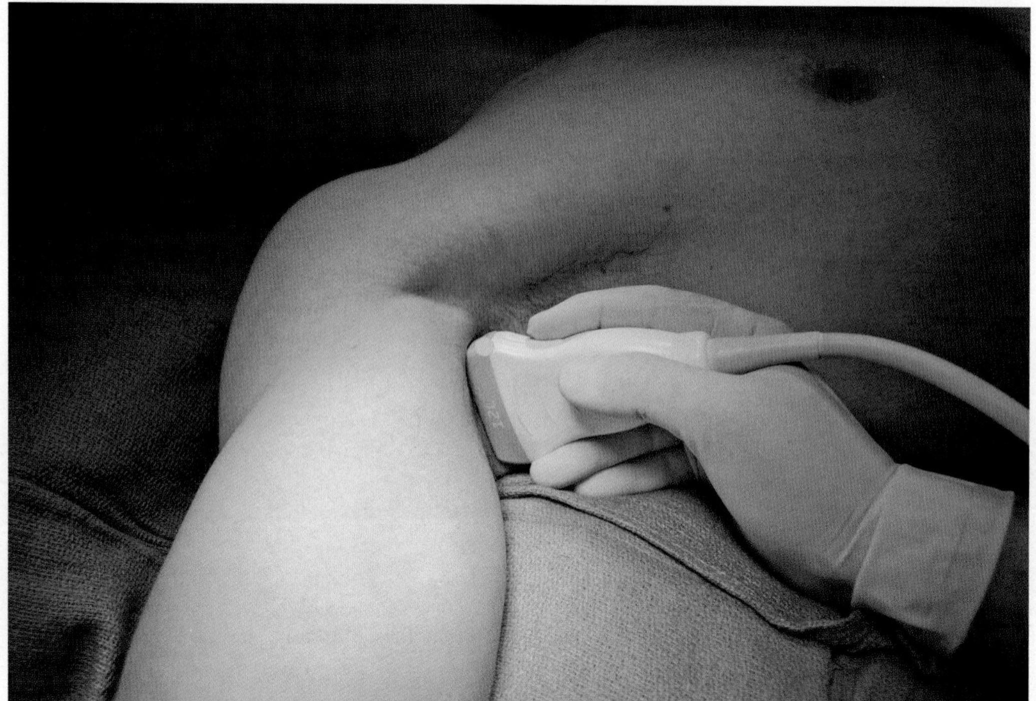

**FIGURE 7.19.1A** Ultrasound transducer position to image the ulnar nerve at the level of the axilla.

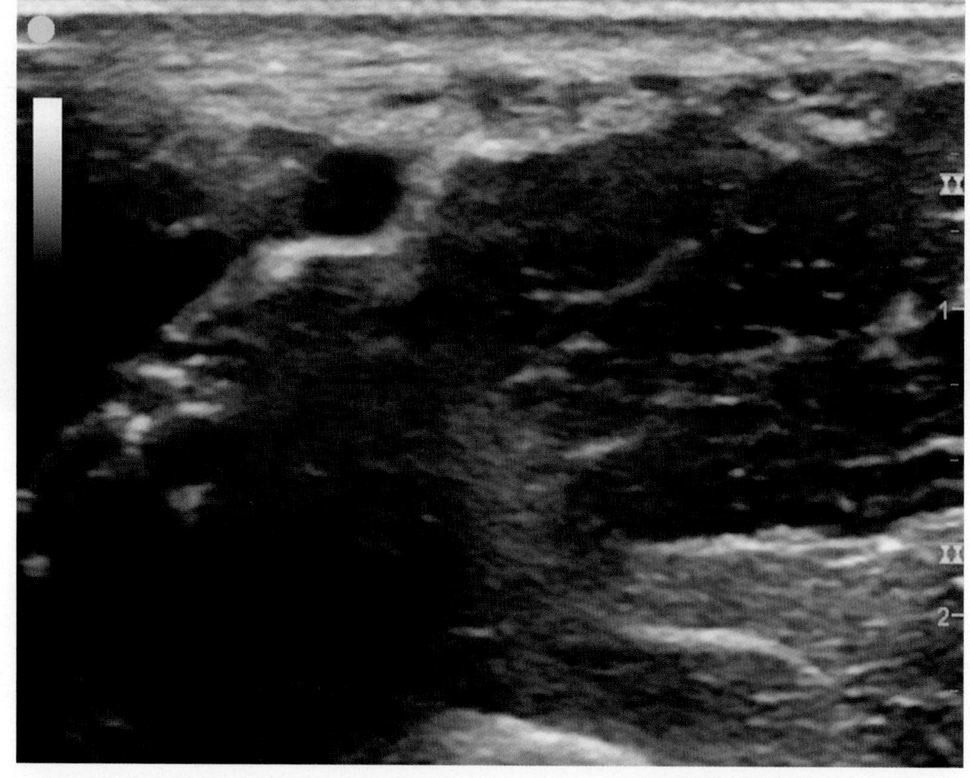


**FIGURE 7.19.1B** Ultrasound image of the ulnar nerve at the level of the axilla.

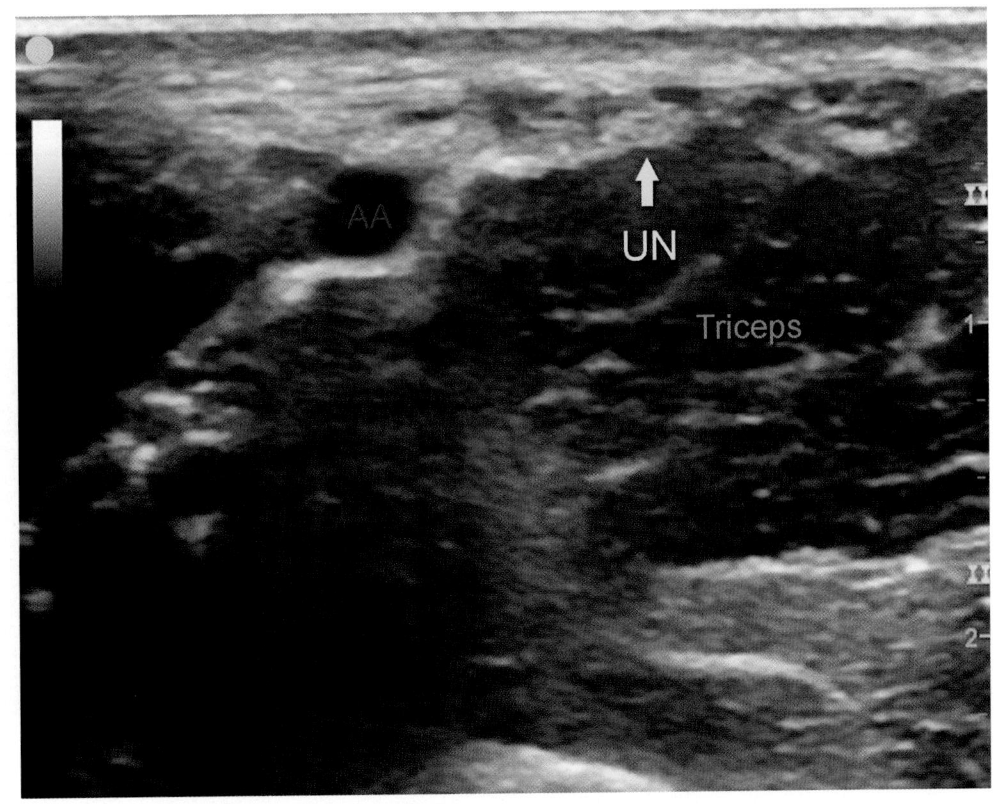


**FIGURE 7.19.1C** Labeled ultrasound image of the ulnar nerve.

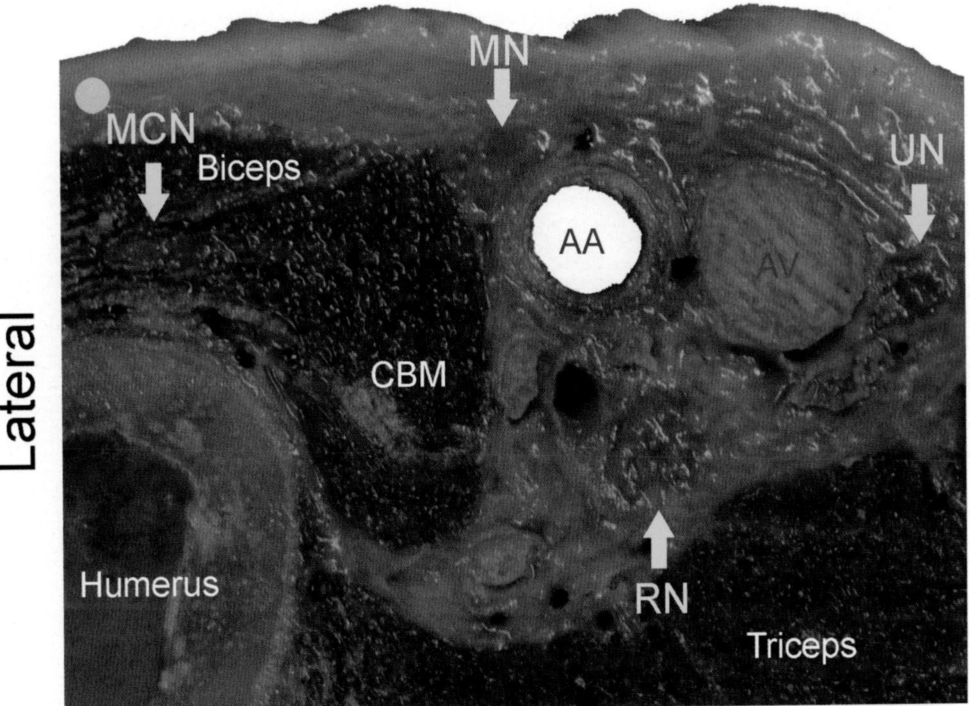


**FIGURE 7.19.1D**

**Abbreviations:** AA, Axillary Nerve; UN, Ulnar Nerve.

# Midhumerus: Posterior Antebrachial Cutaneous Nerve and Radial Nerve

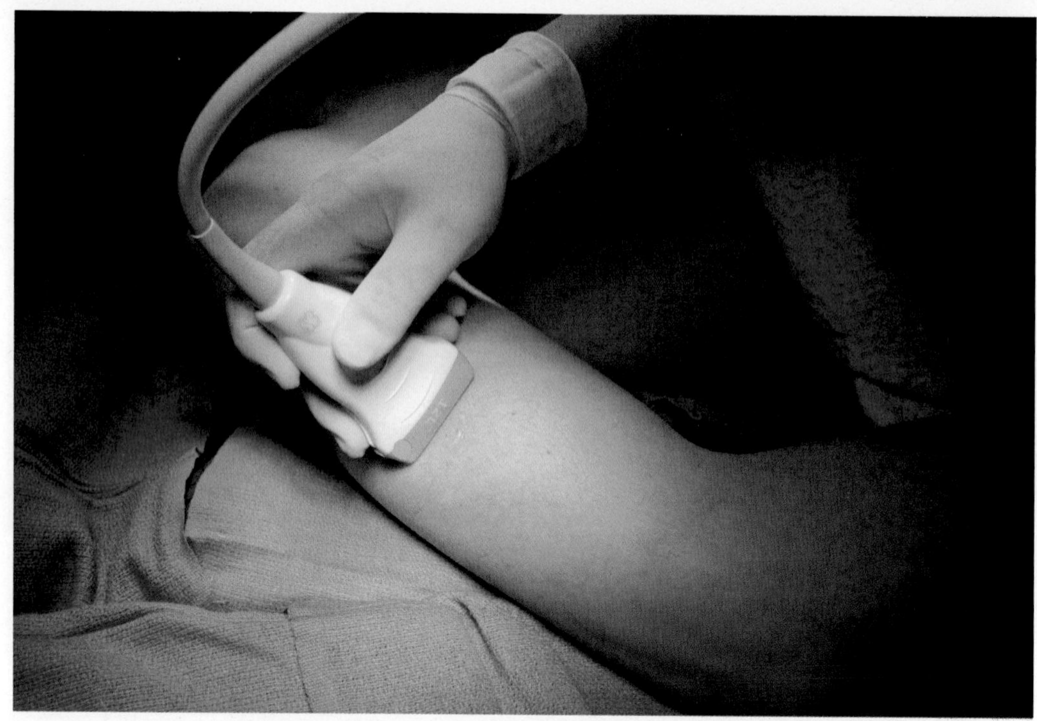

**FIGURE 7.20.1A** Ultrasound transducer position to image the posterior antebrachial cutaneous and radial nerves.

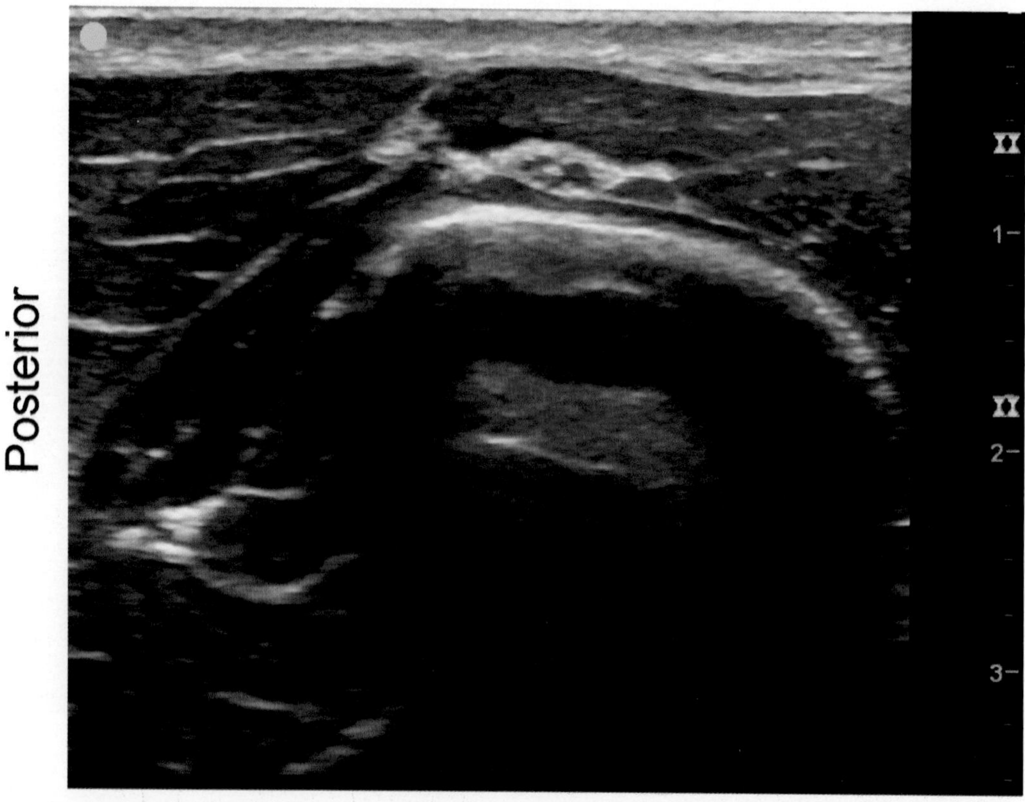


**FIGURE 7.20.1B** Ultrasound image of the midhumerus: posterior antebrachial cutaneous nerve and radial nerve.

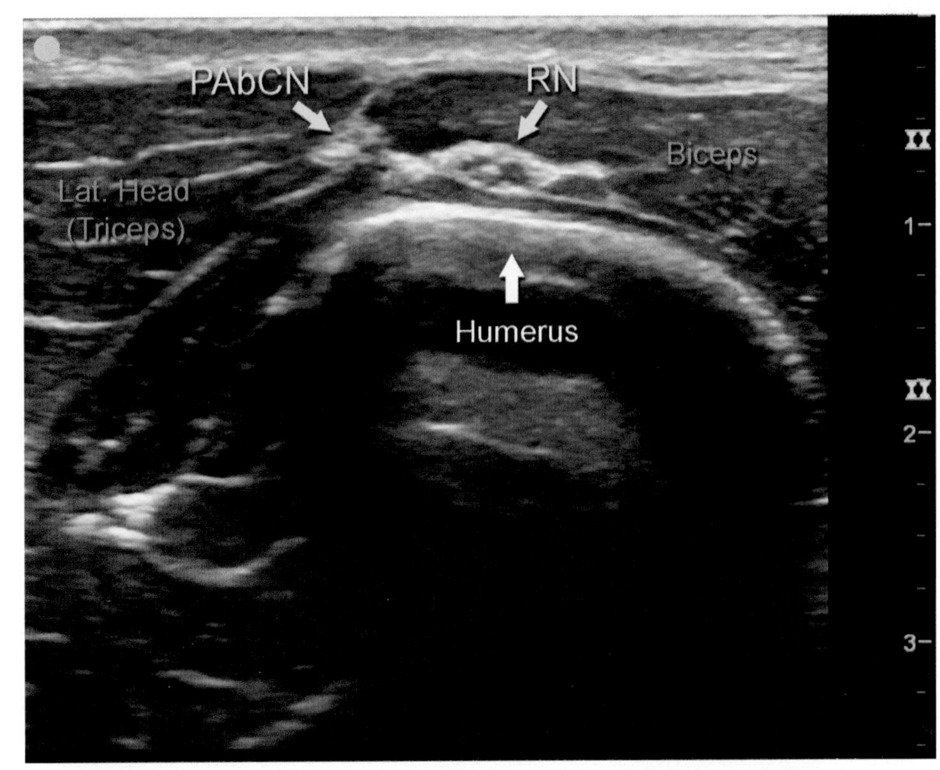


**FIGURE 7.20.1C** Labeled ultrasound image of the midhumerus: posterior antebrachial cutaneous nerve and radial nerve.

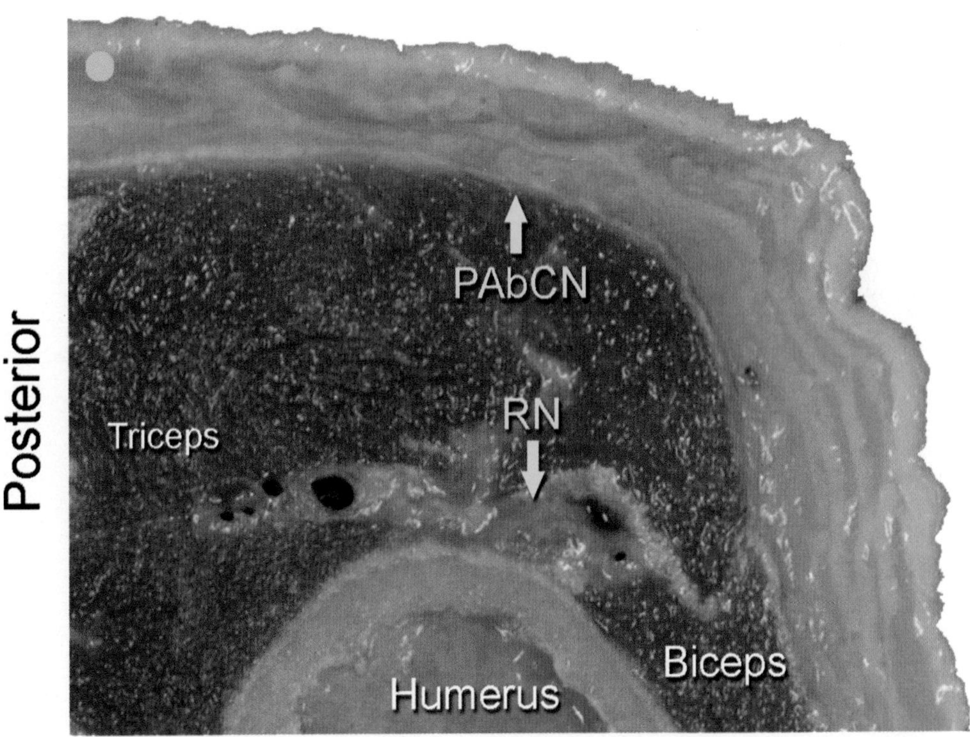


**FIGURE 7.20.1D** Labeled cross-sectional anatomy of the midhumerus: posterior antebrachial cutaneous nerve and radial nerve.

**Abbreviations:** PAbCN, Posterior Antebrachial Cutaneous Nerve; RN, Radial Nerve.

# Ulnar Nerve Above the Elbow

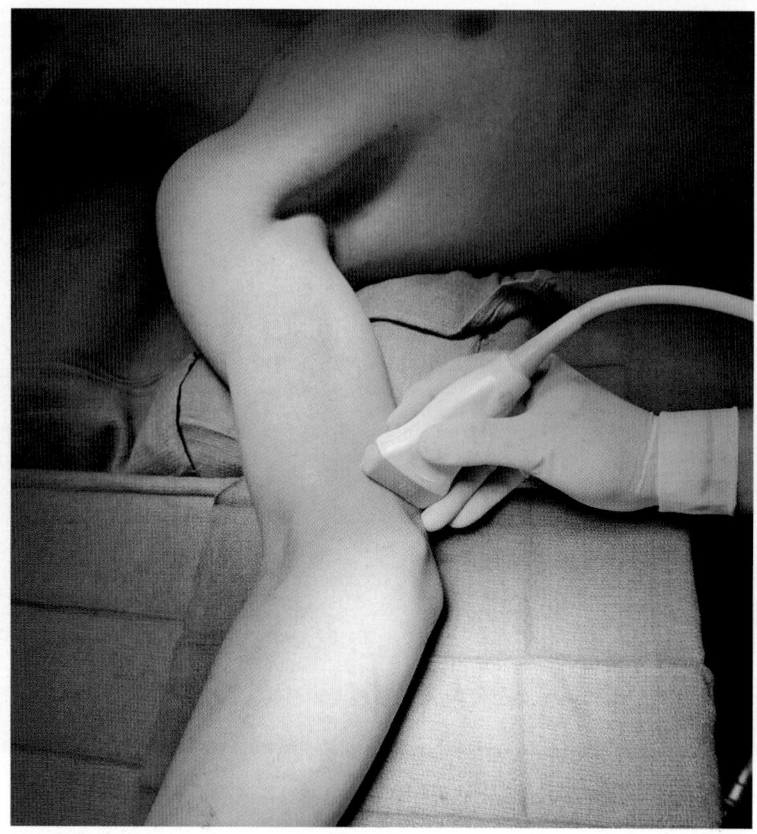

**FIGURE 7.21.1A** Ultrasound transducer position to image the ulnar nerve above the elbow.

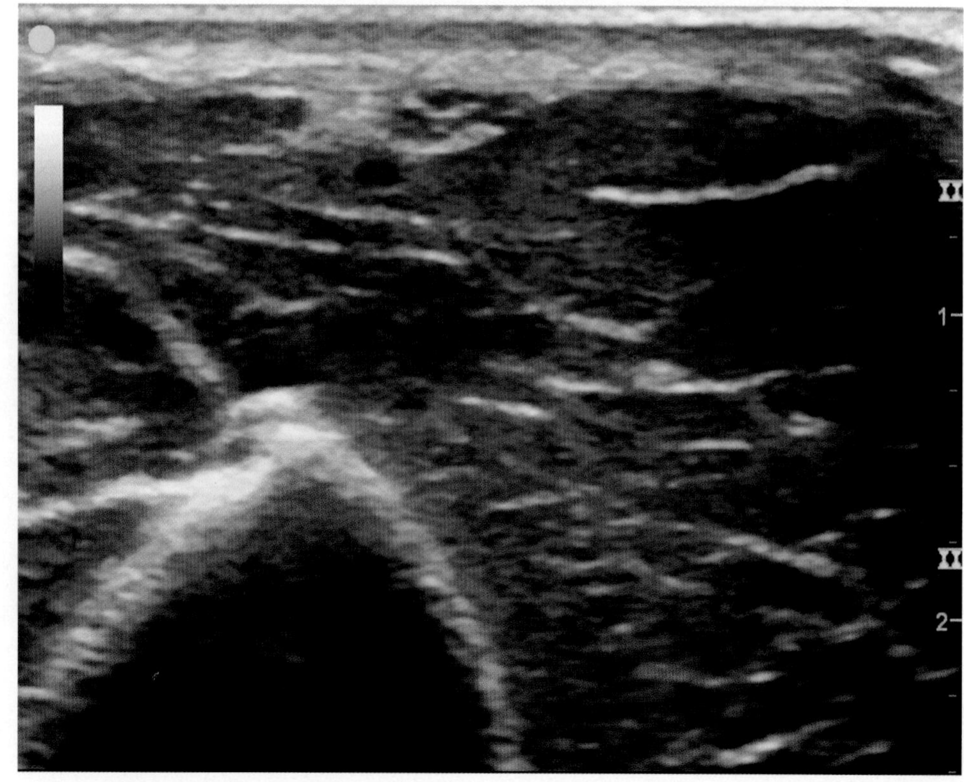


**FIGURE 7.21.1B** Ultrasound image of the ulnar nerve above the elbow.

Anterior

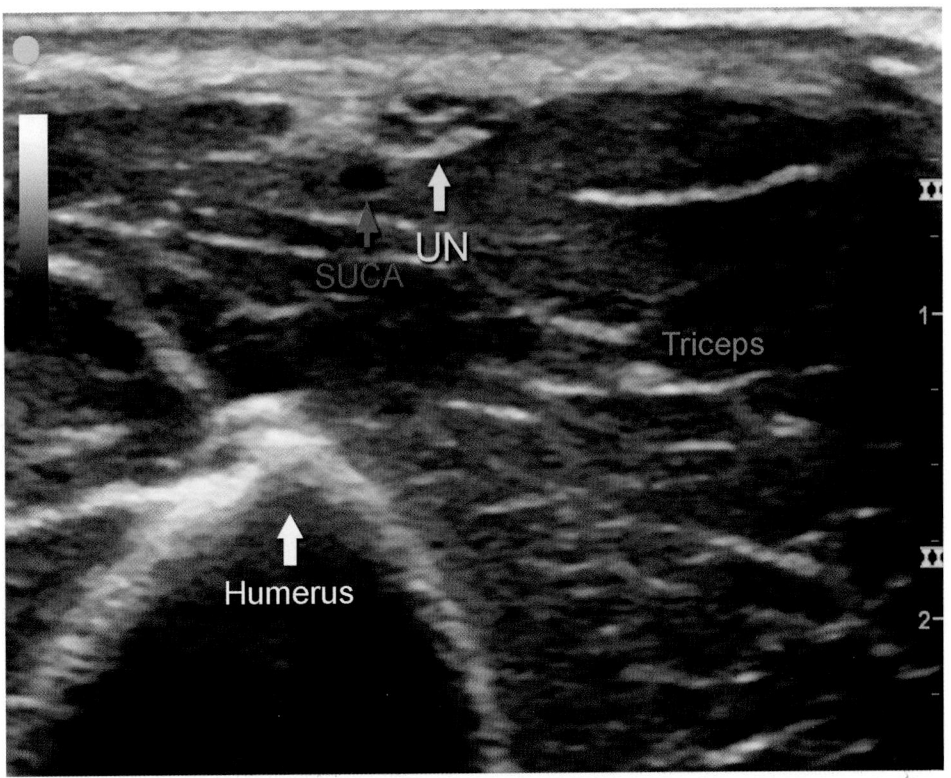


**FIGURE 7.21.1C** Labeled ultrasound image of the ulnar nerve above the elbow.

Anterior

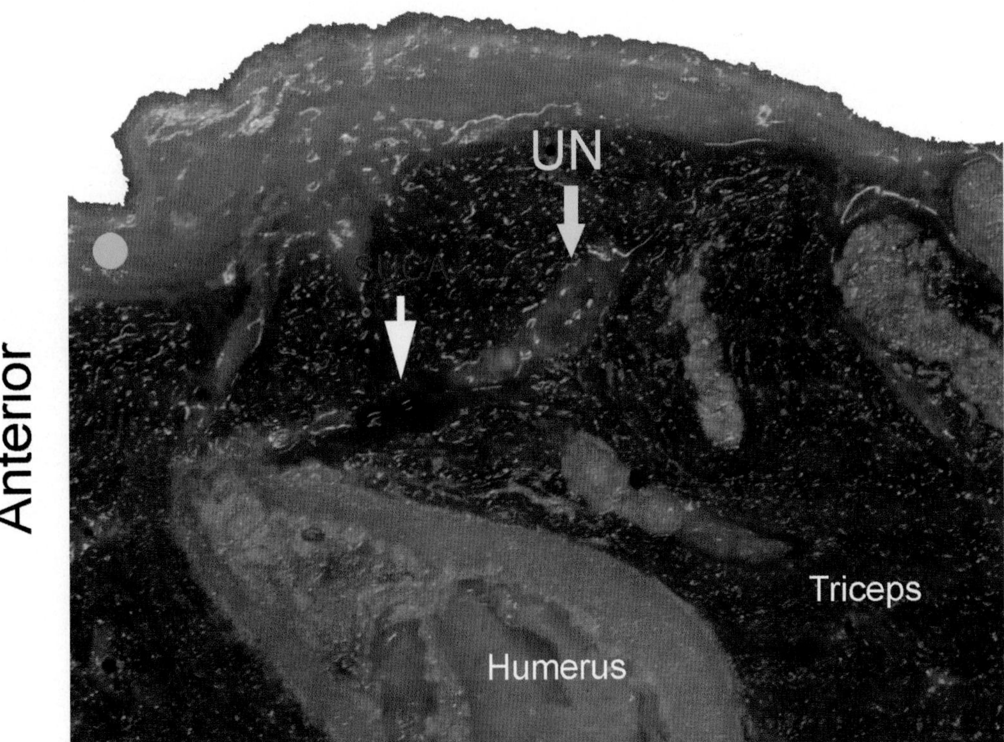


**FIGURE 7.21.1D** Labeled cross-sectional anatomy of the ulnar nerve above the elbow.

**Abbreviations:** UN, Ulnar Nerve; SUCA, Superior Ulnar Collateral Artery.

## Medial Antebrachial Cutaneous Nerve Above the Elbow

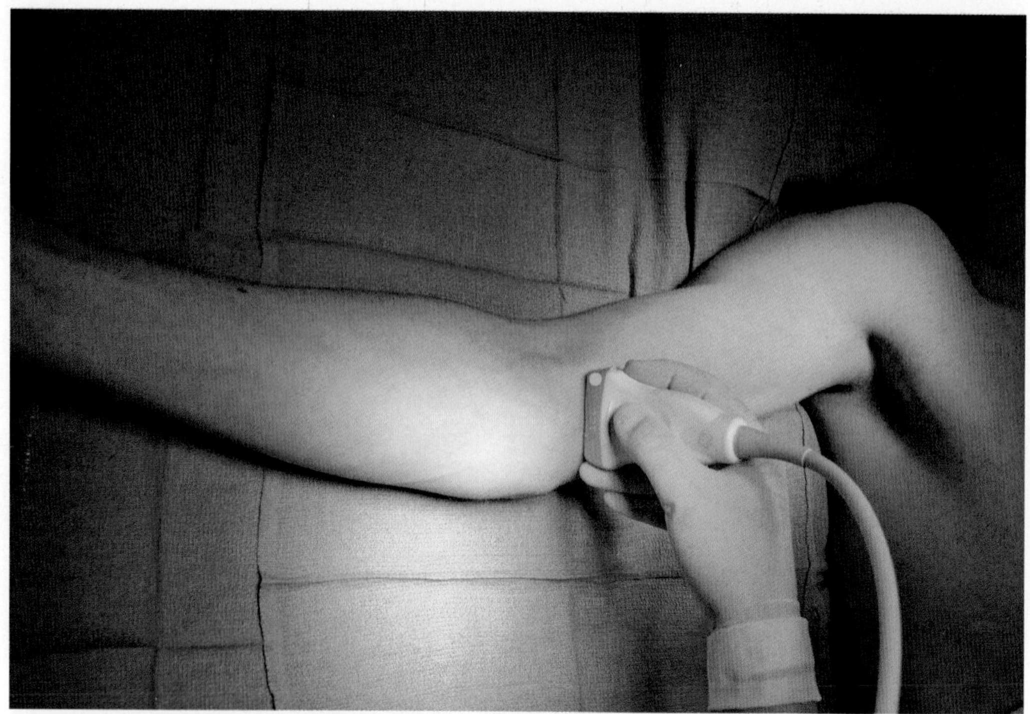

**FIGURE 7.22.1A** Ultrasound transducer position to image the medial antebrachial cutaneous nerve above the elbow.

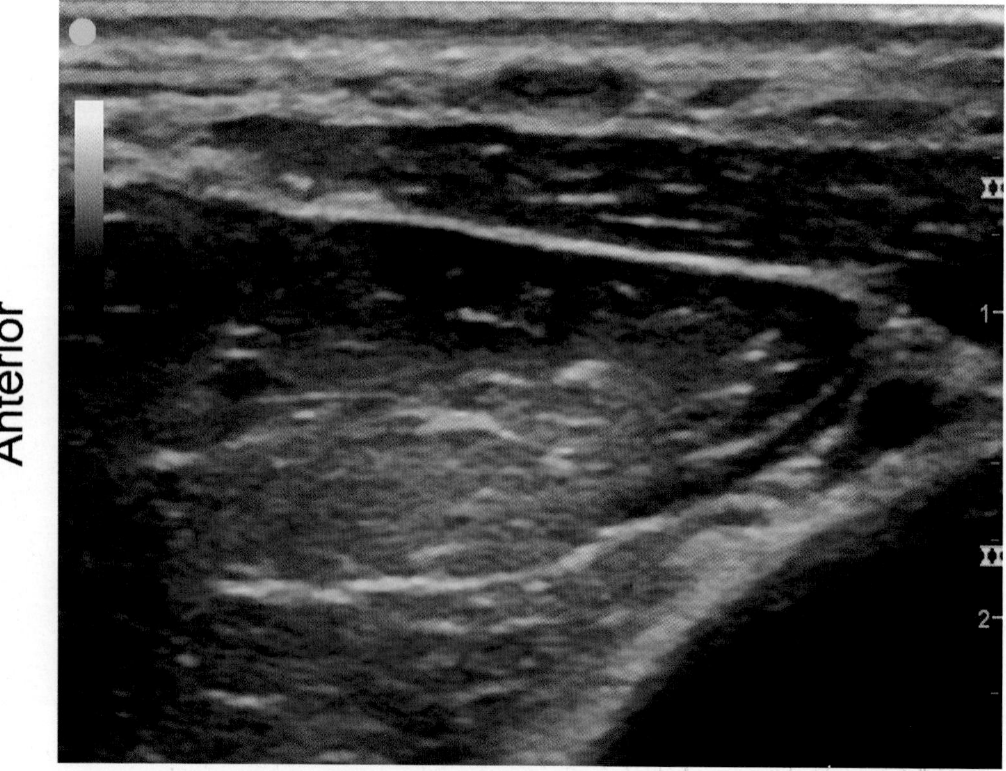


**FIGURE 7.22.1B** Ultrasound image of the medial antebrachial cutaneous nerve above the elbow.

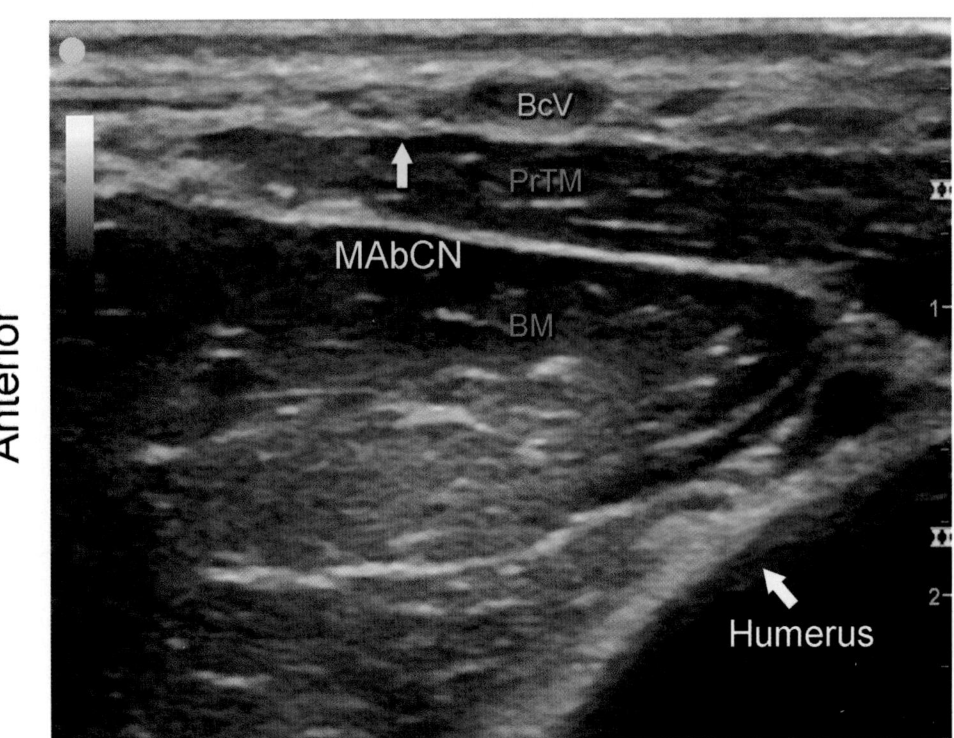


**FIGURE 7.22.1C** Labeled ultrasound image of the medial antebrachial cutaneous nerve above the elbow.

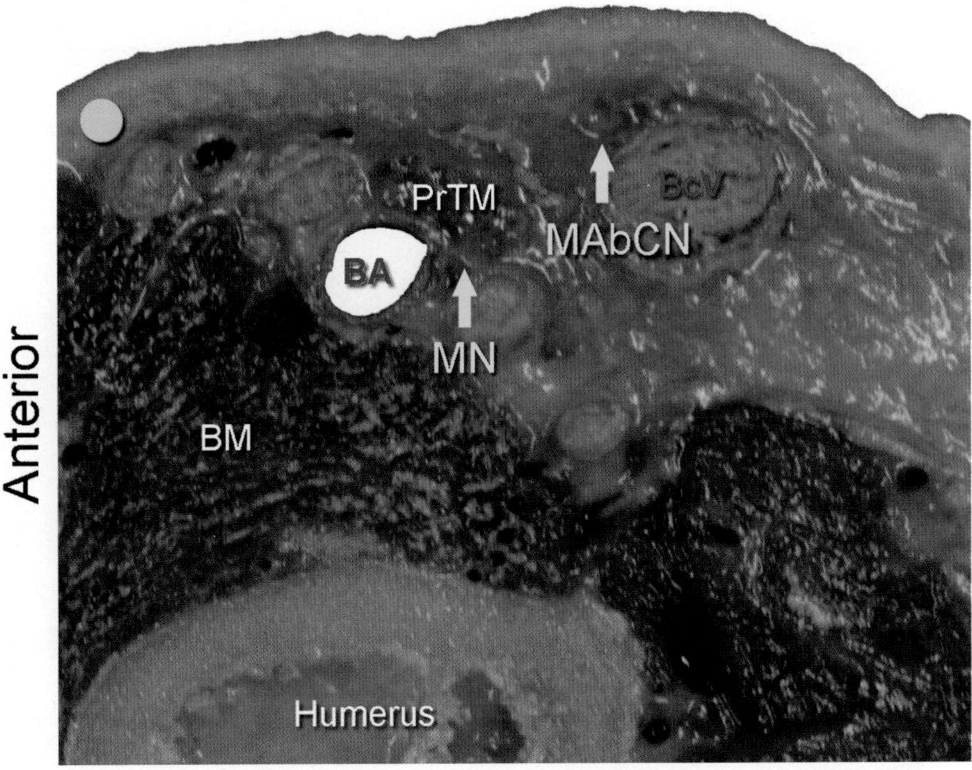


**FIGURE 7.22.1D** Labeled cross-sectional anatomy of the medial antebrachial cutaneous nerve above the elbow.

**Abbreviations:** BcV, Basilic Vein; PrTM, Pronator Teres Muscle; BM, Brachialis Muscle; MAbCN, Medial Antebrachial Cutaneous Nerve; MN, Median Nerve; BA, Brachial Artery.

# Biceps Tendon, Median, and Lateral Antebrachial Cutaneous Nerve at the Elbow

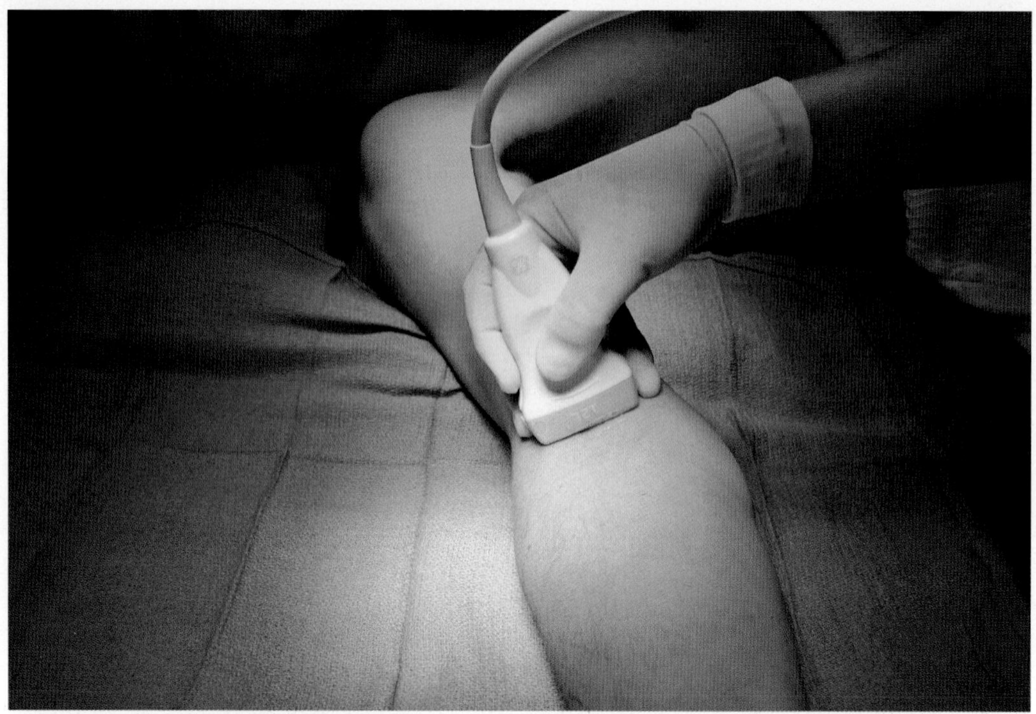

**FIGURE 7.23.1A** Ultrasound transducer position to image the biceps tendon, median, and lateral antebrachial cutaneous nerve at the elbow.

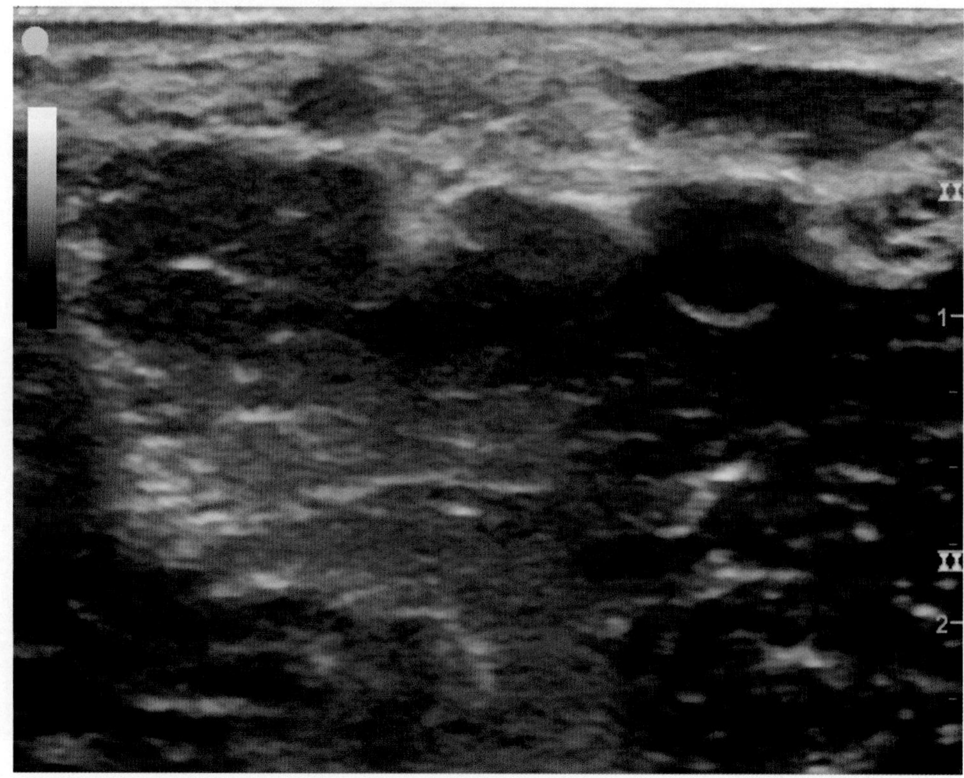


**FIGURE 7.23.1B** Ultrasound image of the biceps tendon, median, and lateral antebrachial cutaneous nerve at the elbow.

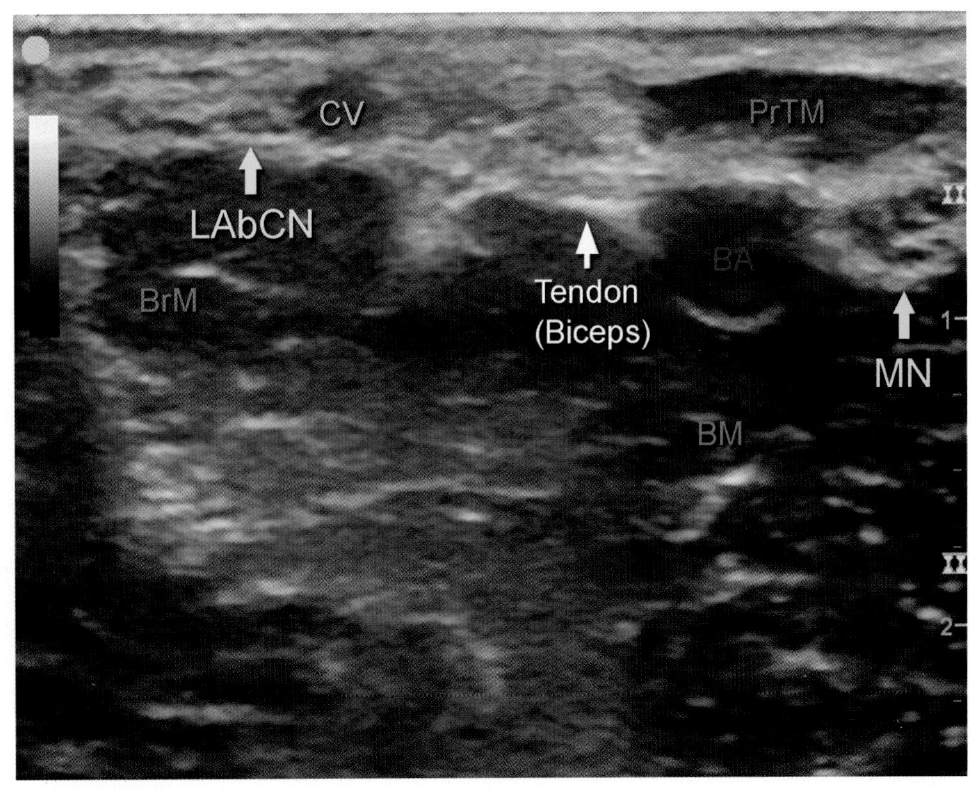


**FIGURE 7.23.1C** Labeled ultrasound image of the biceps tendon, median, and lateral antebrachial cutaneous nerve at the elbow.

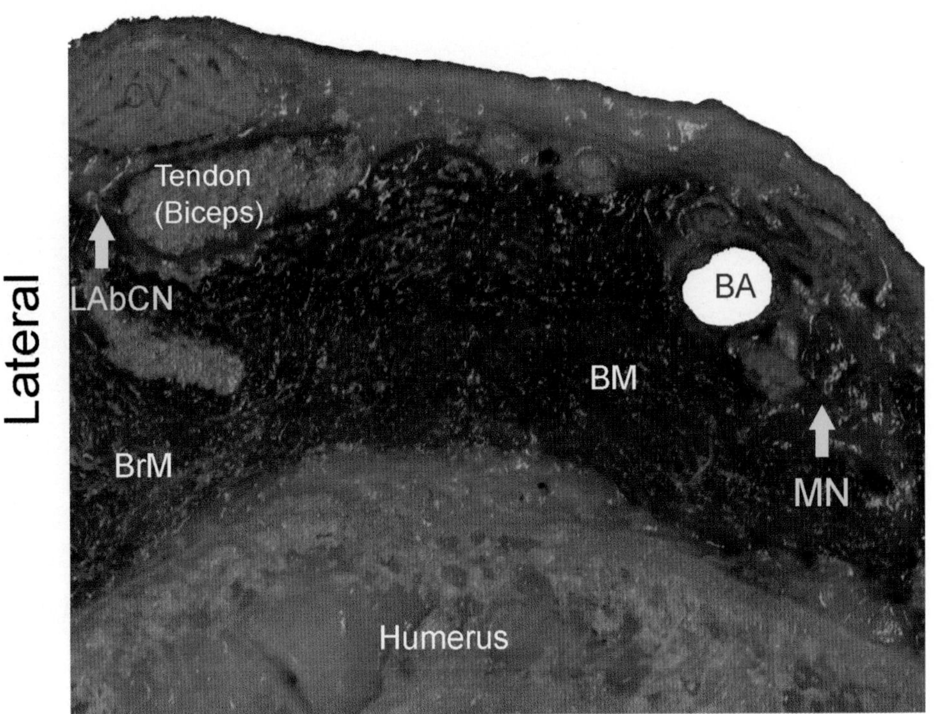


**FIGURE 7.23.1D** Labeled cross-sectional anatomy of the biceps tendon, median, and lateral antebrachial cutaneous nerve at the elbow.

**Abbreviations:** CV, Cephalic Vein; PrTM, Pronator Teres Muscle; BM, Brachialis Muscle; LAbCN, Lateral Antebrachial Cutaneous Nerve; MN, Median Nerve; BA, Brachial Artery; BrM, Brachioradialis Muscle.

# Median Nerve at the Elbow

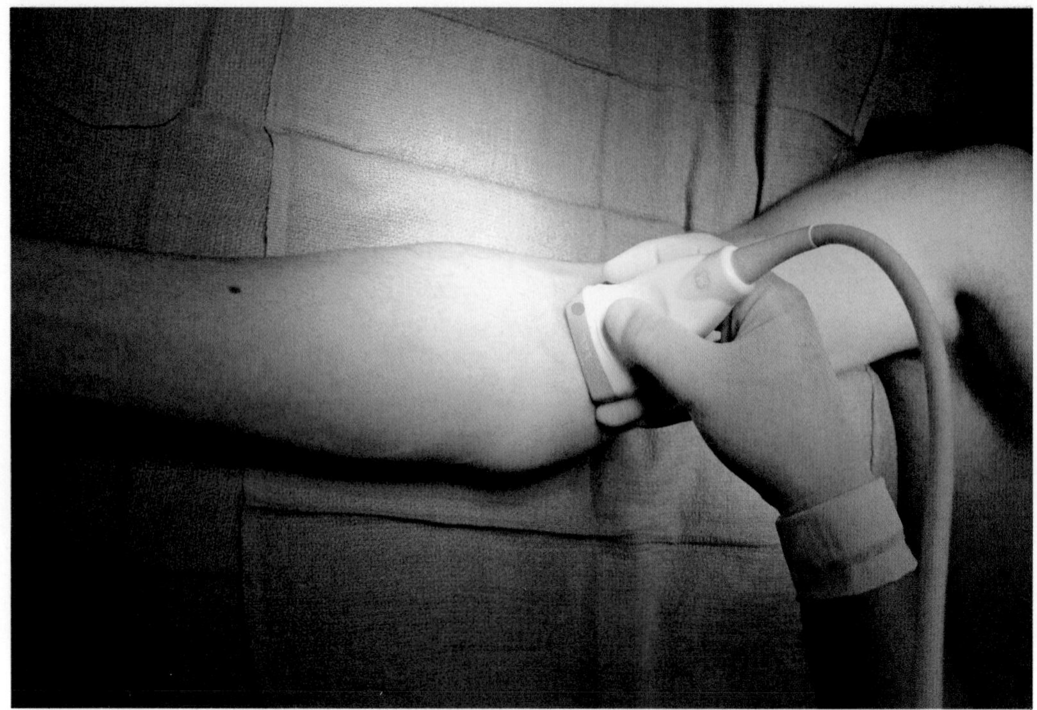

**FIGURE 7.24.1A** Ultrasound transducer position to image the median nerve at the elbow.

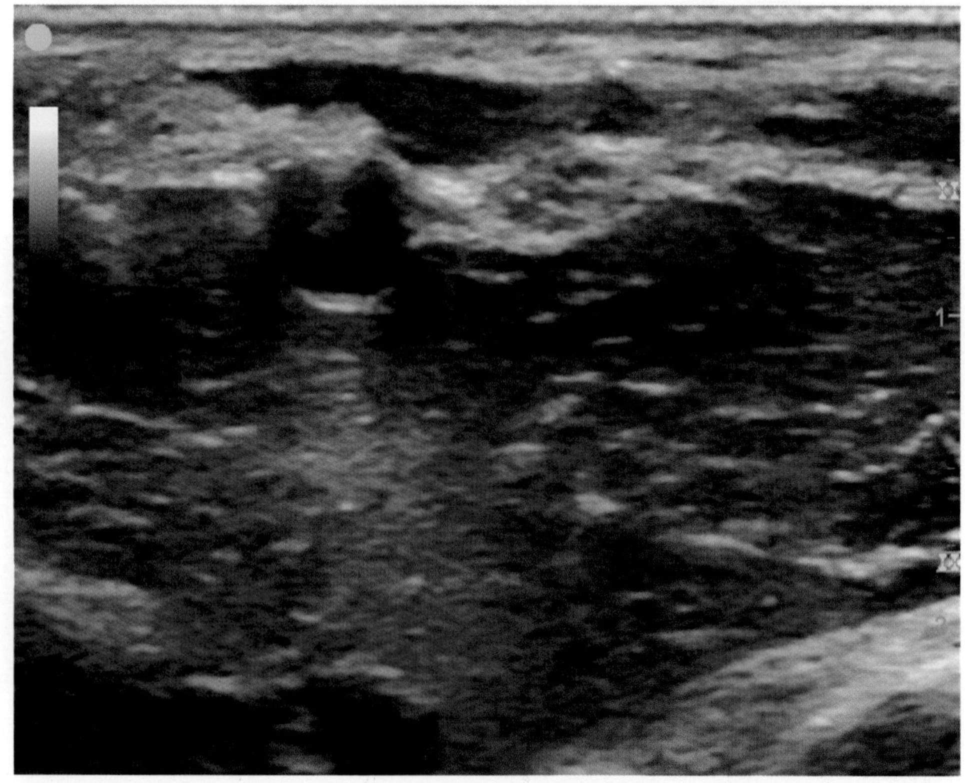


**FIGURE 7.24.1B** Ultrasound image of the median nerve at the elbow.

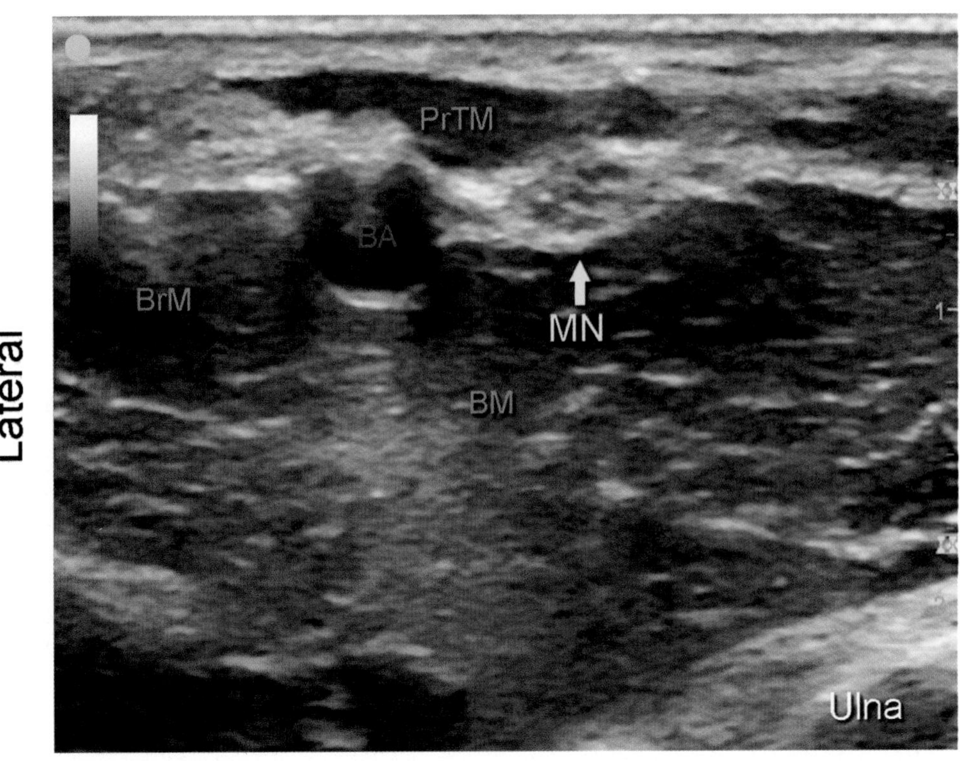


**FIGURE 7.24.1C** Labeled ultrasound image of the median nerve at the elbow.

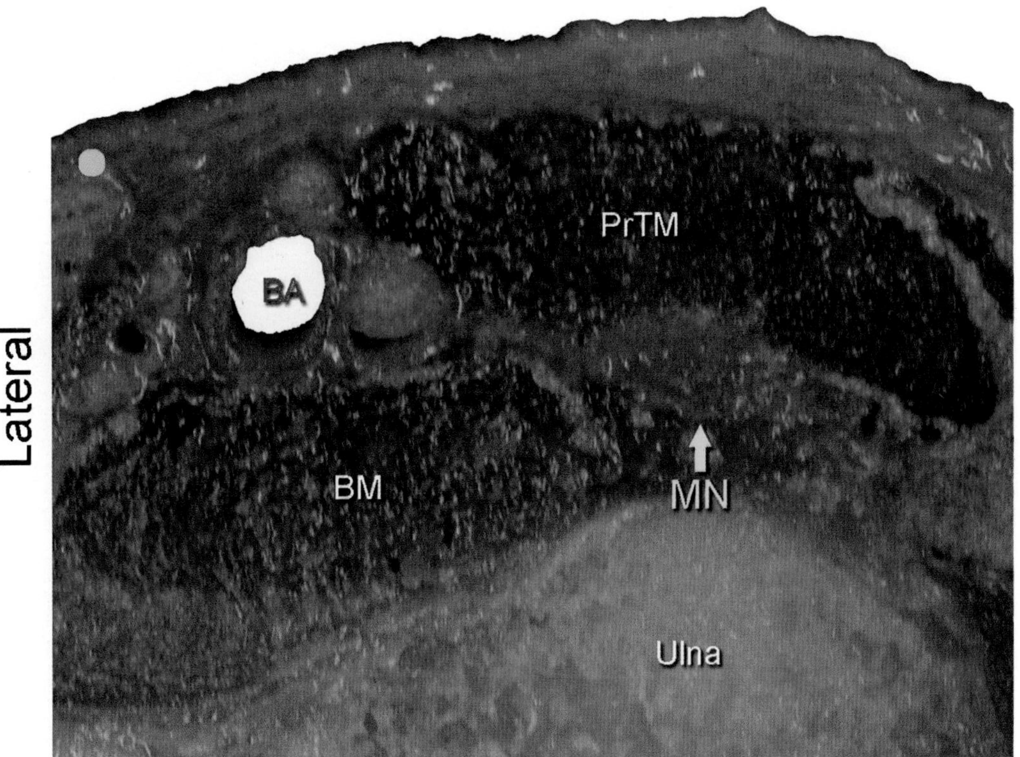


**FIGURE 7.24.1D** Labeled cross-sectional anatomy of the median nerve at the elbow.

**Abbreviations:** MN, Median Nerve; BM, Brachialis Muscle; BA, Brachial Artery; PrTM, Pronator Teres Muscle; BrM, Brachioradialis Muscle.

# Radial Nerve at the Midforearm

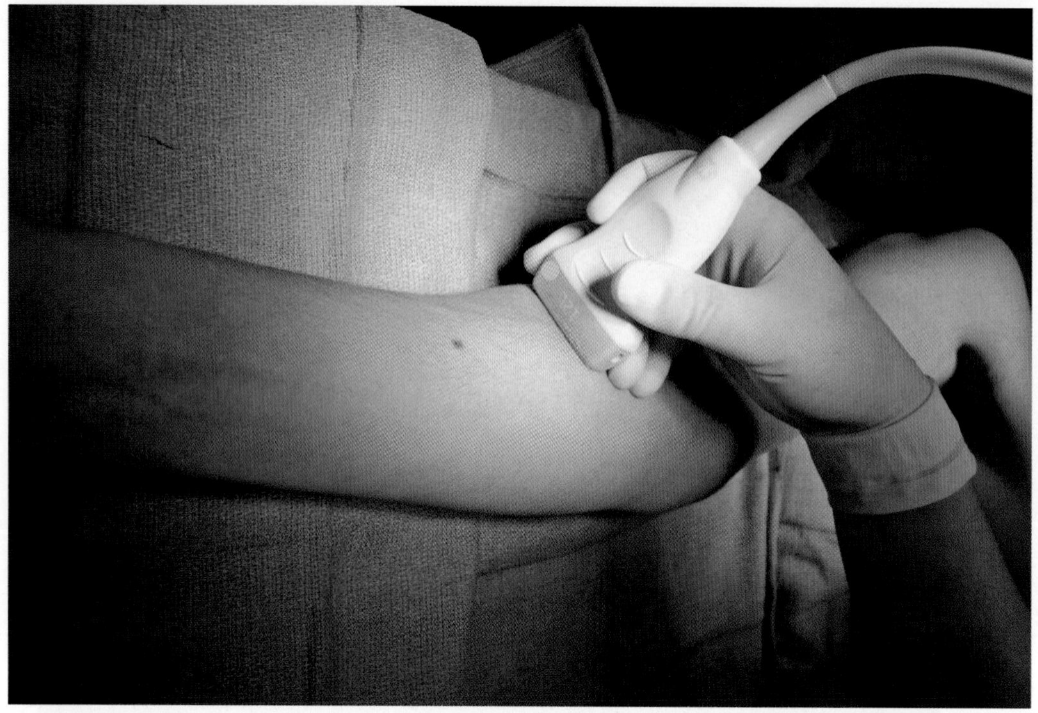

**FIGURE 7.25.1A** Ultrasound transducer position to image the radial nerve at the midforearm.

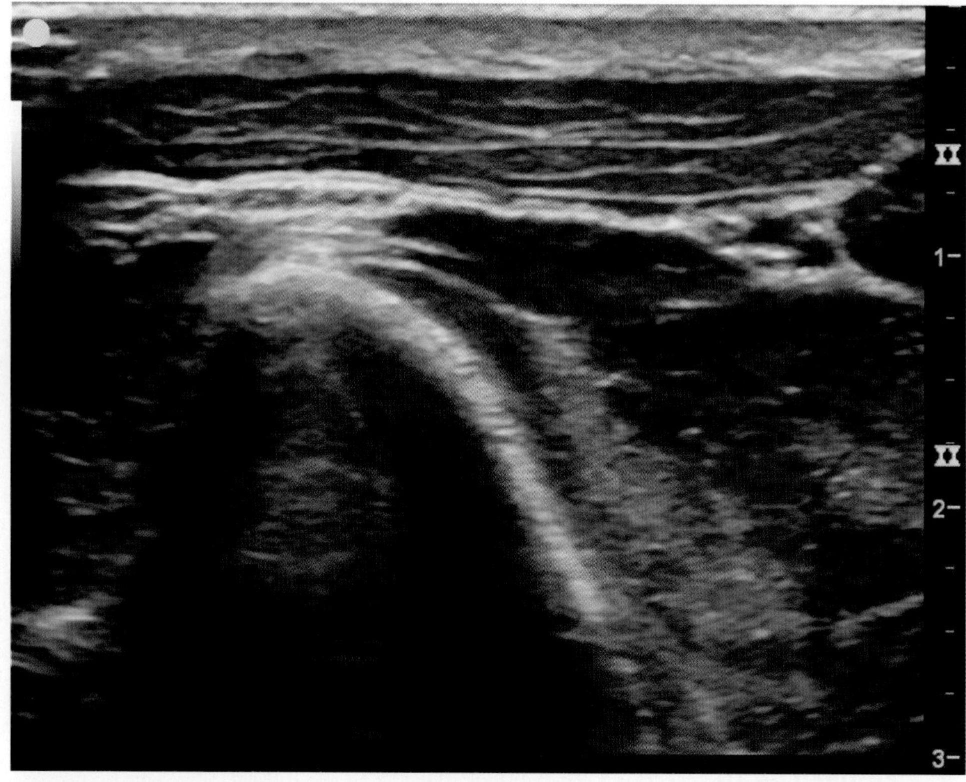


**FIGURE 7.25.1B** Ultrasound image of the radial nerve at the midforearm.

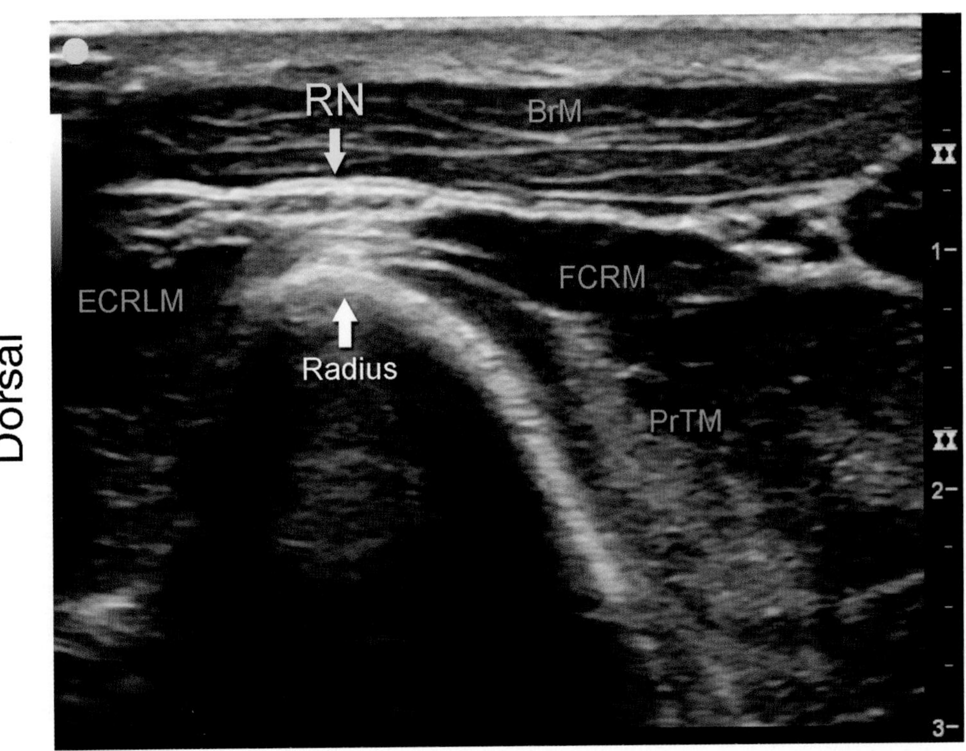


**FIGURE 7.25.1C** Labeled ultrasound image of the radial nerve at the midforearm.

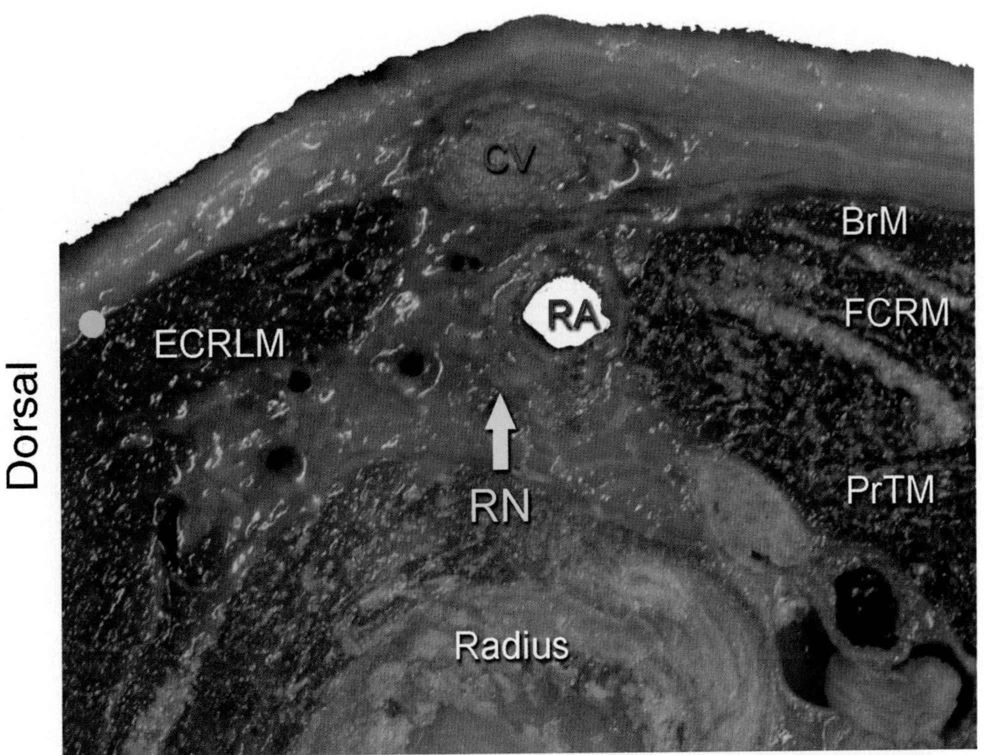


**FIGURE 7.25.1D** Labeled cross-sectional anatomy of the radial nerve at the midforearm.

**Abbreviations:** RN, Radial Nerve; ECRLM, Extensor Carpi Radialis Longus Muscle; FCRM, Flexor Carpi Radialis Muscle; BrM, Brachioradialis Muscle; PrTM, Pronator Teres Muscle, CV, Cephalic Vein; RA, Radial Artery.

# Median and Ulnar Nerve at the Midforearm

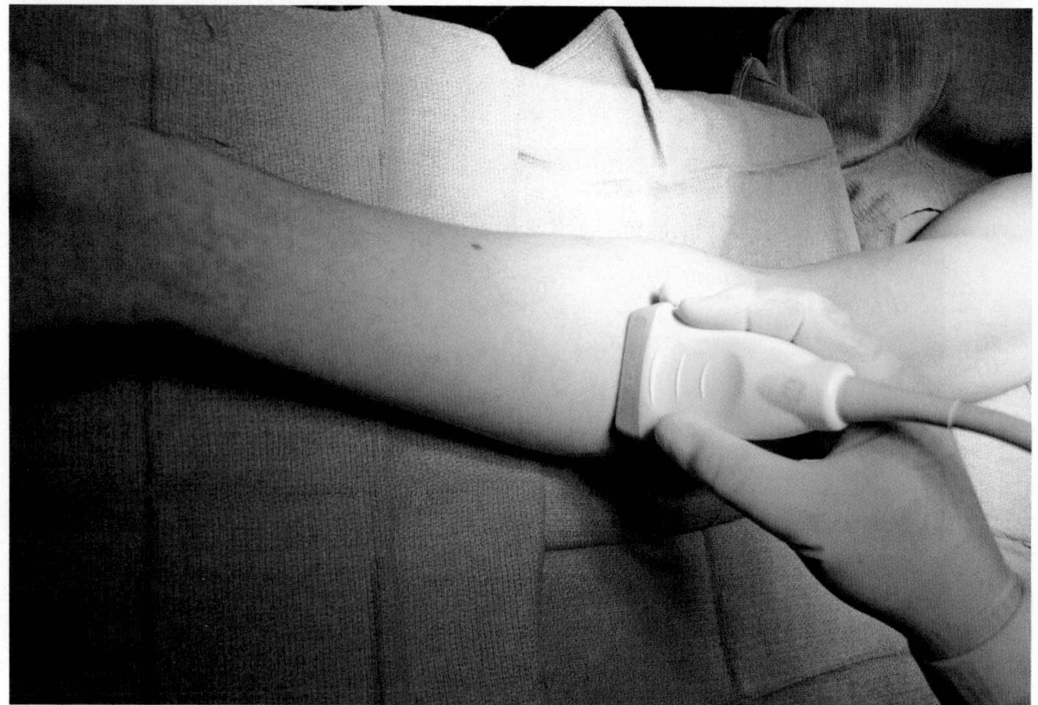

**FIGURE 7.26.1A** Ultrasound transducer position to image the median and ulnar nerve at the midforearm.

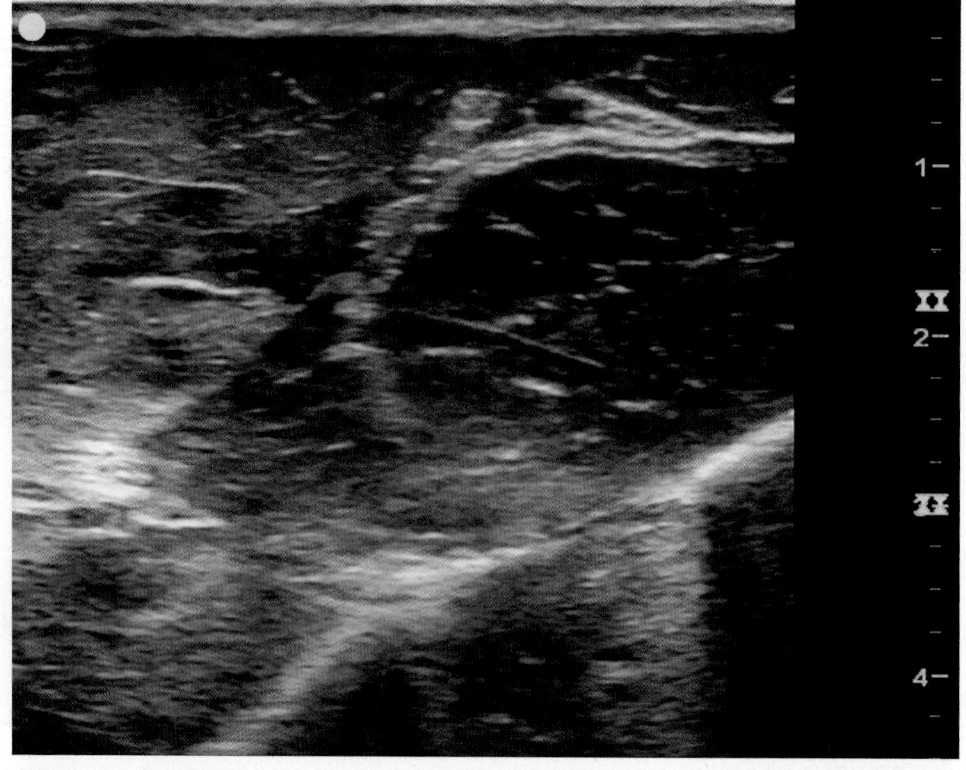


**FIGURE 7.26.1B** Ultrasound image of the median and ulnar nerve at the midforearm.

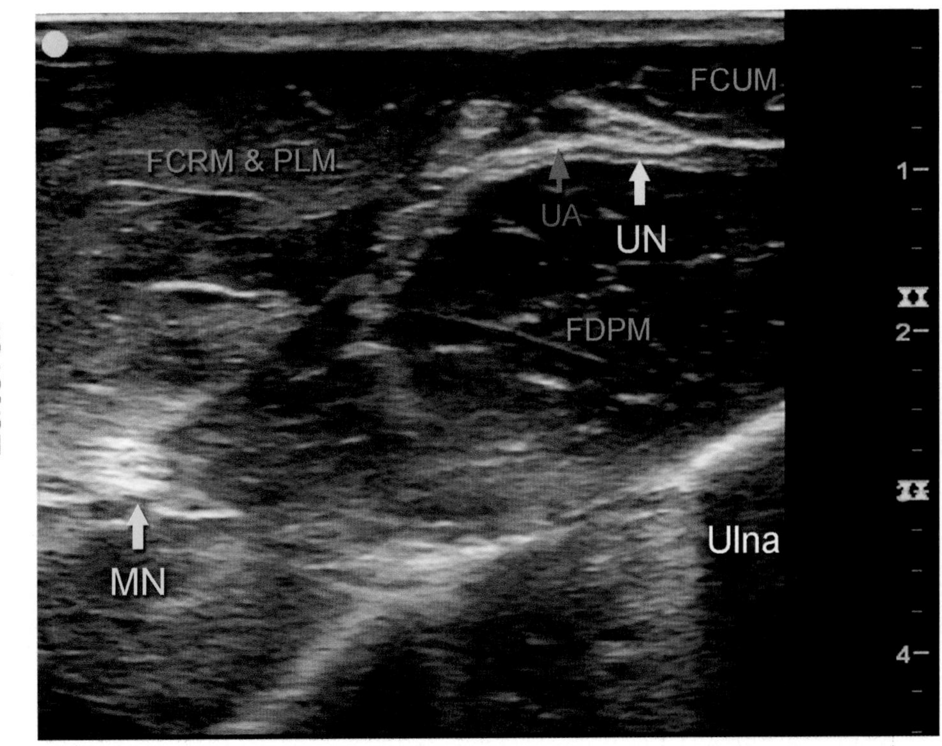


**FIGURE 7.26.1C** Labeled ultrasound image of the median and ulnar nerve at the midforearm.

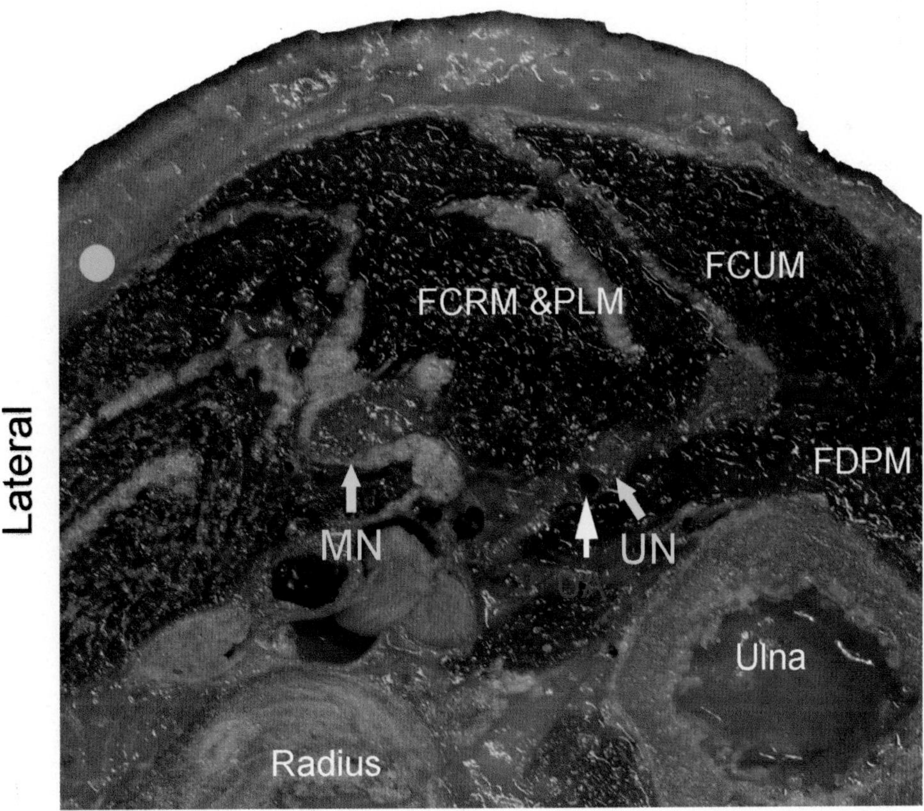


**FIGURE 7.26.1D** Labeled cross-sectional anatomy of the median and ulnar nerve at the midforearm.

**Abbreviations:** MN, Median Nerve; UN, Ulnar Nerve; UA, Ulnar Artery; FDPM, Flexor Digitorum Profundus Muscle; FCUM, Flexor Carpi Ulnaris Muscle; FCRM, Flexor Carpi Radialis Muscle; PLM, Palmaris Longus Muscle.

# Posterior Interosseous Nerve at the Midforearm

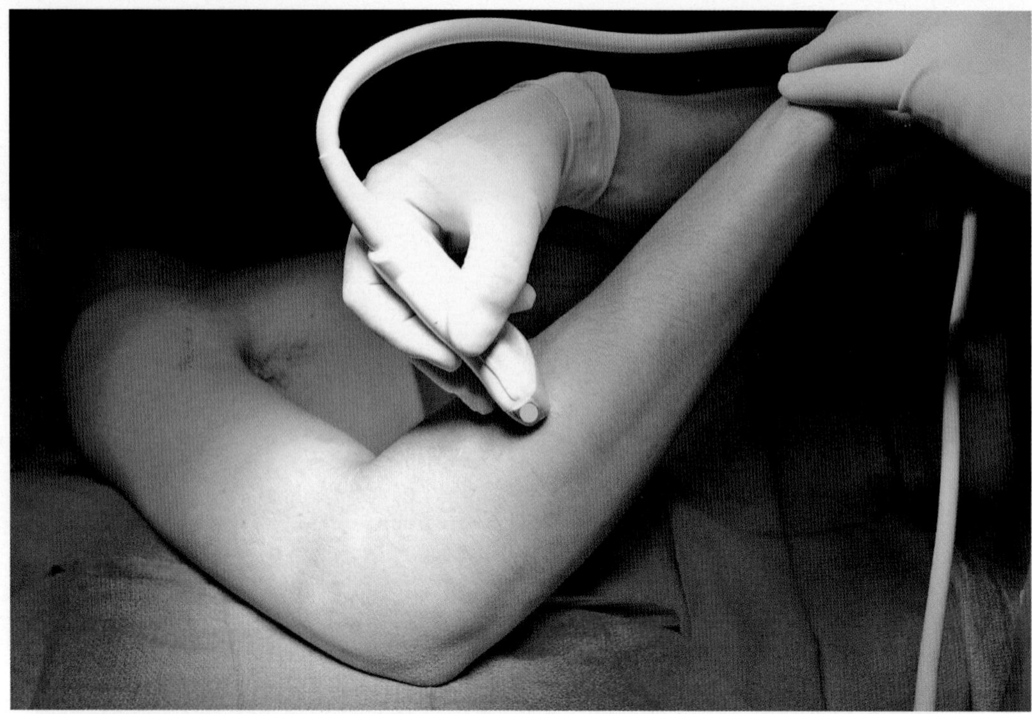

**FIGURE 7.27.1A** Ultrasound transducer position to image the posterior interosseous nerve at the Midforearm.

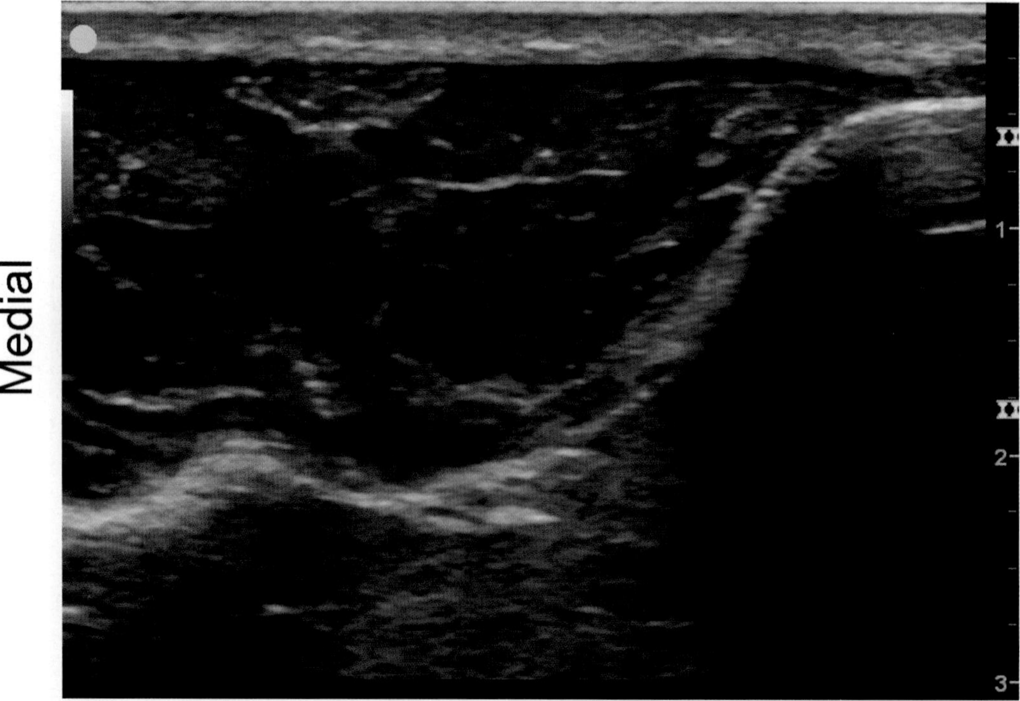


**FIGURE 7.27.1B** Ultrasound image of the posterior interosseous nerve at the Midforearm.

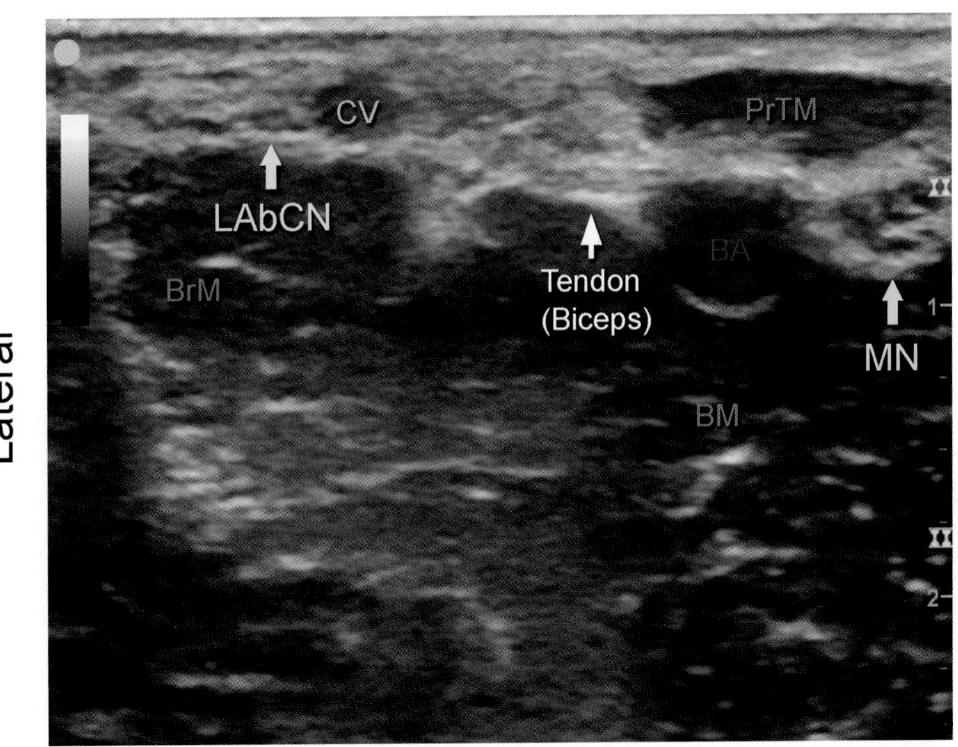


**FIGURE 7.27.1C** Labeled ultrasound image of the posterior interosseous nerve at the midhumerus.

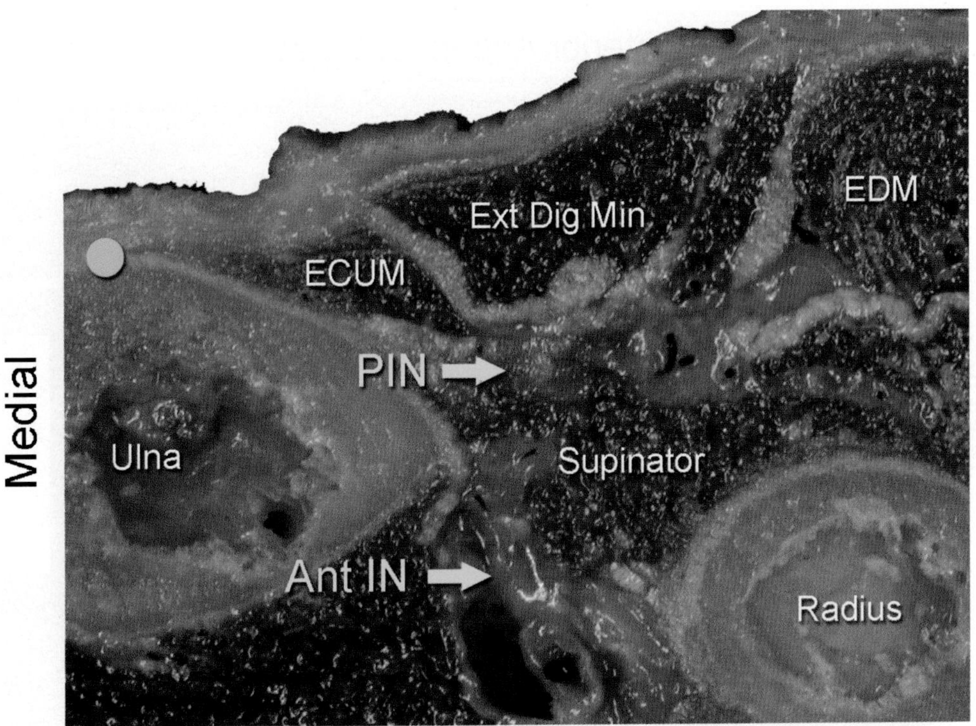


**FIGURE 7.27.1D** Labeled cross-sectional anatomy of the posterior interosseous nerve at the Midforearm.

**Abbreviations:** EDM, Extensor Digitorum Muscle; ECUM, Extensor Carpi Ulnaris Muscle; Ant.IN, Anterior Interosseous Nerve; PIN, Posterior Interosseous Nerve.

## Posterior Interosseous Nerve at the Wrist

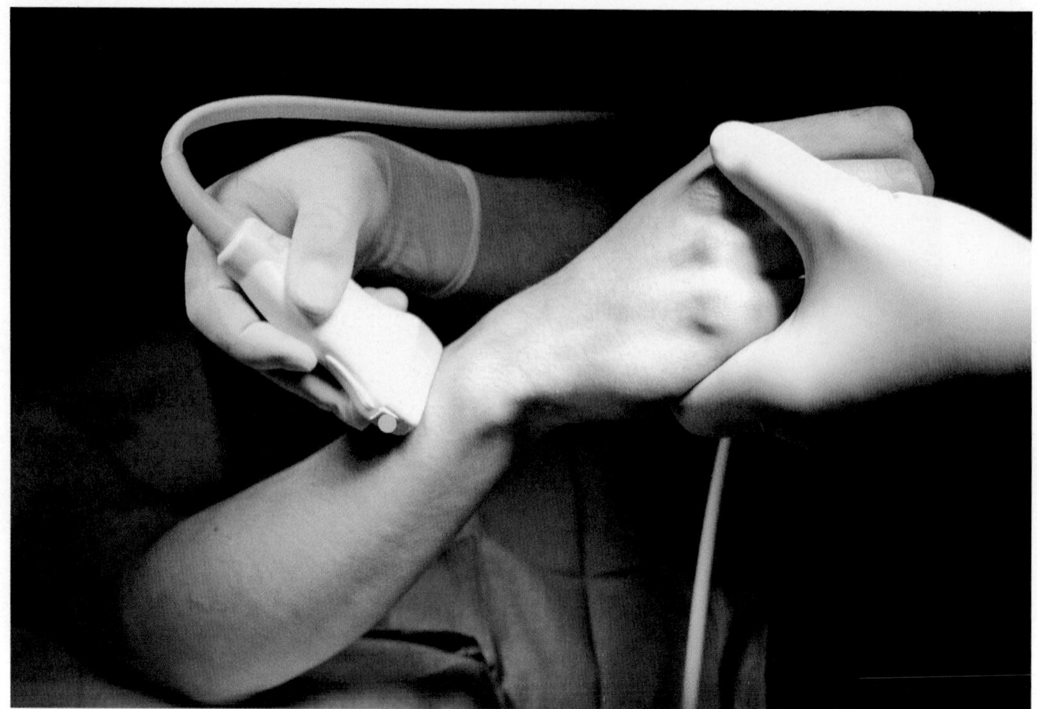

**FIGURE 7.28.1A** Ultrasound transducer position to image the posterior interosseous nerve at the wrist.

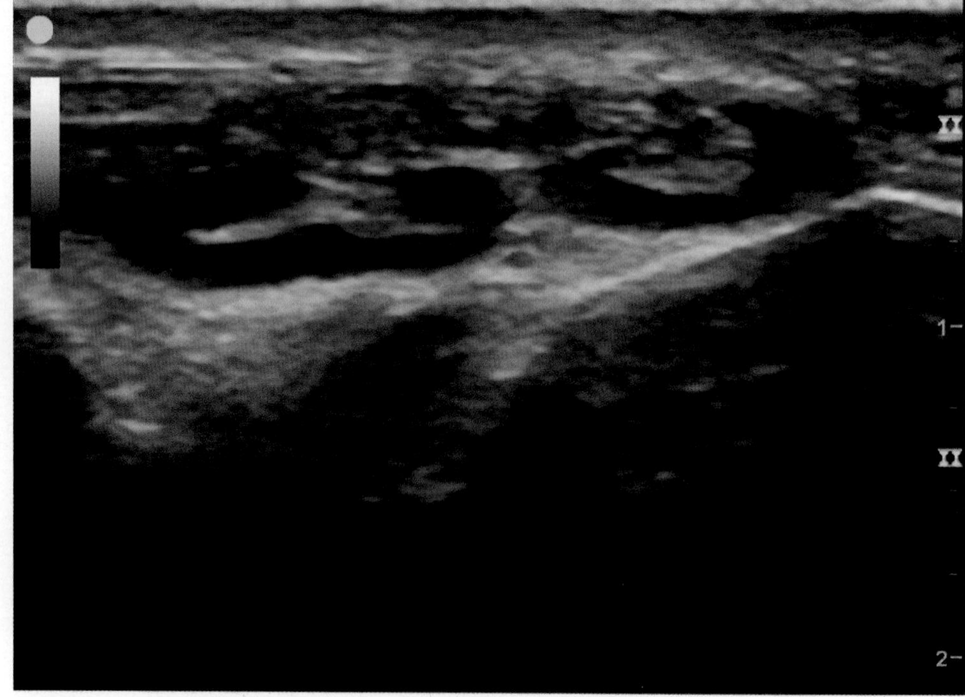


**FIGURE 7.28.1B** Ultrasound image of the posterior interosseous nerve at the wrist.

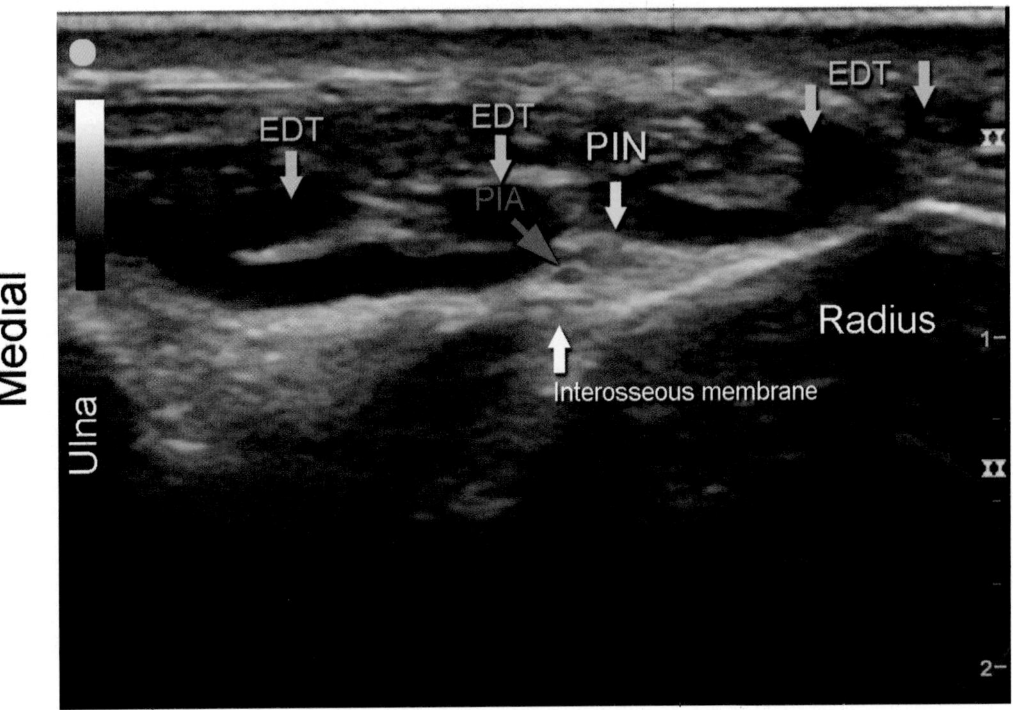


**FIGURE 7.28.1C** Labeled ultrasound image of the posterior interosseous nerve at the wrist.

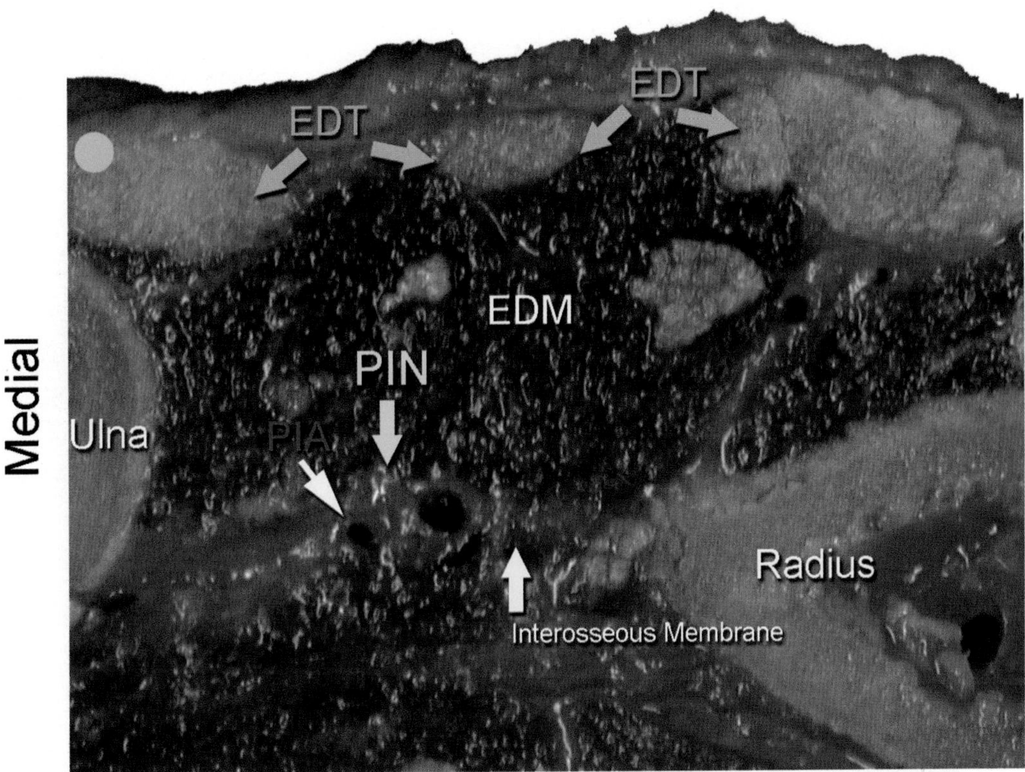


**FIGURE 7.28.1D** Labeled cross-sectional anatomy of the posterior interosseous nerve at the wrist.

**Abbreviations:** PIN, Posterior Interosseous Nerve; PIA, Posterior Interosseous Artery; EDT, Extensor Digitorum Tendon.

# Radial Nerve and Palmar Cutaneous Branches at the Wrist

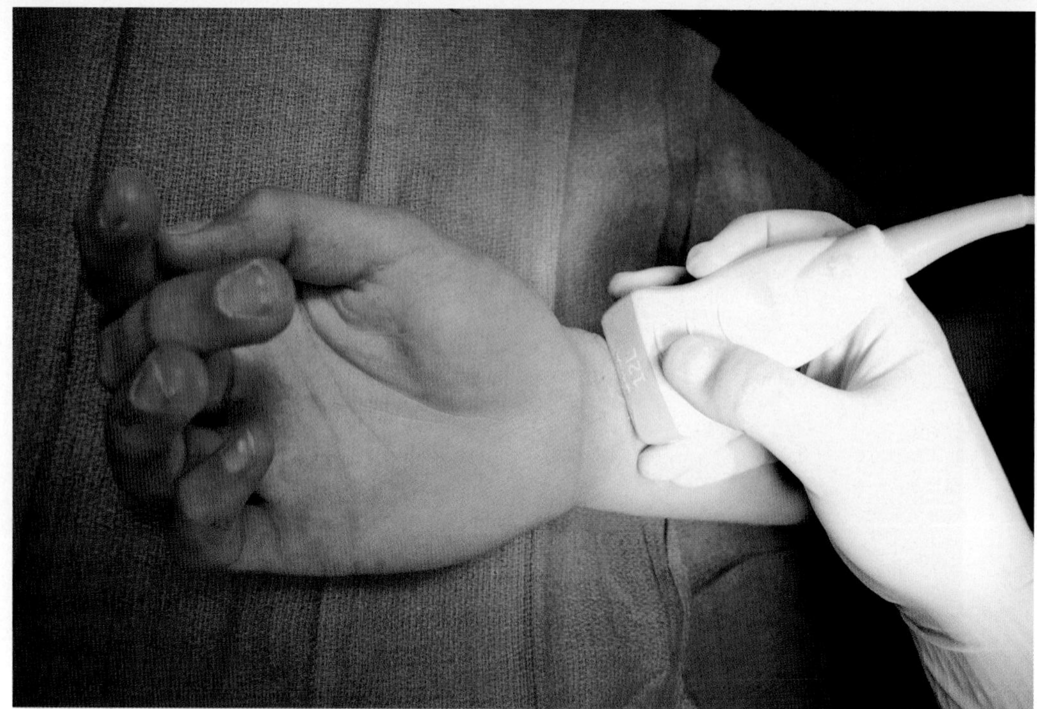

**FIGURE 7.29.1A** Ultrasound transducer position to image the radial nerve and palmar cutaneous branches at the wrist.

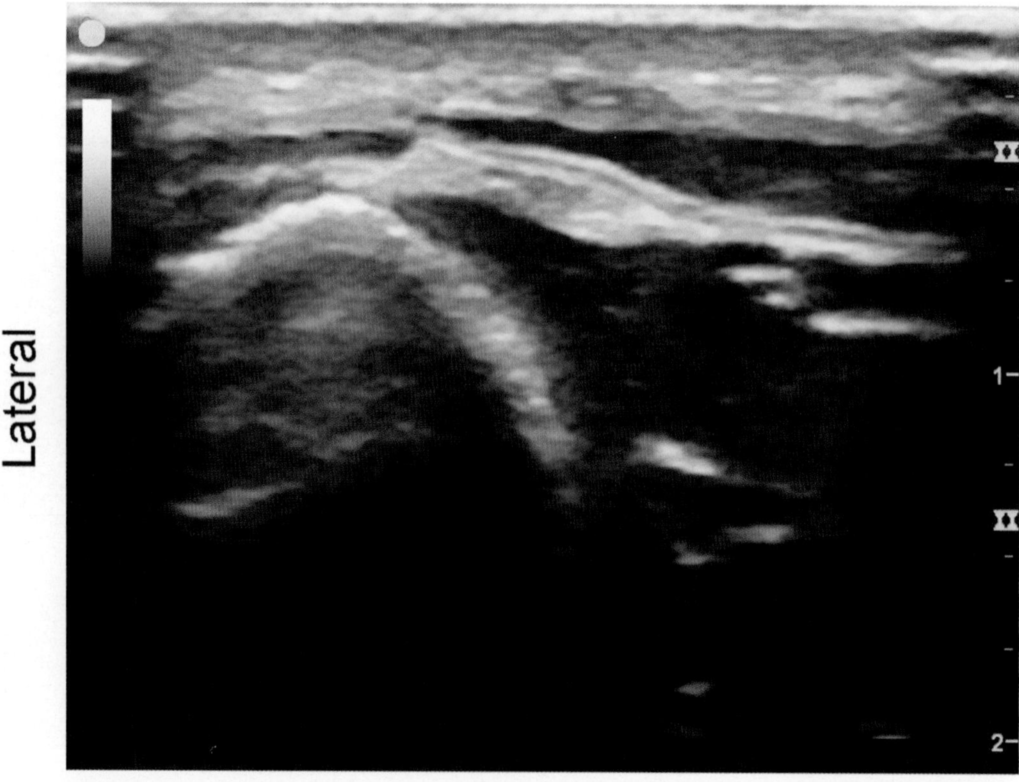


**FIGURE 7.29.1B** Ultrasound image of the radial nerve palmar cutaneous branches at the wrist.

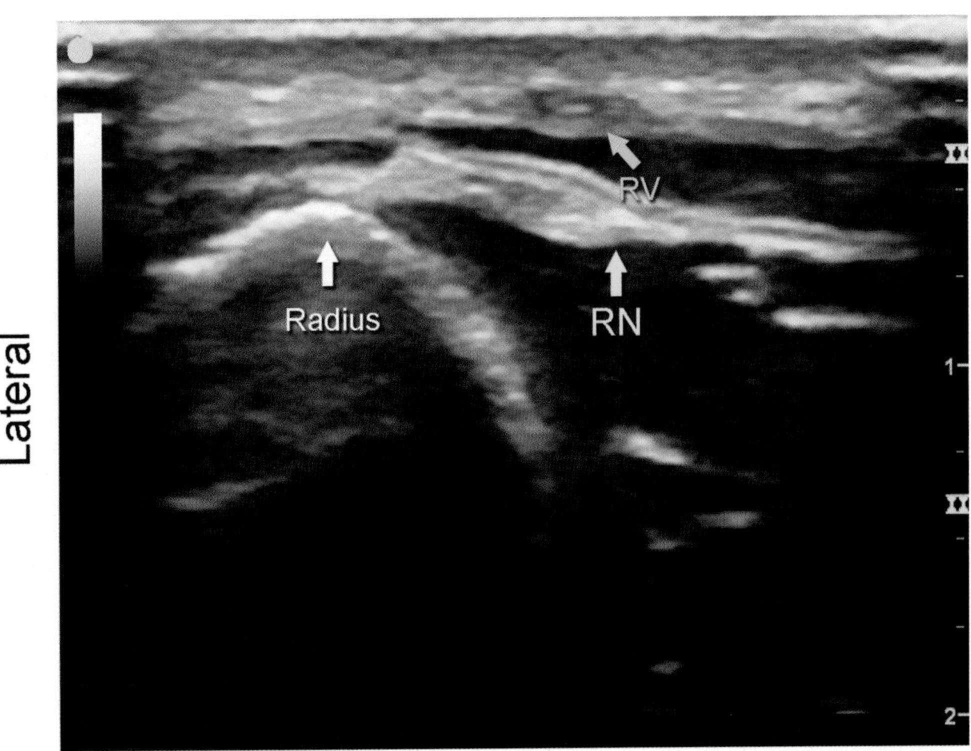


FIGURE 7.29.1C Labeled ultrasound image of the radial nerve and palmar cutaneous branches at the wrist.

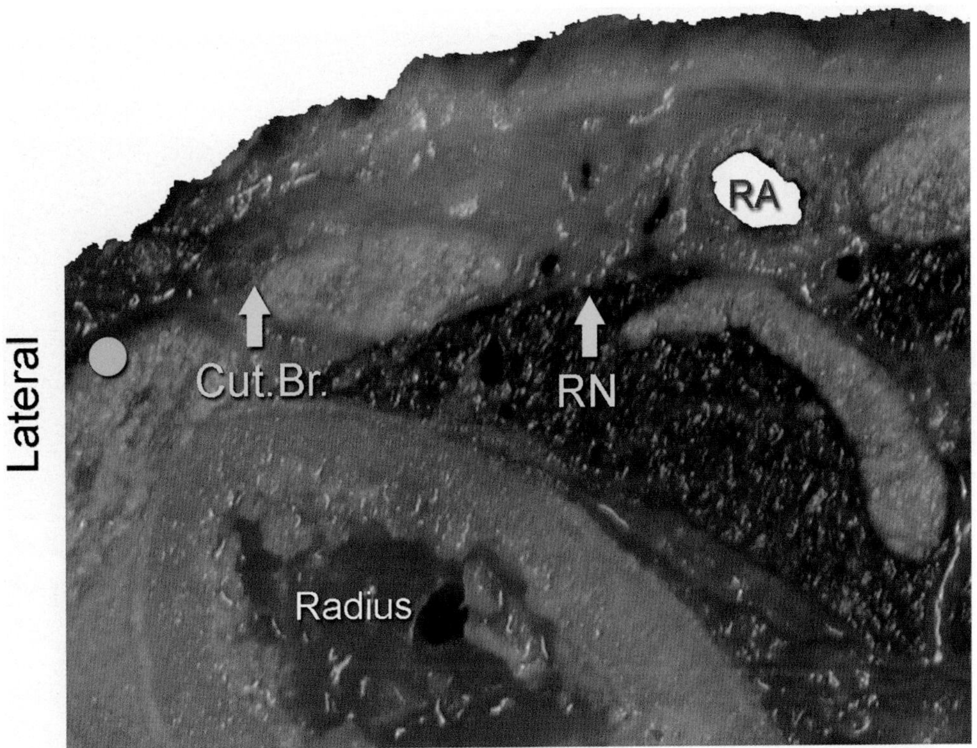


FIGURE 7.29.1D Labeled cross-sectional anatomy of the radial nerve palmar cutaneous branches at the wrist.

**Abbreviations:** Cut. Br., Cutaneous Branche; RN, Radial Nerve; RA, Radial Artery; RV, Radial Vein.

# Radial Nerve

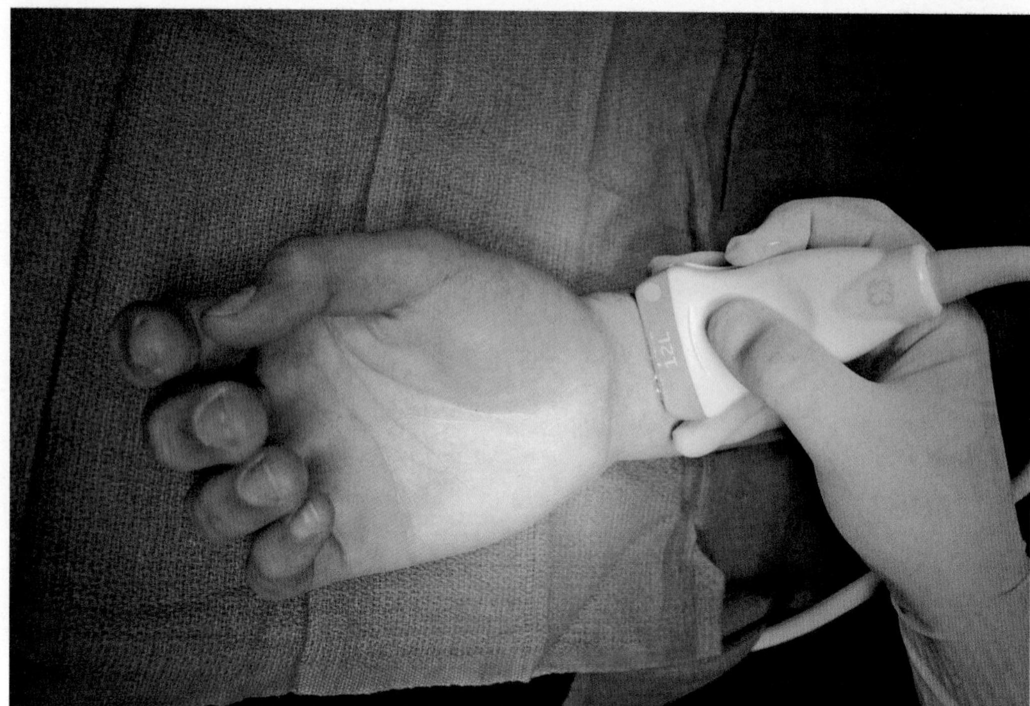


**FIGURE 7.30.1A** Ultrasound transducer position to image the radial nerve.

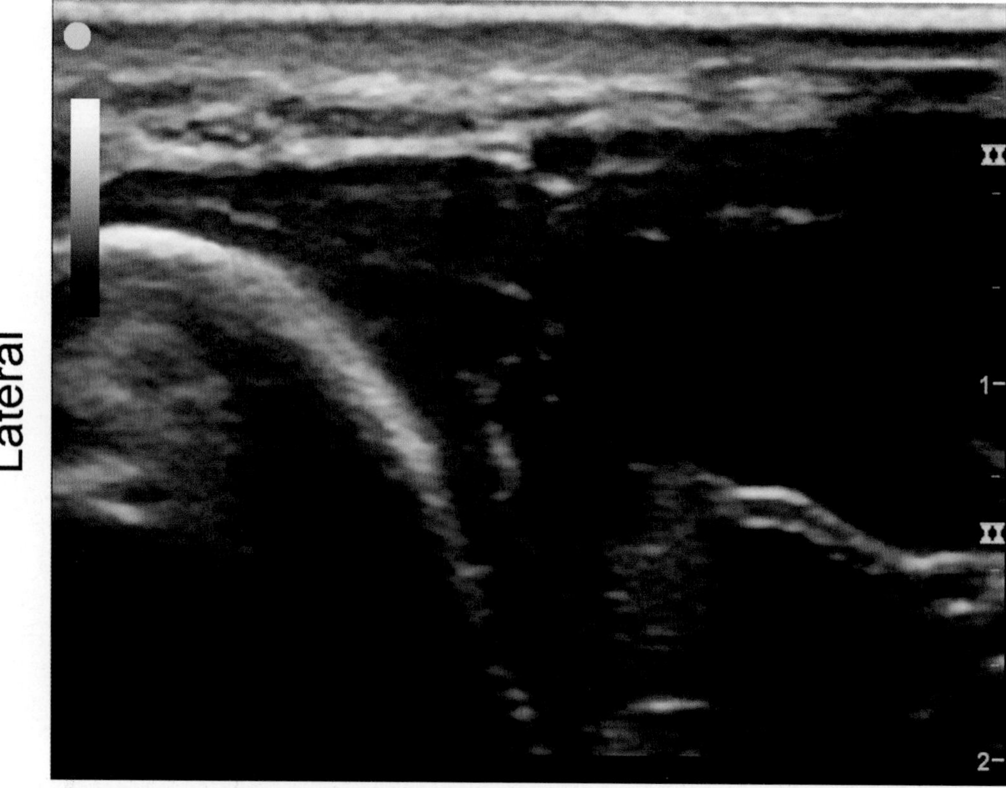


**FIGURE 7.30.1B** Ultrasound image of the radial nerve.

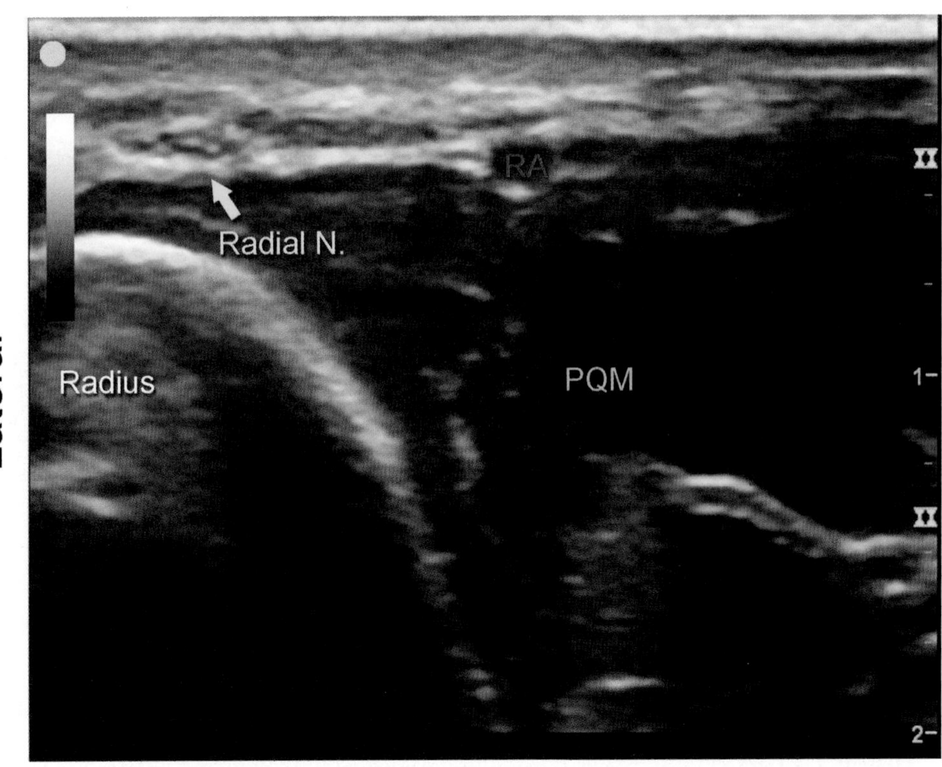


**FIGURE 7.30.1C** Labeled ultrasound image of the radial nerve.

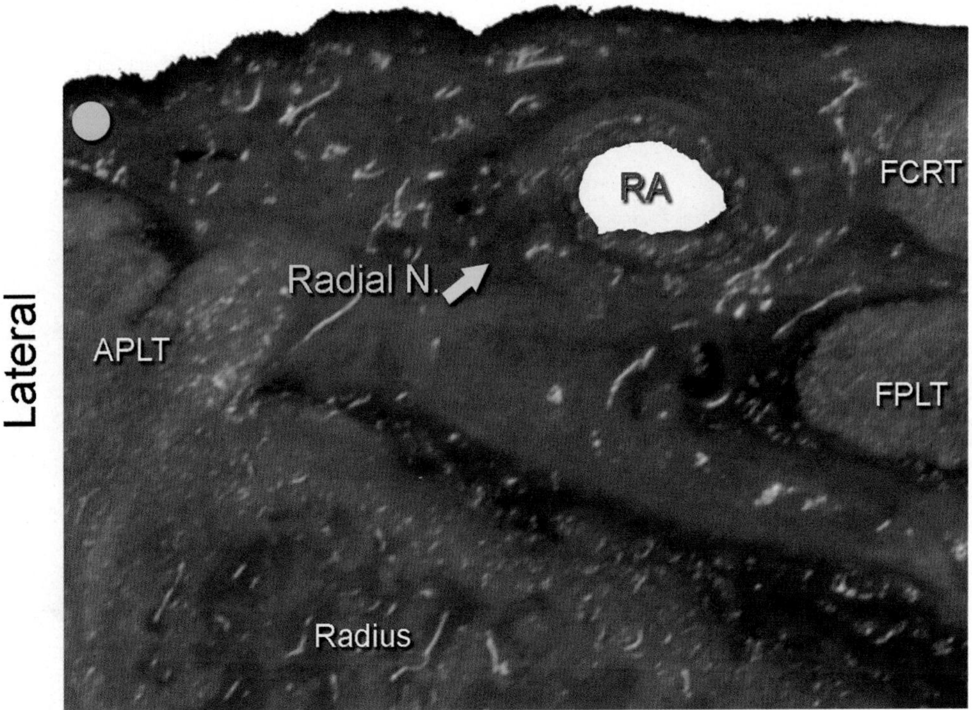


**FIGURE 7.30.1D** Labeled cross-sectional anatomy of the radial nerve.

**Abbreviations:** RA, Radial Artery; PQM, Pronator Quadratus Muscle; FPLT, Flexor Pollicus Longus Tendon; FCRT, Flexor Carpi Radialis Tendon; APLT, Abductor Pollicis Longus Tendon.

## Median Nerve at the Wrist

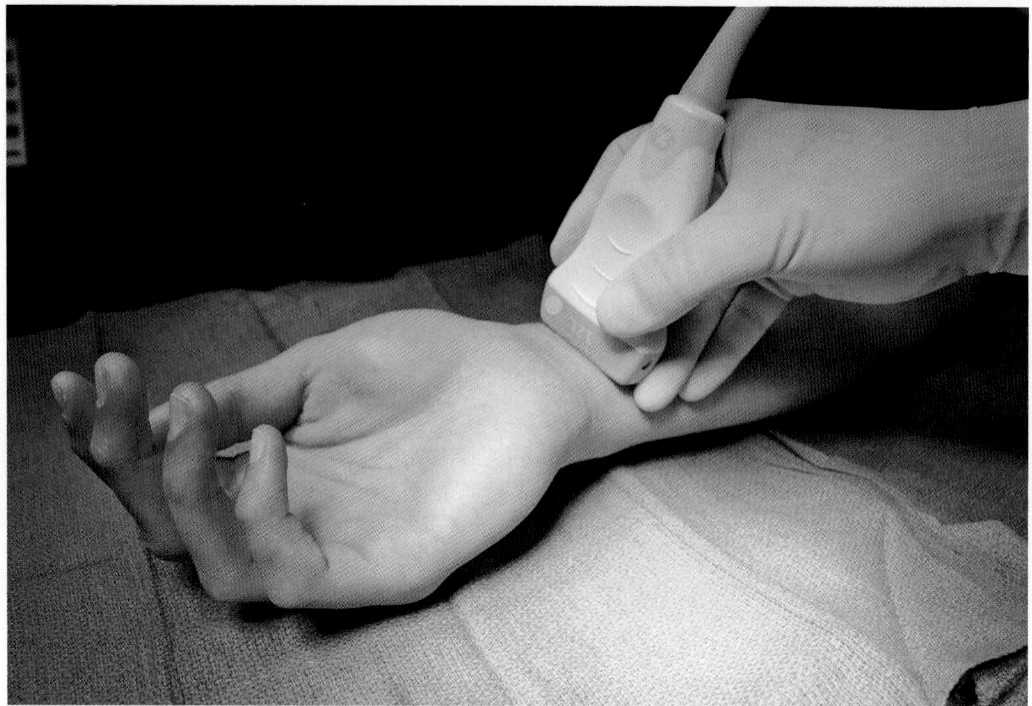

**FIGURE 7.31.1A** Ultrasound transducer position to image the median nerve at the wrist.

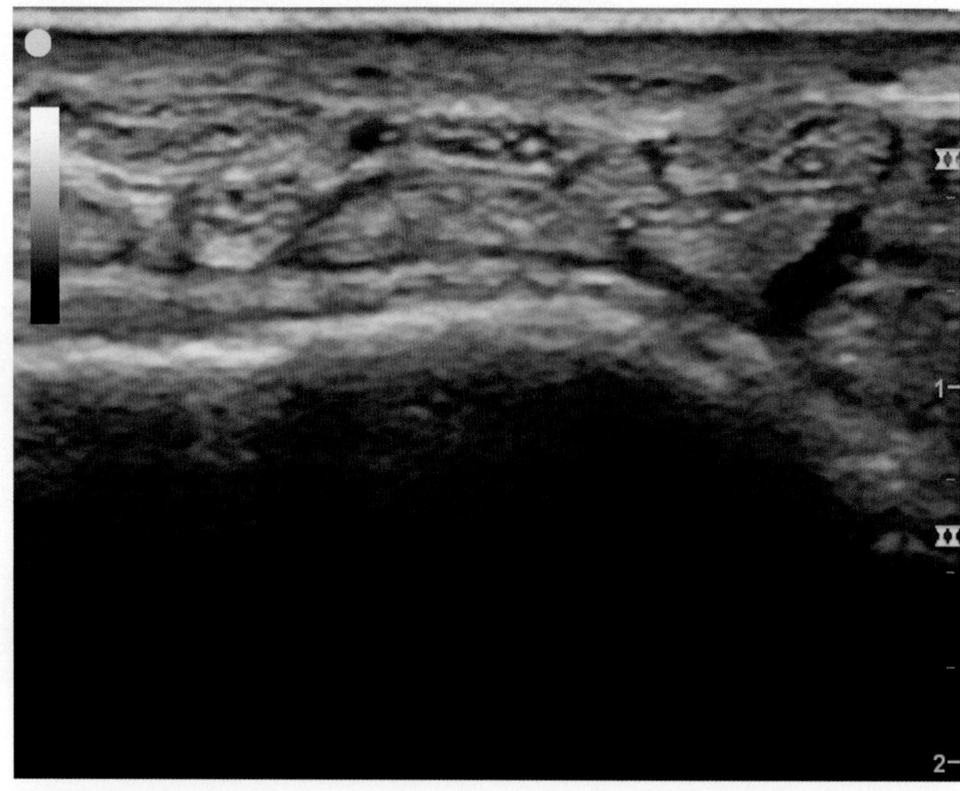


**FIGURE 7.31.1B** Ultrasound image of the median nerve at the wrist.

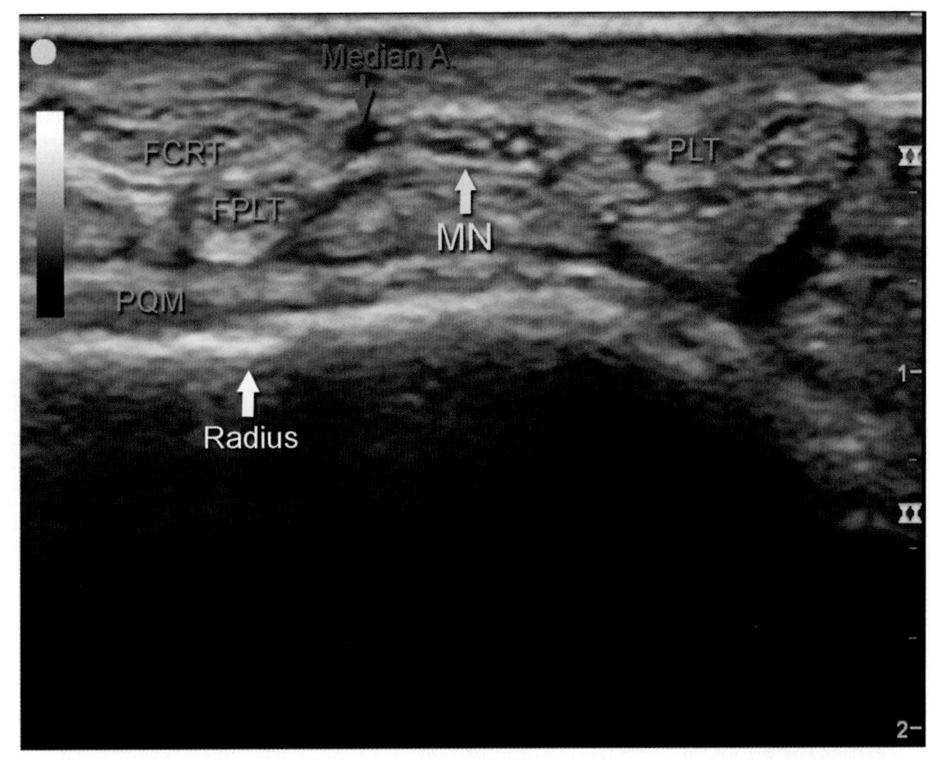


**FIGURE 7.31.1C** Labeled ultrasound image of the median nerve at the wrist.

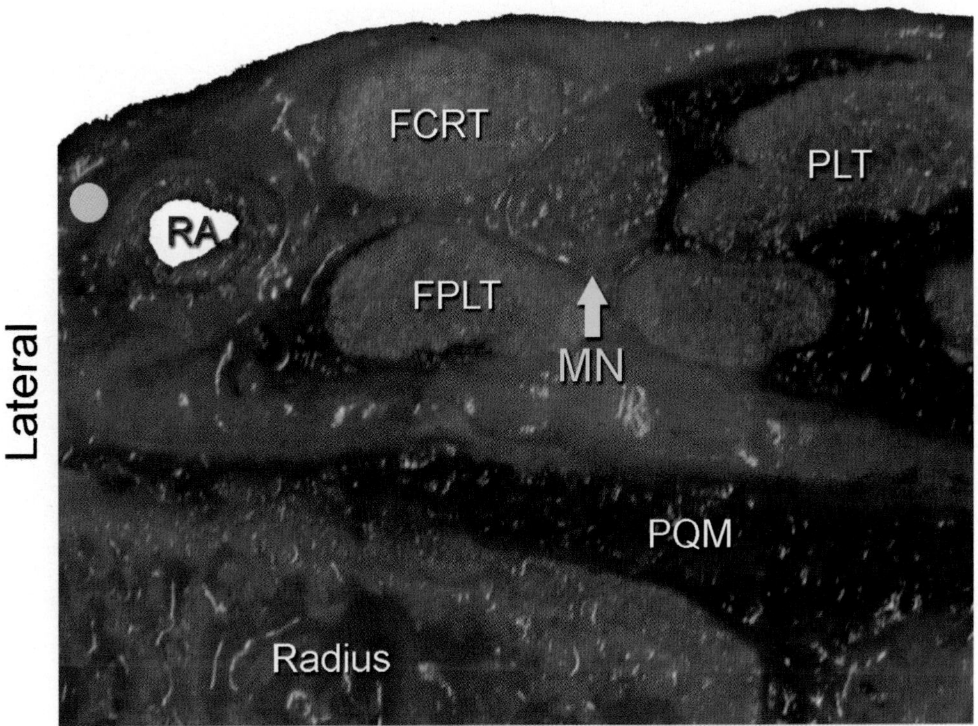


**FIGURE 7.31.1D** Labeled cross-sectional anatomy of the median nerve at the wrist.

**Abbreviations:** RA, Radial Artery; FCRT, Flexor Carpi Radialis Tendon; PLT, Palmaris Longus Tendon; FPLT, Flexor Pollicis Longus Tendon; MN, Median Nerve; PQM, Pronator Quatratus Muscle.

## Ulnar Nerve at the Wrist

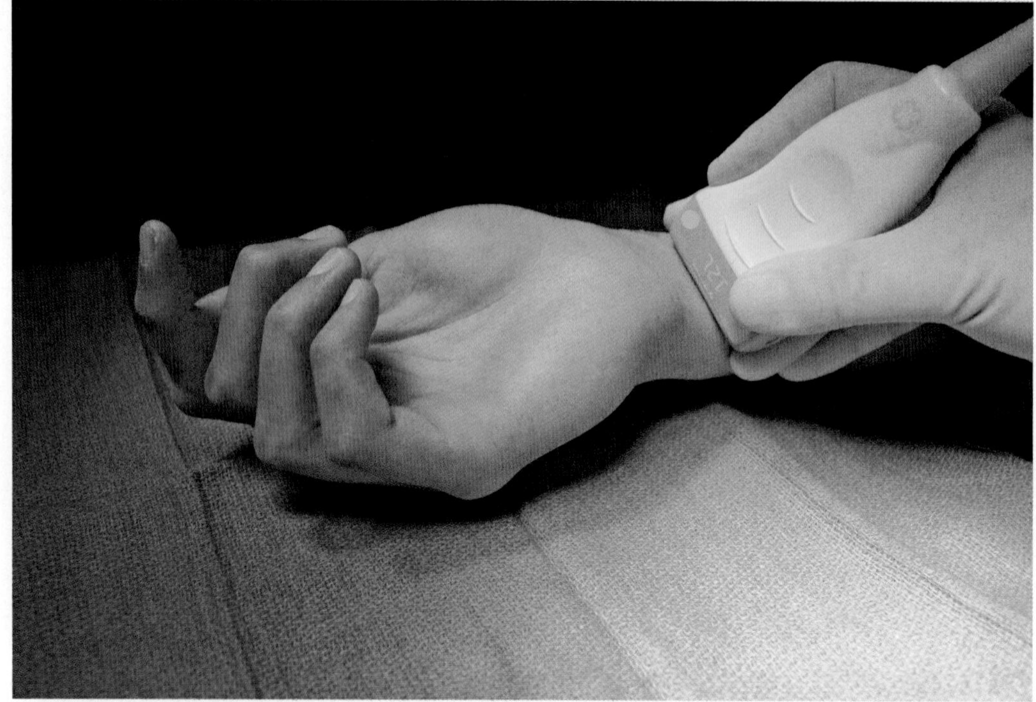

**FIGURE 7.32.1A** Ultrasound transducer position to image the ulnar nerve at the wrist.

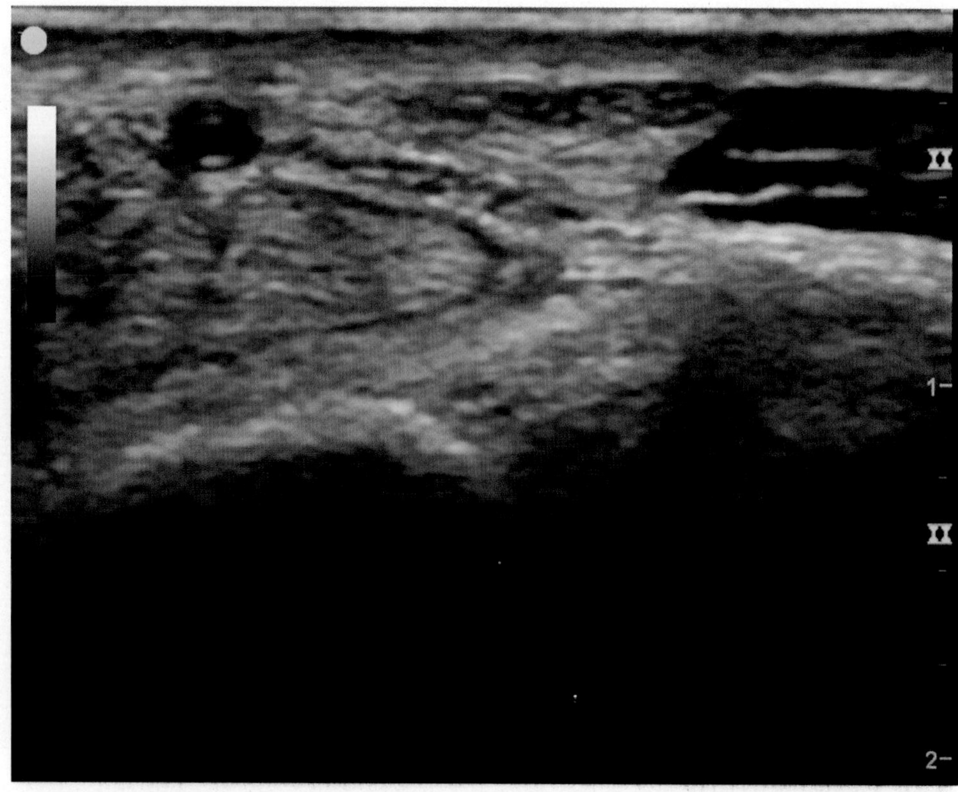


**FIGURE 7.32.1B** Ultrasound image of the ulnar nerve at the wrist.

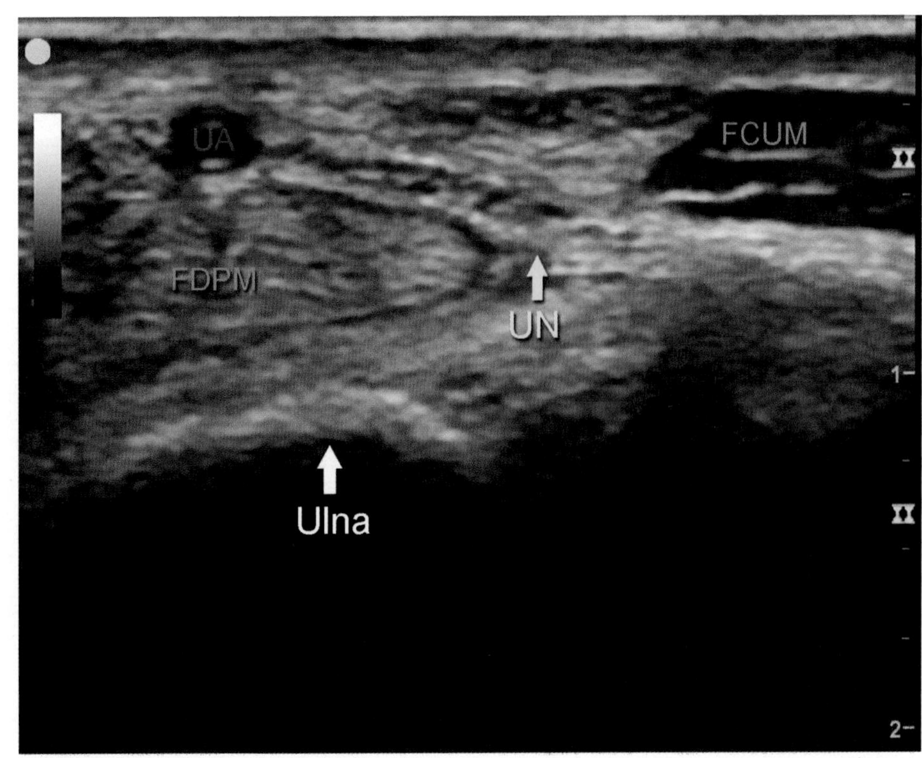


**FIGURE 7.32.1C** Labeled ultrasound image of the ulnar nerve at the wrist.

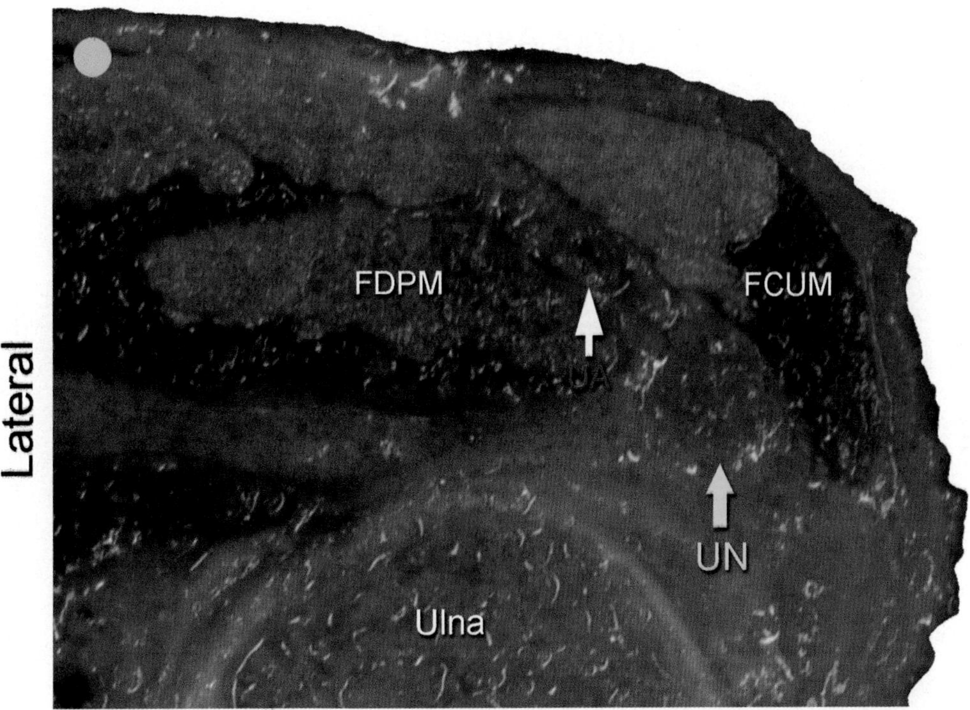


**FIGURE 7.32.1D** Labeled cross-sectional anatomy of the ulnar nerve at the wrist.

**Abbreviations:** UA, Ulnar Artery; UN, Ulnar Nerve; FCUM, Flexor Carpi Ulnaris Muscle; FDPM, Flexor Digitorum Profundus Muscle.

# Posterior Interosseous Nerve at the Wrist

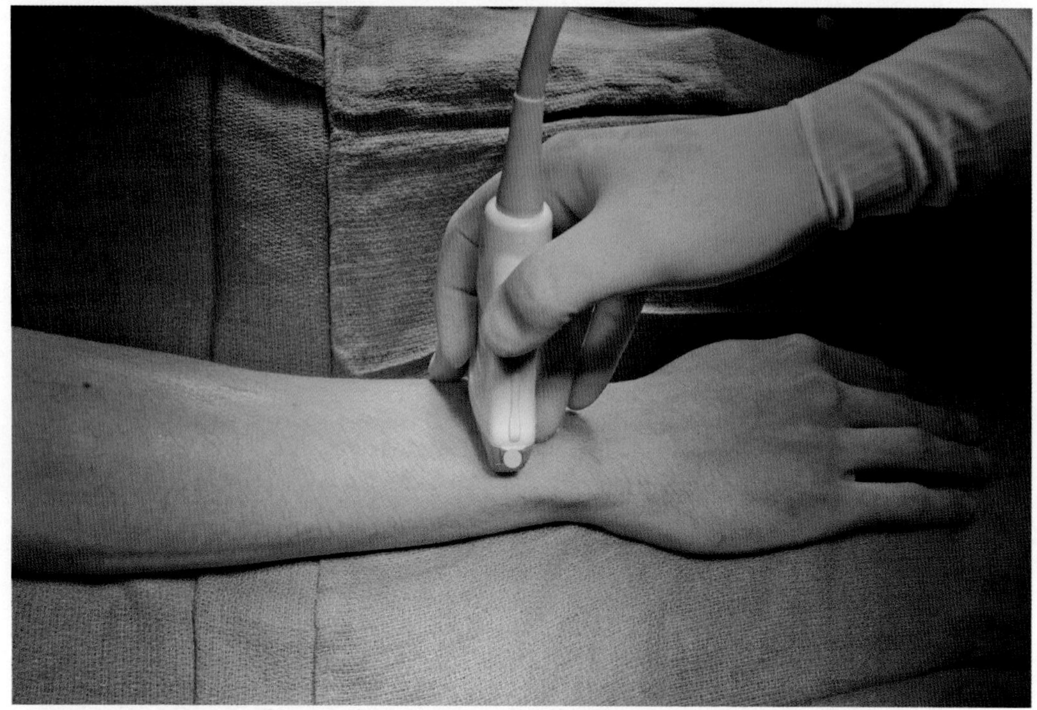

**FIGURE 7.33.1A** Ultrasound transducer position to image the posterior interosseous nerve at the wrist.

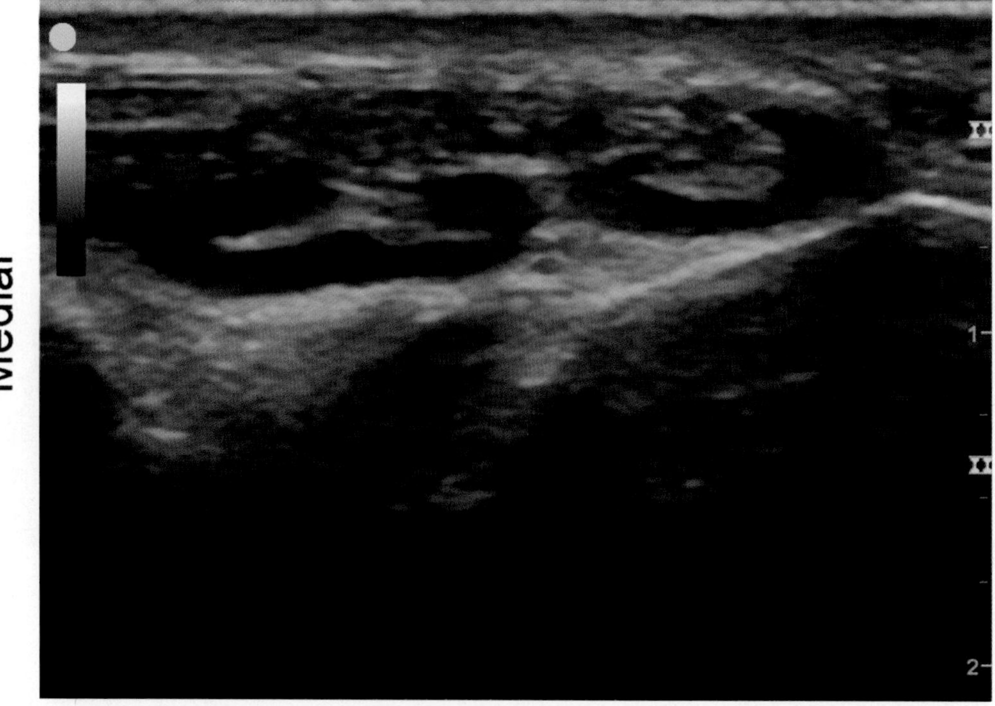


**FIGURE 7.33.1B** Ultrasound image of the posterior interosseous nerve at the wrist.

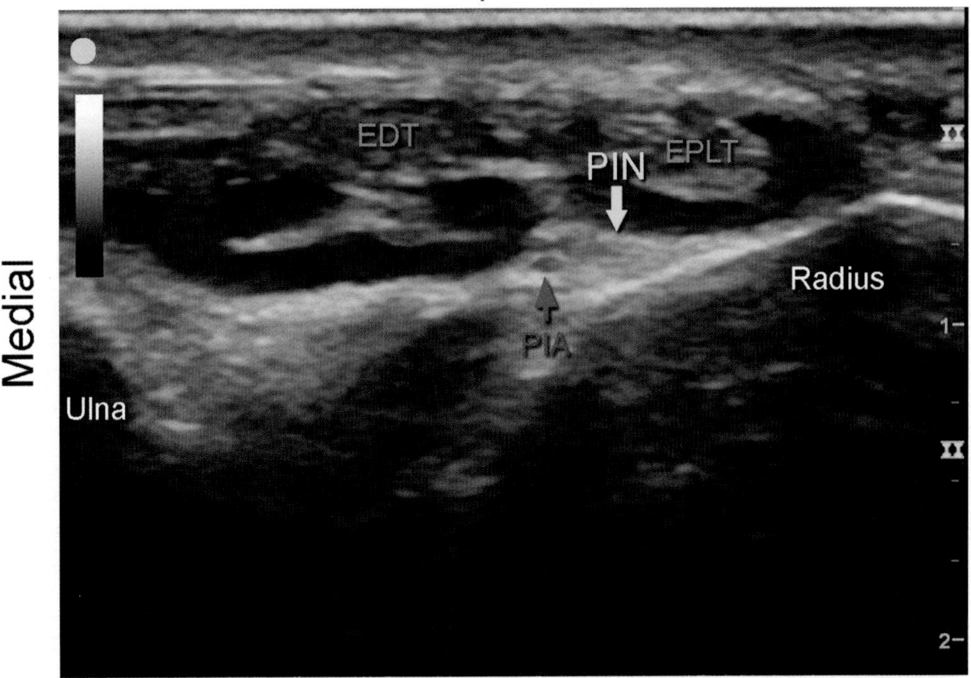


**FIGURE 7.33.1C** Labeled ultrasound image of the posterior interosseous nerve at the wrist.

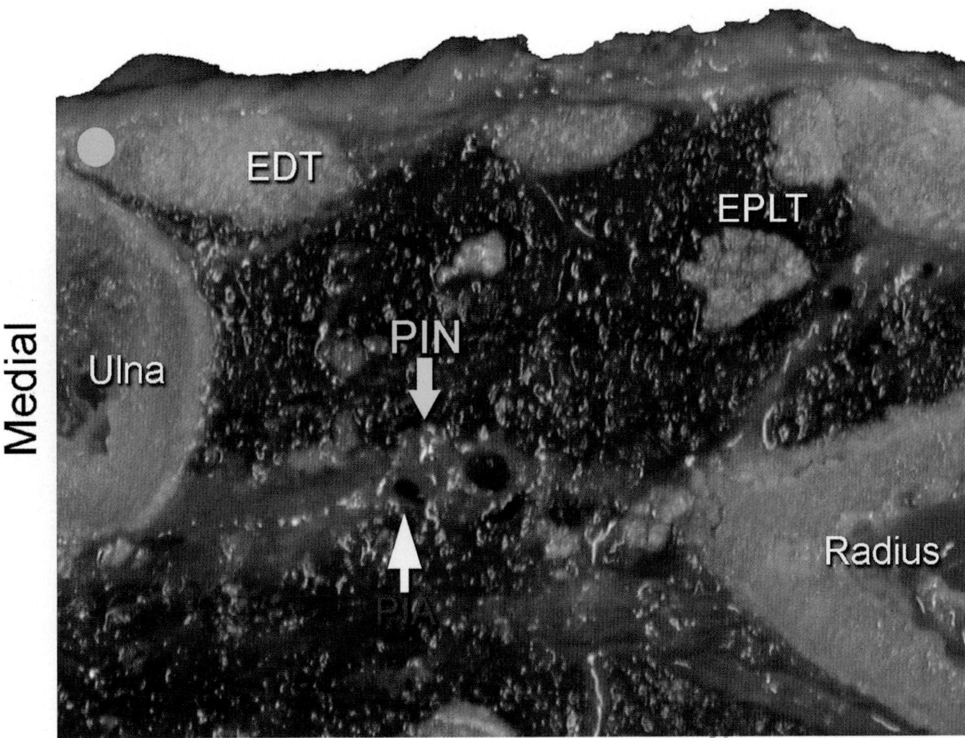


**FIGURE 7.33.1D** Labeled cross-sectional anatomy of the posterior interosseous nerve at the wrist.

**Abbreviations:** EPLT, Extensor Pollicis Longus Tendon; EDT, Extensor Digitorum Tendon; PIN, Posterior Interosseous Nerve; PIA, Posterior Interosseous Artery.

# Iliohypogastric and Ilioinguinal Nerves at the Abdominal Wall

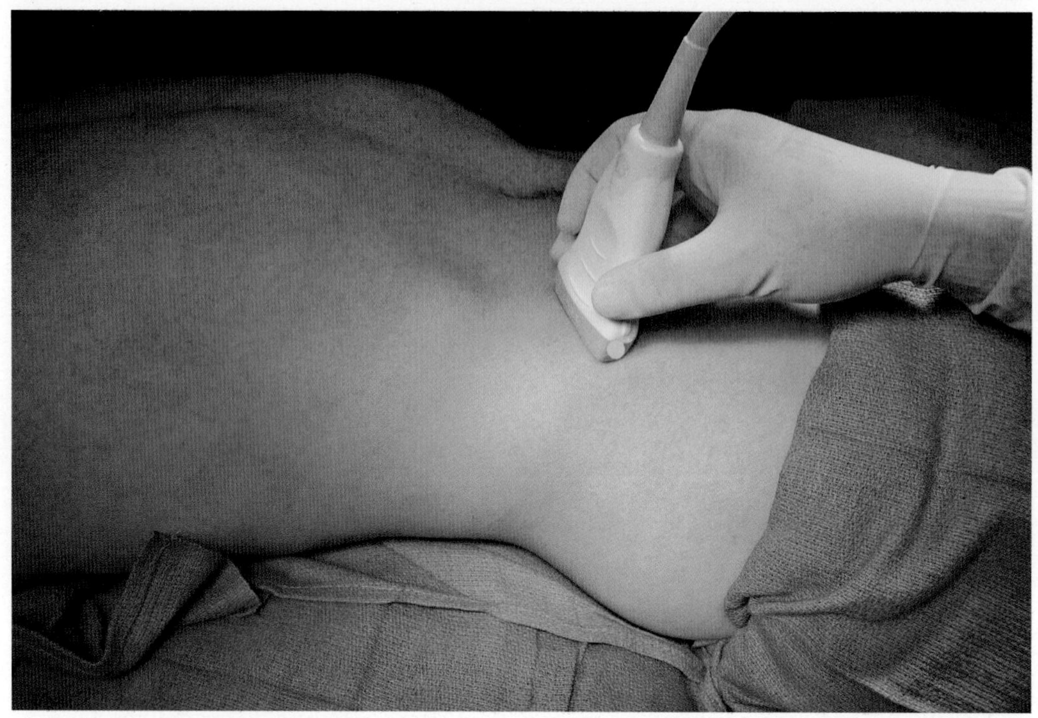

**FIGURE 7.34.1A** Ultrasound transducer position to image the iliohypogastric and ilioinguinal nerves at the abdominal wall.

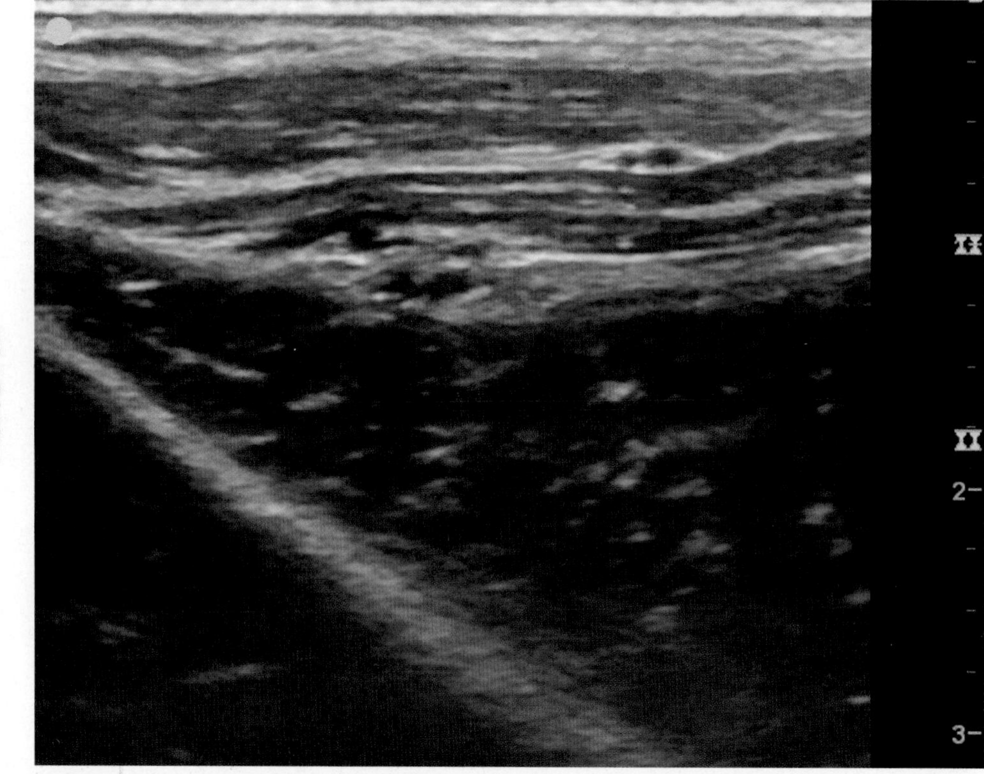


**FIGURE 7.34.1B** Ultrasound image of the iliohypogastric and ilioinguinal nerves at the abdominal wall.

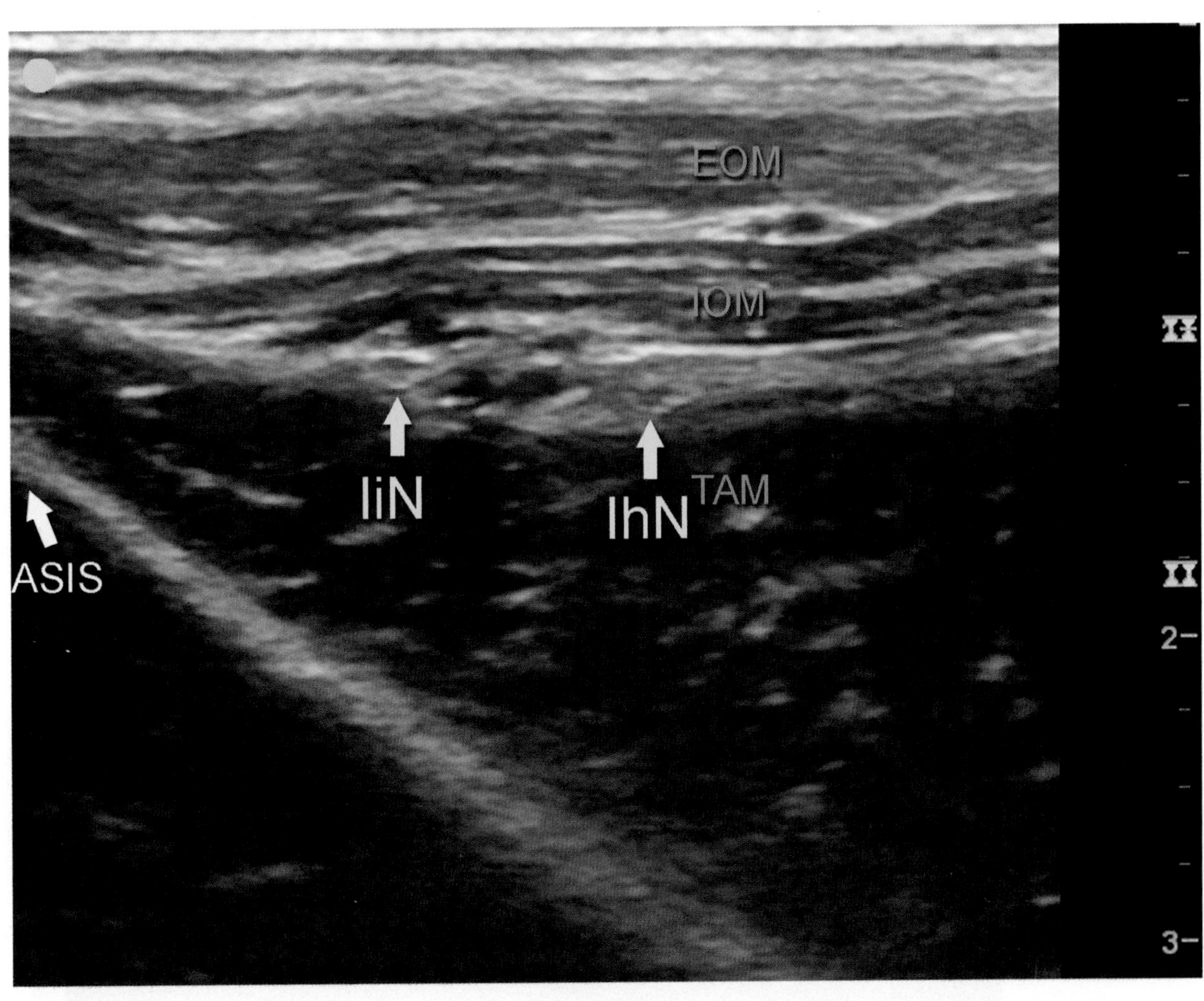


**FIGURE 7.34.1C** Labeled ultrasound image of the iliohypogastric and ilioinguinal nerves at the abdominal wall.

**Abbreviations:** EOM, External Oblique Muscle; IOM, Internal Oblique Muscle; TAM, Transverse Abdominis Muscle; IiN, Ilioinguinal Nerve; IhN, Iliohypogastric Nerve; ASIS, Anterior Superior Iliace Spine.

# Genital Branch of the Genitofemoral Nerve at the Abdominal Wall

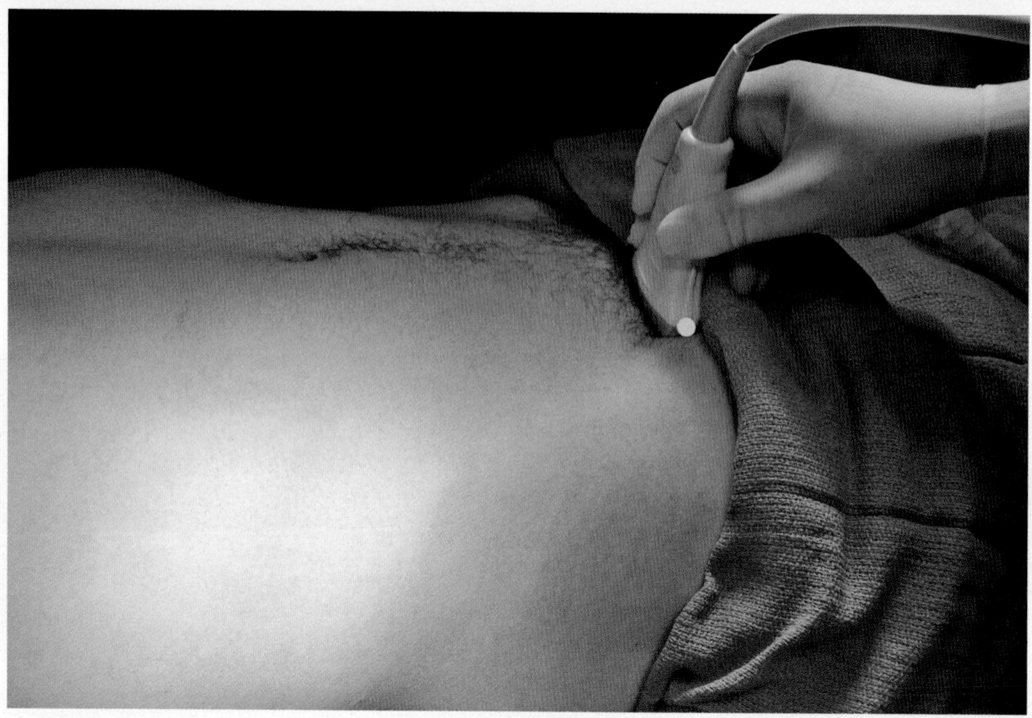

**FIGURE 7.35.1A** Ultrasound transducer position to image the genital branch of the genitofemoral nerve at the abdominal wall.

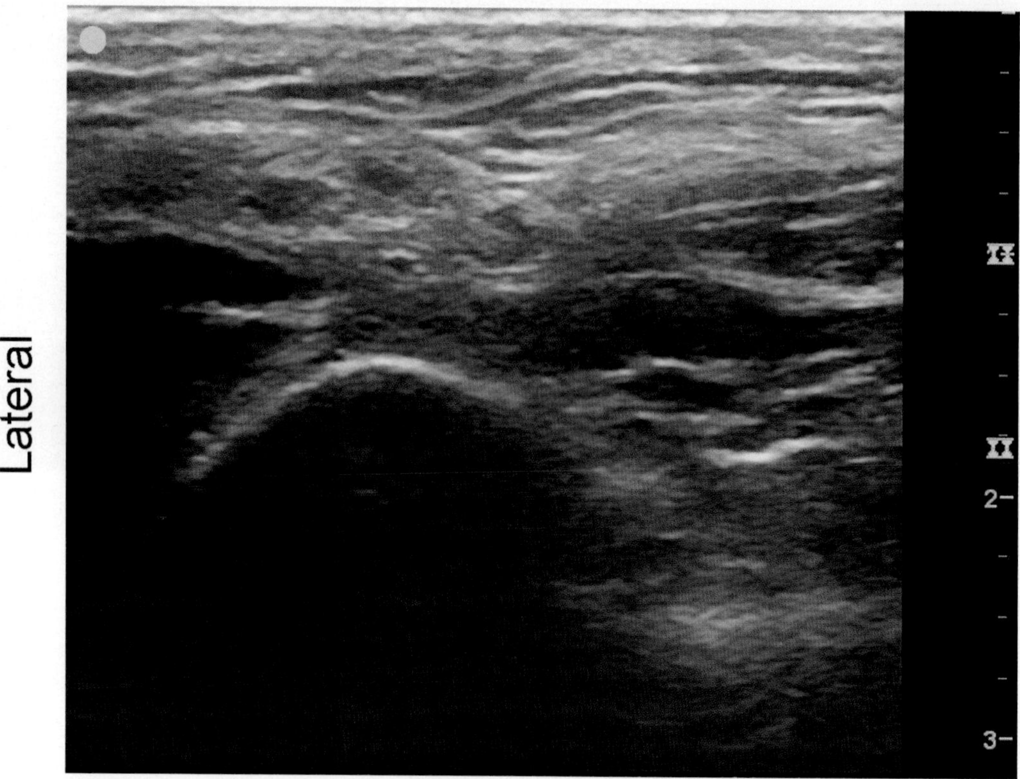


**FIGURE 7.35.1B** Ultrasound image of the genital branch of the genitofemoral nerve at the abdominal wall.

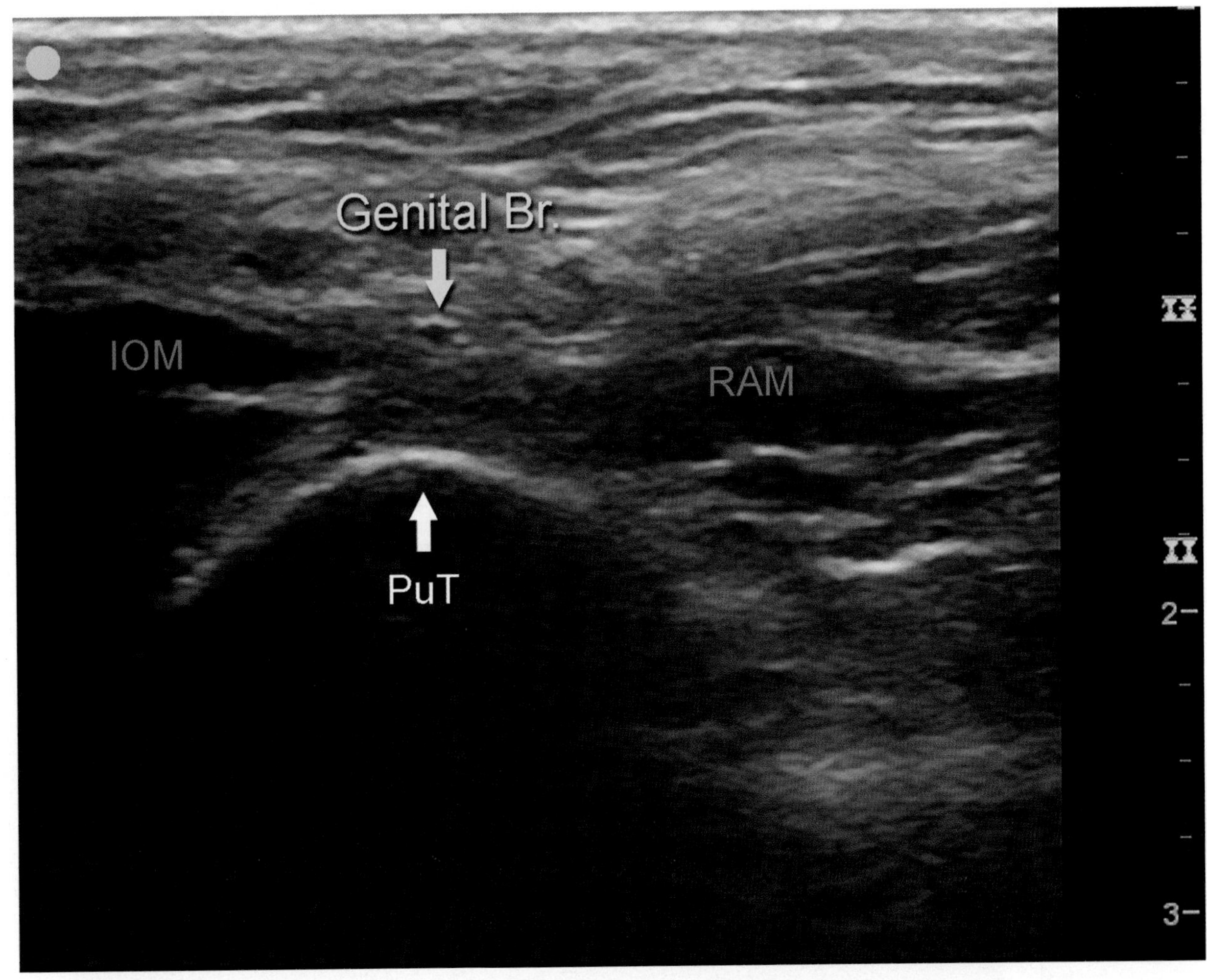


**FIGURE 7.35.1C** Labeled ultrasound image of the genital branch of the genitofemoral nerve at the abdominal wall.

**Abbreviations:** IOM, Internal Oblique Muscle; RAM, Rectus Abdominis Muscle; PuT, Pubic Tubercle.

## Femoral Branch of the Genitofemoral Nerve and Rectus Abdominis Nerve

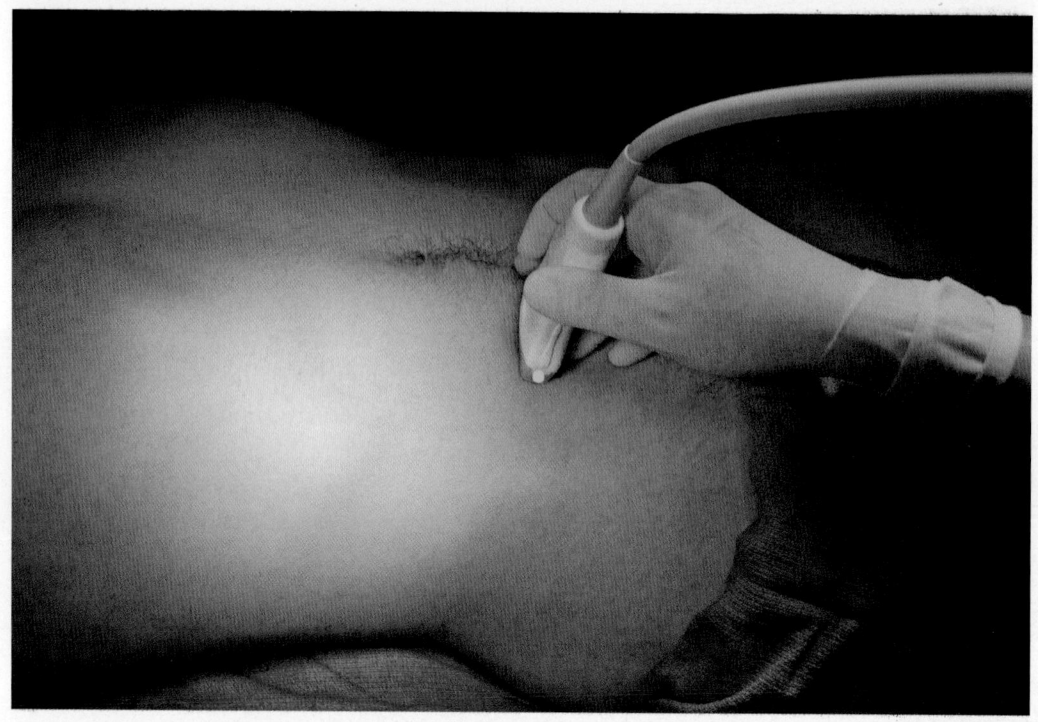

**FIGURE 7.36.1A** Ultrasound transducer position to image the femoral branch of the genitofemoral nerve and the rectus abdominis nerve.

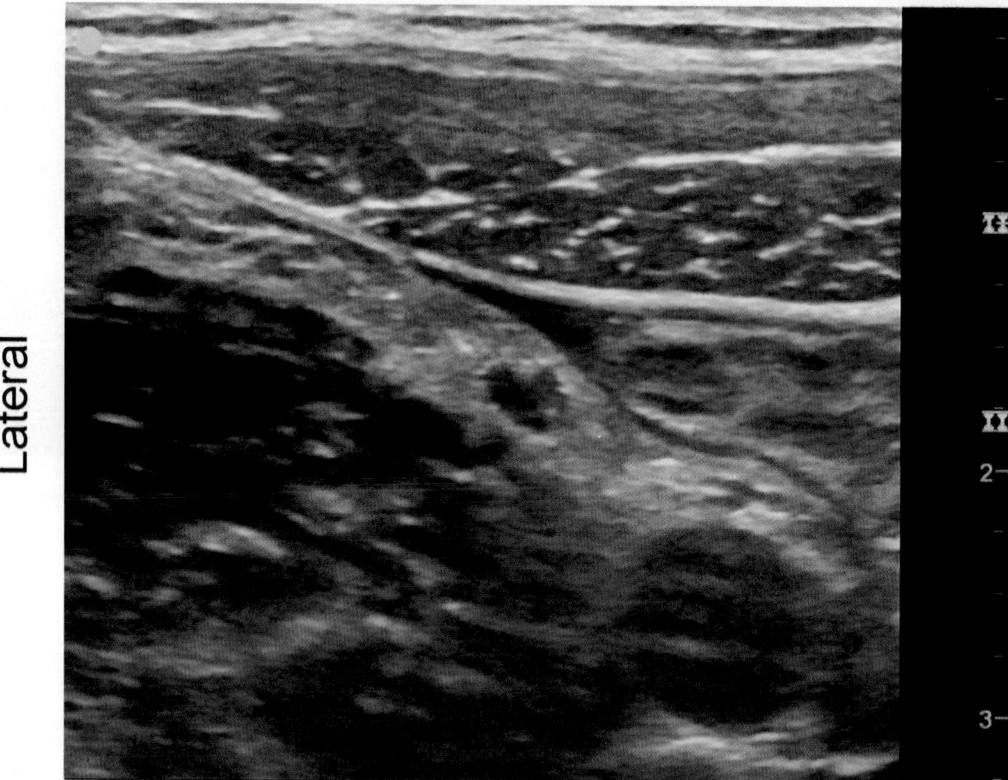


**FIGURE 7.36.1B** Ultrasound image of the femoral branch of the genitofemoral nerve and the rectus abdominis nerve.

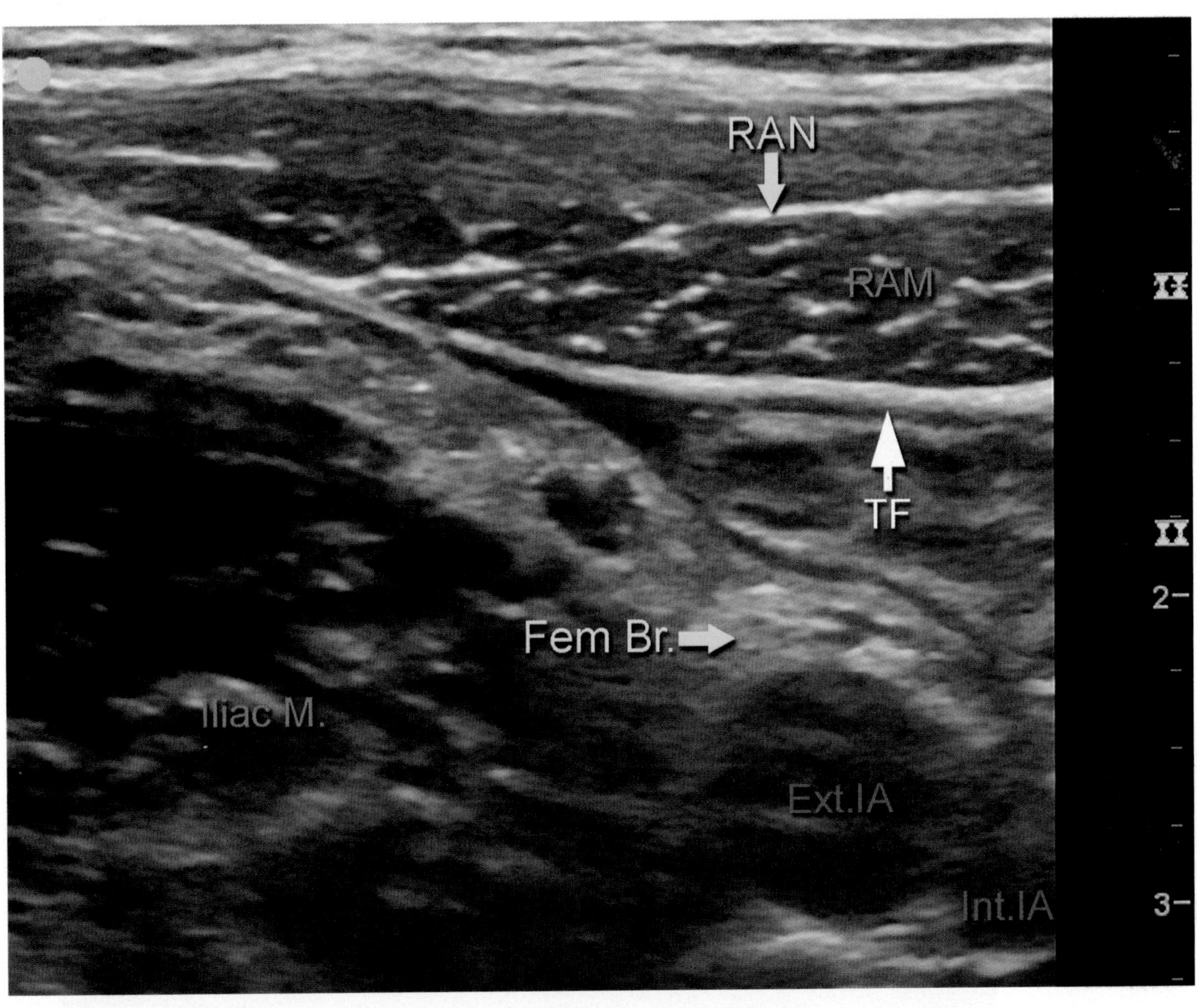


**FIGURE 7.36.1C** Labeled ultrasound image of the femoral branch of the genitofemoral nerve and the rectus abdominis nerve.

**Abbreviations:** RAN, Rectus Abdominis Nerve; RAM, Rectus Abdominis Muscle; TF, Transversalis Fascia; Ext. IA, External Iliac Artery; Int. IA, Internal Iliac Artery.

# Paramedian Epidural Space at the Midthoracic Spine

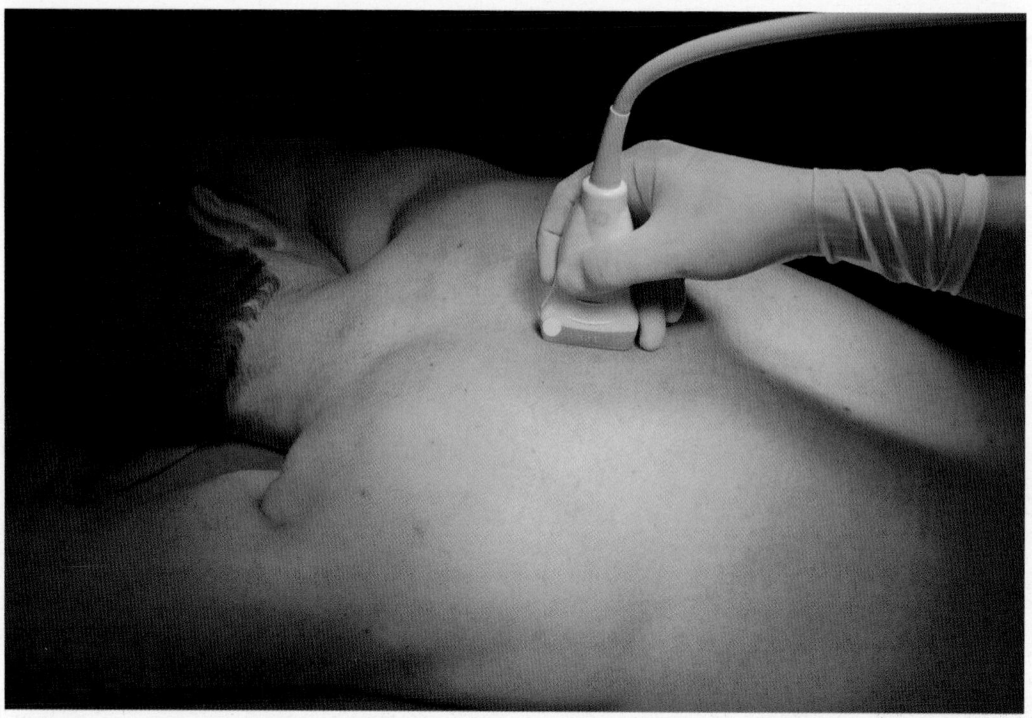

**FIGURE 7.37.1A** Ultrasound transducer position to image the paramedian epidural space at the midthoracic spine.

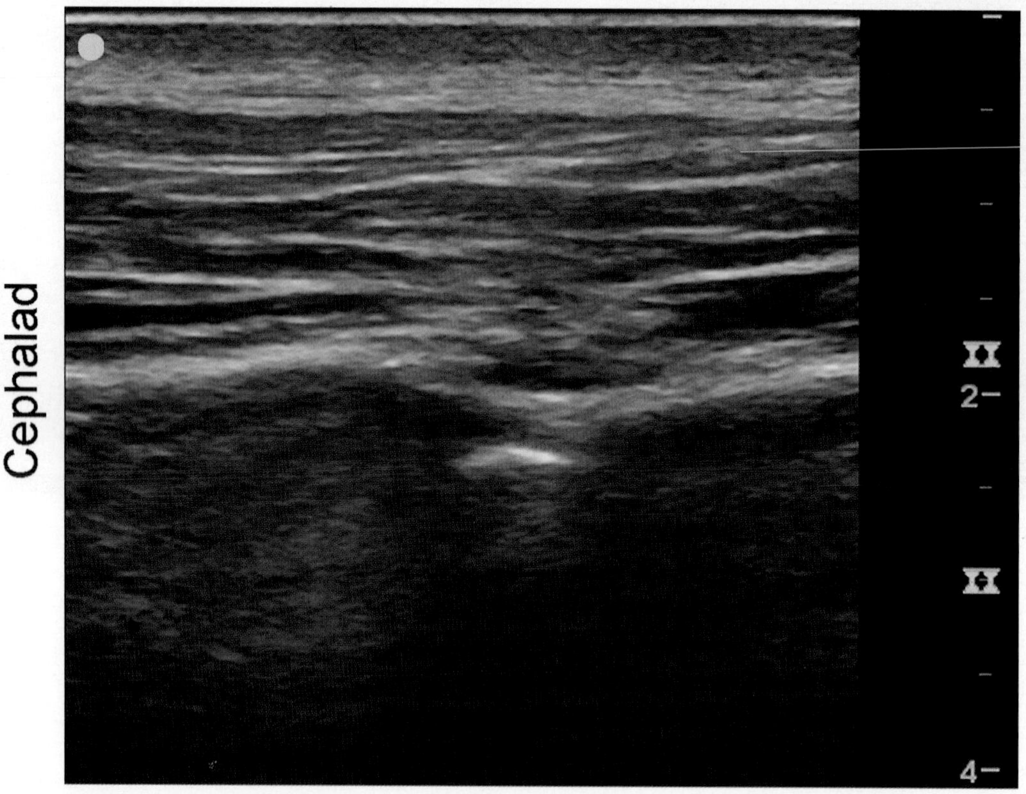


**FIGURE 7.37.1B** Ultrasound image of the paramedian epidural space at the midthoracic spine.

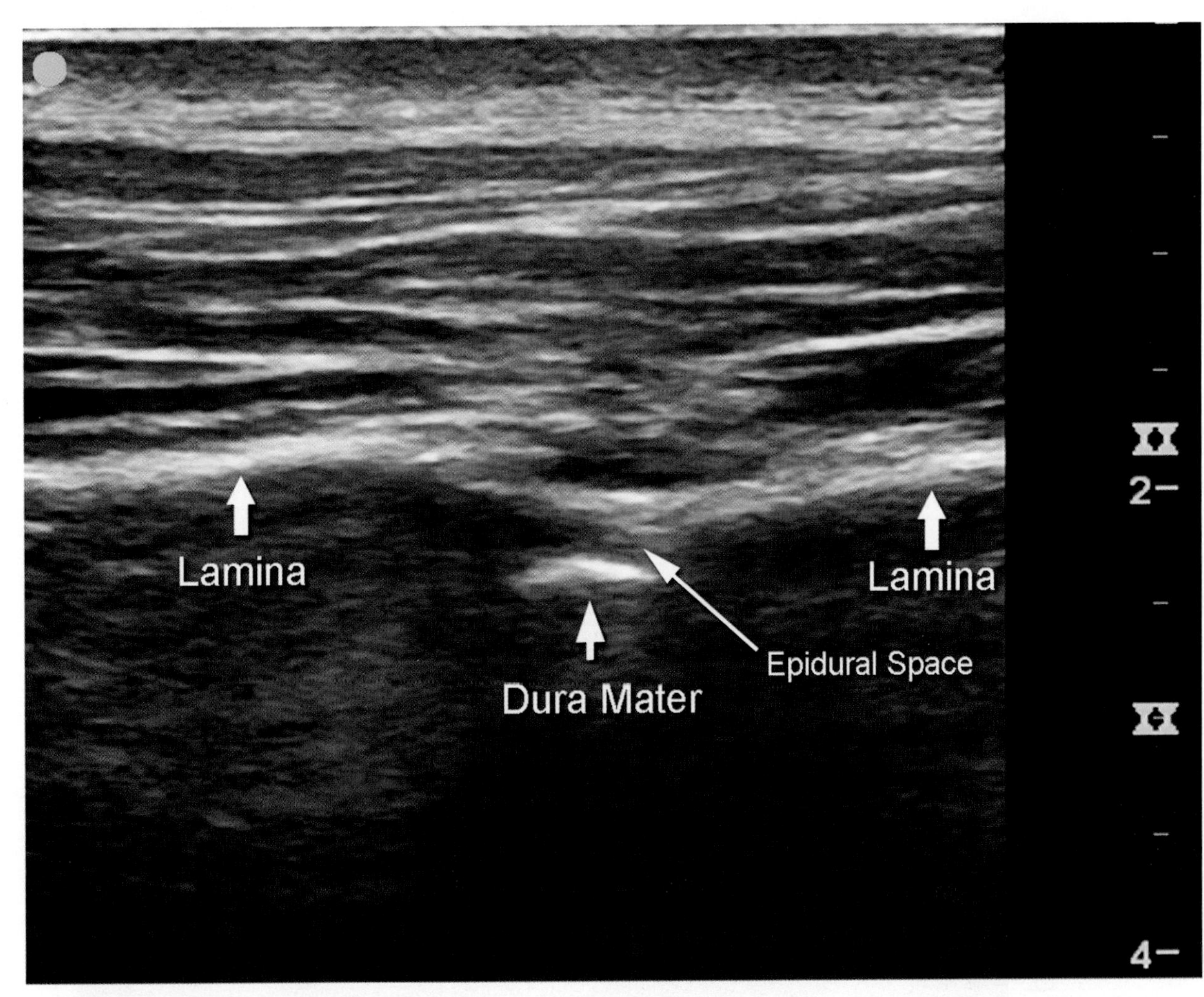


**FIGURE 7.37.1C** Labeled ultrasound image of the paramedian epidural space at the midthoracic spine.

# Paramedian Epidural Space at the Lumbar Spine, Longitudinal View

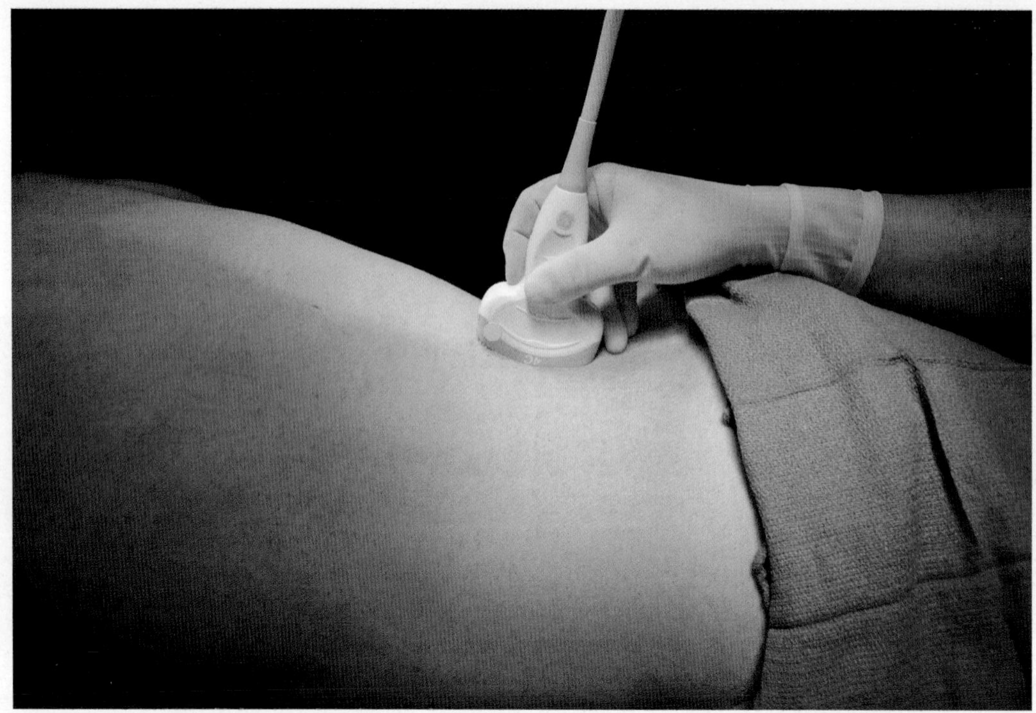

**FIGURE 7.38.1A** Ultrasound transducer position to image the paramedian epidural space at the lumbar spine, longitudinal view.

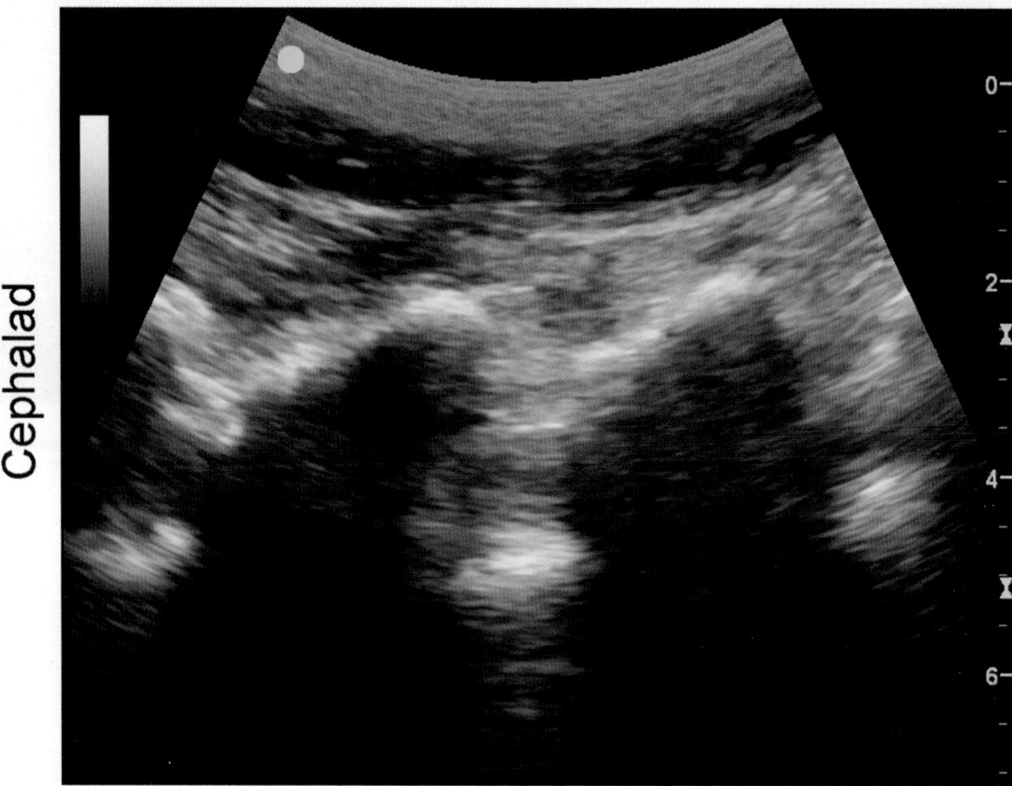


**FIGURE 7.38.1B** Ultrasound image of the paramedian epidural space at the lumbar spine, longitudinal view.

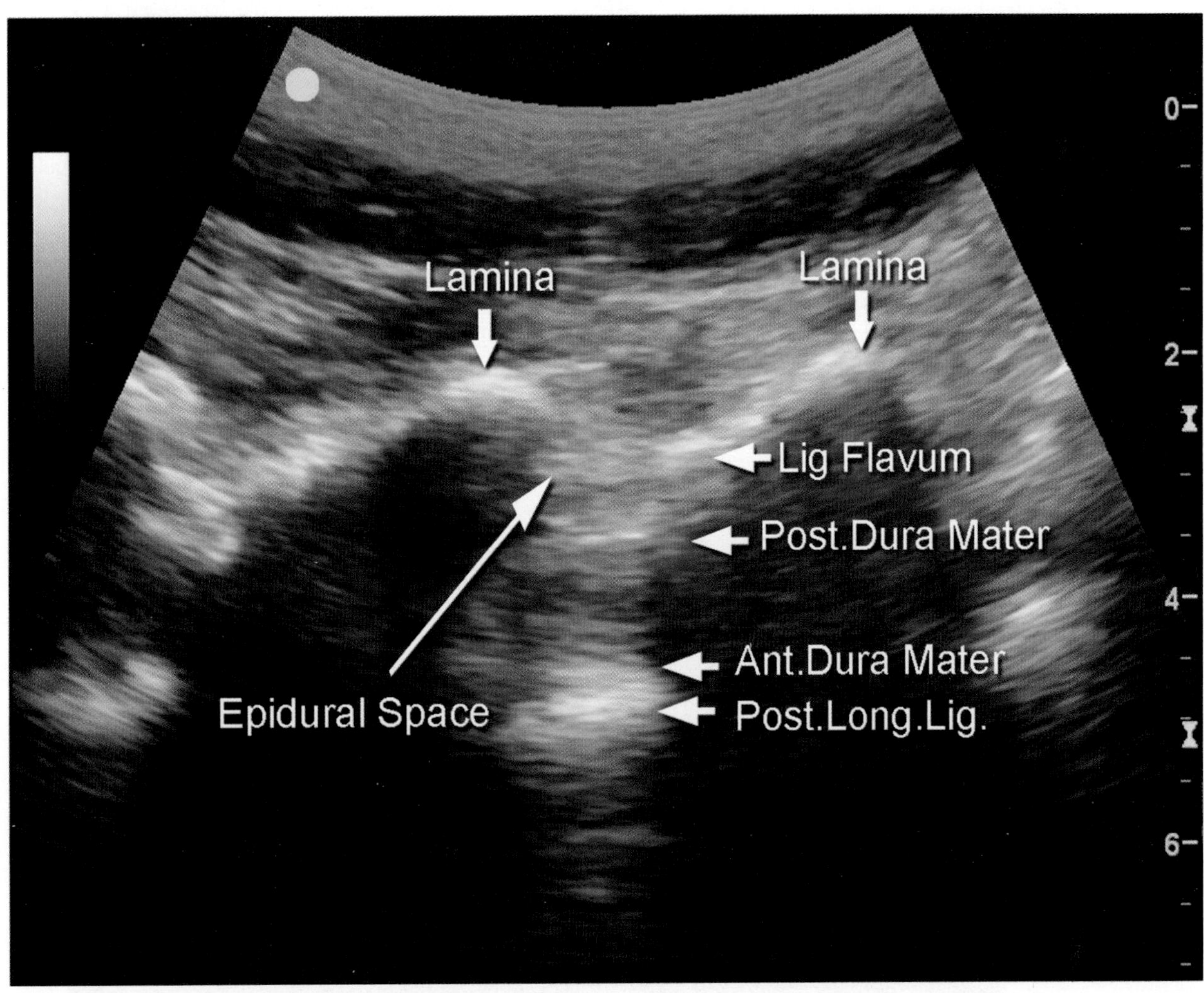


**FIGURE 7.38.1C** Labeled ultrasound image of the paramedian epidural space at the lumbar spine, longitudinal view.

**Abbreviations:** Post. Long. Lig., Posterior Longitudinal Ligament; Lig. Flavum, Ligamentum Flavum; Ant. Dura Mater, Anterior Dura Mater; Post. Dura Mater, Posterior Dura Mater.

## Paravertebral Space, Midthoracic Spine, Transverse View

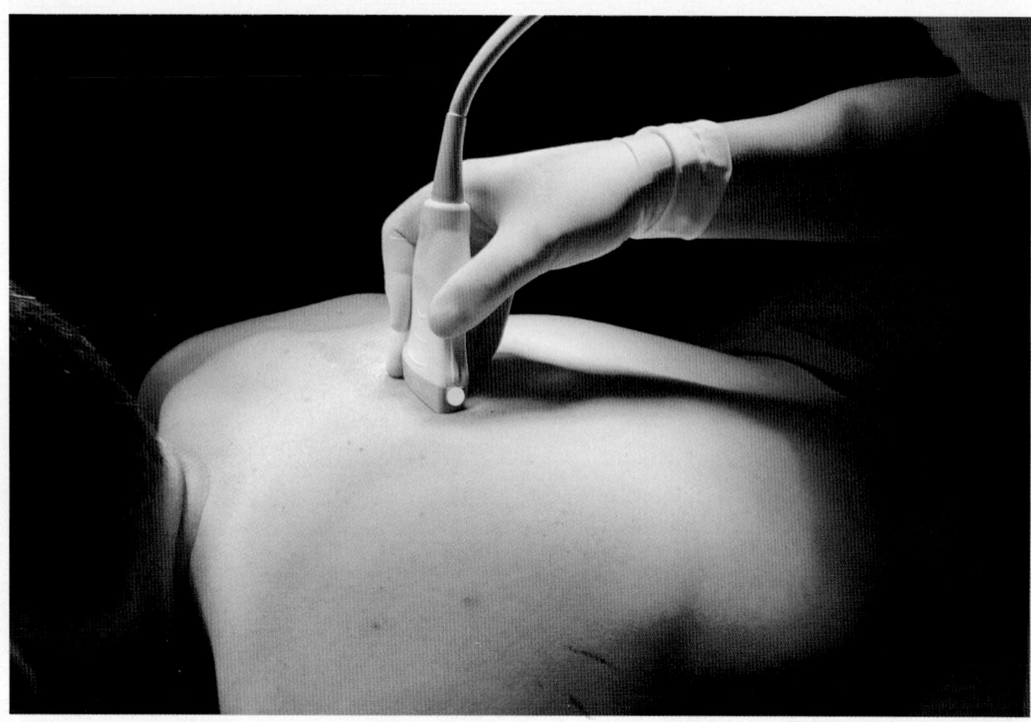

**FIGURE 7.39.1A** Ultrasound transducer position to image the paravertebral space, midthoracic spine, transverse view.

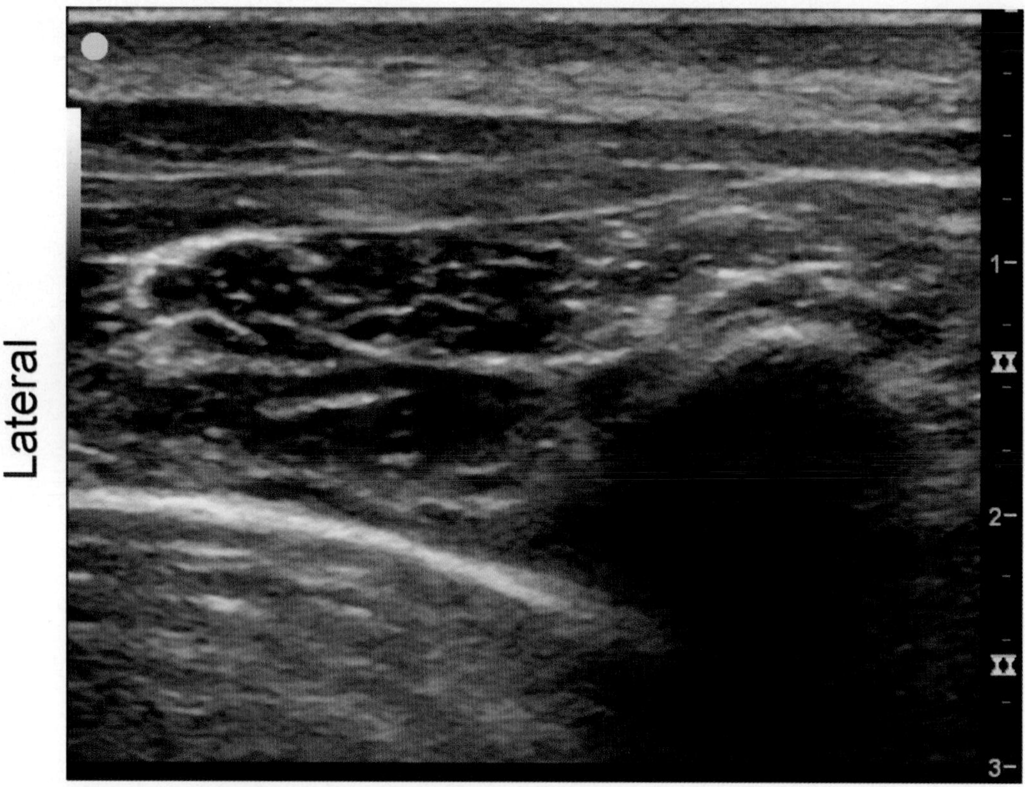


**FIGURE 7.39.1B** Ultrasound image of the paravertebral space, midthoracic spine, transverse view.

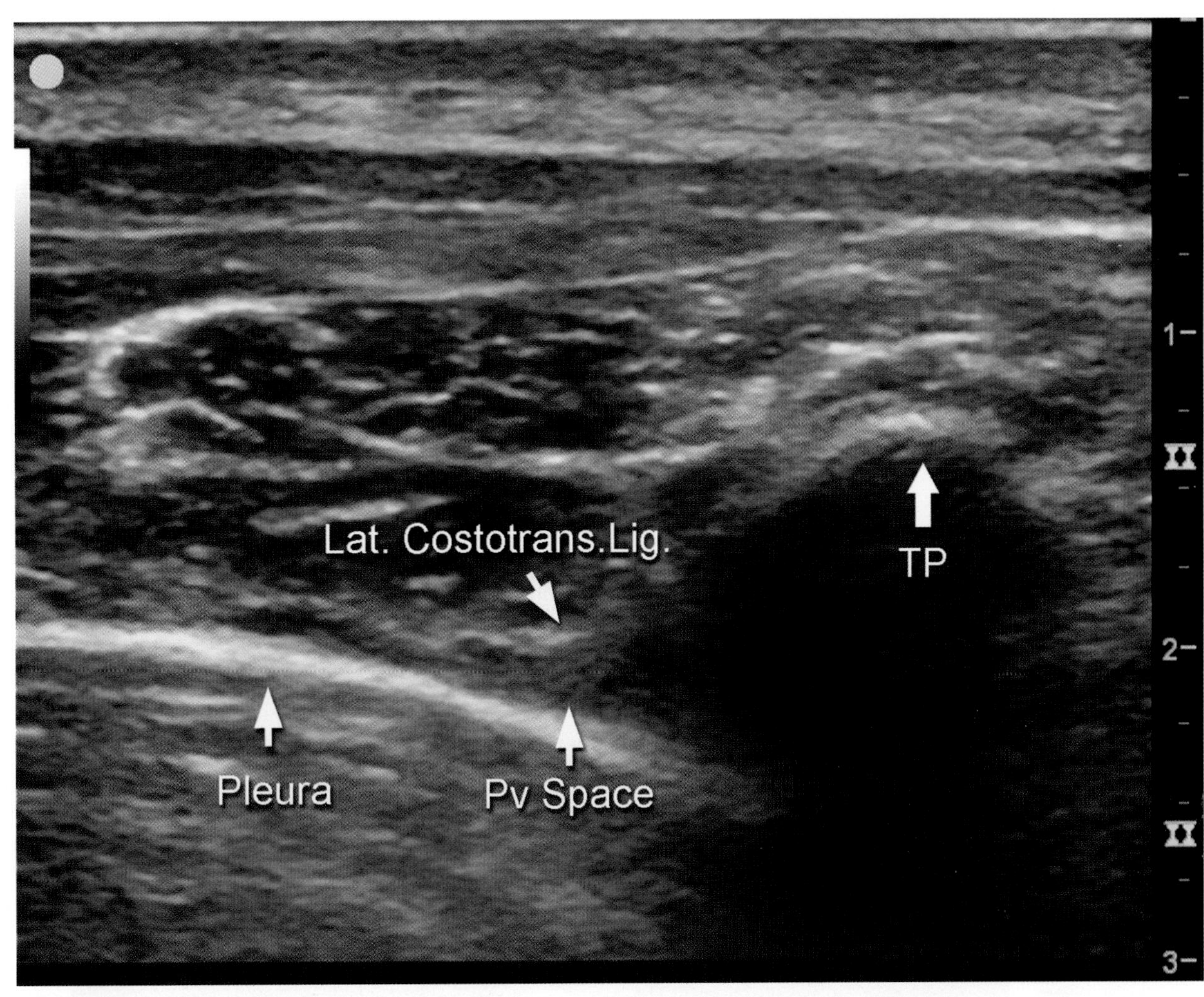


**FIGURE 7.39.1C** Labeled ultrasound image of the paravertebral space, midthoracic spine, transverse view.

**Abbreviations:** Lat. Costotrans. Lig., Lateral Costotransverse Ligament; TP, Transverse Process; Pv Space, Paravertebral Space.

# Lumbar Plexus, Transverse View

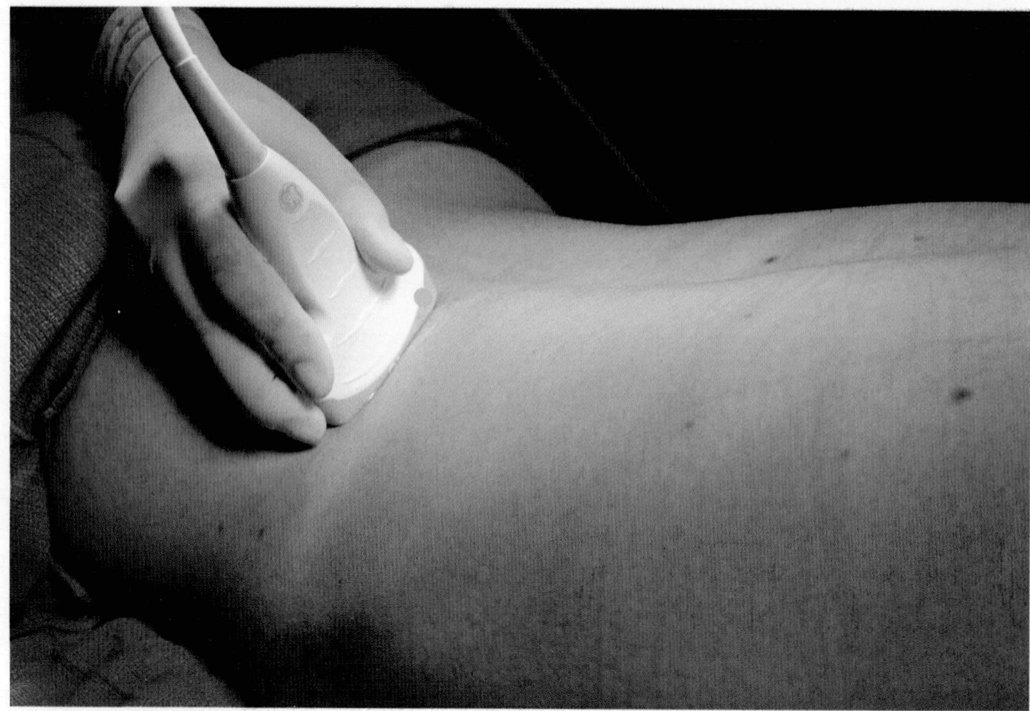

**FIGURE 7.40.1A** Ultrasound transducer position to image the lumbar plexus, transverse view.

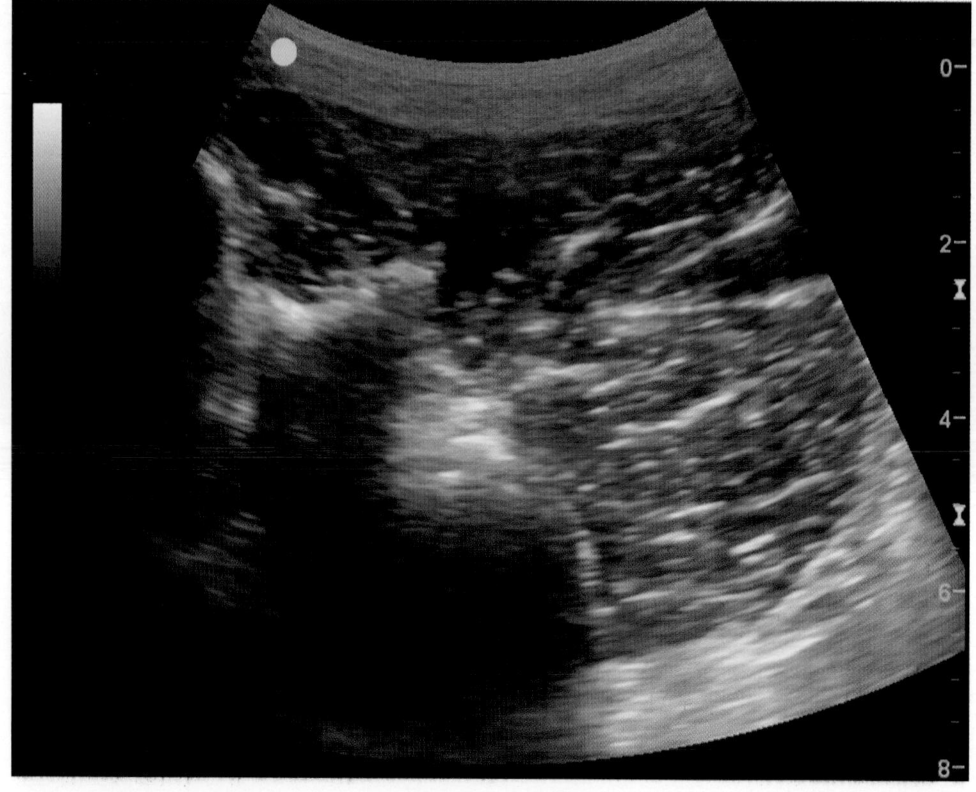


**FIGURE 7.40.1B** Ultrasound image of the lumbar plexus, transverse view.

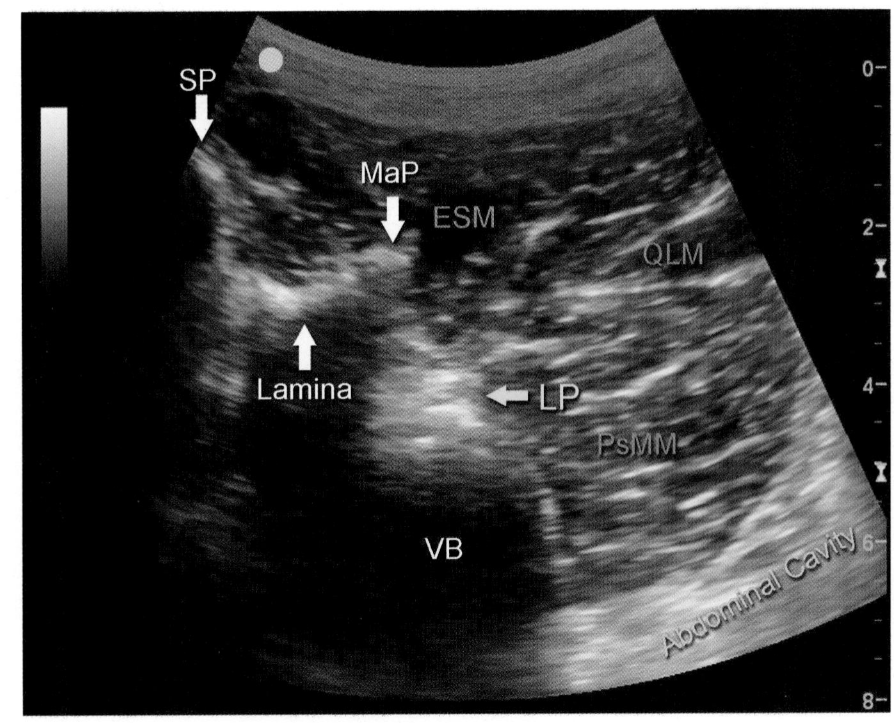


**7.40.1C** Labeled ultrasound image of the lumbar plexus, transverse view.

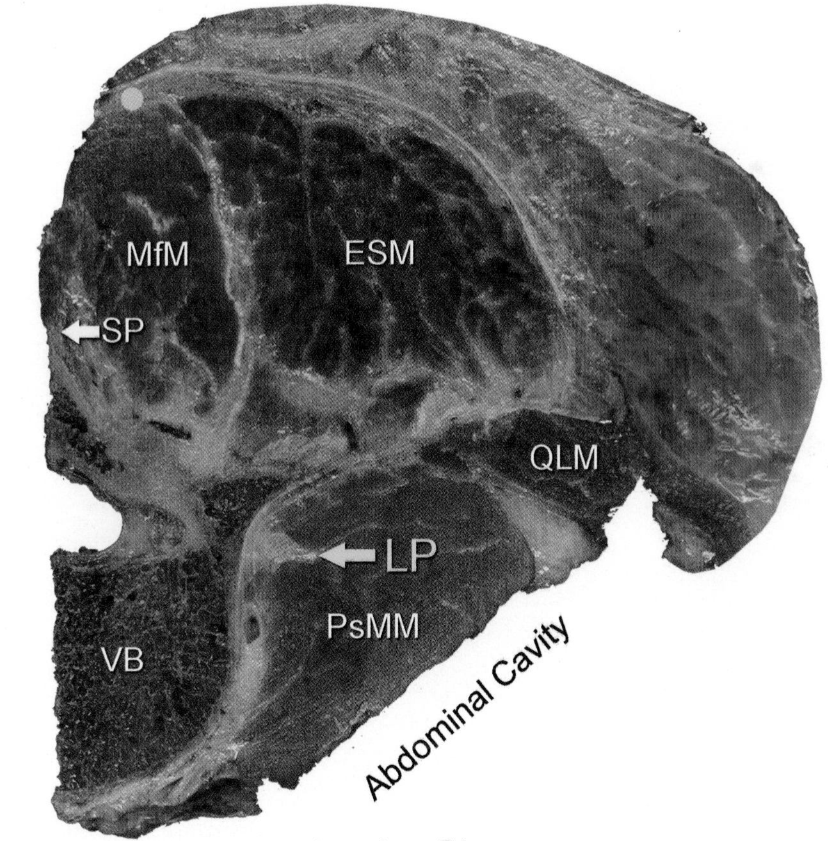


**FIGURE 7.40.1D** Labeled cross-sectional anatomy of the lumbar plexus, transverse view.

**Abbreviations:** SP, Spinous process; Map, Mammillary Process; ESM, Erector Spinae Muscle; QLM, Quadratus Lumborum Muscle; LP, Lumbar Plexus; PsMM, Psoas Major Muscle; VB, Vertebral Body; MfM, Multifidus Muscle; LDM, Longissimus Dorsi Muscle.

# Facet Joints at the Lumbar Level, Transverse View

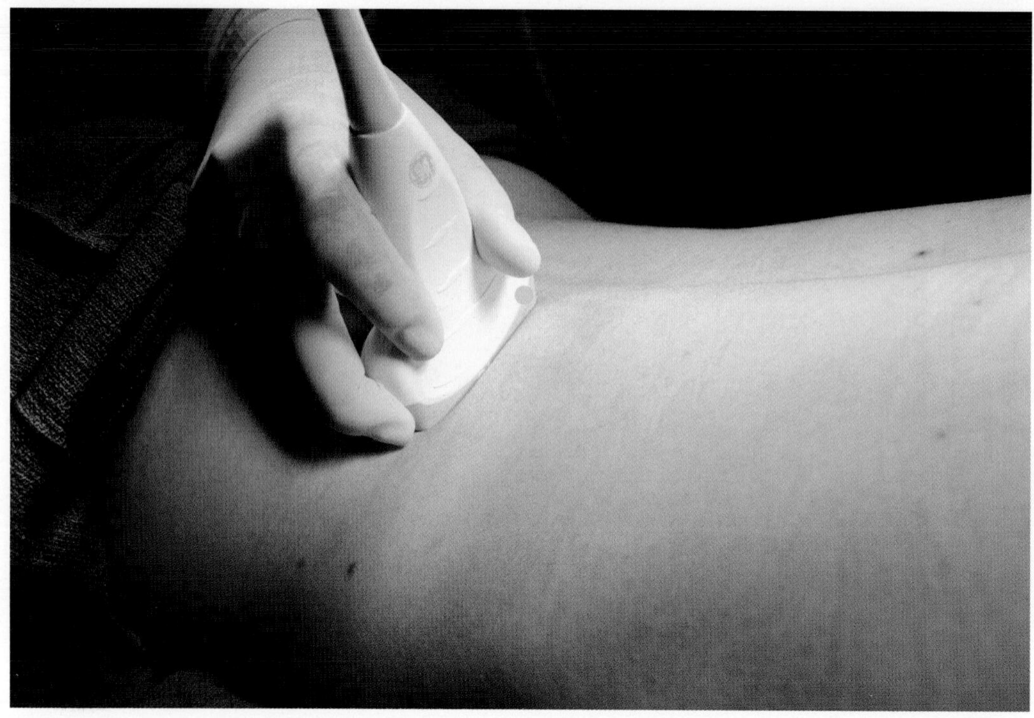

FIGURE 7.41.1A Ultrasound transducer position to image the facet joints at the lumbar level, transverse view.

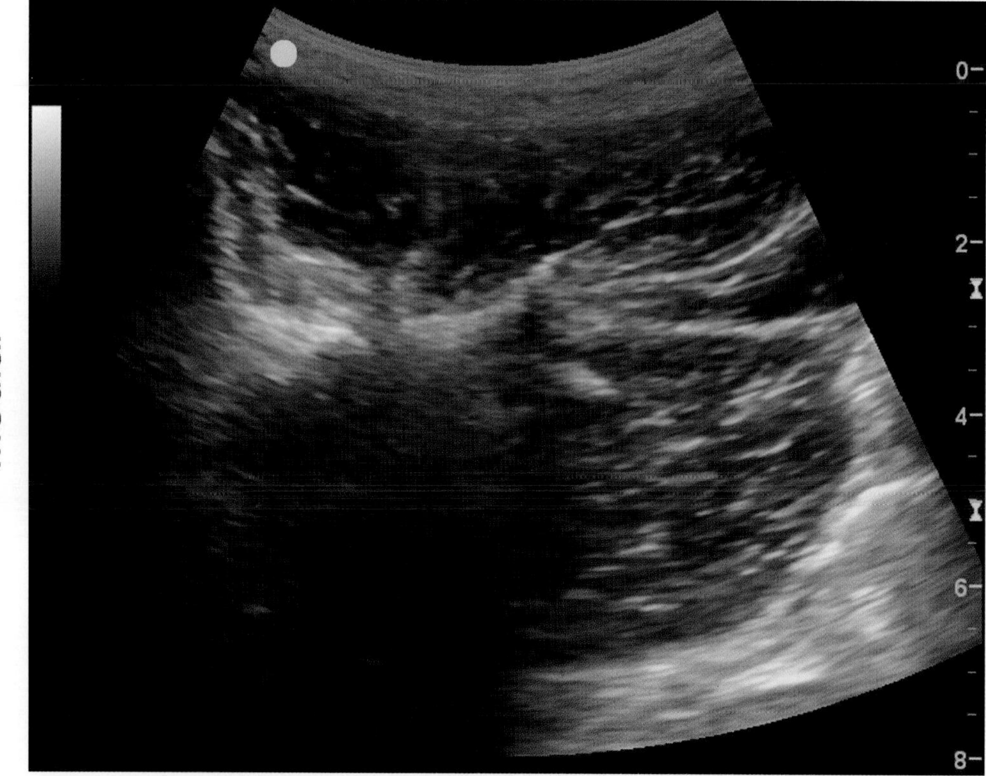


FIGURE 7.41.1B Ultrasound image of the facet joints at the lumbar level, transverse view.

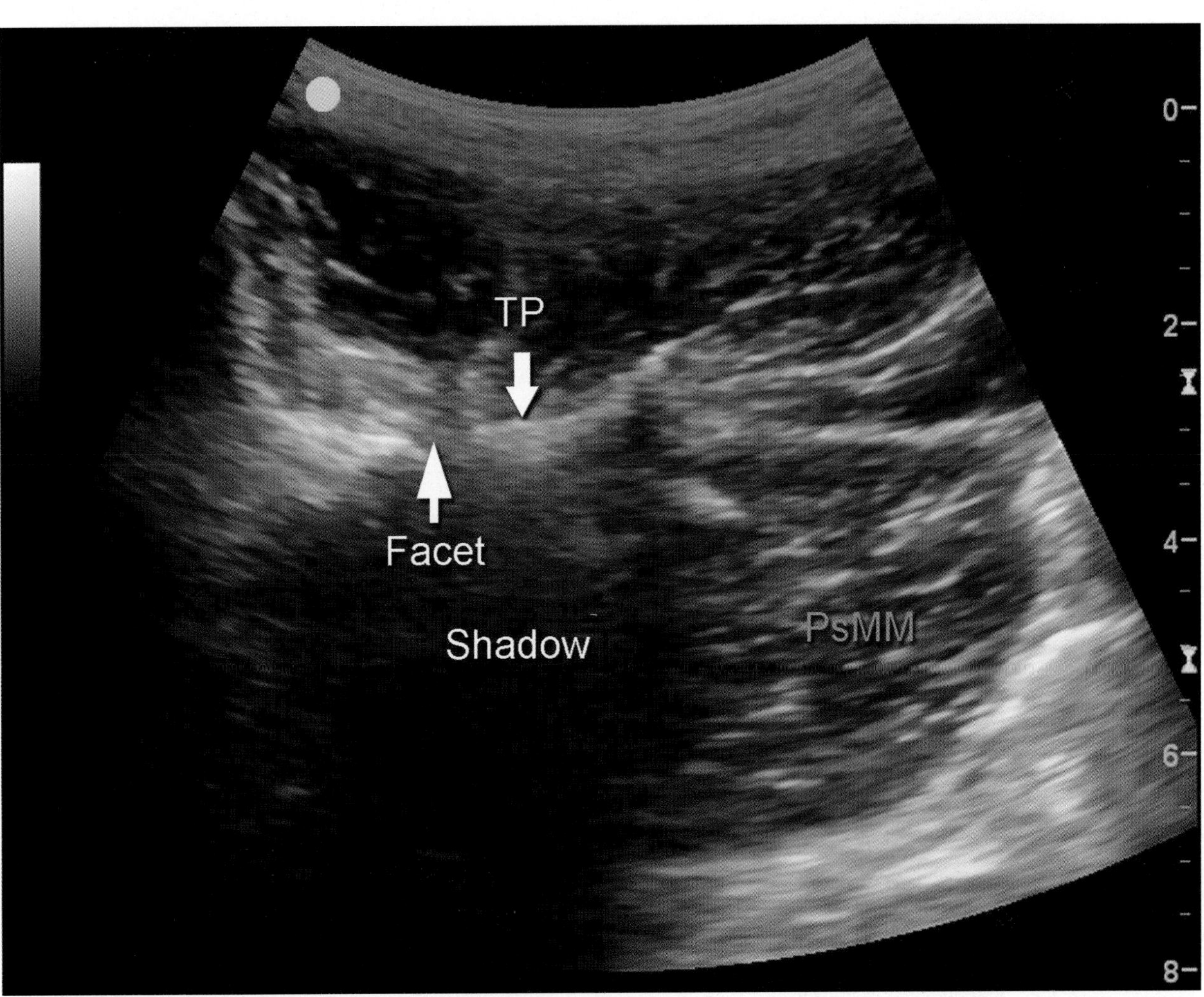


**FIGURE 7.41.1C** Labeled ultrasound image of the facet joints at the lumbar level transverse view.

**Abbreviations:** TP, Transverse Process; PsMM, Psoas Major Muscle.

# Lumbar Plexus, Lateral Transverse View

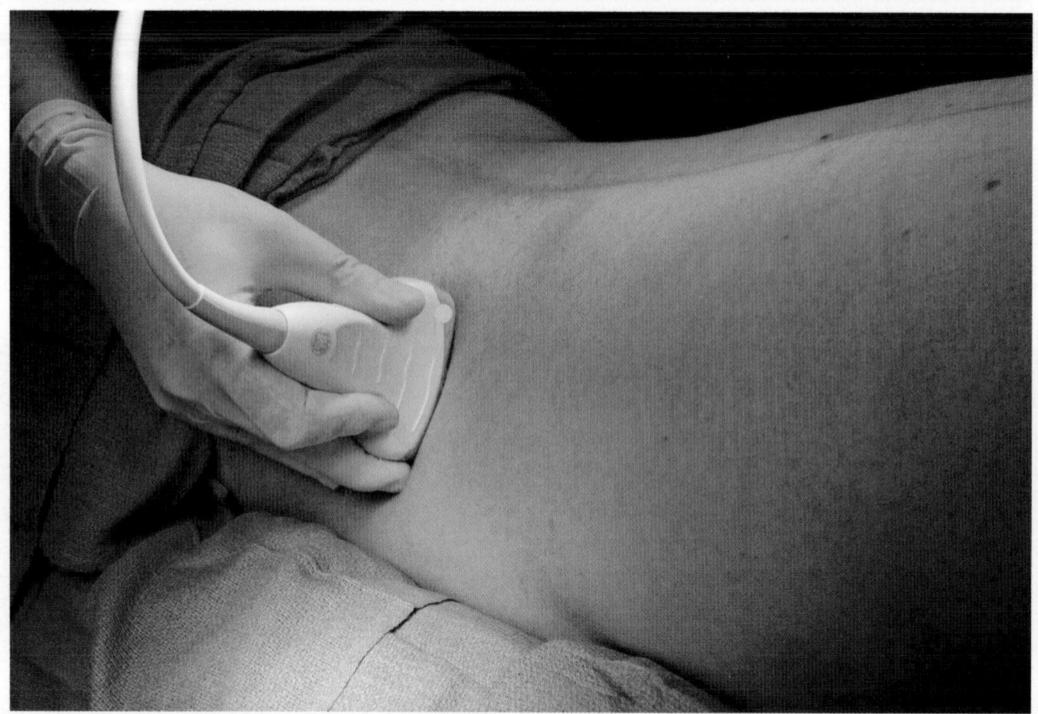

**FIGURE 7.42.1A** Ultrasound transducer position to image the lumbar plexus, lateral transverse view.

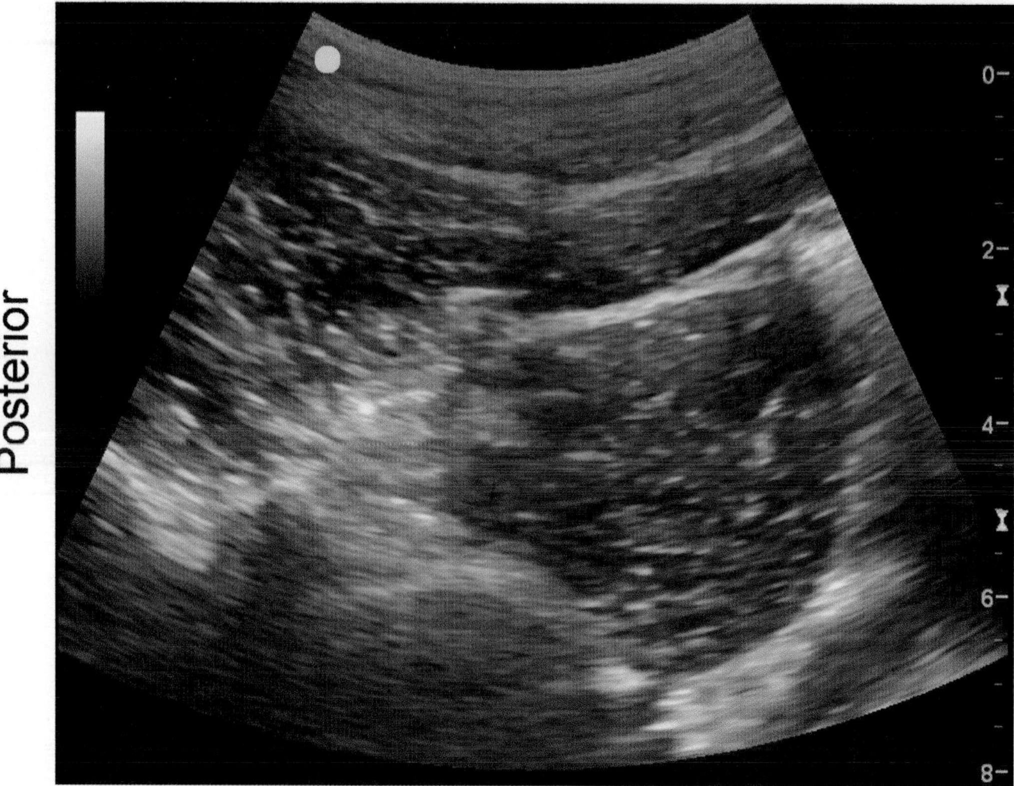


**FIGURE 7.42.1B** Ultrasound image of the lumbar plexus, lateral transverse view.

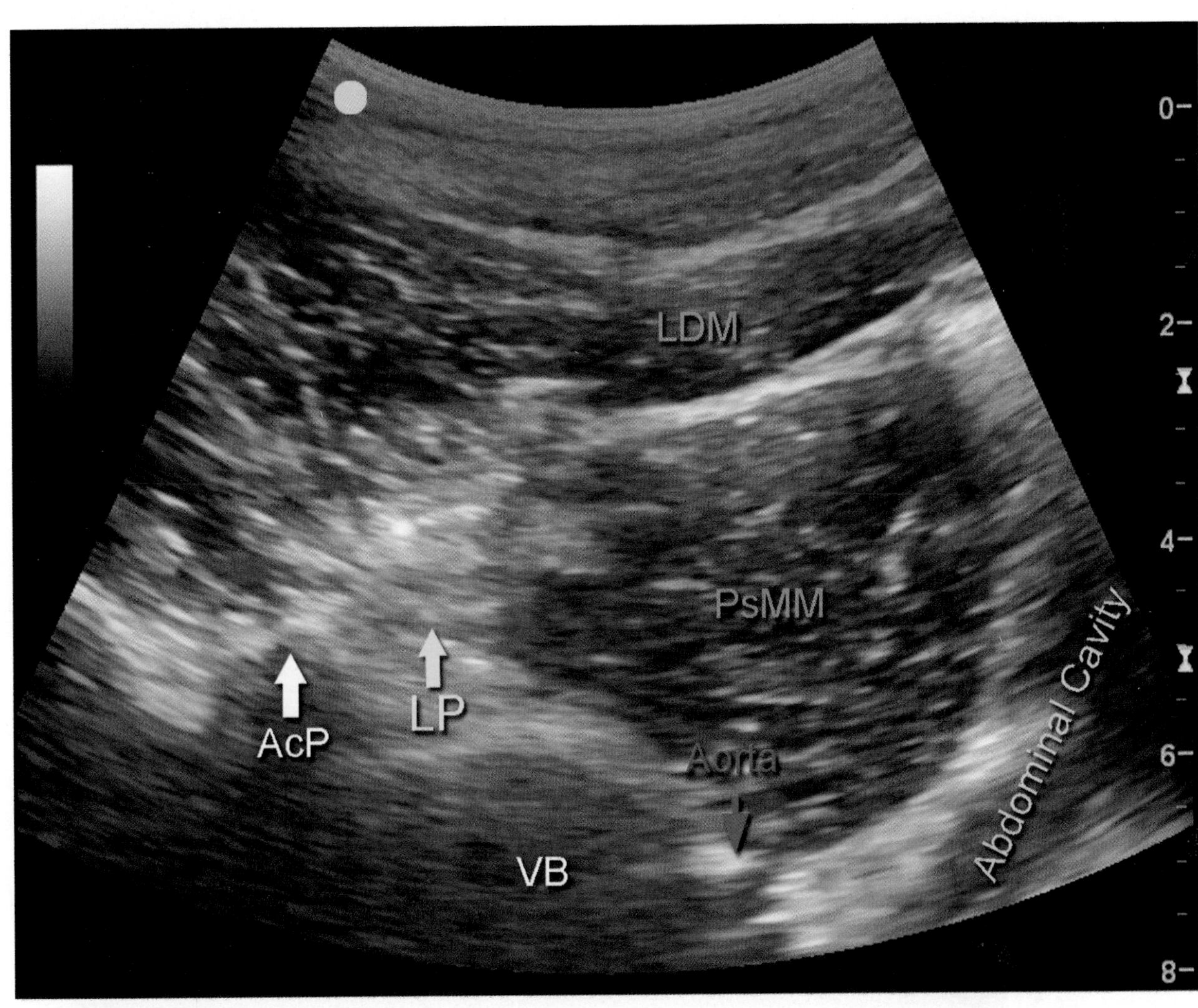


**FIGURE 7.42.1C** Labeled ultrasound image of the lumbar plexus via the lateral approach, transverse view.

**Abbreviations:** AcP, Accessory Process; LP, Lumbar Plexus; B, Vertebral Body; PsMM, Psoas Major Muscle; LDM, Latissumus Dorsi Muscle.

## Lumbar Plexus, Lateral Longitudinal View

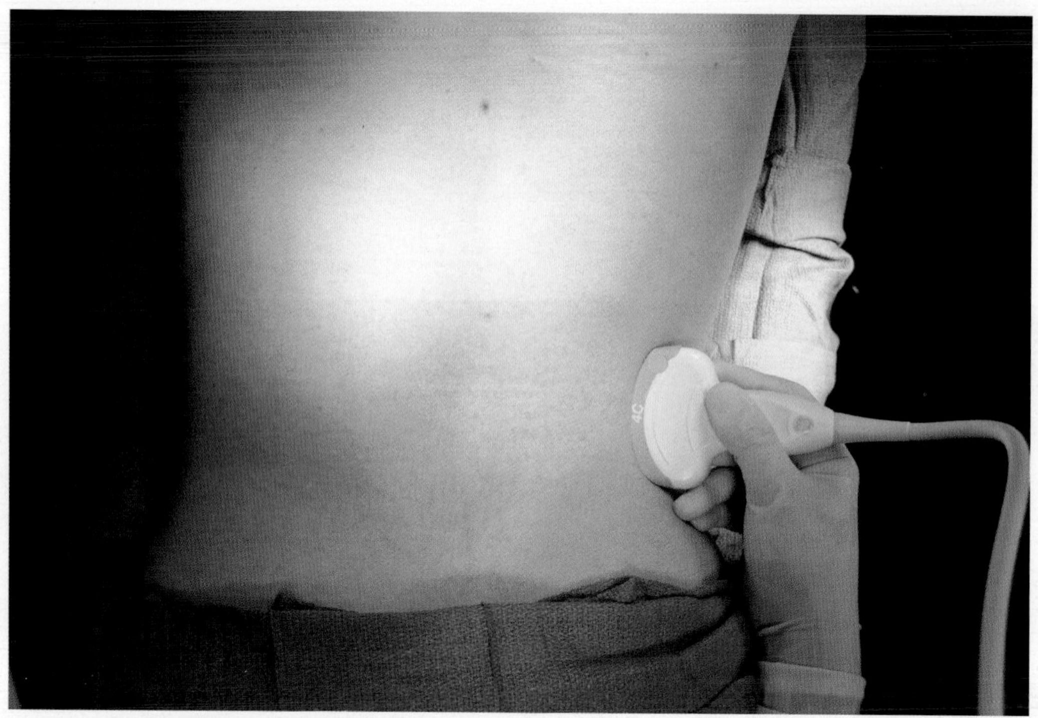

**FIGURE 7.43.1A** Ultrasound transducer position to image the lumbar plexus, lateral longitudinal view.

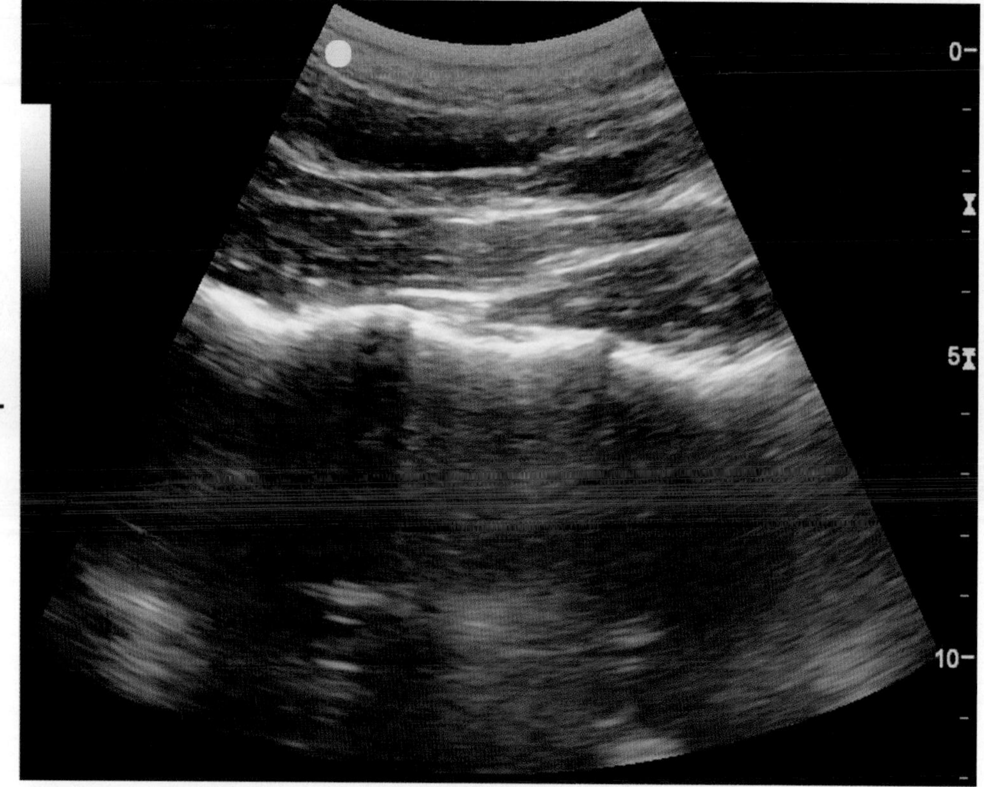


**FIGURE 7.43.1B** Ultrasound image of the lumbar plexus, lateral longitudinal view.

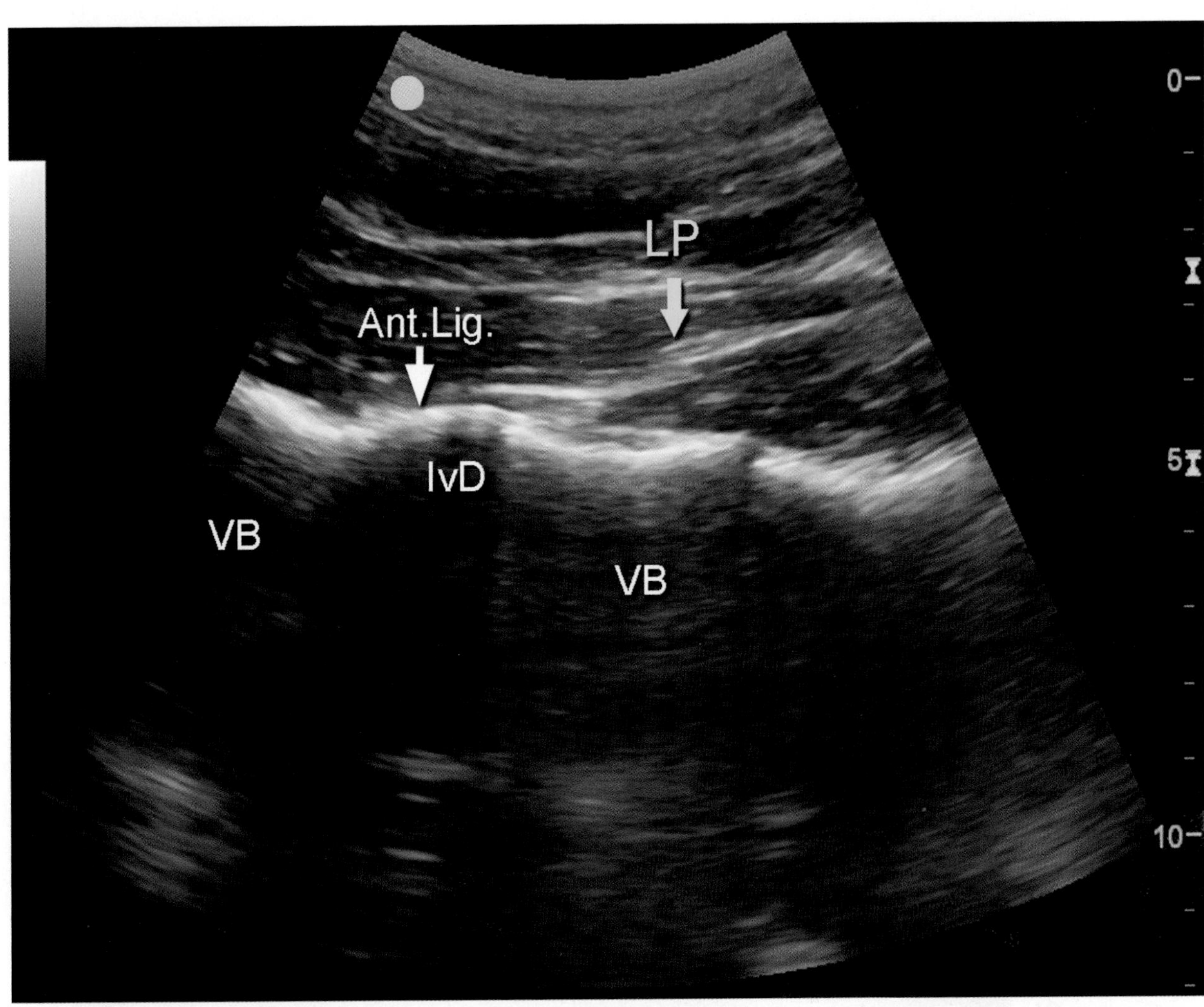


**FIGURE 7.43.1C** Labeled ultrasound image of the lumbar plexus via the lateral approach, longitudinal view.

**Abbreviations:** VB, Vertebral Body; IvD, Intervertebral Disc; Ant. Lig., Anterior Ligament; LP, Lumbar Plexus.

# Lumbar Plexus, Posterior Oblique View

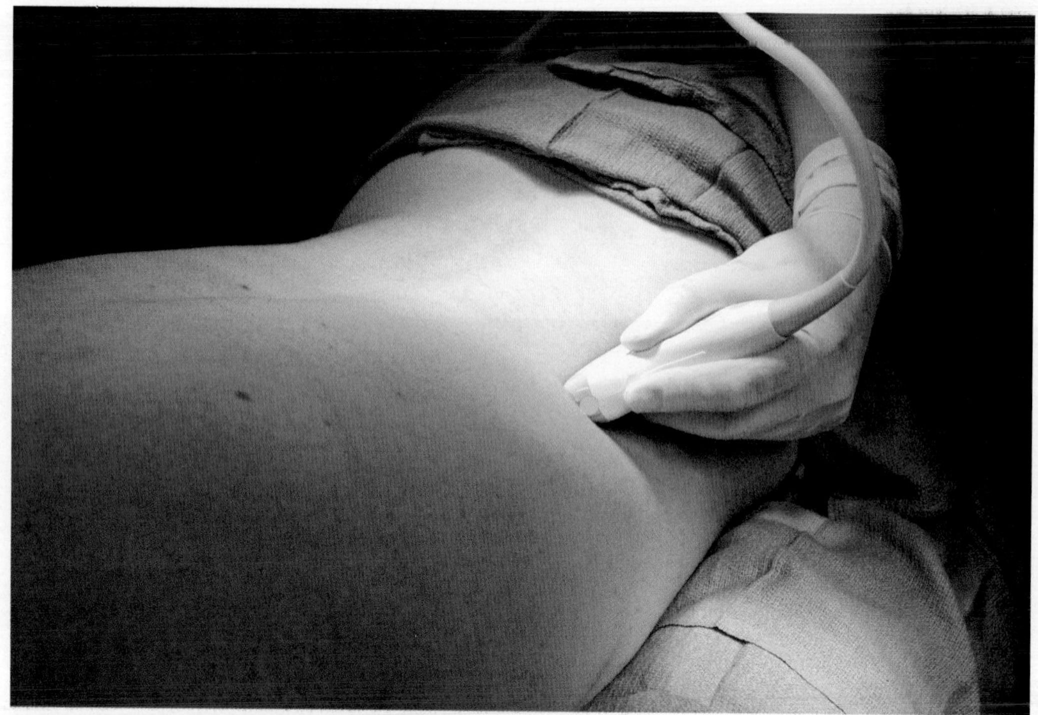

**FIGURE 7.44.1A** Ultrasound transducer position to image the lumbar plexus, posterior oblique view.

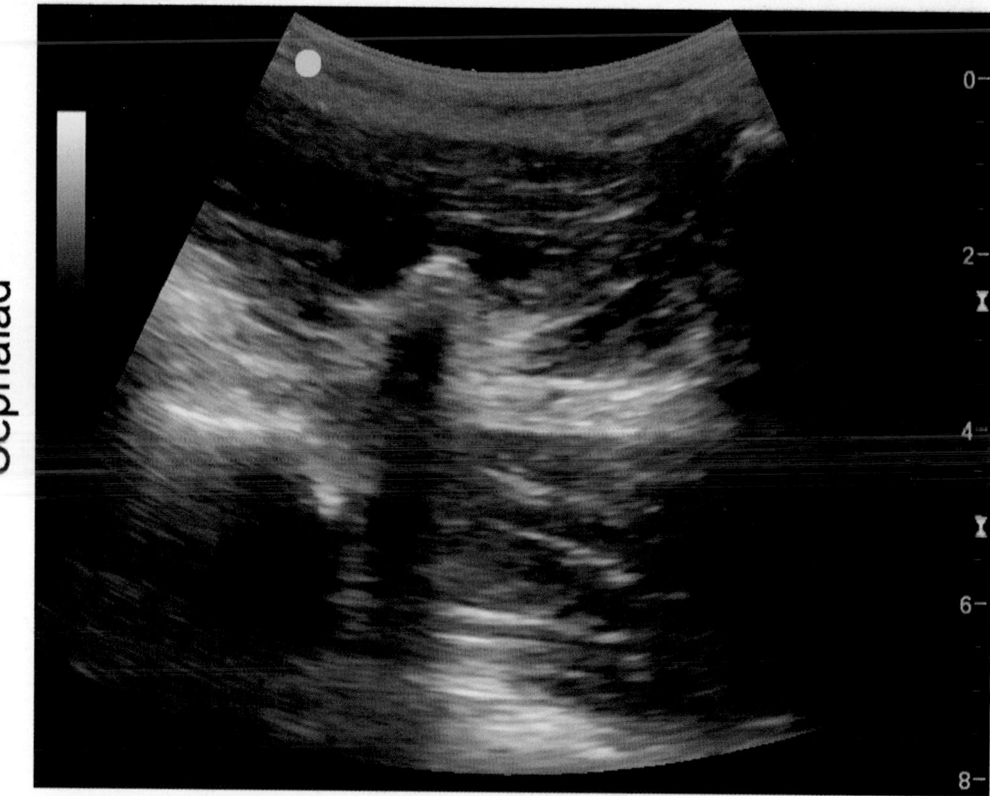


**FIGURE 7.44.1B** Ultrasound image of the lumbar plexus, posterior oblique view.

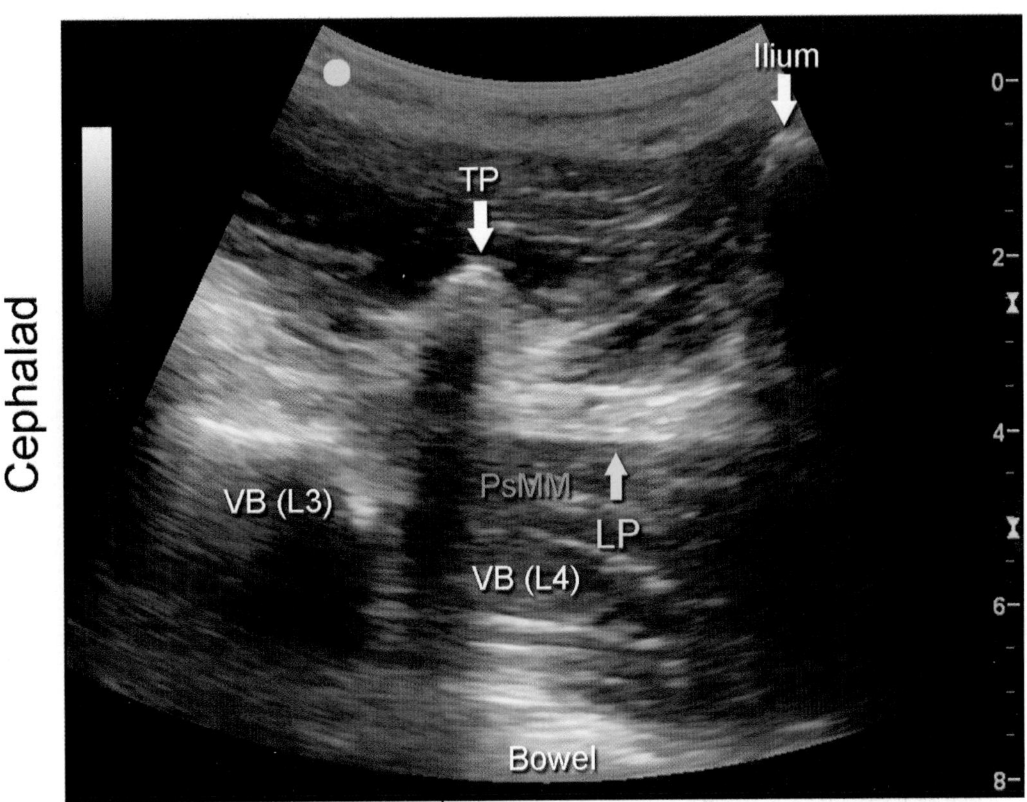


**FIGURE 7.44.1C** Labeled ultrasound image of the lumbar plexus via the posterior, posterior, oblique view.

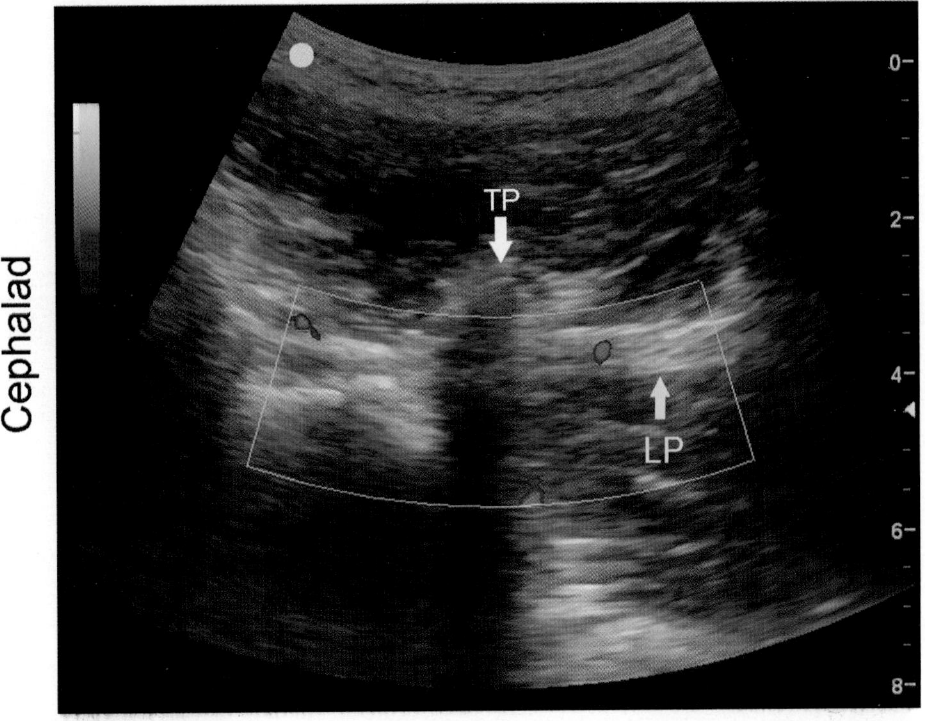


**FIGURE 7.44.1D** Labeled ultrasound image of the lumbar plexus, posterior oblique view with color flow Doppler.

**Abbreviations:** TP, Transverse Process; VB, Vertebral Body; PsMM, Psoas Major Muscle; LP, Lumbar Plexus.

# Anatomy of the Lumbar Spine, Posterior Longitudinal View

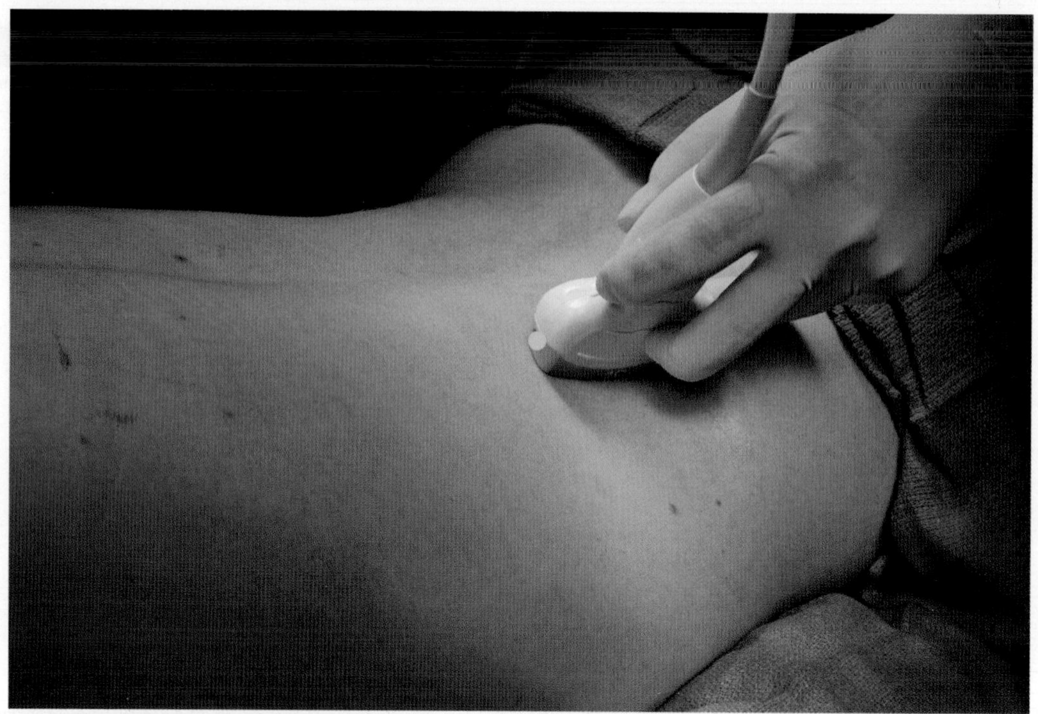

**FIGURE 7.45.1A** Anatomy of the lumbar spine, posterior longitudinal view.

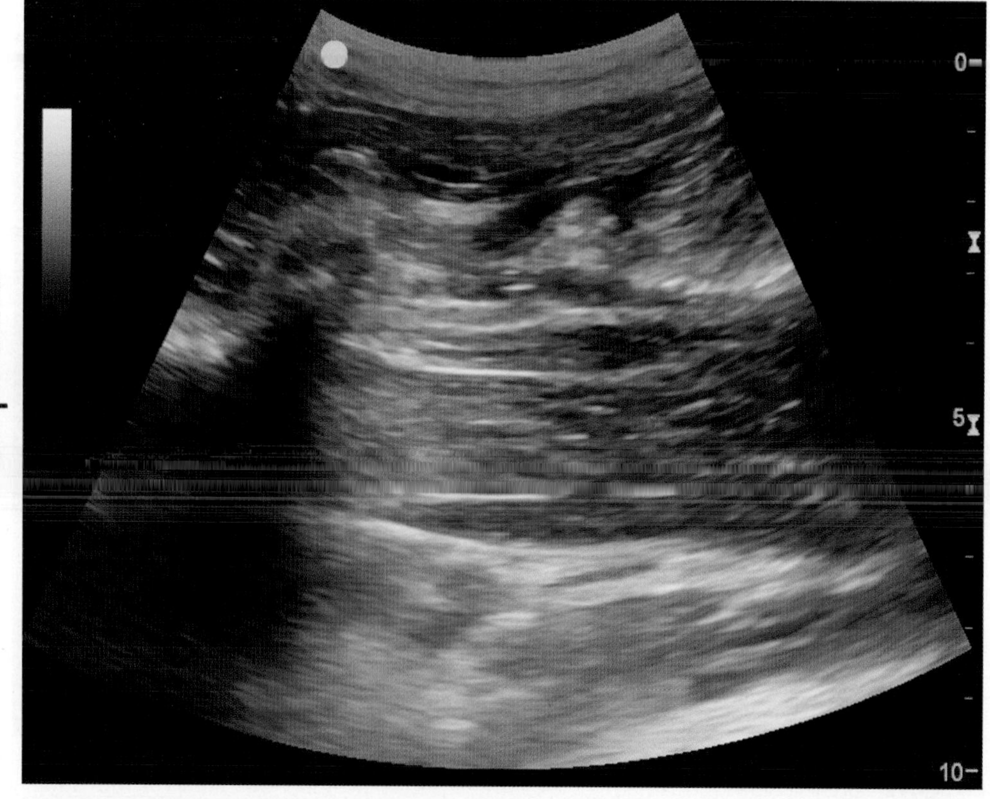


**FIGURE 7.45.1B** Anatomy of the lumbar spine, posterior longitudinal view.

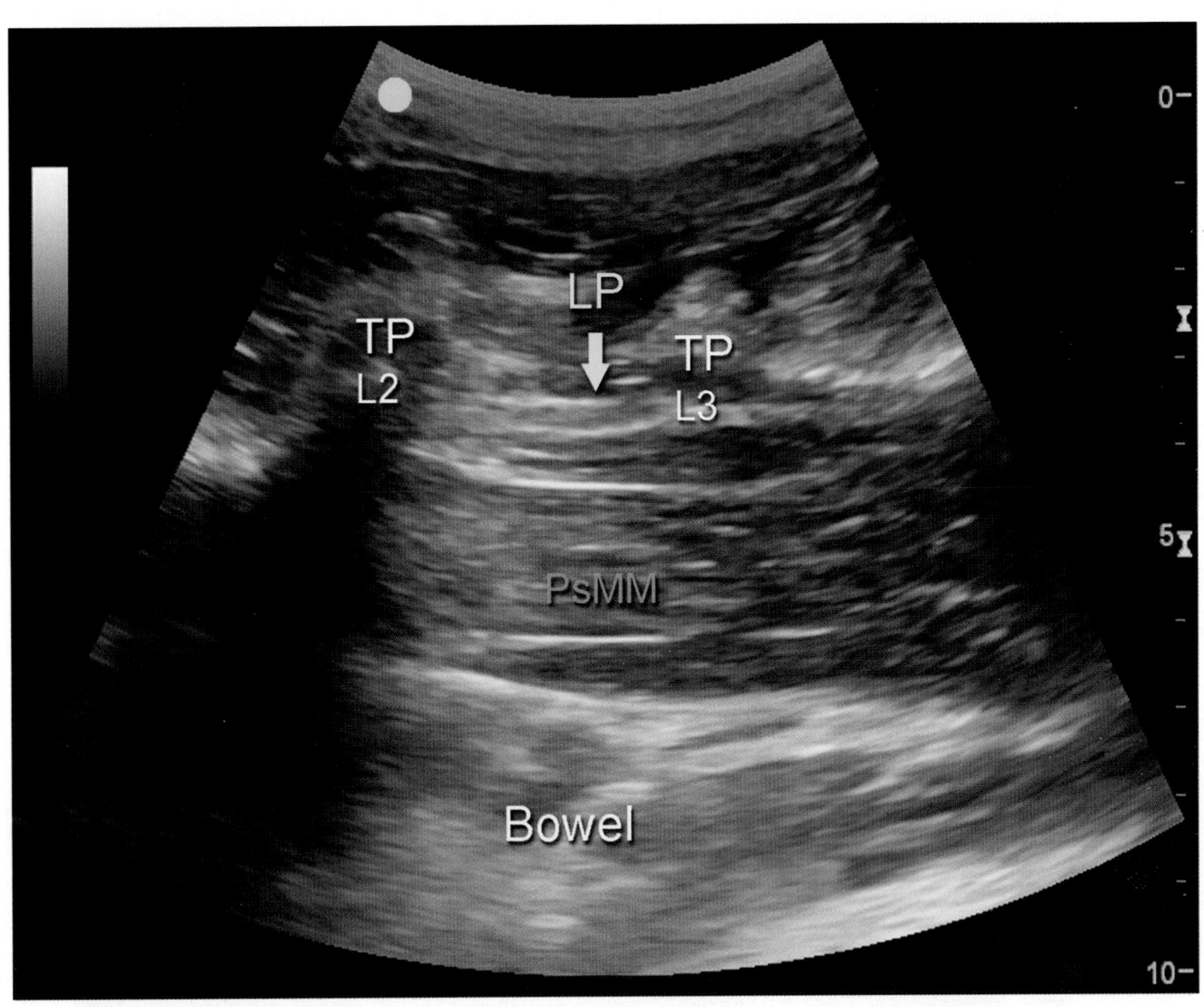


**FIGURE 7.45.1C** Labeled anatomy of the lumbar spine, posterior longitudinal view.

**Abbreviations:** TP, Transverse Process; LP, Lumbar Plexus; PsMM, Psoas Major Muscle.

## Sacral Plexus, Posterior Transverse View

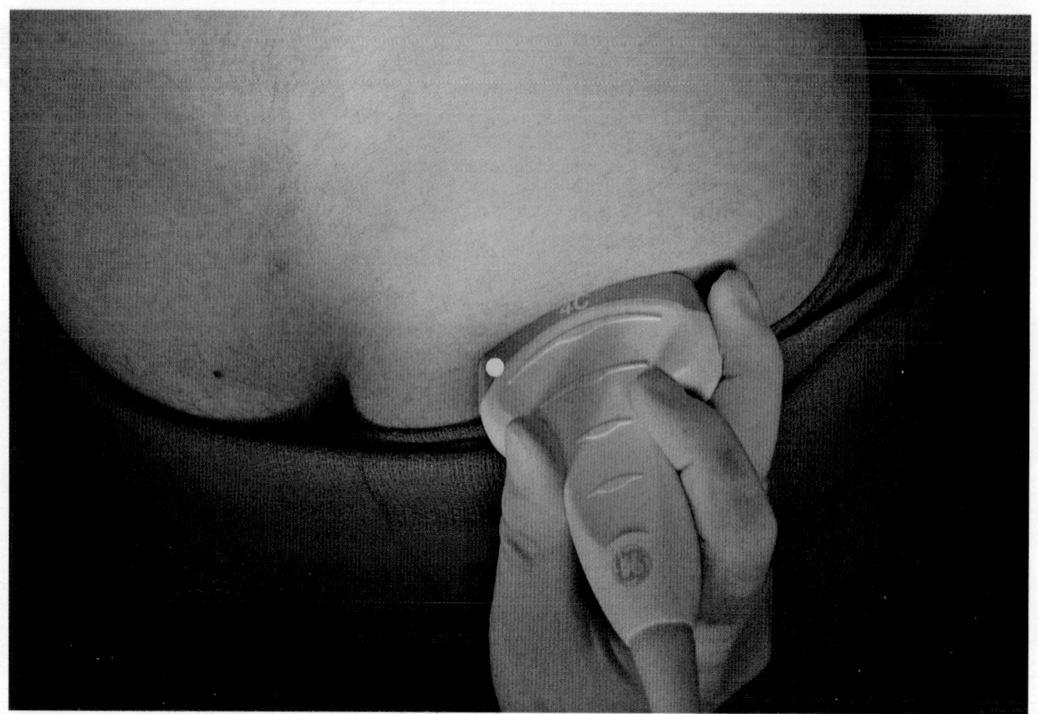

**FIGURE 7.46.1A** Ultrasound transducer position to image the sacral plexus, posterior transverse view.

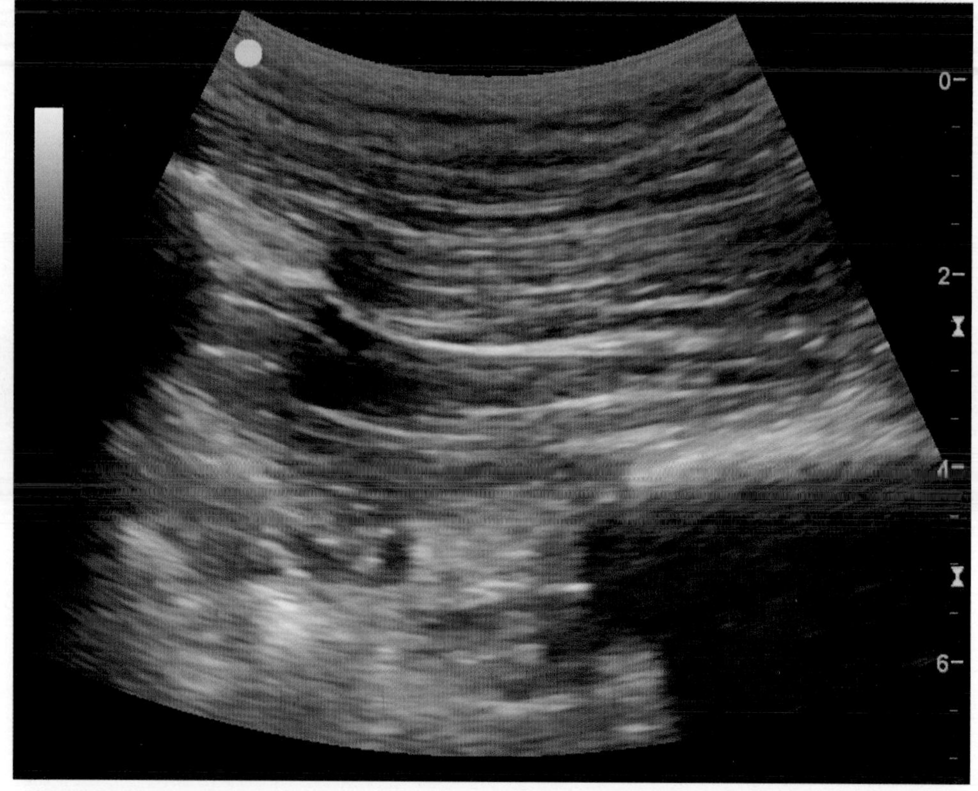


**FIGURE 7.46.1B** Ultrasound image of the sacral plexus, posterior transverse view.

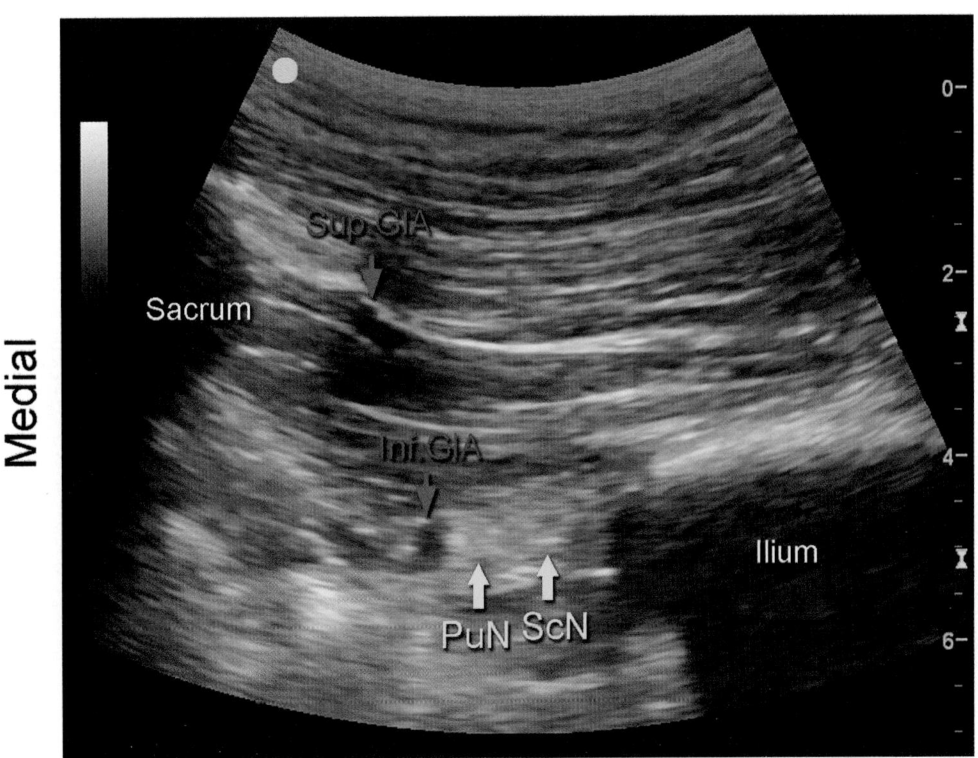


**FIGURE 7.46.1C** Labeled ultrasound image of the sacral plexus, posterior transverse view.

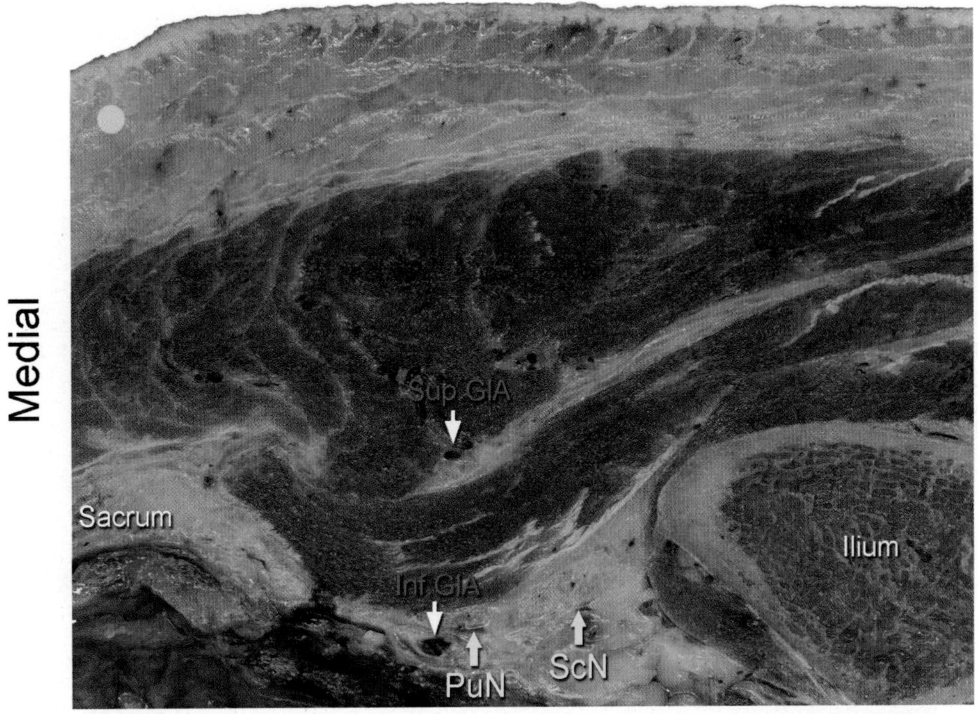


**FIGURE 7.46.1D** Labeled cross-sectional anatomy of the sacral plexus, posterior transverse view.

**Abbreviations:** Sup. GIA, Superior Gluteal Artery; Inf. GIA, Inferior Gluteal Artery; PuN, Pudendal Nerve; ScN, Sciatic Nerve.

# Sciatic Nerve, Anterior Longitudinal View

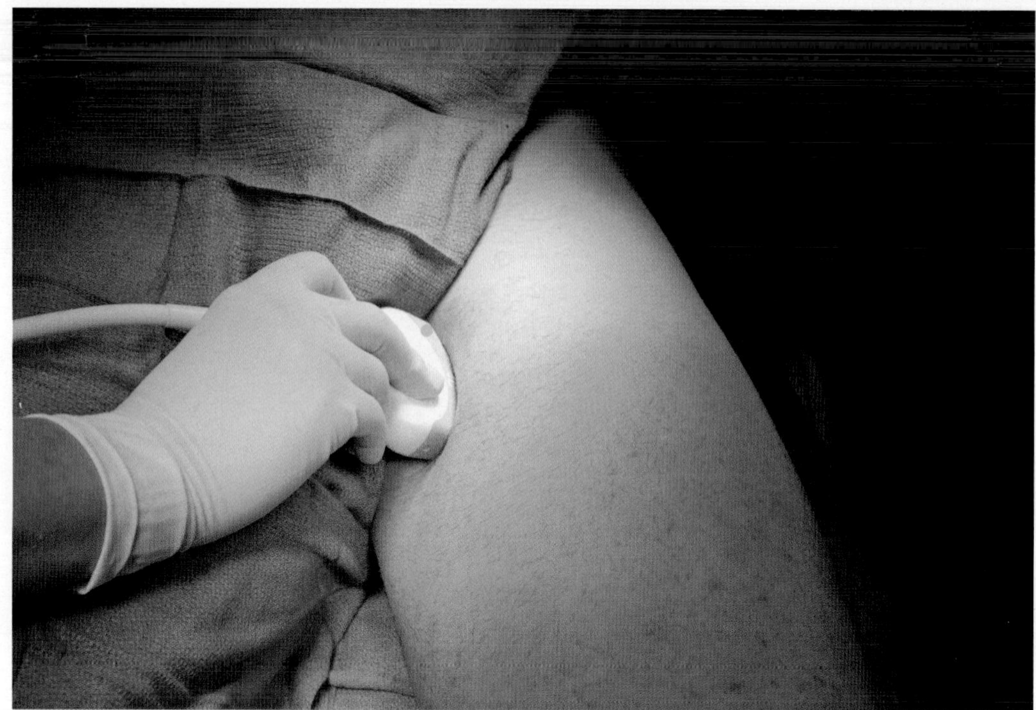

**FIGURE 7.47.1A** Ultrasound transducer position to image the sciatic nerve, anterior longitudinal view.

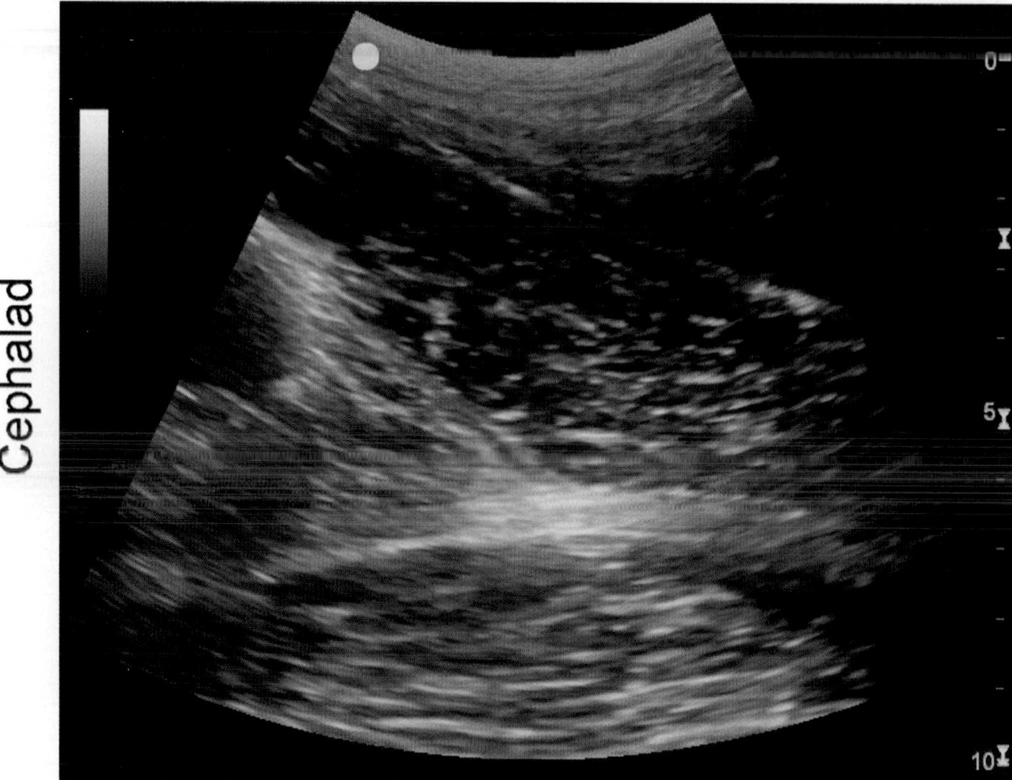


**FIGURE 7.47.1B** Ultrasound image of the sciatic nerve, anterior longitudinal view.

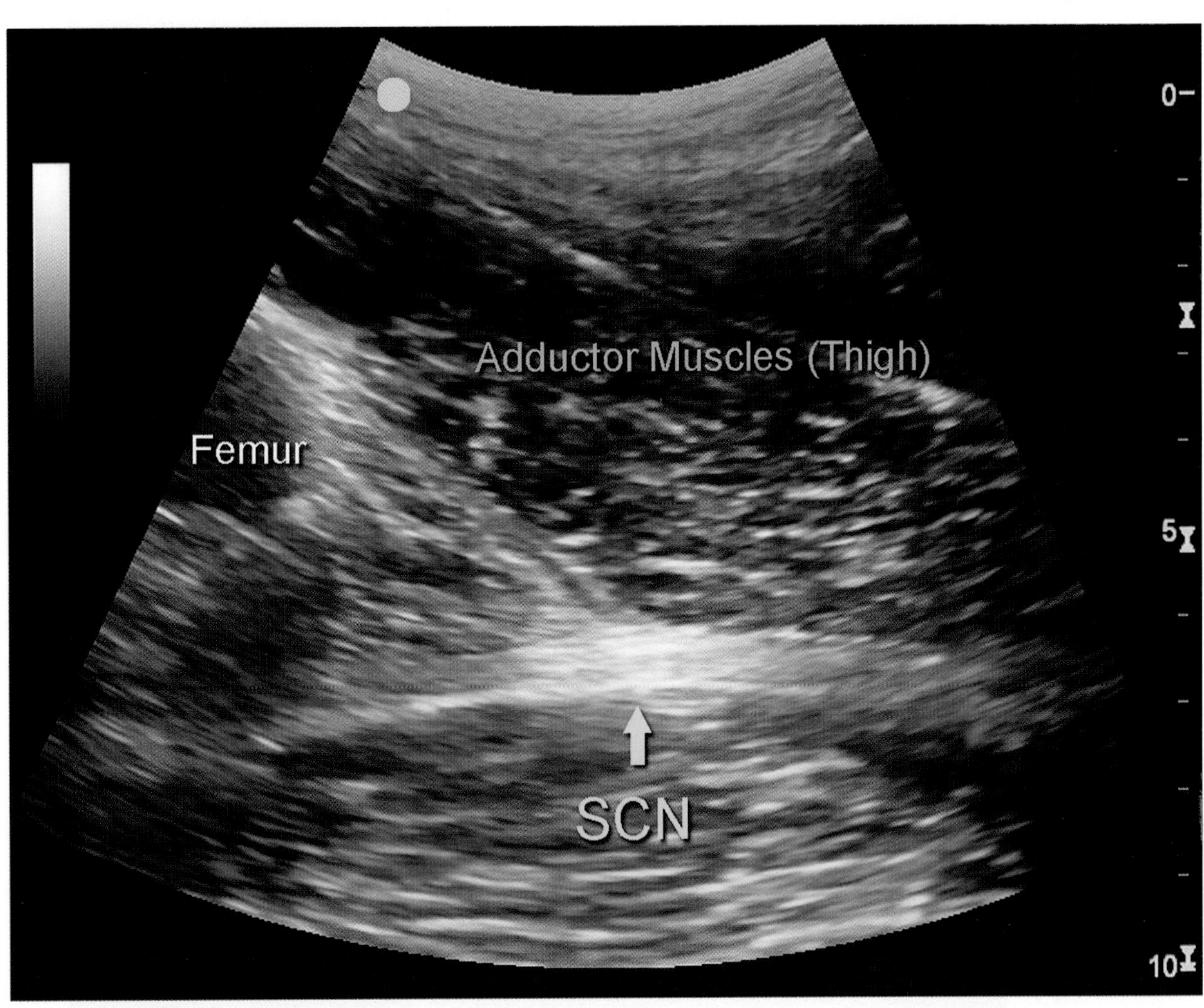


**FIGURE 7.47.1C** Labeled ultrasound image of the sciatic nerve, anterior longitudinal view.

**Abbreviation:** SCN, Sciatic Nerve.

## Sciatic Nerve, Anterior Transverse View

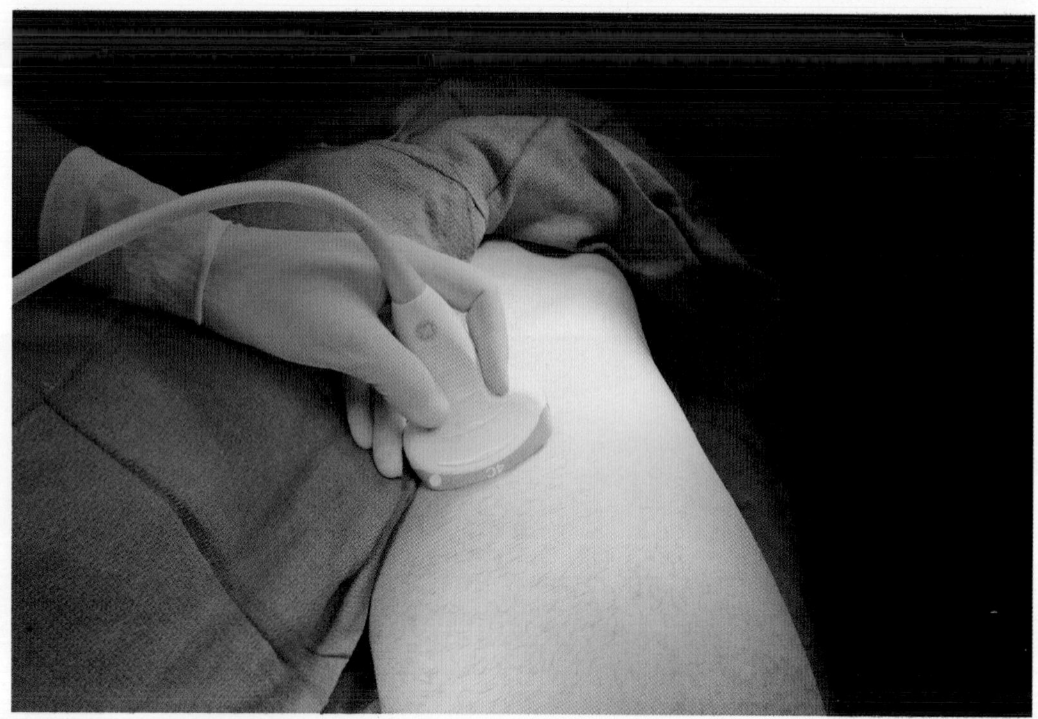

**FIGURE 7.47.2A** Ultrasound transducer position to image the sciatic nerve, anterior transverse view.

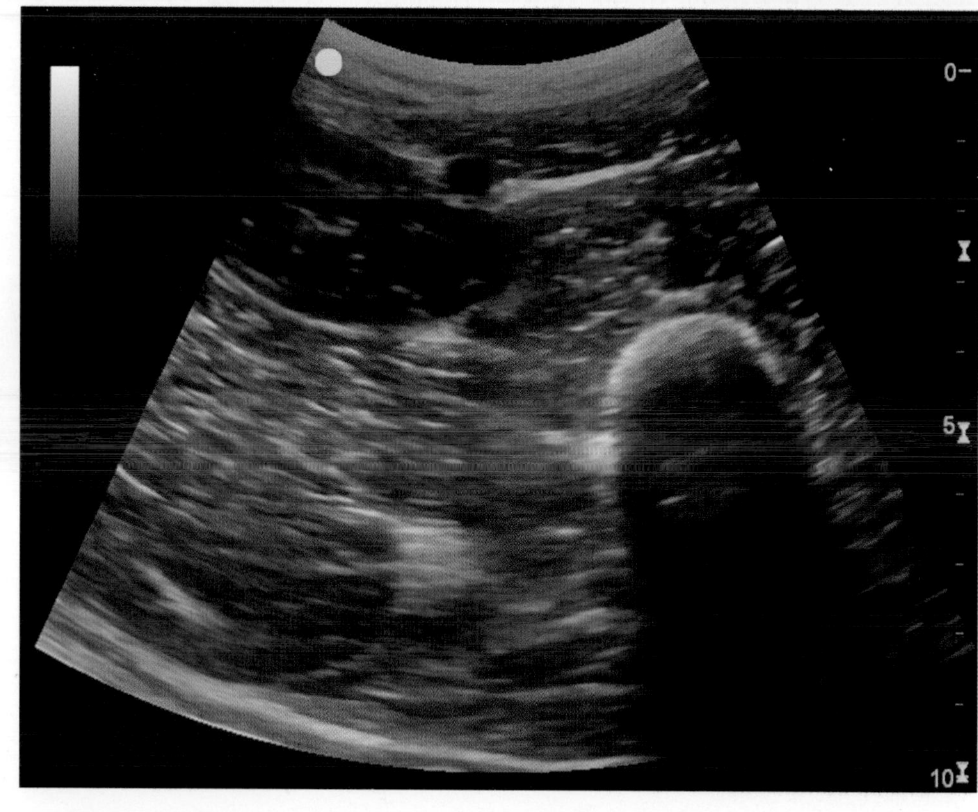


**FIGURE 7.47.2B** Ultrasound image of the sciatic nerve, anterior transverse view.

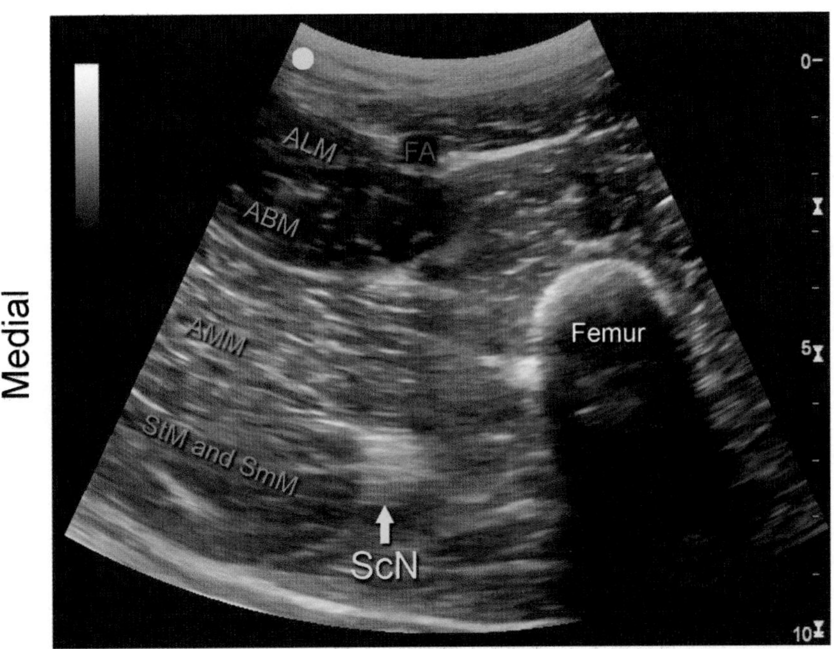


**FIGURE 7.47.2C** Labeled ultrasound image of the sciatic nerve, anterior transverse view.

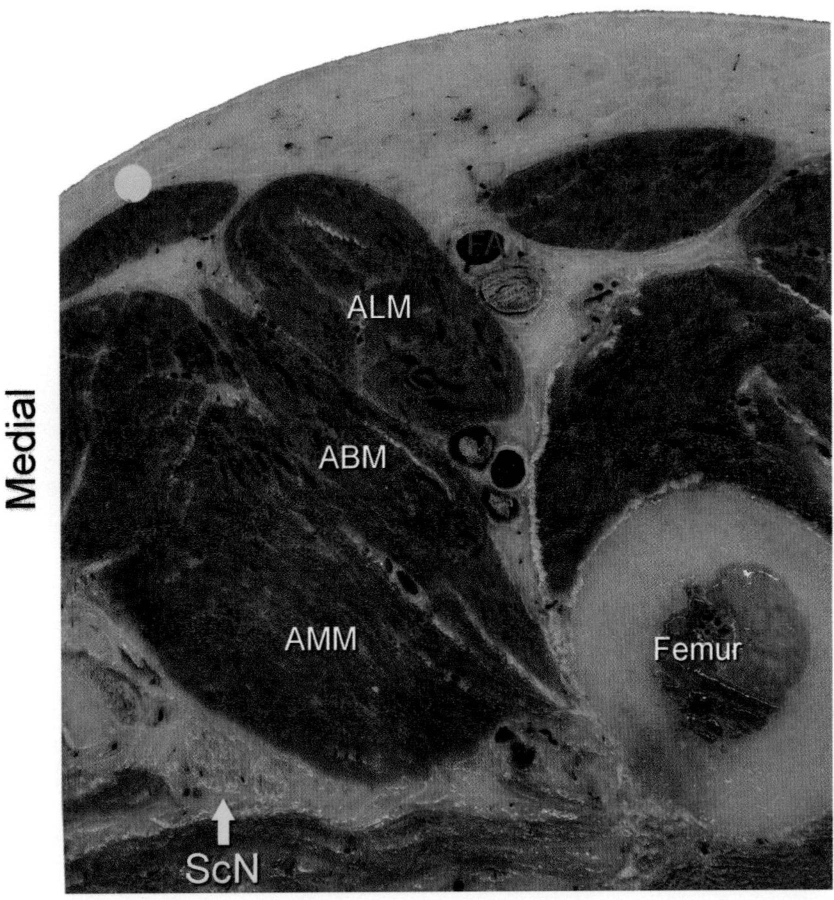


**FIGURE 7.47.2D** Labeled cross-sectional anatomy of the sciatic nerve, anterior transverse view.

**Abbreviations:** FA, Femoral Artery; ALM, Adductor Longus Muscle; ABM, Adductor Brevis Muscle; AMM, Adductor Magnus Muscle; ScN, Sciatic Nerve; StM, Semitendinosus Muscle; SmM, Semimembranosus Muscle.

## Sciatic Nerve, Lateral Transverse View

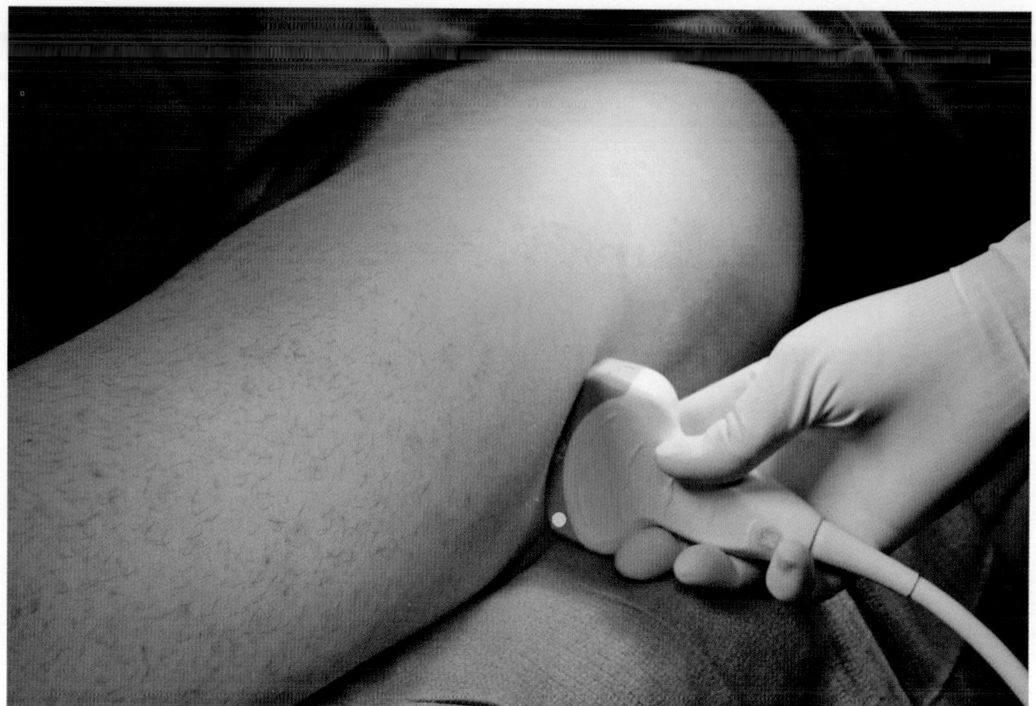

**FIGURE 7.47.3A** Ultrasound transducer position to image the sciatic nerve, lateral transverse view.

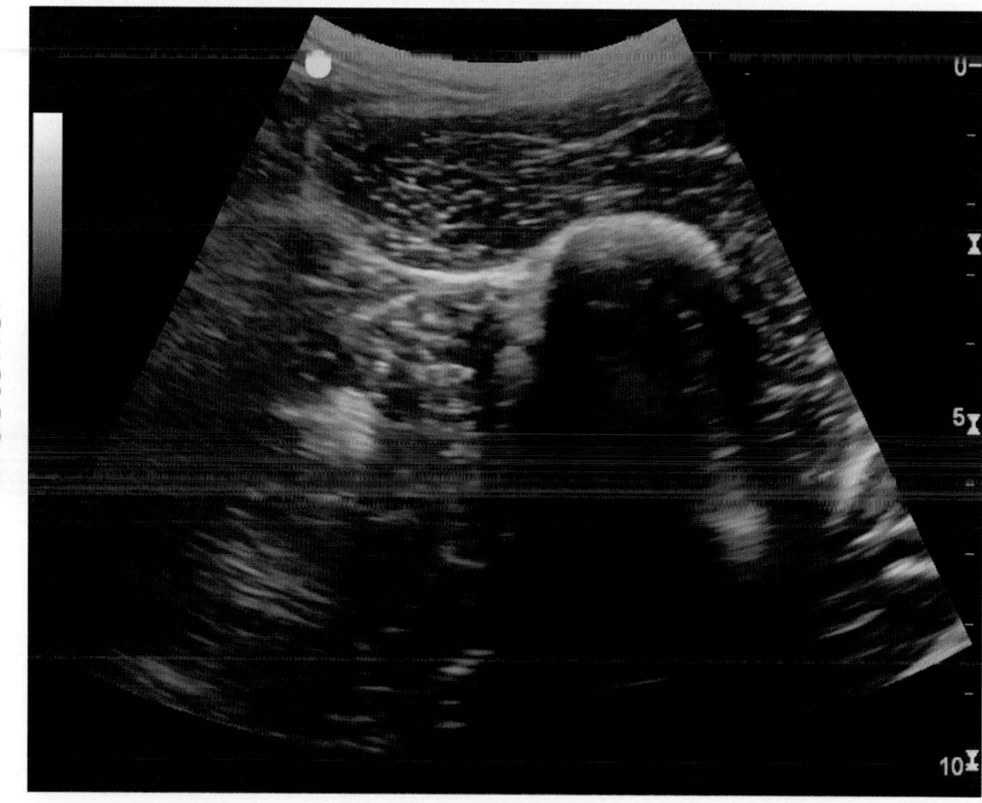


**FIGURE 7.47.3B** Ultrasound image of the sciatic nerve, lateral transverse view.

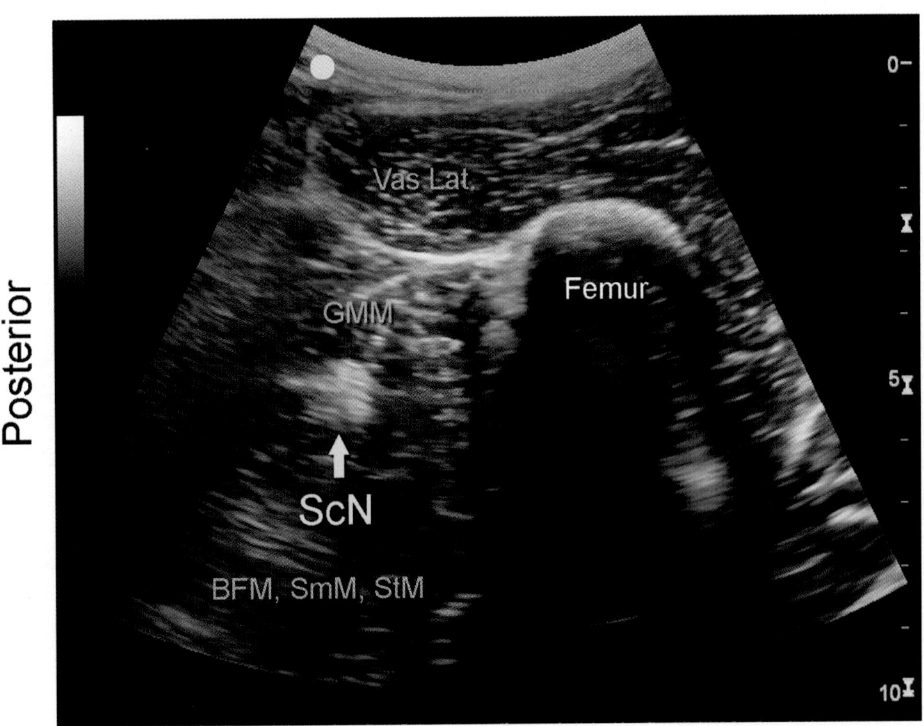


**FIGURE 7.47.3C** Labeled ultrasound image of the sciatic nerve, lateral transverse view.

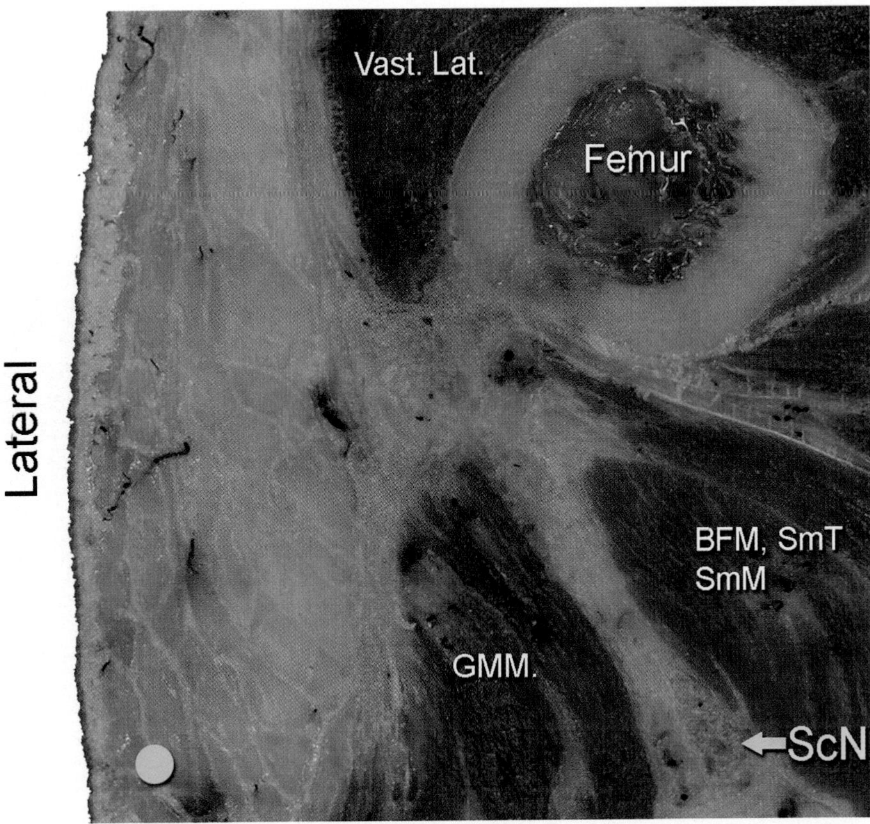


**FIGURE 7.47.3D** Labeled cross-sectional anatomy of the sciatic nerve, lateral transverse view.

**Abbreviations:** ScN, Sciatic Nerve; GMM, Gluteus Maximus; Vast. Lat., Vastus Lateralis Muscle; BFM, Biceps femoris Muscle; SmM, Semimembranosus Muscle; StM, Semitendinosus Muscle.

## Sciatic Nerve at the Popliteal Fossa, Posterior View

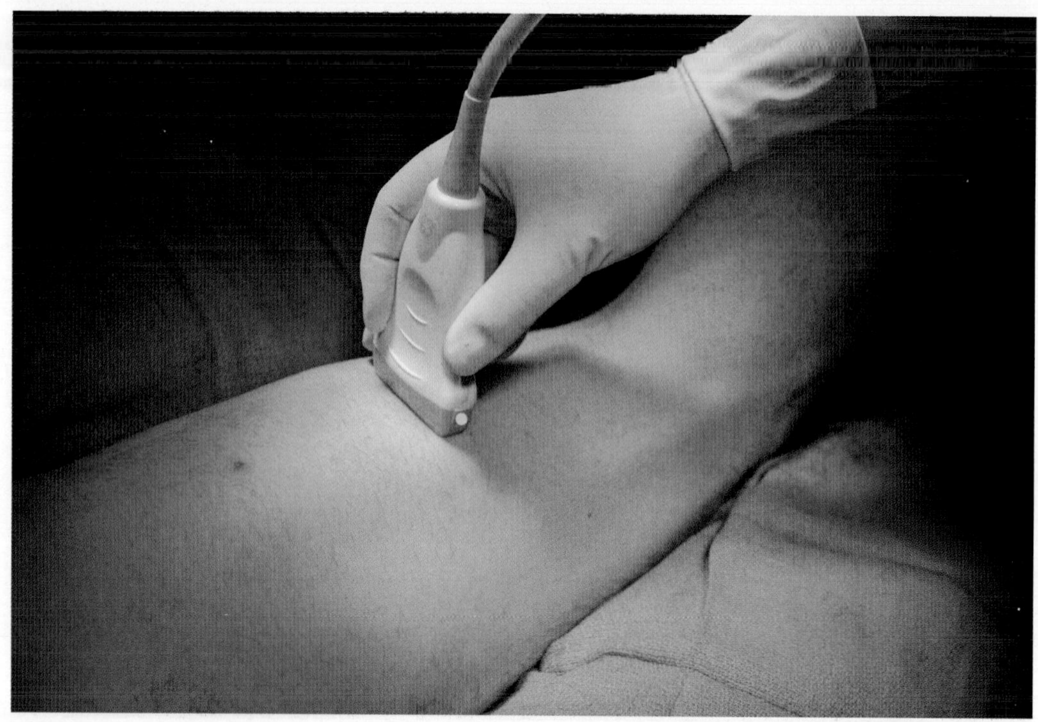

**FIGURE 7.48.1A** Ultrasound transducer position to image the sciatic nerve at the popliteal fossa, posterior view.

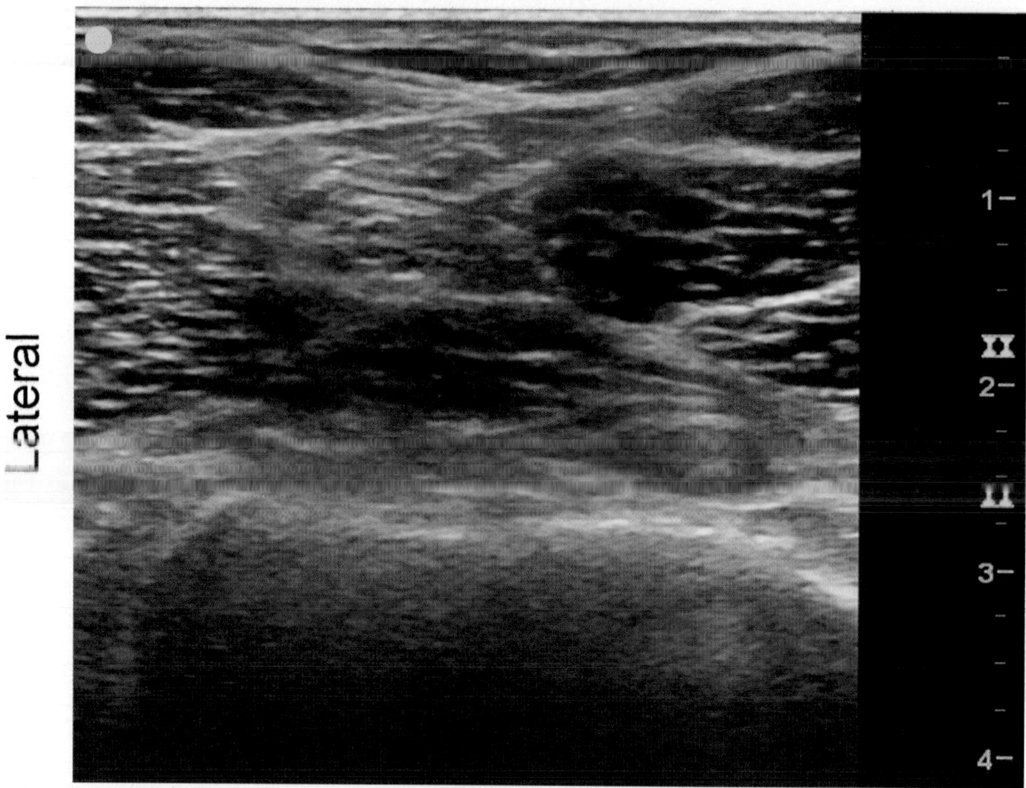


**FIGURE 7.48.1B** Ultrasound image of the sciatic nerve at the popliteal fossa, posterior view.

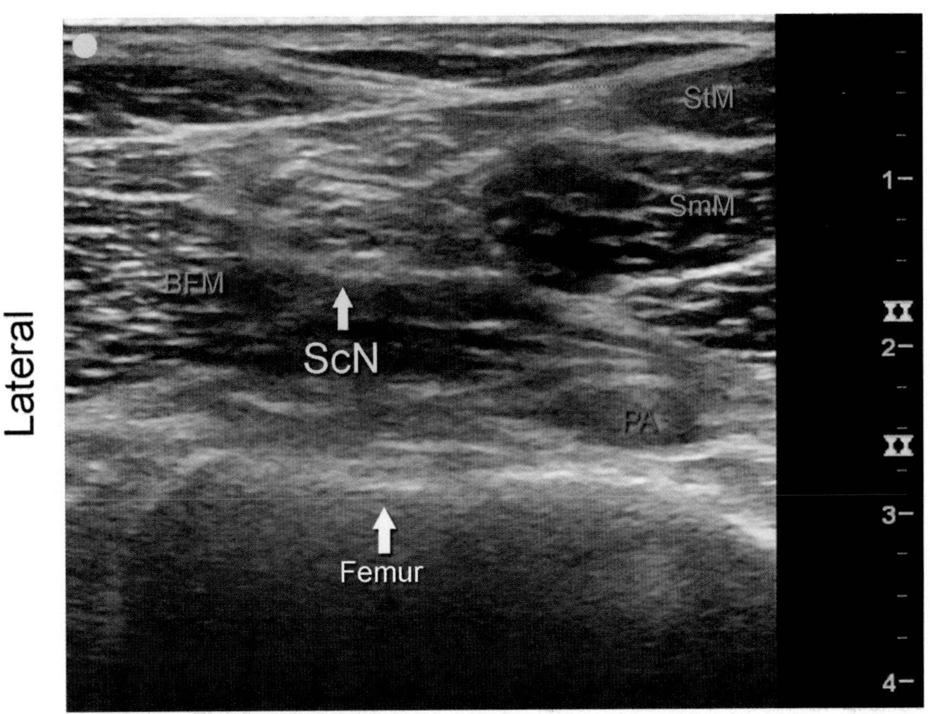


**FIGURE 7.48.1C** Labeled ultrasound image of the sciatic nerve at the popliteal fossa, posterior view.

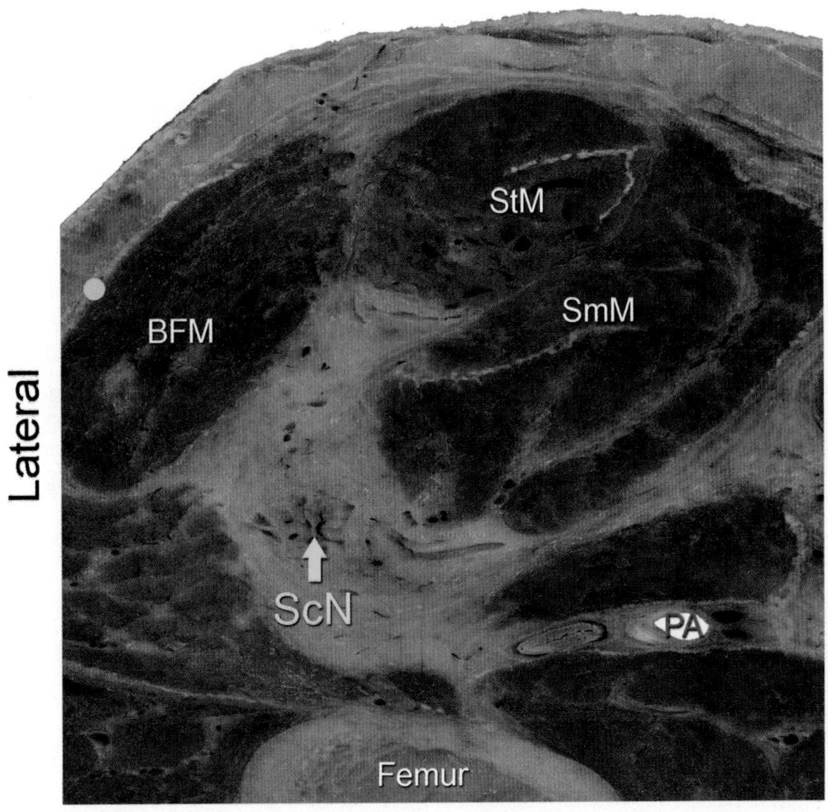


**FIGURE 7.48.1D** Labeled cross-sectional anatomy of the sciatic nerve at the popliteal fossa, posterior view.

**Abbreviations:** StM, Semitendinosus Muscle; SmM, Semimembranosus Muscle; BFM, Biceps Femoris Muscle; ScN, Sciatic Nerve; PA, Popliteal Artery.

## Anatomy of the Sciatic Nerve at the Distal Popliteal Fossa

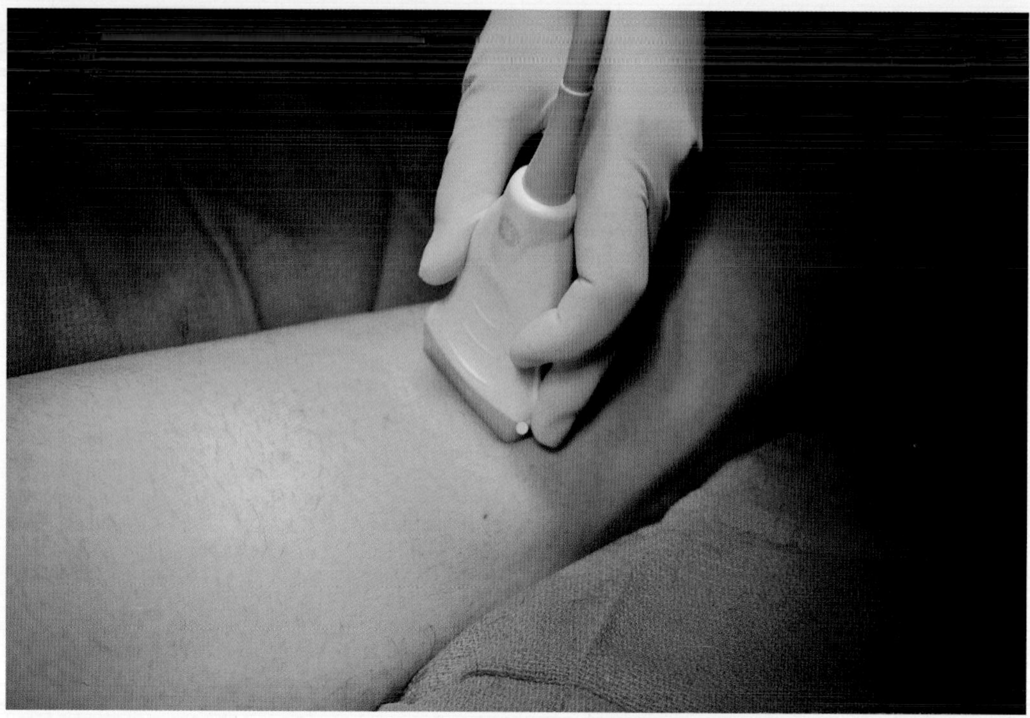

**FIGURE 7.48.2A** Ultrasound transducer position to image the sciatic nerve bifurcation at the popliteal fossa, posterior view.

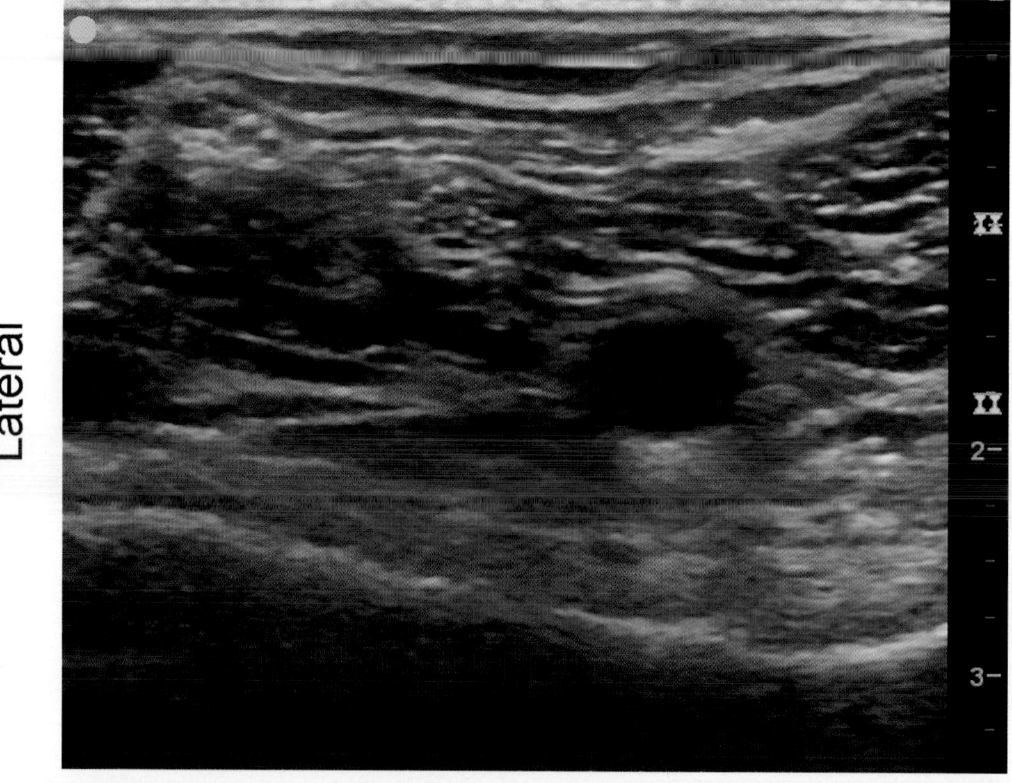


**FIGURE 7.48.2B** Ultrasound image of the sciatic nerve bifurcation at the popliteal fossa, posterior view.

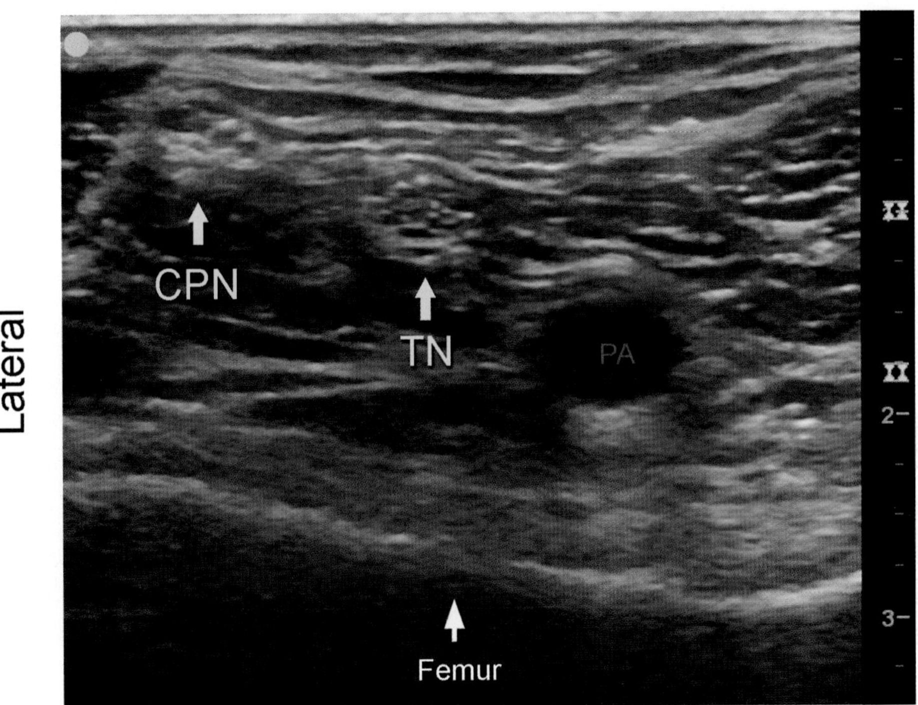


**FIGURE 7.48.2C** Labeled ultrasound image of the sciatic nerve bifurcation at the popliteal fossa, posterior view.

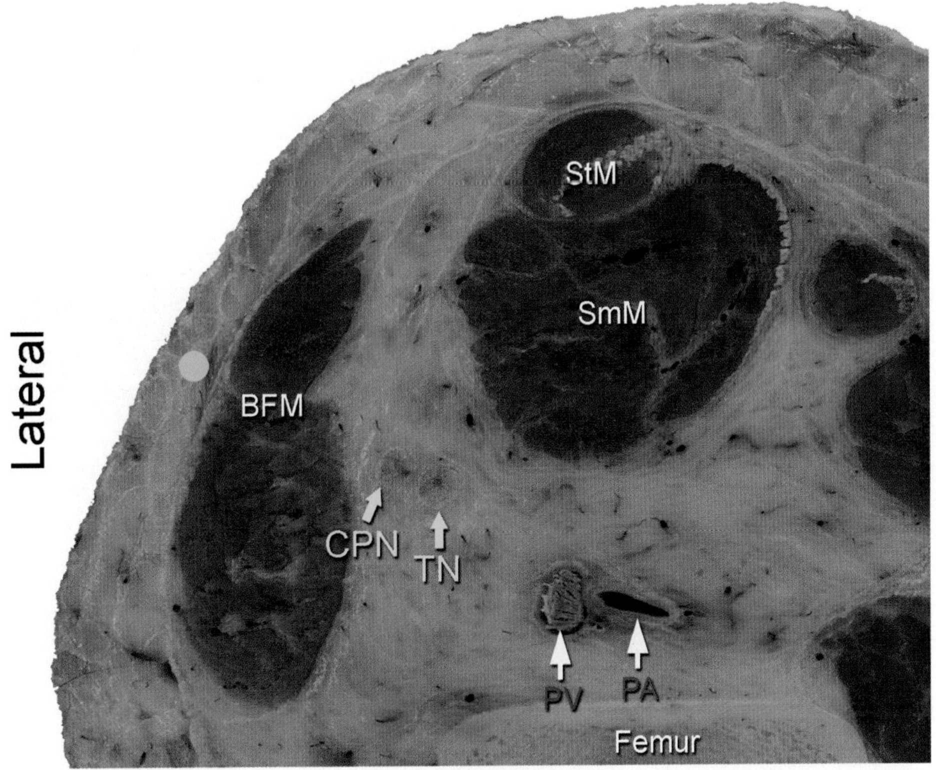


**FIGURE 7.48.2D** Labeled cross-sectional anatomy of the sciatic nerve bifurcation at the popliteal fossa, posterior view.

**Abbreviations:** StM, Semitendinosus Muscle; SmM, Semimembranosus Muscle; BFM, Biceps Femoris Muscle; CPN, Common Peroneal Nerve; TN, Tibial Nerve; PV, Popliteal Vein; PA, Popliteal Artery.

# Femoral Nerve, Transverse View

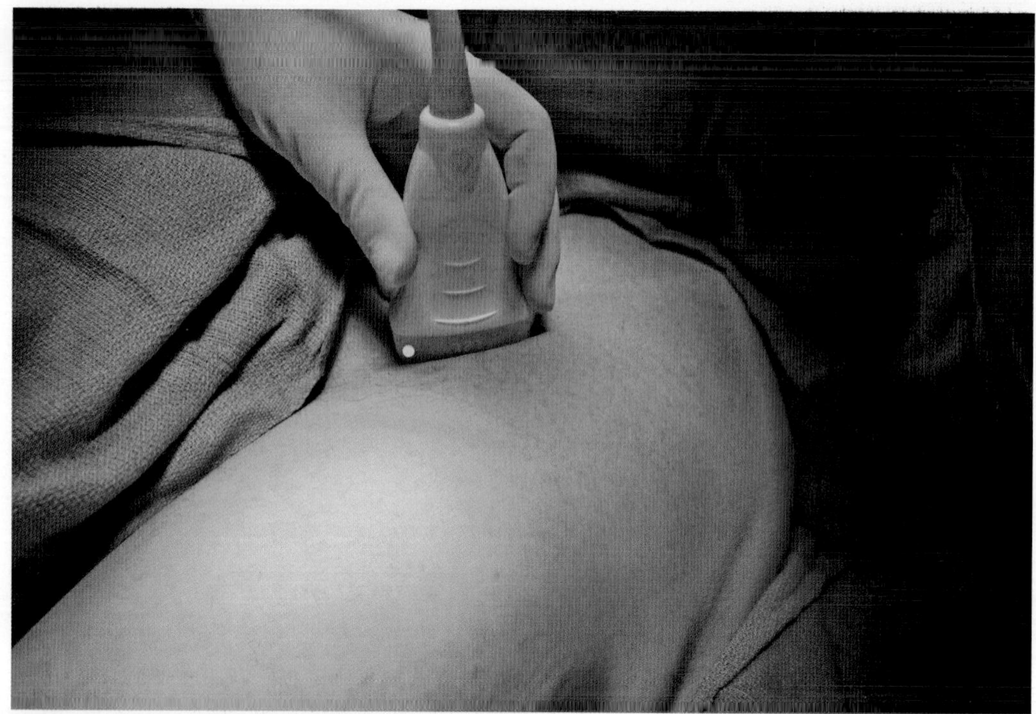

**FIGURE 7.49.1A** Ultrasound transducer position to image the femoral nerve, transverse view.

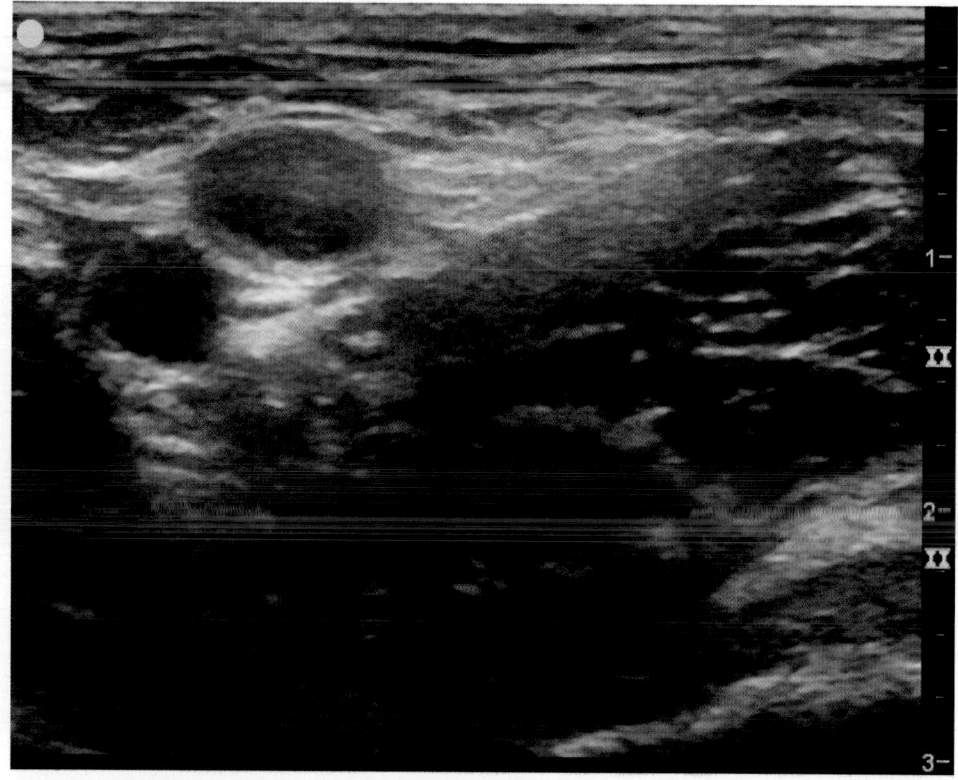


**FIGURE 7.49.1B** Ultrasound image of the femoral nerve, transverse view.

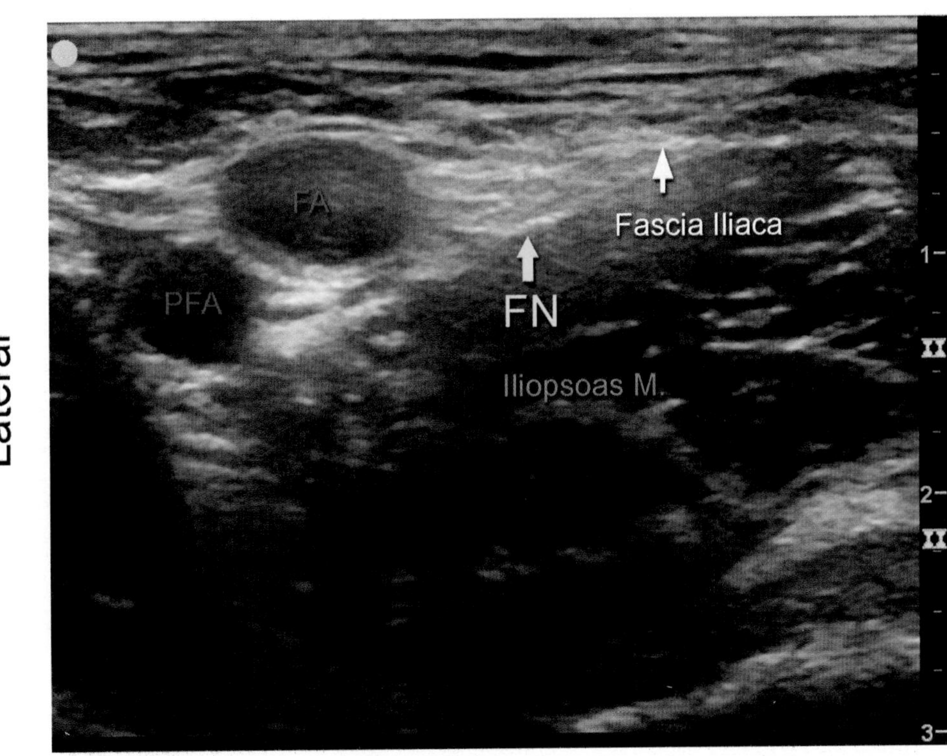


**FIGURE 7.49.1C** Labeled ultrasound image of the femoral nerve, transverse view.

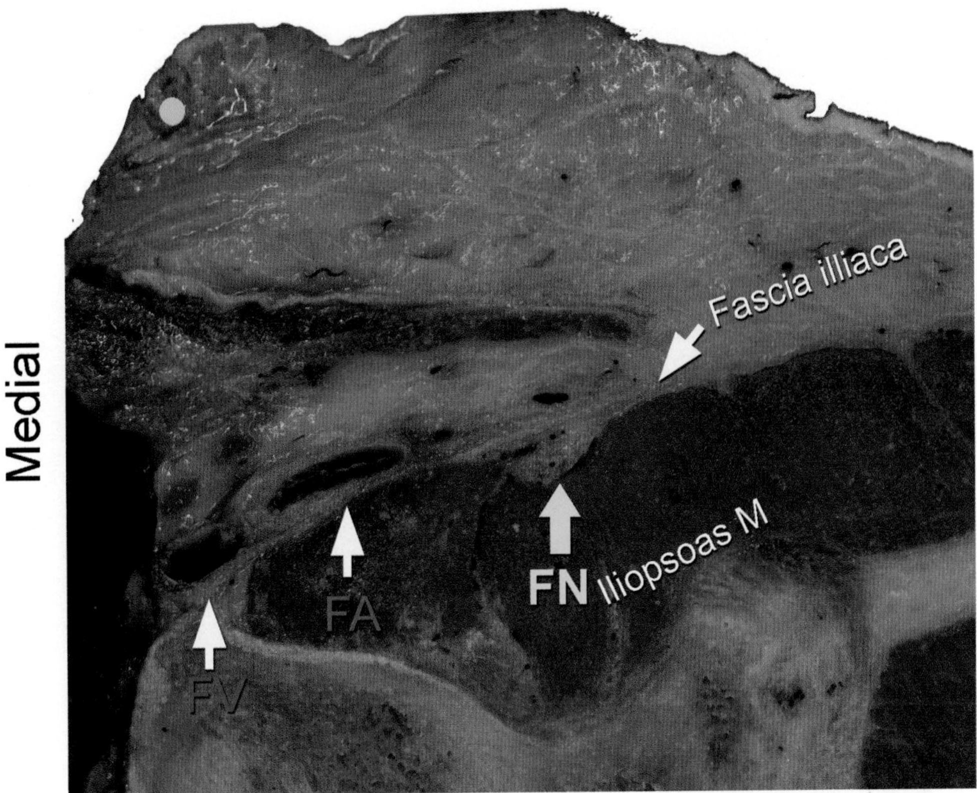


**FIGURE 7.49.1D** Labeled cross-sectional anatomy of the femoral nerve at the level between inguinal ligament and femoral crease.

**Abbreviations:** FA, Femoral Artery; PFA, Profunda Femoris Artery; FN, Femoral Nerve; FV, Femoral Vein.

# Obturator Nerve, Transverse View

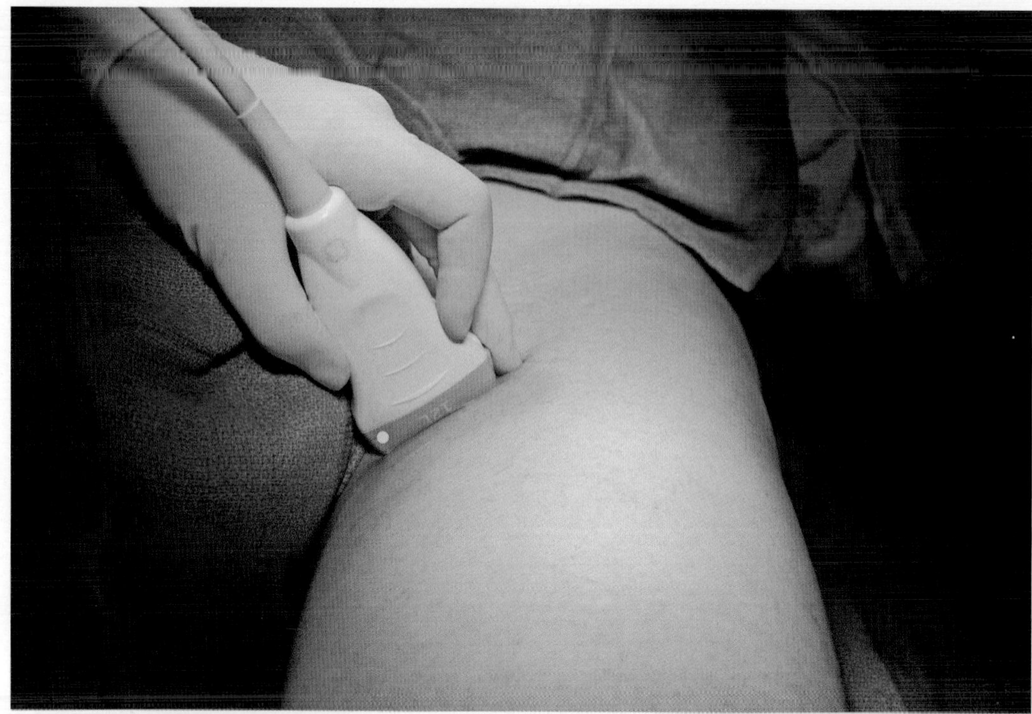

**FIGURE 7.50.1A** Ultrasound transducer position to image the obturator nerve, transverse view.

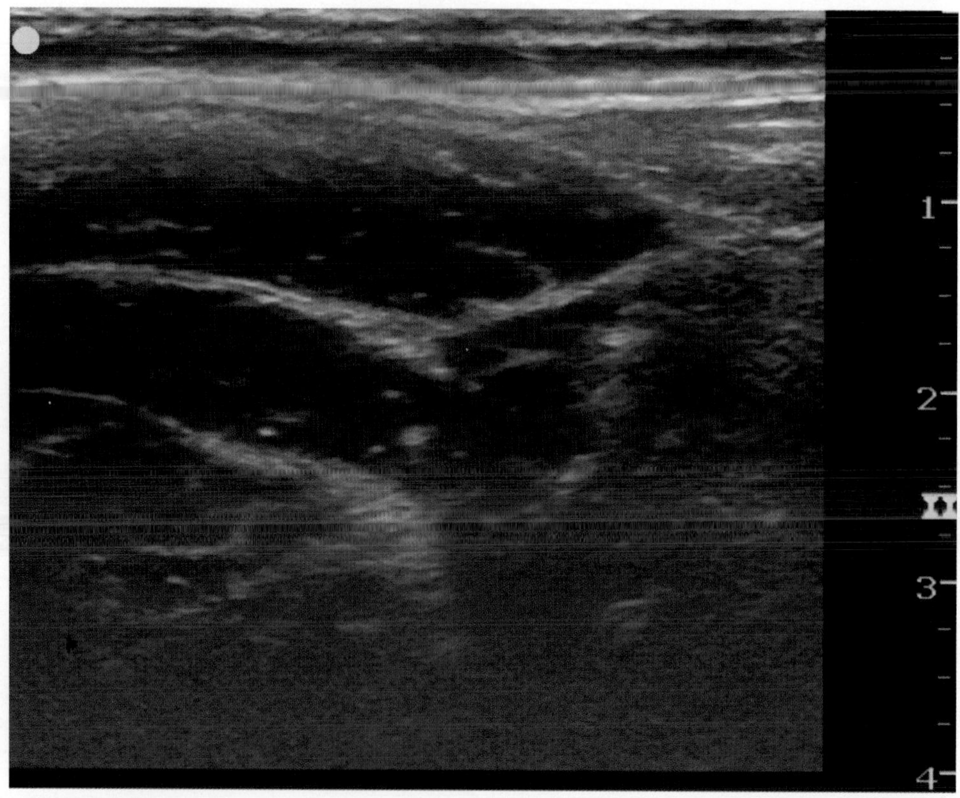


**FIGURE 7.50.1B** Ultrasound image of the obturator nerve, transverse view.

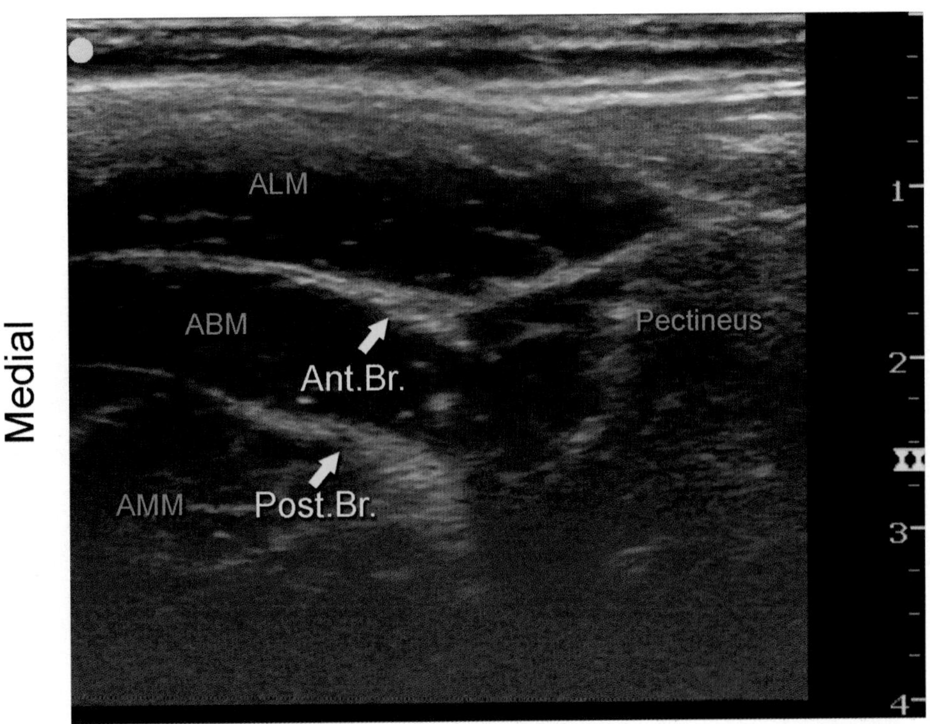


**FIGURE 7.50.1C** Labeled ultrasound image of the obturator nerve, transverse view.

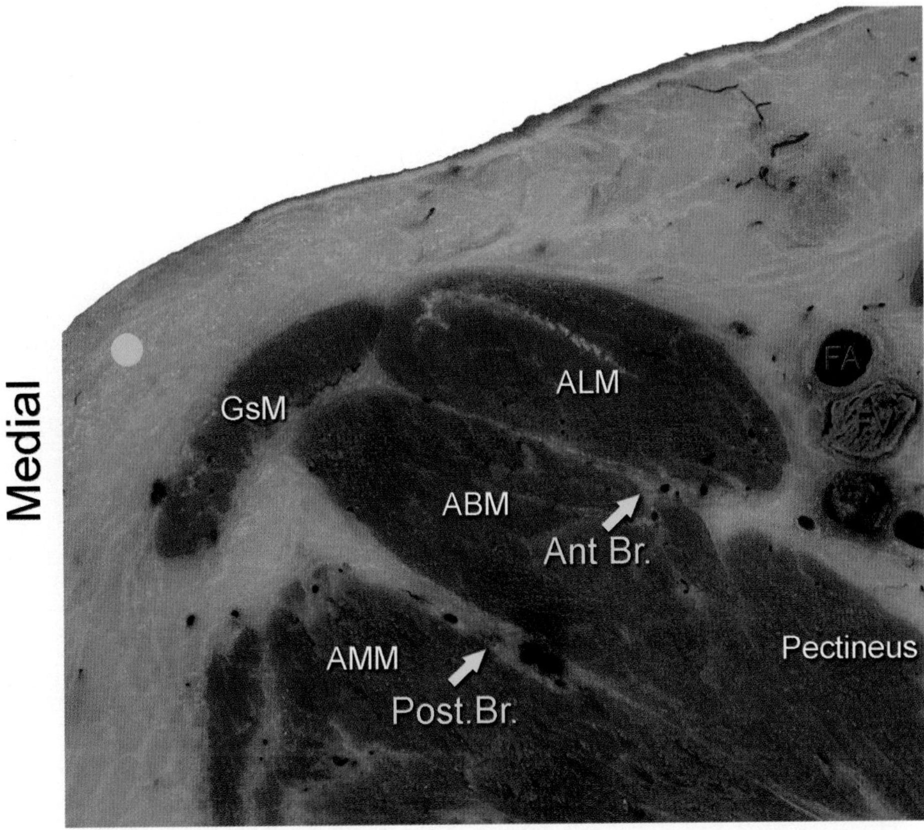


**FIGURE 7.52.1D** Labeled cross-sectional anatomy of the obturator nerve, transverse view.

**Abbreviations:** FA, Femoral Artery; FV, Femoral Vein; ALM, Adductor Longus Muscle; ABM, Adductor Brevis Muscle; AMM, Adductor Magnus Muscle; GsM, Gracilis Muscle; Ant. Br., Anterior Branch of Obturator Nerve; Post. Br., Posterior Branch of Obturator Nerve, Pectineus, Pectineus Muscle.

# Pudendal Nerve and Pudendal (Alcock's ) Canal

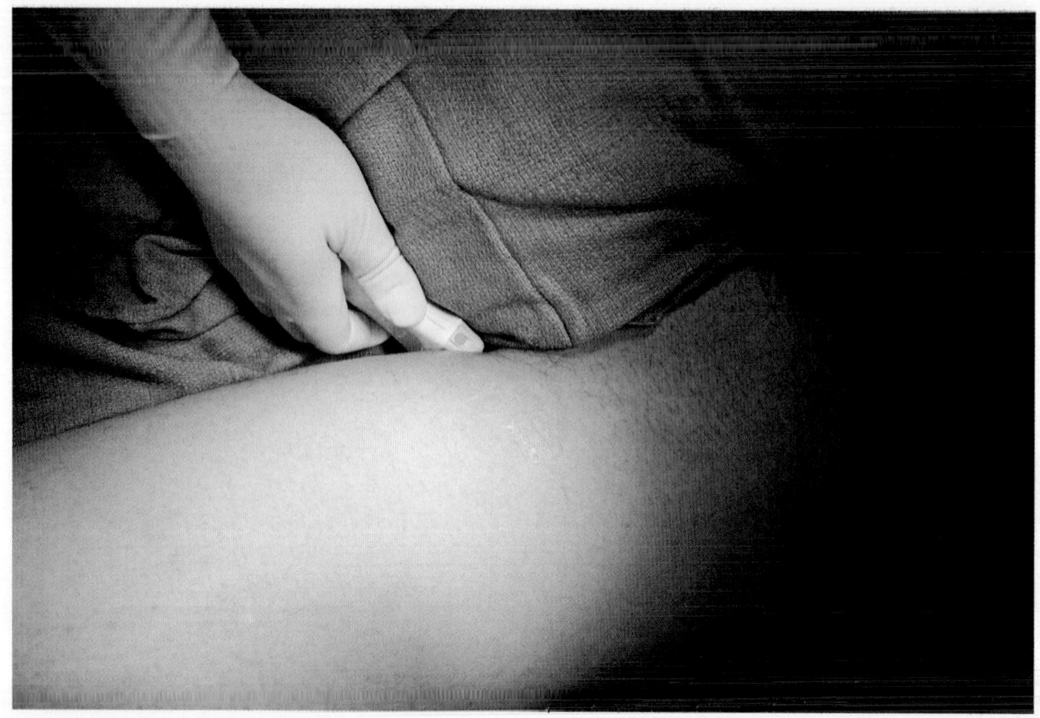

**FIGURE 7.51.1A** Ultrasound transducer position to image the pudendal nerve and pudendal canal.

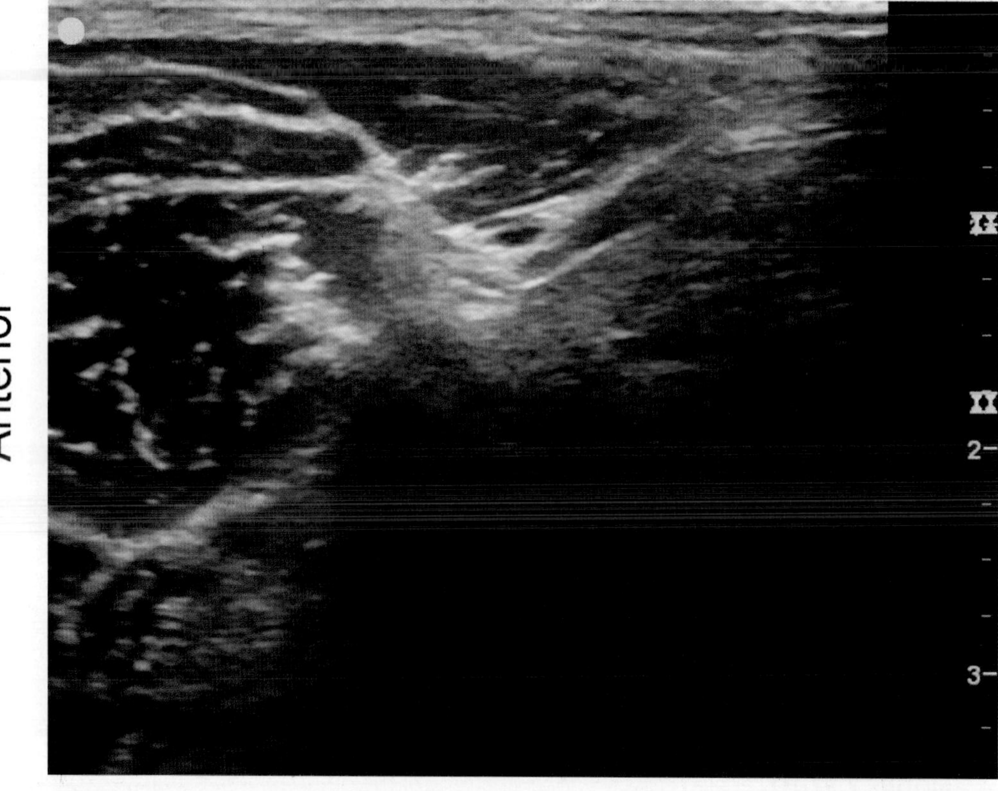


**FIGURE 7.51.1B** Ultrasound image of the pudendal nerve, medial approach, transverse view.

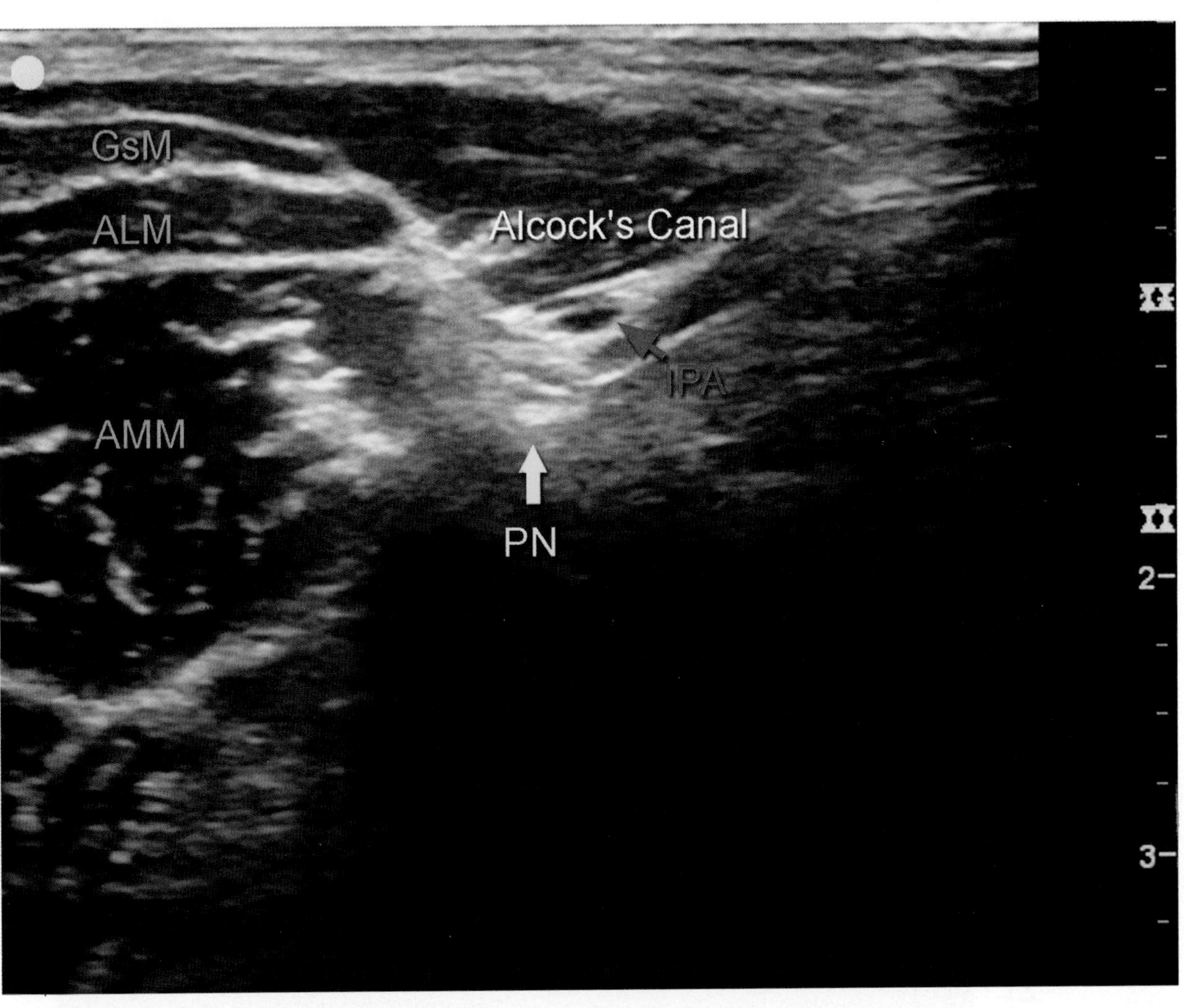


**FIGURE 7.51.1C** Labeled ultrasound image of the pudendal nerve, medial approach, transverse view.

**Abbreviations:** AMM, Adductor Magnus Muscle; ALM, Adductor Longus Muscle; GsM, Gracilis Muscle; IPA, Internal Pudendal Artery; PN, Pudendal Nerve.

## Lateral Femoral Cutaneous Nerve, Transverse View

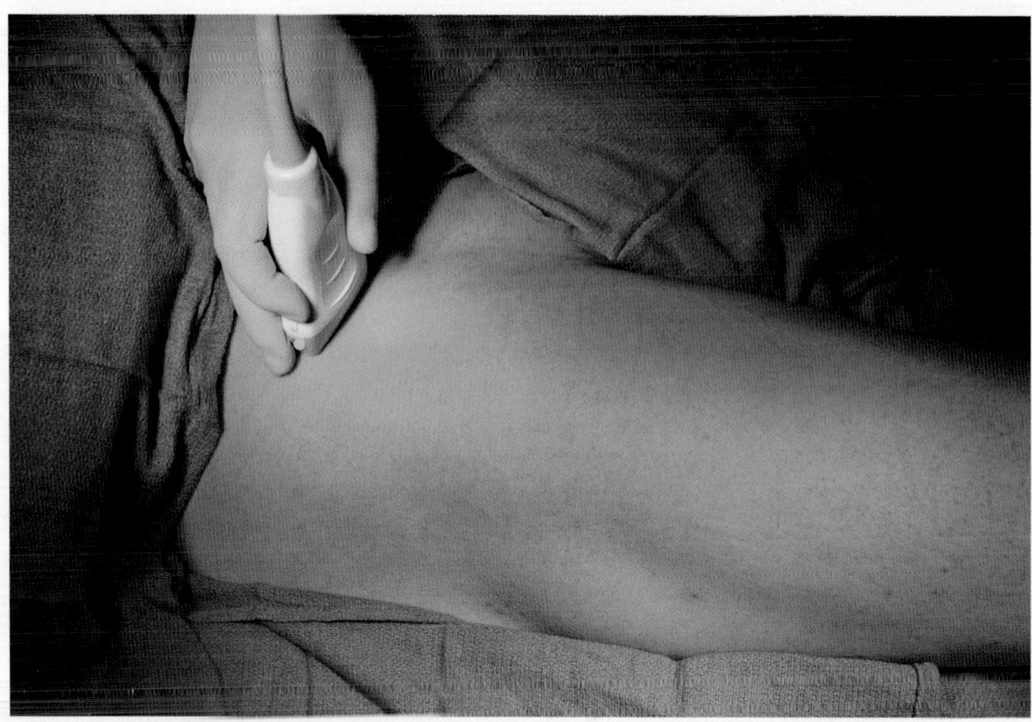

**FIGURE 7.52.1A** Ultrasound transducer position to image the lateral femoral cutaneous nerve, transverse view.

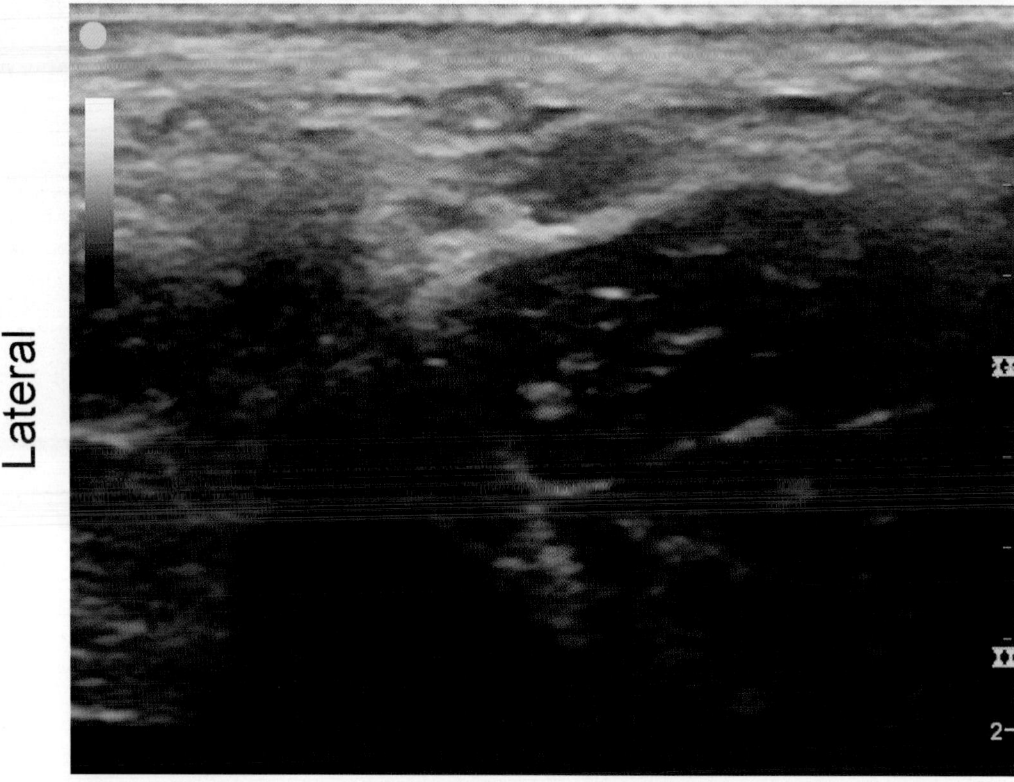


**FIGURE 7.52.1B** Ultrasound image of the lateral femoral cutaneous nerve, transverse view.

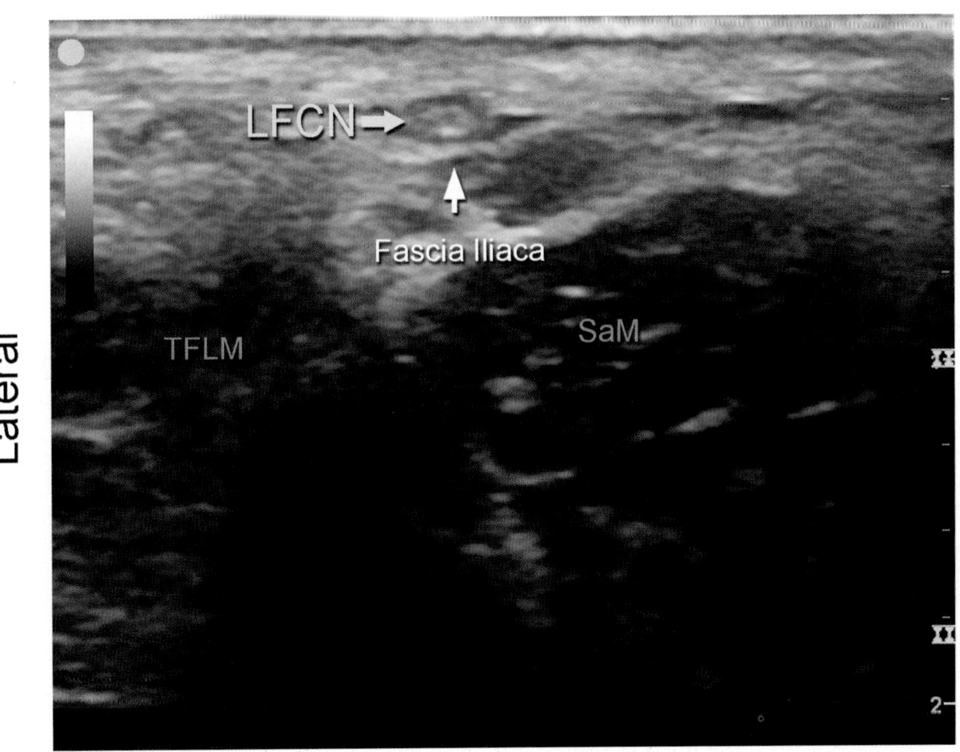


**FIGURE 7.52.1C** Labeled ultrasound image of the lateral femoral cutaneous nerve, transverse view.

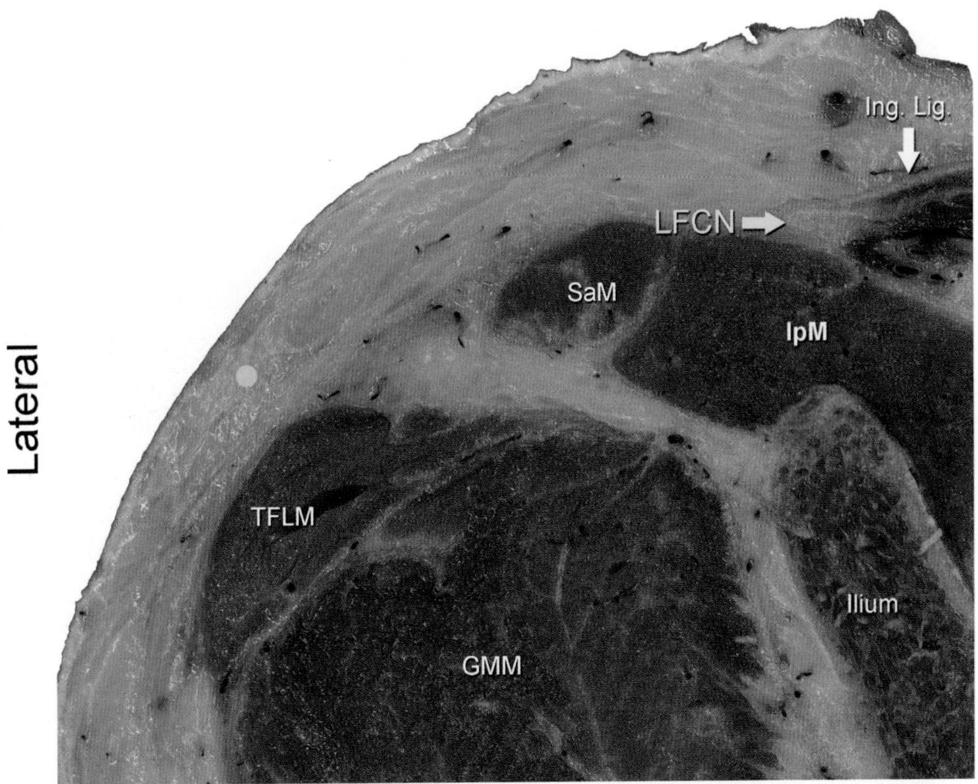


**FIGURE 7.52.1D** Labeled cross-sectional anatomy of the lateral femoral cutaneous nerve, transverse view.

**Abbreviations:** LFCN, Lateral Femoral Cutaneous Nerve; SaM, Sartorius Muscle; IpM, Iliopsoas Muscle; TFLM, Tensor Fasciae Latae Muscle; Glu. Max. M., Gluteus Maximus Muscle.

# Saphenous Nerve at Mid-thigh

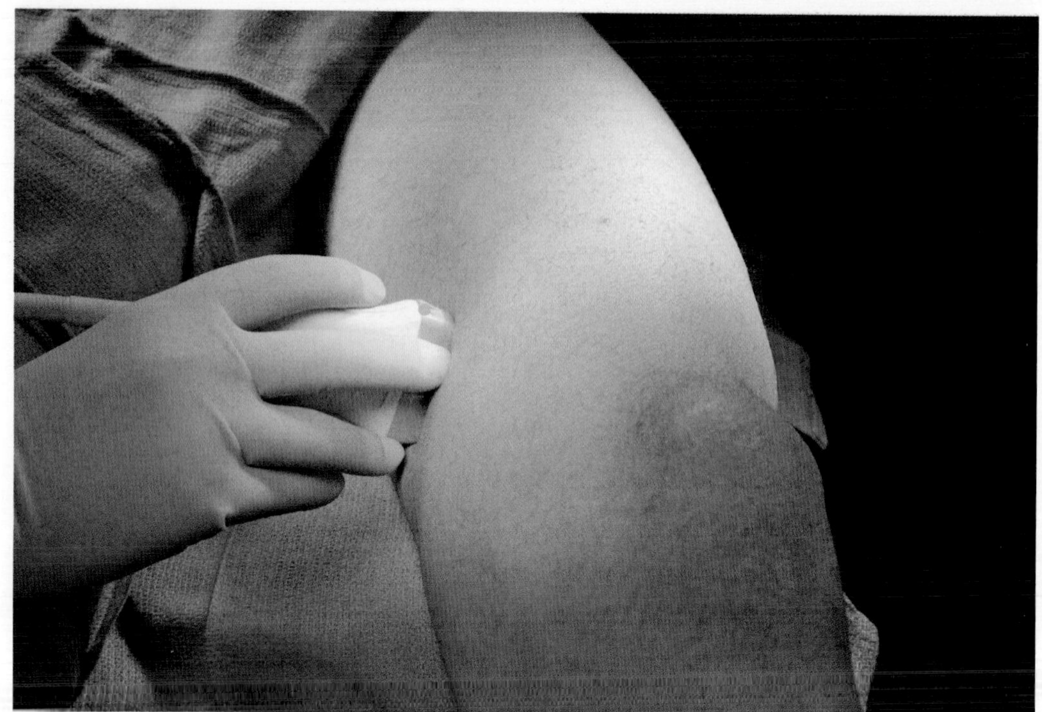

**FIGURE 7.53.1A** Ultrasound transducer position to image the saphenous nerve at mid-thigh.

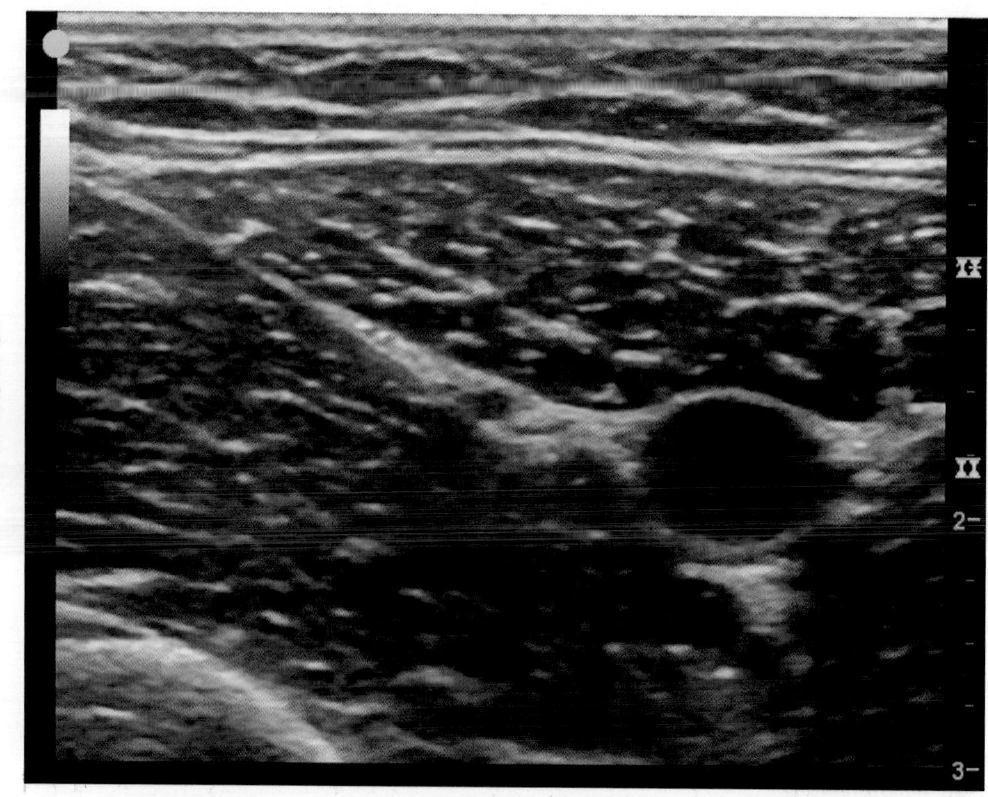


**FIGURE 7.53.1B** Ultrasound image of the saphenous nerve at mid-thigh.

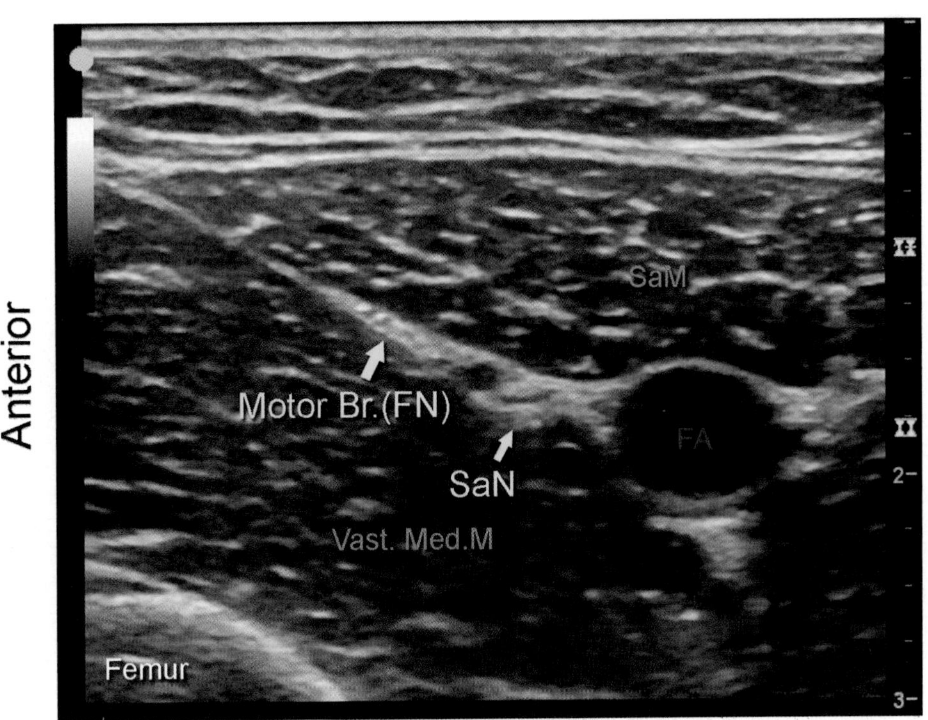


**FIGURE 7.53.1C** Labeled ultrasound image of the saphenous nerve at mid-thigh.

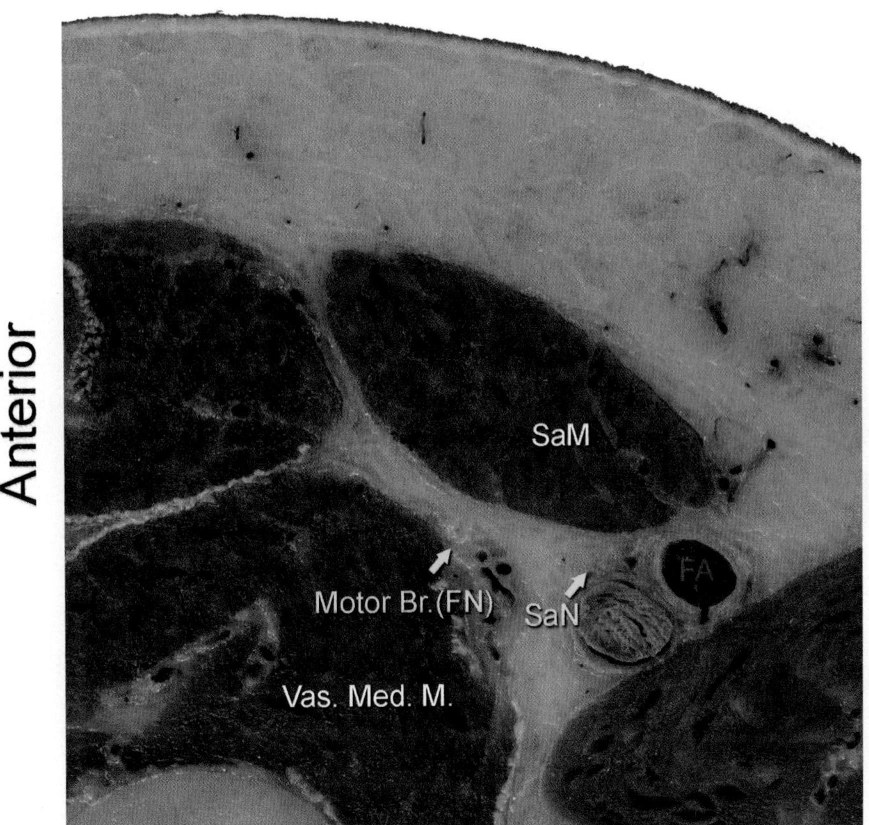


**FIGURE 7.53.1D** Labeled cross-sectional anatomy of the saphenous nerve at mid-thigh.

**Abbreviations:** SaM, Sartorius Muscle; SaN, Sartorius Nerve; FA, Femoral Artery; Motor Br. (FN), Motor Branch of Femoral Nerve.

## Saphenous Nerve at Distal Thigh

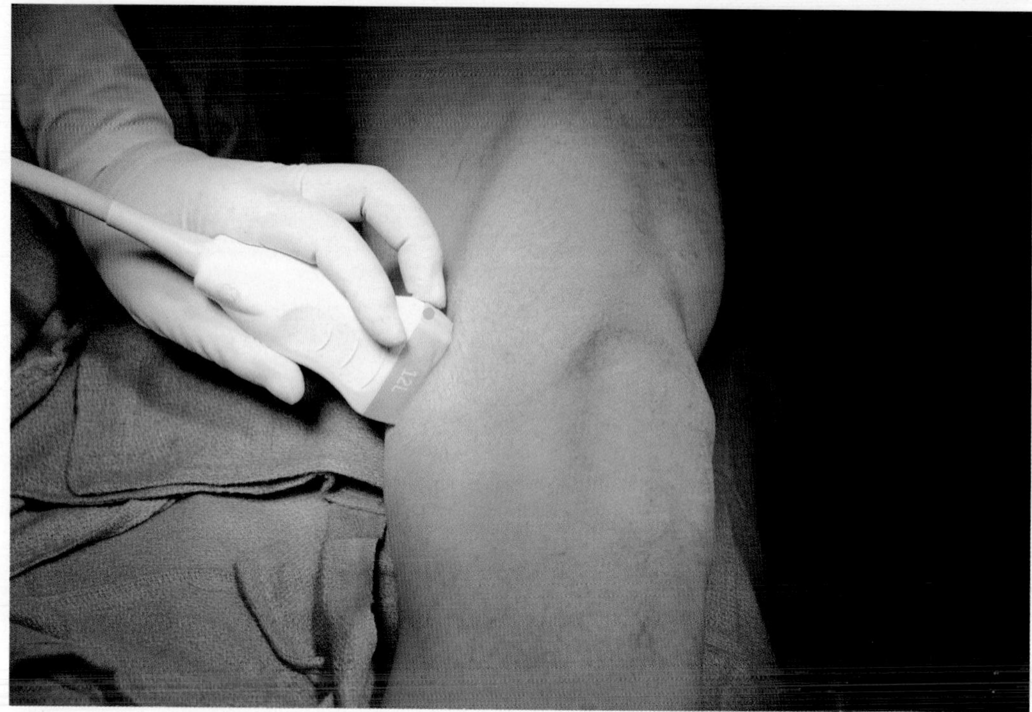

**FIGURE 7.53.2A** Ultrasound transducer position to image the saphenous nerve at distal thigh.

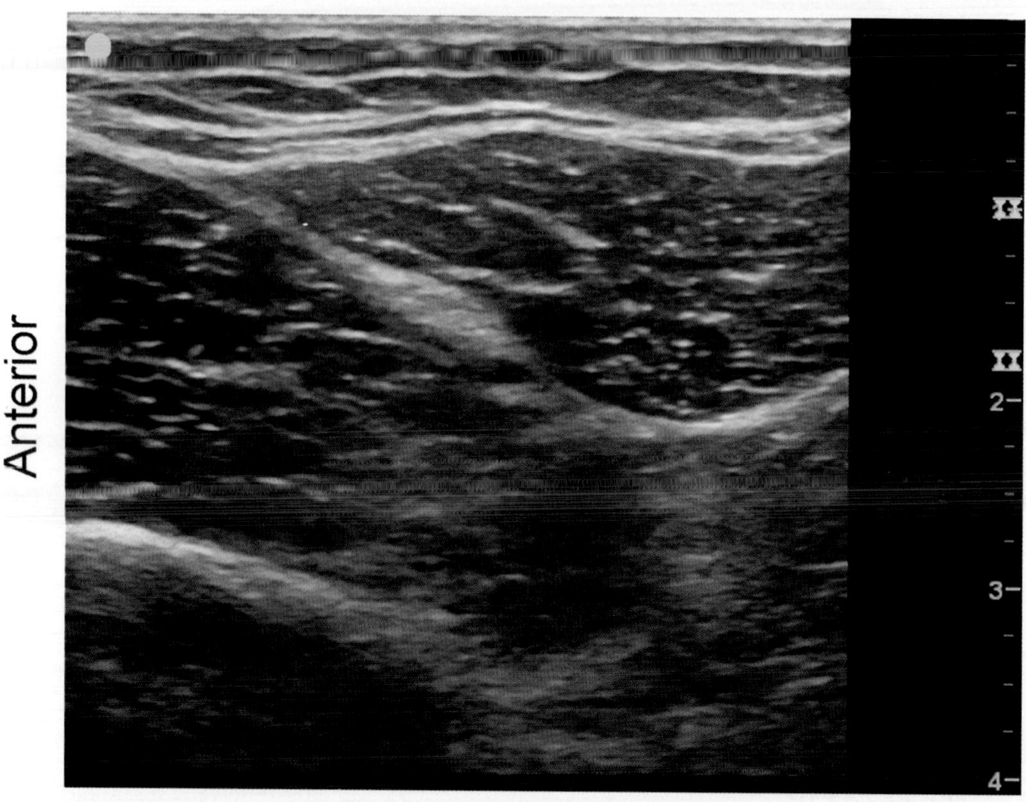


**FIGURE 7.53.2B** Ultrasound image of the saphenous nerve at distal thigh.

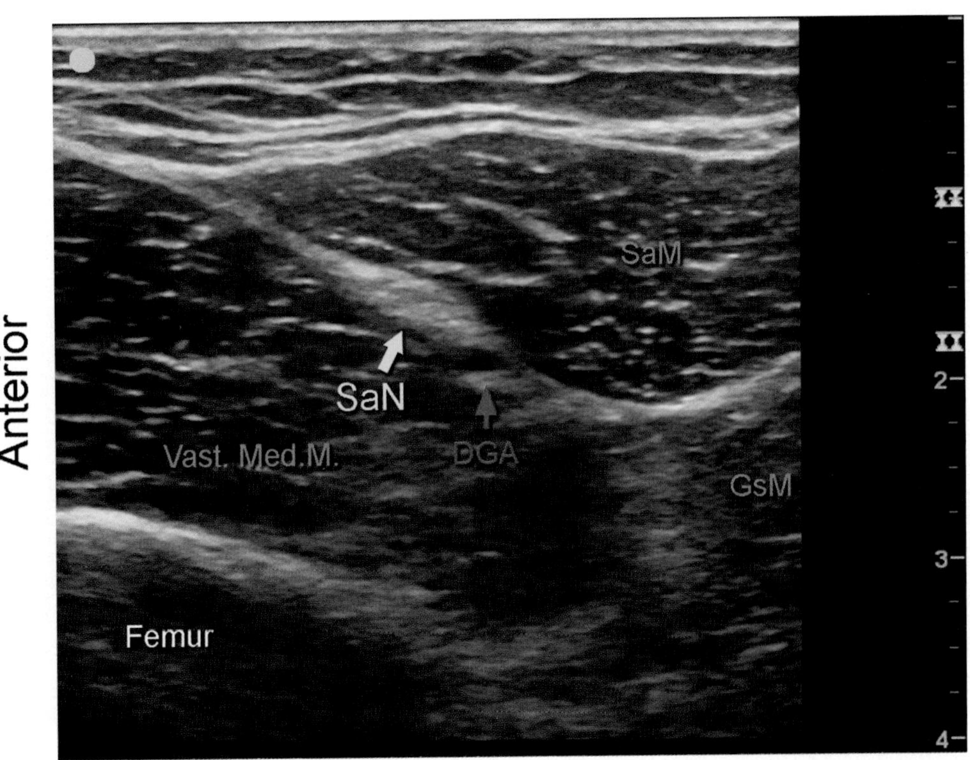


**FIGURE 7.53.2C** Labeled Ultrasound image of the saphenous nerve at distal thigh.

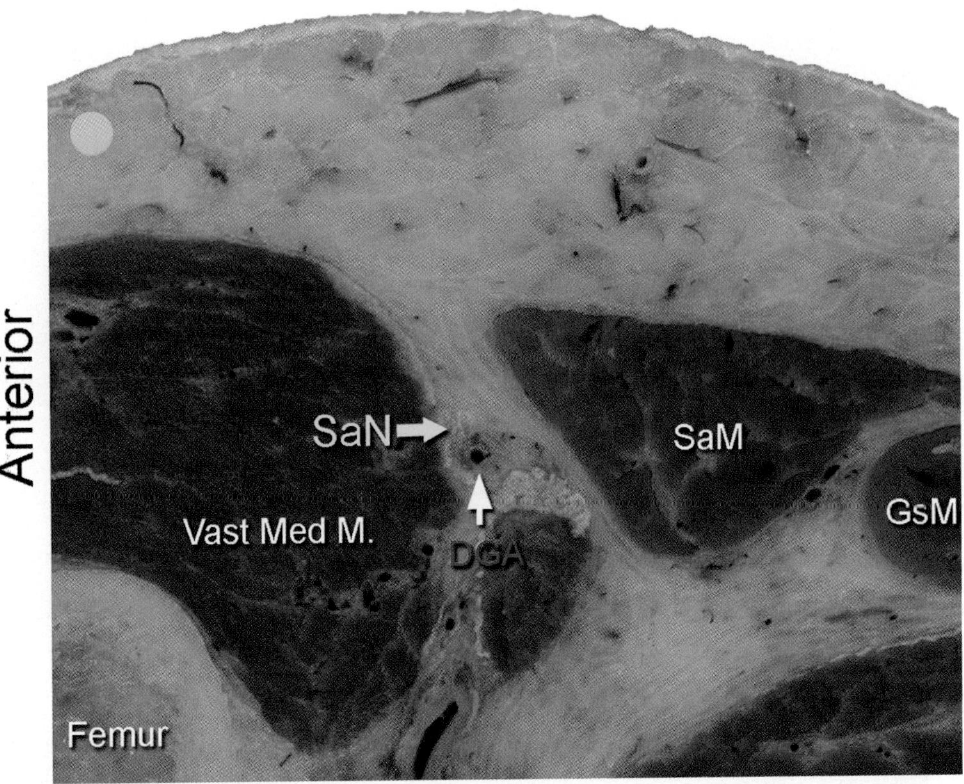


**FIGURE 7.53.2D** Labeled cross-sectional anatomy of the saphenous nerve at distal thigh.

**Abbreviations:** SaN, Sartorius Nerve; DGA, Descending Genicular Artery; SaM, Sartorius Muscle; GsM, Gracilis Muscle.

# Tibial Nerve at the Level of the Calf

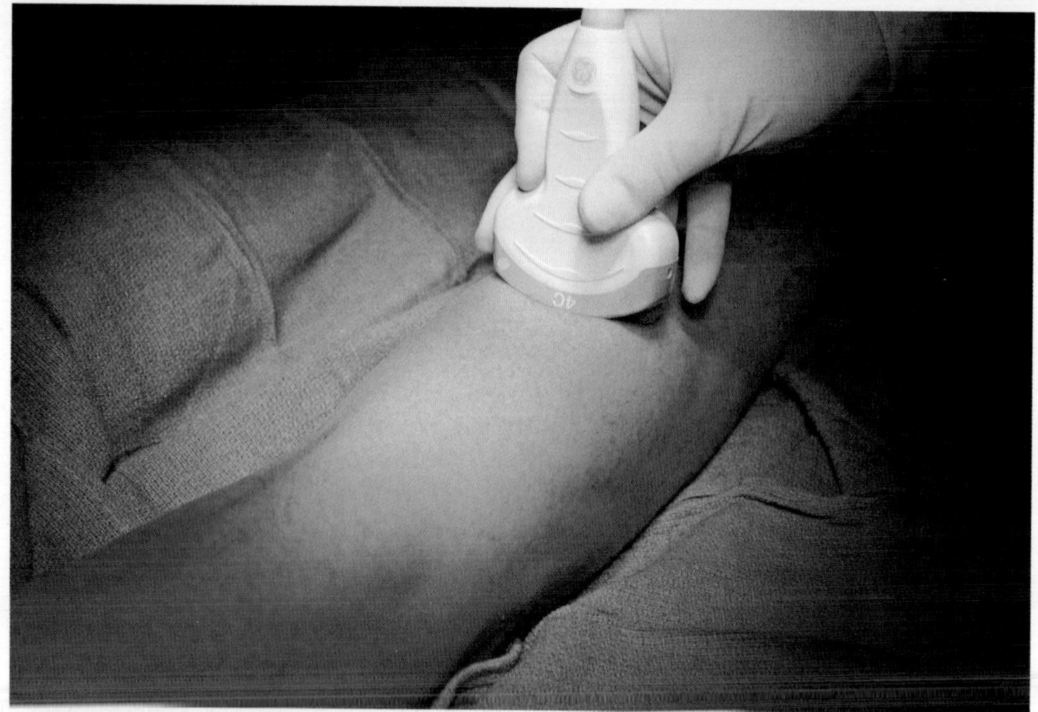

**FIGURE 7.54.1A** Ultrasound transducer position to image the tibial nerve at the level of the calf.

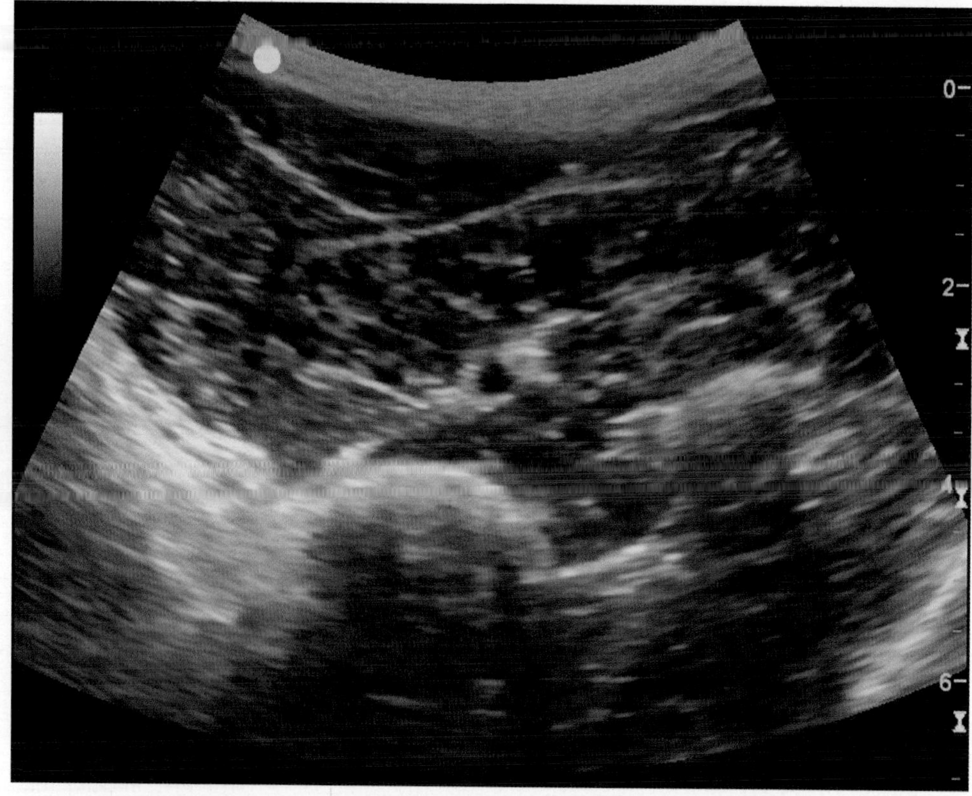


**FIGURE 7.54.1B** Ultrasound image of the tibial nerve at the level of the calf.

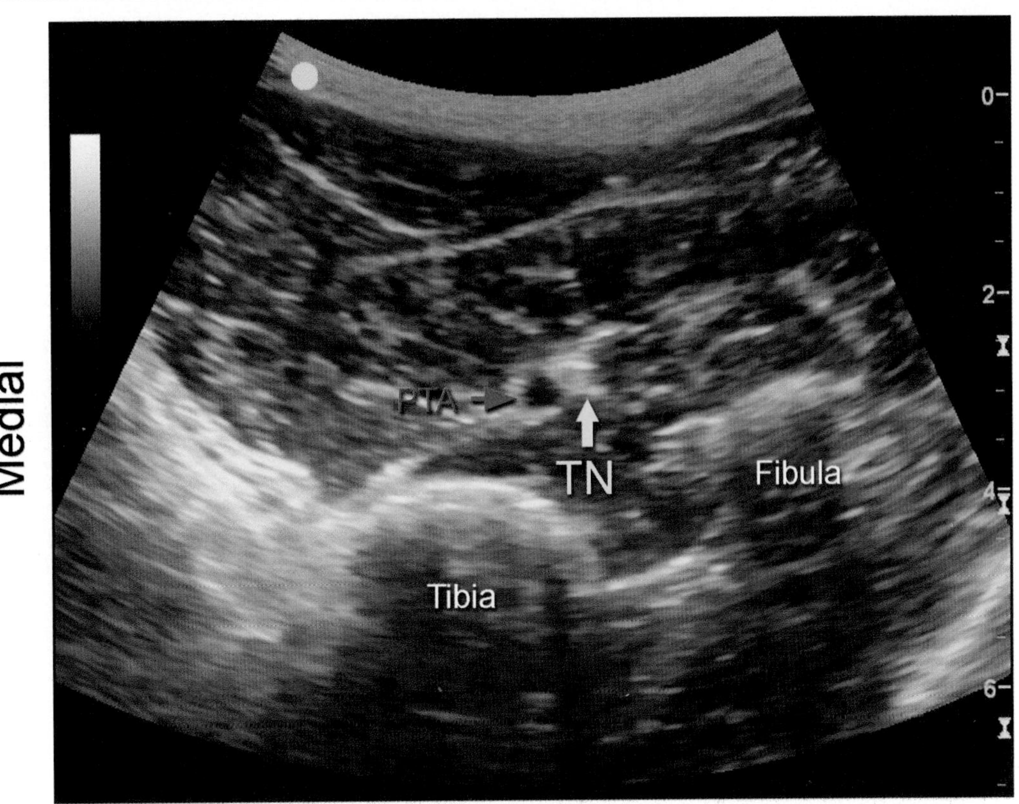


**FIGURE 7.54.1C** Labeled ultrasound image of the tibial nerve at the level of the calf.

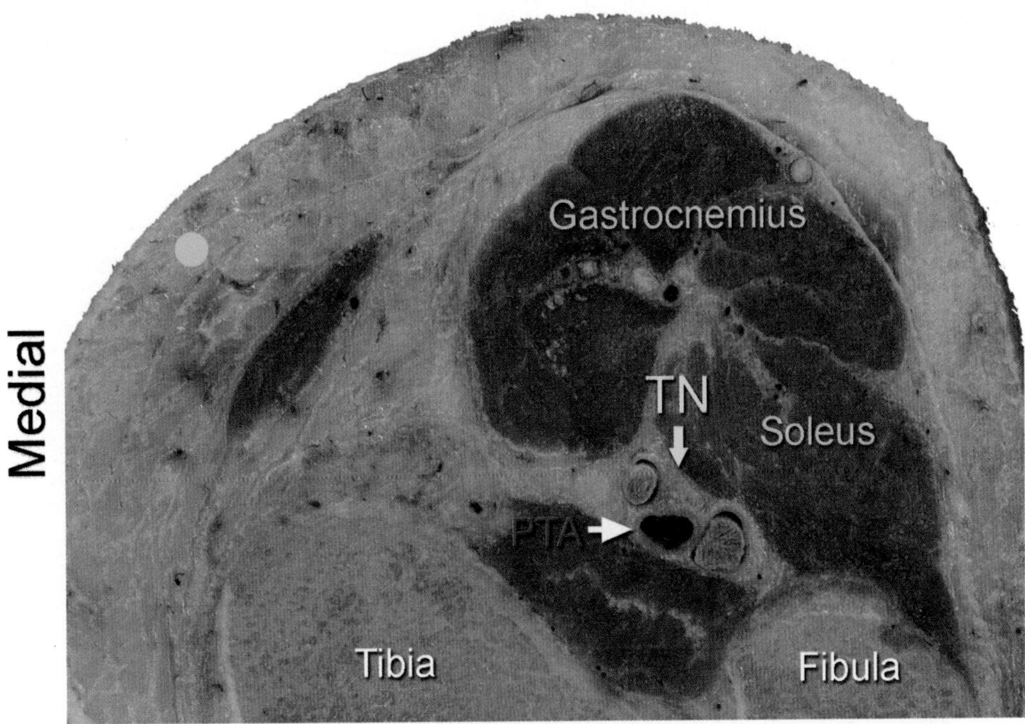


**FIGURE 7.54.1D** Labeled cross-sectional anatomy of the tibial nerve at the level of the calf.

**Abbreviations:** TN, Tibial Nerve; PTA, Posterior Tibial Artery.

# Saphenous Nerve Below the Knee

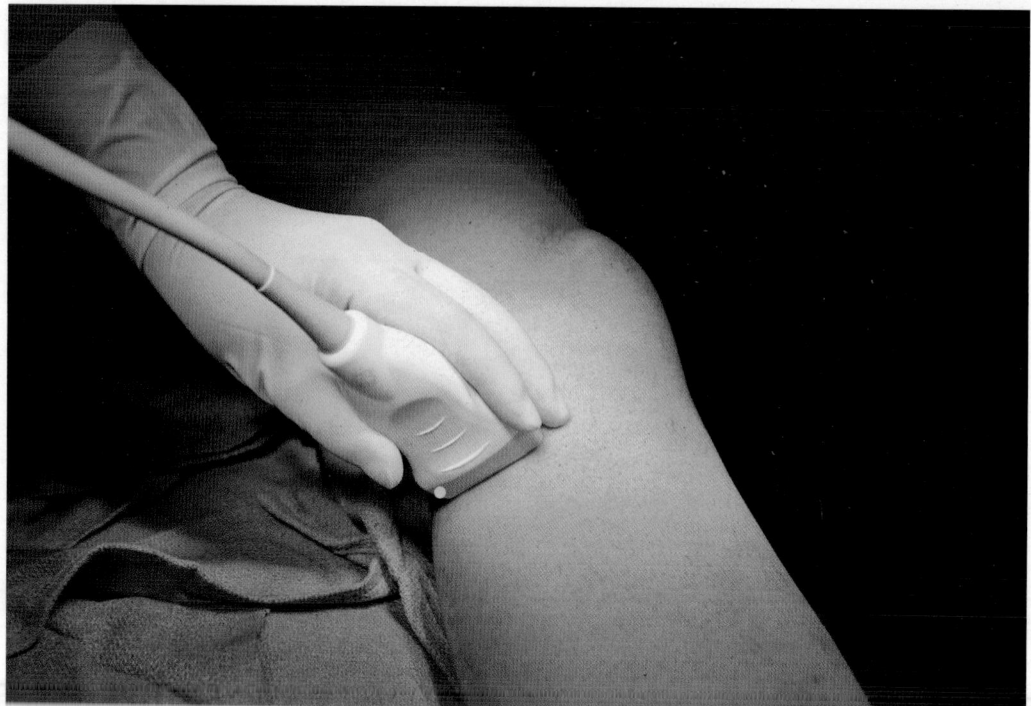

**FIGURE 7.55.1A** Ultrasound transducer position to image the saphenous nerve below the knee.

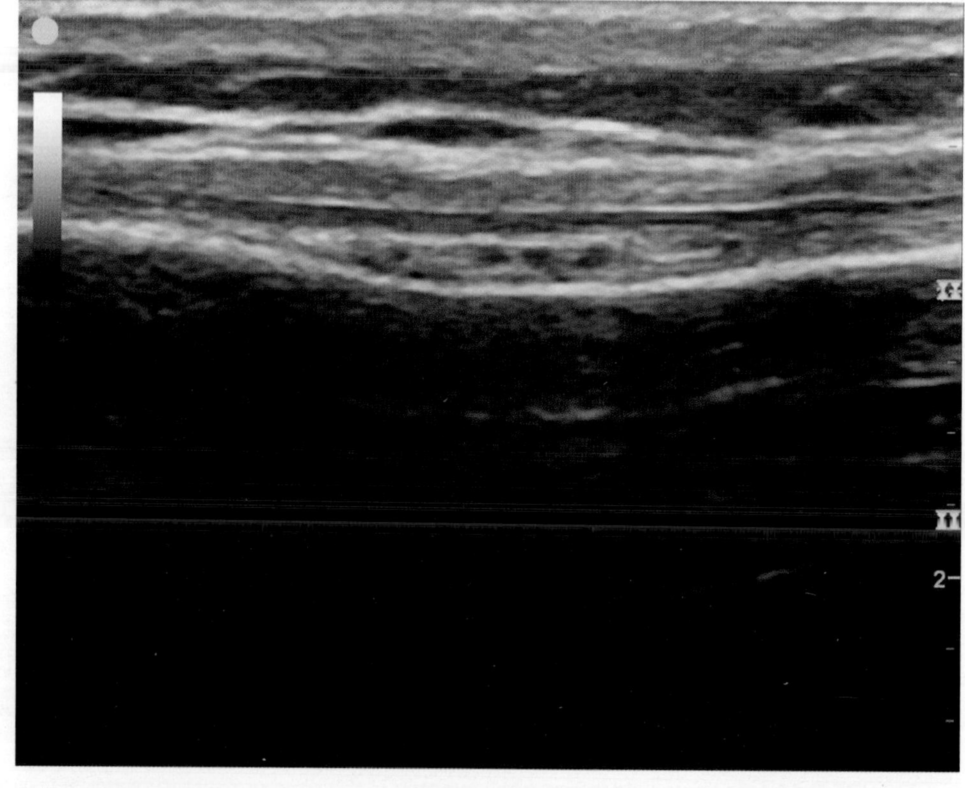


**FIGURE 7.55.1B** Ultrasound image of the saphenous nerve below the knee.

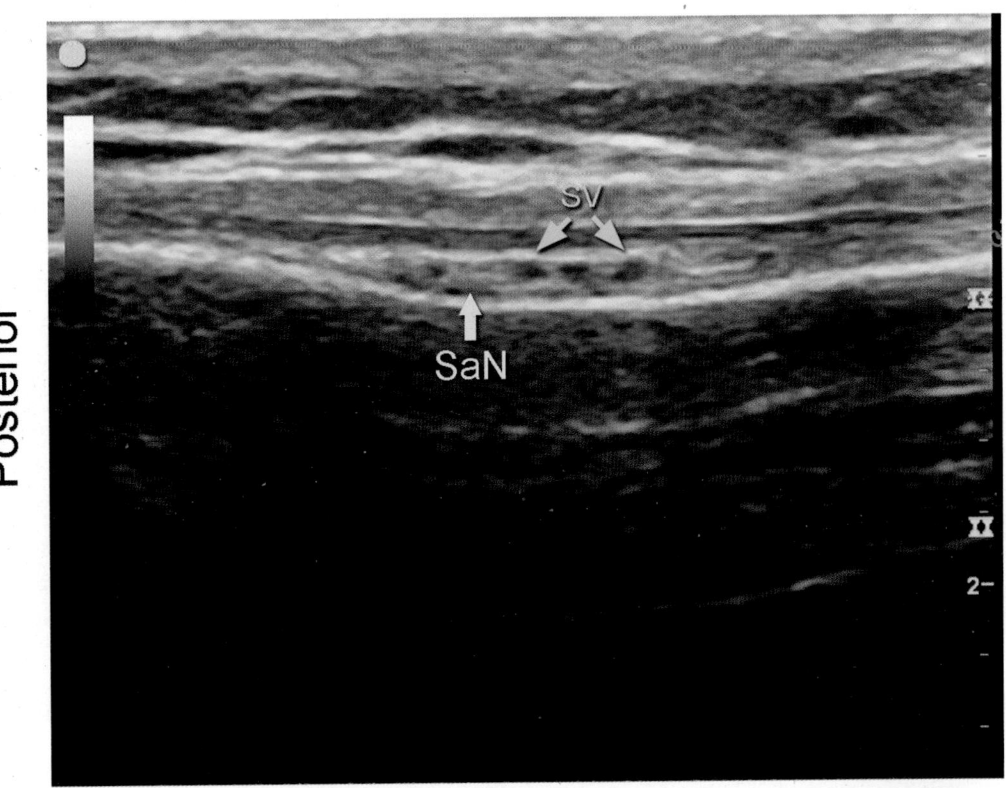


**FIGURE 7.55.1C** Labeled ultrasound image of the saphenous nerve below the knee.

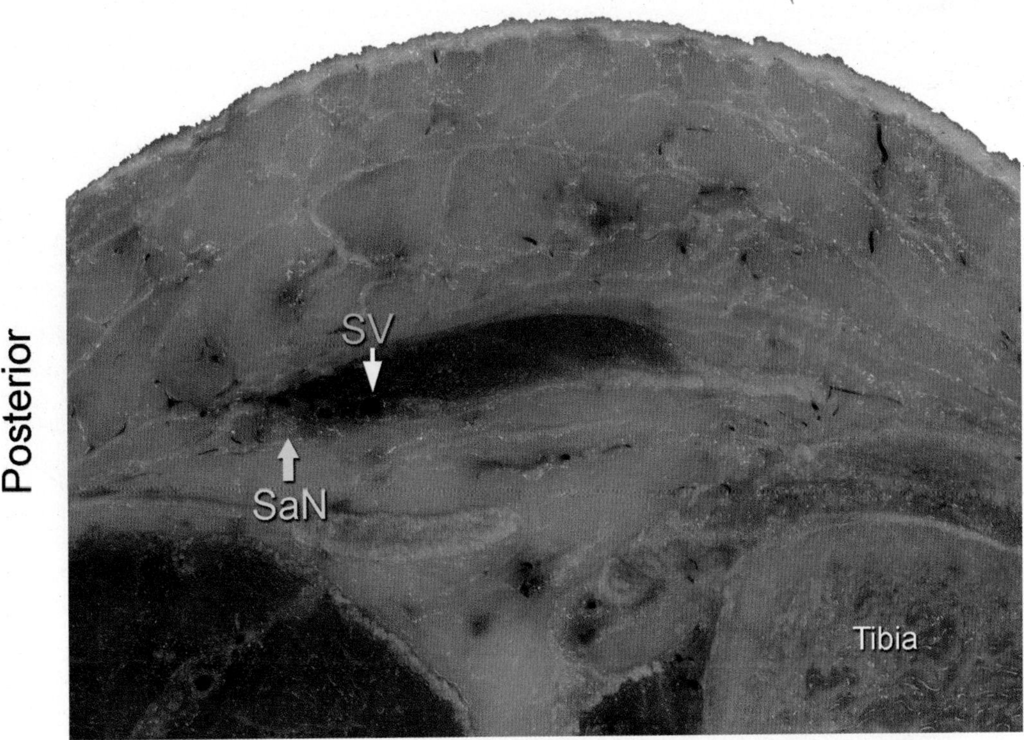


**FIGURE 7.55.1D** Labeled cross-sectional anatomy of the saphenous nerve below the knee.

**Abbreviations:** SaV, Great Saphenous Vein and its contributories; SaN, Saphenous Nerve.

# Common Peroneal Nerve at the Fibular Neck

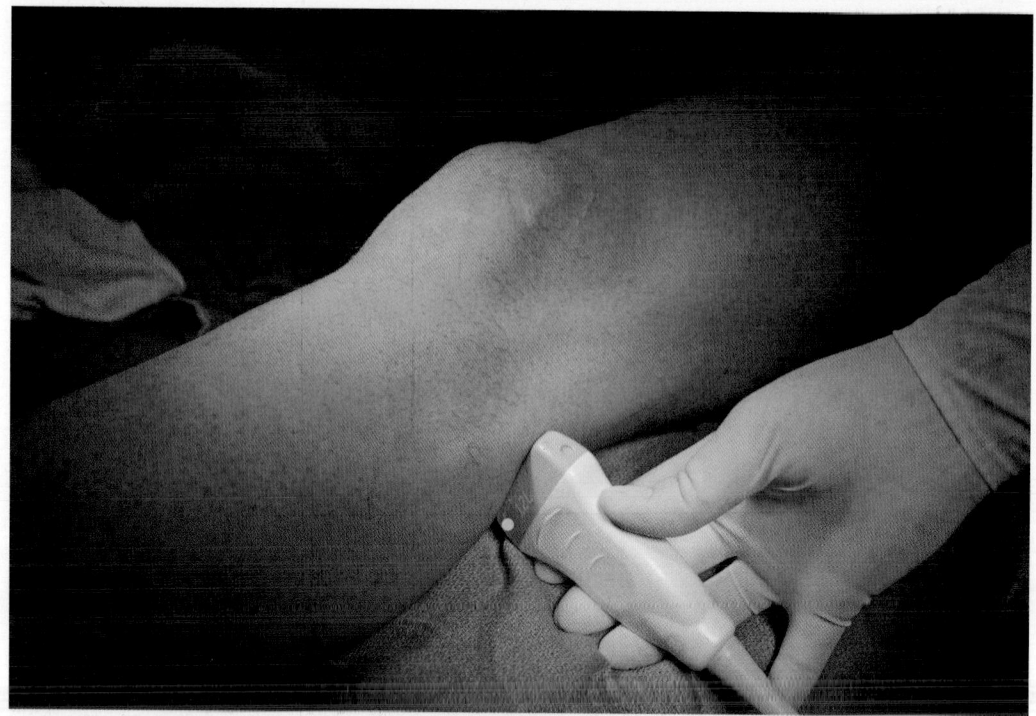

**FIGURE 7.56.1A** Ultrasound transducer position to image the common peroneal nerve at the fibular neck.

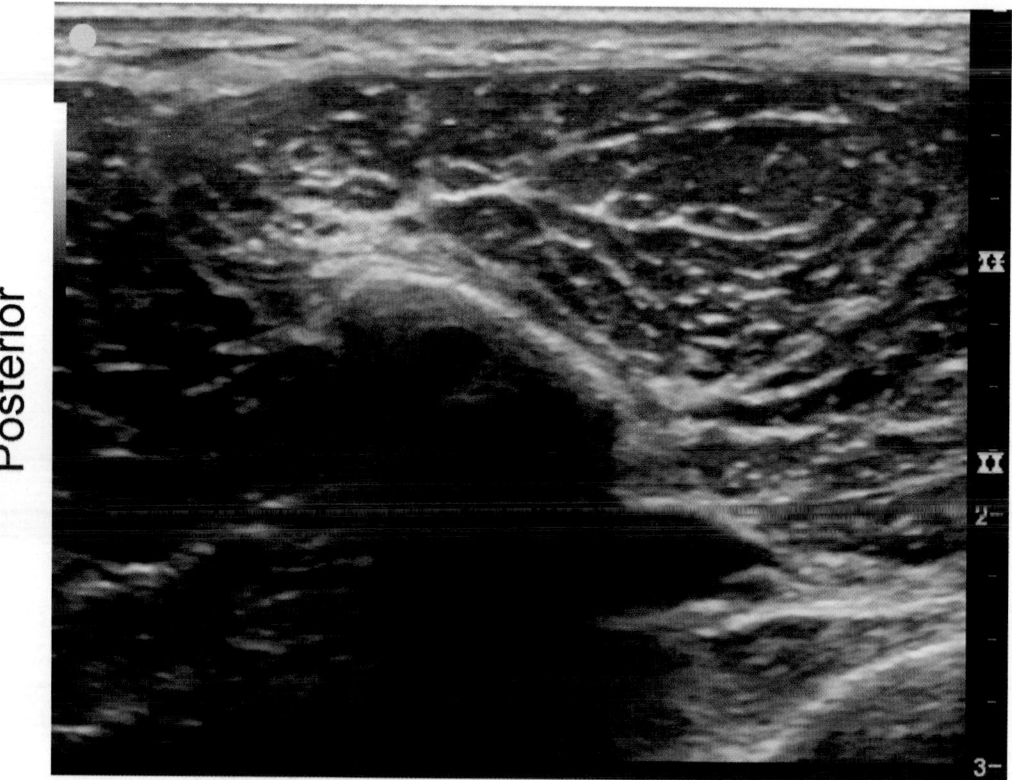


**FIGURE 7.56.1B** Ultrasound image of the common peroneal nerve at the fibular neck.

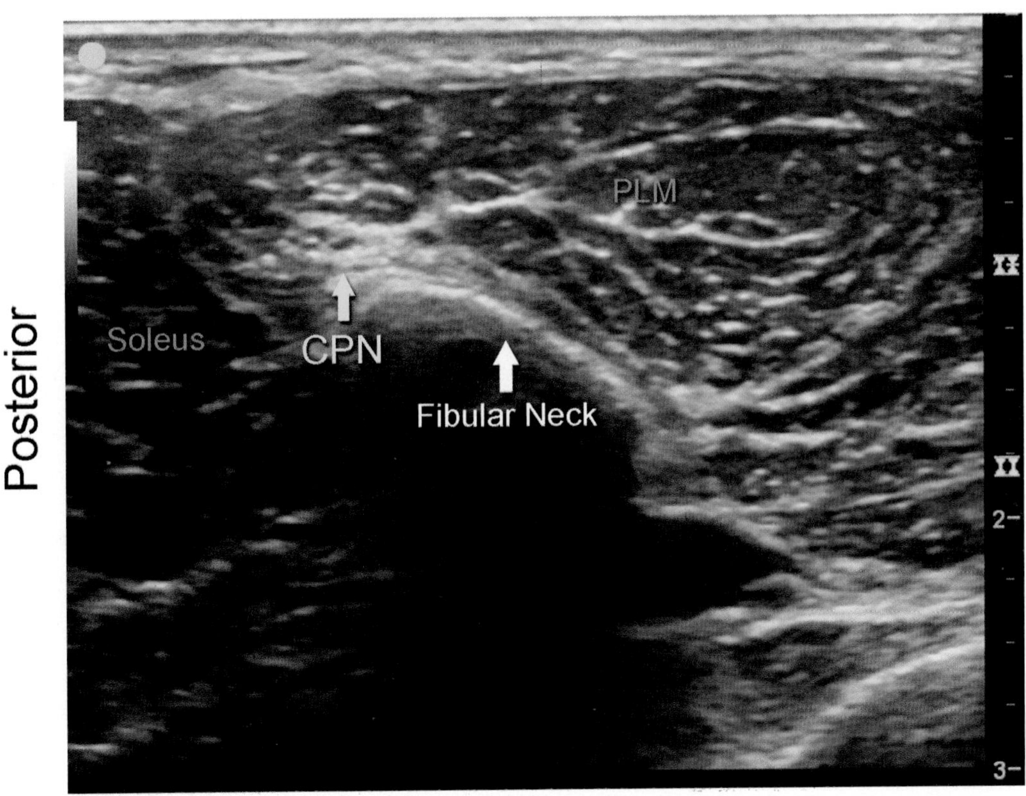


**FIGURE 7.56.1C** Labeled ultrasound image of the common peroneal nerve at the fibular neck.

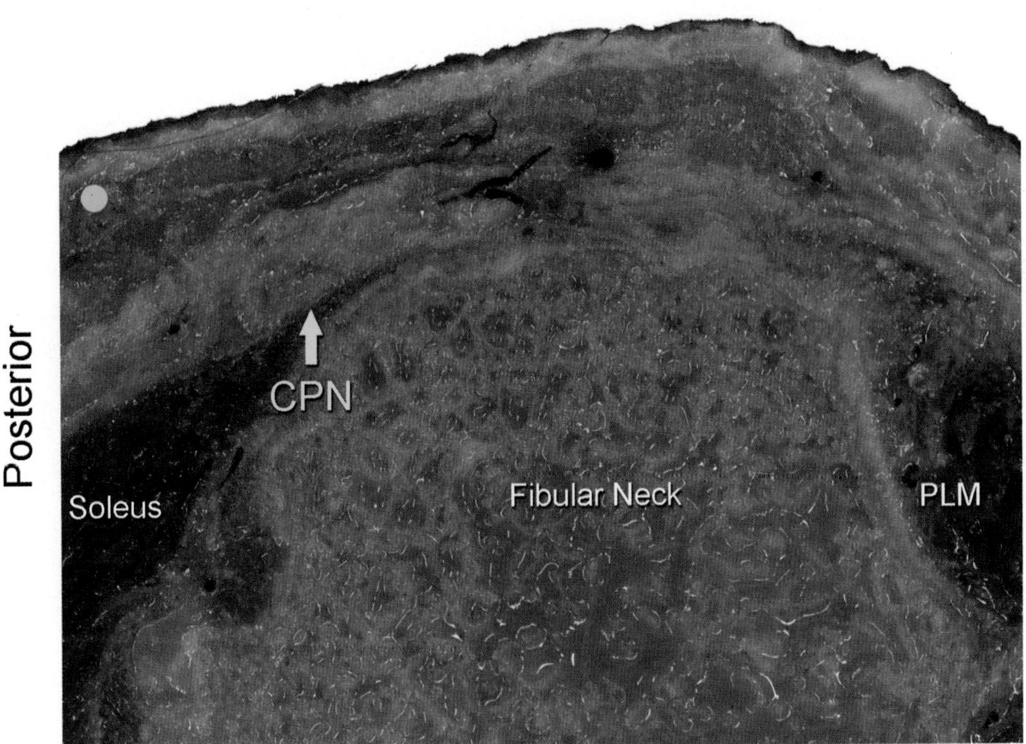


**FIGURE 7.56.1D** Labeled cross-sectional anatomy of the common peroneal nerve at the fibular neck.

**Abbreviations:** CPN, Common Peroneal Nerve; PLM, Peroneus Longus Muscle.

## Peroneal Nerve, Deep and Superficial Branches

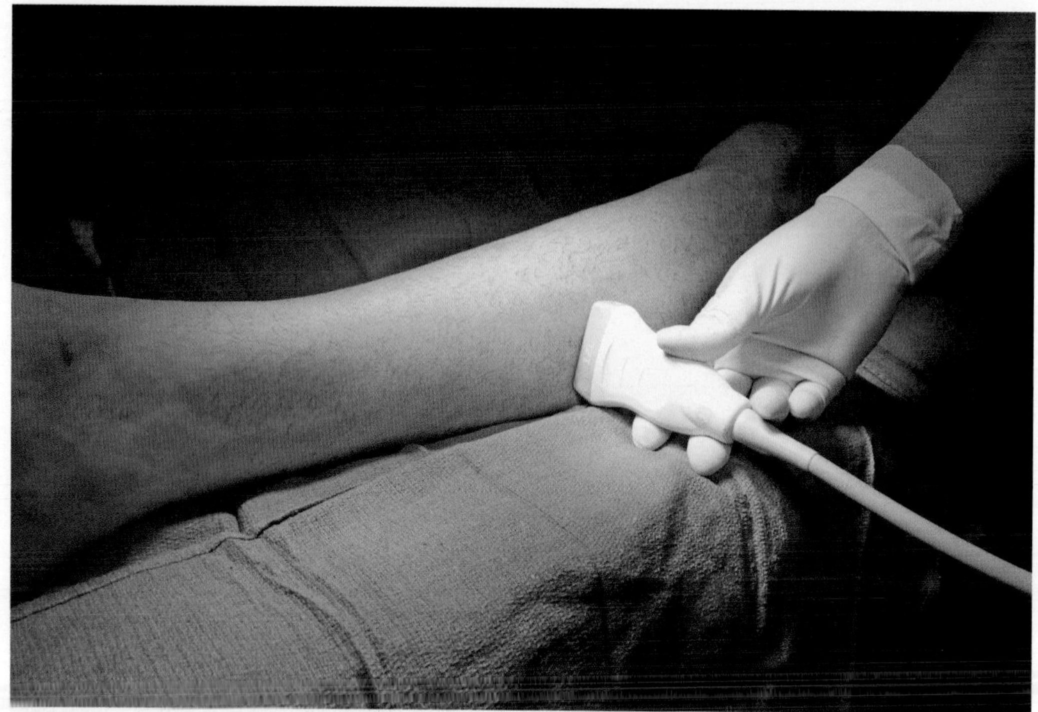

**FIGURE 7.57.1A** Ultrasound transducer position to image the peroneal nerve, deep and superficial branches.

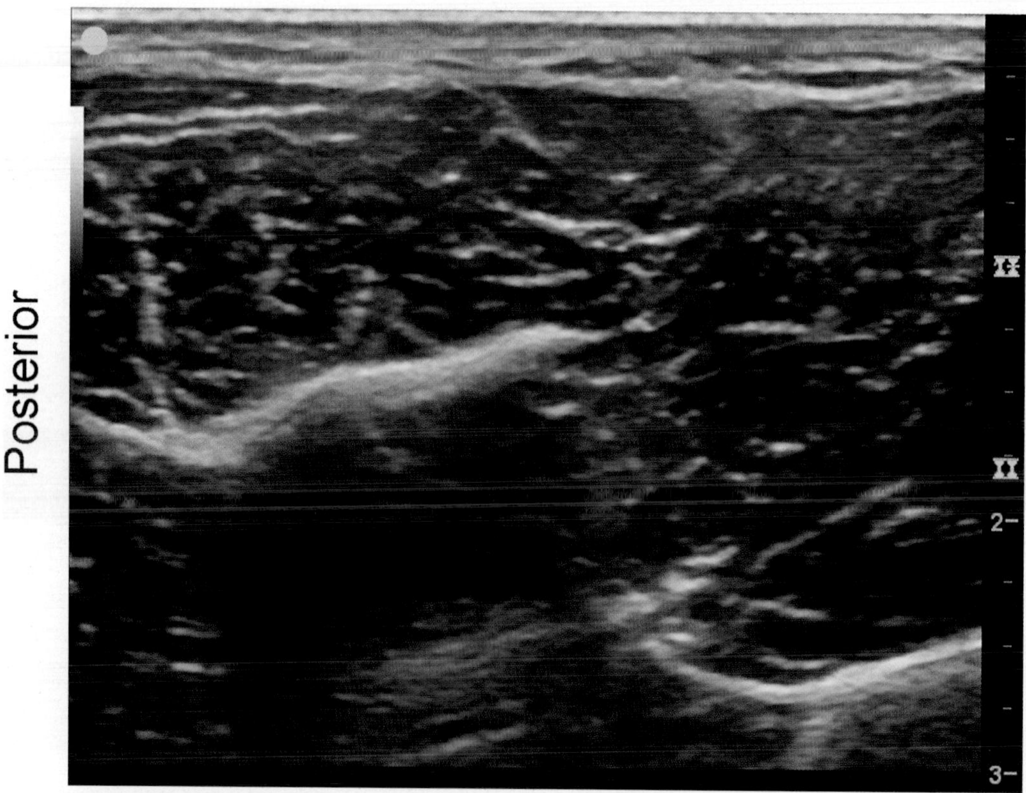


**FIGURE 7.57.1B** Ultrasound image of the peroneal nerve, deep and superficial branches.

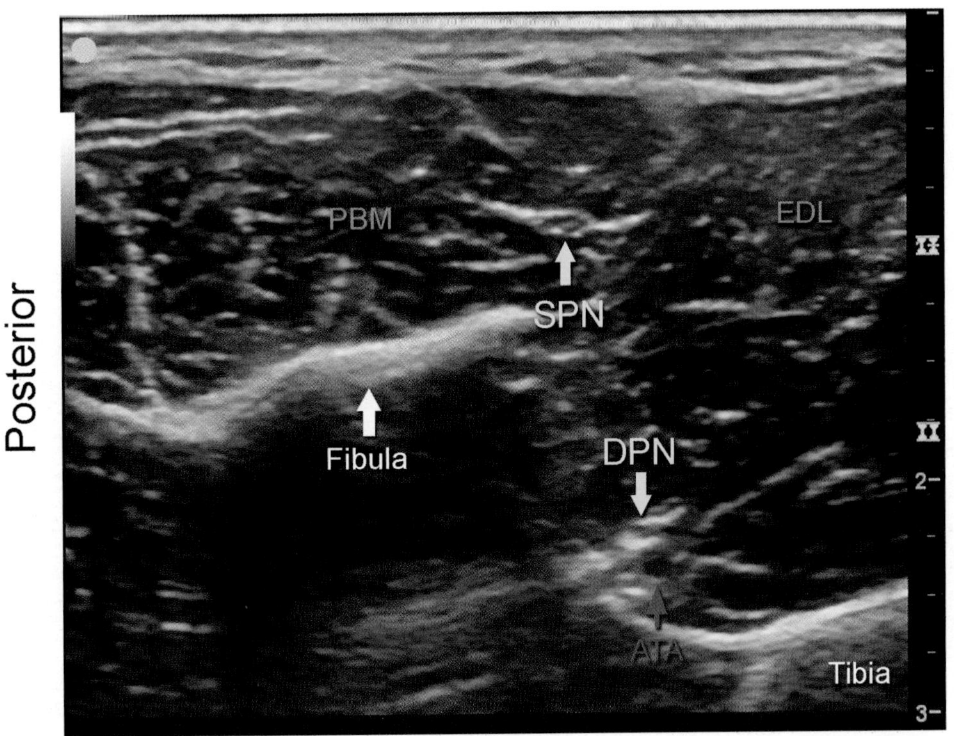


**FIGURE 7.57.1C** Labeled ultrasound image of the peroneal nerve, deep and superficial branches.

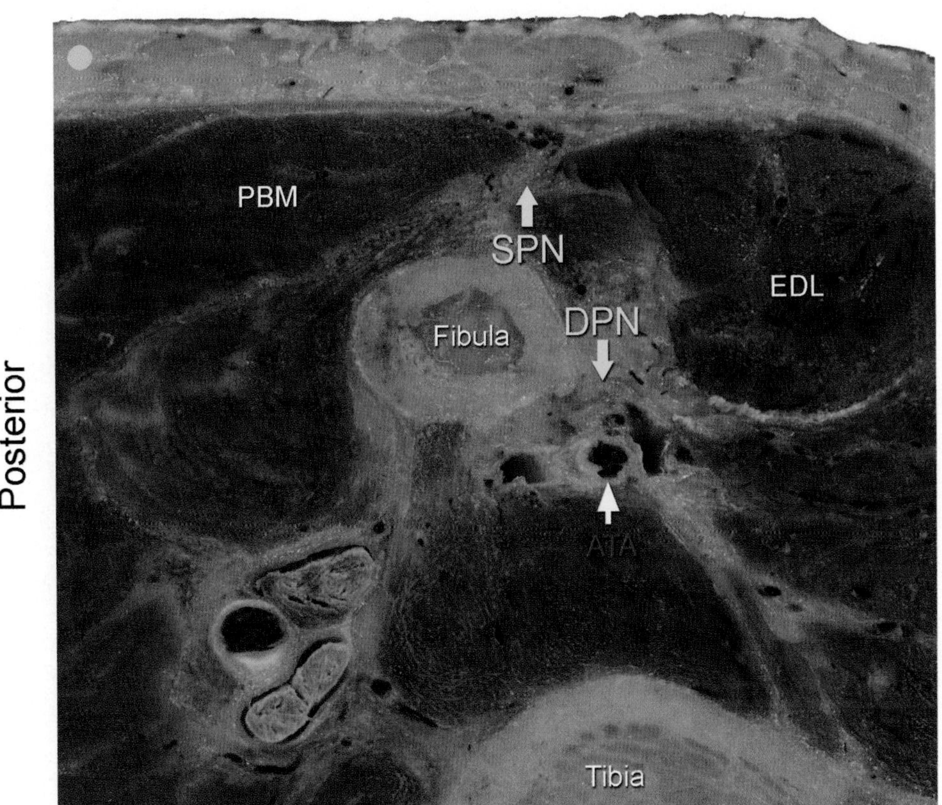


**FIGURE 7.57.1D** Labeled cross-sectional anatomy of the peroneal nerve, deep and superficial branches.

**Abbreviations:** PBM, Peroneus Brevis Muscle; EDL, Extensor Digitorum Longus; SPN, Superficial Peroneal Nerve; DPN, Deep Peroneal Nerve; ATA, Anterior Tibial Artery.

# Peroneal Nerve, Deep and Superficial Branches at the Level of the Ankle

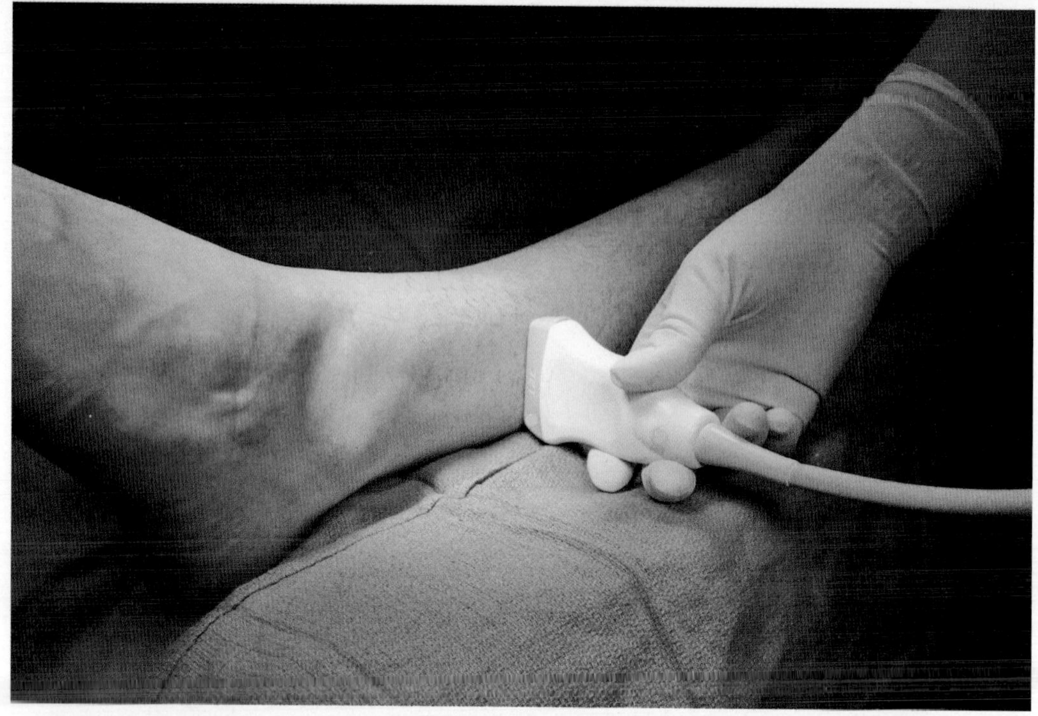

**FIGURE 7.58.1A** Ultrasound transducer position to image the peroneal nerve, deep and superficial branches at the level of the ankle.

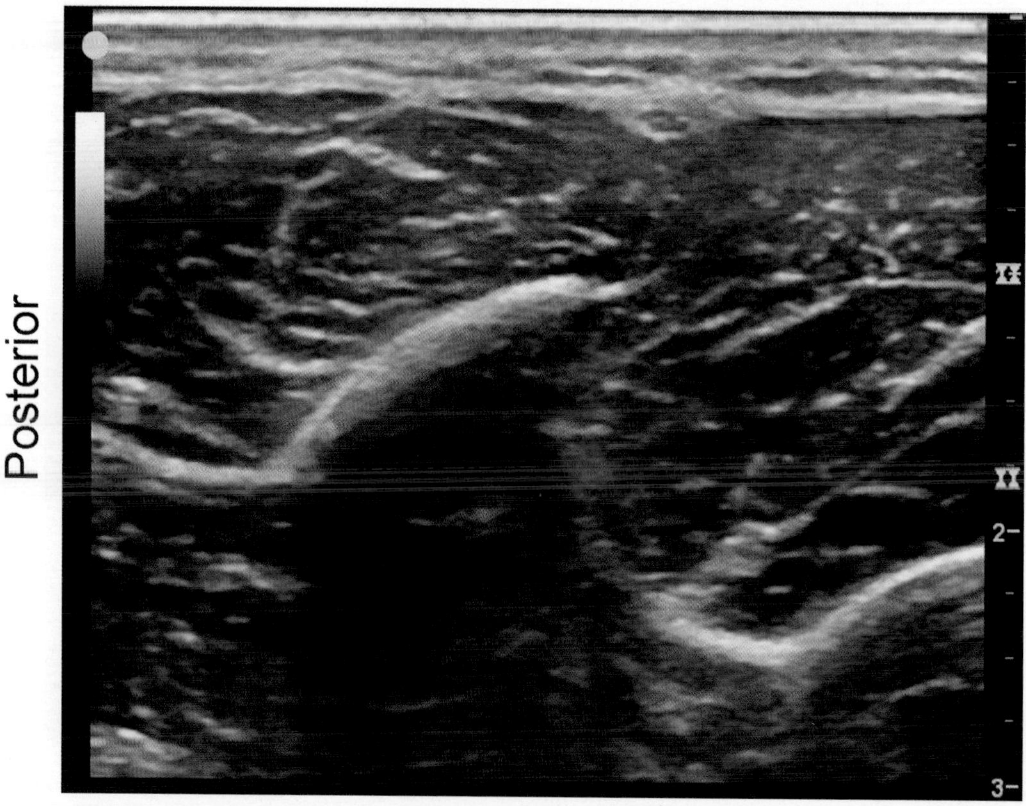


**FIGURE 7.58.1B** Ultrasound image of the peroneal nerve, deep and superficial branches at the level of the ankle.

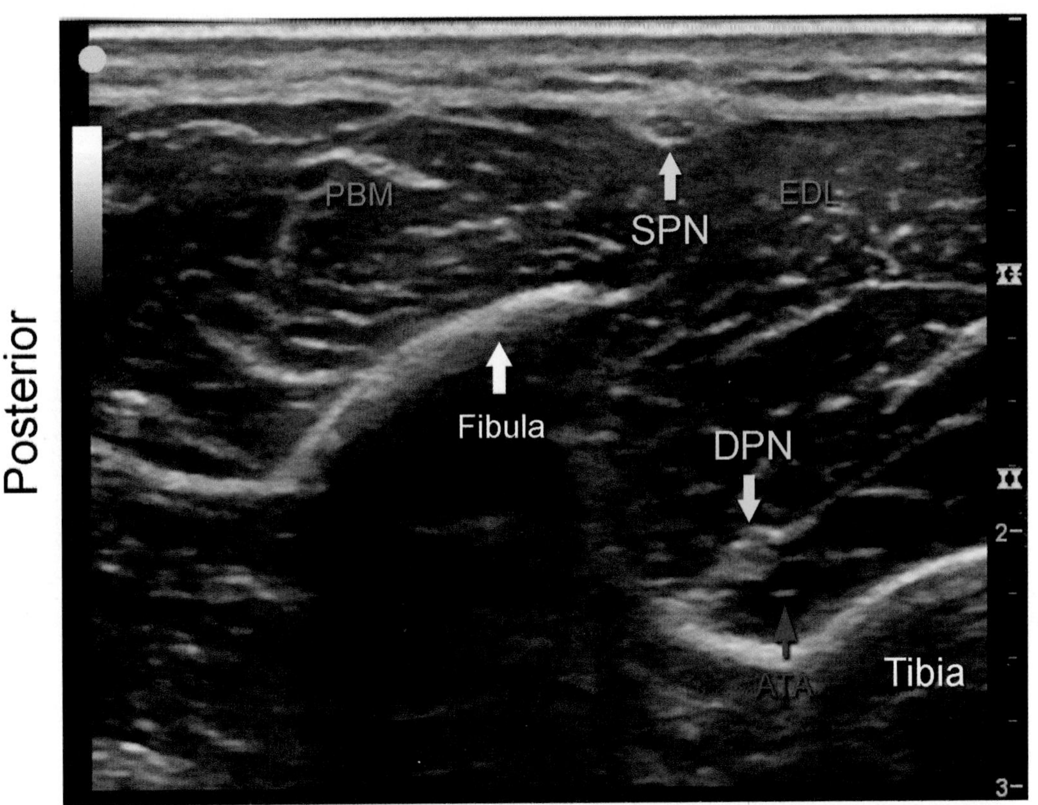


**FIGURE 7.58.1C** Labeled ultrasound image of the peroneal nerve, deep and superficial branches at the level of the ankle.

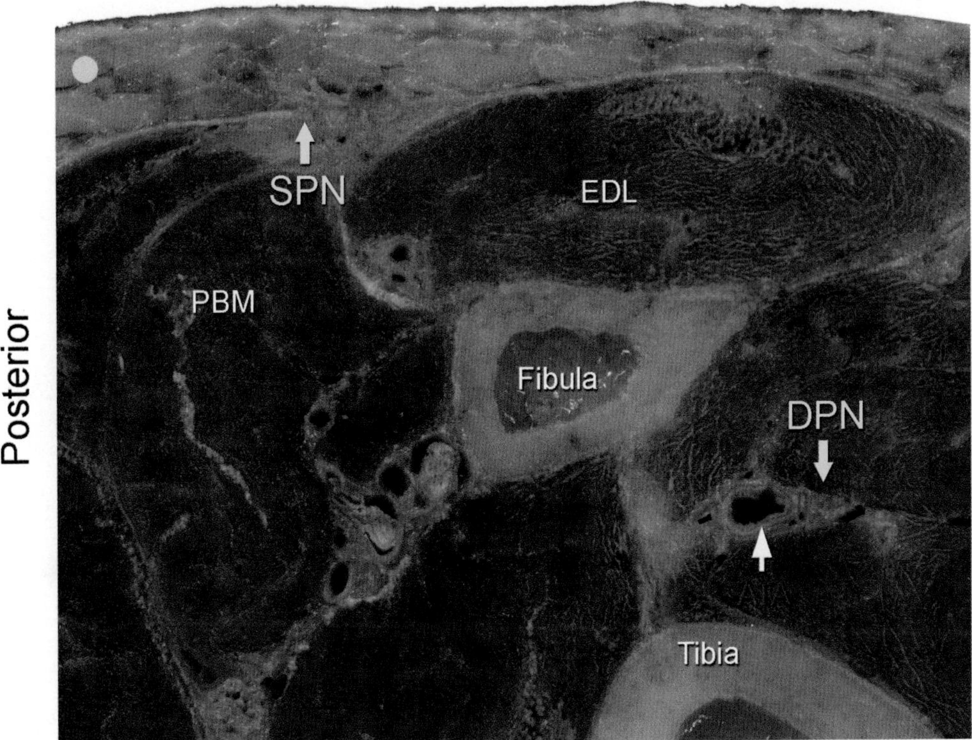


**FIGURE 7.58.1D** Labeled cross-sectional anatomy of the peroneal nerve, deep and superficial branches at the level of the ankle.

**Abbreviations:** PBM, Peroneus Brevis Muscle; EDL, Extensor Digitorum Longus; SPN, Superficial Peroneal Nerve; DPN, Deep Peroneal Nerve; ATA, Anterior Tibial Artery.

# Posterior Tibial Nerve at the Ankle, Medial Aspect

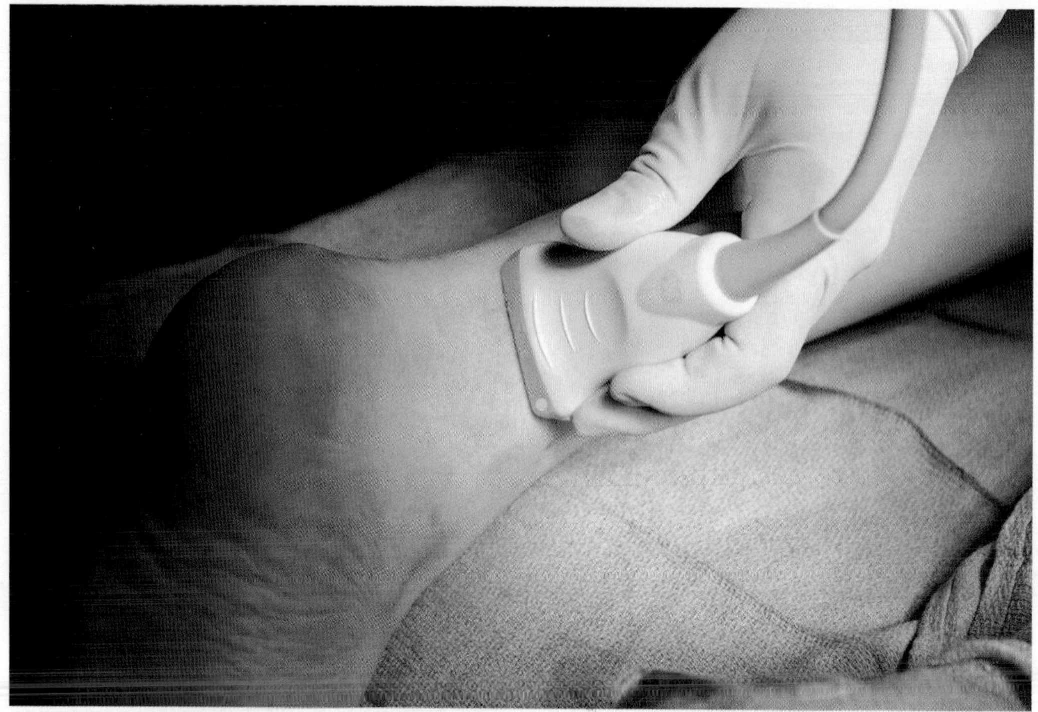

**FIGURE 7.59.1A** Ultrasound transducer position to image the posterior tibial nerve at the ankle, medial aspect.

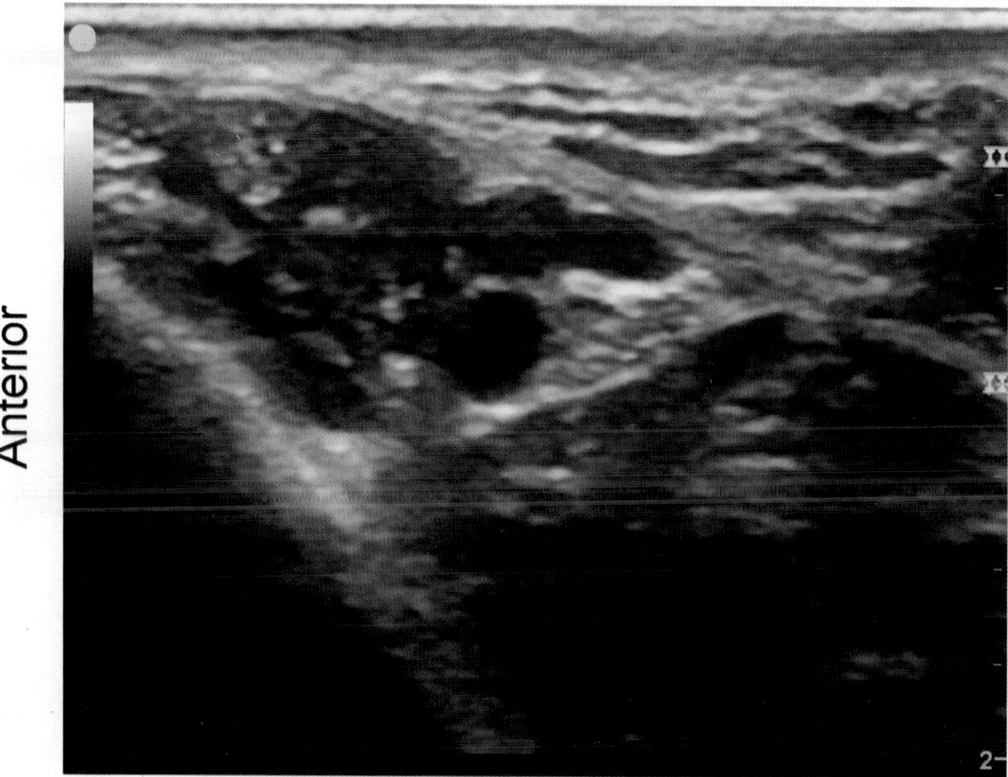


**FIGURE 7.59.1B** Ultrasound image of the posterior tibial nerve at the ankle, medial aspect.

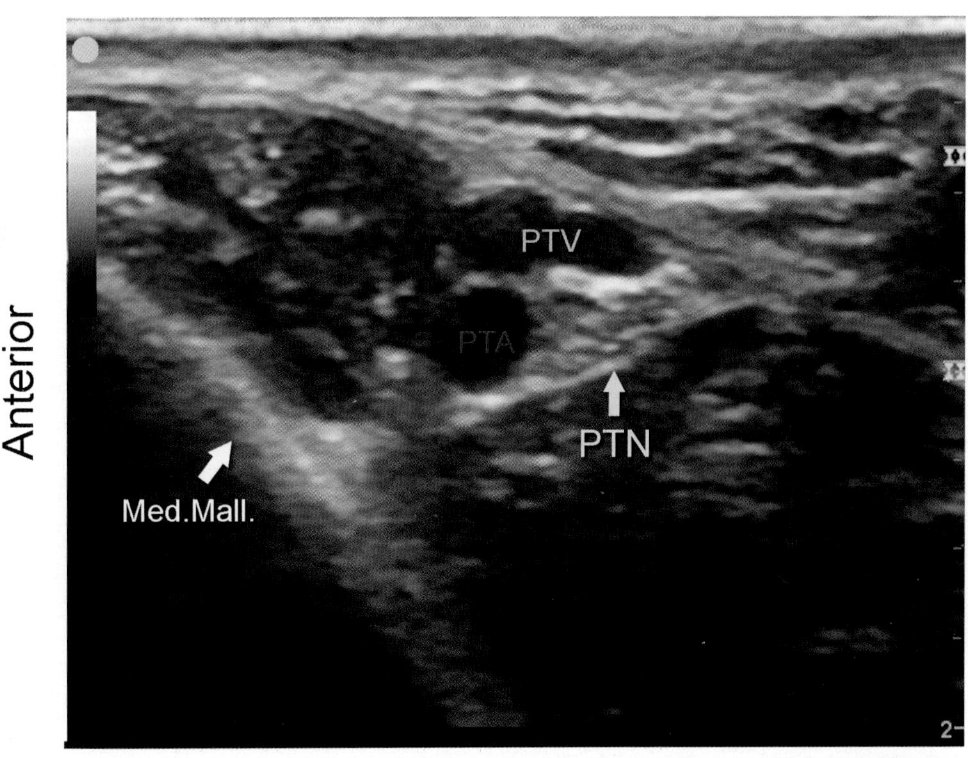


**FIGURE 7.59.1C** Labeled ultrasound image of the posterior tibial nerve at the ankle, medial aspect.

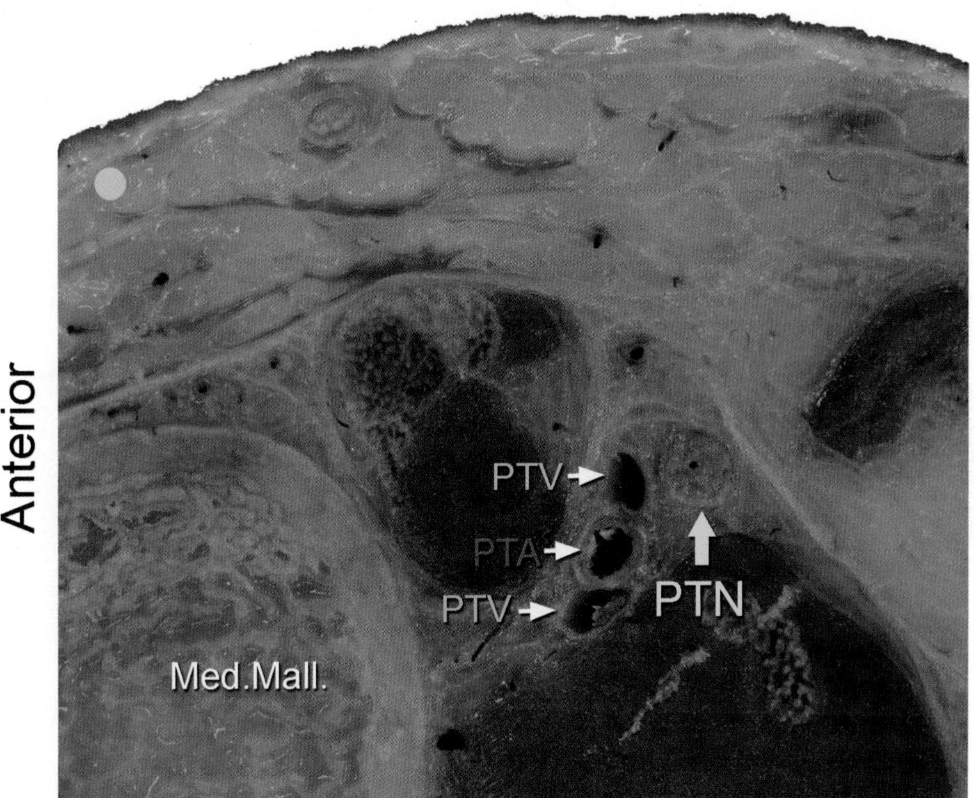


**FIGURE 7.59.1D** Labeled cross-sectional anatomy of the peroneal nerve, deep and superficial branches at the level of the ankle.

**Abbreviations:** PTN, Posterior Tibial Nerve; PTA, Posterior Tibial Artery; PTV, Posterior Tibial Vein; Med. Mall., Medial Malleolus.

## Saphenous Nerve at the Ankle

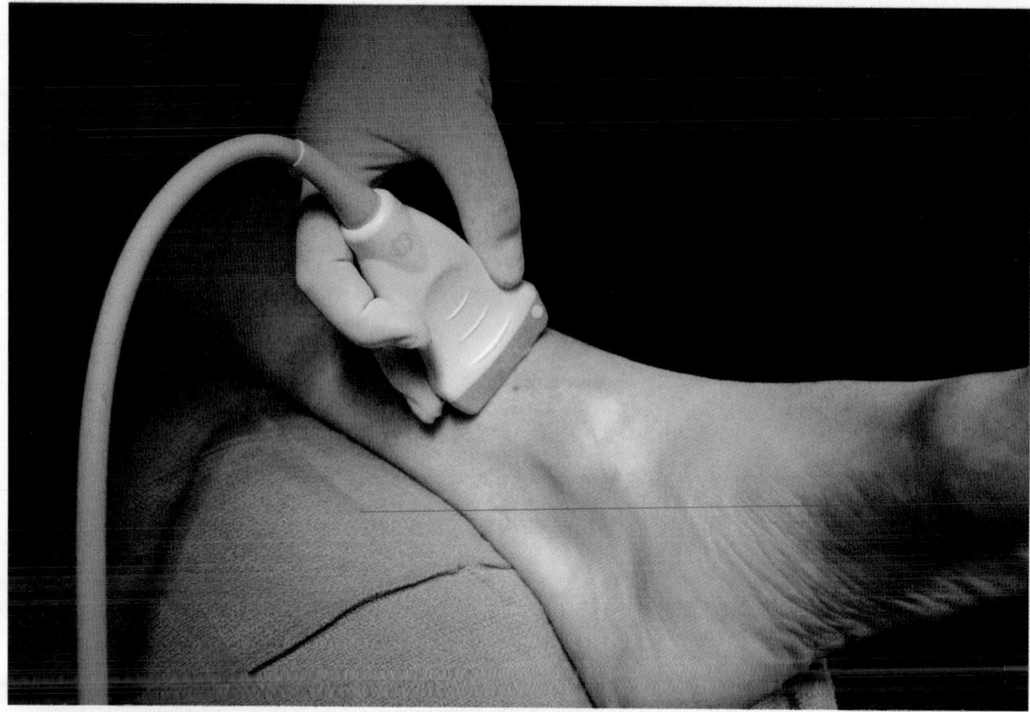

**FIGURE 7.60.1A** Ultrasound transducer position to image the saphenous nerve at the ankle.

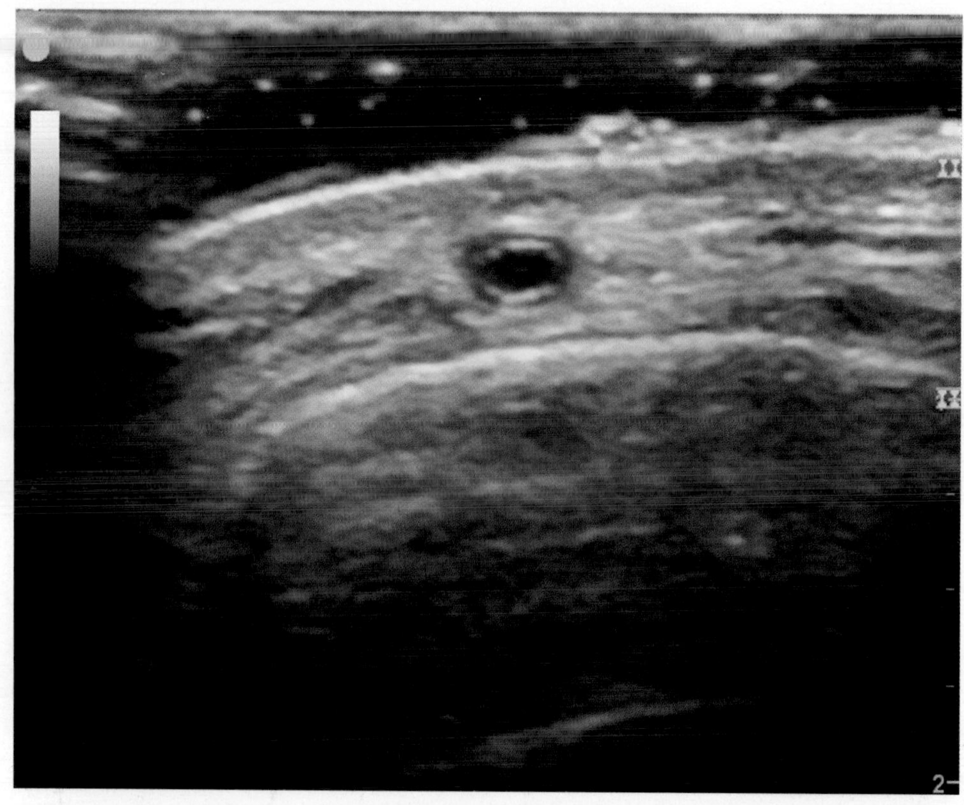


**FIGURE 7.60.1B** Ultrasound image of the saphenous nerve at the ankle.

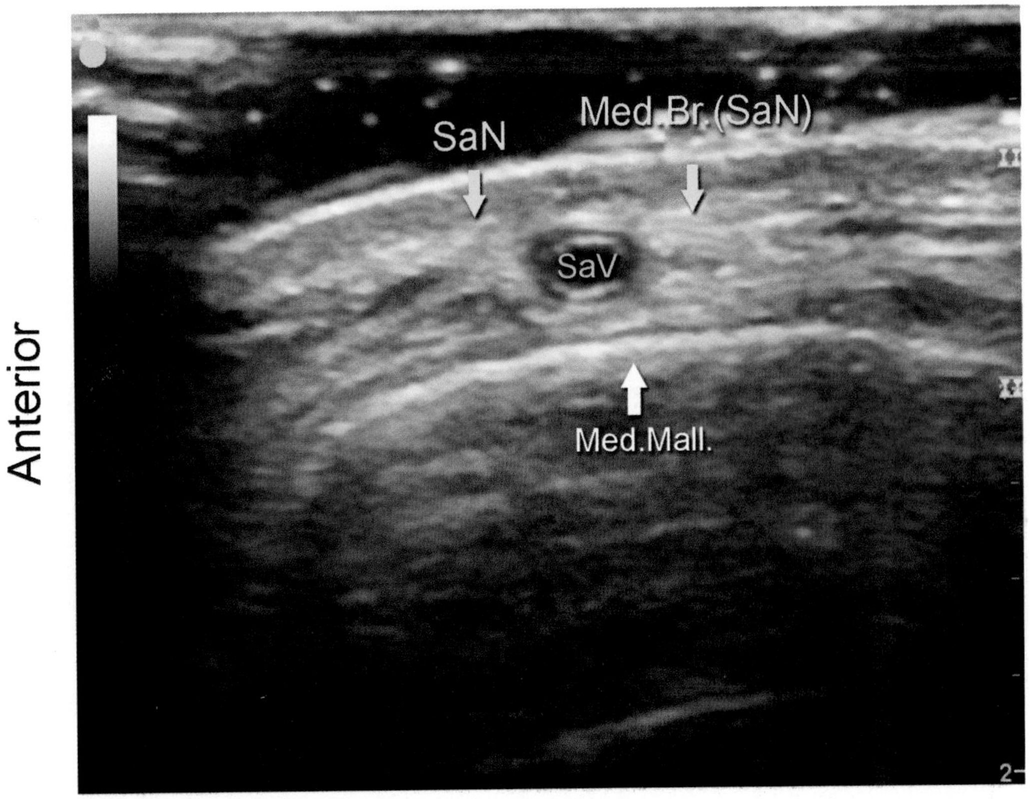

**FIGURE 7.60.1C** Labeled ultrasound image of the saphenous nerve at the ankle.

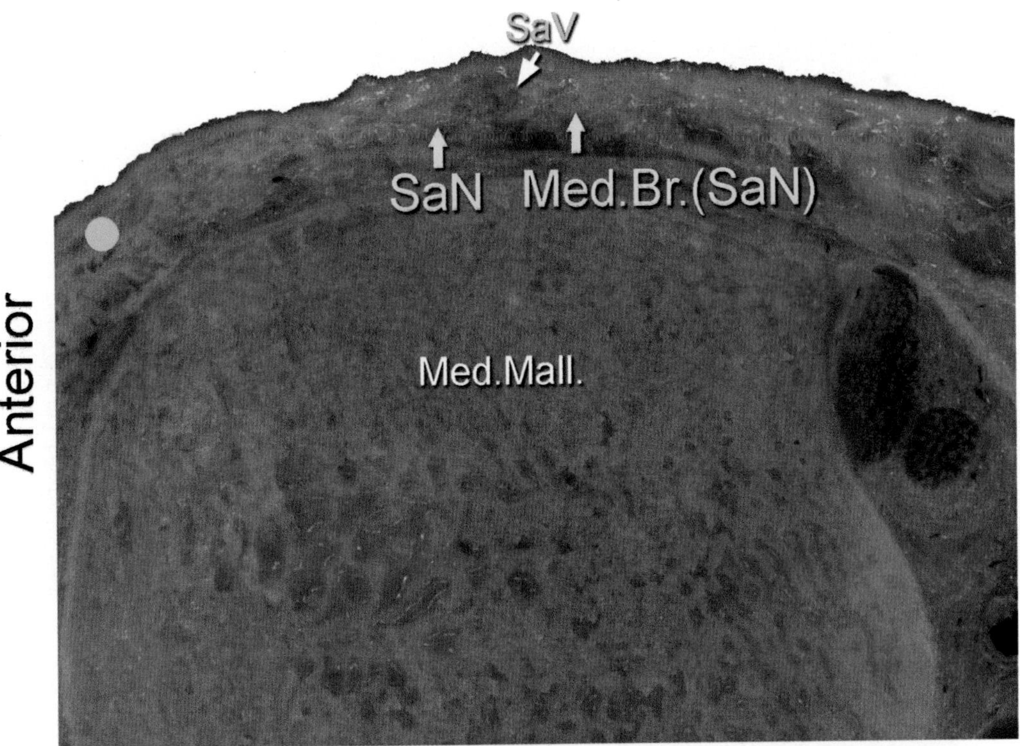


**FIGURE 7.60.1D** Labeled cross-sectional anatomy of the saphenous nerve at the ankle.

**Abbreviations:** SaN, Saphenous Nerve; Med. Br. (SaN), Medial Branch of Saphenous Nerve; SaV, Saphenous Vein; Med. Mall., Medial Malleolus.

## Superficial Peroneal Nerve at the Ankle

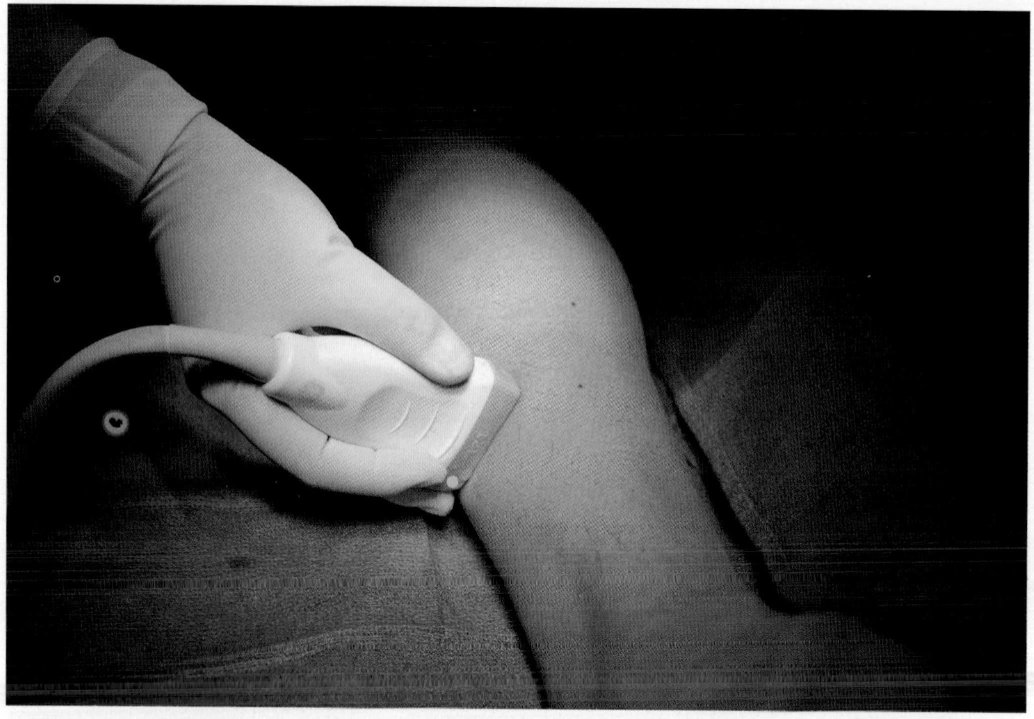

**FIGURE 7.61.1A** Ultrasound transducer position to image the superficial peroneal nerve at the ankle.

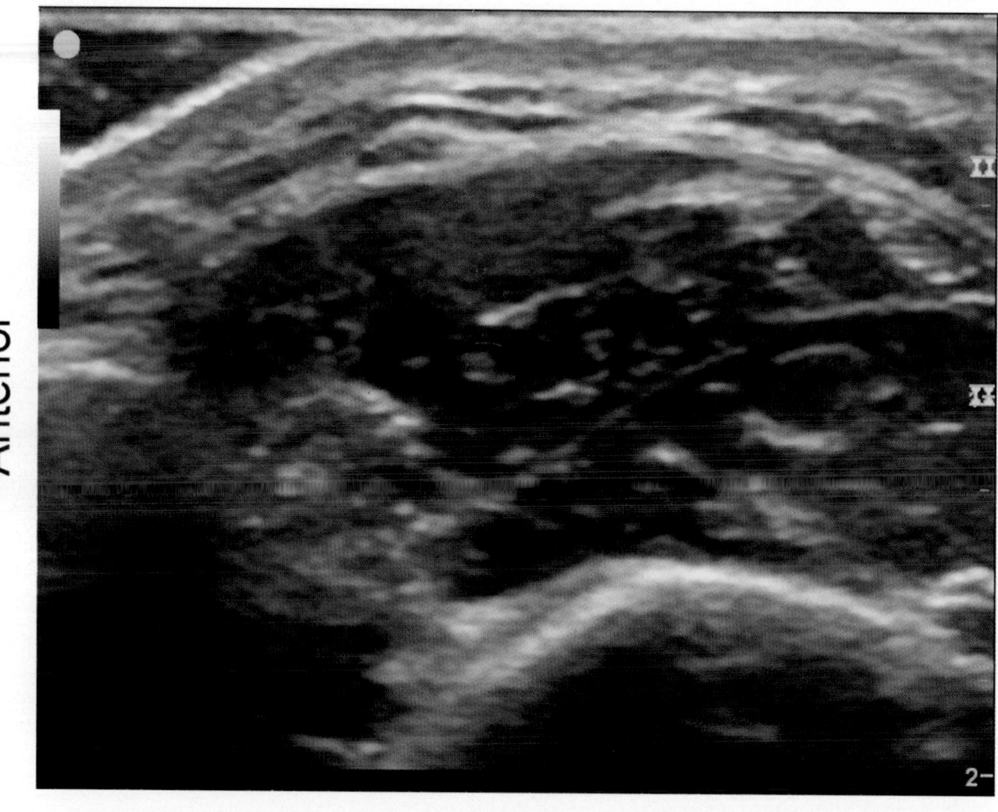


**FIGURE 7.61.1B** Ultrasound image of the superficial peroneal nerve at the ankle.

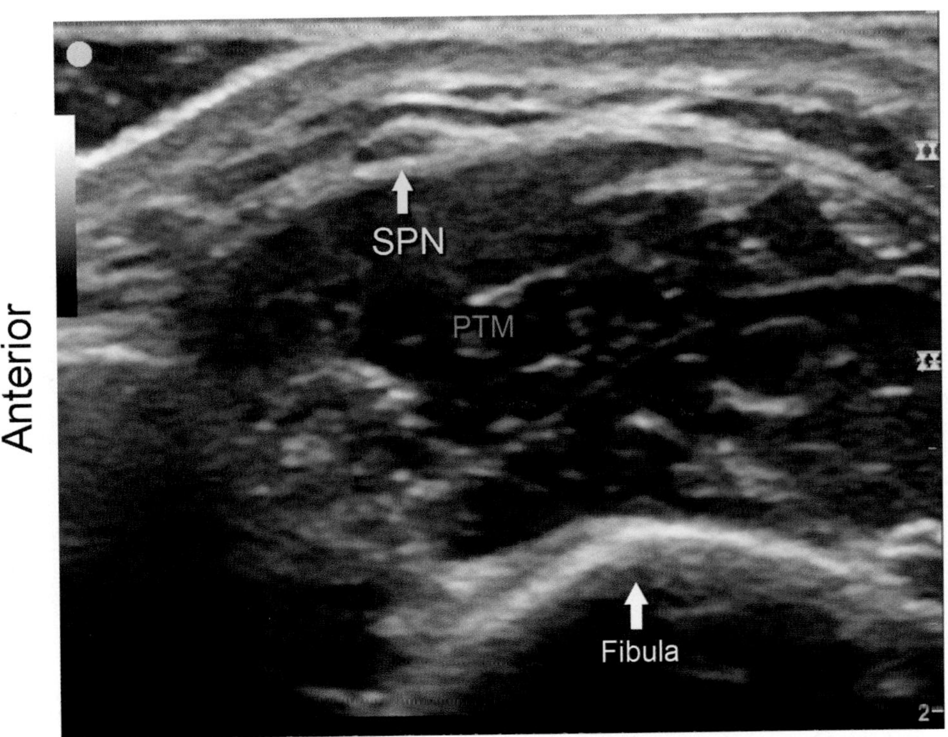


**FIGURE 7.61.1C** Labeled ultrasound image of the superficial peroneal nerve at the ankle.

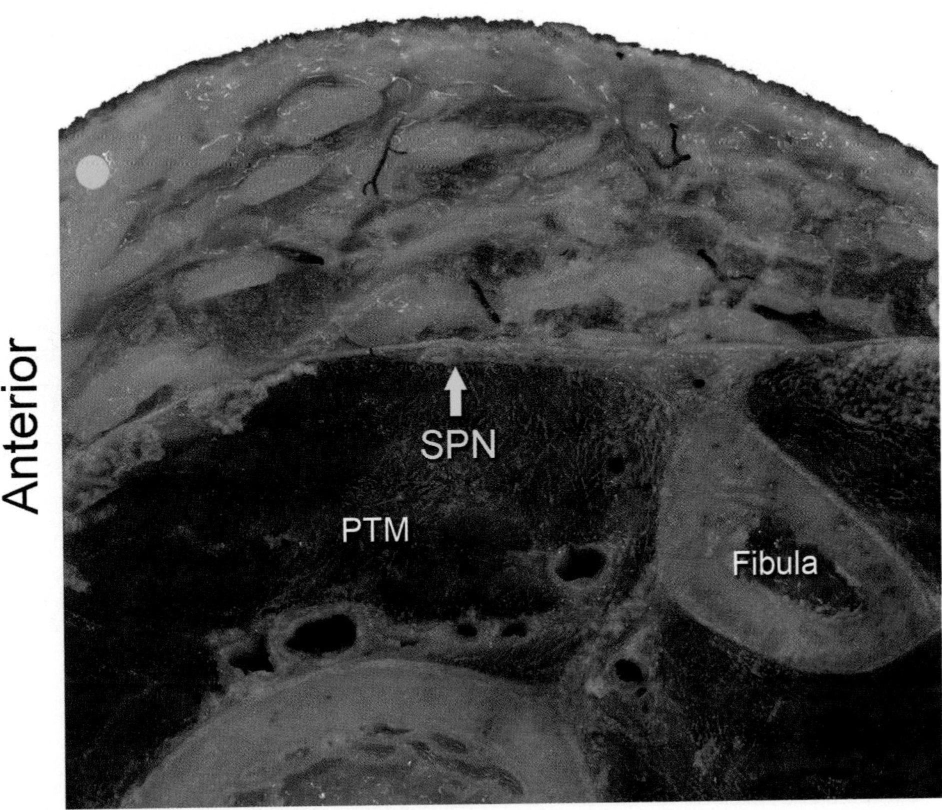


**FIGURE 7. 61.1D** Labeled cross-sectional anatomy of the superficial peroneal nerve at the ankle.

**Abbreviations:** SPN, Superficial Peroneal Nerve; PTM, Peroneus Tertius Muscle.

# Deep Peroneal Nerve at the Ankle

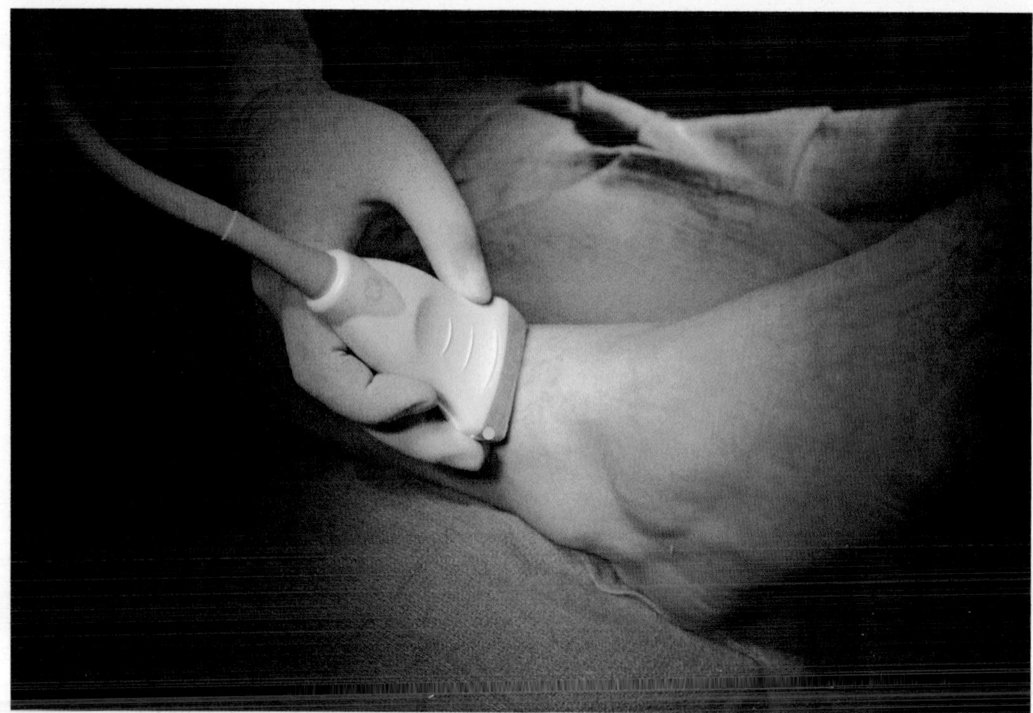

**FIGURE 7.62.1A** Ultrasound transducer position to image the deep peroneal nerve at the ankle.

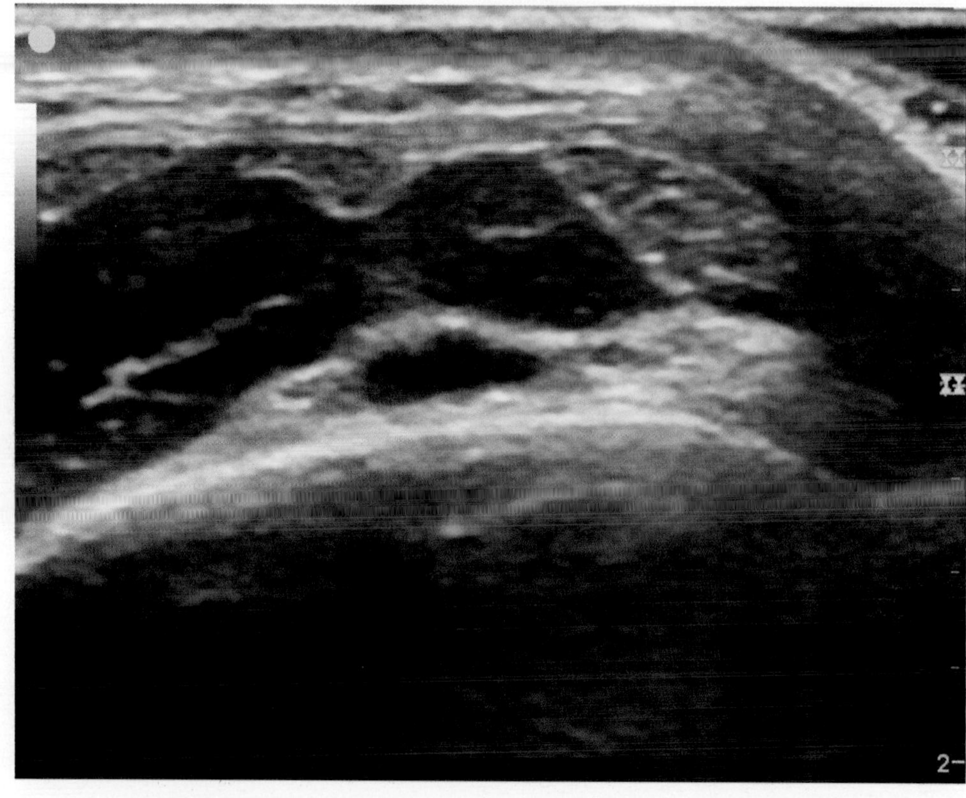


**FIGURE 7.62.1B** Ultrasound image of the deep peroneal nerve at the ankle.

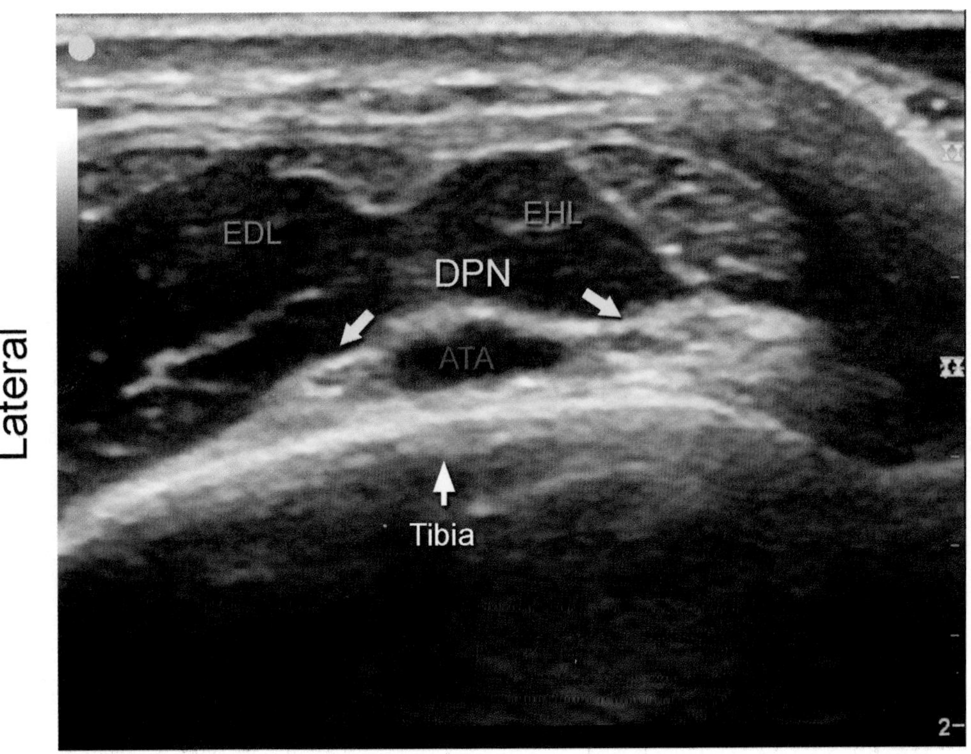


**FIGURE 7.62.1C** Labeled ultrasound image of the deep peroneal nerve at the ankle.

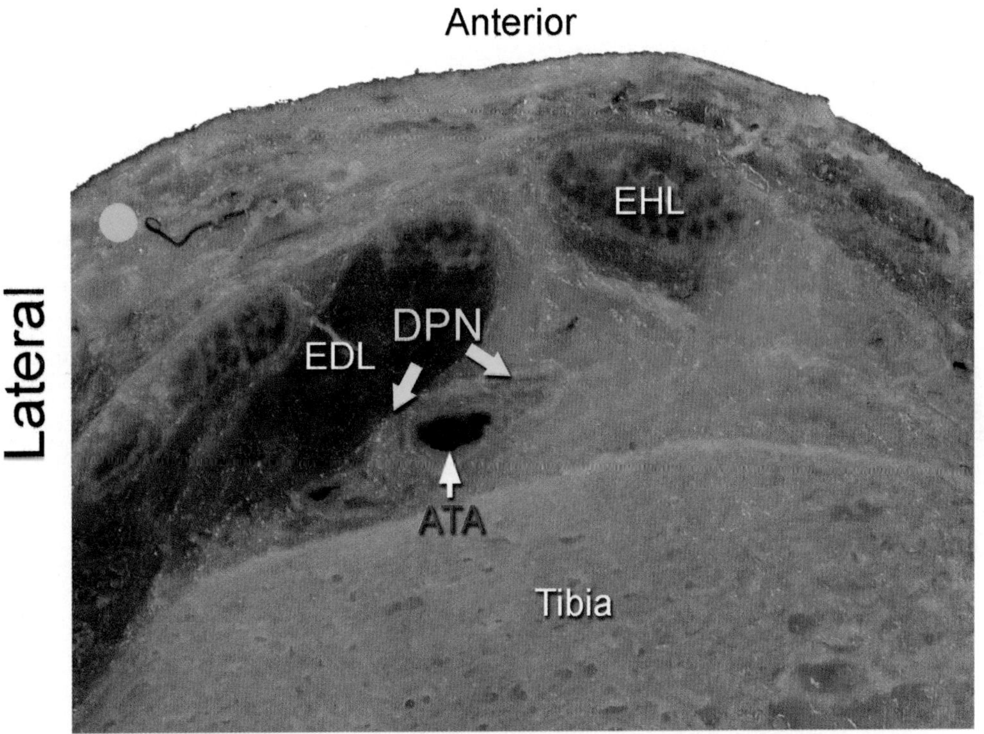


**FIGURE 7.62.1D** Labeled cross-sectional anatomy of the deep peroneal nerve at the ankle.

**Abbreviations:** EHL, Extensor Hallucis Longus; EDL, Extensor Digitorum Longus; DPN, Deep Peroneal Nerve; ATA, Anterior Tibial Artery.

## Sural Nerve at the Ankle

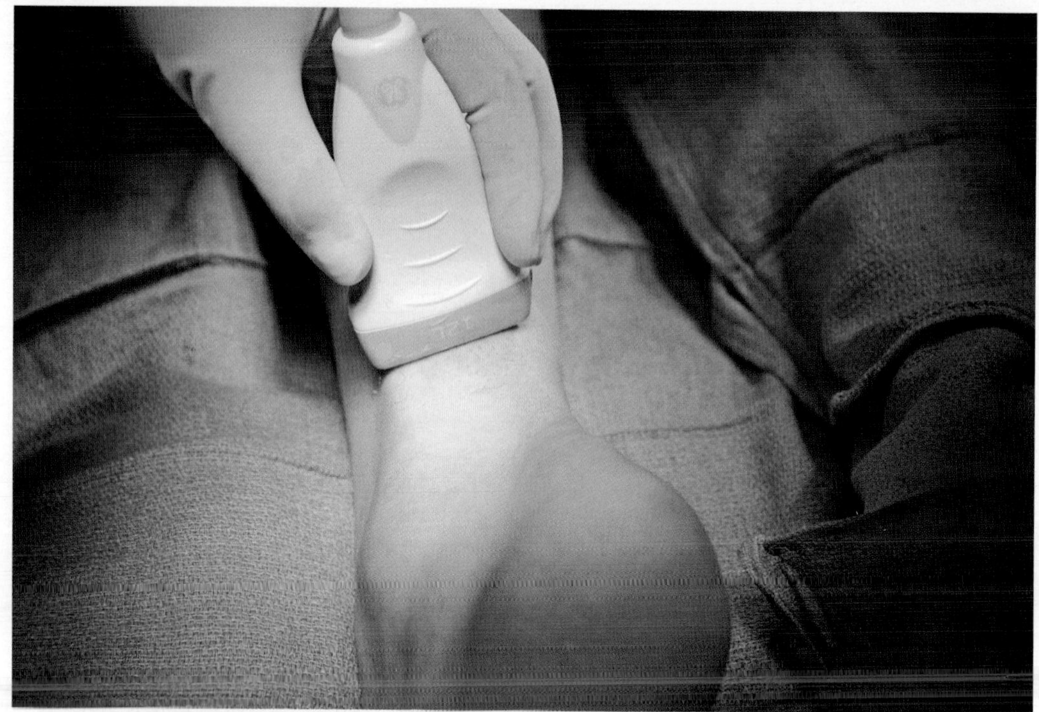

**FIGURE 7.63.1A** Ultrasound transducer position to image the sural nerve at the ankle.

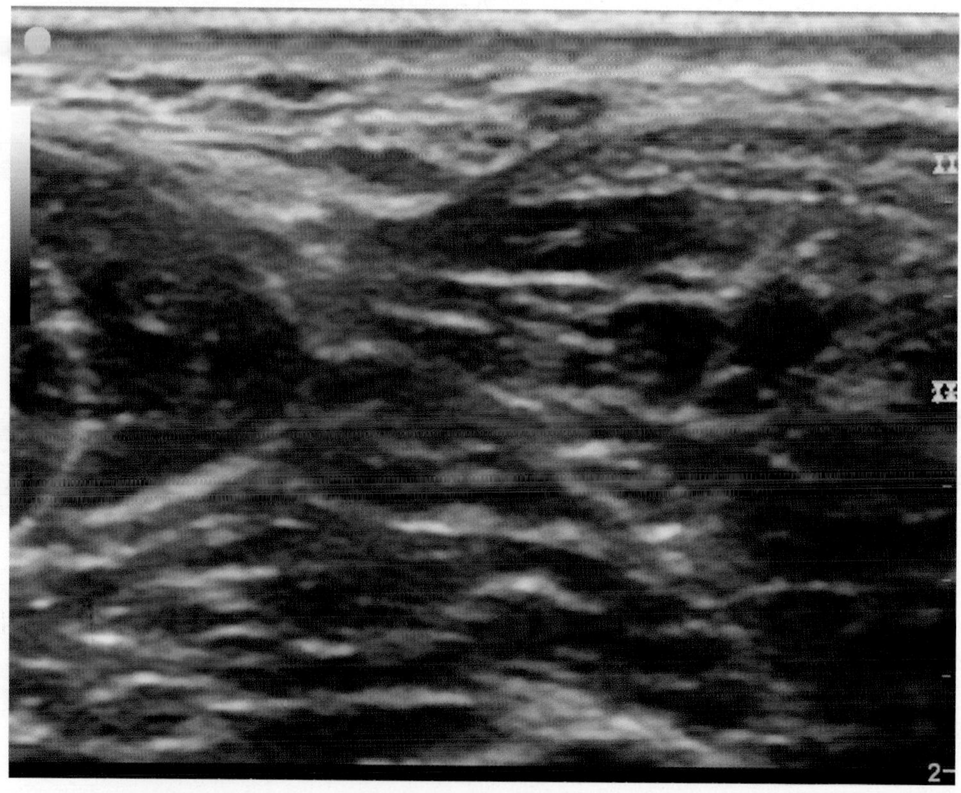


**FIGURE 7.63.1B** Ultrasound image of the sural nerve at the ankle.

Anterior - Lateral

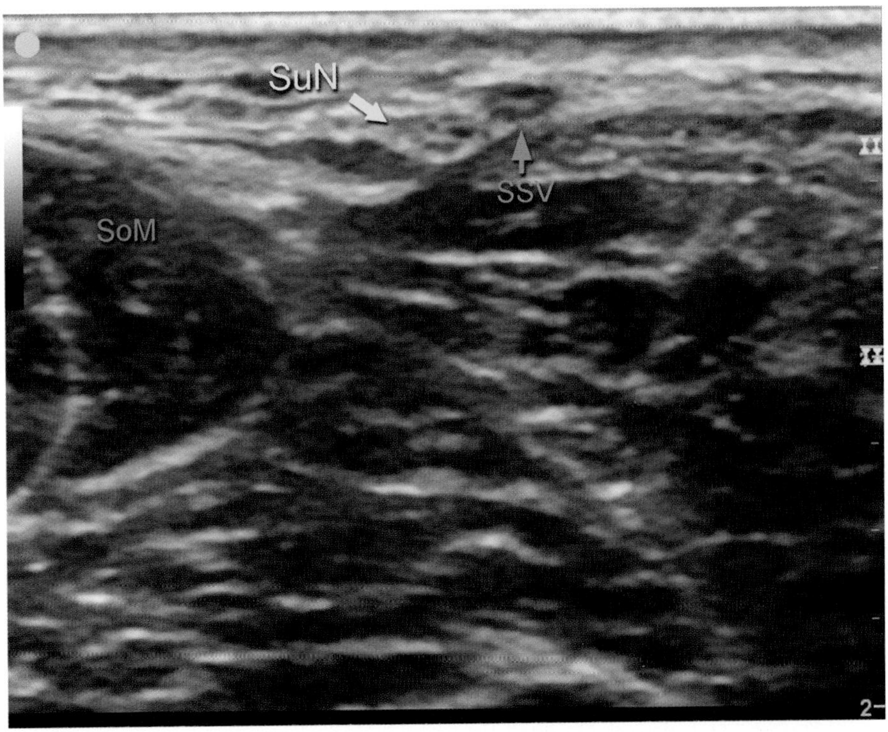


**FIGURE 7.63.1C** Labeled ultrasound image of the sural nerve at the ankle.

Anterior - Lateral

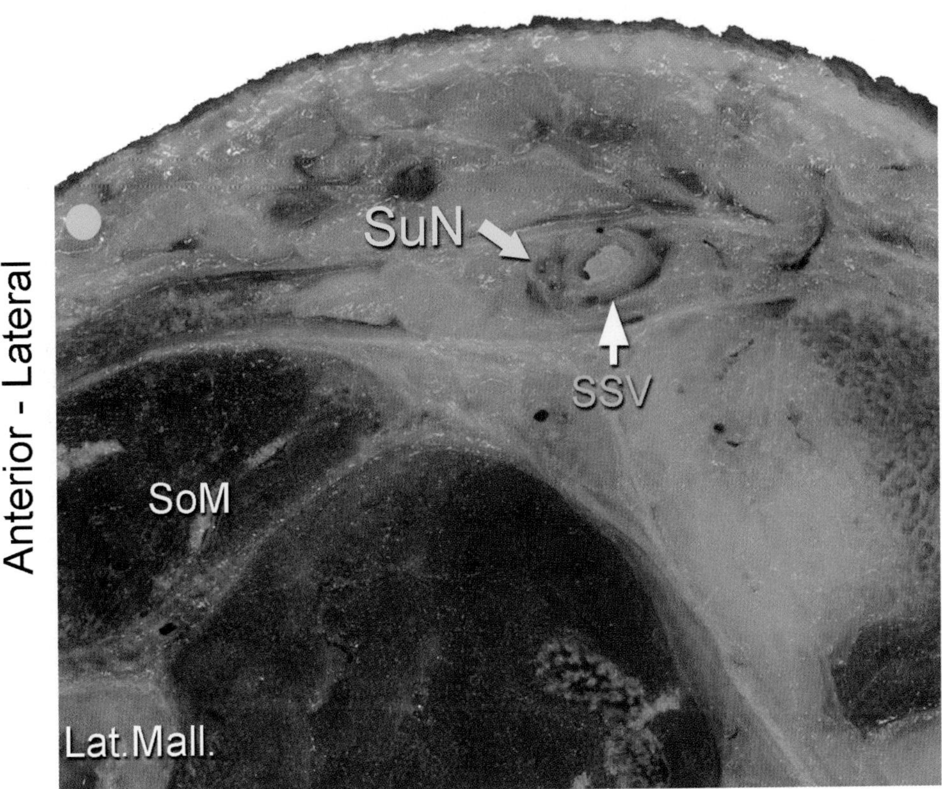


**FIGURE 7.63.1D** Labeled cross-sectional anatomy of the sural nerve at the ankle.

**Abbreviations:** SuN, Sural nerve; SSV, Small Saphenous Vein; SoM, Soleus Muscle; Lat. Mall., Lateral Malleolus.

SECTION 8

# Atlas of Surface Anatomy

# Upper Body Anterior View of Face, Neck, and Upper Chest

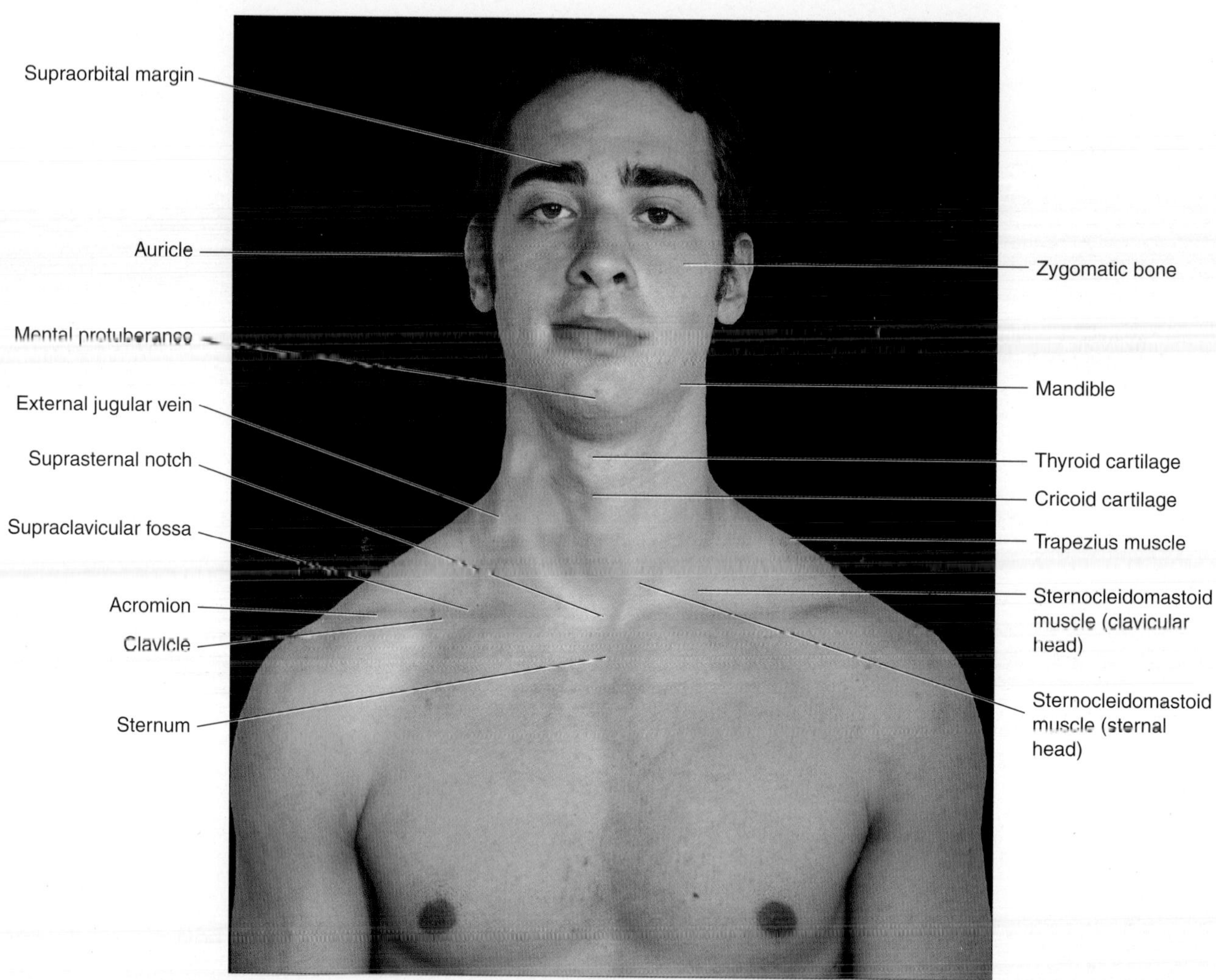


**FIGURE 8.1A** Surface landmarks: Upper body anterior view of face, neck, and upper chest.

## Upper Body Profile View of Face, Neck, and Upper Chest

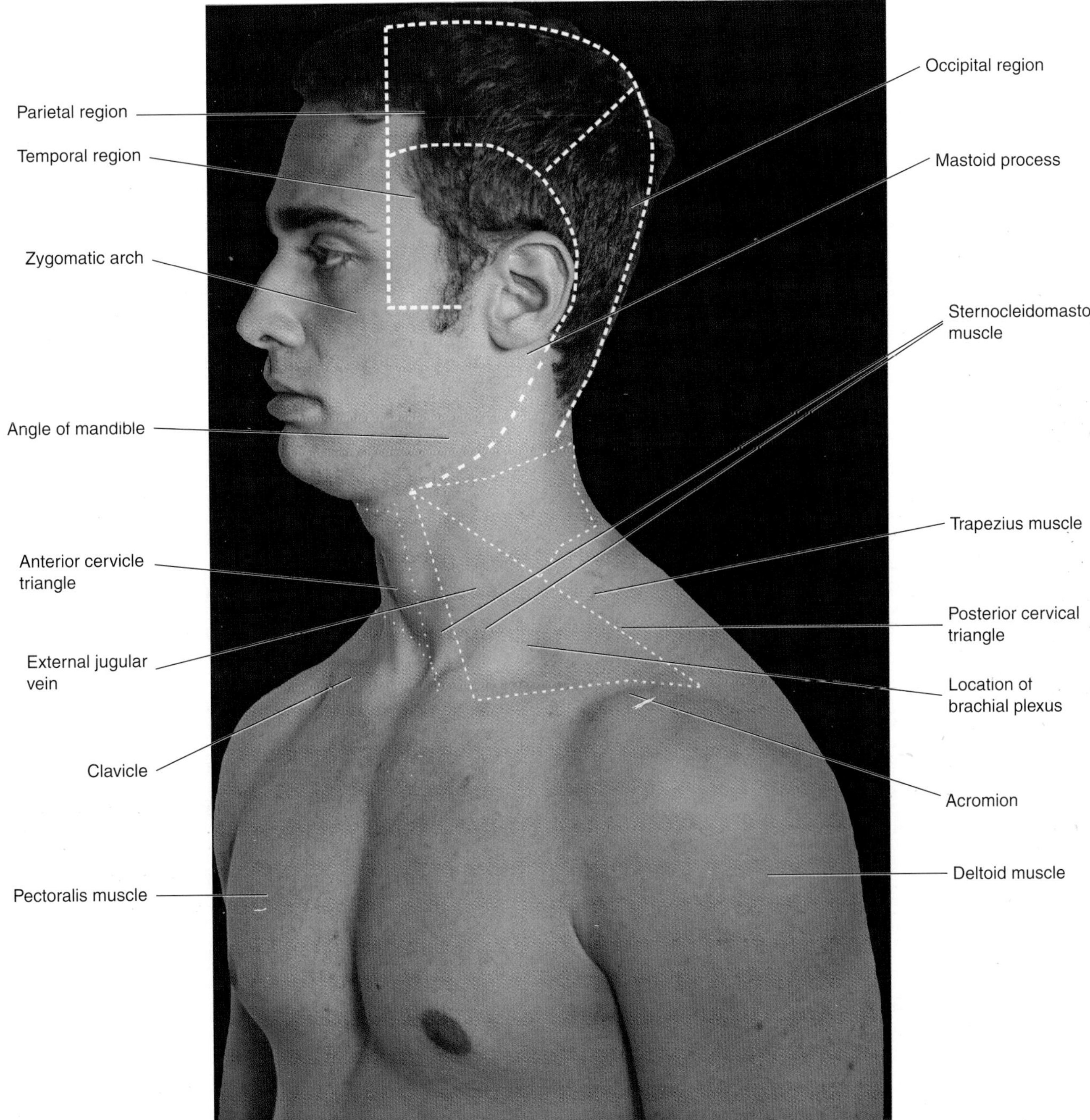


**FIGURE 8.1B** Surface landmarks: Upper body profile view of face, neck, and upper chest.

# Upper Body Including Chest, Torso, and Upper Arms

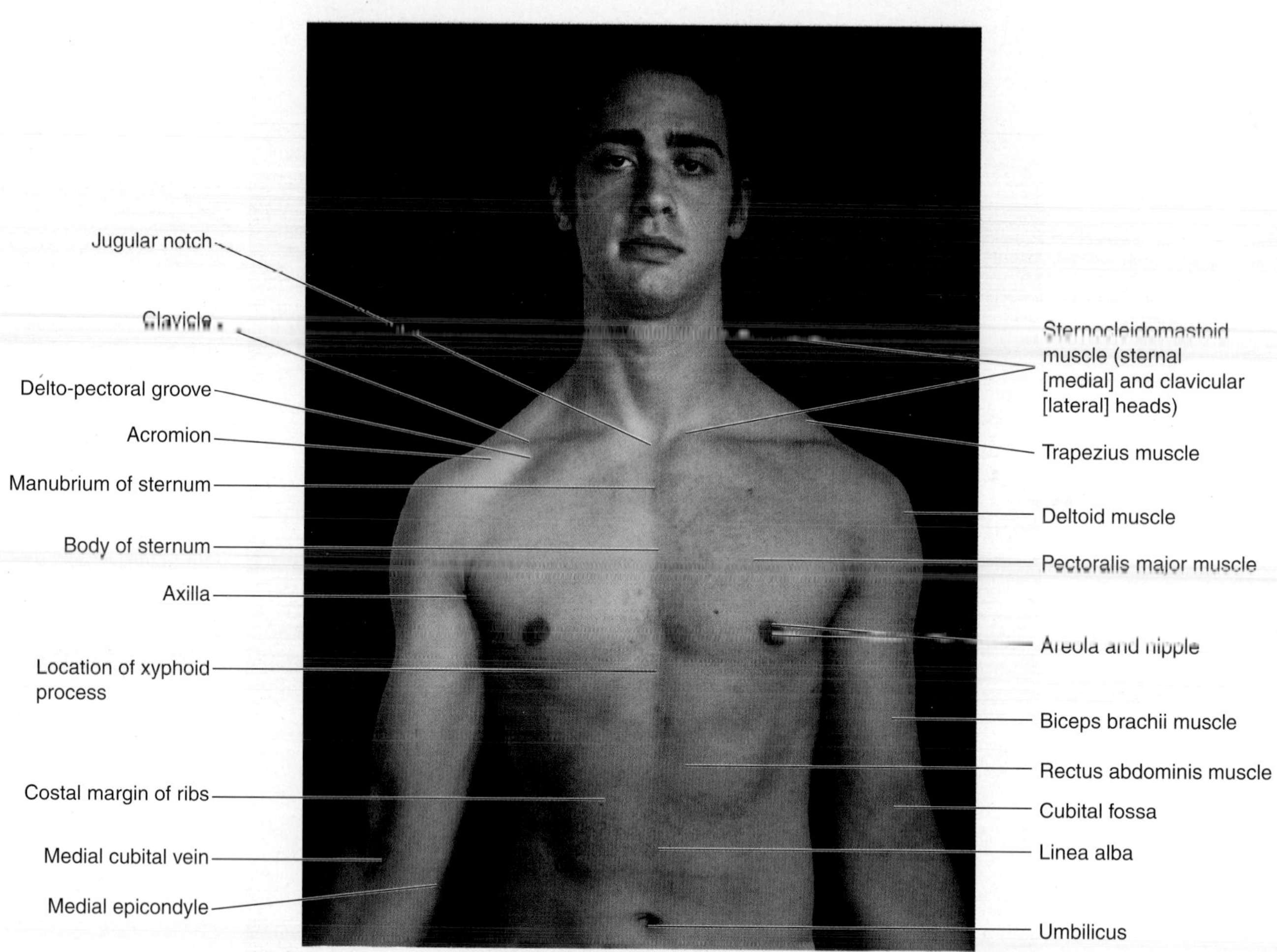


**FIGURE 8.1C** Surface landmarks: Upper body including chest, torso, and upper arms.

# Upper Body Including Back and Posterior Arms

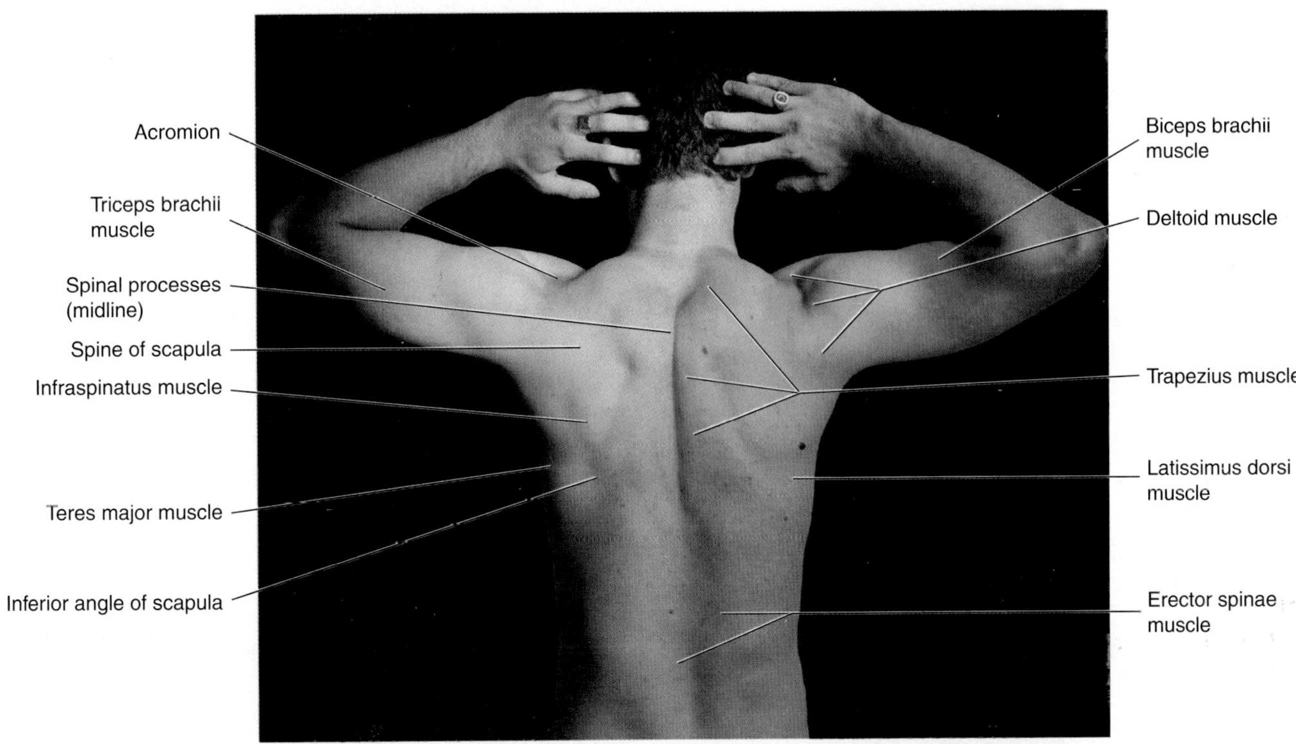


**FIGURE 8.2A** Surface landmarks: upper body including back and posterior arms.

# Upper Body Including Back and Posterior Surface of Arms

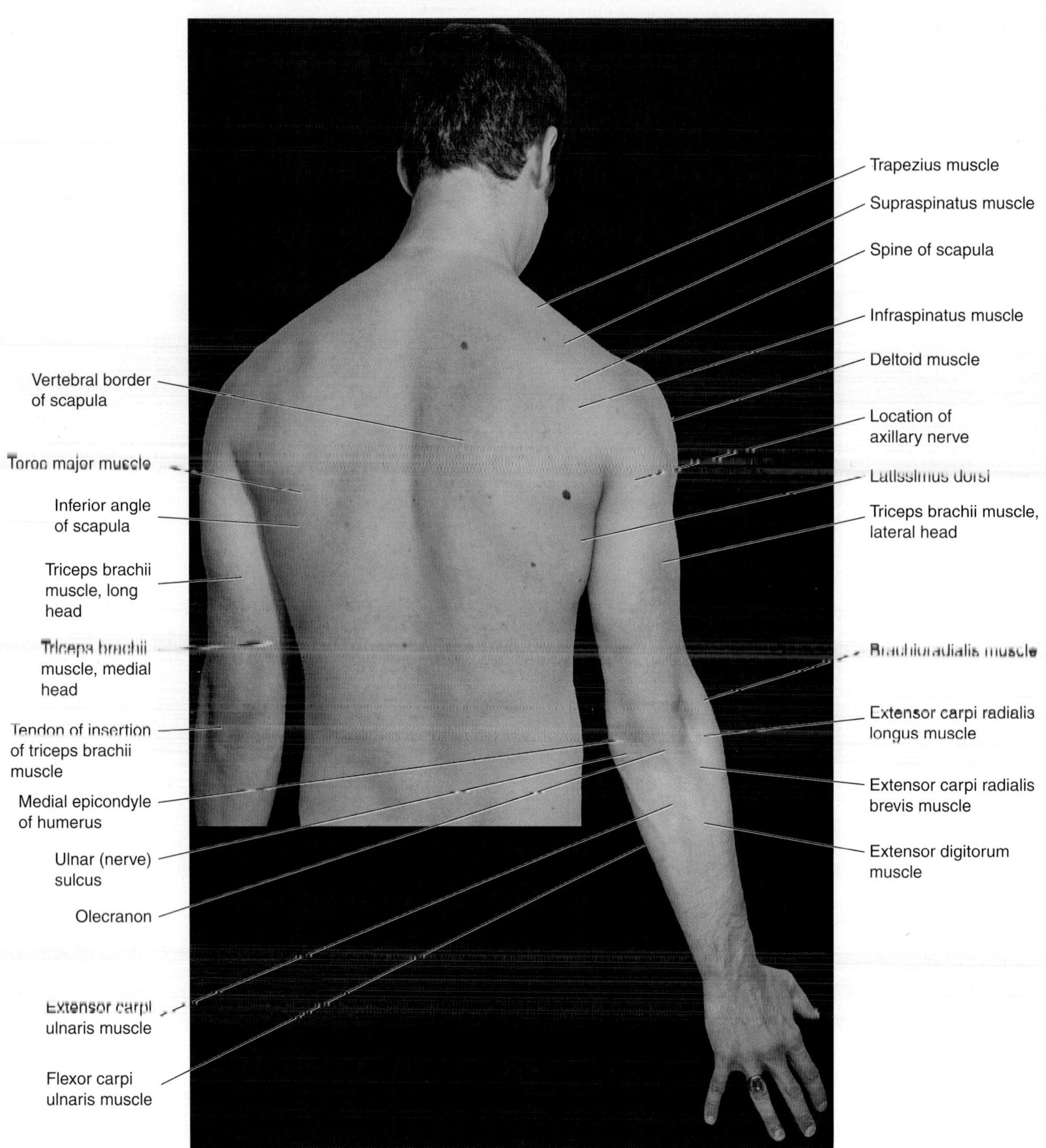


**FIGURE 8.2B** Surface landmarks: Upper body including back and posterior surface of arms.

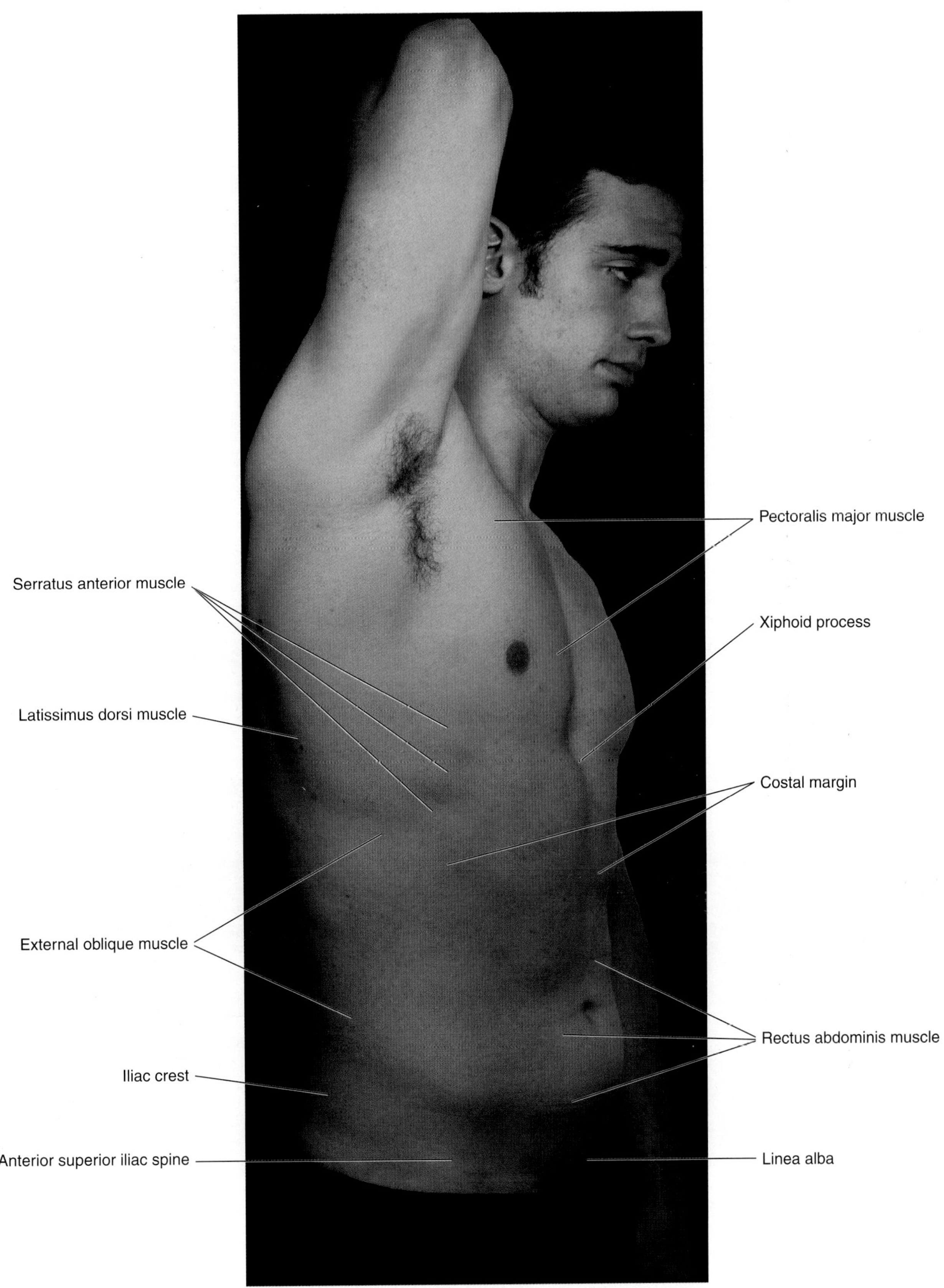


**FIGURE 8.3** Surface landmarks: torso.

# Shoulder and Upper Extremity

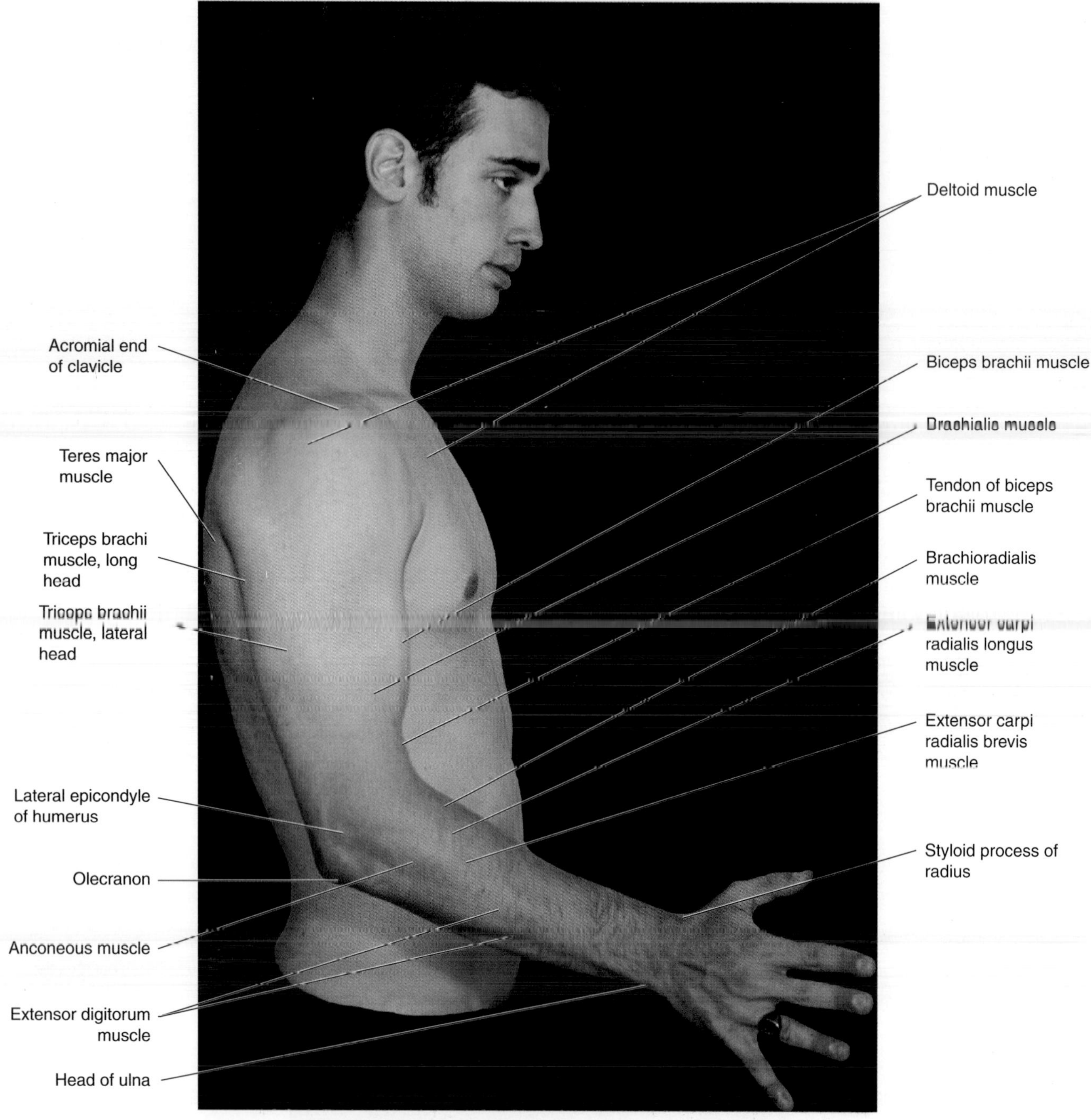


**FIGURE 8.4** Surface landmarks: shoulder and upper extremity.

## Lower Extremity Anterior View

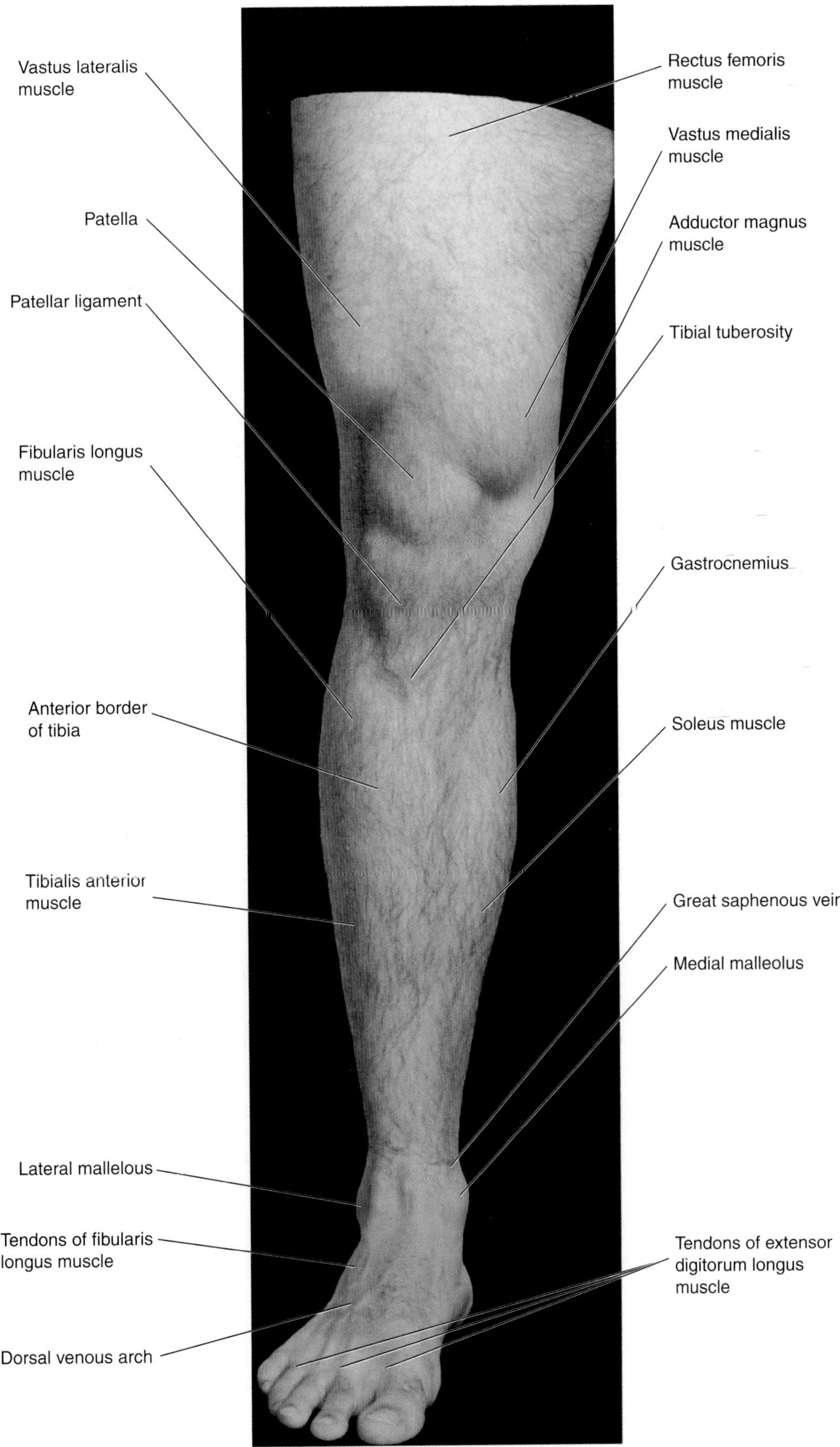


**FIGURE 8.5A** Surface landmarks: lower extremity anterior view.

# Lower Extremity Posterior View

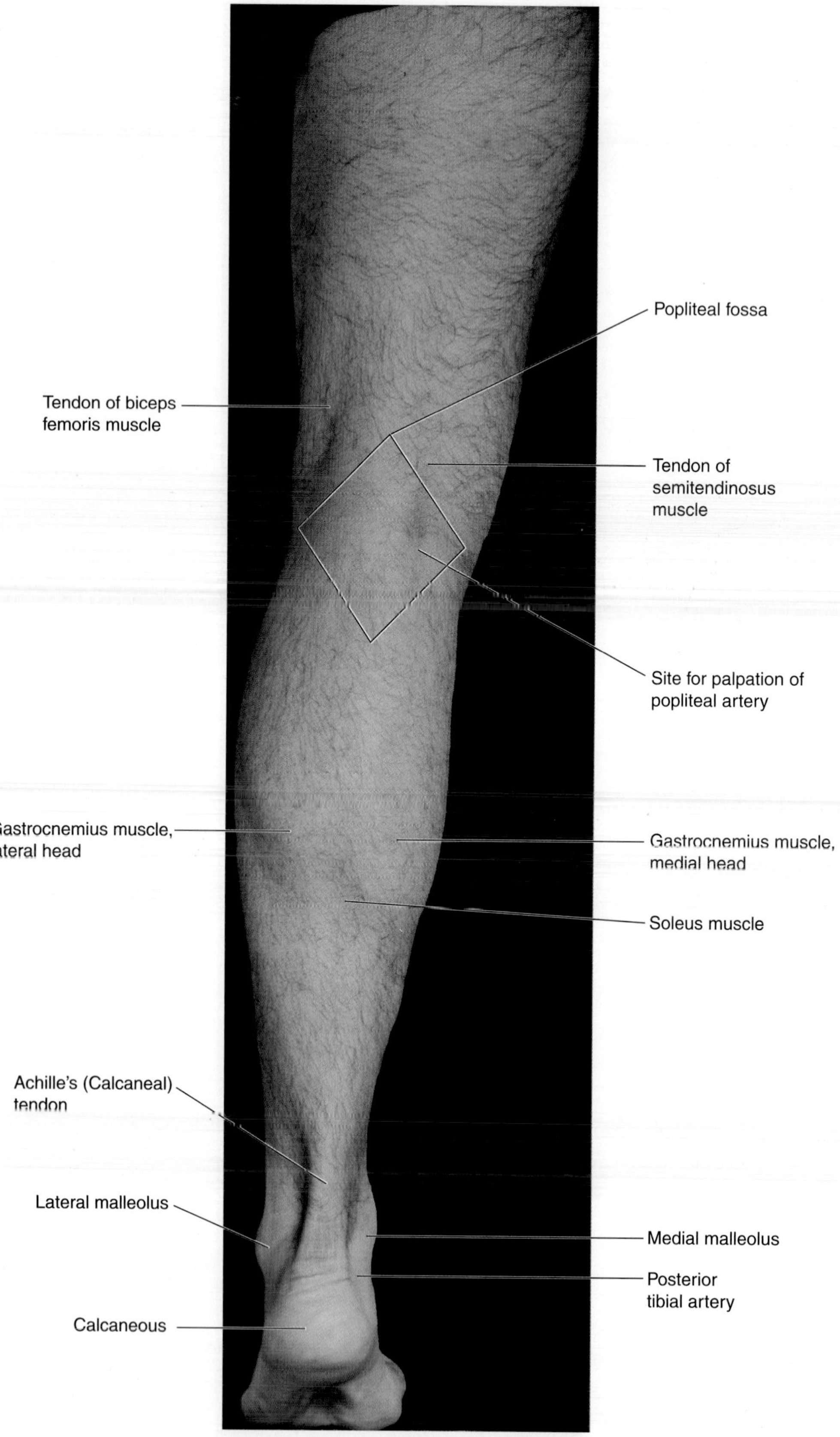


**FIGURE 8.5B** Surface landmarks: Lower extremity posterior view.

# Anterior Ankle and Foot

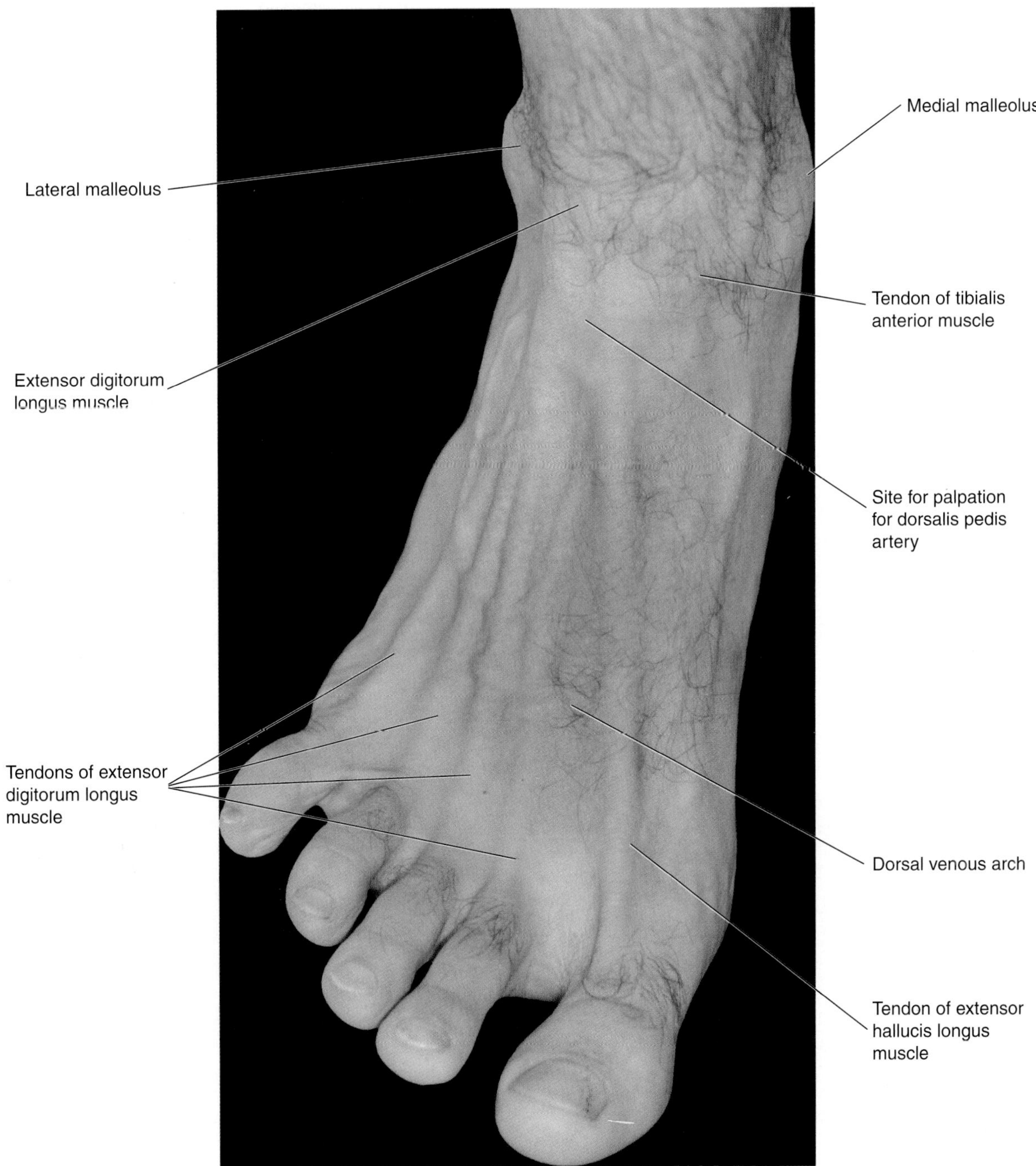


**FIGURE 8.6A** Surface landmarks: anterior ankle and foot.

# Posterior Ankle and Foot

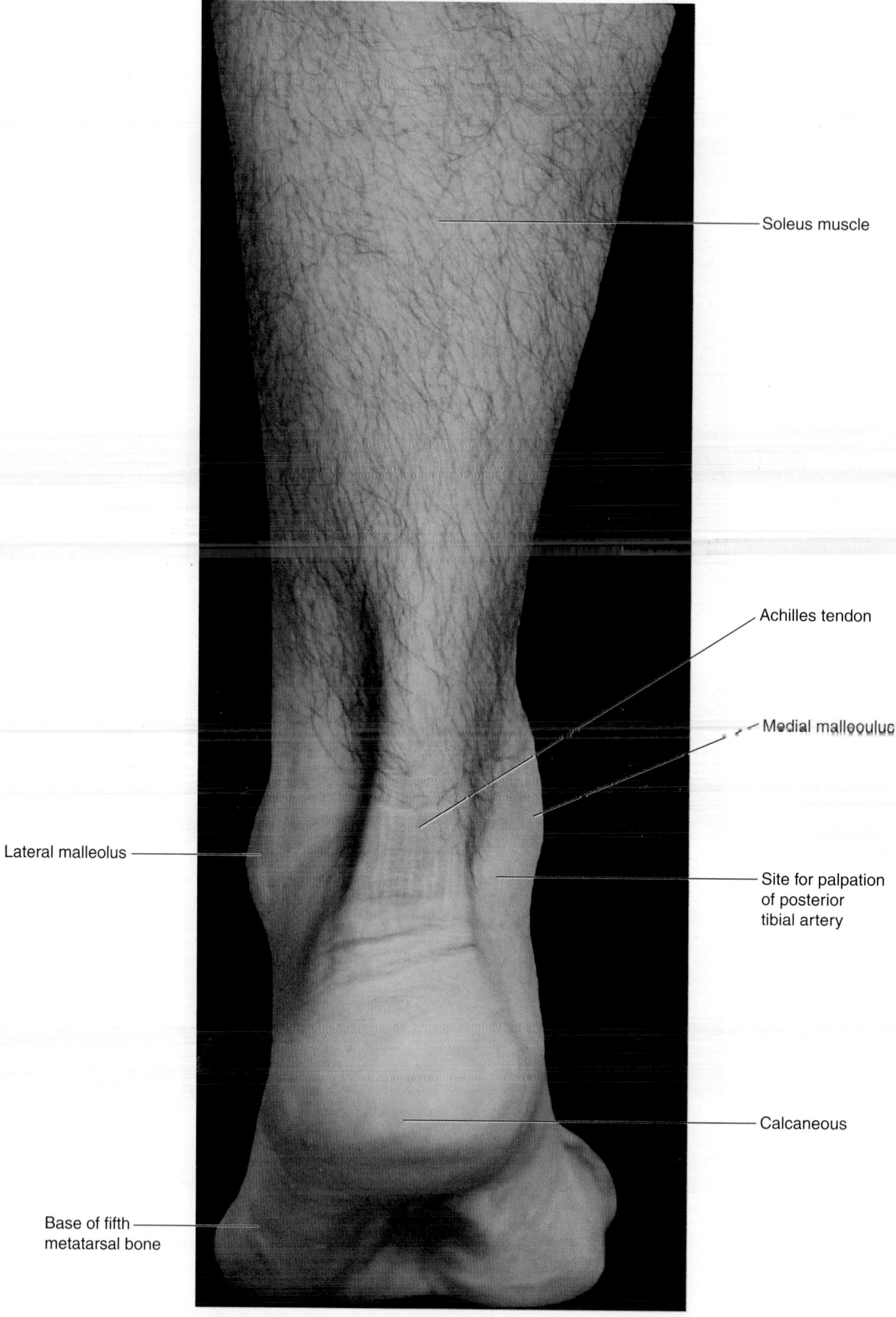


**FIGURE 8.6B** Surface landmarks: Posterior ankle and foot.

# INDEX

Page numbers followed by *f* indicate figures; those followed by *t* indicate tables.

**O**



**P**